Scott-Brown's Otolaryngology

Sixth edition

Laryngology and Head and Neck Surgery

Scott-Brown's Otolaryngology

Sixth edition

General Editor

Alan G. Kerr FRCS

Consultant Otolaryngologist, Royal Victoria Hospital, Belfast and Belfast City Hospital;
Formerly Professor of Otorhinolaryngology, The Queen's University, Belfast

Other volumes

1 **Basic Sciences** *edited by* Michael Gleeson

2 **Adult Audiology** *edited by* Dafydd Stephens

3 **Otology** *edited by* John B. Booth

4 **Rhinology** *edited by* Ian S. Mackay and T. R. Bull

6 **Paediatric Otolaryngology** *edited by* David A. Adams and Michael J. Cinnamond

Laryngology and Head and Neck Surgery

Editor

John Hibbert MA, ChM, FRCS
Consultant ENT Surgeon, Guy's Hospital, London

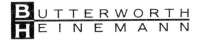

Butterworth-Heinemann
Linacre House, Jordan Hill, Oxford OX2 8DP
A division of Reed Educational and Professional Publishing Ltd

 A member of the Reed Elsevier plc group

OXFORD   BOSTON   JOHANNESBURG
MELBOURNE   NEW DELHI   SINGAPORE

First published 1952
Second edition 1965
Third edition 1971
Fourth edition 1979
Fifth edition 1987
Sixth edition 1997

British Library Cataloguing in Publication Data
A catalogue record for this book is
available from the British Library

Library of Congress Cataloguing in Publication Data
A catalogue record for this book is
available from the Library of Congress

ISBN 0 7506 0595 2 (Volume 1)
        0 7506 0596 0 (Volume 2)
        0 7506 0597 9 (Volume 3)
        0 7506 0598 7 (Volume 4)
        0 7506 0599 5 (Volume 5)
        0 7506 0600 2 (Volume 6)
        0 7506 1935 X (set of six volumes)
        0 7506 2368 3 (Butterworth-Heinemann International Edition, set of six volumes)

Printed and bound in Great Britain by Bath Press, Bath

Contents

List of colour plates in this volume

List of contributors to this volume

Introduction
Alan G. Kerr

Preface
John Hibbert

1 Examination and endoscopy of the upper aerodigestive tract
M. A. Birchall and C. B. Croft

2 Radiological examination
P. D. Phelps

3 Oral cavity
John Hibbert

4 Acute and chronic infection of the pharynx and tonsils
D. L. Cowan and John Hibbert

5 Acute and chronic laryngitis
Paul van den Broek

6 Disorders of the voice
P. H. Damsté

7 Management of the obstructed airway and tracheostomy
Patrick James Bradley

8 Trauma and stenosis of the larynx
A. G. D. Maran

9 Neurological affections of the pharynx and larynx
David Howard

10 Pharyngeal pouches
D. A. Bowdler

11 Tumours of the larynx
P. E. Robin and Jan Olofsson

12   Angiofibroma
      O. H. Shaheen

13   Nasopharynx (the postnasal space)
      Chuan-Tieh Chew

14   Tumours of the oropharynx and lymphomas of the head and neck
      Peter Rhys Evans

15   Tumours of the hypopharynx
      Randall P. Morton and Nicholas P. McIvor

16   Benign diseases of the neck
      A. G. D. Maran

17   Metastatic neck disease
      John Hibbert

18   The thyroid gland
      O. H. Shaheen

19   Non-neoplastic salivary gland disease
      A. G. D. Maran

20   Benign salivary gland tumours
      O. H. Shaheen

21   Malignant salivary gland tumours
      Michael Gleeson

22   Tumours of the infratemporal fossa and parapharyngeal space
      O. H. Shaheen

23   Cysts, granulomas and tumours of the jaws, nose and sinuses
      A. D. Cheesman and P. Jani

24   The oesophagus in otolaryngology
      Janet Ann Wilson

25   Facial plastic surgery
      Michael P. Stearns

26   Plastic and reconstructive surgery of the head and neck
      William R. Panje and Michael R. Morris

27   Terminal care of patients with head and neck cancer
      J. R. Hardy

Volume index

Colour plates in this volume

Between pages 5/5/18 and 5/5/19

Plate 5/5/I   Reinke's oedema on both vocal cords

Plate 5/5/II   Chronic hyperplastic laryngitis with polypoid projections. Microscopically this was a grade I squamous cell hyperplasia

Plate 5/5/III   Contact ulcer, saucer-like lesion on left vocal cord

Plate 5/5/IV   Chronic laryngitis with local squamous cell hyperplasia grade II

Plate 5/5/V   Small lesion on right vocal cord. Microscopically a carcinoma *in situ*

Plate 5/5/VI   Contact granuloma of the left vocal cord

Plate 5/5/VII   Tuberculosis of the right vocal cord and posterior commissure

Between pages 5/11/ 47 and 5/12/1

Plate 5/11/I   (*a*) Keratosis. Extensive hyperplasia and keratosis (leucoplakia) of the left vocal cord and anterior commissure area; (*b*) severe dysplasia. The mucosa of the left vocal cord is red and somewhat oedematous and there is a papillomatous lesion anteriorly. Histological examination showed severe dysplasia

Plate 5/11/II   (*a*) 'Anterior commissure carcinoma'. Squamous cell carcinoma involving the anterior part of the right vocal cord and the anterior commissure; (*b*) exophytic squamous cell carcinoma of the right hemilarynx with a fixed vocal cord; (*c*) supraglottic squamous cell carcinoma involving the epiglottis and left aryepiglottic fold (telescopic view)

Plate 5/13/I   (*a*) Endoscopic view of Henckel's biopsy forceps sampling the tissue in a typical undifferentiated carcinoma with ulcerative polypoidal appearance. (*b*) Posterior rhinoscopic picture of a very early carcinoma arising from the left torus and tubal recess depicting the most common site of tumour origin with minimal anatomical distortion. Such early detection is not common and the tumour can easily be missed without proper endoscopic inspection

Contributors to this volume

M. A. Birchall MD, FRCS, FRCS(Otol)
Senior Lecturer/Honorary Consultant in ENT,
Southmead Hospital, Bristol

D. A. Bowdler FRCS
Consultant ENT Surgeon, Lewisham Hospital,
London

Patrick James Bradley MB, BCh, BAO, DCH, FRCS(Ir),
FRCS(Ed)
Consultant Otolaryngologist/Head and Neck
Oncologist, Queen's Medical Centre, University
Hospital, Nottingham

A. D. Cheesman BSc, MB, BS(Lond), FRCS
Consultant Otolaryngologist, Charing Cross Hospital
and Royal National Throat, Nose and Ear Hospital,
London

Chuan-Tieh Chew MB, BS, FRCS(Ed), FRCS(Glas), FAMS
Consultant Ear, Nose and Throat Surgeon,
Mt Elizabeth Medical Centre, Singapore

D. L. Cowan MB, CHB, FRCS(Ed)
Consultant Otolaryngologist and Honorary Senior
Lecturer, City Hospital and Royal Hospital for Sick
Children, Edinburgh

C. B. Croft MB, FRCS, FRCS(Ed)
Consultant Otolaryngologist, Royal National
Throat, Nose and Ear Hospital, London

P. H. Damsté MD, PhD
Professor of Phoniatry, Medical School, University of
Utrecht, The Netherlands

Michael Gleeson MD, FRCS
Professor of Otolaryngology, UMDS, Guy's Hospital;
Consultant Otolaryngologist and Skull Base Surgeon
to Guy's, St Thomas' and King's College Hospitals

J. R. Hardy MD, BSc, FRACP
Consultant Physician, Department of Palliative
Medicine, Royal Marsden Hospital, London

John Hibbert MA, ChM, FRCS
Consultant ENT Surgeon, Guy's Hospital, London

David Howard BSc, MB, BS, LRCP, FRCS, FRCS(Ed)
Honorary Consultant ENT Surgeon, Royal National
Throat, Nose and Ear Hospital, London; Senior
Lecturer in Laryngology, The Institute of
Laryngology and Otology, University of London

P. Jani BDS, LDSRCS, FDS, MB, BS, FRCS
Senior ENT Registrar, Royal National Throat, Nose
and Ear Hospital, London

Nicholas P. McIvor MB, ChB, FRCS(Ed), FRACS
Consultant Otolaryngologist/Head and Neck
Surgeon, Green Lane Hospital, Auckland, New
Zealand

A. G. D. Maran MD, FRCS, FACS
Head of Department of Otolaryngology, University of
Edinburgh; Consultant Otolaryngologist, Royal
Infirmary/City Hospital, Edinburgh

Michael R. Morris MD, FACS
Consultant Otolaryngologist, Pinehurst Surgical
Clinic, Pinehurst, USA

Randall P. Morton MB, BS, MSc(Med), FRACS
Associate Professor in Otolaryngology, Department
of Surgery, Auckland Medical School, Auckland,

ix

New Zealand; Consultant Otolaryngologist/Head
and Neck Surgeon, Green Lane Hospital, Auckland,
New Zealand

Jan Olofsson MD, PhD
Professor and Head, Department of Otolaryngology/
Head and Neck Surgery, Haukeland University
Hospital, Bergen, Norway

William R. Panje MD, FACS
Professor of Otolaryngology and Director of Head
and Neck Reconstruction and Skull Base Surgery,
St Luke's Medical Centre, Rush University, Chicago,
USA

P. D. Phelps MD, FRCS, FRR, FRCR, DMRD
Consultant Radiologist, Royal National Throat, Nose
and Ear Hospital, London

P. E. Robin MB, ChB, BDS, MD, FRCS
Consultant ENT Surgeon, City Hospital NHS Trust;
Honorary Senior Clinical Lecturer, University of
Birmingham

Peter Rhys Evans DCC, FRCS
Consultant Surgeon (Head and Neck/ENT), Royal
Marsden Hospital, London

O. H. Shaheen MS, FRCS
Consultant ENT Surgeon, London Bridge Hospital,
London

Michael P. Stearns FRCS
Consultant ENT Surgeon, Royal Free Hospital,
London

Paul van den Broek
Professor and Chairman, Department of
Otorhinolaryngology and Head and Neck Surgery,
Catholic University, Nijmegen, The Netherlands

Janet Ann Wilson
Professor of Otolaryngology, Department of Surgery
(Otolaryngology), University of Newcastle, Freeman
Hospital, Newcastle-upon-Tyne

Introduction

When I started work on this Sixth Edition I did so in the belief that my experience with the Fifth Edition would make it straightforward. I was wrong. The production of the Fifth Edition was hectic and the available time short. The contributors and volume editors were very productive and in under two and a half years we produced what we, and happily most reviewers, considered to be a worthwhile academic work. On this occasion, with a similar team, we allowed ourselves more time and yet have struggled to produce in four years. One is tempted to blame the health service reforms but that would be unfair. They may have contributed but the problems were certainly much wider than these.

The volume editors, already fully committed clinically, have again been outstanding both in their work and in their understanding of the difficulties we have encountered. Once again there was an excellent social spirit among the editors. They have been very tolerant of the innumerable telephone calls and it has always been a pleasure to work with them. The contributors have also been consistently pleasant to deal with, even those who kept us waiting.

There have been technical problems in the production of this work and I want to pay tribute to the patience of all those who suffered under these, not least the publishing staff at Butterworth-Heinemann. One of the solutions to the problems has been the use of a system of pagination that I consider to be ugly and inefficient for the user and I wish to apologize in advance for this. Unfortunately anything else would have resulted in undue delay in the publication date.

Medicine is a conservative profession and many of us dislike change. Some will feel that we have moved forward in that most Latin plurals have been replaced by English, for example we now have polyps rather than polypi. We have also buried acoustic neuromata, with an appropriate headstone, and now talk about vestibular schwannomas. It has taken about two decades for this to become established in otological circles and may take even longer again, to gain everyday usage in the world of general medicine.

I am pleased with what has been produced. Some chapters have altered very little because there have been few advances in those subjects and we have resisted the temptation of change for change's sake. There have been big strides forward in other areas and these have been reflected in the appropriate chapters.

Despite, and because of, the problems in the production of these volumes, the staff at Butterworth-Heinemann have worked hard and have always been pleasant to deal with. I wish to acknowledge the co-operation from Geoff Smaldon, Deena Burgess, Anne Powell, Mary Seager and Chris Jarvis.

It would be impossible to name all those others who have helped, especially my colleagues in Belfast, but I want to pay tribute to the forbearance of my wife Paddy who graciously accepted the long hours that were needed for this work.

As I stated in my introduction to the Fifth Edition, I was very impressed by the goodwill and generosity of spirit among my Otolaryngological colleagues and am pleased that there has been no evidence of any diminution of this during the nine years between the editions. I remain pleased and proud to be a British Otolaryngologist and to have been entrusted with the production of this latest edition of our standard textbook.

Alan G. Kerr

Preface

The fact that this volume has changed its name from the Throat (Third Edition) to The Pharynx and Larynx (Fourth Edition) via Laryngology (Fifth Edition) to Laryngology and Head and Neck Surgery is really a reflection of the changes in this part of our speciality. These changes are due mainly to the intelligence, industry and brilliance of a number of Ear, Nose and Throat surgeons who have expanded the throat part of our speciality into what it is today. These individuals have developed the speciality of ENT to include head and neck surgery and subsequent generations of ENT surgeons owe them a great deal

I hope that everybody who reads this volume will enjoy it, will learn a little from it and will forgive me for the deficiencies. The credit for the volume lies with the individual contributors who have given their time, thoughts and experience with little in the way of reward. I thank them warmly for their contributions which I think are excellent reviews of the subject produced by experts in the field.

I would like to thank Alan Kerr for his kindness, wisdom and guidance in the production of this volume. It is a monumental task to be General Editor of such a book and Alan has done the job superbly. I am indebted to Julian McGlashan and Piyush Jani for reading the page proofs and giving me sound advice and also to all the registrars and senior registrars with whom I have worked at Guy's. It has always been a pleasure to be associated with outstanding trainees and I and our patients owe them a great deal. I would like also to thank Sue Sikora, the best secretary in the world, Ann, Jan, Esme and Josie, the best family in the world, and my close friends, the best friends in the world. Thank you for making work and life such a very enjoyable experience.

John Hibbert

1

Examination and endoscopy of the upper aerodigestive tract

M. A. Birchall and C. B. Croft

Look ere thou leap, see ere thou go
Thomas Tusser 1524–1580: *Dialogue of wiving and thriving*

Before a verdict is reached, it is customary to examine all the available evidence. Medieval physicians commonly chose to prognosticate based on Galenical texts, and rarely, if ever, examined anyone. We think we would all now agree that as thorough an examination as possible is an essential prerequisite to diagnosing and treating a patient. In otolaryngology, this means direct inspection, mirror examination and, in many instances endoscopy of the relevant tract. However, to look does not necessarily mean to see: the information conveyed by our eyes needs to be critically appraised in the light of our knowledge (experienced or read) of the normal and the abnormal. Examination and endoscopy require patience and thought, as, in many ways, they are the most important operations that we ever perform.

In the past few years, we have seen great advances in our ability to image the human body. Thus, videoswallows, CT and MRI scanning all contribute to our understanding of the normal and abnormal function of the aerodigestive tract. However, it cannot be stressed too strongly that:

> In the case of mucosal lesions in otolaryngology, even the finest of radiological examinations contributes little when compared to direct visualization techniques.

Advances in flexible and rigid endoscopy together with the increasing use of cameras and recording facilities have necessitated updating earlier accounts of this subject. In addition, we will combine this discussion with that of foreign bodies.

History

The maintenance of an airway, the ability to swallow and to produce voice are the three essential functions performed by the healthy throat. Because these functions are intimately related, impaired performance of one function will often impact on and involve the others. It is therefore important to correlate any presenting complaints of vocal difficulties or alteration of voice with signs or symptoms of respiratory obstruction and change in the patient's swallowing pattern. It is also important to realize that, although significant change in the voice with hoarseness localizes the disease process to the larynx, presenting symptoms such as dysphagia are much less specific in indicating the site of the lesion or pathological change. In the exclusion of major diseases in the upper aerodigestive tract the association of these diseases with the use of tobacco and alcohol are significant and the concept of the 'high risk' patient who both smokes and drinks significantly must be fully appreciated. Such patients require extremely careful analysis of their history and the most diligent evaluation of the upper aerodigestive tract to exclude serious underlying disease.

Examination of the larynx and pharynx

General

An estimate of the patient's general health and degree of nourishment is an essential prelude to regional examination. This includes checking for the signs of anaemia in hands, eyes and mouth. It is worth performing an assessment of the nervous system: as many as 10% of neuromuscular disorders present with dysphagia as the sole initial symptom (Jones, Lannigan and Salama, 1991). The features of myxoedema should also be sought as hoarseness is one of the presenting symptoms of this condition.

Basic examination

External examination of the neck represents an important starting point in the examination of the patient. It is important to remember that some cervical masses may escape the very best surgical palpation. It is essential that an orderly and systematic examination of the lymphatic fields on both sides of the neck is performed (Stell and Maran, 1972). Modern imaging techniques in the neck have supplemented physical examination and have become an important part of patient evaluation and tumour staging (Som, 1987). The mouth is another area that requires thorough and systematic examination. All mucosal surfaces should be examined using two tongue blades and good reflected light. Pulling the buccal mucosa outwards, the sulci and buccal mucosa should be examined carefully, the tongue should be protruded and movement and mobility assessed. All mucosal surfaces are examined, giving attention to such signs as fasciculation and wasting which may be indicative of neurological disease. Labial and lingual control are critical for the manipulation of food and initiation of swallowing (Logemann, 1983).

Where a macroscopic lesion is detected it should be evaluated for mobility, tenderness and palpated with the gloved finger to try to determine submucosal spread. This is particularly important where lesions of the tongue extend posteriorly into the posterior third and tongue base. There is a significant amount of overlap between dental disease and otolaryngological disease, and at least a note should be made with respect to the state of the patient's dentition. In the presence of hoarseness or dysphagia, examination of the larynx should be accompanied by a view of the postnasal space. The insidious nature of postnasal space carcinoma causing dysphagia by involvement of the nerves around the jugular foramen should be borne in mind (see Chapter 13). Examination of the larynx should follow.

Classical mirror examination of the larynx remains the preferred technique, although the ready availability of rigid and flexible laryngoscopes is impinging on the first line mirror examination. It should be noted that the resolution of fibreoptic systems is actually far inferior to that obtained with a simple mirror and rigid endoscopes are not universally available in outpatient primary care facilities. The old art of mirror indirect laryngoscopy must therefore continue to be practised and taught. During indirect laryngoscopy, assessment of the mucosal surfaces of the hypopharynx and larynx is made, mobility of the vocal cords is assessed and any narrowing, web formation or mucosal irregularities within the larynx noted. In approximately 10% of patients, mirror laryngoscopy is not possible because of a brisk or uncontrollable gag reflex. These patients will require fibreoptic flexible laryngoscopy. Cranial nerve function should be assessed.

Speech and swallowing are very complex activities involving more than 30 muscles and six cranial nerves. By now the examining physician will have a good idea of the nature of the patient's problems and the plan of diagnosis and proposed investigations can be presented to the patient. Radiological examination of the upper aerodigestive tract is covered elsewhere, but the role of the video-swallow in the functional investigation of the pharynx and larynx is stressed (Logemann, 1983).

Flexible endoscopy

Nasendoscopy/nasolaryngoscopy

Technological advance is producing increasingly smaller diameter fibreoptic endoscopes for examination of the human body. Nowhere is this more useful than in the head and neck. Using local anaesthesia, it is possible to use the flexible nasendoscope to examine the postnasal space, pharynx and larynx, down to the level of the vocal cords. Although the view is not as good as with direct laryngoscopy or as clear as with a mirror, it is possible to obtain a satisfactory view in almost every patient (even children above the age of 4 years). In addition, flexible nasendoscopy is generally carried out in a normal anatomical position and with normal respiration, unlike the rather distorted position achieved by indirect laryngoscopy or the use of the Hopkins rods. The procedure may be performed at the bedside with a suitable portable light source. Local anaesthesia, lubrication and the application of a de-misting agent are required for flexible nasendoscopy.

Additionally, flexible endoscopy may be used to observe directly the pharyngeal phase of swallowing, giving complementary information to that obtained by videofluoroscopy. Test swallows of milk or coloured food may be observed (Logemann, 1983).

An important point for flexible endoscopes is that of sterility. This has been controversial for some time: glutaraldehyde soaking may damage the endoscope and is sometimes ineffective. Ethylene oxide is very effective but requires 24 hours to work properly. Simply wiping the endoscope with a swab between procedures may not protect against the transmission of some important infectious conditions such as tuberculosis. While these issues are far from resolved, reasonable options are, first, to have more than one nasendoscope available in outpatients, and second the use of protective disposable sheaths (Silbermann, Hampel and Kominsky, 1993).

Wherever there remains doubt about the appearance of the larynx following flexible endoscopy, and in any case if instrumentation is planned, it is best to proceed to direct laryngoscopy under general anaesthesia. Despite the assurances of some practitioners who feel that many forms of laryngeal surgery can be performed under stroboscopic control and local anaesthesia (Bastian *et al.*, 1989), biopsy in the outpatients remains a relatively uncontrolled, and therefore unsafe, procedure.

Oesophagogastroduodenoscopy

Where the clinical picture suggests lower oesophageal disease, it is advisable to perform flexible oesophagogastroduodenoscopy. Modern flexible instruments have a wide field of view, excellent photographic capability (Figure 1.1), may be used under local anaesthetic and sedation, and may be the only method of examination possible in some patients (Howard and Croft, 1992). Flexible endoscopy may also be performed under general anaesthesia as part of a 'panendoscopy' procedure.

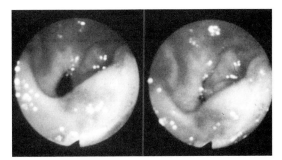

Figure 1.1 An example of a view down a flexible oesophagoscope: oesophageal candidiasis in an immunosuppressed patient

In some areas, however, the rigid instruments remain superior: the removal of foreign bodies is easier and biopsies are substantially larger. In addition, it has been well-demonstrated that flexible endoscopes are poor at visualizing the pharynx, hypopharynx and postcricoid regions. Lesions in these sites may be completely missed, but it is more common for them to cause difficulty in passing the endoscope satisfactorily, and this sign should indicate the need for rigid examination (Bingham *et al.*, 1986).

The use of Lugol's solution (iodine) combined with oesophagogastroduodenoscopy is the best way to detect early oesophageal cancer. Early lesions stain lividly and may then be biopsied (Adachi *et al.*, 1993). In cases of oesophageal carcinoma, however, the larger biopsies obtained by rigid endoscopy lead to a greater diagnostic yield (99% for rigid endoscopy as opposed to 80% for oesophagogastroduodenoscopy: Ritchie *et al.*, 1993). The sensitivity of barium swallow for identifying oesophagitis is low at around 33%. The definitive modern test for oesophagitis is oesophagoscopy and biopsy. However, reports vary in how well endoscopic findings correlate with the clinical symptoms of reflux disease (33–72% correlation: Koufman, 1991). Peptic strictures may be easily identified and dilated, for example using Eada-Puesto dilators along a guidewire, at the same sitting if indicated.

Bronchoscopy

The indications for bronchoscopy are diagnostic (haemoptysis, suspected bronchial obstruction, obscure chest symptoms) and therapeutic (toilet, palliation, foreign bodies). Relative contraindications relate to biopsy and include bleeding diatheses and pulmonary hypertension (Gaer, 1992). The main strength of the flexible method is the ability to visualize and biopsy relatively peripheral lesions compared to the rigid method, but it is also practicable in the case of cervical spine abnormalities or thoracic aneurysms. It is, of course, perfectly possible to use the flexible bronchoscope via a tracheostomy or end-stoma, if required.

The most patent nasal airway is selected and anaesthetized with 4% lignocaine spray or 10% cocaine. The pharynx and vocal cords are anaesthetized via the mouth. It is helpful to provide oxygen via a cannula passed through the other nostril. Once through the cords, further lignocaine is delivered into each main bronchus via the endoscope. During the examination, aspirates should be taken for cytology and culture, using sputum traps (at least two: one for each main bronchus). It is to be remembered in the latter context that tuberculosis is enjoying something of a resurgence in many places, and that Grocutt staining for pneumocystis should be requested if there is a suspicion of retrovirus infection (AIDS). Pathological findings should be recorded on a sketched (or pre-printed) plan of the bronchial tree (Figure 1.2).

Hopkins rod

The use of the 70° or 90° Hopkins rod telescope allows a high resolution view of the larynx to be obtained in most adult and many paediatric patients. An 83% rate of visualization (compared to 52% for mirror examination) has been claimed for this method (Barker and Dort, 1991). It allows assessment of vocal cord function, high quality photography, and is the ideal instrument for videostroboscopy of the larynx. In patients with tracheostomies, an angled telescope provides an excellent view of the trachea, carina and the inferior aspect of the glottis (Howard and Croft, 1992).

However, it is difficult for prolonged phonation to occur during this procedure, and normal swallowing

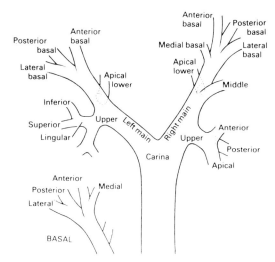

Figure 1.2 Diagram of the bronchial tree demonstrating the typical arrangement of bronchi as visible at bronchoscopy. In reality there is a wide normal variation of this pattern

is impossible, limiting its usefulness in the dynamic assessment of dysphagia. Some authors (Bastian *et al.*, 1989) have suggested that indirect videostrobolaryngoscopy performed as an outpatient procedure is an accurate means of staging laryngeal tumours. We do not feel that this is necessarily the case, as subglottic and pharyngeal detail may be easily missed. Furthermore, it does not allow a search for synchronous primary tumours, and it becomes difficult to manage bleeding from biopsy sites.

Stroboscopy

Oertel first performed stroboscopy in 1878. In the modern application, 2 Hz flashes of light 2 ms out of synchronization with phonation, are applied to the larynx via an endoscope, and the rigid instrument is to be preferred (Soderstan and Lindestad, 1992). This gives the illusion of slowness of movement, revealing features that are otherwise lost by the persistence of vision (Von Leyden, 1961). Stroboscopy is generally performed with video equipment for instant replay and frame-by-frame analysis (video stroboscopy). Parameters to measure are symmetry, amplitude, speed and phase difference of waves compared on the two cords.

It is useful for the differentiation of functional from anatomical defects (Sercarz *et al.*, 1992) and has been employed in the early detection of glottic cancer. In the latter setting, preservation of the mucosal wave suggests that a lesion is not invasive (Zhao, 1992). Unfortunately, the flashes do not synchronize so well in the very hoarse larynx, where shimmer may be marked. In patients with a cord palsy, the

first sign of recovery may be the return of a visible travelling wave on stroboscopy even before clinical signs become evident (Bless, Hirano and Feder, 1987). Similarly, in subtle abnormalities, such as isolated superior laryngeal nerve paralysis, an abnormality of the travelling wave may be the easiest finding to elicit (Sercarz *et al.*, 1992).

Photography

There are a number of methods for still photography and videography of the upper aerodigestive tract (Yanagisawa and Yanagisawa, 1991). While still photography via the flexible endoscope is best for the bronchi and oesophagus, videography is increasingly the method of choice for recording laryngeal abnormalities, especially when combined with stroboscopy. This enables detailed records of laryngeal structure and function that still photography rarely reveals. Colour videoprinters may now be attached to endoscopic equipment and give instant images for inclusion in patient records. Although, currently, their quality appears inferior to that achieved with still photography, further improvements are likely.

Rigid endoscopy
Preparation of the patient

Preoperative procedures

The procedure is carefully explained to the patient. Consent should include warnings about possible trauma to lips and teeth. A chest radiograph and any contrast studies or scans should be obtained and carefully examined preoperatively: the surgeon is often better placed to put the films into clinical context than the radiologist, however good the latter may be!

It is important, especially when contemplating biopsy of the larynx or bronchial tree, to ascertain that the patient's clotting is normal (Lewis and Treasure, 1993). Patients should be fasted for a minimum of 4 hours, and appropriate premedication should be administered. For laryngoscopy and bronchoscopy, this should include an anticholinergic agent, such as atropine, otherwise secretions can become a major problem. False teeth should be removed. If lymphoma is suspected, warn the pathology department, well in advance if possible, that a fresh specimen may be imminent.

Positioning

The patient is placed supine on the operating table. For oesophagoscopy, the head is placed on a ring on the upper hinged area of the table, with the head initially flexed slightly. As the procedure progresses, the table and head area are extended until the patient is in the classical 'sword swallowing' position (Howard and Croft, 1992). For bronchoscopy, the head is initially placed on a head ring or pillow, which is removed after the bronchoscope has passed through the cords (Lewis, and Treasure, 1993) (Figure 1.3). Draping the body is unnecessary for these procedures and restricts observation of respiratory movements.

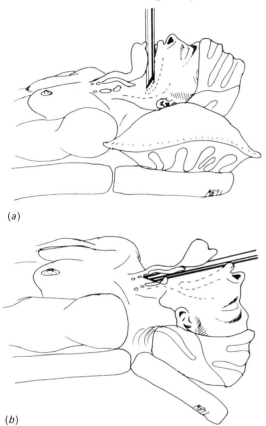

(a)

(b)

Figure 1.3 (*a*) and (*b*) Method of insertion of the rigid bronchoscope

Teeth and lips

Of course, false teeth should be removed prior to any of these procedures. In dentate individuals, however, protection of the teeth is essential for two reasons: first, to prevent dislodging crowns, caps or whole teeth, which may then be aspirated causing bronchial obstruction; second, to prevent disfigurement and associated litigation. Hence, the preoperative state of the teeth should be noted carefully, and the patient warned about possible damage. Protection involves the use of meticulous surgical technique and in addition, the use of a mouth guard. Metal guards are very much more protective in this regard than the commonly seen silastic devices.

In all rigid endoscopy, the non-dominant hand should be used to protect teeth or gums and to keep the lips from being crushed between teeth and endoscope.

Anaesthesia for endoscopy

Local

For outpatient nasendoscopy, the application of co-caine hydrochloride solution (1 ml of 10%; maximum 3 mg/kg) to the nose via a suitable spray is advocated. In addition, a benzocaine lozenge may be used to facilitate examination of the larynx in certain patients, with either flexible or Hopkins rod instruments. The use of a lignocaine and xylometazoline mixture is a useful alternative to cocaine and avoids the problems of toxicity occasionally seen with the latter. It is important to note that vagal attacks and cocaine reactions have been reported with these techniques, so suction and resuscitation equipment should be to hand if required.

For oesophagogastroduodenoscopy, a 10 mg benzo-caine lozenge is given half an hour before the procedure, and intravenous benzodiazepine is titrated during the procedure. A similar routine is followed for flexible bronchoscopy, but the more patent nasal fossa is also anaesthetized. Direct laryngoscopy is rarely performed under local anaesthetic now, but is enjoying a resurgence in some areas and is preferred by some for Teflon injection of the vocal cords as the patient may be instructed to phonate at various times. Again titrated sedation is given, after anaesthetizing the larynx with a combination of cocaine on pledgets (external laryngeal nerve) and 4% lignocaine spray. This procedure should ideally be performed with an anaesthetist present and monitoring equipment in place.

General

An anaesthetist and surgeon share a common airway for much of the above, and additional problems, such as the intense cardiovascular response to suspension microlaryngoscopy, are additionally encountered. Therefore, despite the fact that modern general anaesthetic examination of the aerodigestive tract is in many ways safer than a local one, problems may still occur and hence partnership with an anaesthetist skilled in these techniques is essential.

Premedication with a short half-life benzodiazepine is useful in adults, while an anticholinergic agent is helpful to reduce secretions in all age groups. Intravenous induction (e.g. thiopentone or propofol) may be used unless airway obstruction is suspected, when an inhalational agent (e.g. halothane) is preferred. Potential airway problems on induction should be anticipated, so that the surgeon is standing by in the anaesthetic room and tracheostomy facilities are available if urgently required. Topical anaesthesia of the larynx and trachea with 4% lignocaine reduces unwanted reflex activity prior to endoscopy.

A variety of techniques is used for general anaesthesia, and the choice should be carefully matched to the individual patient. Apnoeic oxygenation with oxygen insufflated down a Harris catheter is adequate for brief (less than 10 minutes) examinations in adults, while spontaneous respiration is very valuable in children, allowing collapse of the upper airway to be observed. For most laryngoscopies, small-bore endotracheal intubation is used: the obstructed view of the posterior larynx is rarely a problem, and the anterior larynx is well seen. The Venturi jet system provides ventilation via a cannula attached to or built into the endoscope. It permits a wholly unobstructed view, which is particularly valuable for laser surgery. The flow is regulated by a hand-held device or ventilator. An alternative for laser work is the metal Oswald-Unton tube, which requires the use of moist neurosurgical patties packed around it to attain a seal (Howard and Croft, 1992).

The sharing of the airway becomes of particular importance when one is attempting a detailed examination of the larynx. It is possible to observe most of the larynx around a small bore endotracheal tube, but the examination can never be complete in this setting. In adults, it is preferable to replace the tube with either a Venturi device or a jet ventilator which may be attached to the laryngoscope. In infants, the tube is withdrawn into the pharynx while examination is performed, anaesthetic gases continuing to be applied down the tube, and spontaneous ventilation being maintained throughout.

A recent innovation is the use of the laryngeal mask as an alternative to intubation. This method, for example combined with Venturi insufflation and a Dedo-Pilling laryngoscope, has made even the most difficult of laryngoscopies more practical (Briggs, Bailey and Howard, 1992).

Indications

Rigid endoscopy is mandatory in any patient with hoarseness or dysphagia who falls into a high risk group for upper aerodigestive tract malignancy, especially smokers and drinkers over 40 years of age. It should also be performed on lower-risk patients, such as younger non-smokers, in the presence of persistent symptoms or a suspicious clinical picture. The use of rigid endoscopes is the only reliable way to assess mucosal lesions of this region (Phelps, 1992), and more often enables adequate biopsies to be taken than is the case with flexible techniques (Ritchie *et al.*, 1993).

When a tumour is detected, its limits in all directions should be determined by both sight and palpation. These findings should be recorded immediately

the procedure is completed in the form of both words and drawings, indicating spread in all three dimensions. Many departments have standard sheets of drawings on which even the least artistic of surgeons may accurately outline the disease in a standardized form (Figure 1.4.)

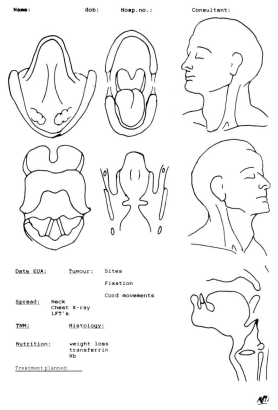

Figure 1.4 A standard sheet for the recording of tumour extent following endoscopy

When obtaining material for histology, it is important to biopsy any *viable* area. This has two implications: first, there is little point in sending necrotic material from the centre of a lesion; second, in most cases it will be necessary to send more than one biopsy, carefully labelling the site of origin of each. When obtaining biopsies of leukoplakic lesions, it is important to biopsy any red raised areas, which are more likely to harbour invasive disease than the flatter white areas. Biopsies should be taken as atraumatically as possible, using cutting forceps, and should be placed directly into formalin without the aid of a needle, rather than onto a swab (this distorts tissues). Where a lymphoma is suspected, part of the tissue should be forwarded fresh to the pathologist, who should be alerted of the possibility beforehand.

'Panendoscopy'

In most patients, pharyngoscopy, laryngoscopy and oesophagoscopy comprise an adequate assessment in the hoarse or dysphagic patient. The detection rate of synchronous primary tumours in this way is about 3–13% (Levine and Nielson, 1992). Rigid broncho-scopy should be added if there is a suggestion of bronchial disease. However, where there is an obvi-ous cancer of the laryngopharynx, the place of rigid bronchoscopy in 'panendoscopy' as part of a hunt for synchronous primary tumour is probably not merited on current evidence, since there is less than a 1% probability of discovering a bronchial tumour (Parker and Hill, 1984). Where bronchial tumours do coexist, an abnormal preoperative chest radiograph is almost universal in any case (Neal, 1984).

Direct laryngoscopy

Suitable laryngoscopes for routine purposes are the Negus and Storz varieties. For microlaryngoscopy, the Royal National, Throat, Nose and Ear Hospital variant is useful, while that designed by Benjamin is more suited to children. The Dedo-Pilling modifica-tion is helpful for those with difficult teeth and jaws. In any case, the laryngoscope chosen should be the largest that will comfortably fit the individual patient. The number of accessory instruments employed should be restricted to the minimum compatible with achieving adequate biopsy and manipulation, and should be those with which the surgeon is most comfortable.

The laryngoscope is inserted until its tip lies a few millimetres above the anterior commissure. En route, the uvula, epiglottis and arytenoids are noted (Figure 1.5). The use of 'BURP' (backward, upward and rightward pressure) on the thyroid cartilage by an assistant facilitates the view in many patients (Knill, 1993). If it is still not possible to view the anterior commissure satisfactorily, the straight-sided, broad tipped anterior commissure laryngoscope is used.

In the past, the latter instrument has also been advocated to obtain views into the ventricles and subglottis, but the advent of Hopkins rods enables us to perform a far more satisfactory examination of these regions. In addition, there is a subglottiscope available if detailed examination and biopsy of the subglottis and upper trachea is required (Ossoff, Dun-cavage and Dere, 1991). For lesions slightly further down, a tracheoscope may be used, but a better view may be obtained with a Storz bronchoscope.

If examination of vocal fold movement is required, this should be planned with the anaesthetist at the start of the procedure, so that interference from muscle relaxants may be minimized. In order to observe cord movements in uncooperative, anatomi-cally difficult or very young patients, it is possible to pass a flexible nasendoscope through the recently

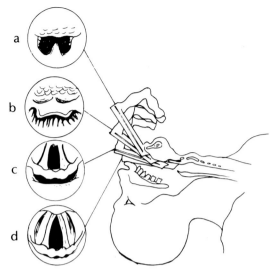

Figure 1.5 Method of insertion of the laryngoscope; a–d represent sequential views down the laryngoscope. (Modified, with permission from Parker, R. (1992) Laryngoscopy, microlaryngoscopy and laser surgery. In: *Rob and Smith's Operative Surgery: Head and Neck*, part 2, 4th edn, edited by I. A. McGregor and D. J. Howard. Oxford: Butterworth)

developed 'laryngeal mask' in theatre or as the pa-tient is waking in the recovery room (Briggs, Bailey and Howard, 1992; Dich-Nielson and Nagal, 1993).

A complete examination of the larynx involves:

1 A systematic review of all areas, including the epiglottis
2 Examination of the laryngeal ventricles and sub-glottis using 90° Hopkins rods via the laryngoscope
3 Assessment of vocal cord and arytenoid mobility using a straight probe (passive mobility test)
4 In infants, additionally checking for the presence of a laryngeal cleft posteriorly by stroking a probe between the arytenoids
5 Assessment of vocal fold movements or laryngeal collapse on waking
6 Carefully recording all of the above with the use of suitable drawings (see Figure 1.4).

Although little will be missed by performing the above with traditional direct laryngoscopy, the most detailed examinations should nowadays employ the operating microscope.

Microlaryngoscopy

The introduction of the operating microscope has facilitated both detailed examination of the larynx (Kleinsasser, 1965) and a whole new area of otolaryngology: phonosurgery. Only the former will be dealt with in the present chapter. A high quality operating microscope is employed with a 400 mm focal length lens in place. The use of the Loewy-type laryngostat support enables the endoscopist to use both hands in the examination of the patient. Initially, the support was placed on the patient's chest, and indeed this is still sometimes done as minimal pressure is, in fact, exerted. However, to give the anaesthetist access and to allow observation of the chest and, in any case, in infants and children, it is better to rest the laryngostat on a Mayo table attached to the operating table (Matt, 1993) (Figure 1.6). The broad-lumen Kleinsasser laryngoscope is used for adults, while Storz paediatric or Benjamin laryngoscopes give excellent access in children. The laryngoscope is first placed with the tip at the petiolus (adults) or in the valleculae (infants), then the laryngostat is attached and the tension tightened until the view is just adequate (Parker, 1992). The microscope is then brought into position and focused. Special techniques are used for laser surgery to the larynx and will not be described here.

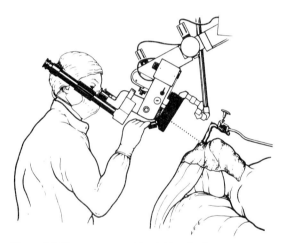

Figure 1.6 The arrangement for stable microlaryngoscopy. (Reproduced, with permission, from Parker, R. (1992) Laryngoscopy, microlaryngoscopy and laser surgery. In: *Rob and Smith's Operative Surgery: Head and Neck*, part 2, 4th edn, edited by I. A. McGregor and D. J. Howard. Oxford: Butterworth)

Oesophagoscopy

The oesophagoscope is held between the finger and thumb of the dominant hand like a pen, and at no stage should even firm pressure be required to negotiate the lumen. If the endoscope will not pass in this way, then either it is not being directed correctly, or there is a pathological obstruction. In either case, continued pressure may result in perforation.

Introduction is with the head initially slightly flexed, and the instrument facing backwards and upwards. The head is then extended and the endoscope brought round in an arc until its tip lies behind the anaesthetic tube and epiglottis. It is then passed behind or to the right of the larynx. Negotiating the cricopharyngeus (14–16 cm from the teeth) is an important step, and is aided by further extension, temporary deflation of the endotracheal tube cuff and external advancement of the larynx by an assistant. These manoeuvres are particularly important where osteophytes compress the lumen. At all times, steady pressure should be maintained and any sudden advances avoided.

Throughout the procedure the lumen must be kept in the middle of the field of view, and suction used to maintain vision. Further restrictions occur at 23–25 cm (aortic arch on the left) and 38–40 cm (lower oesophageal sphincter). It is often easier to observe the lumen on withdrawal of the instrument rather than on passage, so this part of the procedure should be performed deliberately and slowly.

Pharyngoscopy

As mentioned above, both contrast studies and the flexible oesophagoscope are notoriously poor at diagnosing lesions of the pharynx and postcricoid region. These may be adequately viewed with the rigid oesophagoscope as above, but the best view is obtained with the traditional Negus pharyngoscope. This is passed as for a laryngoscope, but placed into each pyriform fossa, laryngopharynx and postcricoid region in turn.

Rigid bronchoscopy

Even in skilled hands, flexible bronchoscopy under local anaesthetic and sedation is an uncomfortable procedure. Additionally, as with the oesophagus, more substantial biopsies may be obtained and foreign bodies better removed using a rigid endoscope under general anaesthesia (Gaer, 1992).

The older, hollow Negus instruments have been superseded by instruments using Hopkins rod facilities for increased visualization, such as those manufactured by Storz. In adults, 7 or 8 mm gauges are used with telescopes of 0°, 30° or 90°. For most purposes, however, the 0° telescope suffices, and is easier to interpret. The choice of the size of the bronchoscope in infants and children is discussed elsewhere. Side ports are used for introducing anaesthetic gas, and channels exist for suction, biopsy or manipulation.

The bronchoscope is introduced into the right side of the mouth between thumb and forefinger, held like a pen, with the beak anteriorly. The left hand is used to hold the position of the patient's head, and to keep the patient's lips from being crushed under the instrument. As with other rigid instruments, it is essential not to lever on the teeth. The beak is used to elevate the epiglottis and then advanced to the cords where it is rotated through 90°, so that the beak passes through sideways. At this stage, the pillow or head ring is removed (see Figure 1.3). When it is difficult to pass the bronchoscope the use of the Negus laryngoscope, with its sliding blade removed, may facilitate access to the larynx. At this point, ventilation via the sidearm may be commenced.

Examination of the bronchial tree is accomplished in a systematic manner:

1 Rotating the head to the left, right main and lower lobe (0°), right upper (90°) and right middle (30°) lobe bronchi
2 Rotating the head to the right, left main and lower lobe (0°), and left upper (90°) lobe bronchi.

At each site note:

1 Appearance of mucosa
2 Nature of secretions
3 Mass lesions
4 Compression or collapse
5 Mobility or blunting of the carina.

Only after all the above observations have been done are washings and biopsies, preferably with optical forceps, carried out as appropriate.

Laser bronchoscopy is useful in a number of settings. It is now standard practice to use a rigid instrument connected to a carbon dioxide laser for removal of tracheobronchial papillomas and granulomas, e.g. at the tip of tracheostomy tubes. Unfortunately, the view obtained with a rigid laser bronchoscope is more limited than that with a standard telescope, and is easily obscured by smoke and debris. In addition, palliation of obstructing bronchial carcinomas is possible by this route, although the Nd-YAG laser combined with the flexible endoscope is probably superior in this regard. For vascular lesions using the argon laser via flexible fibres is also a possibility.

Complications of endoscopy

As with all surgical procedures much of the morbidity and mortality is related to the underlying health of the patients concerned, and this is avoided as far as possible by careful pre-endoscopic assessment by surgical and anaesthetic teams.

General complications resulting from anaesthesia will not be discussed.

Perforation of the oesophagus

The overall perforation rate from simple diagnostic rigid oesophagoscopy is in the order of 1% (as, incidentally is mortality). In one series of 50 oesophageal perforations (White and Morris, 1992), 52% were iatrogenic. Perforation was more common in the thoracic oesophagus (54%), as it is more commonly associated with attempted dilatation of strictures than simple diagnostic endoscopy.

Diagnosis is based on clinical findings, a plain chest radiograph which may show free gas in the mediastinum, contrast studies, and flexible endoscopy. The presence of postoperative pain, especially if radiating to the back and shoulders and requiring more than simple analgesia, should alert the surgeon to the possibility of a perforation. Other features are surgical emphysema, pyrexia and dysphagia (often even to saliva). Diatrizoate (Gastrograffin) contrast studies are particularly useful in diagnosing perforations of the cervical oesophagus, while flexible endoscopy appears equally useful for thoracic injury (White and Morris, 1992).

Oesophageal perforation is an emergency with significant morbidity and mortality. Minor leaks in the neck are fortunately the majority of those seen after purely diagnostic oesophagoscopy. If only a small leak is detected, conservative treatment with the passage of a nasogastric tube and administration of antibiotics is advocated. For anything larger, and in any case in an unwell patient, exploration of the neck with the insertion of a neck drain should be performed.

Intrathoracic leaks require thoracotomy, and in these patients, particularly if associated with a pre-existing carcinoma, resection and reconstruction are probably required (Moghissi and Pender, 1988). There is significantly increased mortality for thoracic tears if there is a delay of more than 24 hours before thoracotomy (White and Morris, 1992). Referral should therefore be as soon as the diagnosis has been made. The mortality for cervical and thoracic tears is about 5% and 50% respectively (White and Morris, 1992).

Laryngeal spasm, mucosal haemorrhage and oedema

In a series of 204 endoscopic laryngeal procedures, Robinson (1991) found a 1% incidence of respiratory obstruction severe enough to require tracheostomy, due to oedema. One patient developed laryngospasm requiring reintubation. In the same series, 31% of examinations resulted in mucosal haemorrhage or oedema that was visible on indirect laryngoscopy, but neither of these was found to be a significant problem. It is concluded that endoscopy of the upper airway is a relatively safe procedure, that may, in selected patients be suitable for day-case surgery.

Teeth

Should damage to teeth occur, this should be carefully noted, the patient informed at an early stage, and referred to a dental surgeon. Where a tooth is removed, it should not be discarded but retained for replacement by the dentist. If there is any doubt as to whether a tooth is aspirated into the bronchial tree, bronchoscopy should be performed immediately, without waiting for a chest radiograph.

Cervical spine

Abnormalities of the cervical spine such as fusion of vertebrae, or severe osteophyte formation may prevent rigid endoscopy and special techniques are required for flexible instrumentation in these individuals (Welsh, Welsh and Chinnici, 1989). In addition, osteophytes may predispose to tearing of the cervical oesophagus. However, it is very important to remember that atlantoaxial dislocation may occur, particularly in rheumatoid arthritis, and can lead to paralysis or death. Thus, great care is needed in the preoperative evaluation of these patients.

Complications of bronchoscopy

The mortality for bronchoscopy is less than 0.01% and is usually related to massive bleeding. This is a particular risk if biopsying around the spurs of bronchial orifices, where large vessels lie in close proximity, and this should therefore be avoided whenever possible. If bleeding does occur, local adrenalin application, pressure or cautery may be applied (Lewis and Treasure, 1993). Other possible complications are laryngospasm, bronchial rupture, pneumothorax and cardiac arrhythmias.

Foreign bodies in the aerodigestive tract

Hand in hand with experience of endoscopy of the upper aerodigestive tract, there inevitably comes experience of foreign bodies. Many are easily removed, sometimes in outpatients, but many are not, and the technique for removal in each patient needs to be carefully tailored.

Acute foreign body airway obstruction: 'cafe coronary'

Acute foreign body airway obstruction is said to cause some 3000 deaths per annum in the USA. The object, classically a bolus of food 'bolted' in a restaurant, lodges in the larynx or pharynx causing acute respiratory embarrassment. If the airway is not restored, irreversible cerebral ischaemia occurs within 6 minutes. Survival is thus often dependent on the actions of passers-by, rather than on trained medical staff (Kitay and Shafer, 1989).

Attempts to retrieve the foreign material with the fingers are to be avoided, as they can cause further impaction. However, the Heimlich manoeuvre may be life saving: the rescuer stands behind the subject and places a clenched fist below the xiphisternum. This is followed by a rapid subdiaphagramatic, upwards thrust, producing an artificial cough of some force. If this step fails, it is necessary to perform cricothyrotomy. Here, while one hand steadies the larynx, the groove between the thyroid and cricoid cartilages is sought. A sharp knife is then used to cut horizontally into the larynx and rotated through 90° to maintain the airway. Any convenient tube is then placed through into the lumen until the patient can be transferred to a hospital. An alternative temporary airway may also be rapidly created by passing a minimum of three large (14 gauge) intravenous cannulae through the cricothyroid membrane should obstruction occur in a hospital setting.

Other types of foreign body

A careful history is important. Usually there is a clear history of symptoms dating from the time of ingestion of a foreign body or bolus. Occasionally, however, particularly in the case of bronchial foreign bodies in children, the history may be vague: there may be a history of a choking attack, followed by a symptomless interval of days or weeks. In the case of pharyngo-oesophageal foreign bodies, patients are generally able to indicate the level and side of obstruction with some accuracy (Connolly *et al.*, 1992).

Examination includes an assessment of the patient's general health and a full otolaryngological appraisal. The degree of oesophageal obstruction may be assessed from the ability to swallow saliva, and the presence of pharyngeal pooling of secretions. If the foreign body is in the larynx or tracheobronchial tree, the degree of respiratory embarrassment is important and is indicated by stridor, wheeze and chest signs: a unilateral wheeze is especially indicative, and it is to be remembered that the lower right lobe is the preferential site for such foreign bodies. Perforation of the oesophagus is indicated by surgical emphysema, back pain and pyrexia.

Although the routine role of radiography in the detection of fishbones is controversial (Knight and Lesser, 1989), we would still recommend a plain lateral neck film in all patients with a suspected foreign body where no acute airway obstruction is present. Many foreign bodies are clearly shown by plain films: most meat bones, certain fish (cod, haddock and mullet; Ell and Parker, 1992) and items of metal. It is important to note that most modern dentures are in fact radiolucent (Willsher, Clarke and Danile, 1993). Contrast studies rarely add much, but if perforation is suspected, a diatrizoate swallow can be contributory. Widening of the prevertebral shadow and air in the soft tissues are important signs. Where bolus obstruction exists, it is often possible to see air pockets in the upper oesophagus, a rare finding in the absence of obstruction. Chest radiographic abnormalities may be absent in the early stages of bronchial obstruction. There may be shifting of the mediastinum to the obstructed side early on (collapse), but classically this later gives way to hyperexpansion of the affected side due to a 'ball-valve' effect. Lobar pneumonia unresponsive to antibiotics is sometimes a later presenting feature, especially in the elderly.

Management

Larynx

Occlusion of the larynx may cause acute respiratory obstruction, the management is dealt with above. Where obstruction is subtotal, extreme care must be exercised: it is not necessary to image the larynx and indeed many obstructing bodies are radiolucent. On no account should attempts be made to remove the obstruction with fingers or forceps in the accident department. Rather, the patient should be immediately transferred by an otolaryngological surgeon to the operating theatre, where preparations for removal are made with tracheostomy equipment standing by if required (Kent and Watson, 1990). Under these conditions, removal often becomes straightforward.

Pharynx and oesophagus

Foreign bodies tend to lodge in sites of constriction in the oesophagus. These are usually the points of natural narrowing at 15 and 25 cm, but the reason for impaction at these levels may have more to do with motility patterns than anatomy *per se* (Stein *et al.*, 1992). A significant proportion of impactions, particularly in the elderly, occur at benign or malignant, strictures. This should always be borne in mind, and facilities for biopsy must be available when removing foreign bodies.

Foreign bodies may conveniently be divided into fishbones and 'others' in terms of their sites of impaction and management (O'Flynn and Simo, 1993). Of all those presenting with a history of pain after fishbone ingestion, only 20% are subsequently found to have a bone impacted (Knight and Lesser, 1989). In some parts of the world, fishbones are by far the commonest form of foreign body. Experience in these places has shown that 73% may be removed perorally or with the use of the laryngeal mirror and appropriate curved forceps, while half of the remainder may be removed with the use of the flexible nasendoscope under local anaesthetic (Choy *et al.*, 1992). If these measures fail, general anaesthesia is required. Fishbones rarely cause serious perforations, but may migrate and lead to cervical abscess formation.

Meat boluses and dentures are more commonly swallowed in the elderly. Peristaltic changes in the oesophagus with age, decrease in psychological function and reduction in the tactile functions of the palate consequent on the wearing of dentures are all contributory. In addition, about one-third of food bolus obstructions are due to underlying abnormalities of the oesophagus, and half of these will be carcinomas (Stadler *et al.*, 1989). Occasionally, bizarre ingested foreign bodies, sometimes multiple, are found in the psychologically disturbed, the mentally retarded and prisoners.

Removal of most foreign bodies should be preferably performed with rigid instruments under general anaesthesia. Some pharyngeal foreign bodies, particularly coins in children may be removed in the anaesthetic room as soon as intubation is accomplished. If not the patient should be positioned and endoscoped as outlined above. Some foreign bodies, particularly bones and dental plates, may not be removed whole and cutting forceps and shears exist to enable their piecemeal removal. There are, in addition, special forceps for the removal of safety pins.

On removing the foreign body, there is sometimes an obvious underlying lesion such as a benign or malignant structure. These should be biopsied, and appropriate investigations instituted. On removing the endoscope, a careful check should be made for mucosal tears that may have occurred during extraction. If there is any doubt about this, a nasogastric tube should be carefully passed, and nothing given by mouth until a chest radiograph has been performed, and the patient observed for 24 hours. If there is a history of recurrent impaction, videofluoroscopy should be performed to rule out motility disorders, or a psychiatric assessment arranged if appropriate. Jones, Lannigan and Salama (1991) advocated a follow-up barium swallow in all patient with bolus obstruction.

Where impaction is severe, rather than risk perforation, it is preferable to refer the patient to a thoracic surgeon for removal by thoracotomy. In addition, some lower oesophageal foreign bodies may be better removed by gently delivering into the stomach and referring for consideration of gastrotomy. Flexible endoscopes allow only delicate forceps to be passed, and so foreign body removal is rather limited. We therefore advocate that where the expertise exists, removal with rigid instruments under general anaesthesia should be performed.

Complications of foreign body ingestion are airway obstruction, perforation and cervical abscess formation. The first two are dealt with above, while half of all cervical abscesses are due to foreign body migration (Sethi and Chew, 1991). These latter should be dealt with by external exploration and drainage.

Alternatives to rigid endoscopy

Where there is a history of foreign body ingestion, but the patient is asymptomatic, it is sometimes possible to pursue a conservative course. This is particularly the case with asymptomatic coin ingestion in children, where simple serial radiographs may be sufficient to allay parental anxiety (Caravati, Bennett and McElwee, 1989). Of course, should dysphagia develop at any stage, endoscopy should be undertaken without delay and in any case where the foreign body fails to pass.

Disimpaction of meat boluses with spasmolytic agents such as hyoscine butylbromide (Buscopan, 20 mg q.d.s., i.v./i.m.) has been reported to be successful in up to two-thirds of patients (Tibling and Stanquist, 1991). Contraindications to its use are related to its anticholinergic properties and include glaucoma, urinary retention and heart failure. Recently, successful attempts have been made to dislodge boluses with gas-forming agents such as tartaric acid and bicarbonate mixtures. These are yet to be fully evaluated (Zimmers *et al.*, 1988).

The passage of a catheter under radiological control beyond the foreign body, inflation of the balloon and subsequent withdrawal has been advocated for the removal of coins in children (Campbell and London, 1989). However, it is a blind procedure, and in the authors' opinion is far inferior to rigid endoscopy.

Flexible endoscopy may be used for the removal of foreign bodies from the oesophagus, and indeed is often successful. Where rigid endoscopy is contraindicated (see above), it is the method of choice, but in other contexts, rigid instrumentation is superior. An occasional alternative to thoracotomy for the removal of severely impacted foreign bodies is retrograde flexible oesophagoscopy via a surgical gastrostomy (Winkler *et al.*, 1989).

Ingestion of corrosives

This commonly occurs in children or suicidal adults. The nature of the ingested substances should be immediately ascertained. Alkali ingestion, e.g. that produced by lye, is, in general, more severe than that produced by acids. Injury varies from oral burns requiring simple analgesia, to oesophageal and gastric perforation requiring resection and replacement. Immediate management includes securing the airway, with emergency room intubation if necessary, intravenous fluid resuscitation and adequate analgesia. The role of steroids in this context is undetermined. Early endoscopic assessment is required to determine the depth and extent of burns. Where burns are extensive, the decision lies between early excision and replacement or temporary jejunostomy. Repeat endoscopy is required to assess healing and to check for stricture formation (Meredith, Kon and Thompson, 1988).

An increasingly recognized form of caustic ingestion is in the form of swallowed batteries (Thompson *et al.*, 1990). If left for a period of time, the acid may leak with resultant burns and stricture formation.

Thus, an aggressive approach to management is required.

Bronchial foreign bodies

In Holinger and Holinger's series of more than 2000 patients with tracheobronchial foreign bodies (Holinger and Holinger, 1978), only 6% were over the age of 14 years. While their referral population may have been somewhat skewed, it is certainly the case that these are more common in children. With modern bronchoscopic equipment, especially optical forceps (Figure 1.7), thoracotomy with bronchotomy and segmental resection as part of the management of bronchial foreign bodies has been largely confined to the past. Some respiratory units possess experience of using the flexible bronchoscope for removal of bronchial foreign bodies, but most authors agree that modern rigid telescopes are far preferable in this regard and should be employed wherever possible (Lewis and Treasure, 1993).

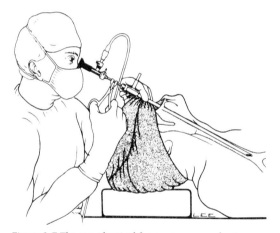

Figure 1.7 The use of optical forceps to remove foreign body. (Reproduced with permission from Howard, D. J. and Croft, C. B. (1992) Endoscopy. In: *Rob and Smith's Operative Surgery: Head and Neck*, part 2, 4th edn, edited by I. A. McGregor and D. J. Howard. Oxford: Butterworth)

In the bronchi, vegetable matter, such as peanuts, produces a rapid, severe chemical bronchitis. This makes removal after any period of time somewhat hazardous. Inflammation may cause bleeding, and the foreign body frequently fragments, distributing foreign matter further down the bronchial tree. Hence, in all cases, especially children, bronchoscopy for the removal of foreign bodies must not be taken lightly. The most senior available anaesthetic and surgical staff should perform the procedure, which should be done on the first available list, rather than under suboptimal conditions of a night-time emergency theatre. Adequate antibiotic cover

Table 1.1 Summary of the typical clinical features, radiographic findings and treatment of the common pharyngo-oesophageal foreign bodies

Foreign body	Age group	Radiopaque	Conservative treatment	Surgical treatment
Coins	Children	Yes	30% expectant	Endoscopy
Dentures	Elderly	If wires attached	No	Endoscopy/thoracotomy
Fishbones	Any	50%	Outpatient removal most	Endoscopy, remainder
Meat bones	Elderly	75%	No	Endoscopy/thoracotomy
Food bolus	Elderly	No	Hyoscine/? gas formers	Endoscopy
Batteries	Children	Yes	No	Endoscopy/burn treatment

should be given. The equipment to be used should be thoroughly checked and some centres have models of the tracheobronchial tree (Storz) that may be used to rehearse the procedure beforehand.

First, the appropriately angled bronchoscope is introduced to identify the site and nature of the obstruction. Careful use of suction is essential. It is very helpful at this stage to instill small amounts of 1:200 000 adrenalin solution into the affected bronchus, especially if significant impaction has occurred. This has the effect of releasing the foreign material by vasoconstriction of the inflamed mucosa, and also reduces bleeding, which may otherwise obstruct the view. However, careful cardiovascular monitoring is required, as adrenalin is rapidly absorbed from the lungs. Various optical forceps exist for the actual extraction, and the correct choice depends on the shape and constitution of the item. As it is gradually removed, there is often a gush of pus from beyond. The optical forceps are then removed from the airway, continuing to grasp the foreign body.

Where a foreign body has been in place for some time, it is wise for the patient to remain in hospital, with intravenous antibiotics and intensive physiotherapy, for many days. The radiological resolution of chest signs is an encouraging but rather late, sign. If doubt remains at any stage about the complete clearance of the obstruction, repeat bronchoscopy should be performed without hesitation.

References

ADACHI, Y., KITAMURA, K., TSUTSUI, S., IKEDA, Y., MATSUDA, H. and SUGIMACHI, K. (1993) How to detect early carcinoma of the oesophagus. *Hepatogastroenterology*, **40**, 207–211

BARKER, M. and DORT, J. C. (1991) Laryngeal examination: a comparison of mirror examination with a rigid lens system. *Journal of Otolaryngology*, **20**, 100–103

BASTIAN, R. W., COLLINS, S. L., KANIFF, T. and MATZ, G. J. (1989) Indirect videolaryngoscopy versus direct endoscopy for larynx and pharynx cancer staging. *Annals of Otology, Rhinology and Laryngology*, **98**, 693–698

BINGHAM, B. J., DRAKE-LEE, A., CHEVRETTON, E. and WHITE, A. (1986) Pitfalls in the assessment of dysphagia by fibreoptic oesophagogastroscopy. *Annals of the Royal College of Surgeons of England*, **68**, 22–23

BLESS, D. M., HIRANO, M. and FEDER, R. J. (1987) Videostroboscopic evaluation of the larynx. *Ear, Nose and Throat Journal*, **66**, 48–58

BRIGGS, R. J., BAILEY, P. and HOWARD, D. J. (1992) The laryngeal mask: a new type of airway in anaesthesia for direct laryngoscopy. *Otolaryngology – Head and Neck Surgery*, **107**, 603–605

CAMPBELL, J. B. and CONDON, V. R. (1989) Catheter removal of blunt oesophageal foreign bodies in children. Survey of the Society for Paediatric Radiology. *Paediatric Radiology*, **19**, 361–365

CARAVATI, E. M., BENNETT, D. L. and MCELWEE, N. E. (1989) Paediatric coin ingestion. A prospective study on the utility of routine roentgenograms. *American Journal of Diseases of Children*, **143**, 549–551

CHOY, A. T., GLUCKMAN, P. G., TONG, M. C. and VAN HASSALT, C. A. (1992) Flexible nasopharyngoscopy for fishbone removal from the pharynx. *Journal of Laryngology and Otology*, **106**, 709–711

CONNOLLY, A. A. P., BIRCHALL, M. A., WALSH-WARING, G. P. and MOORE-GILLON, V. (1992) Ingested foreign bodies: patient-guided localisation is a useful clinical tool. *Clinical Otolaryngology*, **17**, 520–524

DICH-NIELSON, J. O. and NAGAL, P. (1993) Flexible bronchoscopy via the laryngeal mask. *Acta Anaesthesiologica Scandinavica*, **37**, 17–19

ELI, S. R. and PARKER, A. J. (1992) The radio-opacity of fishbones. *Clinical Otolaryngology*, **17**, 514–516

GAER, J. (1992) Thoracic diagnosis. *Surgery*, **10**, 6–8

HOLINGER, P. H. and HOLINGER, L. D. (1978) Use of open tube bronchoscope in the extraction of foreign bodies. *Chest*, **73**(S), 721–724

HOWARD, D. J. and CROFT, C. B. (1992) Endoscopy. In: *Rob and Smith's Operative Surgery: Head and Neck* part 2 4th edn, edited by I. A. McGregor and D. J. Howard. Oxford: Butterworth. pp. 417–440

JONES, N. S., LANNIGAN, F. J. and SALAMA, N. Y. (1991) Foreign bodies in the throat: a prospective study of 388 cases. *Journal of Laryngology and Otology*, **105**, 104–108

KENT, S. E. and WATSON, M. G. (1990) Laryngeal foreign bodies. *Journal of Laryngology and Otology*, **104**, 131–133

KITAY, G. and SHAFER, N. (1989) Cafe coronary: recognition, treatment and prevention. *Nurse Practitioner*, **14**, 35–38

KLEINSASSER, O. (1965) Weitere Technische Entwicklung und erste Ergebnisse der 'endolaryngealen Mikrochirurgie'. *Zeitschrift für Laryngologie, Rhinologie und Otologie*, **44**, 711–727

KNILL, R. L. (1993) Difficult laryngoscopy made easy with a 'BURP'. *Canadian Journal of Anaesthesia*, **40**, 279–282

KNIGHT, L. C. and LESSER, T. H. (1989) Fish bones in throat. *Archives of Emergency Medicine*, **6**, 13–16

KOUFMAN, J. A. (1991) The otolaryngologic manifestations of gastroesophageal reflux disease (GERD): a clinical investigation of 225 patients using ambulatory 24 hour pH monitoring and an experimental investigation of the role of acid and pepsin in the development of laryngeal injury. *Laryngoscope*, **101** (suppl. 53), 1–78

LEVINE, B. and NIELSON, E. W. (1992) The justifications and controversies of panendoscopy – a review. *Ear, Nose and Throat Journal*, **71**, 335–343

LEWIS, M. P. N. and TREASURE, T. (1993) Rigid bronchoscopy. *Surgery*, **11**, 430–431

LOGEMANN, J. A. (1983) *Evaluation and Treatment of Swallowing Disorders*. San Diego: College Hill Press

MATT, B. H. (1993) Suspension platform for stable microlaryngoscopy. *Otolaryngology – Head and Neck Surgery*, **108**, 199–200

MEREDITH, J. W., KON, N. D. and THOMPSON, J. N. (1988) Management of injuries from liquid lye ingestion. *Journal of Trauma*, **28**, 1173–1180

MOGHISSI, K. and PENDER, D. (1988) Instrumental perforations of the oesophagus and their management. *Thorax*, **43**, 642–646

NEAL, H. B. (1984) Routine panendoscopy: is it necessary every time? *Archives of Otolaryngology*, **110**, 531–532

O'FLYNN, P. and SIMO, R. (1993) Fish bones and other foreign bodies. *Clinical Otolaryngology*, **18**, 231–233

OSSOFF, R. H., DUNCAVAGE, J. A. and DERE, H. (1991) Microsubglottoscopy: an expansion of operative microlaryngoscopy. *Otolaryngology – Head and Neck Surgery*, **104**, 842–848

PARKER, J. J. and HILL, J. H. (1984) Panendoscopy in screening for synchronous primary malignancies. *Laryngoscope*, **94**, 147–149

PARKER, R. (1992) Laryngoscopy, microlaryngoscopy and laser surgery. In: *Rob and Smith's Operative Surgery: Head and Neck*, part 2, 4th edn, edited by I. A. McGregor and D. J. Howard. Oxford: Butterworth. pp. 451–463

PHELPS, P. D. (1992) Carcinoma of the larynx – the role of imaging in staging and pre-treatment assessments. *Clinical Radiology*, **46**, 77–83

RITCHIE, A. J., MCGUIGAN, J., STEVENSON, H. M. and GIBBONS, J. R. (1993) Diagnostic rigid and flexible oesophagoscopy in carcinoma of the oesophagus: a comparison. *Thorax*, **48**, 115–118

ROBINSON, P. M. (1991) Prospective study of complications of endoscopic laryngeal surgery. *Journal of Laryngology and Otology*, **105**, 356–358

SERCARZ, J. A., BERKE, G. S., MING, Y., GERRATT, B. R. and NATIVIDED, M. (1992) Videostroboscopy of human vocal fold paralysis. *Annals of Otology, Rhinology and Laryngology*, **101**, 567–577

SETHI, D. S. and CHEW, C. T. (1991) Retropharyngeal abscess – the foreign body connection. *Annals of the Academy of Medicine Singapore*, **20**, 581–588

SILBERMANN, H. D., HAMPEL, A. and KOMINSKY, A. H. (1993) New techniques for the sterile introduction of flexible nasopharyngolaryngoscopes. *Annals of Otology, Rhinology and Laryngology*, **102**, 687–689

SODERSTAN, M. and LINDESTAD, P. A. (1992) A comparison of vocal fold closure in rigid telescopic and flexible fibreoptic laryngostroboscopy. *Acta Otolaryngologica*, **112**, 144–150

SOM, P. M. (1987) Lymph nodes of the neck. *Radiology*, **165**, 593–600

STADLER, J., HOLSCHER, A. H., FAUSSNAR, H., DITTLER, J. and SIEWART, R. (1989) The steakhouse syndrome. Primary and definitive diagnosis and therapy. *Surgical Endoscopy* **3**, 195–198

STEIN, H. J., SCHWIZER, W., DEMEESTER, T. R., ALBERTUCCI, M., BONAVINA, L. and SPIRAS-WILLIAMS, K. J. (1992) Foreign body entrapment in the oesophagus of healthy subjects – a manometric and scintigraphic study. *Dysphagia*, **7**, 220–225

STELL, P. M. and MARAN, A. G. D. (eds) (1972) Pre-operative considerations. In: *Head and Neck Surgery*. London: William Heinnemann Medical. p.6

TIBLING, L. and STANQUIST, M. (1991) Foreign bodies in the oesophagus: a study of causative factors. *Dysphagia*, **6**, 224–227

THOMPSON, N., LOWE- PONSFORD, F., MANT, T. G. and VOLAN, G. N. (1990) Button buttery ingestion: a review. *Adverse Drug Reactions and Acute Poisoning Review*, **9**, 157–180

VON LEYDEN, H. (1961) The electronic synchron-stroboscope. Its value for the practising laryngologist. *Annals of Otology, Rhinology and Laryngology*, **70**, 881–893

WELSH, L. W., WELSH, J. J. and CHINNICI, J. C. (1989) Endoscopic problems due to cervical vertebral disease. *Annals of Otology, Rhinology and Laryngology*, **98**, 597–601

WHITE, R. K. and MORRIS, D. M. (1992) Diagnosis and management of oesophageal perforations. *American Surgeon*, **58**, 112–119

WILLSHER, P. C., CLARKE, C. P. and DANILE, F. J. (1993) Dentures: difficult oesophageal foreign bodies. *Australian and New Zealand Journal of Surgery*, **63**, 736–738

WINKLER, A. R., MCCLANATHAN, D. T., BORGER, J. A. and AHMED, N. (1989) Retrograde oesophagoscopy for foreign body removal. *Journal of Paediatric Gastroenterology and Nutrition*, **8**, 536–540

YANAGISAWA, E. and YANAGISAWA, R. (1991) Laryngeal photography. *Otolaryngology Clinics of North America*, **24**, 999–1022

ZHAO, R. (1992) Diagnostic value of stroboscopy in early glottic carcinoma. *Chung Rua Ehr Pi Yan Hou Ko Tsa Chih*, **27**, 175–176

ZIMMERS, T. E., CHAN, S. B., KOUCHOUKOS, P. L., MIRANDA, H., NOY, Y. and VAN LAUVAN, B. (1988) Use of gas forming agents in oesophageal food impactions. *Annals of Emergency Medicine*, **17**, 693–695

2

Radiological examination

P. D. Phelps

Radiological evaluation of the mucosal surfaces of the upper aerodigestive tract has always been secondary to clinical examination, but can be useful for showing foreign bodies or the lower limits of a tumour when this cannot be assessed endoscopically. Traditionally the radiographic techniques used have been (a) plain film to show the air/soft tissue interface and surrounding bony structures, (b) intraluminal contrast examinations. High kilovolt techniques, tomography and xeroradiography, single or in combination, are used to give a better demonstration of the outlines of these air-filled cavities; the first two techniques by partially eliminating the overlying bony structures from the image, and xeroradiography by the edge enhancement effect. However, interpretation is fraught with difficulty because of variations in airway contour, poor radiographic contrast and superimposition of areas of interest. The barium swallow remains the most important radiological examination for the oro- and hypopharynx, especially when combined with cineradiography and videofluoroscopy. It is a simple and easy means of examination, although obviously of more value for lesions below the cricopharyngeus which cannot be assessed with a laryngeal mirror.

High resolution computerized tomography (CT) has greatly improved and extended the imaging capabilities in this region. Not only is the clearest demonstration of the air/soft tissue interface given in axial sections, but also shown are the surrounding fascial planes, muscles and vessels in the parapharyngeal region. Thus anatomy which formerly could not be assessed, except by invasive contrast examinations such as angiography or sialography, can be seen and CT has proved capable of showing deep abnormalities undetectable by physical examination and sometimes even by biopsy.

The radiographic anatomy and a brief account of some features of disease of the mucosal surface of the nasopharynx are considered in Volume 4, Chapter 3. The demonstration of infiltration by nasopharyngeal carcinoma into the deep tissue planes of the parapharyngeal region is the most significant advance made by CT. The parapharyngeal space bridges the nasopharynx and oropharynx and so a discussion of the CT anatomy and the fascial spaces and compartments below the skull will be considered, together with a brief account of the relations of the salivary glands to these spaces.

Magnetic resonance (MR) gives even better demonstration of these soft tissue structures. Differentiation between mucosal and lymphoid tissue and muscle is possible (Figure 2.1) and there is clear delineation of tumours from surrounding soft tissues. The

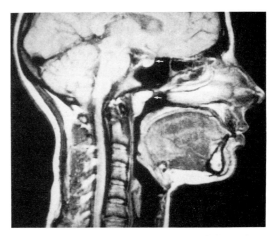

Figure 2.1 Magnetic resonance in the sagittal plane. The white arrows indicate the pituitary gland above and a small adenoid pad below

relationship of a mass to major blood vessels is also shown better with MR than by enhanced CT. Above all, direct three-plane imaging is a major advantage especially in the demonstration of the limits of the tumour, but an anterior or wrap-around surface coil is really necessary to obtain high signal to noise images of the larynx: the standard head or spine coils are rarely satisfactory.

Imaging techniques

Plain radiography

The best plain film view of the nasopharynx, larynx and pharynx is given by the lateral projection with the pharynx and larynx clear of the cervical spine. The film is placed against the shoulder and the incident beam is centred on the angle of the jaw if the nasopharynx is the region of interest, or the thyroid cartilage if the larynx is being examined. Xerograms give a clearer demonstration. Alternatively, a high kilovolt technique may be used utilizing 'low dose' film with screens, or a wedge filter to allow visualization of the range of densities from the neck to the thoracic inlet.

To show the structures low in the neck and upper mediastinum, the central ray is directed to a point below the middle of the clavicle at the level of the thoracic inlet and to the centre of the film, placed in the Bucky tray.

Even with xeroradiography or high kilovolt techniques the anteroposterior projection is usually less informative as the air-filled structures of the nasopharynx and larynx are largely obscured by the cervical spine, but it may show tracheal displacement or compression, or a fluid level in a pouch or abscess. To demonstrate a laryngocoele the exposure is made during the Valsalva manoeuvre, but tomography may be necessary. Long ossified styloid processes are best shown on an anteroposterior view taken through the open mouth. If possible all examinations should be performed erect to show any fluid levels.

Structures demonstrated (Figure 2.2)

On the lateral projection, air in the upper respiratory passages outlines the vallecula and cavities of the larynx and trachea. Soft tissue structures such as the soft palate, base of tongue, epiglottis and aryepiglottic folds are silhouetted against this air background. Occasionally, enlarged tonsils may be seen as oval densities, and the cartilaginous eustachian tube may present as a narrow dark slit when filled with air having a rim around it due to the eustachian cushion. The hyoid bone and, if ossified, the thyroid and cricoid cartilages, can usually be clearly seen. Careful note should be made of the thickness of the soft tissues in the nasopharynx and of the prevertebral

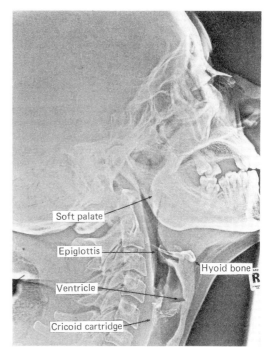

Figure 2.2 Lateral xerogram showing larynx, pharynx and nasopharynx. (From *Sutton's Textbook of Radiology*, Edinburgh: Churchill Livingstone, with permission). Because of the high radiation dose involved xeroradiography is now no longer used

soft tissues. These are important, as a bulge or increase in thickness may indicate oedema, abscess, haematoma, cyst or tumour. Loss of the normal spinal curvature should also be noted. Surgical emphysema shows as linear streaks of air in the prevertebral plane. In adults the soft tissues in the roof of the nasopharynx should measure not more than 1 cm; they should be regular in outline and thickness. In children, hypertrophy of the adenoid may be so pronounced as to obliterate the air space between the posterosuperior wall and the soft palate, and enlarged adenoids may be visible into early adult life. Imaging of the adenoids is considered in Volume 6, Chapter 18.

In infants, particularly in the first weeks of life, the prevertebral soft tissues normally look thick, especially on full expiration, and this should not be mistaken for a retropharyngeal infection. Films should always be taken on inspiration and, if there is any doubt, the films should be repeated on expiration, or a cine run taken with the infant held in an erect lateral position.

The depth of the cervical prevertebral soft tissues normally increases slightly from the level of the anterior arch of the atlas down to the lower border of the fifth and sixth cervical vertebrae, where it blends with the thicker soft tissue shadow of the cricopharyngeus and upper oesophagus. After the age of 2 or 3 years it should not measure more than 4 mm in depth. Below the cricoid the soft tissue thickness between the air-filled trachea and the spine should not normally exceed three-quarters of the diameter of the corresponding cervical vertebra, and should it do so a tumour or inflammation in the postcricoid region or upper oesophagus should be suspected.

Foreign bodies and growths in the larynx or trachea may be silhouetted against intraluminal air. At the thoracic inlet the trachea usually lies centrally in the anteroposterior projection. On the lateral view, it normally lies equidistant between the anterior vertebral border and the posterior profile of the upper manubrium. These relationships may be disturbed by scoliosis or kyphosis, the trachea being displaced towards the concavity of the scoliosis, and forwards with kyphosis. With a straight cervical spine, displacement of the air-filled trachea (or barium-filled oesophagus) indicates extrinsic pressure.

Ossification commonly occurs in one or more of the laryngeal cartilages, although there is considerable individual variation both in age of onset and extent. It is uncommon before the third decade. Ossification occurs more commonly in the thyroid cartilage in which it starts posteriorly and slowly extends forwards and upwards. The cricoid tends to ossify from behind forwards. The stylohyoid ligament not infrequently ossifies in its upper part, and occasionally throughout its whole extent. The styloid processes are best shown on an anteroposterior view taken through the open mouth. Rarely, ossification occurs in the epiglottis and occasionally the cricothyroid ligament is ossified. Compression of the trachea is usually obvious.

The arytenoids may ossify in the absence of ossification in other laryngeal cartilages and present as dense triangular opacities. If superimposed they should not be mistaken for a swallowed foreign body when the examination has been performed to try to demonstrate one. The same applies to ossified triticeous cartilages. The corniculate and cuneiform cartilages are unlikely to be so mistaken because they lie more anteriorly.

The region of the anterior commissure is often difficult to assess endoscopically and lesions of this part of the larynx may be shown best by lateral xerography (Figure 2.3) or by CT or MR which can also demonstrate extension of a tumour into the pre-epiglottic space.

Tomography

Conventional tomography still has a place in the examination of the larynx especially in the frontal projection, although a similar demonstration may be obtained by high-kilovolt techniques. Anteroposterior

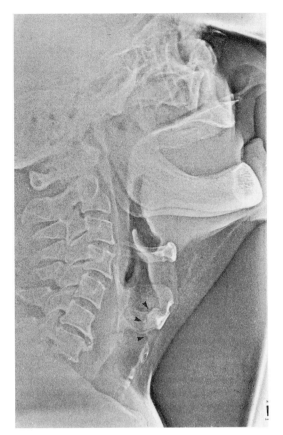

Figure 2.3 Lateral xerogram of a patient with a small carcinoma of the anterior commissure of the glottis (arrow heads)

tomographic studies of the larynx demonstrate the true and false vocal cords and the laryngeal ventricle between them. The cords should be demonstrated in full adduction by obtaining a picture with the patient phonating 'ee' (Figure 2.4) and as near as possible in full abduction in the phase of quiet respiration. Linear tomography is preferred because of the short exposure time and good radiographic contrast. Further views may be obtained in inspiratory phonation to distend the laryngeal ventricles, or with the patient performing a Valsalva manoeuvre which produces distension of the supraglottic larynx and hypopharynx.

Immobility of one vocal cord due to paralysis or fixation shows loss of the normal acute angle between the undersurface of the cord and the subglottis when the patient phonates 'ee' (Figure 2.5), but such immobility is of course normally assessed clinically. Tomography is of more value for lesions below the cords, especially when there is narrowing as by a tumour (Figure 2.6) or previous intubation. Laryngocoeles which may be difficult to diagnose clinically are also well shown by tomography.

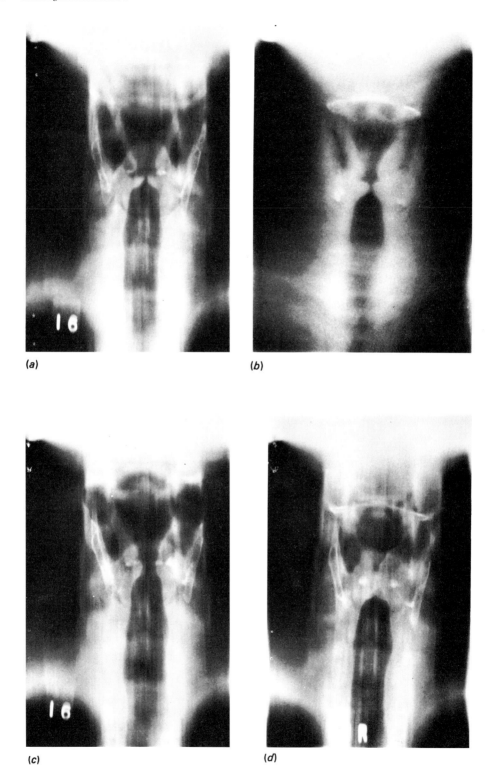

Figure 2.4 Tomogram of the larynx (*a*) phonating 'ee' (linear), (*b*) phonating 'e' (spiral), (*c*) quiet breathing (linear), (*d*) Valsalva manoeuvre (linear)

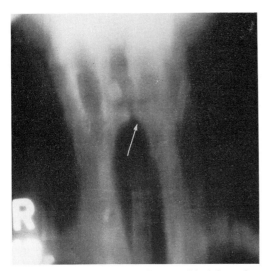

Figure 2.5 Tomogram showing fixation of the left vocal cord (arrow), as well as obliteration of the left pyriform fossa by a tumour

Computerized tomography

Computerized tomography of the larynx is now a valuable addition to available imaging techniques. The axial CT sections produce an image similar to the one seen by the surgeon. Respiratory movement is less of a problem with the new fast scanners, but acceptable images can be obtained in quiet respiration with long scanning times. Scanning is begun at the level of the hyoid bone and sequential scans of 5-mm slices are made in a caudal direction. The shape of the airway alters as sequential scans are viewed. Above the rounded hypopharynx it is bisected by the crescentic epiglottis. Further down the median and lateral glosso-epiglottic folds delineate the vallecula. Below this the airway assumes a triangular shape and the pyriform fossae are seen as two lateral appendages separated by the aryepiglottic folds. At the level of the cords the shape changes to the characteristic glottic chink or boat shape with the sharp anterior commissure extending right up to the thyroid cartilage in the midline (Figure 2.7). In the

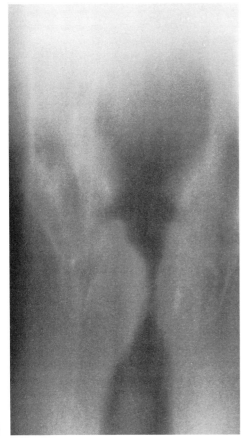

(a)

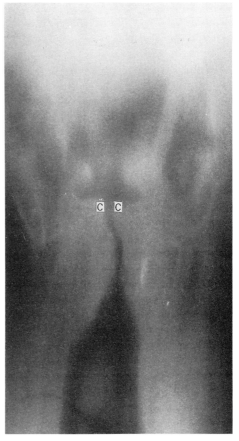

(b)

Figure 2.6 Subglottic carcinoma with much narrowing of the airway. Note, however, the normal movement of the vocal cords (*c*). Tomogram (*a*) was performed with the cords in full abduction and (*b*) in adduction

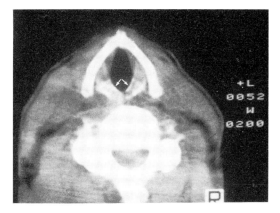

Figure 2.7 CT of the larynx at the level of the glottis. The arrows point to the arytenoid cartilages

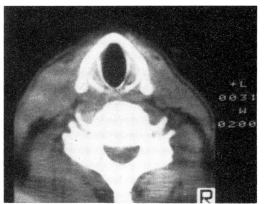

Figure 2.8 CT of the larynx at the subglottic level. The thyroid and cricoid cartilages are shown and the airway has an oval shape. (From *Sutton's Textbook of Radiology*, Edinburgh: Churchill Livingstone, with permission)

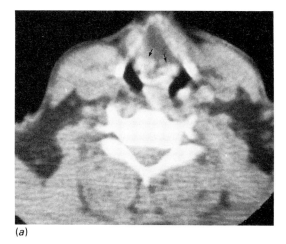

(*a*)

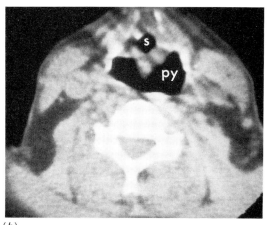

(*b*)

Figure 2.9 CT of the larynx during Valsalva manoeuvre: (*a*) at the level of the adducted cords showing the arytenoid cartilages (arrows) with air in the pyriform fossae behind, (*b*) at supraglottic level showing air in the larynx (S), and in the pyriform fossae (py)

subglottic area there is an even symmetrical oval shape (Figure 2.8) which gives way at the level of the first tracheal ring to an oval, flattened posteriorly, which may be likened to the shape of a horseshoe. Further sections may be taken with the patient holding his breath or performing a modified Valsalva manoeuvre. A good demonstration of the distended pyriform fossae and the supraglottic structures may be obtained (Figure 2.9).

Computerized tomography provides a non-invasive, quick and effective radiological investigation of the larynx, and is not uncomfortable for the patient. It can be carried out without risk in the face of respiratory obstruction or after suspected laryngeal injury. It gives an accurate assessment of laryngeal anatomy and involvement by tumour, particularly at the glottic level. The value of such an assessment is greatly increased if partial laryngectomy is contemplated, but this is an unusual operation in the UK where carcinoma of the larynx is treated by radiotherapy

and/or total laryngectomy. Because CT and conventional tomography present images in different planes, the two are complementary. Whereas CT is better for showing the laryngeal cartilages and structures at the glottic level, conventional tomography is superior for showing subglottic extension of growths, and gives a more satisfactory demonstration than reformatted CT images in the coronal plane.

Fractures of the larynx, as from direct contact with the steering wheel of a motor vehicle, are difficult to demonstrate radiologically and even harder to assess clinically. Xeroradiography may be useful but CT is now the best method for showing fractures of the thyroid cartilage, displacement of the arytenoids and the size and state of the airway (Figure 2.10).

Computerized tomography can assist the endoscopic assessment of tumours, both benign and malignant,

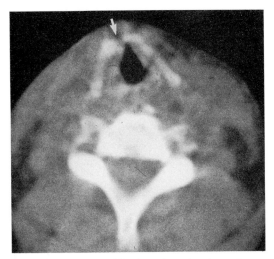

Figure 2.10 Fracture of the thyroid cartilage (arrow)

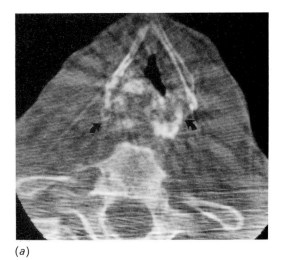

(a)

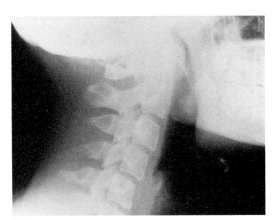

(b)

Figure 2.11 (*a*) A calcified mass at the glottic level shows areas of calcification and proved to be a chondroma. (*b*) Plain lateral radiograph of neck showing a subglottic plasmacytoma

although it is not required routinely. Some rare benign tumours may show characteristic features. Chondromas arise from one of the laryngeal cartilages and show a typical appearance on CT with speckled calcification (Figure 2.11a). A plasmacytoma appears radiologically as a smooth rounded tumour, homogeneous in consistency and often indistinguishable from carcinoma of the larynx (Figure 2.11b). A lipoma is a very rare tumour which may be suspected preoperatively because of low attenuation of the fat (Figure 2.12).

Malignant tumours are nearly always squamous cell carcinomas, and CT may help to evaluate deep laryngeal and paralaryngeal soft tissue invasion, thereby altering the staging of the disease. The paraglottic space, that is the space between the mucosa and the cartilage, is well demonstrated and is seen as a translucent line just deep to the thyroid lamina. When this line is absent on one side, it contrasts with the normal side and indicates tumour infiltration of the thyroarytenoid muscle, up to the thyroid cartilage. The most important role for CT is for showing invasion of the cartilaginous skeleton of the larynx by the tumour (Figure 2.13). Such involvement is a strong indication for total laryngectomy. Gross involvement of the thyroid laminae is usually obvious on CT, but minor degrees of destruction by tumour invasion may be difficult to evaluate, since the thyroid laminae may show considerable unevenness of density in the normal. This may give rise to both false positives and false negatives in interpretation (Lloyd, Michaels and Phelps, 1981). Another feature which has been associated with invasion of the cartilages, confirmed after surgical excision of the larynx, has been the presence of increased density and ossification. This may involve the arytenoid, cricoid and thyroid lamina. In the author's series of 26 cases, increase in the density of the cartilage was shown to be

due to increased ossification and was most often seen in the arytenoid. Previous radiotherapy appeared to be an important factor in most but not all cases.

Magnetic resonance

The most important role of imaging in the assessment of laryngeal tumours is to show:

1 Extension into the pre-epiglottic space and base of tongue
2 Extension into the paraglottic region
3 Cartilage erosion.

After the injection of contrast most tumours show significant enhancement. However, the normal mucosa lining the upper airway will also enhance and unfortunately it is not possible to differentiate

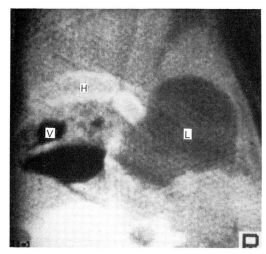

Figure 2.12 A section at the level of the hyoid (H) and the vallecula (V) proved to be a lipoma (L) bulging into the neck. Radiological differentiation from a laryngocoele is difficult

tumour from radiation necrosis following radiotherapy. Accurate plain T1-weighted images, contrast enhanced images and the subtraction technique allow good or at least sufficient judgement of cartilage invasion in all cases. The subtraction technique improves visualization of tumour spread beyond the larynx and hypopharynx, classified T4 (Vogl, 1992).

Magnetic resonance would seem to be the imaging investigation of choice for cancer of the larynx and can improve the accuracy of the staging, although CT may be easier for the patient and MR is not always necessary. In a previous review of current practice in the UK I came to the following conclusions (Phelps, 1992):

1 There is general agreement that endoscopy is the primary and most important investigation for cancer of the larynx and imaging is not required for the mucosal surfaces, except occasionally in subglottic tumours, very bulky tumours, or tumours arising in the ventricle when endoscopic assessment is difficult.

2 Glottic cancer is assessed entirely by endoscopy, especially if the treatment is to be by radiotherapy and subsequent salvage surgery (total laryngectomy) if required. Magnetic resonance shows cartilage destruction and pre-epiglottic space invasion and can therefore upstage the tumour, but this has little relevance to management unless some form of partial laryngectomy is envisaged.

3 Pre-epiglottic space invasion is a feature in the majority of supraglottic infrahyoid carcinomas and for these T3 and T4 lesions imaging confirmation may assist the decision to perform total laryngec-

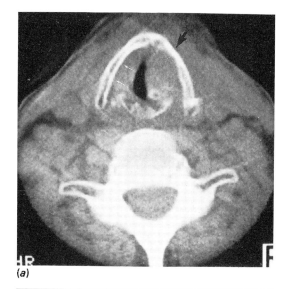

(a)

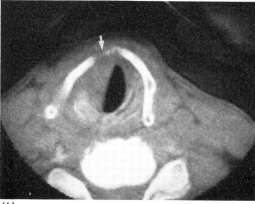

(b)

Figure 2.13 Carcinoma of the larynx at the level of the vocal cords: (*a*) there is some swelling of the right vocal cord with loss of the normal radiolucent line that lies inside the thyroid cartilage (small white arrows). There is also questionable erosion of the thyroid lamina on the right (black arrow); (*b*) more definite erosion of the thyroid cartilage (white arrow)

tomy as the primary procedure. MRI with gadolinium enhancement and subtraction studies is the investigation of choice (Vogl *et al.*, 1991). However, there is a high incidence of invasion of the pre-epiglottic space not recognized by imaging but confirmed by histological study of the resected larynx (Sulfaro *et al.*, 1989). Moreover, Zeitels and Vaughan (1991) showed that in 50% of their patients with invasion of the pre-epiglottic space, cervical node metastases were present despite a preoperative staging of T1 or T2. Hopefully improvements in MRI will enable more of such extensions of disease to be recognized (Figure 2.14).

4 Imaging after radiotherapy to assess the need for salvage surgery is most unsatisfactory as tumour recurrence cannot be differentiated from inflammatory disease by current imaging methods. Occasionally the demonstration of cartilage destruction by imaging in the presence of persistent oedema and negative biopsy can help the decision to remove the larynx.

Soft tissue imaging in the parapharyngeal region

An axial CT scan with 5-mm contiguous sections forms the basis of the examination. Contrast enhance-ment, by bolus injection or infusion, is usual to show the position of the major vessels or the presence of a vascular tumour. There is normally clear delineation of the parotid gland from the muscles and from fat in the parapharyngeal space (Figure 2.15), but sialography may help to define the limits of the deep lobe of the parotid. Magnetic resonance shows the position of the vessels more clearly and is now the imaging investigation of choice.

Infratemporal and pterygopalatine fossae

The infratemporal fossa is an irregularly-shaped space behind the maxilla and medial to the ramus of the mandible. It is situated below the zygoma, the greater

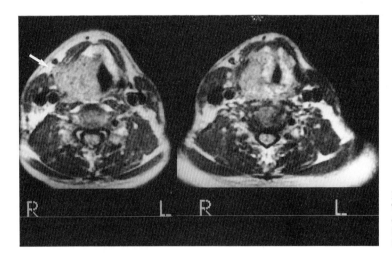

Figure 2.14 Axial T1-weighted MR. Two sections showing a supraglottic carcinoma that has eroded through the thyroid cartilage into the superficial tissues (arrows)

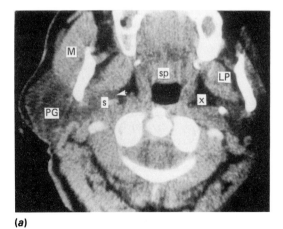

(a)

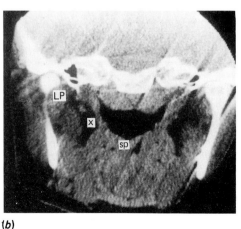

(b)

Figure 2.15 Normal CT of the parapharyngeal region: (*a*) axial scan at the level of the soft palate (SP). The parotid gland (PG) is well shown and also the extent of the deep lobe. The arrow points to the separation of the deep lobe from the fat in the parapharyngeal space (x). M = Masseter, LP = lateral pterygoid, S = styloid process. (*b*) Section in coronal plane

wing of the sphenoid and part of the squamous temporal bone. The medial wall of the fossa is the lateral pterygoid plate. The anterior and medial walls meet below, but are separated above by the pterygomaxillary fissure through which the infratemporal fossa communicates with the pterygopalatine fossa. The upper end of the pterygomaxillary fissure is continuous with the inferior orbital fissure. The pterygopalatine fossa is well shown by axial CT and the sphenopalatine foramen, which is an opening in its medial wall, that is the lateral wall of the nasal cavity, can sometimes be seen (Figure 2.16). The normal fossa contains fat.

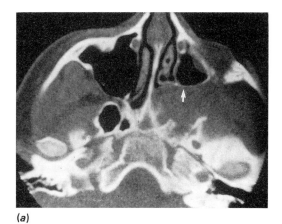

(a)

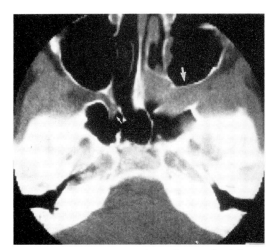

Figure 2.16 Normal pterygopalatine fossa on the right, with sphenopalatine foramen shown (small arrow). On the left side the pterygopalatine fossa is expanded and the posterior wall of the antrum displaced forwards (large white arrow) by a juvenile angiofibroma

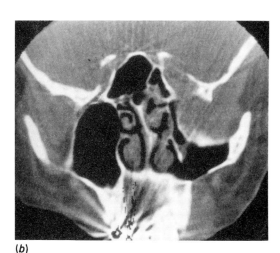

(b)

Figure 2.17 (*a*) Axial scan shows much forward bowing of the posterior wall of the left antrum (antral wall sign). (*b*) Coronal scan shows that there is also inferior bowing of the back of the antrum. This latter feature is not typical of an angiofibroma and, in fact, the tumour was a neurofibroma

Spread of tumours along the axis of the pterygomaxillary fissure with expansion of the walls is an important concept, particularly in the natural history of juvenile angiofibroma. This tumour arises in the region of the sphenopalatine foramen and spreads through the fissure into the infratemporal fossa (Lloyd and Phelps, 1986). This is a much more important sign than the traditional 'bowing' of the posterior wall of the antrum (Figure 2.17), and erosion of bone in the region of the sphenopalatine foramen appears to be diagnostic.

The infratemporal fossa contains all the muscles of mastication except the laterally placed masseter and the small depressors of the mandible. Most laterally and superiorly is the head of the temporalis muscle which inserts onto the coronoid process of the mandible. The pterygoid muscles are protractors of the mandible and fill the bulk of the infratemporal fossa.

A significant portion of the maxillary artery also lies within the infratemporal fossa.

The 'spaces' that have been considered so far have some bony boundaries, although inferiorly they are continuous with other described potential spaces whose boundaries are not bony but the deep fascial planes of the neck. Unfortunately these fascial boundaries are not demonstrated by imaging techniques, neither do they interfere with the spread of malignant neoplasms. Nevertheless they must be considered, as expansion of benign tumours and the resultant CT and MR appearances depend very much on the site of origin of the tumour. The two most important of these spaces will be referred to as the parapharyngeal space and the carotid space.

The parapharyngeal space

This is the most anterior space and extends from the base of the skull to the hyoid bone. The fat in the space is a prominent feature of axial CT scans at this level. The lateral wall of the parapharyngeal space is formed by the pterygoid muscles. The medial wall is made up of the muscles of deglutition. At the level of the nasopharynx, these are principally the tensor and levator palati, but below this the medial wall is formed by the constrictor muscles of the pharynx. The muscles arising from the styloid process form the posterior wall (Figure 2.18).

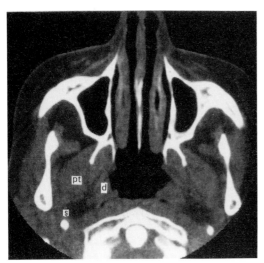

Figure 2.18 Axial CT scan showing the nasopharynx and soft tissue structures in the parapharyngeal region. The parapharyngeal space is bounded by the pterygoids (pt), swallowing muscles (d) and the muscles of the styloid process (s)

MRI (either spin-echo or gradient echo pulse sequences) readily demonstrates most vascular structures as well as tumour vascularity. Differentiation of the parotid from extraparotid masses is also more reliable by MRI. A head coil is usually satisfactory and T1-weighted axial views are used in the first instance. T2-weighted protocols usually give a stronger signal from tumour and are better able to differentiate tumour from muscle. Coronal images are best for demonstrating any intracranial extension of tumour, especially with gadolinium. Sagittal and coronal views are helpful in discerning the position of the mass in relation to the carotid and jugular vessels.

Parapharyngeal masses in the anterior compartments in front of the styloid process and styloid muscle are usually salivary in origin. They arise in the deep lobe of the parotid, from a minor pharyngeal salivary gland or from ectopic salivary cell rests. The important differentiation between a mass in the deep lobe of the parotid and an extra-parotid mass depends upon whether or not a fat plane can be identified between the mass and the parotid gland, although this sign is unreliable if the tumour is very large (Figure 2.19). All these masses in the anterior compartment tend to push the carotid artery posteriorly.

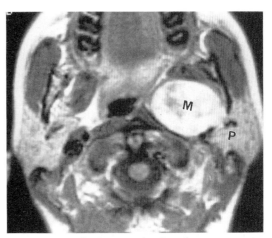

Figure 2.19 Axial MR section showing a large inhomogeneous pleomorphic adenoma (M) which appears contiguous with the parotid (P) and has probably arisen in the deep lobe

The carotid space

The carotid space or sheath is a potential fascial space containing the internal jugular vein, the carotid arteries, and the lower four cranial nerves as well as the sympathetic chain and various lymph nodes. Benign tumours arising in this space are usually vagal neuromas or rarely glomus tumours. These tumours tend to respect the fascial margins of the carotid space and to separate the major blood vessels (Figure 2.20). The relationship of the blood vessels to the mass is better shown by MRI (Figure 2.21). Lower down at the hyoid level, a densely enhancing but smoothly outlined mass shown by CT is almost certain to be a carotid body tumour. Neuromas typically are relatively homogeneous and show peripheral enhancement, while glomus tumours, being very vascular, show intense enhancement on both CT and MRI. The areas of signal void on the MR

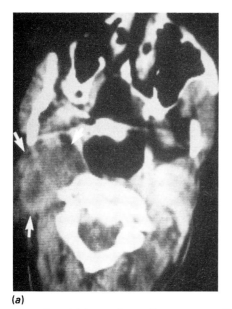
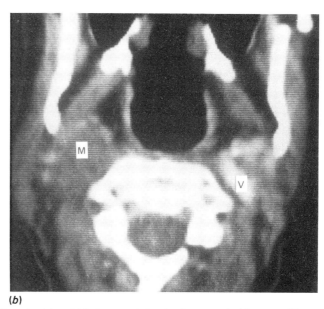

(a)   **(b)**

Figure 2.20 (*a*) A typical neurofibroma, presumably of vagal origin, which shows peripheral enhancement of the mass; (*b*) the vessels are displaced around the mass (M). Note the normal vessels (V) on the other side

scan representing blood vessels are almost pathognomonic of a glomus tumour.

Rarely a mass may arise more posteriorly in the so-called 'paraspinal space' and displace all the vessels as well as the anterior scalene muscle anteriorly (Figure 2.22).

Regimen for investigating parapharyngeal masses

At the present time CT in the axial plane with 5-mm contiguous sections and contrast enhancement, preferably by infusion, is the usual means of investigating these lesions. In selected cases, further sections in the coronal plane may be an advantage. However MR is now becoming the preferred means of investigating these tumours with both contrast enhancement and MR angiography (MRA) being used.

Further discrimination can be made by the degree and timing of the contrast enhancement by plotting attenuation against time curves. Immediate enhancement followed by rapid washout is a feature of vascular anomalies and vascular tumours with little stroma such as glomus tumours, whereas meningiomas show a less rapid but more persistent degree of enhancement. Neuromas almost always enhance less but the degree of enhancement is very variable and difficulty may be encountered in distinguishing between extraparotid benign mixed tumours and the neuromas that do not show enhancement. Their similar appearances on CT scans and the dynamic scan findings do not, in most cases, allow a confident distinction to be made. The inter-

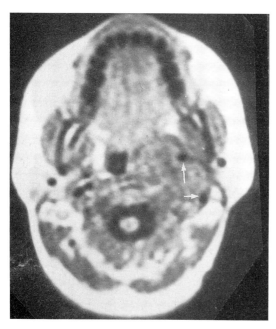

Figure 2.21 Axial MR scan. A mass in the carotid sheath displaces the carotid artery forwards and the internal jugular vein laterally (white arrows)

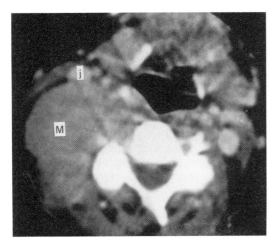

Figure 2.22 Mass (M) in the paraspinal space displacing all vessels, styloid and anterior scalene muscles forwards; j = internal jugular vein which is usually displaced backwards and laterally by masses arising in the more anterior compartments

nal carotid artery is usually, but not always, displaced anteromedially by neuromas and posteriorly by minor salivary gland tumours.

Imaging nodal metastatic disease

Although positron emission tomography appears to promise a significant role in the future, the demonstration of nodal metastases is generally agreed to be slightly but significantly better by CT or MR than by clinical examination alone. At present both CT and MR are used for staging, neither having a definite advantage. CT is quicker and gives a good demonstration of 'ring enhancement', spread outside the node and other signs of neoplasia. The optimum protocols for MR have not been fully agreed and Gd enhancement tends to make the edge of the enhanced node indistinguishable from the surrounding fat. However, the fat suppression technique may well prove the most useful and post-contrast fat suppressed T1-weighted images can show clearly the thickened enhancing necrotic walls of metastatic nodes. An excellent review of current imaging practice for metastatic adenopathy is given by Som (1992).

The usual criteria for malignancy are:

1 Lymph node greater than 1 cm in size (1.5 cm for jugulodigastric and submandibular nodes)
2 A node with central necrosis regardless of size in the absence of clinical infection
3 A group of three or more nodes, each smaller than 1 cm in the primary drainage station of the primary tumour as sometimes enlarged nodes may be

demonstrated replacing the parotid gland or within the carotid sheath obscured by the overlying sternomastoid muscles (Figure 2.23). Extracapsular nodal spread is diagnosed when there is enhancement of the nodal capsule and poorly defined margins around the node (Figure 2.24).

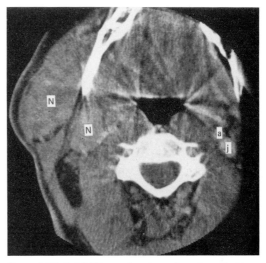

Figure 2.23 Axial CT scan showing enlarged neoplastic lymph nodes (N) both replacing the parotid gland and situated within the carotid sheath. This axial CT section with contrast enhancement illustrates several points. The patient has an anaplastic carcinoma from an unknown primary. On the left, the bolus injection has demonstrated the normal carotid (a) and internal jugular vein (j). On the right the parotid gland has largely been replaced by an affected node which is isodense with the surrounding musculature. Another large clinically inapparent node lies medially with compressed vessels surrounding it, thus indicating that this is a node lying within the fascial sheath surrounding the neurovascular bundle. A neuroma of the vagus will produce similar vessel displacement

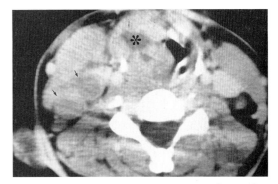

Figure 2.24 A large supraglottic carcinoma with central necrosis (∗) and adjacent metastatic nodes with central necrosis and poorly defined margins indicating extracapsular spread (arrows)

Barium swallow examination

Assessment of the mucosal surfaces of the oro- and hypopharynx is, as with the nasopharynx, almost entirely by inspection. Barium swallow is of more value for showing lesions of the oesophagus, pharyngeal pouches, fistulae, and for neurological swallowing problems especially when cine or video is used.

Normally barium flows rapidly through the pharynx and down the oesophagus (Figure 2.25). It may coat the sides of the pharynx for a short time and, after the first swallow, a little may remain in the vallecula and pyriform fossae only to be quickly cleared by a subsequent swallow. Any degree of stasis beyond this should be suspect. The normal larynx will appear as a 'filling defect' in the frontal projection with contrast in the pyriform fossa on either side. This is well shown on the oblique projection, obtained with the patient swallowing while the head is turned to one side. Tumours of the pharynx will be well outlined by a coating of barium and masses demonstrated in the pyriform fossae, which are sometimes difficult to see with a mirror (Figure 2.26).

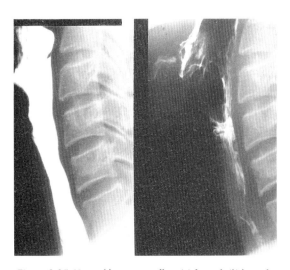

Figure 2.25 Normal barium swallow (*a*) frontal; (*b*) lateral showing full distension with contrast and subsequently contrast coating the mucosa

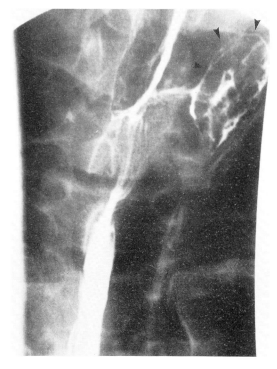

Figure 2.26 Barium swallow in the oblique position. Carcinoma of the pyriform fossa (arrows)

When the larynx fails in its primary function as a protective sphincter for the lungs, 'spillover' will occur to give a 'barium laryngogram' (Figure 2.27). This problem is seen more and more in an ageing population when dysphagia is often the result of a mild stroke. Cineradiography at four frames per second gives a good demonstration of deglutition. Passage of the bolus across the back of the tongue, with elevation of the larynx and tilting of the epiglottis down over the closed larynx, is shown. Contrast then passes through the open cricopharyngeus into the oesophagus. Minor functional disorders of swal-

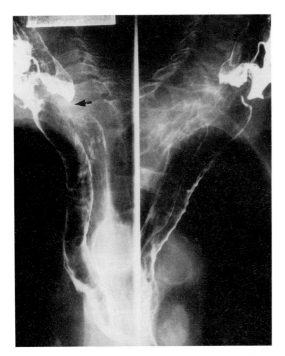

Figure 2.27 Barium swallow in the oblique position. There is spillover into the larynx and trachea. The arrow points to the position of the cricopharyngeus

lowing can only be shown by this technique (Figure 2.28), but it is wasteful of film and should probably only be used to try to solve a particular swallowing problem. A good account of pharyngeal deglutition in patients with functional disorders of the act of swallowing, compared with a group of volunteers with no complaint of dysphagia, is contained in two papers from Malmo, Sweden (Ekberg and Nylander, 1982a, b). These authors, using cineradiography at 50–100 frames per second, found a high incidence of epiglottic dysmotility and cricopharyngeal incoordination in the patients with dysphagia. Although only a small percentage had severe disturbance, such as complete paralysis of the pharyngeal constrictors or aspiration into the trachea, nevertheless contrast was frequently seen to enter the vestibule of the larynx.

Oesophagus

This is a tubular organ the diameter of which varies from a potential space to the size needed to accommodate whatever can be swallowed. It normally contains no air, although occasionally a small triangular air shadow can be seen on a lateral film just below the level of the cricopharyngeus. Air is almost always visible in this region when there is a foreign body present in the pharynx or upper oesophagus.

The conventional radiological examination is the barium swallow. It is often stated that barium should never be used if it is thought that spillover into the trachea may occur, but provided small amounts only are used, there seems to be little danger, especially if postural drainage is used afterwards.

Barium is inert and less irritating than most water-soluble contrast media, and usually provides better radiographic detail. In infants, if atresia or a fistula is suspected, it is better to pass a soft rubber tube and to inject a water-soluble opaque fluid, of the kind used for bronchography, only if necessary. Communication between the oesophagus and trachea involves the anterior wall of the oesophagus so that injection of opaque fluid should be made in prone and prone oblique positions under radiographic screen control and films taken as required.

When undertaking a screen examination of the oesophagus, the patient is usually given barium fluid to swallow, although occasionally barium paste is used. The radiologist follows the passage of a mouthful of barium from the mouth to the stomach. The situation, extent, and form of physiological and pathological constrictions or filling defects, or any hesitation, hold-up or diversion of the normal flow are noted. Attention is paid to the form and amplitude of peristaltic waves. Some authorities test the lower oesophageal sphincter for competence by watching the patient swallowing prone while abdominal compression is applied. However, such an unphysiological manoeuvre has little relevance as a test for reflux. Reflux of barium into the oesophagus when the patient swallows water in the supine position is probably a better test.

Zaino and colleagues (1970) have demonstrated that there is a sphincter, 1–2 cm long, at the upper end of the oesophagus, below the cricopharyngeus, in which increased pressure can be measured manometrically, and stated that this provides the true sphincter mechanism for the upper oesophagus and not the circular fibres of the cricopharyngeus. At times the cricopharyngeus muscle may produce a pronounced indentation of the posterior outline of the filled oesophagus as barium passes through, and this is often especially marked when there is neuromuscular incoordination present, as with bulbar lesions.

Foreign bodies in the upper aerodigestive tract are usually fish or meat bones lodged in the upper oesophagus (Figure 2.29). It may be difficult to differentiate the foreign body from ossification in the laryngeal cartilages. Air in the soft tissues or in the oesophagus, held open by a non-opaque foreign body, is an important sign. Less often objects such as pins, coins, dentures, buttons, etc. may lodge in the pyriform fossa, the nasopharynx or between the cords. Perforation, either by the foreign body or by

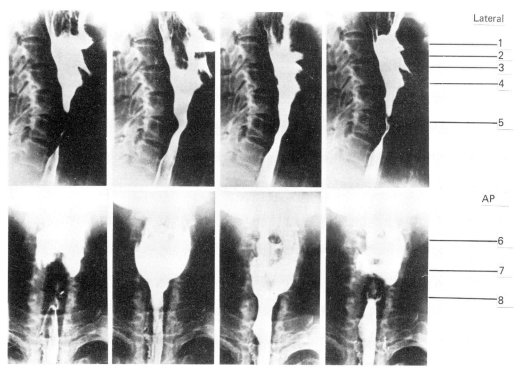

Lateral
— 1
— 2
— 3
— 4
— 5

AP
— 6
— 7
— 8

Figure 2.28 Cine barium swallow. Four frames in one second, frontal and lateral. The patient has mild dysphagia due to unilateral vagal paralysis. Various normal and abnormal features are demonstrated. Lateral view: (1) the vallecula fills with barium and is then partially affected by the normal backward compression of the tongue. (2) The epiglottis is partially immobile and only tilts down to the transverse position, not fully covering the laryngeal inlet. (3) Barium enters the vestibule of the larynx. This may occasionally be observed in asymptomatic subjects but is usually an indication of failure of the laryngeal sphincters ('spillover'). (4) At the same time the relation of the posterior pharyngeal wall to the cervical spine does not change, indicating paralysis of the middle pharyngeal constrictor. (5) Cricopharyngeus contracts and relaxes normally. Anteroposterior (AP) view: (6) the epiglottis shows little movement. (7) The right side of the pharynx contracts normally but the left remains flaccid and filled with barium. (8) Cricopharyngeus contracts and relaxes normally. (From *Sutton's Textbook of Radiology*, Edinburgh: Churchill Livingstone, with permission)

instrumentation, can lead to inflammatory changes in the para- and retropharyngeal tissue planes. Widening of the retropharyngeal soft tissue space is seen in such cases, sometimes with surgical emphysema or an abscess cavity.

When one attempts to demonstrate or localize a non-opaque swallowed foreign body such as a fish bone, success can sometimes be achieved by persuading the patient to swallow a sandwich of teased-out dry cotton wool with a centre of cotton wool soaked in barium. The patient should try to swallow this without mouthing it and saturating it with saliva and, should it be impaled on the fish bone, the site is immediately shown.

The upper oesophagus normally deviates a little to the left at the level of the thoracic inlet. It may be indented, compressed or displaced by an enlarged thyroid, or parathyroid gland, or enlarged lymph nodes, as well as by mediastinal tumours or aneurysms of the aortic arch. It is indented anteriorly, and on its left side, by the normal aortic arch and left main bronchus and, when present, the oblique indentation of an anomalous right subclavian artery above the level of the aortic impression is diagnostic. Malformations of the aortic arch, such as a right-sided aorta or double aorta, may be suspected or diagnosed by the different impressions they produce on the barium-filled oesophagus.

The oesophagus is usually loosely attached to the descending aorta and tends to maintain this relationship throughout life, so that when the aorta becomes elongated and unfolded with atheroma, the oesophagus tends to be displaced with it. An atheromatous aorta may compress the oesophagus at its lower end where they cross, and this is particularly liable to happen when the thoracic aorta is tortuous and heavily calcified.

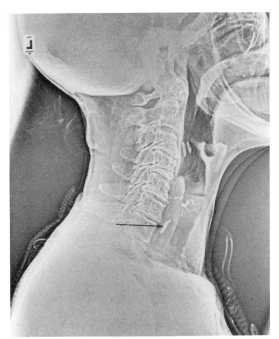

Figure 2.29 The arrow points to a fish bone in the upper oesophagus

Subsidiary imaging techniques

Other imaging techniques which have a minor or obsolete role in the examination of the pharynx, larynx and oesophagus have been briefly considered in Volume 1, Chapter 17.

Sinography

Cysts of congenital origin in the neck arise laterally from branchial cleft remnants or in the midline along the course of the thyroglossal duct. On CT scans they will appear as well circumscribed low density lesions with normal fascial planes around them unless the cyst has become infected. When a cyst breaks through to the skin it produces a sinus or fistula. Valuable information about the situation and extent of fistulae, sinuses and tracts in the neck can be obtained by injecting an oily contrast medium (Lipiodol Ultra Fluid) through a small catheter (Figure 2.31).

Barium swallow is complementary to oesophagoscopy in the diagnosis of obstructive lesions at the lower end of the oesophagus and is the principal means of identifying achalasia of the cardia (Figure 2.30).

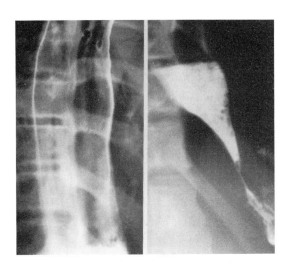

Figure 2.30 Barium swallow showing the typical appearance of achalasia of the cardia

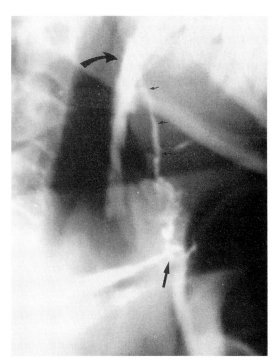

Figure 2.31 Patent thyroglossal duct. Contrast medium injected into a sinus in the front of the neck (large arrow) passes up through the base of the tongue (small arrows) and emerges into the pharynx (curved arrow)

Imaging the salivary glands

Pathological changes in the salivary glands are traditionally investigated by plain radiography (Figure 2.32), or after injection of a contrast medium into the parotid or submandibular ducts. The technique of sialography and its importance for showing abnormalities of the duct systems (Figure 2.33) are discussed in Volume 1, Chapter 17.

Mass lesions within or around the salivary glands can be demonstrated by CT. The precise location of a

mass within the parotid gland can be shown, and the position of the facial nerve inferred. CT demonstrates whether a mass is circumscribed or invasive and suggests the histological nature of a cyst or lipoma. It can differentiate masseter muscle hypertrophy (Figure 2.34) from diffuse non-inflammatory enlargement of the parotid gland. It is not, however, reliable for differentiating benign from malignant neoplasms. Most intraparotid masses, even those differing little in density from the surrounding gland, are detectable by CT, but intravenous or intraductal contrast injection may be helpful to delineate the tumour more clearly and confirm that the deep lobe is not involved.

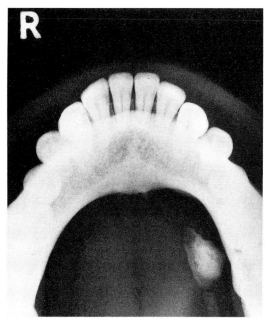

Figure 2.32 An intraoral view of the floor of the mouth showing two calculi in the left submandibular duct

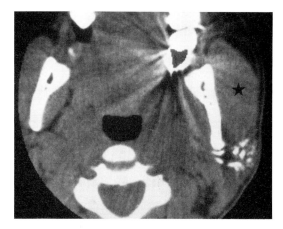

Figure 2.34 Axial CT section with parotid sialogram. There is hypertrophy of the masseter (∗) and this 'swelling' is shown to be quite separate from the parotid gland

Adenolymphoma (Warthin's tumour) tends to have multiple lobules and is often wholly or partially outside the gland. Isotope studies with technetium-99m (^{99m}Tc) may be diagnostic as Warthin's tumour accumulates the radionuclide intensely. This differs from other tumours which show as areas of decreased activity in the concentration of isotope which occurs in normal salivary glands. Malignant tumours may be well defined (Figure 2.35), or they may have indistinct margins at their interface with the parotid tissue and may infiltrate outside the gland into the surrounding fat if they are invasive.

These features are demonstrated much better by MRI, which is now the imaging investigation of choice for tumours of the salivary glands. Like the Guy's Hospital authors (Chaudhuri *et al.*, 1992) we prefer a routine regimen of axial T1-weighted spin echo and coronal STIR (short tau inversion recovery) without contrast enhancement (Figure 2.36). The STIR sequence produces an image with greater tissue contrast than its T2-weighted spin-echo equivalent and therefore will show an area of abnormal tissue not immediately obvious on a T1 image, although the latter gives the best spatial resolution and defines

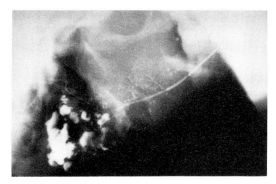

Figure 2.33 Sialadenitis: this parotid sialogram shows gross peripheral ductal dilatation and saccular accumulation of contrast material, although the proximal part of the gland appears normal. No cause of obstruction was found at surgery, but this was considered to be the most likely pathogenesis

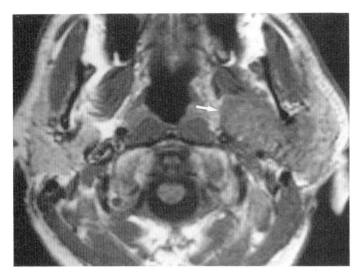

Figure 2.35 An adenocarcinoma of the left parotid gland is poorly demarcated from normal gland tissue and has extended into the parapharyngeal space (arrow). The mass has lower signal than the parotid gland on this T1-weighted axial image

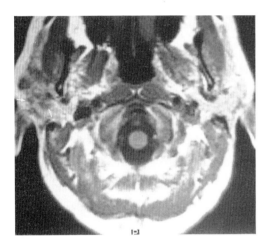
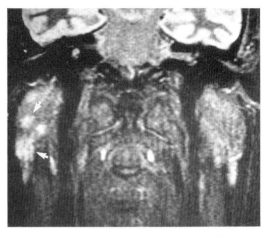

Figure 2.36 Axial T1-weighted (*a*) and coronal STIR (*b*) images of small recurrent pleomorphic adenomas from spillage of neoplastic cells during removal of the original tumour. Note the low signal on the T1-weighted images and high signal on the STIR

best the surgical relations especially to the retromandibular vein and the external carotid artery. However it is not usually possible to differentiate benign from malignant neoplasms or to distinguish from inflammatory infiltration. T2-weighted images are required if a cystic lesion is suspected.

We have not found gadolinium enhancement helpful for the investigation of most masses in the parotid gland although other authors have (Vogl, 1992).

Generally a tumour which enhances thereby becomes less distinguishable from the surrounding normal gland which will itself show some degree of enhancement. Gadolinium enhancement should be used if a malignant tumour is suspected and also for a suspected recurrence when use of a chemical shift fat suppression sequence rather than STIR is indicated (see Volume 1, Chapter 17).

The commonest benign tumour of the salivary glands is the pleomorphic adenoma which may reach a large size in the parotid gland and occurs in both superficial and deep lobes (Figure 2.37). On T1-weighted images adenomas appear as areas of low signal intensity within the parenchyma of the gland. The margins are distinct and without infiltration.

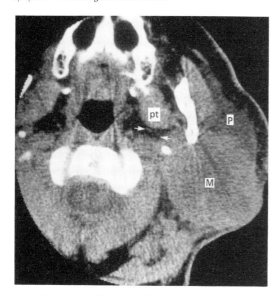

Figure 2.37 Axial CT scan of a large parotid mass (M) displacing the normal part of the gland (P) forwards. The small white arrows point to the junctions between the deep lobe of the gland and the fat in the parapharyngeal space and the deep extent of the tumour. pt = pterygoid muscles

Oropharynx and tongue

Tumours of the oropharynx, particularly the tongue and floor of the mouth, can be difficult to assess clinically and their extent hard to define. Computed tomography has proved valuable particularly for showing erosion of the cortical bone of the mandible but despite the use of contrast enhancement does not clearly define the margins of the tumour. Standard spin-echo MR sequences give similar information to that provided by CT and the T1-weighted sequences show the tumour as an area of low signal distinguished from the fat of the tissue planes between the muscles of the floor of the mouth and between the muscle fasciculi of the tongue. However the tumour is not well differentiated from muscle. The biggest advance in MR imaging of the oropharynx has been the use of fast gradient echo techniques such as FISP (fast imaging with steady state precession) and FLASH (fast low angle shot) in which a gradient reversal is used instead of the second 180° refocusing pulse of the spin echo sequence. Using a reduced flip angle, heavily T1-weighted images are produced and this is of great value when enhancement with gadolinium is used, as with these sequences tumour can be differentiated from both muscle *and* fat. The reduced time for the examination is another advantage. The tumours, almost always squamous cell carcinomas, need to be staged accurately so that the best combination of surgery and radiotherapy treatment can be planned. Involvement of the tongue base and evidence that the tumour crosses the mid-

line are particularly important. Conventional imaging and CT can show erosion of the cortical bone indicating invasion of the body of the mandible. Often beam hardening artefacts from dental fillings make CT unsatisfactory. Thus MR is the investigation of choice for cancers of the floor of the mouth (Figure 2.38).

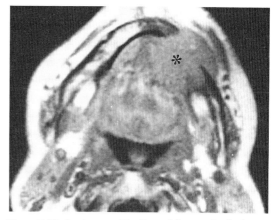

Figure 2.38 Carcinoma of the floor of the mouth which has eroded through the body of the mandible into the buccal sulcus. A standard T1-weighted MR image in the axial plane shows the tumour as an area of low signal (∗)

The basic examination consists of T1-weighted spin-echo images in the axial plane when the tumour will be seen as an area of low signal contrasted against the high signal from the fat in the floor of the mouth, the bone marrow in the mandible and between the muscle bundles in the tongue. This spin-echo protocol is then followed by a fast gradient echo sequence before and after enhancement with gadolinium (FISP or FLASH). The tumour shows marked enhancement with this regimen but unfortunately lymphoid tissue also shows higher signal after contrast and there is high signal from blood flowing in the major vessels (Figure 2.39). A similar regimen is

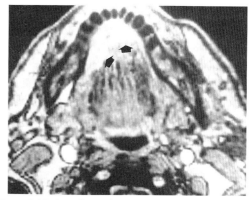

Figure 2.39 A gradient echo FLASH sequence with Gd enhancement of a carcinoma of the floor of the mouth showing marked enhancement (arrows)

used to examine cancers of the tongue and tonsil which may not appear initially to be malignant on CT. A useful alternative protocol, also involving gradient echo sequences before and after Gd, is the chemical shift fat suppression sequence (Figure 2.40). Often zones of necrosis in the centre of the tumour give a halo effect. High signal from the tumour is usually seen on the STIR sequence.

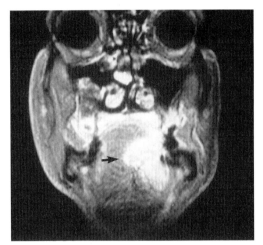

Figure 2.40 Chemical shift fat suppression sequence after Gd enhancement showing a carcinoma of the tongue which has crossed the midline

Angiography

Angiography, by means of transfemoral catheterization, is now largely replaced for the study of neck masses by enhanced CT, MR and MR angiography. There seems to be little point in performing angiography unless the lesion shows significant contrast enhancement on CT scanning. A sparsely vascularized mass, such as a neurofibroma, will show some 'puddling' of contrast on the angiogram, and characteristically there is anteromedial displacement of the internal carotid artery. The paragangliomas or glomus tumours make up the next most common group of enhancing extraparotid parapharyngeal masses (Som *et al.*, 1984). They may also displace the internal carotid artery anteriorly (Figure 2.41), but the angiogram will demonstrate the intense and typical vascularity of the lesion. Carotid body tumours occur lower in the neck. They arise medial to the carotid bifurcation and displace the carotid artery laterally, or at a higher level splay the carotid bifurcation. Although the internal jugular vein can usually be recognized, displaced posteriorly on the CT scan, the carotid arteries are usually incorporated in the hyperdense mass (Figure 2.42).

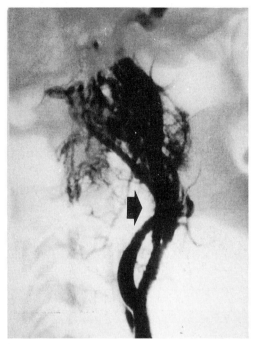

(a)

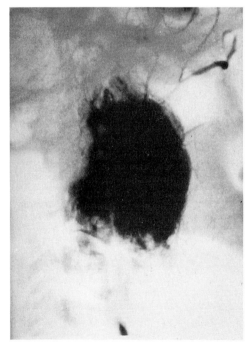

(b)

Figure 2.41 (*a*) Carotid angiogram showing anterior displacement of the internal carotid artery (arrow) by a vascular mass. (*b*) The mass shows intense vascularity and staining typical of a glomus tumour

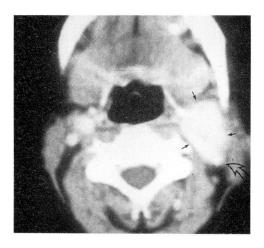

Figure 2.42 Axial CT scan of the neck showing a typical carotid body tumour (arrows). The curved arrow points to the internal jugular vein displaced backwards. Note the normal vessels on the other side on this enhanced scan

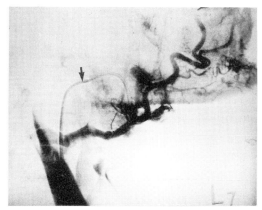

Figure 2.43 (*b*) Subtraction selective external carotid angiogram in the venous phase following embolization of a haemangioma of the base of the tongue. Little pathological circulation remains and the lingual vein and its tributaries can be seen draining into the internal jugular vein. The arrow points to the catheter which introduced the contrast. (Courtesy of Dr Brian Kendall, The National Hospital, London)

Vascular masses such as glomus tumours and haemangiomas, which also occur in the neck, in the salivary glands or the base of the tongue, are extremely difficult to excise and embolization techniques may be necessary to reduce the blood supply prior to surgery (Figure 2.43b). These techniques are described briefly in Volume 1, Chapter 17.

tract, for showing foreign bodies and occasionally for cysts and tumours, especially those presenting problems of assessment by endoscopy (Figures 2.44 and

Summary

Imaging will continue to have a limited role for assessing the outlines of the upper aerodigestive

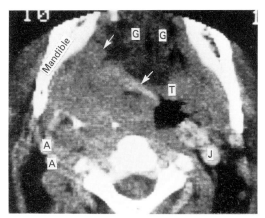

Figure 2.43 (*a*) Haemangioma of the base of the tongue shown on an axial CT scan with contrast infusion (arrows). The major vessels, as well as the lingual tonsil (T), are shown, G = genioglossus muscles. (Courtesy of Dr Brian Kendall, The National Hospital, London)

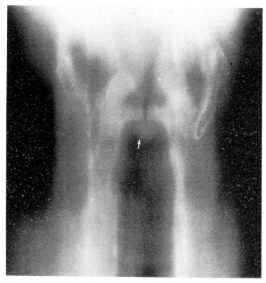

Figure 2.44 Frontal tomogram with the true cords in full adduction. Patient phonating 'ee'. There is a small polyp on the underside of the cords in this case (arrow)

2.45). Barium swallow examination still has a most important role for the study of the oesophagus and for some swallowing problems in the hypopharynx as well as in the diagnosis of pharyngeal pouches and achalasia of the cardia. Computerized tomography has a limited role in the investigation of laryngeal abnormalities. It is rarely required to assist the endoscopic assessment of tumours but may help to confirm persistence of disease and erosion of the laryngeal cartilages after radiotherapy. Assessment of laryngeal trauma by CT (see Figure 2.10) may be of value. Severe injuries to the framework of the larynx require open exploration, but CT may show that this is not required in less severe cases (Schaefer and Brown, 1983). MRI is especially useful for demonstrating the anatomical relations and extent of deep neck masses, but has frequently proved unreliable for distinguishing between benign and malignant tumours. Nevertheless, the combination of physical

examination and MRI gives the opportunity to stage these lesions more accurately than before (Figure 2.46).

Magnetic resonance gives better discrimination of such masses and normal structures in the soft tissues below the skull (Figures 2.47 and 2.48). Malignant tumours of the oropharynx seem particularly well suited to assessment by magnetic resonance imaging, especially those in the base of the tongue. The extent of local deep infiltration should be demonstrated along with any spread to adjacent areas such as the hypopharynx or pre-epiglottic space (Figure 2.49). The lateral projection possible with MR, but not directly with CT, is particularly useful. The biggest problem is the difficulty in distinguishing radiation necrosis from neoplasia. Even positron emission tomography, which seems to show excellent prospects as a marker for neoplastic disease, is unsatisfactory in this respect.

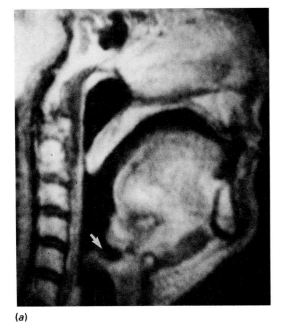

(a)

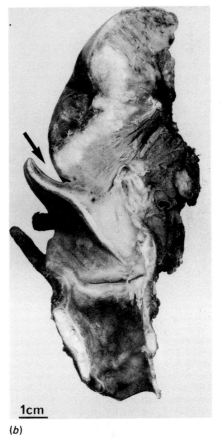

1cm

(b)

Figure 2.45 (*a*) Lateral MR scan showing a carcinoma of the base of the tongue. The arrow points to the vallecula. (*b*) An operative specimen from a different patient, but showing a similar lesion in a similar site

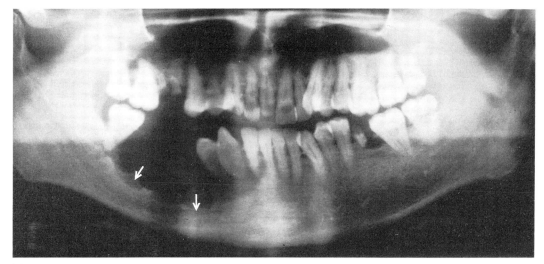

(*a*)

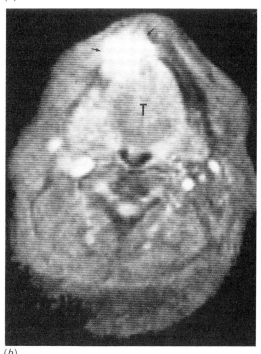

(*b*)

Figure 2.46 (*a*) Carcinoma of the floor of the mouth, eroding the mandible. The orthopantogram shows extensive erosion of one side of the mandible (arrows). It is only when bony involvement by a carcinoma is quite extensive that it will be demonstrated by conventional imaging. (*b*) Carcinoma of the floor of the mouth, eroding into the mandible. This axial MR scan is a hybrid image mixing both T1-weighted inversion recovery data with saturation proton density data. The tumour appears as an intense white area in front of the tongue (T). The mandible appears black. (Courtesy of Dr Graham Cherryman and the Department of Bio-Medical Physics and Bio-Engineering, University of Aberdeen)

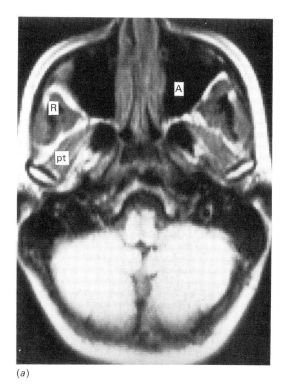

(*a*)

Figure 2.47 (*a*) Normal MR of the parapharyngeal region in the axial plane A = Antrum, R = ramus of mandible, pt = pterygoid muscles

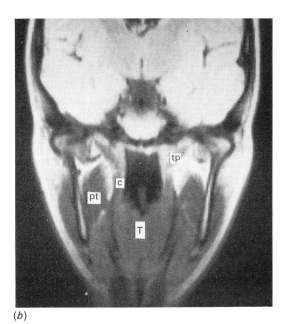

(*b*)

Figure 2.47 (*b*) Normal MR of the parapharyngeal region in the coronal plane. pt = pterygoid muscles, tp = tensor palati, c = constrictor muscles of the pharynx, T = tongue

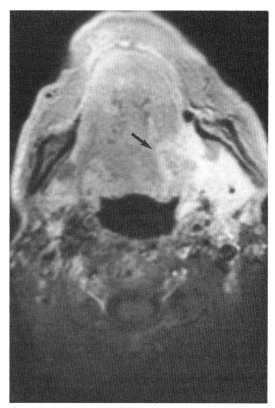

Figure 2.49 Chemical shift fat suppressed sequence after Gd enhancement showing a carcinoma of the tonsil which has invaded the base of the tongue (arrow)

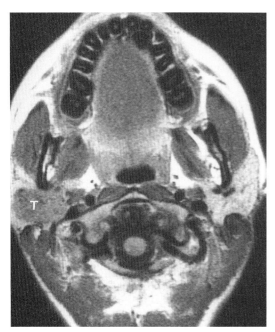

Figure 2.48 A pleomorphic salivary adenoma of the deep lobe of the parotid gland (T) shown by fast spin echo MRI. Note the excellent soft tissue detail of the parapharyngeal region shown on this T2-weighted image

References

CHAUDHURI, R., BINGHAM, J. B., CROSSMAN, J. E. and GLEESON, M. J. (1992) Magnetic resonance imaging of the parotid gland using the STIR sequence. *Clinical Otolaryngology*, **17**, 211–217

EKBERG, O. and NYLANDER, G., (1982a) Cineradiography of the pharyngeal stage of deglutition in 250 individuals without dysphagia. *British Journal of Radiology,* **55**, 253–257

EKBERG, O. and NYLANDER, G. (1982b) Cineradiography of the pharyngeal stage of deglutition in 250 patients with dysphagia. *British Journal of Radiology*, **55**, 258–262

LLOYD, G. A. S., MICHAELS, L. and PHELPS, P. D. (1981) The demonstration of cartilaginous involvement in laryngeal carcinoma by computerized tomography. *Clinical Ortolaryngology*, **6**, 171–177

LLOYD, G. A. S. and PHELPS, P. D. (1986) The demonstration of tumours of the pharyngeal space by magnetic resonance imaging, *British Journal of Radiology*, **59**, 679–683

PHELPS, P. D. (1992) Carcinoma of the larynx – the role of imaging in staging and pre-treatment assessments. *Clinical Radiology*, **467**, 77–83

SCHAEFER, S.D. and BROWN, O. E. (1983) Selective application of CT in the management of laryngeal trauma. *Laryngoscope*, **93**, 1473–1475

SOM, P. M. (1992) Detection of metastases in cervical lymph nodes: CT and MR criteria and differential diagnosis. *American Journal of Radiology*, **158**, 961–969

SOM, P. M., BILLER, H. F., LAWSON, W., SACHER, M. and LANZIERI, C. F., (1984) Pharapharyngeal space masses: an updated protocol based upon 104 cases. *Radiology*, **153**, 149–156

SULFARO, P., BARZAN, L., QUERIN, F., LUTMAN, M., CARUSO, G., COMORETTO, R. *et al.* (1989) CT staging of laryngohypopharyngeal carcinoma. *Archives of Otolaryngology, Head and Neck Surgery*, **115**, 613–619

SUTTON, D. (1993) *A Textbook of Radiology and Imaging*, 5th edn. Edinburgh: Churchill Livingstone

VOGL, T. J. (ed.) (1992) *MRI of the Head and Neck*. Berlin: Springer-Verlag, p. 167

VOGL, T. J. STEGER, W., GREVERS, G., SCHREINER, M., DRESEL, S. and LISSNER, J. (1991) MRI with Gd-DTPA in tumors of larynx and hypopharynx. *European Radiology*, **1**, 58–64

ZAINO, C., JACOBSON, H. G., LEPOW, H. and OZTURK, C. H. (1970) *The Pharyngo-oesophageal Sphincter*, Springfield, Illinois: Charles C Thomas, p. 102

ZEITELS, S. M. and VAUGHAN, C. W. (1991) Preepiglottic space invasion in 'early' epiglottic cancer. *Annals of Otology, Rhinology and Laryngology*, **100**, 789–792

3

Oral cavity

John Hibbert

The variety of diseases both local and systemic which can affect the mouth or oral cavity is remarkable. For example, the number of conditions which can lead to oral ulceration is staggering and classification of diseases of the oral cavity is difficult. In theory, because of the sensitive nature of the oral cavity, because lesions of the oral cavity interfere with speech and swallowing and because examination both by the patient and the physician is easy, one would expect early diagnosis of oral conditions. Unfortunately this is far from the case and oral cancers are notorious for their late presentation.

Surgical anatomy

The detailed anatomy of the oral cavity is given in Volume 1 but the most important points are worth summarizing.

The oral cavity begins anteriorly at the vermilion border of the lips, i.e. the junction between skin which is keratinizing and mucous membrane which is non-keratinizing and pink. Posteriorly the limits of the oral cavity are the anterior pillars of the fauces, the junction of the anterior two-thirds and posterior one-third of the tongue (i.e. the circumvallate papillae) and the junction of the hard and soft palate superiorly. The soft palate and the tonsil are therefore part of the oropharynx. There is a certain amount of dispute regarding the soft palate. Anatomists see it as belonging to the oral cavity with the junction between oral cavity and oropharynx being the lower free border of the soft palate. Clinicians would classify the soft palate as part of the oropharynx. Disease processes unlike anatomists and clinicians are less aware of somewhat arbitrary anatomical boundaries and many conditions which affect the oral cavity will also involve the oropharynx.

Within the oral cavity are important anatomical areas such as the floor of the mouth with the sublingual glands and openings of the submandibular ducts, the buccal mucosa lining the cheeks with the openings of the parotid ducts, the anterior two-thirds of the tongue, the upper and lower jaws and dentition and the hard palate.

The oral cavity is lined by a mucous membrane which is a non-keratinizing stratified squamous epithelium and is therefore pink. It contains taste buds and many minor salivary glands.

Congenital conditions affecting the oral cavity

The most important congenital conditions affecting the oral cavity are cleft lip and palate and congenital abnormalities of the jaws (e.g. Pierre Robin syndrome). Other congenital conditions are relatively minor and include the following.

Mucosal abnormalities

Dyskeratosis congenita is a rare ectodermal abnormality which can give rise to dyskeratotic white patches in the mouth. In addition there are abnormalities of the skin, nails, cornea and the hair, which may be absent.

Fordyces spots are atopic sebaceous glands in the buccal and labial mucosa giving small yellowish lesions of no significance. They seem to increase in occurrence with age and may be seen in up to 80% of the population (Halperin *et al.*, 1953).

White sponge naevus is a condition transmitted in an autosomal dominant fashion giving rise to raised white lesions of the oral mucosa, particularly inside the cheek. They are of no significance (Banoczy, Sugar and Frithiof, 1973).

Hereditary haemorrhagic telangiectasia (Osler-Weber-Rendu disease) is a dominantly inherited condition in which telangiectases may be present in the lips and oral mucosa.

Congenital lesions of the tongue

Macroglossia can occur in Down's and Beckwith's syndromes and cretinism. Lymphangiomas can give rise to this appearance and, although not congenital, macroglossia is also seen in acromegaly and amyloidosis.

Ankyloglossia or tongue tie is related to a short lingual frenulum close to the tip of the tongue. The incidence depends upon the criteria used to make the diagnosis but may be as much as 1–2% (Catlin and De Haas, 1971). It is rare that this condition is severe enough to affect suckling or later speech. Surgical division with a horizontal incision and vertical repair is usually sufficient.

Median rhomboid glossitis is a condition of no significance in which there is an area on the dorsum of the tongue anterior to the circumvallate papillae which is devoid of papillae and therefore flat and pink. It is due to a failure of the lateral halves of the tongue to fuse in the midline with the tuberculum impar.

Lingual thyroid

This actually occurs in the posterior one-third of the tongue behind the circumvallate papillae and is therefore not in the oral cavity but in the oropharynx. Treatment is only necessary if the lesion is enlarging and leading to change in speech, dysphagia and later airway obstruction. Radionuclide scans (technetium or iodine) will establish the nature of the tissue as thyroid and will determine whether this is the only thyroid tissue present. A lingual thyroid can be the site of a thyroid neoplasm.

Stomatitis and oral ulceration

The causes of ulceration of the mouth are numerous and the condition may be confined to the mouth or upper aerodigestive tract, may be part of a mucocutaneous condition, or may be part of a generalized disorder. The causes may vary from a trivial condition which can be safely ignored to acute life-threatening diseases. Although stomatitis implies a more florid condition with widespread inflammation and multiple ulcers there seems little point in trying to separate stomatitis and oral ulceration as there is a great deal of overlap between the two. Classification of the causes of oral ulceration is difficult and many conditions must be considered. The diagnosis in some

conditions is easily made on history and clinical examination. In others bacteriological examination of a smear, blood film or serological tests are necessary. If there is any doubt whatsoever biopsy is easy to perform and should never be neglected.

Oral manifestations of systemic disease

Numerous systemic diseases may give rise to signs and symptoms within the oral cavity. Usually, but not always, the appearances are non-specific but taken with other signs and symptoms may help to make the diagnosis.

Haematological disorders

Agranulocytosis, which may be a hypersensitivity reaction to certain drugs (e.g. sulphonamides, chloramphenicol, carbimazole, isoniazid) or a normal response to chemotherapeutic agents (bleomycin, methotrexate), gives rise to acute ulceration and slough formation in the oral cavity. The patient is usually pyrexial and ill and the diagnosis is made on the blood picture. In acute leukaemia the first presentation may be ulceration and bleeding from the gingival margins. The acquired immune deficiency syndrome (AIDS) may present with oral symptoms and of these hairy leukoplakia, oral candidiasis (very rare in young adult males), herpetic stomatitis and Kaposi's sarcoma are the most frequent.

Acute exanthems

Chickenpox may give rise to vesicles in the oral cavity, acute streptococcal tonsillitis gives rise to the strawberry tongue, measles to Koplik spots and glandular fever to a petechial rash on the hard palate.

Drug reactions

As well as those drugs causing agranulocytosis, phenytoin causes gingival hyperplasia and gold may produce gingivitis and, in addition, agranulocytosis. Acute erythema multiforme (see below) may be due to penicillin, sulphonamides or barbiturates.

Vitamin deficiency

Vitamin C deficiency produces a gingivitis, iron, folate and B_{12} deficiency produce a glossitis, riboflavin (B_2) and nicotinic acid deficiency produce angular chelitis and glossitis.

Autoimmune diseases

Chronic discoid lupus and systemic lupus erythematosus may be associated with vesicular and ulcerative lesions of the oral mucosa; less commonly scleroderma and polyarteritis nodosa may give oral ulceration (see below). Sjögren's syndrome and rheumatoid arthritis often cause xerostomia. Behçet's syndrome (see below) is a condition of unknown aetiology but may be autoimmune as may pemphigus and benign mucous membrane pemphigoid (see below).

Oral pigmentation

Although not an ulcerative condition the causes of oral pigmentation may be listed here. Oral pigmentation is more common and entirely normal in black races but may be seen in haemochromatosis, Albright's disease, Peutz-Jeghers syndrome, von Recklinghausen's disease and Addison's disease. Melanomas of the oral cavity are rare and initially may appear as a non-ulcerative pigmented lesion. Mercury, bismuth and lead poisoning give rise to areas of discoloration of the oral mucosa.

Infective conditions of the oral mucosa

Many different microorganisms can give rise to oral lesions which may be acute or chronic.

Virus infections

Primary herpetic gingivostomatitis (Figure 3.1)

This is the most frequent cause of acute stomatitis in children. (The differential diagnosis includes herpangina, chickenpox, hand foot and mouth disease and acute erythema multiforme.) The infection is due to the herpes simplex virus and while most often affecting children is now more frequent in adults than it used to be, presumably because they were not exposed to the virus in childhood. The condition gives rise to fever and malaise and vesicular lesions 2–4 mm in size which break down to form ulcers with a yellowish base and erythematous halo very similar to the lesions of aphthous ulcers. The condition lasts for 1 or 2 weeks and the diagnosis can be made by scrapings or smears from the lesion. The virus can be identified by immunofluorescent staining, exfoliative cytology which shows typical multinucleated giant cells, or may be cultured.

Recurrent oral herpes is very unusual but recurrent herpes labialis (cold sores) is very common.

Herpes zoster

When herpes zoster affects the trigeminal nerve there may be intraoral lesions, always unilateral and often painful. There may be cervical lymphadenopathy and occasionally there may be an associated facial palsy, i.e. Ramsey Hunt syndrome.

Hand, foot and mouth disease

This is a condition caused by a group A coxsackie virus and may occur in epidemics among school children. It gives rise to vesicles on the hands, feet and occasionally buttocks together with intraoral vesicles and later ulcers. The patient may be febrile and have a generalized malaise. The incubation period of the disease is about a week and the illness lasts a variable amount of time but rarely more than a week.

Herpangina

This is again a condition mainly of children which may be due to different viruses including different coxsackieviruses and enteric cytopathogenic human orphan (ECHO) viruses. The disease is very similar to herpes simplex except the lesions are more commonly in the oropharynx than oral cavity.

Bacterial infections

Perhaps the most common oral infections are those associated with predominantly dental conditions, gingivitis, periodontitis and dental abscesses.

Acute necrotizing gingivitis (Vincent's angina)

This condition is an infection with the spirochaete *Borrelia vincentii* and an anaerobic organism *Bacillus fusiformis*. It occurs in adults who are generally debilitated or who have poor dental hygiene and is essentially a gingivitis affecting the interdental papillae, producing ulceration and a necrotic membrane. The lesions are painful, associated with foetor and the patient may be pyrexial with tender enlarged cervical glands. The lesions may spread to involve the tonsil and oropharynx but on occasions the tonsil may be

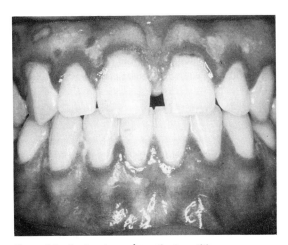

Figure 3.1 Acute primary herpetic stomatitis

involved alone. The diagnosis can be made from a smear stained with gentian violet to identify the spirochaete and fusiform bacillus. Treatment is both local, with mouth washes, and systemic with benzylpenicillin and metronidazole given intravenously.

Gangrenous stomatitis (cancrum oris)

This is a rare condition in the western world but still a problem in countries where there is little access to health care. It usually affects children and results in a rapidly enlarging ulcer with much necrosis involving the oral cavity and upper or lower jaws. There is widespread local tissue destruction. The condition is most common in debilitated children and though no specific microorganisms are involved mixed bacterial growths (rather like Vincent's angina) are implicated. Local hygiene and the systemic antibiotics, benzylpenicillin and metronidazole, are successful if the condition is treated in an early phase.

Syphilis

Syphilis, due to the spirochaete, *Treponema pallidum*, is acquired by sexual intercourse apart from the congenital form of the disease. The disease progresses through a primary stage, which is at the site of the initial inoculation, and through secondary and tertiary stages. The secondary stage is the one most likely to affect the oral cavity but any of the stages may give rise to oral lesions. The disease manifests itself in a great many ways, and particularly in the tertiary stage, virtually any organ system may be involved. The pathological process in syphilis is an endarteritis with an increase in adventitial cells, proliferation of endothelial cells and an inflammatory cell infiltrate with lymphocytes, plasma cells and monocytes. In the tertiary phase of the disease there is a granulomatous reaction with giant cells surrounding a necrotic centre. Organisms can be isolated from the lesions of the primary and secondary stages and the disease can be transmitted in these stages.

Primary syphilis

The lesion of primary syphilis is the chancre and the most frequent extragenital sites are the lips, buccal mucosa, tongue and tonsil. After an incubation period of 3 weeks a papule forms and breaks down to a painless ulcer which heals within 2–6 weeks. The ulcer may be accompanied by painless lymphadenopathy.

Secondary syphilis

The secondary stage occurs 4–6 weeks after the primary stage and 30% of patients in the secondary stage will have signs of a healing chancre. The secondary stage is associated with malaise, headache and fever with generalized lymphadenopathy, a mucocutaneous rash and sore throat. The lesions in the oral cavity particularly affect the tongue and palate and consist of ulcers covered by a greyish membrane. Because of their configuration they are known either as snail-track ulcers or mucous patches (which are circular areas). The secondary stage of the disease lasts for a few weeks.

Tertiary syphilis

This develops many years after the initial infection and is characterized by lesions which may be widespread throughout the body affecting any organ system or may be restricted to one or two organs. In the upper respiratory tract the lesion is the gumma which begins as a nodule which breaks down to form a necrotic ulcer. It can occur in the hard palate, the nasal septum, tonsil, posterior pharyngeal wall or larynx. The gumma is painless and causes marked tissue destruction which in the palate produces an oronasal or oroantral fistula.

In the primary or secondary stages syphilis can be diagnosed by identifying spirochaetes taken from smears of the lesions. Spirochaetes can also be identified in biopsy specimens from primary and secondary lesions using silver stains or immunofluorescent techniques. Although microorganisms cannot be identified in the tertiary lesions, biopsies of these lesions give a typical histopathological appearance. Serological tests for syphilis fall into two main groups: those used to identify non-specific antibodies to cardiolipin (VDRL tests), and those to detect specific treponemal antibodies (TPI and FTA). The VDRL (Venereal Disease Research Laboratory) test uses a beef heart antigen and becomes positive about 1–2 weeks after the development of the chancre. About 99% of patients with secondary and tertiary syphilis will give a positive reaction. However, a number of other diseases will also give a positive reaction including non-syphilitic treponemal disease (yaws, bejel, pinta), other infections (atypical pneumonia, malaria, leprosy, smallpox) and autoimmune diseases (systemic lupus erythematosus, rheumatoid arthritis). The *Treponema pallidum* immobilization (TPI) test depends upon a specific antibody in the patient's serum which immobilizes spirochaetes observed by dark ground illumination. It is 100% positive in patients with secondary and tertiary syphilis and is 100% specific. The fluorescent treponemal antibody (FTA) test involves the absorption of antibodies onto dried *Treponema pallidum* preparations and their identification by fluorescent labelled antihuman gammaglobulin. The FTA test is 100% positive in secondary and tertiary syphilis but not 100% specific as occasionally patients with systemic lupus erythematosus and rheumatoid arthritis will give a positive reaction.

In primary and secondary syphilis a single or perhaps two deep intramuscular injections of 2.4 megaunits of benzathine penicillin will cure the disease. In tertiary syphilis three injections of 2.4 megaunits of benzathine penicillin at weekly or 2-weekly intervals are given.

Tuberculosis

Tuberculosis only affects the oral cavity in patients with sputum positive pulmonary tuberculosis and gives rise to multiple superficial and painful ulcers on the tongue and elsewhere in the oral cavity.

Fungal infections

Candidiasis

Candida albicans is a normal commensal organism in the mouth of many patients and only usually becomes pathogenic when there is a predisposing factor such as general debilitating illness (e.g. AIDS), antibiotic therapy, anticancer chemotherapy and steroids (local and systemic).

Acute candidiasis gives rise to multiple small white patches on the oral mucosa which when wiped off leave an erythematous patch. The lesions are often quite painful and seen particularly in the buccal mucosa and soft palate (Figure 3.2). The diagnosis can be made by staining a smear using the periodic acid-Schiff method. Local treatment with nystatin or amphotericin is usually sufficient providing the underlying cause is also corrected.

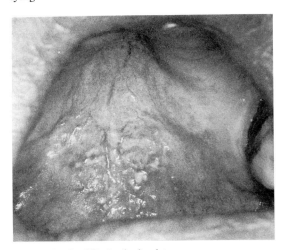

Figure 3.2 Candidiasis of soft palate

In chronic candidiasis a white lesion appears which cannot be rubbed off and gives the appearance of leukoplakia, hence the term candidal leukoplakia (Cawson and Lehner, 1968). These lesions may be widespread and particularly affect the buccal mucosa just inside the corner of the mouth. The presence of candida in biopsies of these lesions may be overlooked. Although these lesions may respond to local

or systemic antifungal agents such as ketoconazole, excision may be the only way of removing them.

Histoplasmosis

This fungal infection due to *Histoplasma capsulatum* gives rise to granular-looking ulcers in the oral cavity usually only in patients with widespread systemic histoplasmosis and responds to systemic chemotherapy with ketoconazole.

Traumatic oral ulceration

Trauma can cause oral ulceration, particularly hard food, rough dentures, sharp rough dentition, the patient biting his tongue or buccal mucosa. However, many patients with an oral carcinoma relate this to an ill-fitting denture or to trauma. A traumatic ulcer will heal within 2 weeks and if it does not, it should be biopsied.

Miscellaneous conditions causing oral ulceration

A large number of conditions of unknown aetiology will produce oral ulceration. It is difficult to classify these lesions, some are of little significance, others may be serious.

Aphthous ulceration (Figure 3.3)

Aphthous ulcers are very common and of unknown aetiology though many factors have been suggested

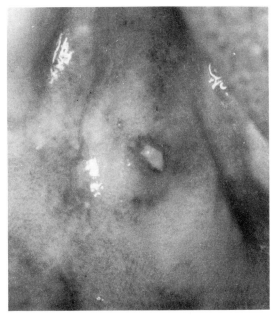

Figure 3.3 Recurrent aphthous ulcers

as causative such as hypersensitivity reactions, hormonal or vitamin deficiency and stress (Antoon and Miller, 1980). Susceptible individuals usually have an episode of single or multiple ulcers (2–10 mm in size) which lasts a few weeks. Each individual ulcer will heal in about 10 days. The frequency of episodes is very variable. Occasional patients will have larger ulcers 2–3 cm in diameter which may take much longer to heal. Typically the edges of these ulcers are not indurated but biopsy may be necessary to distinguish them from a carcinoma. Although patients with aphthous ulcers are often given local steroids in an attempt to reduce inflammation and assist healing, there is no evidence that steroids help.

Behçet's syndrome

This is a condition of unknown aetiology in which oral ulceration is associated with genital ulceration, uveitis, vasculitis of the skin, synovitis and meningo-encephalitis. It is a relapsing condition and the oral ulcers are very similar to aphthous ulcers, often of the larger type. Oral steroids are valuable in treatment.

Pemphigus vulgaris

This is a serious condition which, before the use of oral steroids, was often fatal. The disease is one in which bullae are formed on the skin and in the oral cavity, particularly palate, buccal mucosa and tongue (Laskaris, Sklavounou and Straligos, 1982). The disease affects patients in late middle age and the elderly and is a disease in which periods of quiescence and relapses are common. The bullae in the oral cavity break down to form irregular very painful erosions and histologically acantholysis is present in the epithelium and immunofluorescence will demonstrate IgG. Nikolsky's sign is said to be diagnostic: stroking the mucous membrane induces a vesicle or bulla to appear. Long-term steroids are the treatment of choice.

Benign mucous membrane pemphigoid

This is a less serious disease than pemphigus vulgaris but, nevertheless, it is often chronic, and scarring, particularly of the conjunctiva, can occur. The disease affects an older age group than pemphigus and women more than men. The vesicles occur most often in the oral cavity, occasionally in the pharynx and larynx and also affect the conjunctiva. Skin lesions are rare. The vesicles rupture to give a ragged ulcer but the condition is usually much less florid and painful than pemphigus. Histologically the lesions can be distinguished from pemphigus in that acantholysis does not occur, there being only subepi-

thelial clefts. Immunofluorescence demonstrates IgG and compliment C3 in the basement membrane. Benign mucous membrane pemphigoid may require no treatment although sometimes systemic steroids are necessary.

Erythema multiforme (Figure 3.4)

This is a condition of unknown aetiology which affects young people, usually between the ages of 10 and 30 years. Although the cause is unknown erythema multiforme may be secondary to infections like herpes and mycoplasma or due to a reaction to drugs such as penicillin, sulphonamides or barbiturates. Usually the skin is involved in this disease with erythematous nodular lesions with a bluish centre but bullae and vesicles are also seen. Oral lesions are more common in the major form of the disease (Stevens-Johnson syndrome) than the minor form. In one-quarter of patients lesions are restricted to the oral cavity. In both forms of the disease the illness usually lasts 2–3 weeks though relapses are common. In Stevens-Johnson syndrome the patient may be pyrexial and severely ill and steroids are necessary. The oral lesions consist of macules, bullae and extensive erosions covered by a slough. Often the lips are covered with a haemorrhagic crust which is characteristic of the condition.

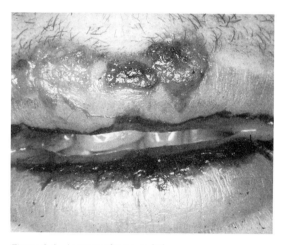

Figure 3.4 Acute erythema multiforme

Necrotizing sialometaplasia

This is an uncommon condition leading to ulceration of the hard palate or oropharynx and consisting of ductal metaplasia or hyperplasia of salivary tissue with very extensive inflammatory changes. The condition is self-limiting and spontaneous healing takes place in a few weeks. The diagnosis and the differentiation from carcinoma is made by biopsy (Grillon and Lally, 1981).

Lichen planus (Figure 3.5)

This was originally described as a skin disease. Patients may have both the skin disease and the oral disease but usually they are separate. The disease most commonly affects adults in middle age, women more frequently than men. The aetiology is unknown and although several different types of oral lesion have been described the two usual types are described as reticular and erosive. The reticular type gives rise to slightly raised lesions which are white, with a slightly bluish tinge with a reticular pattern of striae, particularly affecting the buccal mucosa. The erosive type gives rise to erythematous lesions, often ulcerated and painful. These lesions often need to be biopsied to distinguish them from leukoplakia, erythroplakia or early carcinoma. Histologically lichen planus shows keratosis, parakeratosis with pointed or saw-toothed rete pegs and accumulation of fluid along the basement membrane. There is a cellular inflammatory infiltration usually of T lymphocytes. Local steroids are helpful in erosive lichen planus and these patients should be kept under observation with biopsy if necessary. There may be an increased incidence of oral cancer in patients with lichen planus particularly of the erosive type.

Leukoplakia (Figure 3.6)

White patches in the oral mucosa are abnormal and represent an epithelial abnormality because normally the epithelium is not keratinizing. The cause of leukoplakia is unknown. The important thing about it is its relationship with carcinoma. Few would dispute that a relationship exists but the risk of a patient with leukoplakia actually developing carcinoma is small (see below). In leukoplakia there are a number of histological changes: there is accumulation of keratin, i.e. keratosis, there is thickening of the superficial layer of the epithelium, the stratum corneum known as hyperkeratosis, increase in the proportion of nucleated cells, i.e. parakeratosis, abnormality of the basal layer of the epithelium, the stratum granulosum, with elongation of the rete pegs called acanthosis. The most important factor in leukoplakia is the degree of abnormality or dyskeratosis with nuclear hyperchromatism, nuclear pleomorphism, mitoses and loss of the normal maturation of cells seen throughout the epithelium, i.e. loss of polarity and loss of intercellular adherence. These changes vary from mild atypia through to a frankly carcinomatous appearance in which no cellular invasion deep to the basal layer is seen, i.e. intraepithelial carcinoma or carcinoma *in situ*. The term erythroplakia is reserved for areas of mucosal abnormality which are erythematous and represent dysplasia without keratosis. It is generally accepted that the lesions showing severe dysplasia have the greatest potential for malignant change. Candidal leukoplakia has been described above and is felt to be due to a chronic candidiasis in which dysplasia is present.

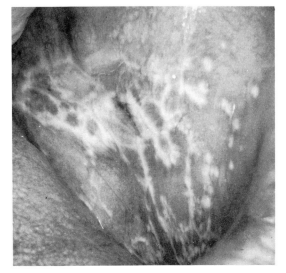

Figure 3.5   Lichen planus

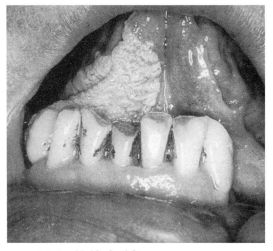

Figure 3.6   Speckled leukoplakia

Geographical tongue

This condition also known as migratory glossitis or erythema migrans is entirely benign and of unknown aetiology. The appearance resembles that of a map with flattened erythematous areas where the papillae have been lost, surrounded by a margin of keratosis. Usually the condition is asymptomatic though occasionally there may be a mild burning pain. The areas of loss of papillae regress and increase hence the use of the adjective migratory in the name. No treatment influences the condition.

Hairy tongue

The coated tongue due to elongation and accumulation of keratin associated with the filiform papillae gives a thickened appearance to the epithelium which is often white but may be blackened in smokers. The cause of these changes is unknown and the only treatment is to scrape off the keratin with a brush.

Benign swellings of the oral cavity

As well as benign tumours, developmental swellings and inflammatory swellings should be considered in this group. When considering tumours of the oral cavity the tissues present in the mouth should be borne in mind, namely lining epithelium, salivary tissue, lymphoid tissue, connective tissue, muscle and bone.

Cysts in the mouth

Developmental cysts

These occur in the lines of fusion of the elements which make up the upper jaw. They may be in the midline or laterally where the maxillary and premaxillary elements fuse. Also of developmental origin is the nasopalatine cyst. Dermoid cysts are of developmental origin and contain elements of ectodermal and mesodermal origin. Thus they are lined by squamous epithelium and contain sebaceous glands and connective tissue. They occur in the submental region and give rise to an external swelling in this region but also may elevate the floor of the mouth and tongue.

Cysts associated with a tooth

These include primordial cysts (due to maldevelopment of a tooth), cysts of eruption, dentigerous cysts and dental cysts (Figures 3.7 and 3.8).

Cysts and tumours of the jaws

These are considered in Chapter 23.

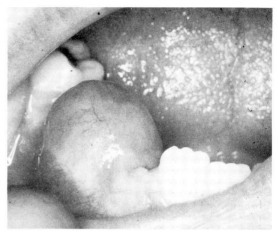

Figure 3.7 Eruption cyst

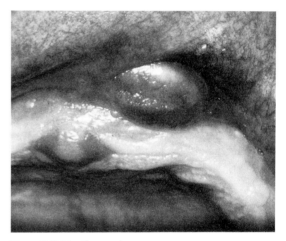

Figure 3.8 Maxillary cyst

Retention cysts

Occlusion of the opening of minor salivary glands can result in small cysts anywhere in the oral cavity (Figure 3.9). A ranula is a cyst in the floor of the mouth usually on one side which arises from the sublingual salivary gland. A ranula may arise as a rare complication of transposition of the submandibular ducts in the treatment of drooling and may in this case either arise from the submandibular duct or from the sublingual gland. A ranula gives rise to a bluish semitranslucent cyst which resembles the belly of a frog and is treated by excision to include the sublingual gland (Black and Croft, 1982).

Inflammatory swellings

Most of the inflammatory swellings which occur in the oral cavity are associated with the teeth and

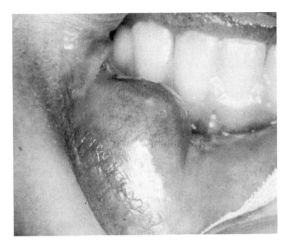

Figure 3.9 Mucous retention cyst

jaws. Dental caries, gingivitis (inflammation of the gums) and periodontal disease (inflammation and destruction of the periodontal membrane) are all probably related to dental plaque. Dental plaque is a deposit forming on the teeth consisting of an organic matrix containing bacteria such as streptococci, lacto-bacilli, actinomyces, diphtheroids and anaerobic organisms of which *Bacillus melaninogenicus* is probably the most important. Plaque can be removed by cleaning but if it persists results in destruction of the enamel, dentine and eventually a dental abscess and also chronic inflammatory disease of the gums, i.e. gingivitis, inflammation and abscess formation in the periodontal membrane (Figures 3.10 and 3.11). The inflammatory processes and abscesses spread in a variety of directions depending on the thickness of the adjacent bone and the adjacent muscle attachments (Figure 3.12). Thus odontogenic abscesses give

rise to a variety of inflammatory swellings in the mouth. The most frequent is the vestibular abscess on the labial side of the jaw. The infection may spread to involve the maxillary spaces (the buccal space or the canine space) or the mandibular spaces (submental, sublingual and submandibular spaces) from which deep neck space infections may arise.

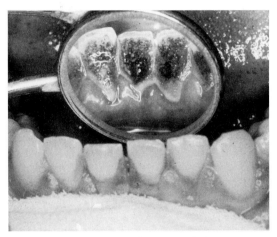

Figure 3.11 Gingivitis and subgingival calculus

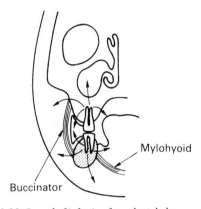

Figure 3.12 Spread of infection from dental abscesses

Epulis

Epulis means on the gums and thus any swelling on the gum is theoretically entitled to be called an epulis (Figure 3.13). In practice the term epulis is usually restricted to inflammatory swellings in relation to the teeth. Thus the fibrous epulis is usually seen protruding between two teeth and is a chronic inflammatory lesion (Figure 3.14). The swelling should be removed and any underlying infection dealt with. The giant cell epulis gives a similar appearance but is somewhat

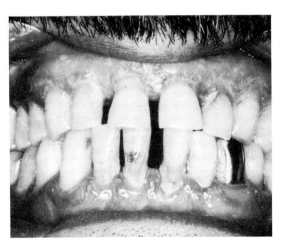

Figure 3.10 Gingivitis

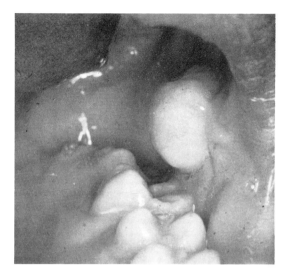

Figure 3.13 Fibroepithelial polyp

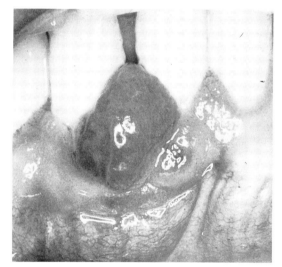

Figure 3.14 Recurring epulis

more vascular. It contains multinucleated giant cells and is usually related to the eruption of secondary dentition and shedding of deciduous teeth.

The pregnancy tumour is a type of epulis when there is gingival inflammation and hypertrophy in pregnancy. Phenytoin also produces hypertrophy of the gingiva.

Benign tumours of the oral cavity

Odontogenic tumours and cysts are dealt with in Volume 4.

Papilloma

Squamous papillomas arise from the stratified squamous epithelium lining the oral cavity. They are more common in the oropharynx than oral cavity but do occur on the tongue.

Pleomorphic adenoma

This is by far the most frequent benign salivary gland tumour arising within the oral cavity. The vast majority occur on the hard palate extending to involve the soft palate (Isaacson and Shear, 1983) (Figure 3.15). Parapharyngeal pleomorphic adenomas either arise in the deep lobe of the parotid gland or from a minor salivary gland in the oropharynx. Pleomorphic adenomas should be completely excised. This may be difficult in the oral cavity but since this is a benign tumour mutilating surgery has no place in the initial management. Although there is often a false capsule of compressed normal tissue around these tumours the characteristic of the surface of a pleomorphic adenoma is that it is nodular or bosselated and small projections of the tumour may penetrate the capsule. If after the operation and as a result of histological examination there seems a real risk that the excision has been incomplete then the options are either radiotherapy or close observation with further surgery if the lesion recurs.

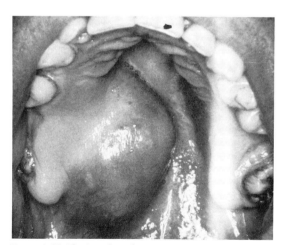

Figure 3.15 Pleomorphic adenoma

Connective tissue tumours
Haemangioma

Most oral haemangiomas are probably of developmental origin and are a mixture of haemangiomatous and lymphangiomatous elements. Many of these lesions are present at birth or appear soon after and the oral tumours may be solely restricted to the oral cavity or may be part of a larger lesion arising in the neck. Of the lesions restricted to the oral cavity the tongue and floor of mouth are the usual sites. The lesions are soft, irregular and bluish or purple in colour. Often they regress and a conservative approach to management is preferable. Large lesions and those increasing in size are a difficult problem. Resection is difficult and should be as conservative as possible. Embolization may be helpful (Thompson, Fierstein and Kohut, 1979). Pure lymphangiomas are somewhat easier to deal with because they are less vascular but, because these lesions can be so widespread with finger-like processes extending into surrounding tissues, complete excision is very difficult (Goldberg, Nemarick and Danielson, 1977). Again the oral part of the lesion may be an extension of a lymphangioma (cystic hygroma) of the neck (Ward, Harris and Downey, 1970).

Neurogenic tumours

Neurilemmomas (schwannomas) occur rarely in the oral cavity, mostly in the tongue (Gallo, Moss and Shapiro, 1977). Neurofibromas may be single or part of von Recklinghausen's disease. On occasions they may be very extensive and surgery is difficult (Maceri and Saxon, 1984).

Miscellaneous connective tissue tumours

Rarely leiomyomas, rhabdomyomas and lipomas occur in the oral cavity.

Granular cell myoblastoma

This is probably not a true neoplasm but its exact nature is unknown. It is a rare lesion of the tongue which presents as a firm non-ulcerated nodule. The lesion is composed of a mass of large cells with a granular eosinophilic cytoplasm. The important thing about this swelling is that in 50% of patients the overlying epithelium shows pseudoepitheliomatous hyperplasia, i.e. shows changes which could be mistaken for a squamous carcinoma. Treatment is by conservative surgery (Strong, McDivitt and Brasfield, 1970).

Xerostomia

It must be stated at the outset that the complaint of a dry mouth by a patient is quite a common one and in a large proportion of patients no cause is found. In those patients without demonstrable abnormality additional symptoms may be a burning pain in the mouth or tongue and, although careful examination and investigation is always necessary, many times no abnormality is found (Stell, 1982). There are however some well-recognized causes of a dry mouth.

Sjögren's syndrome

This is probably an autoimmune disorder which affects the salivary glands, the lacrimal glands and less obviously other exocrine glands. In addition a number of these patients also have an autoimmune connective tissue disorder. The condition usually affects patients in middle age and is much more common in women than in men. The presenting symptoms are a dry mouth, painful tongue and itching, gritty and dry eyes. Examination of the oral cavity may show obvious xerostomia particularly when the condition is of long standing and there may be glossitis. Schirmer's test will be abnormal in a high proportion of patients and the diagnosis can usually be made by removing a minor salivary gland from the mucosa inside the lower lip and demonstrating lymphocytic infiltration (Daniels, 1984). Over half of the patients with Sjögren's syndrome will have an associated connective tissue disorder mainly rheumatoid arthritis but also systemic lupus erythematosus, polymyositis or polyarteritis nodosa. Autoantibodies are present in the serum of patients with Sjögren's syndrome and include antinuclear antibodies, positive latex fixation, antilacrimal and antithyroid antibodies. The major salivary glands in Sjögren's syndrome may be diffusely enlarged with a lymphocytic infiltration and a discrete mass may be palpable within a salivary gland. There is an association between Sjögren's syndrome and non-Hodgkin's lymphoma.

Radiotherapy

Radiotherapy to the head and neck region produces marked xerostomia due to its effects on the major salivary glands and also on the minor salivary glands in the oral and pharyngeal mucosa. If possible fields should be designed so that one or more major salivary gland is protected from radiation. In both Sjögren's syndrome and radiation-induced xerostomia artificial saliva may be of value, recently pilocarpine has been investigated in this context. Most patients however, find that the most useful measure is to carry a bottle of water around with them.

Drug-induced xerostomia

Atropine-like drugs produce xerostomia of which the most widely used are the tricyclic antidepressants. In addition, rarely, other drugs such as thiouracil, phenylbutazone and some antibiotics (sulphonamides, tetracycline) can produce sicca syndromes and salivary gland enlargement.

Cancer of the oral cavity

The oral cavity is easy to examine both by the patient and by medical and dental practitioners and therefore in theory early diagnosis should be the rule; unfortunately this is far from being the case and quite lengthy delays in treatment are common. Brunn (1976) showed that in Denmark the average delay between the diagnosis and treatment of patients with mouth cancer was 10.5 months. This was divided into 5 months due to patient delay and 5.5 months' delay between the patient first seeing a medical or dental practitioner and referral to a specialist. This is unfortunate because there is no doubt that patients with an early mouth cancer have an excellent prognosis, whereas those diagnosed late not only have a poor prognosis but also often need extensive and mutilating surgery. Much of the delay in diagnosis is because the patient ignores the lesion but also since mouth cancer is relatively rare many general practitioners will only see the occasional patient and will fail to diagnose early lesions. Somewhat surprisingly perhaps this seems also to be true of dental practitioners. Bruun found that the average delay in referral was greater if the patient saw a dental practitioner rather than a medical practitioner. The effects of delay of diagnosis on the prognosis was discussed in a leading article in *The Lancet* (1972) and in one series of patients with cancer of the floor of the mouth there was a direct correlation between delay in treatment and prognosis (Ballard, Guess and Pickren, 1978). Thus patients treated within 1 month of the onset of symptoms had a 5-year survival of 86%, those treated between 7 and 12 months had a survival of 47% and when the delay in treatment was more than 12 months no patients survived.

Applied anatomy

In both the AJC and UICC classifications the oral cavity is separated from the oropharynx by the anterior pillar of the fauces laterally, the junction of the hard and soft palate above, and the line of the circumvallate papillae below. This means that both the soft palate and the posterior one-third of the tongue are excluded from the oral cavity and are part of the oropharynx.

The anterior limit of the oral cavity is the junction between the mucosa and skin of the lips and the vermilion or red part of the lip is included in the oral cavity. This is the source of some confusion and difficulty in reporting mouth cancers. Cancer of the vermilion, although strictly speaking part of the oral cavity is usually reported separately as cancer of the lip. In most patients with a lip cancer it is difficult and probably irrelevant to decide where the lesion

originated. The oral cavity is divided into a number of sites for the localization of mouth cancers: the anterior two-thirds of the tongue, the floor of the mouth, upper and lower alveolar ridges including the gingiva, the hard palate, buccal mucosa, and the lip. The retromolar trigone is an area in which a mouth cancer may arise; it is difficult to see on clinical examination and difficult to visualize anatomically. It is an area of mucosa covering the ascending ramus of the mandible, roughly triangular in shape. The base of the triangle is the posterior surface of the last lower molar tooth and the apex is the tuberosity of the maxilla. Above its lateral border is the lateral margin of the ascending ramus of the mandible joining the gingivobuccal sulcus and medially is the mucosa of the gingivolingual sulcus and the mucosa on the inner surface of the lower alveolus. Clinically the area is exposed by using two tongue depressors, one to retract the tongue medially and the other to retract the cheek laterally. Cancer is no more frequent in the retromolar trigone than in other areas on the lower alveolus or buccal mucosa but, because of the difficulty in seeing this area clinically, an early cancer in this site may be missed.

There are a number of details of normal anatomy which are important not only in understanding the spread of cancers of the oral cavity but when considering the surgery of this area.

1 Cancers spread along the lines of tissue planes and also spaces created by the passage of normal anatomical structures. Particularly important in the oral cavity are the channels in bone for the passage of nerves. Not only do adenoid cystic carcinomas spread along the nerve trunks themselves but squamous carcinoma spreads adjacent to the nerves in bone. Thus in the mandible the inferior alveolar nerve runs in the inferior dental canal from the mandibular foramen to the mental foramen. In the edentulous mandible when alveolar bone is absorbed the mandible may be as thin as a pencil and the mandibular canal may be only a few millimetres from the surface. This allows early spread of a carcinoma of the lower alveolus into the mandibular canal and hence along it. Paraesthesia or anaesthesia of an area of skin to one side of the midline of the chin may indicate invasion of the inferior alveolar nerve.

The hard palate is perforated by a number of canals for the passage of blood vessels and nerves. These canals provide channels for the spread of malignancies of the hard palate. The greater palatine foramina are situated one on each side of the hard palate close to its posterior border. These foramina are the lower openings of the greater palatine canal and transmit the anterior palatine nerves (branches of Vb) and vessels. An adenoid cystic carcinoma of the hard palate is particularly liable to spread along the anterior palatine nerve eventually reaching the pterygopalatine ganglion in the pterygopalatine fossa. The lesser palatine foramina are usually two openings just behind the greater foramina and transmit the middle and posterior palatine nerves and vessels.

The incisive fossa lies in the midline of the hard palate anteriorly and is pierced by lateral incisive foramina which lead via the incisive canals to the nasal cavity. There may also be median incisive foramina. These foramina in the incisive fossa transmit the terminal branches of the greater palatine vessels and nasopalatine nerve.

2 The floor of the mouth consists of a mucosal covering for a muscular diaphragm formed by the mylohyoid, geniohyoid, genioglossus and hyoglossus muscles. The duct of the submandibular gland runs submucosally on the mylohyoid muscle and tumours or scarring due to surgery or radiotherapy may obstruct the duct or its opening to cause swelling of the submandibular salivary gland. Classically this swelling is intermittent and occurs with meals but, when the obstruction is longstanding, the swelling may be persistent and confused wth a metastatic lymph node in the submandibular triangle. Carcinomas of the tongue and floor of the mouth can penetrate deeply into the adjacent muscles growing between the muscle bundles. In the tongue what appears to be a fairly superficial lesion may spread deeply into the substance of the tongue and isolated nodules of tumour are often found distinct from the main tumour mass. Spread can occur along the hyoglossus muscle to the region of the hyoid bone and into the pre-epiglottic space. Floor of mouth tumours do not often penetrate all the way through the mylohyoid muscle but spread along it and may grow around its posterior border into the submandibular triangle. The medial pterygoid muscle inserting into the angle of the mandible may be infiltrated by tumour which spreads along it and into the lateral pterygoid muscle. Invasion of these muscles gives rise to trismus which is prognostically a bad sign in mouth cancer.

Invasion of the mandible by mouth cancers

Squamous carcinomas invade the cortex of the mandible usually on the alveolar ridge (Carter, 1990). Occasionally more posterior lesions in the floor of the mouth, retromolar trigone or oropharynx may gain access along the inferior alveolar nerve as it enters the mandible. The surface of the mandible is irregular with clefts to which the periosteum is attached. An infiltrative squamous carcinoma can spread into these clefts and invade the cortical bone. This stimulates osteoclasts to resorb bone (Carter, Tsao and Burman, 1983; O'Brien, Carter and Soo, 1986) which facilitates the spread of the tumour. Once the cortex has been invaded spread can occur into the inferior dental canal allowing rapid spread of tumours forwards and backwards. As has already been stated, in the edentulous mandible the inferior dental canal lies very close to the surface of the mandible.

Lymphatic drainage of the oral cavity

Lymphatic vessels in the buccal mucosa, tongue and floor of the mouth form an extensive submucosal plexus which eventually drains into the deep cervical nodes. The vessels of the floor of the mouth and tongue freely communicate across the midline and so drainage of lymph from regions close to the midline is bilateral. The drainage of lymph may be direct to the deep cervical nodes or through intermediate lymph nodes. The deep cervical nodes receiving lymph from the oral cavity may be the jugulodigastric or the jugulo-omohyoid nodes. In general the more anterior the location in the mouth the lower in the neck that the lymph may drain (Figure 3.16). Anteriorly lymphatic vessels in the floor of the mouth and tongue pierce the mylohyoid muscle and enter submental nodes. Further posteriorly the nodes within the submandibular triangle receive lymph before it passes to the upper deep cervical nodes. The pattern of lymph drainage from the normal mouth is variable with bilateral drainage to the upper and lower deep cervical nodes but when the patient has undergone radiotherapy or surgery the lymphatic drainage is even more unpredictable and variable. This has practical applications affecting the likely site of metastases from mouth cancers when the possibilities of bilateral or high or low metastases in the neck need to be considered. Using submucosal injections of dye and intralymphatic injections of radiopaque material Larson, Lewis and Rappaport (1965) studied the lymphatic drainage of the tongue. They confirmed earlier anatomical studies and also demonstrated that lymph channels bypassed groups of lymph nodes and passed from the tongue directly to lymph nodes in the lower neck.

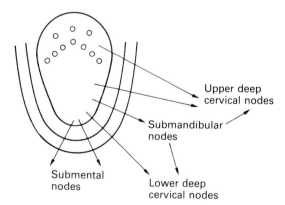

Figure 3.16 Spread of cancer to cervical lymph nodes

Epidemiology and aetiology of mouth cancer

One of the great difficulties in correlating epidemiological studies is that classification of the site of disease is often not rigorous. Thus in the case of mouth cancer many publications include disease of the oropharynx, and other regions of the pharynx. Some include lip and others exclude this site from mouth cancer. This results in tremendous artificial variation in the figures for the incidence of the disease. In the USA the incidence of mouth cancers is about 10 cases per 100 000 per year (20 per 100 000 for men and 5 per 100 000 for women), representing 6% of all cancers in men and 3% in women (Hamner, 1986) (compared with cancer of the lung in men and cancer of the breast in women which each form about 20% of the total cancers). In the UK the incidence of the disease is probably lower than this and Powell and Robin (1987) quoted figures of 2.3 cases per 100 000 per year for men and 1.2 cases per 100 000 per year for women. These figures can be compared with those for laryngeal cancer with 4.8 per 100 000 for men and 0.7 per 100 000 for women. To put this in perspective the figures for carcinoma of the lung in men are 80 per 100 000 in Birmingham and for all mucosal head and neck cancers the figure is 7.6 per 100 000 (Waterhouse *et al.*, 1982). Oral cancer ranks as the sixth most common cancer worldwide (Parkin, Laara and Muir, 1988).

Population figures are also dependent on the age of the population sampled because there is a progressive increase of the incidence of mouth cancer with age, the elderly showing a much increased rate of susceptibility. There is no doubt that marked geographic variations in the incidence of mouth cancer do occur and although the figures for absolute values may be exaggerated definite trends do exist. Study of the trends is important in the implication of aetiological factors. Table 3.1 shows the death rates from oral cancer for various countries and although India is not quoted in this table the rates for India are probably the highest in the world. Even within India

tremendous geographical variation occurs and the incidence varies from 14 to 26 per 100 000. Perhaps more interesting are the changes in incidence which occur with time. Overall in the present century the incidence of mouth cancer is falling slightly and what also is apparent is that the difference between the rates for men and women is decreasing (Russell, 1955; Binnie and Rankin, 1984).

Smoking and alcohol are the two most strongly implicated factors in the aetiology. Either alone increases the incidence of the disease and together there is a greatly increased incidence, in fact the risk is roughly the multiple of the risks of each factor individually (Wynder, Bross and Feldman, 1957).

Quoted figures for alcohol and tobacco alone indicate that they individually increase the risk of developing a cancer of the mouth about sixfold (Silverman and Griffiths, 1972). This is the figure also quoted when comparing the chances of developing a second mouth cancer after the successful treatment of the first. Patients who continue to smoke are six times as likely to develop a second cancer as those who stop smoking (Moore, 1971; Silverman and Griffiths, 1972; Kissin *et al.*, 1973).

Although the relation between mouth cancer and smoking seems fairly well established it remains to be explained why, in the first half of the present century, the incidence of mouth cancer has remained static or fallen slightly yet during this time the consumption of tobacco has greatly increased (Smith, 1982; Morton *et al.*, 1983). It may suggest that alcohol has the more important role (Rothman and Keller, 1972). Certainly the trends in mouth cancer are not similar to those in lung cancer which has increased markedly this century and has been shown to be closely related to tobacco consumption.

The increased incidence of oral cancer in India is felt to be at least in part related to two habits peculiar to that area. The habit of chewing a betel quid in India is widespread. The quid consists of betel leaf, areca palm nut, slaked lime and catechu in addition to certain other additives and flavourings. The most common additional constituent is tobacco. Similarly in India the habit of reverse smoking with the lighted end of the cigarette in the mouth is thought to increase the incidence of cancer of the hard palate (Reddy, 1974).

In the past syphilis has been implicated in the aetiology of mouth cancer and early reports related an increased prevalence of syphilis in patients with mouth cancer (Martin, Munster and Sugarbaker, 1940). More recent reports have failed to show this association (Myer and Abbey, 1970).

Although poor oral hygiene, sharp jagged teeth, chronic gingivitis and ill-fitting dentures have often in the past been implicated in the aetiology of mouth cancer there is no objective evidence that this is the case (Wynder, Bross and Feldman, 1957).

Table 3.1 Age adjusted death rate for oral cancer rates per 100 000

Country	Men	Women
USA	5.8	2.0
Australia	5.3	1.5
England and Wales	3.7	1.7
Hong Kong	21.2	7.1
Japan	2.2	0.8
Norway	4.3	1.1
Singapore	18.9	6.3

From Hamner (1986)

The role of premalignant conditions in the development of oral cancer has been mentioned previously. In Banoczy's study (1977) of 670 patients with oral leukoplakia followed up for 30 years, 6% of patients developed squamous carcinoma and there was a strong association between the type of leukoplakia and the potential for development of cancer. In those patients with histological evidence of dysplasia 13% developed a carcinoma and in patients with erosive leukoplakia the risk was 26%. It seems that leukoplakia with severe epithelial dysplasia is the most likely to undergo malignant change and Waldron and Shafer (1975) showed that 17% of lesions clinically diagnosed as leukoplakia had epithelial dysplasia and 43% invasive carcinoma. Erythroplakia, which in the WHO (1978) definition is described as an oral mucosal lesion which appears as a red velvety plaque which cannot be clinically or pathologically ascribed to any other predetermining condition, is the most strongly implicated premalignant condition in the oral cavity. Maskberg (1978) stated that rather than being premalignant a large proportion of lesions clinically diagnosed as erythroplakia are, in fact, invasive carcinomas from the start. Lichen planus of the oral cavity has also been implicated as a condition which may predispose to oral cancer, in a small proportion of patients. In one study of 725 patients with oral lichen planus (Vas Kovskaia and Abramova, 1981) followed up for up to 32 years 4% of patients developed an oral squamous carcinoma.

Pathology

The vast majority of malignant oral tumours are squamous cell carcinomas. Malignancies do arise from minor salivary glands within the oral cavity and rarely sarcomas and melanomas occur in the mouth.

Squamous cell carcinoma

The gross pathological appearance of squamous cell carcinoma of the oral cavity is said to be exophytic, ulcerative or infiltrative (Figure 3.17). In fact, most cancers show more than one of these characteristics. The vast majority of mouth cancers are both ulcerative and infiltrative and exophytic tumours are less common.

The histological grading of squamous cell carcinoma of the mouth was first applied to the lip by Broders (1920) and later he applied the same classification to the oral cavity proper (Broders, 1941). He classified the tumours into four groups depending on the degree of differentiation of the cells. Well-differentiated tumours show few mitoses and little pleomorphism of the cells whereas poorly differentiated tumours show much pleomorphism, many mitoses and very little keratinization. Broders used two intermedi-

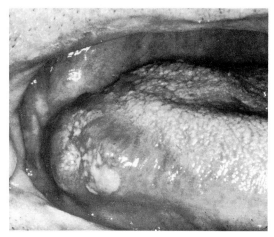

Figure 3.17 Squamous cell carcinoma of the tongue

ate grades, moderately well differentiated and moderately differentiated. Arthur and Farr (1972) using the same histological classification related the degree of differentiation to prognosis and felt it to be a significant factor. Lesions classified histologically as high grade were more advanced on presentation and palpable lymph nodes were more often present in patients with high grade as opposed to low grade tumours.

A much more sophisticated and detailed grading system was introduced by Jacobson *et al.* (1973). In this system the tumour cell population is graded 1–4 depending upon the degree of differentiation, the nuclear pleomorphism and the frequency of mitotic figures. The tumour–host relationship is also estimated on a scale of 1–4 by the mode and stage of invasion. The relationship between grading and prognosis has given conflicting results. Holm *et al.* (1982) found a positive correlation as did Willen *et al.* (1975), although Lund *et al.* (1975) found no significant prognostic predictive value. A further attempt to identify histological characteristics important in prognosis is the attempt to relate the mode of invasion of a mouth cancer (i.e. whether it is plump or expansive or reticular or finger-like) and the depth of invasion (Platz, Fries and Hudec, 1982). There is some evidence that the depth of invasion of the tumour is related to prognosis (Lederer and Managetta, 1982). More recent work has suggested that if histological grading is applied to the invasive margin of the tumour there is a closer correlation to prognosis (Bryne *et al.*, 1992; Odell *et al.*, 1994).

Variants of squamous carcinoma

Verrucous carcinoma

Verrucous carcinoma is a very well-differentiated squamous carcinoma. It forms a flat warty tumour which is slow growing and may have been present for some years. It is a rare tumour comprising only 2–4% of all squamous carcinomas of the oral cavity (Jacobson and Shear, 1972). The lesion consists of highly differentiated squamous cells with only occasional mitoses. The surface of the lesion is covered by layers of keratin. The invasive deep margin of the lesion is a blunt pushing one. Histopathologically the diagnosis is difficult to make unless the biopsy specimen is large and deep enough to include the deep margin. Superficial biopsies will be reported as showing keratinization but no evidence of malignancy. The clinical features of the lesion with soft tissue and bone invasion are important in making a diagnosis. Within a verrucous carcinoma there may be an area of less differentiated squamous carcinoma and this occurred in 20% of verrucous carcinomas in one series (Medina, Diechtel and Luna, 1984). One other often quoted characteristic of verrucous carcinoma is the suggestion that if irradiated they undergo malignant transformation (Demian, Bushkin and Echevarria, 1973). The evidence for this is not strong (Batsakis, Hybels and Crissman, 1982) and in one report of 10 patients (Fonts, Greenlaw and Rush, 1969) the diagnosis of verrucous carcinoma was in doubt in six of these. Verrucous carcinomas are slow growing, undoubtedly malignant but only locally so and rarely if ever metastasize to local lymph nodes.

Sarcomatoid or spindle cell carcinoma

The spindle cell carcinoma is a carcinoma arising from epithelium which shows spindle-shaped cells resembling sarcoma cells but with a definite squamous carcinoma component. They may be polypoidal or infiltrative, the former carrying a better prognosis but the latter are highly malignant (Ellis and Cario, 1980; Leventon and Evans 1981; Batsakis, Rice and Howard, 1982) and few patients survive.

Malignant oral salivary gland tumours

These are uncommon forming less than 10% of intraoral malignancies. They are most frequent on the hard palate (Frable and Elzay, 1970; Spiro, Koss and Hajdu, 1973).

Adenoid cystic carcinoma

This is the most frequent intraoral salivary gland malignancy (about 50% of the total) and is very similar in histopathology and behaviour to the same tumour in the parotid gland. Thus the microscopic patterns of tubular, cribriform, cylindromatous, solid and mixed are found with the tubular forms being low grade and the solid high grade in terms of their behaviour.

Spread of the disease from the primary site occurs in a somewhat different pattern to that in squamous carcinoma. The incidence of metastatic nodes in the neck is lower than in squamous carcinoma. About 10–15% of patients have palpable nodes on presentation and a further 10% develop nodes at some time after presentation. Distant metastases are, however, much more frequent than in squamous carcinoma and were present in 25% of patients in Spiro, Koss and Hajdu's series (1973). The true incidence is thought to be much higher than this. Pulmonary metastases are most frequent but widespread dissemination to other sites including bone also occurs.

Adenocarcinoma

This forms 30% of malignant oral salivary gland tumours and may be low grade with a good prognosis or high grade with a very poor prognosis.

Mucoepidermoid carcinoma

This carcinoma is similar to its counterpart in the parotid gland and most of them are low grade.

Melanoma of the oral cavity

These are rare forming less than 10% of all melanomas and 30% of mucosal melanomas. In general they are most frequent on the hard palate and mucosa of the upper and lower alveolus (Batsakis *et al.*, 1982). They carry a worse prognosis than cutaneous melanoma and occur in an older age group, being rare below the age of 30 years. There is some evidence that they arise in pre-existing pigmented areas within the oral cavity, at least one-third of patients having long-standing oral melanosis prior to the development of malignant melanoma (Takagi, Ishikawa and Mori, 1974). Although cutaneous melanoma is less common in Japanese patients compared with Caucasians mucosal melanoma is relatively common in Japan.

Clinical features and diagnosis of mouth cancer

Most patients with a mouth cancer present with a painful ulcer. Other complaints may be of pain in a tooth or loose teeth or an ill-fitting denture with ulceration which is thought to be related to the denture. Occasionally the patient will present with referred earache unaware of a lesion in the mouth and this will only be found by careful examination using two tongue depressors. In a similar way a patient may present with a metastatic node in the neck with no complaints related to the oral cavity. Oral salivary tumours may present as a nodule, a non-ulcerative swelling or more usually as an ulcerative lesion. Oral melanomas similarly may present as a nodule but more usually as an ulcerated swelling. More often than not the lesion will be pigmented.

Examination

Examination is performed with a head mirror and with two tongue depressors to examine difficult areas such as the retromolar trigone and floor of the mouth. Palpation is an essential part of the examination of the oral cavity, both to determine the true extent of the lesion and also to diagnose recurrence of disease if it is not visible. Palpation of the neck is of course essential in the assessment of a patient with mouth cancer as perhaps the single most important factor determining the method of treatment and also prognosis is the presence of metastatic nodes. Biopsy of a lesion can be performed under local anaesthetic but is better combined with careful examination under general anaesthetic. It is striking how many times the size of a lesion is underestimated even by careful examination unless it is done under anaesthesia. Another reason for anaesthesia is to allow examination of other regions in the upper respiratory tract to exclude synchronous primary tumours.

Sites of mouth cancer

Exact rates for the various sites in the mouth are impossible to determine between series because classification systems differ so widely. Thus until recently the AJC classification has included lip cancer in the oral cavity whereas this is separately classified in the UICC system. Many studies include the soft palate and oropharynx which of course is incorrect and further confusion is added because some series quote all cancers; others restrict the figures to squamous carcinoma. Extrapolating the figures from various studies and excluding cancer of the lip, the site distribution of mouth cancer is shown in Table 3.2. Lip cancer is discussed as a separate section at the end of this chapter.

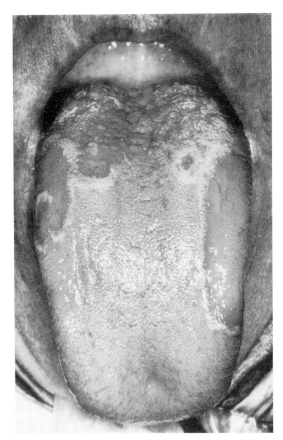

Figure 3.18 The lateral border of the tongue is the most common site inside the mouth for squamous cell carcinoma to occur

Table 3.2 Site distribution of oral cavity squamous carcinomas (%)

Tongue	45
Floor of mouth	25
Upper and lower alveolus	20
Buccal mucosa	7.5
Hard palate	2.5

Carcinoma of the anterior two-thirds of the tongue is the most frequent site for a mouth cancer and the lateral border is the most common location (Figure 3.18). Next most frequent is the undersurface of the tongue and tip of the tongue. A carcinoma arising on the dorsum of the tongue is least frequent.

Carcinoma of the floor of the mouth most commonly occurs anteriorly either in the midline or more usually to one side of the midline. Extension to the tongue or lower alveolus occurs so that in large lesions the site of origin may be difficult to determine. Squamous carcinoma of the alveolar ridges occurs more frequently in the lower jaw than the upper jaw. Squamous carcinoma of the hard palate is unusual and very much less frequent than malignant salivary tumours at this site.

Radiology

Radiology certainly has a place in the investigation of a patient with mouth cancer but only as an adjunct to careful clinical examination.

Orthopantomograms of the mandible will show bone erosion usually as an irregular defect with a moth-eaten appearance around it.

CT scanning has a limited place in the assessment of a patient with mouth cancer. It is particularly useful in lesions of the upper jaw demonstrating for example extension into the pterygopalatine or infratemporal fossa. Also assessment of the extension of an oral cancer into the firmer tissue of the base of the tongue can be very difficult clinically. In this situation CT may show the true extent of the tumour (Larsson, Hoover and Juillard, 1987). In the presence of many dental fillings the CT image will be streaked due to scatter of radiation and impossible to interpret.

MR scanning has yet to be evaluated fully in oral cancer. It may, however, be particularly useful in the assessment of the extent of soft tissue invasion (Bootz *et al.*, 1992).

Bone scanning with technetium-99 has been thought useful in assessing involvement of the mandible by tumour but in fact the scans have very poor specificity as periodontal disease, inflammation and trauma all result in uptake of the tracer.

Staging of mouth cancer

Over the years there have been changes in the classification of mouth cancers in the TNM classification. In the past lip cancer has sometimes been included and sometimes excluded, three T stages only were recognized and the N staging has recently been changed. This means that when reviewing the literature the changes which have occurred must be borne in mind. Although perhaps some would argue with the present N staging system it is of major importance that the most recent AJC (1988), and UICC (1987) classifications are now identical (apart from the spelling) and this is a great advantage. Although the lip is included within the oral cavity it is usual to report lip cancer separately from oral cancer because these tumours do behave differently. The classifications are shown in Tables 3.3 and 3.4. It should be remembered that these are clinical classifications and when pathological examination is used then the prefix p should be added i.e. pT, pN and pM. The stage grouping of lip and oral cavity cancer is shown in Table 3.5. Essentially stage I and stage II are T1 and T2 tumours respectively with no palpable metastases. Stage III includes T3 tumours with no metastases and T1, T2

Table 3.3 Primary tumour

Tx	Primary tumour cannot be assessed
T0	No evidence of primary tumour
Tis	Carcinoma *in situ*
T1	Tumour 2 cm or less in greatest dimension
T2	Tumour more than 2 cm but not more than 4 cm in greatest dimension
T3	Tumour more than 4 cm in greatest dimension
T4	Tumour invades adjacent structures, e.g. through cortical bone, into deep (extrinsic) muscle of tongue, maxillary sinus, skin

Table 3.4 TNM classification of regional nodes

Nx	Regional lymph nodes cannot be assessed
N0	No regional lymph node metastases
N1	Metastasis in a single ipsilateral lymph node 3 cm or less in greatest dimension
N2	Metastasis in a single ipsilateral lymph node, more than 3 cm but not more than 6 cm in greatest dimension, or in multiple ipsilateral lymph nodes none more than 6 cm in greatest dimension, or in bilateral or contralateral lymph nodes, none more than 6 cm in greatest dimension
N2a	Metastasis in a single ipsilateral lymph node, more than 3 cm but not more than 6 cm in greatest dimension
N2b	Metastasis in multiple ipsilateral lymph nodes, none more than 6 cm in greatest dimension
N2c	Metastasis in bilateral or contralateral lymph nodes, none more than 6 cm in greatest dimension
N3	Metastasis in a lymph node more than 6 cm in greatest dimension

Table 3.5 Stage grouping for oral cavity cancer

Stage I	T1N0M0
Stage II	T2N0M0
Stage III	T3N0M0
	T1N1M0
	T2N1M0
	T3N1M0
Stage IV	T4N0M0
	T4N1M0
	Any T N2 or N3M0
	Any T or NM1

and T3 tumours with N1 glands. Everything else is included as stage IV. This still may be slightly illogical as for example the prognosis of patients with a T4 N0 M0 tumour differs considerably from those classified T2 N3 M0 or T2 N3 M1.

Metastases in mouth cancer

Perhaps the single most important factor in determining prognosis in mouth cancer is the presence or absence of palpable nodes at presentation. A number of series have shown a very significant difference in survival between patients with no palpable metastases at presentation compared with those patients with palpable nodes (Farr and Arthur, 1972; Krause, Lee and McCabe, 1973; Hibbert *et al.*, 1983). The factors which affect the presence or absence of palpable nodes on presentation are variable and the rate varies from series to series. The site of the primary tumour is an important factor, tongue and floor of mouth cancer having the highest rate of palpable nodes on presentation (Yves and Ghossein, 1981) and Table 3.6 shows representative rates.

Table 3.6 Frequency of palpable metastases on presentation related to site of oral cancer (%)

Tongue	40
Floor of mouth	40
Buccal mucosa	30
Alveolus	15
Lip	10

The size of the primary tumour is a significant factor in the presence of nodes on presentation. Patients with larger tumours are more likely to have nodes than those with smaller tumours (Krause, Lee and McCabe, 1973; Crissman *et al.*, 1980; Hibbert *et al.*, 1983).

The histology of the primary lesion may have a bearing on the incidence of palpable or impalpable metastatic disease. Certainly in the studies of Arthur and Farr (1972), Willen *et al.* (1975) and Holm *et al.* (1982), patients with high grade lesions were more likely to have a palpable metastasis on presentation and also a greater tendency to develop nodal disease after primary treatment.

Of equal or even more prognostic significance than the presence of nodes on presentation is the presence of occult nodes, i.e. nodes containing squamous carcinoma but not clinically detectable. The exact figures for occult nodes are difficult to determine because many patients have prophylactic treatment. The rate of occult nodes in general is higher in sites with a high incidence of palpable nodes on presentation and the rates quoted vary from series to series (Lyall and Schetlin, 1952; Ward *et al.*, 1959; Leipzig *et al.*, 1982; Meikle *et al.*, 1985). In the tongue and floor of mouth a figure of 30–40% is probably a reasonable estimate of the number of patients who have occult metastases and who will subsequently develop nodes in the neck if the primary tumour alone is treated with no treatment to the neck. The site of cervical metastases in mouth cancer is important. Most nodes on presentation or which develop subsequently are ipsilateral and in the submandibular or jugulodigastric regions. Contralateral or bilateral nodes are more likely in lesions close to the midline in the floor of the mouth and dorsum of the tongue and nodes low in the neck, i.e. in the jugulo-omohyoid region, are more common with lesions anteriorly placed in the floor of the mouth and tip of the tongue.

Metastatic disease in the lower neck in the jugulo-omohyoid region may occur in the absence of obvious disease higher in the neck (Droulias and Whitehurst, 1976). In one series of patients with anterior tongue cancers, 6.3% of patients had metastatic neck disease outside the submandibular and jugulodigastric regions (Donegan, Gluckman and Crissman, 1982). This is certainly of prognostic significance. The survival figures for patients with cervical metastases in the upper neck are significantly better than for patients with disease in the lower neck (Farr and Arthur, 1972). Another well known characteristic of mouth cancer is the tendency to spread to nodes on both sides of the neck and this occurs at least 20% of the time (Droulias and Whitehurst, 1976; Leipzig and Hikanson, 1982).

Systemic metastases in mouth cancer are rare. Very few patients have clinically apparent metastases on presentation and even in patients dying of their local disease clinically detectable metastases are rare. In a series of 5019 patients with squamous carcinoma of the head and neck who had no clinical evidence of distant metastases on presentation 11% of patients subsequently developed distant metastases which were clinically detectable (Merino, Lindberg and Fletcher, 1977). The lungs and bones were the most common sites and 80% of metastases became evident within 2 years. Metastases were more common in patients with advanced disease on presentation and in those with a recurrence of the primary or nodal disease. The true incidence of metastases in patients who have died of disease and identified at post mortem is much higher and figures from 17 to 47% have been reported (Peltier, Thomas and Crawford, 1951; O'Brien *et al.*, 1971).

Treatment of mouth cancer

Any treatment plan for mouth cancer must take into consideration the cure rates for various modalities and the functional and cosmetic effects of treatment. It is logical to identify those factors which have a significant prognostic influence and treatment should be modified accordingly. This is one of the purposes of a TNM classification system and thus it is to be expected that prognosis falls as one passes from stage I to stage IV and studies of mouth cancer have shown this to be the case (Harrold, 1971; Arthur and Farr, 1972; Panje, Smith and McCabe, 1980; Yves and Ghossein, 1981; Leipzig and Hikanson, 1982; Leipzig *et al.*, 1982; Hibbert *et al.*, 1983). Within the classification system the most salient factor seems to be the absence or presence of palpable nodes (Farr and Arthur, 1972; Krause, Lee and McCabe, 1973; Hibbert *et al.*, 1983). The size of nodes, their number and whether they are ipsilateral, contralateral or bilateral are also important. Similarly the spread of disease outside the capsule of the lymph node is prognostically significant (Noone, Bonner and Raymond, 1974; Johnson *et al.*, 1981; Snow *et al.*, 1982). This is a factor which cannot be determined by clinical examination but, for example, if a neck dissection specimen shows extracapsular spread of disease additional treatment with radiotherapy should be considered.

When formulating a treatment plan for mouth cancer it goes without saying that one is treating patients and not disease and this must be an important factor when deciding on treatment. A general treatment plan for mouth cancer is shown in Table 3.7. This does not take into consideration the fact that some patients should not be offered curative treatment. Thus the very elderly, patients with very significant cardiovascular or pulmonary disease and patients with far advanced local disease may well be better off having no curative treatment rather than overenthusiastic futile attempts at cure.

Table 3.7 Treatment of mouth cancer

T1 and T2N0	Surgery or radiotherapy
T3 T4	Surgery
T1–4 N1–3	Surgery + radiotherapy

Early lesions

In this category are the T1 and T2 lesions with no palpable cervical metastases at presentation. In general 5-year survival figures of about 80% have been obtained with this group. The treatment options are surgery or radiotherapy and survival figures are probably equivalent (Chu and Fletcher, 1973; Chu, Litwin and Strawitz, 1978; Johnson, Leipzig and Cummings, 1980; Yves and Ghossein, 1981; Meikle *et al.*, 1985). There are strong advocates for each modality which probably means there is little to choose between them. The advantages of surgery are that for small early accessible lesions the surgery is simple and uncomplicated, the patient is in and out of hospital rapidly and there are none of the long-term sequelae and complications of radiation therapy. The advocates of radiotherapy draw attention to the impairment of function which accompanies surgery. The options for radiotherapy are either external beam treatment or interstitial treatment, i.e. an implant. The advantages of an implant are that a higher local dose is possible with fewer and more localized complications. In general, if the lesion is implantable (accessible and not adjacent to bone) the results are better than with external beam therapy (Pierquin, Chassagne and Baillet, 1971; Declos, Lindberg and Fletcher, 1976; Fu *et al.*, 1976; Seagren, Syed and Byfield, 1979; Yves and Ghossein, 1981).

The argument as to what is the best form of treatment for these early lesions cannot be considered fully in isolation. It is also relevant when deciding on therapy to consider whether the cervical lymphatics should be treated prophylactically and this certainly has a bearing on the treatment modality chosen. The question of prophylactic treatment of the neck is considered below.

The present author favours treatment of early accessible mouth cancer with an iridium implant if this is technically possible (i.e. anteriorly placed lesions not adjacent to bone). Surgery is reserved for more posterior lesions, those adjacent to the mandible or maxilla or recurrence following failure of an implant to cure the primary.

Surgery

The disadvantage of surgery in the treatment of early lesions in the mouth is that in order to excise the lesion adequately a margin of normal tissue must also be excised. This macroscopically normal margin should be of the order of 2 cm, sometimes slightly less (Stell, Wood and Scott, 1982) and particularly in the tongue this does affect function, namely speech and deglutition. The surgery of mouth cancer is discussed later but in general the access to a small lesion will be entirely peroral and the defect will be closed either directly, i.e. by approximation of the edges of the defect, or by a split skin graft sutured to the bed of the defect (McGregor, 1975). Occasionally a flap repair will be necessary and this may be a lingual flap (Chambers, Jacques and Maloney, 1969) or possibly a nasolabial flap (Cohen and Theogaraj, 1975).

Radiotherapy

As has been said already external beam radiation is probably less effective than an implant for an early mouth cancer mainly because the dose to the tumour can rarely be as high. In addition the complications and long-term effects of external beam radiation to the oral cavity are significant and are discussed later.

Interstitial irradiation in the oral cavity can either take the form of a gold grain implant or an iridium implant. Gold grains are rarely applicable because they only treat a superficial volume and one of the great advantages of an implant is that it can be used to treat a fairly deep volume of tissue. This is particularly valuable in the floor of the mouth when it is difficult with local surgery to achieve a satisfactory deep margin on the tumour. Iridium implants are hairpins of iridium wire inserted into the tumour at about 1 cm intervals under general anaesthesia. It is usual to deliver a local tumour dose of 7000–8000 cGy and, depending on the activity of the iridium, the hairpins are removed several days later. The main disadvantage of an implant is that the area treated is very susceptible to recurrent painful ulceration. This is a sufficient disadvantage alone but is also a source of anxiety when radiation induced ulceration must be distinguished from local recurrence. This can be difficult but if the area of ulceration is soft and not indurated a policy of observation is advised. If the area persists biopsy is essential but of course leads to further ulceration and pain. Local recurrence after a technically satisfactory implant is not common being about 5% (Meikle *et al.*, 1985).

Management of metastatic neck disease

One of the major controversies in the treatment of mouth cancer is the management of possible neck disease in patients who have T1 and T2 tumours with no palpable nodes at presentation. Such patients have a very high risk, of the order of 30–40%, of developing neck metastases following successful treatment of the primary disease. The controversy is whether these patients should have prophylactic treatment to their necks and if so what form this treatment should take. The policy of not treating the neck, waiting until palpable disease is present and then performing neck dissection has a significant failure rate. Radical neck dissection in this situation is successful between 35% and 60% of the time (Spiro and Strong, 1971; Johnson, Leipzig and Cummings, 1980; Meikle *et al.*, 1985). In other words one has at least a 40–60% chance of failure. Martin *et al.* (1951) and also Harrold (1971) in reviewing a series of patients with mouth cancer were opposed to prophylactic neck dissection because the proportion of patients who would benefit was small, i.e. after excluding failures at the primary site, patients who never developed nodes, patients with contralateral nodes and patients successfully treated by neck dissection for palpable disease, only 20% of patients remained. This figure of patients who may possibly benefit varies from 5% to 20% in other series (Cade and Lee, 1957; Frazell and Lucas, 1962; Jesse *et al.*, 1970). The fact that tongue cancer metastasizes to both sides of the neck in possibly 20% of patients is further argument against prophylactic neck dissection. Two prospective trials (Van den Brouck *et al.*, 1980; Ferrara *et al.*, 1982) have failed to show any difference in survival between patients treated with prophylactic neck dissection and those treated by observation and neck dissection when disease becomes palpable.

Despite these theoretical arguments, in many centres, particularly in the USA where surgery is perhaps favoured for early mouth tumours, there is a tendency to include a conservative neck dissection as part of the treatment when resecting early mouth cancers. The alternative prophylactic therapy for occult neck disease is radiotherapy and this has the distinct advantage that both sides of the neck can be treated at the same time. There is no doubt that prophylactic neck irradiation does reduce the development of nodes in those patients at high risk of developing nodes after successful treatment of the primary tumour (Fletcher, 1972; Million, 1974; Jesse and Fletcher, 1977). The morbidity of treating both sides of the neck with radiotherapy is not negligible and many of these patients, i.e. those who would not anyway have gone on to develop nodes will have been treated unnecessarily and this amounts to some 60%. Another argument used against prophylactic irradiation is that this group of patients has a high risk of developing a second primary tumour and previous irradiation will have removed the option of treating subsequent tumours with radiotherapy. What is needed is an accurate predictor of which patients are particularly at risk of developing nodes following treatment of the primary tumour and, at the moment, this is not available.

Treatment of stage III and stage IV disease

All the major series dealing with the treatment of patients with oral cancer demonstrate that survival is markedly worse with larger tumours and with metastatic neck disease. These patients therefore must be treated aggressively and most authorities feel that radiotherapy alone is inadequate treatment for the larger lesions (Cade and Lee, 1957; Guillamondegui, Oliver and Haden, 1980; Panje, Smith and McCabe, 1980). Those patients with large lesions (T3 and T4), with palpable neck disease on presentation and with lesions involving bone should have surgical treatment. Because the prognosis in these patients is poor many centres also add radiotherapy to surgery in an attempt to improve survival. The evidence that combined therapy is more effective than surgery alone in mouth cancer is not strong. The radiotherapy can be given preoperatively or postoperatively. Most authorities favour the latter because at least following surgery the areas of greatest risk of recurrence will be known and the radiotherapy can be designed accordingly.

In a study of preoperative radiotherapy in patients with advanced cancers, Rosuit, Spiro and Kolson (1972) showed that preoperative radiotherapy was a feasible proposition. Disease in most of the patients responded to the radiation and the complication rate of the subsequent surgery was not increased. However, survival rates at 2 and 5 years were not felt to be improved by the preoperative radiation. In a study of postoperative radiation using historical controls, Robertson, McGregor and Souttar (1986) showed that the incidence of recurrence of disease at 18 months was reduced by the addition of radiation. At the present time in many centres it is usual to give patients who have had surgical resection for advanced cancer of the mouth a course of postoperative radiation. There is no evidence that this in fact improves survival figures and what is really needed is a randomized trial.

Neck dissection for mouth cancer

The subject of prophylactic neck dissection has been discussed above. The question of conservation neck dissection is a complicated subject which is discussed in Chapter 17. In mouth cancer the type of conservation neck dissection which is advocated is the subject of debate. Certainly it is unusual for disease to be found in the posterior triangle and so preservation of the accessory nerve is probably an acceptable procedure. Suprahyoid neck dissection has been advocated in the past for patients with mouth cancer, particularly when the neck dissection is elective or prophylactic in patients with no palpable disease. Certainly on anatomical grounds, with the known lymphatic drainage of the tongue and floor of the mouth to the lower neck, suprahyoid neck dissection is not logical. Mendelson, Hodgkinson and Woods (1977) reported that 20% of patients having radical neck dissection for mouth cancers had metastatic disease in the middle or lower jugular nodes and these would not be removed by a suprahyoid neck dissection. Chu and Strawitz (1978) studied a series of patients having suprahyoid, modified radical and radical neck dissection for head and neck cancers and found a recurrence rate for disease in the neck of 29% after suprahyoid dissection compared wth 3.5% after radical dissection. There is no place for suprahyoid neck dissection in the treatment of patients with mouth cancer.

Surgical treatment of mouth cancer

The surgical procedure when treating a mouth cancer can be divided into three phases, namely exposure of the disease, excision of the disease and reconstruction of the defect. Although these three phases are interdependent they can be usefully considered in isolation.

Exposure of the disease

The single most important factor in determining survival in patients treated surgically is adequate excision of the primary tumour. There is no doubt that residual cancer after surgical treatment is almost always fatal and there is evidence that leaving macroscopic disease within 0.5 cm of the surgical margin results in a high incidence of recurrence of disease (Looser, Shah and Strong, 1978). Adequate excision of the primary tumour by the surgeon is very much dependent on adequate exposure of the disease. A number of approaches is available depending on the size and site of the tumour.

Peroral approach

This approach to a mouth cancer without any external incision gives the most limited access. It is entirely satisfactory for small anteriorly placed lesions such as those in the anterior floor of the mouth, anterior portion of the tongue and for lesions of the buccal mucosa. It can also be combined with a marginal mandibulectomy for small anterior lesions of the lower alveolus and is perfectly satisfactory for lesions of the upper jaw treated by palatal fenestration.

Pull-through procedure

This term was originally devised to describe the procedure whereby a mouth cancer, say of the lateral border of the tongue, was excised by a combination of a peroral and external approach in which a cheek and upper neck flap was elevated but the mandible and lip were not divided. In this way, after neck dissection, the primary lesion was excised in continuity with the neck dissection specimen partly through a peroral approach and partly from below. The great advantage of this technique is that the lip and mandible remained intact and so cosmesis is excellent. Many modifications of this approach have been devised and it is not important whether the neck dissection specimen is pulled through the mouth or the primary tumour pulled into the neck. In fact, the basis of this operation is the cheek flap so that the excision of the primary tumour is done partly though the neck and partly perorally. It can be combined with marginal mandibular resection or hemimandibulectomy. When the mandible is excised the approach is very much easier and it is probably the approach of choice for lateral tongue tumours and floor of mouth tumours when the mandible needs to be resected. The access is more limited for posterior lesions. For anterior lesions preserving the mandible the visor flap has been devised. Basically this involves lifting the lower lip and skin of the chin over the mandible by dividing the buccal and labial mucosa. The disadvantage of the technique is the anaesthesia of the lower lip caused by division of the mental nerves and this probably increases the problem of drooling postoperatively.

Lip split

This approach in which the lower lip is split in the midline and a cheek flap is elevated gives by far and away the best exposure for excision of a mouth cancer. It can be combined with hemimandibulectomy or, if resection of the mandible is not necessary, a mandibulotomy can be done either in the midline or laterally and this improves the access. This approach is to be recommended if the surgeon is uneasy about his ability to excise a mouth cancer adequately with a good margin by one of the more limited approaches. It is particularly recommended for posterior lesions. The main disadvantage is the scar of the lower lip but if the junction of vermilion to skin is marked accurately before the incision is made and the repair is done carefully the scar is acceptable.

Excision of the disease

This is the most important phase of the operation and as has been stated above adequate exposure is the key to adequate excision. The surgical margin of macroscopically normal tissue to be included around the tumour is the subject of debate. A 2 cm margin is the minimum requirement and particularly in the tongue larger margins may be necessary.

It is essential that a mouth cancer be visualized in three dimensions and that the margin of normal tissue excised around the tumour should be adequate in all three dimensions. Often the most difficult margin to estimate is the deep one because the extent of a deeply infiltrative tumour is most difficult to assess. Palpation of the tumour is most important in assessing this deep extent. At the time of surgery frozen section control of the margins may be helpful (Byers, Gland and Waxler, 1978; Looser, Shah and Strong, 1978), particularly in areas where the surgeon is doubtful about the adequacy of his margins. On the other hand, the cynics among us would say that if a microscope is necessary to judge the adequacy of a surgical margin in the mouth then it is bound to be inadequate.

Management of the mandible in mouth cancer

Invasion of the mandible by a squamous carcinoma of the oral cavity occurs immediately adjacent to the primary tumour and thus is much more common and occurs earlier in carcinoma of the alveolar ridge. Recently there has been enthusiasm for surgical procedures which preserve the mandibular arch with major advantages for cosmesis and function. Invasion of the inferior dental canal or cancellous bone of the mandible necessitates full thickness removal of the mandible. This may also be necessary in the edentulous mandible which is very thin. Fixation of the tumour to the mandibular periosteum or minimal invasion may allow a marginal resection with preservation of the mandibular arch (Som and Nussbaum, 1971; Flynn and Moore, 1974; Wald and Calcaterra, 1983). Thus the bone immediately adjacent to the tumour must be excised together with a margin of non-invaded normal bone. In a cancer of the alveolar ridge the superior border of the mandible will be resected leaving an inferior strut of bone. In a floor of mouth or tongue cancer the lingual plate of the mandible is excised. The problem of whether to perform a full thickness excision or marginal resection is yet to be solved. The usual guideline is that when there is radiological evidence of bone erosion a full thickness segment should be taken but this almost certainly means that some mandibles will be excised unnecessarily.

Reconstruction of the defect

The major changes in the surgery of mouth cancer which have occurred in the last 20 years have all related to changes in reconstruction. This of course does not influence the chances of curing the disease but the newer techniques have made reconstruction more reliable with better functional and cosmetic results. The basic principles of reconstruction within the mouth have been stated by Myers (1972) and are summarized below:

1 The reconstructive technique should not interfere with or limit the excisional surgery
2 Form and function should be quickly restored
3 The morbidity or mortality should not be increased by the reconstruction. (This of course is impossible but it should be minimized)
4 A secondary cosmetic defect should not be produced
5 The reconstructive phase should be completed as quickly as possible (i.e. multistaged procedures should be avoided if possible)
6 Prolonged reconstructive procedures should be avoided if a prosthesis would provide an adequate alternative.

The options available in reconstruction of the oral cavity are:

1 A split skin graft
2 Primary closure
3 Local or distant flap.

Split skin graft

Split skin grafts have limited use. They are obviously only appropriate if there is a vascular bed into which the graft can be sutured. Thus they are useful to cover the raw area remaining after excision of a superficial tongue tumour, buccal tumour or a small lesion in the floor of the mouth. The technique of suturing the split skin graft into the defect by quilting was originally described by McGregor (1975).

Primary closure

Primary closure of the defect following excision of a mouth cancer can be performed for almost any lesion varying from the defect resulting from excision of a small tongue tumour to that after composite resection. Certainly after excision of a small tumour of the tongue it is perfectly reasonable. The criticism of primary closure after the excision of more major defects is that it is felt to compromise function. An extreme example of this would be excision of the anterior floor of mouth to include the mylohyoid and genioglossus. This defect could be closed by suturing the anterior part of the tongue to the lower lip. Although this is the simplest way to close such a defect the functional result is unsatisfactory and speech would be greatly impaired. Loss of the sulcus between the lip and tongue which the floor of the mouth provides would result in very severe drooling of saliva and food and tethering of the lower lip would result in an unsatisfactory cosmetic result. Similarly it is felt that the tethering of the tongue in other situations which results when a primary closure is carried out results in poor speech due to poor tongue mobility. In fact, this is a very poorly understood subject and although flap repair is felt to be superior to primary closure the effect on tongue mobility of a large, immobile, bulky flap sutured to the tongue is probably equal to primary closure. The most important factors affecting intelligibility of speech following resection of oral cavity tumours are:

a The amount of mobile tongue remaining
b The degree of fixation of the tongue
c A soft palate defect.

Certainly up to about half the tongue can be excised without affecting speech in a major way (De Fries, 1974; Bradley, Hoover and Stell, 1982) providing that the tongue remnant retains its mobility. The effect of a significant soft palate defect on articulation is very dramatic and failure to close the nasopharynx from the oropharynx results in almost unintelligible speech. This is one situation where filling the defect with a flap is essential. Although the flap is immobile, nevertheless, its bulk fills the defect and intelligible speech is preserved. In the past when no reconstruction was the rule primary closure after for example, hemiglossectomy and hemimandibulectomy involved suturing the tongue remnant to the buccal mucosa. Because this is a simple method of closure it is certainly quick and avoids the complications associated with flap surgery. There is no real evidence that tongue mobility is less after such a procedure but it has two other disadvantages. First, if the mandibular arch is preserved the tension resulting from suturing the tongue to the cheek is such that the repair line is liable to break down and a fistula result. This is particularly true if the patient has had radiotherapy. The second consideration is that if the mandible has been excised, primary closure results in a very marked sinking in of the cheek with a most noticeable cosmetic defect. A bulky flap in this situation helps to provide support and a more symmetrical external appearance. Most head and neck surgeons have abandoned primary closure except for the smallest defects and, although we should not be too enthusiastic about the functional superiority when using a flap there are advantages. It must be borne in mind however, that flap repair carries additional morbidity and creates a cosmetic defect elsewhere.

Flap repair

Although flaps are considered in detail in Chapter 26, some flaps are specific to oral cavity repair and will be considered in detail here.

Local flaps

a Buccal flaps

A local flap can be constructed from the buccal mucosa and rotated into a small defect (Craft, 1961). These are of limited size and little used at the present time because more satisfactory alternatives are available.

b Lingual flaps

The use of the tongue to close a defect resulting from excision of a mouth cancer is only possible when the excision does not involve the tongue. The tongue is divided to one side of the midline and the resulting flap can be rotated into quite a large defect (Chambers, Jacques and Mahoney, 1969). Thus the oropharynx on one side can be replaced and also the full thickness of the floor of mouth can be replaced. The latter is probably the most valuable use of a lingual flap providing a mobile and very satisfactory floor of mouth.

c Nasolabial flaps

These flaps are discussed in Chapters 25 and 26. They are of limited value in the oral cavity.

Distant flaps

In 1978 in a Chapter in '*Recent Advances in Otolaryngology*' (Stell and Hibbert, 1978) it was stated that, 'Two axial flaps have proved extremely useful for reconstruction of large defects in the mouth and the oropharynx: the temporal flap and the deltopectoral flap'. Fifteen years later the whole field has been totally changed and these two flaps have almost disappeared from reconstruction of the oral cavity to be replaced by a variety of myocutaneous flaps and free flaps.

Myocutaneous flaps

Because of their reliability and the fact that they provide one stage reconstruction, the myocutaneous flaps are the most commonly used flaps in oral cavity reconstruction. Their bulk at times is an advantage, filling major defects particularly after resection of the mandible, but can be a disadvantage, for example in the floor of the mouth where a thin, pliable flap is required.

The pectoralis major flap is the most widely used flap in oral cavity reconstruction at the present time (Baek, Lawson and Biller, 1982). Its main disadvantage is sometimes that it is extremely bulky, particularly in women, and does not lend itself to reconstruction of defects of the floor of the mouth where the tongue and mandible are intact.

The trapezius myocutaneous flap can be based inferiorly on the transverse cervical vessels or superiorly on the occipital artery (Panje, 1980; Shapiro, 1981). Its main disadvantage is that the XIth nerve must be sacrificed. It is less popular than the pectoralis major flap having a less reliable blood supply, particularly when based superiorly.

The latissimus dorsi flap is not as popular as the two previously described flaps, mainly because the patient must be repositioned to mobilize the flap. Also it is probably more prone to necrosis because the vascular pedicle is very long and more likely to be damaged. It is less reliable than the previous two flaps but does provide a massive area of skin which is less bulky than the pectoralis major flap (Maves, Panje and Shagets, 1984).

The sternomastoid myocutaneous flap is occasionally used in intraoral reconstruction (Ariyan, 1979). It provides a limited amount of skin, is contraindicated when there are palpable metastases in the neck and is much less reliable than any of the above flaps. Similarly a platysma myocutaneous flap using cervical skin has been described for intraoral use (Cannon *et al.*, 1982) but is less reliable than the other myocutaneous flaps.

Free flaps

The use of a free flap with microvascular anastomosis of its artery and vein is the most recent reconstructive technique in head and neck surgery. Its role in reconstruction has yet to be defined but free flaps offer a variety of methods for reconstruction. The main disadvantage of free flaps is that the microvascular anastomosis requires expertise and regular practice and a separate team of surgeons. The main reason microvascular anastomosis fails is technical and for the same surgeon to attempt such a procedure after performing a composite resection is unwise. As techniques improve, microvascular anastomosis will become more reliable. At the present time it is only in the very best hands that the success rate of free flaps even approaches that of myocutaneous flaps. The scope for free flaps is immense. Skin alone can be moved, the usual donor site being the forearm or the groin (Ackland and Flynn, 1978; Panje, 1982). This provides thin flexible skin without the advantages or sometimes disadvantages of bulk. Perhaps more usefully free flaps can also include bone either from the radius (Souttar *et al.*, 1983) or from the iliac crest or from the spine of the scapula (Taylor, Townsend and Corlett, 1979). This is perhaps the major future use of free flaps in oral cavity surgery.

Reconstruction of the mandible

It has already been said that wherever possible an operation should be performed which preserves the mandibular arch because reconstruction is difficult. On many occasions however, the correct surgical procedure will remove a full thickness segment of mandible. If this is lateral mandible as in hemimandibulectomy the defect is best left not reconstructed. This is because of the unsatisfactory and unreliable methods of reconstruction which are at present available. If a myocutaneous flap is used in the intraoral repair the bulk of the muscle pedicle together with the skin in the mouth fills out the defect to some extent making it cosmetically acceptable. With time the muscle pedicle atrophies and there is always a certain amount of sinking in of the cheek after hemimandibulectomy. Functionally the flap adds nothing and the segment of mandible swings to one side (to the side of excision) every time the patient opens his mouth. This can be partially corrected if the patient can wear a lower denture by using a dental prosthesis with a glide bar to restore reasonable occlusion. Removal of the anterior portion or body of the mandible leaves a defect which is cosmetically and functionally unacceptable. So far as function is concerned lack of an anterior mandible leads to severe drooling, great difficulty in swallowing and the loss of support for the tongue may lead to respiratory difficulties, particularly during sleep. Reconstruction of the mandible is essential in this situation but a variety of methods is in use at the present time which is good evidence that none is satisfactory. Reconstruction may be immediate, i.e. at the same time as the excision of tumour or it may be delayed. An important consideration here is the size of the soft tissue defect. If large amounts of oral mucosa have been resected immediate reconstruction is generally felt to be bound to fail because the bone graft will be contaminated by saliva and bacteria if the suture lines are not totally watertight. If the resection is limited to excision of a lesion of the mandible with minimal soft tissue loss immediate reconstruction may be possible. The condemnation of immediate reconstruction is really based upon experience of reconstruction using less reliable flaps for soft tissue replacement. It may be that since the advent of myocutaneous flaps and free flaps with microvascular anastomosis immediate replacement of mandibular defects will regain popularity. If delayed grafting is performed the remaining mandibular fragments must be immobilized to prevent contraction and scarring which results in each mandibular remnant rotating upwards and medially. This fixation is usually external with an acrylic bar fixed to screws in the mandibular fragments. The material and methods used to reconstruct the mandible are many and varied, detailed discussion of all methods is beyond the scope of the present chapter but the five main methods currently in use will be discussed briefly.

Replacement with iliac crest graft

The mandible can be replaced by a bone graft from the iliac crest to include cortical and cancellous bone. This is usually done as a delayed procedure following immobilization of the fragments by external fixation until intraoral healing has taken place. Alternatively an iliac crest graft can be performed immediately and fixed to the mandibular fragment with compression plates. This fixation is so stable that an external device is probably unnecessary.

Cancellous bone and a tray

In this technique, after immobilization of the fragments at a second operation a prosthetic tray is used. It is fixed to both mandibular fragments and has a space in it which is filled with cancellous bone and bone marrow from the iliac crest (Maisel, Hilger and Adams, 1983). The tray may be cobalt-chromium, titanium or dacron urethane. It is usual to leave the external fixation device in position for 6–12 weeks.

Using AO plate

A similar method to the above uses a compression plate which provides internal fixation and the bone graft of cortical and cancellous bone is fixed to the plate between the mandibular fragments (Hilger and Adams, 1985).

Using osseomyocutaneous flaps

This technique involves the incorporation of a bone graft as part of a myocutaneous flap. Thus the spine of the scapula can be included on a trapezius myocutaneous flap (Maisel and Adams, 1983; Panje, 1985) or a rib can be included on a pectoralis major or latissimus dorsi flap.

Free microvascular bone grafts

Although yet to be evaluated fully the use of microvascular anastomosis and bone grafts is probably going to prove to be the most valuable method of mandibular reconstruction. Rib has been used (Serafin, Villarreal-Rios and Georgiade, 1977), as has the iliac crest (Taylor, Townsend and Corlett, 1979), but perhaps the most valuable method in this group is a segment of radius on the radial forearm free flap (Souttar *et al.*, 1983). These flaps with microvascular anastomosis are used as an immediate reconstruction.

Radiotherapy of mouth cancer

As has been discussed, radiotherapy is a most valuable modality in the treatment of mouth cancer. The radiotherapy can be delivered by an implant or by external beam, the advantages of the implant being a higher local tumour dose with therefore a greater chance of cure. The complications and side effects of an implant are probably less than external beam therapy. The main complication of irradiation to the oral cavity is osteoradionecrosis of the mandible which is said to occur in up to 20% of patients (Coffin, 1983). Patients with severe dental caries are felt to be more liable to such a complication and removal of decayed teeth (with antibiotic cover) is generally advised before irradiation, allowing 10 days before the start of treatment (Starke and Shannon, 1977). Irradiation of tumours involving bone increases the incidence of osteoradionecrosis and since the chances of cure in this situation are small radiotherapy is best avoided as primary treatment.

The dryness of the mouth which accompanies irradiation is almost invariable after external beam therapy. Artificial salivas are occasionally helpful but many patients carry with them a bottle of water with which to moisten their mouth. Loss of taste occurs immediately after external beam therapy but usually recovers.

Other treatment modalities for mouth cancer

Cryotherapy was popular for a short time for treating mouth cancers. It is however, difficult to control the depth of freezing and therefore the surgical margins around the tumour are imprecise and unknown. It has almost totally been abandoned as a method of treatment.

The same criticism is valid for the treatment of mouth cancer by electrocoagulation (Paterson, 1979).

The CO_2 laser has been used for resection of primary mouth tumours (Strong *et al.*, 1979) and good results have been reported (Carruth, 1982). It should be remembered however, that the CO_2 laser is simply another way of destroying or dividing tissue. Technically it is more difficult to handle than a knife or diathermy. Perhaps its value in the mouth lies in the removal of superficial dysplastic lesions.

Treatment of non-squamous malignant lesions

Minor salivary gland malignancies

These lesions, although all arising from minor salivary glands, are a heterogeneous group and great variations in their malignant potential are seen. It is therefore very difficult to compare survival figures. There is no doubt that 5-year survival in this disease, compared with squamous carcinoma is not a reliable measure of cure; some recurrences occur well after this time. Thus in Spiro, Koss and Hajdu's series (1973) the 5-, 10- and 15-year survival figures were 45%, 33% and 21%, respectively.

In general all these lesions should be treated by wide surgical excision. In the high grade lesions this should be followed by external beam irradiation. In the case of adenoid cystic carcinoma since there is a particular tendency to spread along the perineural lymphatics the main nerve supply to the areas should be excised with the lesion. Thus in lesions of the hard palate the greater palatine canals should be included in the block of tissue removed and, in the floor of the mouth, the lingual nerve must be included. Neck dissection in minor salivary gland malignancies should only be performed for palpable metastases as the proportion of patients who develop neck disease after successful treatment of the primary disease is small.

Melanoma

This is a rare disease so reports of survival are scanty. However, the prognosis in patients with this disease is poor. They should be treated by wide surgical excision with neck dissection only for palpable disease. Survival figures are about 10% for 5 years (Shah, Huvos and Strong, 1977) and late recurrence and distant spread does occur after this 5 years.

Sarcomas

Sarcomas are very rare in the oral cavity. They most frequently arise from bone and carry a very poor prognosis. A combination of surgery, followed by radiotherapy and then chemotherapy is generally advised and in some instances, e.g. rhabdomyosarcoma, reasonable (40%) 5-year survival figures will be obtained.

Cancer of the lip

The lip is included as one of the sites in the oral cavity in both the AJC and UICC classifications. It only includes the mucosal or vermilion surface and the anterior limit is the junction of mucosa and skin. Because cancers of the lip behave somewhat differently to cancer of the oral cavity proper it is reasonable to consider them separately.

The mucosa of the lip is squamous epithelium and contains accessory salivary tissue. The junction between mucosa and skin is well marked, the latter being a different colour because it is heavily keratinized. The blood supply to the lips is from the facial artery on each side supplying the superior and inferior labial arteries which encircle the lips and anastomose near the midline. The labial arteries lie in the submucosa between the mucosa and the orbicularis oris. The lymphatic drainage of the lower lip is to the submental and submandibular nodes. The upper lip, as well as draining to the submental and submandibular nodes, also drains to the preparotid and parotid lymph nodes.

The incidence of lip cancer is approximately the same as tongue cancer, representing about 25–30% of all oral cancers (Waterhouse *et al.*, 1982; American Cancer Society, 1982). It is eight times more common in men as in women. Smoking is felt to predispose to lip cancer though the major factor in the aetiology of lip cancer is felt by many to be exposure to sunlight, over 30% of patients with a lip cancer having an outdoor occupation (Baker and Krause, 1980) and exposure to sun (Baker, 1980). However, not all studies support the view that sunlight is the main aetiological factor and Lindquist and Teppo (1978) felt that sunlight was not a risk factor. In the USA the disease is much more common in the white population compared with the black. Ninety-five per cent of lip cancers occur on the lower lip with only 5% on the upper lip.

The vast majority of lip cancers are squamous cell cancers with a small proportion of salivary tissue tumours. There is some debate as to whether basal cell carcinomas can arise from the vermilion of the lips and Edmonson, Browne and Potts (1982) have reviewed this subject. The skin beyond the vermilion border can of course be the site of a keratoacanthoma as well as basal cell carcinomas and melanomas. Dyskeratotic epithelium can occur on the lip and the so-called actinic cheilitis is felt to be related to exposure to the sun and to be a premalignant epithelial change.

Since the lip is readily visible and most patients are conscious of a lesion on their lips, diagnosis of lip cancer is relatively early. It presents with an ulcerative lesion with some bleeding and crusting. The diagnosis is made by incisional biopsy. Most lesions are well differentiated and slow growing and therefore carry a good prognosis. There is some evidence (Knabel *et al.*, 1982) that lesions of the upper lip are more aggressive and carry a worse prognosis. The rate of lymph node metastasis in lip cancer is lower than that for the oral cavity in general with less than 10% of patients presenting with nodes (MacKay and Sellas, 1964) and about the same proportion developing nodes following successful treatment of the primary tumour (Jorgensen, Elbrand and Anderson, 1973).

The nodes involved in lip cancer depend upon the site of the lesion. In midline lesions of the lower lip the submental and the submandibular nodes are involved. Tumours on the lateral part of the lower lip tend to metastasize to the submandibular nodes. An upper lip cancer may give rise to nodes in the submandibular and jugulodigastric regions but a proportion of patients will have nodes in the preauricular or parotid groups.

The staging of lip cancer is the same as for oral cavity cancer and has been discussed previously. The staging system reflects survival accurately with survival falling with increased T stage partly due to the difficulty in curing the primary when it is very large and also due to the increased incidence of cervical nodes. Thus the 5-year survival rates for T1 and T2 tumours is 95% (Modlin, 1950; Baker and Krause 1980) falling to about 50% when positive nodes are present.

Treatment

The survival rates for T1 and T2 tumours are the same at 95% for both surgery and external beam radiation. The choice between the two lies with the clinician and the patient. If a lead shield is used to protect the oral cavity from external beam irradiation the side effects are minimal. An alternative is to implant the primary lesion. Surgical excision for T1 and T2 lesions is preferred by many as being quicker than radiation with only a very minor cosmetic defect. The larger lesions and those with metastatic nodes are probably best treated by surgery followed by radiation if there are doubts about the margins of excision or if extracapsular spread or more than one node is involved. The larger lesions clearly result in a more significant cosmetic defect when treated surgically but most believe that radiotherapy does not offer the same rates of cure.

Surgery of lip lesions

Excision of a lip cancer should be done with a margin of normal tissue of between 5 and 10 mm and this margin should be based on appearance and particularly on palpation. More superficial lesions require a smaller margin than the infiltrative ones. The very large lesions may require a 2 cm margin for safety.

Reconstruction of a lip defect depends upon the site of the defect as well as its size. If at all possible the commissure of the lip should be preserved as satisfactory reconstruction of this area is very difficult. A defect of one-third of the lip can be closed primarily either as a V or by converting the defect into a W a more satisfactory closure may be obtained. When the defect is larger than one-third, primary closure results in an unsatisfactory discrepancy between the upper and lower lip and this is avoided by a flap procedure which depends upon the site of the defect. The most common procedure involves a myocutaneous flap from the upper lip to replace the defect. This can be reversed so that an upper lip defect can be filled from the lower lip. These myocutaneous flaps are now collectively known as Abbe Estlander flaps, but Estlander (1872) originally de-

scribed a flap to close a defect near the commissure and Abbe (1898) reported a similar procedure for a midline defect. Other methods of closing large defects of the upper and lower lip involve local advancement flaps. These are described under a variety of names. Karapandzic flaps are used for the lower lip when 50% of the lower lip in the midline has been removed (Bernard 1853; Karapandzic, 1974). The Bernard procedure can be used for the upper and lower lip. It depends upon the excision of Burow's triangles to facilitate advancement of the flap. The vermilion in these operations is reconstructed by advancement of a mucosal flap from the buccal mucosa and these procedures are well described by Webster (1955) and Webster, Coffey and Kelleher (1960).

Another method of reconstructing the lower lip is the Gilles fan flap. If the commissure on one side has been removed it is reconstructed at a later date by two Z-plasties.

References

ABBE, R. (1898) A new plastic operation for the relief of deformity due to hare lip. *Medical Record*, **52**, 477

ACKLAND, R. D. and FLYNN, M.B. (1978) Immediate reconstruction of oral cavity and oropharyngeal defects using microvascular free flaps. *American Journal of Surgery*, **136**, 419–423

AJC (1988) American Joint Committee for cancer staging and end result reporting. In: *Manual for Staging Cancer*, 3rd edn, edited by O. H. Beahrs, D. E. Henson, R. V. P. Hutter and M. H. Myers. Philadelphia: P. Lippincott Co

American Cancer Society (1982) *Facts and Figures*. New York: American Cancer Society

ANTOON, J. W. and MILLER, R. L. (1980) Aphthous ulcers – a review of the literature on aetiology, pathogenesis, diagnosis and treatment. *Journal of the American Dental Association*, **101**, 803–808

ARIYAN, S. (1979) One stage reconstruction for defects of the mouth using a sternomastoid myocutaneous flap. *Plastic and Reconstructive Surgery*, **63**, 618–625

ARTHUR, K. and FARR, H. W. (1972) Prognostic significance of histologic grade in epidermoid cancer of the mouth and pharynx. *American Journal of Surgery*, **124**, 489–492

BAEK, S., LAWSON, W., and BILLER, H. F., (1982) An analysis of 133 pectoralis major flaps. *Plastic and Reconstructive Surgery*, **69**, 460–467

BAKER, S. R. (1980) Risk factors in multiple carcinoma of the lip. *Otolaryngology Head and Neck Surgery*, **88**, 248–251

BAKER, S. R., and KRAUSE, J. (1980) Carcinoma of the lip. *Laryngoscope*, **90**, 19–27

BALLARD, B. R., GUESS, G. R. and PICKREN, J. W. (1978) Squamous cell carcinoma of the floor of the mouth. *Journal of Oral Surgery*, **45**, 568–579

BANOCZY, J. (1977) Follow up studies in oral leukoplakia. *Journal of Maxillofacial Surgery*, **5**, 69–75

BANOCZY, J., SUGAR, L. and FRITHIOF, L (1973) White sponge naevus: leukoedema exfoliativum mucosae oris – a report on 45 cases. *Swedish Dental Journal*, **66**, 481–483

BATSAKIS, J. G., HYBELS, R. J. and CRISSMAN, J. D. (1982) The pathology of head and neck tumours: verrucous carcinoma. *Head and Neck Surgery*, **5**, 29–38

BATSAKIS, J. G., REGEZI, J. A., SOLOMON, A. R. and RICE, D. H. (1982) The pathology of head and neck tumours: mucosal melanomas. *Head and Neck Surgery*, **4**, 404–418

BATSAKIS, J. G., RICE, D. H. and HOWARD, D. R. (1982) The pathology of head and neck tumours: spindle cell lesions. *Head and Neck Surgery*, **4**, 499–513

BERNARD, C. (1853) Cancer de la levre inferieure operee par un procede nouveau. *Bulletin et Memoires de la Societé des Chirurgiens de Paris*, **3**, 357–359

BINNIE, W. H. and RANKIN, K. V. (1984) Epidemiological and diagnostic aspects of oral squamous cell carcinoma. *Journal of Oral Pathology*, **13**, 333–341

BLACK, R. J. and CROFT, C. B. (1982) Ranula: pathogenesis and management. *Clinical Otolaryngology*, **1**, 299–303

BOOTZ, F., LENZ, M., SKALEJ, M. and BONGERS, H. (1992) Computed tomography (CT) and magnetic resonance imaging (MRI) in T stage evaluation of oral and oropharyngeal carcinomas. *Clinical Otolaryngology*, **17**, 421–429

BRADLEY, P. J., HOOVER, L. A. and STELL, P. M. (1982) Assessment of speech after treatment of patients with a tumour of the mouth. *Folia Phoniatrica (Basel)*, **34**, 17–20

BRODERS, A. C. (1920) Squamous cell epithelioma of the lip: a study of five hundred and thirty seven cases. *Journal of the American Medical Association*, **74**, 656–661

BRODERS, A. C. (1941) The microscopic grading of cancer. *Surgery Clinics of North America*, **21**, 947–952

BRUNN, J. P. (1976) Time lapse by diagnosis of oral cancer. *Oral Surgery*, **42**, 139–149

BRYNE, M., KOPPANG, H. S., LILLENG, R. and KJAERHEIM, A. (1992) Malignancy grading of the deep invasive margins of oral squamous cell carcinomas has high prognostic value. *Journal of Pathology*, **166**, 375–381

BYERS, R. M., GLAND, K. I. and WAXLER, J. (1978) The prognostic and therapeutic value of frozen section determinations in the surgical treatment of squamous cell carcinoma of the head and neck. *American Journal of Surgery*, **136**, 525–528

CADE, S., and LEE, E. S. (1957) Cancer of the tongue. *British Journal of Surgery*, **44**, 433–446

CANNON, R. C., JOHNS, M. E., ATKINS, J. P., KEANE, W. M. and CANTRELL, R. W. (1982) Reconstruction of the oral cavity using the platysma myocutaneous flap. *Archives of Otolaryngology*, **108**, 491–494

CARRUTH, J. A. S. (1982) Resection of the tongue with a carbon dioxide laser. *Journal of Laryngology and Otology*, **96**, 529–543

CARTER, R. L., (1990) Patterns and mechanisms of spread of squamous carcinoma of the oral cavity. *Clinical Otolaryngology*, **15**, 185–191

CARTER, R. L., TSAO, S. W. and BURMAN, J. F. (1983) Patterns and mechanisms of bone invasion by squamous carcinoma of the head and neck. *American Journal of Surgery*, **146**, 451–455

CATLIN, F. L. and DE HAAS, V. (1971) Tongue tie. *Archives of Otolaryngology*, **94**, 548–557

CAWSON, R. A. and LEHNER, T. (1968) Chronic hyperplastic candidiasis – candidal leukoplakia. *British Journal of Dermatology*, **80**, 9–16

CHAMBERS, R. G., JACQUES, D. A. and MAHONEY, W. D. (1969) Tongue flaps for intra-oral reconstruction. *American Journal of Surgery*, **118**, 783–786

CHU, W. and FLETCHER, G. H. (1973) Incidence and causes of failure to control by irradiating the primary lesions in squamous cell carcinomas of the anterior two thirds of the tongue and floor of mouth. *American Journal of Roentgenology, Radium Therapy and Nuclear Medicine*, **117**, 502–508

CHU, W. and STRAWITZ, J. G. (1978) Results in suprahyoid modified radical and standard radical neck dissections for metastatic squamous cell carcinoma recurrence and survival. *American Journal of Surgery*, **136**, 512–515

CHU, W., LITWIN, S. and STRAWITZ, J. G. (1978) The comparison of resection and radiation in the control of cancer within the mouth. *Surgery, Gynecology, and Obstetrics*, **146**, 38–42

COFFIN, F. (1983) The incidence and management of osteoradionecrosis of the jaws following head and neck radiotherapy. *British Journal of Radiology*, **56**, 851–857

COHEN, K. and THEOGARAJ, D. (1975) Nasolabial flap reconstruction of the floor of the mouth. *Plastic and Reconstructive Surgery*, **48**, 8–10

CRAFT, J. W. (1961) Immediate reconstruction of the pharynx using rotated mucous membrane flaps. *Plastic and Reconstructive Surgery*, **28**, 26–42

CRISSMAN, J. D., GLUCKMAN, J., WHITELEY, J. and QUENELL, E. D. (1980) Squamous carcinoma of the floor of the mouth. *Head and Neck Surgery*, **3**, 2–7

DANIELS, T. E. (1984) Labial salivary gland biopsy in Sjogren's syndrome: assessment as a diagnostic criterion in 362 suspected cases. *Arthritis and Rheumatism*, **27**, 147–156

DE FRIES, H. O. (1974) Reconstruction of the tongue. *Annals of Otology*, **83**, 471–475

DECLOS, L., LINDBERG, R. D. and FLETCHER, G. H. (1976) Squamous cell carcinoma of the oral tongue and floor of mouth. *American Journal of Roentgenology, Radium Therapy and Nuclear Medicine*, **126**, 223–228

DEMIAN, S. D. E., BUSHKIN, F. L. and ECHEVARRIA, R. A. (1973) Perineural invasion and anaplastic transformation of verrucous carcinoma. *Cancer*, **32**, 395–401

DONEGAN, J. O., GLUCKMAN, J. L. and CRISSMAN, M. D. (1982) The role of suprahyoid neck dissection in the management of cancer of the tongue and floor of mouth. *Head and Neck Surgery*, **4**, 209–212

DROULIAS, C. and WHITEHURST, J. O. (1976) The lymphatics of the tongue in relation to cancer. *American Journal of Surgery*, **42**, 670–674

EDMONSON, H. D., BROWNE, R. M. and POTTS, A. J. C. (1982) Intraoral basal cell carcinoma. *British Journal of Oral Surgery*, **20**, 239–247

ELLIS, G. L. and CARIO, R. L. (1980) Spindle cell carcinoma of the oral cavity: a clinicopathologic assessment of fifty nine cases. *Oral Surgery*, **50**, 523–533

ESTLANDER, J. A. (1872) Eine methode aus der einen lippesubstanzverluste der anderen zu ersetzen. *Archiv für Klinischer Chirurgie*, **14**, 622–624

FARR, H. W. and ARTHUR, K. (1972) Epidermoid carcinoma of the mouth and pharynx. *Journal of Laryngology and Otology*, **86**, 243–253

FERRARA, J., BEAVER, B. L., YOUNG, D. and JAMES, A. G. (1982) Primary procedure in carcinoma of the tongue. Local resection versus combined local resection and radical neck dissection. *Journal of Surgery and Oncology*, **21**, 245–248

FLETCHER, G. H. (1972) Elective radiation of subclinical disease in cancers of the head and neck. *Cancer*, **29**, 1450–1454

FLYNN, M. B. and MOORE, C. (1974) Marginal resection of the mandible in the management of squamous cancer of the floor of the mouth. *American Journal of Surgery*, **128**, 490–493

FONTS, E. A., GREENLAW, R. H. and RUSH, B. F. (1969) Verrucous squamous cell carcinoma of the oral cavity. *Cancer*, **23**, 152–160

FRABLE, W. J. and ELZAY, R. P. (1970) Tumours of minor salivary glands, a report of 73 cases. *Cancer*, **25**, 932–941

FRAZELL, E. L. and LUCAS, J. C. (1962) Cancer of the tongue. *Cancer*, **15**, 1085–1099

FU, K. K., RAY, J. W., CHAN, E. K. and PHILLIPS, T. L. (1976) External and interstitial radiation therapy of carcinoma of the oral tongue. *American Journal of Roentgenology*, **126**, 107–115

GALLO, W. J., MOSS, M. and SHAPIRO, D. N. (1977) Neurilemmoma: review of the literature and report of five cases. *Journal of Oral Surgery*, **35**, 235–236

GOLDBERG, M. H., NEMARICK, A. N. and DANIELSON, P. (1977) Lymphangioma of the tongue: medical and surgical therapy. *Journal of Oral Surgery*, **35**, 841–844

GRILLON, G. L. and LALLY, E. T. (1981) Necrotising sialometaplasia: literature review and presentation of five cases. *Journal of Oral Surgery*, **39**, 747–753

GUILLAMONDEGUI, O. M., OLIVER, B. and HADEN, R. (1980) Cancer of the floor of the mouth. Selective choice of treatment and analysis of failure. *American Journal of Surgery*, **140**, 560–562

HALPERIN, V., KOLAS, S., JEFFERIS, K. R., HUDDLESTON, S. O. and ROBINSON, B. G. (1953) The occurrence of Fordyce's spots, benign migratory glossitis median rhomboid glossitis and fissured tongue in 2478 dental patients. *Oral Surgery*, **6**, 1072–1079

HAMNER, J. E. (1986) Aetiology and epidemiology of oral cancer. In: *Cancer and the Oral Cavity*, edited by L. W. Carr and K. Sako. Chicago: Quintessence. pp. 17–30

HARROLD, C. C. (1971) Management of cancer of the floor of the mouth. *American Journal of Surgery*, **122**, 487–493

HIBBERT, J., MARKS, N. J., WINTER, P. J. and SHAHEEN, O. H. (1983) Prognostic factors in oral squamous carcinoma and their relation to clinical staging. *Clinical Otolaryngology*, **8**, 197–203

HILGER, P. and ADAMS, G. (1985) Mandibular reconstruction with the A-O plate. *Archives of Otolaryngology*, **111**, 469–471

HOLM, L. E., LUNDQUIST, P. G., SILVERSVAARD, C. and SOBIN, A. (1982) Histological grading of malignancy in squamous cell carcinoma of the oral tongue. *Acta Otolaryngologica*, **94**, 185–192

ISSAACSON, G. and SHEAR, M. (1983) Intraoral salivary gland tumours: a retrospective study of 201 cases. *Journal of Oral Pathology*, **12**, 57–62

JACOBSON, P. A., ENEROTH, C. M., KILLANDER, D., MOBERGER, G. and MARLENSSON, B. (1973) Histological classification and grading of malignancy in cancer of the larynx. *Acta Radiologica*, **12**, 1–9

JACOBSON, S. and SHEAR, M. (1972) Verrucous carcinoma of the mouth. *Journal of Oral Pathology*, **1**, 66–75

JESSE, R. H. and FLETCHER, G. H. (1977) Treatment of the neck in patients with squamous cell carcinoma of the head and neck. *Cancer*, **39**, 868–872

JESSE, R. H., BARKELY, H. T., LINDBERG, R. D. and FLETCHER, G. H. (1970) Cancer of the oral cavity: is elective neck dissection beneficial? *American Journal of Surgery*, **120**, 505–509

JOHNSON, J. T., LEIPZIG, B. and CUMMINGS, C. W. (1980) Management of T1 carcinoma of the anterior aspect of the tongue. *Archives of Otolaryngology*, **106**, 249–251

JOHNSON, J. T., BARNES, L., MYERS, E. N., SCHRAMM, V. L., BOROCHOVITZ, D. and SIGLER, B. D. (1981) The extracapsular spread of tumours in cervical node metastases. *Archives of Otolaryngology*, **107**, 725–729

JORGENSON, K., ELBRAND, O. and ANDERSON, A. P. (1973) Carcinoma of the lip: a series of 869 cases. *Acta Radiologica*, **12**, 177–190

KARAPANDZIC, M. (1974) Reconstruction of lip defects by local arterial flaps. *British Journal of Plastic Surgery*, **27**, 93–97

KISSIN, B., KALEY, M. M., SU, W. H. and LERNER, R. (1973) Head and neck cancer in alcoholics, the relationship of drinking, smoking and dietary patterns. *Journal of the American Medical Association*, **224**, 1174–1175

KNABEL, M. R., KORANDA, F. C., PANJE, W. R. and GRANDE, D. J. (1982) Squamous cell carcinoma of the upper lip. *Journal of Dermatology and Surgical Oncology*, **8**, 487–491

KRAUSE, C. J., LEE, J. G. and MCCABE, B. F. (1973) Carcinomas of the oral cavity. *Archives of Otolaryngology*, **97**, 354–358

LANCET (1972) Oral cancer: a stubborn problem. i, 299–300

LARSON, D. L., LEWIS, S. R. and RAPPAPORT, A. S. (1965) Lymphatics of the mouth and neck. *American Journal of Surgery*, **110**, 625–630

LARSSON, S. G., HOOVER, L. A. and JUILLARD, G. J. F. (1987) Staging of base of tongue carcinoma by computed tomography. *Clinical Otolaryngology*, **12**, 25–32

LASKARIS, G., SKLAVOUNOU, A. and STRALIGOS, J. (1982) Bullous pemphigoid, cicatrial pemphigoid and pemphigus vulgaris. *Oral Surgery*, **54**, 656–662

LEDERER, B. and MANAGETTA, J. B. (1982) Morphological aspects of minimal invasive carcinomas (microcarcinoma) of the oral mucosa. *Clinical Oncology*, **1**, 475–481

LEIPZIG, B. and HIKANSON, J. A. (1982) Treatment of cervical lymph nodes in carcinoma of the tongue. *Head and Neck Surgery*, **5**, 3–9

LEIPZIG, B., CUMMINGS, C. W., JOHNSON, J. T., CHUNG, T. C. and SAGERMAN, R. H. (1982) Carcinoma of the anterior tongue. *Annals of Otology, Rhinology and Laryngology*, **91**, 94–97

LEVENTON, G. S. and EVANS, H. L. (1981) Sarcomatoid squamous cell carcinoma of the mucous membranes of the head and neck: a clinicopathologic study of 20 cases. *Cancer*, **48**, 994–1003

LINDQUIST, C. and TEPPO, L. (1978) Epidemiological evaluation of sunlight as a risk factor of lip cancer. *British Journal of Cancer*, **37**, 983–989

LOOSER, K. G., SHAH, J. P. and STRONG, E. W. (1978) The significance of positive margins in surgically resected epidermoid carcinomas. *Head and Neck Surgery*, **1**, 107–111

LUND, C., SOGAARD, H., ELBROND, D., JORGENSEN, K. and PETERSEN, A. P. (1975) Epidermoid carcinoma of the tongue. Histologic grading in the clinical evaluation. *Acta Radiologica Therapy, Physics, Biology*, **14**, 513–521

LYALL, D. J. and SCHETLIN, C. F. (1952) Cancer of the tongue. *Annals of Surgery*, **135**, 489–493

MACERI, D. R. and SAXON, K. G. (1984) Neurofibromatosis of the head and neck. *Head and Neck Surgery*, **6**, 842–850

MCGREGOR, I. A., (1975) Quilted skin grafting in the mouth. *British Journal of Plastic Surgery*, **28**, 100–102

MACKAY, E. N. and SELLAS, A. H. (1964) A statistical review of carcinoma of the lip. *Canadian Medical Association Journal*, **90**, 670–673

MAISEL, R. H. and ADAMS, G. L. (1983) Osteomyocutaneous reconstruction of the oral cavity. *Archives of Otology*, **109**, 731–734

MAISEL, R. H., HILGER, P. A. and ADAMS, G. L. (1983) Reconstruction of the mandible. *Laryngoscope*, **93**, 1122–1126

MARTIN, H., DEL VALLE, B., EHRLICH, H. and CAHAN, W. (1951) Neck dissection. *Cancer*, 4, 441–449

MARTIN, H. E., MUNSTER, H. and SUGARBAKER, E. D. (1940) Cancer of the tongue. *Archives of Surgery*, 41, 888–896

MASKBERG, A. (1978) Erythroplasia – earliest sign of asymptomatic oral cancer. *Journal of the American Dental Association*, 96, 615–619

MAVES, M. D., PANJE, W. R. and SHAGETS, F. W. (1984) Extended latissimus dorsi myocutaneous flap reconstruction of major head and neck defects. *Otolaryngology Head and Neck Surgery*, 92, 551–557

MEDINA, J. E., DIECHTEL, W. and LUNA, M. A. (1984) Verrucous squamous carcinomas of the oral cavity. A clinicopathological study of 104 cases. *Archives of Otology*, 110, 437–440

MEIKLE, D., HIBBERT, J., WINTER, P. J., TONG, D. and SHAHEEN, O. H. (1985) Interstitial irradiation for squamous carcinoma of the oral cavity. *Clinical Otolaryngology*, 10, 171–176

MENDELSON, B. C., HODGKINSON, D. J. and WOODS, J. E. (1977) Cancer of the oral cavity. *Surgery Clinics of North America*, 57, 585–596

MERINO, O. R., LINDBERG, R. D. and FLETCHER, G. H. (1977) An analysis of distant metastases from squamous cell carcinoma of the upper respiratory and digestive tracts. *Cancer*, 40, 145–149

MILLION, R. R. (1974) Elective neck irradiation for treatment of the squamous cell carcinoma of the oral tongue and floor of mouth. *Cancer*, 34, 149–155

MODLIN, J. (1950) Neck dissections in cancer of the lower lip: five year results in 179 patients. *Surgery*, 28, 404–409

MOORE, C. (1971) Cigarette smoking and cancer of the mouth pharynx and larynx. *Journal of the American Medical Association*, 218, 553–558

MORTON, R. P., PHAROAH, P. O. D., STELL, P. M. and RAMADAN, M. F. (1983) Epidemiology of tongue cancer in England and Wales. *Clinical Otolaryngology*, 8, 142

MYER, I. and ABBEY, L. M. (1970) The relationship of syphilis to primary carcinoma of the tongue. *Oral Surgery*, 30, 678–681

MYERS, E. N. (1972) Reconstruction of the oral cavity. *Otolaryngologic Clinics of North America*, 5, 413–433

NOONE, R. B., BONNER, H. JR. and RAYMOND, S. (1974) Lymph node metastases in oral carcinoma: a correlation of histopathology with survival. *Plastic and Reconstructive Surgery*, 53, 158–166

O'BRIEN, C. Y., CARTER, R. L. and SOO, K. C. (1986) Invasion of the mandible by squamous carcinomas of the oral cavity and oropharynx. *Head and Neck Surgery*, 8, 247–256

O'BRIEN, P. H., CARLSON, R., STEILBNER, E. A. and STALEY, C. T. (1971) Distant metastases in epidermoid carcinoma of the head and neck. *Cancer*, 27, 304–307

ODELL, E. W., JANI, P., SHERRIF, M., AHLUWALIA, S. M., HIBBERT, J., LEVISON, D. A. *et al.* (1994) Prognostic value of individual histological grading parameters in lingual carcinoma. *Cancer*, 74, 789–794

PANJE, W. R. (1980) Myocutaneous trapezius flap. *Head and Neck Surgery*, 2, 206–212

PANJE, W. R. (1982) Free flaps vs myocutaneous flaps in head and neck reconstruction. *Otolaryngologic Clinics of North America*, 15, 111–121

PANJE, W. R. (1985) Mandible reconstruction with the osteomusculocutaneous flap. *Archives of Otology*, 111, 223–229

PANJE, W. R., SMITH, B. S. and MCCABE, B. F. (1980) Epidermoid carcinoma of the floor of the mouth: surgical therapy vs combined therapy vs radiation therapy. *Otolaryngology Head and Neck Surgery*, 88, 714–118

PARKIN, D. M., LAARA, E. and MUIR, C. S. (1988) Estimates of the world-wide frequency of sixteen major cancers in 1980. *International Journal of Cancer*, 41, 184–197

PATERSON, W. B. (1979) The treatment of intraoral cancer by electric coagulation. *Cancer*, 43, 821–824

PELTIER, L. F., THOMAS, L. B. and CRAWFORD, R. H. (1951) The incidence of distant metastases among patients dying with head and neck cancers. *Surgery*, 30, 827–833

PIERQUIN, B., CHASSAGNE, D., and BAILLET, F. (1971) The place of implantation in tongue and floor of mouth cancer. *Journal of the American Medical Association*, 215, 961–963

PLATZ, H., FRIES, R. and HUDEC, M. (1982) Prognostic relevance of minimal invasion of the oral cavity. A retrospective Dosak study. *Clinical Oncology*, 1, 467–471

POWELL, J. and ROBIN, P. E. (1987) Cancer of the head and neck: the present state. In: *Head and Neck Cancer*, edited by P. H. Rhys-Evans, P. E. Robin and W. W. L. Fielding. Tunbridge Wells: Castle House

REDDY, C. R. (1974) Carcinoma of the hard palate in India in relation to reverse smoking of Chuttas. *Journal of the National Cancer Institute*, 53, 615–619

ROBERTSON, A. G., MCGREGOR, I. A. and SOUTTAR, D. S. (1986) Post-operative radiotherapy in the management of advanced intra-oral cancers. *Clinical Radiology*, 37, 173–178

ROSUIT, B., SPIRO, R. H. and KOLSON, H. (1972) Planned pre-operative irradiation and surgery for advanced cancer of the oral cavity pharynx and larynx. *American Journal of Roentgenology*, 114, 59–62

ROTHMAN, K. and KELLER, A. (1972) The effect of joint exposure to alcohol and tobacco and risk of cancer of the mouth and pharynx. *Journal of Chronic Diseases*, 25, 711–716

RUSSELL, M. H. (1955) Diverging sex morbidity trends in cancer of the mouth, hospital morbidity study. *British Medical Journal*, 2, 823–827

SEAGREN, S. L., SYED, A. M. N. and BYFIELD, J. E. (1979) Interstitial implant radiotherapy in upper aerodigestive tract malignancy. *Head and Neck Surgery*, 1, 409–416

SERAFIN, D., VILLARREAL-RIOS, A. and GEORGIADE, N. W. (1977) A rib containing free flap to reconstruct mandibular defects. *British Journal of Plastic Surgery*, 30, 263–266

SHAH, J. P., HUVOS, A. G. and STRONG, E. W. (1977) Mucosal melanomas of the head and neck. *American Journal of Surgery*, 134, 531–535

SHAPIRO, M. J. (1981) Use of trapezius myocutaneous flaps in the reconstruction of head and neck defects. *Archives of Otolaryngology*, 107, 333–336

SILVERMAN, J. and GRIFFITHS, M. (1972) Smoking characteristics of patients with oral carcinoma and the risk for a second oral primary carcinoma. *Journal of the American Dental Association*, 85, 637–640

SMITH, E. M. (1982) An analysis of cohort mortality from tongue cancer in Japan, England and Wales and the United States. *International Journal of Epidemiology*, 11, 329–335

SNOW, G. B., ANNYAS, A. A., VAN SLOOTEN, E. A., BARTELINK, H. and HART, A. A. M. (1982) Prognostic factors of neck node metastasis. *Clinical Otolaryngology*, 7, 185–192

SOM, M. L. and NUSSBAUM, M. (1971) Marginal resection of the mandible with reconstruction by tongue flap for carcinoma of the floor of the mouth. *American Journal of Surgery*, **121**, 679–686

SOUTTAR, D. S., SCHEKER, L., TANNER, N. S. B. and MCGREGOR, A. (1983) The radial forearm flap. A versatile method for intraoral reconstruction. *British Journal of Plastic Surgery*, **36**, 1–8

SPIRO, R. H. and STRONG, E. W. (1971) Epidermoid carcinoma of the mobile tongue: treatment by partial glossectomy alone. *American Journal of Surgery*, **122**, 707–710

SPIRO, R. H., KOSS, L. G. and HAJDU, S. I. (1973) Tumours of minor salivary gland origin: a clinico-pathologic study of 492 cases. *Cancer*, **31**, 117–129

STARKE, E. N. and SHANNON, I. L. (1977) How critical is the interval betwen extractions and irradiation in patients with head and neck malignancy. *Oral Surgery*, **43**, 333–337

STELL, P. M. (1982) Editorial: patients with burning mouths. *Clinical Otolaryngology*, **7**, 143–144

STELL, P. M. and HIBBERT, J. (1978) Flaps in head and neck surgery. In: *Recent Advances in Otolaryngology*, edited by T. R. Bull, J. Ransome and H. B. Holden. London: Churchill Livingstone. pp. 141–169

STELL, P. M., WOOD, G. D. and SCOTT, M. H. (1982) Early oral cancer: treatment by biopsy excision. *British Journal of Oral Surgery*, **20**, 234–238

STRONG, E. W., MCDIVITT, R. W. and BRASFIELD, R. D. (1970) Granular cell myoblastoma. *Cancer*, **25**, 415–422

STRONG, M. S., VAUGHAN, C. W., HEALY, G. B., SHAPSHAY, S. and SAKO, G. J. (1979) Transoral management of localised carcinoma of the oral cavity using the CO_2 laser. *Laryngoscope*, **89**, 897–905

TAKAGI, M., ISHIKAWA, G. L. and MORI, W. (1974) Primary malignant melanoma of the oral cavity in Japan with special reference to mucosal melanosis. *Cancer*, **34**, 358–370

TAYLOR, G., TOWNSEND, P. and CORLETT, R. (1979) Superiority of the deep circumflex iliac vessels as the supply for free groin flaps: clinical work. *Plastic and Reconstructive Surgery*, **64**, 745–759

THOMPSON, J. N., FIERSTEIN, S. B. and KOHUT, R. I. (1979) Embolisation techniques in vascular tumours of the head and neck. *Head and Neck Surgery*, **2**, 25–34

UICC (1987) *International Union Against Cancer TNM Classification of Malignant Tumours*, 4th edn, edited by P. Hermanek and L. H. Sobin. Berlin: Springer Verlag

VAN DEN BROUEK, C., SANCHO-GARNIER, H., CHASSAGNE, D., SARAVANE, D., CACHIN, Y. and MICHEAU, C. (1980) Elective versus therapeutic radical neck dissection in epidermoid carcinoma of the oral cavity – results of a randomised clinical trial. *Cancer*, **46**, 386–390

VAS KOVSKAIA, G. P. and ABRAMOVA, E. I. (1981) Cancer development from lichen planus on the oral and labial mucosa. *Stomatologiia*, **60**, 46–51

WALD, R. M. and CALCATERRA, T. C. (1983) Lower alveolar carcinoma. Segmental vs. marginal resection. *Archives of Otolaryngology*, **109**, 578–582

WALDRON, C. A. and SHAFER, W. G. (1975) Leukoplakia revisited, a clinico-pathologic study of 3256 oral leukoplakias. *Cancer*, **36**, 1386–1392

WARD, G. E., EDGERTON, M. T., CHAMBERS, R. G. and MCKEE, D. M. (1959) Cancer of the oral cavity and pharynx and results of treatment by means of the composite operation in continuity with radical neck dissection. *American Journal of Surgery*, **150**, 202–220

WARD, P. H., HARRIS, P. F. and DOWNEY, W. (1970) Surgical approach to cystic hygroma. *Archives of Otology*, **91**, 508–513

WATERHOUSE, J., MUIR, C. S., SHANMUGARATNAM, K. and POWELL, J. (1982) Cancer incidence in five continents. vol IV *IARC Scientific Publications no. 42*, Lyons: IARC

WEBSTER, J. P. (1955) Crescentic peri-alar cheek excision for upper lip flap advancement with a short history of upper lip repair. *Plastic and Reconstructive Surgery*, **16**, 434–439

WEBSTER, R. C., COFFEY, R. J. and KELLEHER, R. E. (1960) Total and partial reconstruction of the lower lip with innervated muscle bearing flaps. *Plastic and Reconstructive Surgery*, **25**, 360–371

WHO (1978) Collaborating centre for oral precancerous lesions: leukoplakia and related lesions: an aid to studies on oral precancer. *Oral Surgery*, **46**, 518–521

WILLEN, R., NATHANSON, A., MOBERGER, G. and ANNEROTH, G. (1975) Squamous cell carcinoma of the gingiva. Histological classification and grading of malignancy. *Acta Otolaryngologica*, **79**, 146–154

WYNDER, E. L., BROSS, I. J. and FELDMAN, R. (1957) A study of the aetiological factors of cancer of the mouth. *Cancer*, **10**, 1300–1323

YVES, D. and GHOSSEIN, N. A. (1981) Experience of the Curie Institute in treatment of cancer of the mobile tongue. Management of neck nodes. *Cancer*, **47**, 503–507

4

Acute and chronic infection of the pharynx and tonsils

D. L. Cowan and John Hibbert

Although acute infection of the pharynx and tonsils must be one of the most common conditions encountered in medicine, it is one of the most poorly understood. Certain well-defined clinical entities do exist but many others are described for which there is little or no scientific basis. Many difficulties arise and several questions remain unanswered.

1 Do virus infections in the pharynx and tonsils predispose to bacterial infection?
2 Is it possible to have an infective condition involving the pharyngeal lymphoid tissue without affecting the tonsils?
3 Is there such a condition as chronic tonsillitis?
4 Is there an infective condition called chronic pharyngitis?
5 Why are some patients susceptible to acute pharyngitis and acute tonsillitis and others not?
6 Does the tonsil become irreversibly diseased after many episodes of acute tonsillitis?
7 Does removal of the tonsils predispose the patient to more frequent attacks of pharyngitis?

One of the most confusing aspects of diagnosing and treating acute infections of the tonsils and pharyngeal lymphoid tissue is the part played by and hence interpretation of the results of throat swabs. Publications on the subject are far from unanimous with some (Surow et al., 1989) showing poor correlation between surface culture swab results and culture of tonsil core and others (Almadori et al., 1988) showing excellent correlation between the two.

The presence of an organism in a patient's throat and its culture from a swab does not mean that it is pathogenic. Studies comparing bacteriological isolates from the throat swabs of patients with acute tonsillitis and acute pharyngitis, and from asymptomatic controls, show very little difference (Box, Cleveland and Willard, 1961; Reilly et al., 1981). This particularly applies to aerobic organisms such as streptococci and Haemophilus. Similarly, virus cultures, when positive, do not imply that the organism is actually causing an infection; conversely patients with a clinically obvious infection may not have a positive culture from a throat swab. It has therefore been suggested that many infections may be caused by anaerobic organisms (Reilly et al., 1981; Toner et al., 1986) or by viruses (Everett, 1979). It has also been suggested that most sore throats are initiated by a virus infection which gives little in the way of signs in the throat and that secondary bacterial infection prolongs the illness and produces more in the way of signs, e.g. pus in the tonsillar crypts. Most authorities distinguish between acute pharyngitis and acute tonsillitis; others talk of streptococcal pharyngitis, to include infection of both.

In general, acute pharyngitis is most often felt to be an acute viral infection involving the pharyngeal lymphoid tissue and including the tonsil. Acute tonsillitis is reserved for infection with most of the signs seen in the tonsil, but it is likely that the pharyngeal lymphoid tissue is also involved. It seems unlikely that infection of some lymphoid tissue of the pharynx can occur without infection of the remainder. There is no doubt that patients who have had their tonsils removed are still susceptible to infections, both viral and bacterial.

One of the other areas of confusion in this whole field is the appearance of the throat on clinical examination. In healthy people there is a very wide variation in the appearance of the anterior pillar, the tonsillar lymphoid tissue and the posterior pharyngeal wall lymphoid tissue. These tissues may vary from being quite pale in colour to being quite pink and apparently injected. Similarly, in healthy people, there may be visible hyperplasia of the pharyngeal lymphoid tissue including the lateral pharyngeal bands. These appearances may be found in either symptomatic or asymptomatic patients and hence are not diagnostic. The appearances of acute follicular tonsillitis are unmistakable and easily diagnosed as abnormal, but many patients who complain of a sore throat may have little in the way of physical signs in the throat.

Some surgeons claim to be able to diagnose 'diseased or chronically infected' tonsils by inspection alone but this tends to be anecdotal and has never been put to the test of a trial. In general terms, the appearance alone of the tonsils when they are not acutely infected is not of diagnostic assistance and certainly the size of the tonsils is not directly related to their infective status. Some surgeons in fact suggest that small sunken tonsils are immunologically incompetent and hence are more likely to be the source of the problem rather than the large immunologically active ones. Certainly it has been shown (Weir, 1972) that the size of the tonsils is not related to the frequency of previous infection.

In this chapter the discussion is restricted to well-defined clinical entities for which there is at least a sound clinical, if not scientific, basis and conditions such as parenchymatous tonsillitis, chronic tonsillitis, streptococcal pharyngitis and chronic hypertrophic pharyngitis will be assigned to a non-proven category.

Acute tonsillitis

Acute infection of the tonsils is most frequent in childhood, presumably because immunity to common organisms has not been established. Acute tonsillitis, however, does occur in adults, but one should always be aware of the differential diagnosis and any predisposing factors.

Causative organisms

There has been a large amount written on this subject and it remains controversial. As has already been mentioned, organisms grown from superficial swabs may not be the same as those obtained from the centre of the tonsil (referred to as 'tonsil core') and there is almost certainly a difference between children and adults. Ylikoski and Karjalainen (1989) studied 257 young men in military service with acute tonsillitis and found group A beta-haemolytic streptococci in 38%, while Gaffney *et al.* (1991) found that *Haemophilus influenzae* was the single most common bacterium isolated from the tonsil core in 262 patients with recurrent tonsillitis. However, in this series mixed pathogens were found in 48%, with the commonest mixture being beta-haemolytic streptococci, *H. influenzae* and *Staphylococcus aureus*. The significance of anaerobes remains uncertain, as in this same series anaerobes were present in moderate to heavy numbers in 32% of superficial swabs but were only isolated in significant numbers from the

tonsil core in 5%. The number of specimens containing a beta-lactamase producer was 42% of those studied.

The part played by viruses in acute tonsillitis is unknown and certainly in children it has been felt that an initial viral tonsillitis may predispose to a superinfection by bacteria (Everett, 1979) or that viruses alone may be responsible for tonsillitis on many occasions. In Ylikoski and Karjalainen's (1989) study 42% of young military men showed a fourfold rise in viral antibody titres. Adenovirus was the most frequent non-streptococcal agent (31%) followed by Epstein-Barr virus (6%) and influenza virus (5%).

Despite the fact that tonsillitis is so common, consensus seems to be lacking as to the main causative organisms.

Clinical features

Prior to the onset of sore throat there may be a day or so of a prodromal illness with pyrexia, malaise and headache. The predominant symptom, however, is a sore throat which is made worse by swallowing. The voice may change, partly due to the accumulation of saliva but also due to the patient's efforts to restrict movement of the soft palate and tongue. Pain may radiate to the ears or may occur in the neck due to enlargement of the jugulodigastric lymph nodes. In classical acute follicular tonsillitis, the tonsils are hyperaemic and pus accumulates in the tonsillar crypts (it should be noted that an identical appearance may occur in infectious mononucleosis). Rarely, the debris in the crypts coalesces to form a purulent membrane. Tonsillitis does occur without pus in the crypts and, in this case, the tonsil is very hyperaemic. Untreated acute tonsillitis will subside over the course of about 1 week, but with appropriate treatment the illness is shorter.

Differential diagnosis

Scarlet fever is a streptococcal tonsillitis in which the streptococcus produces the erythrogenic toxin which results in an erythematous rash. Infectious mononucleosis or acute diphtheria are the conditions most likely to be mistaken for acute tonsillitis and, of course, they do produce an acute tonsillitis. The tonsillitis and pharyngitis associated with leukaemia, or agranulocytosis should always be considered.

Treatment

Benzylpenicillin 600 mg 6-hourly intramuscularly or ideally intravenously is the most effective treatment for acute tonsillitis. After an initial response it is usual to discontinue the parenteral antibiotic and continue with penicillin V by mouth. More commonly antibiotics are given only by mouth.

Analgesics should also be given and soluble aspirin gargles are suitable. Many consider paracetamol to be a more suitable analgesic as this avoids gastric irritation in adults and Reye's syndrome in children. In a patient allergic to penicillin, erythromycin (500 mg 6-hourly) should be given. Ampicillin should never be used to treat acute tonsillitis in case the patient has infectious mononucleosis (see below).

Increasing interest is being shown in the part played by beta-lactamase producing bacteria and hence, in resistant infections, consideration should be given to the use of clindamycin or ciprofloxacin with or without metronidazole.

Complications

These are best considered as either local or general.

Local

Severe swelling with spread of infection and inflammation to the hypopharynx and larynx may occasionally produce increasing respiratory obstruction, although this is very rare in uncomplicated acute tonsillitis. Peritonsillar abscess is one of the complications of acute tonsillitis and its development means that the infection has spread outside the tonsillar capsule.

Spread of infection from the tonsil or more usually from a peritonsillar abscess through the superior constrictor muscle of the pharynx results first in a cellulitis of the tissues of the neck and, later, in a parapharyngeal abscess. Alternatively, such an abscess in the parapharyngeal space can arise following suppuration in a cervical lymph node. Once infection has spread to involve the tissue spaces in the neck it can spread rapidly through these tissue spaces and into the mediastinum. These infections are often due to a number of organisms together (see below) and surgical drainage is as important in the management of the patient as are antibiotics. These neck space infections following acute tonsillitis occasionally occur in fit young patients, but are much more common in debilitated patients with conditions which predispose to infection, e.g. diabetes mellitus and immunosuppressed states such as lymphoma or cytotoxic therapy.

General

Systemic complications of acute tonsillitis such as septicaemia are excessively rare in adults as are the complications of acute glomerulonephritis and rheumatic fever. These are discussed under the section Tonsillitis in Volume 6.

Peritonsillar abscess (quinsy)

A peritonsillar abscess (quinsy) is a collection of pus between the fibrous capsule of the tonsil, usually at its upper pole, and the superior constrictor muscle of the pharynx. It usually occurs as a complication of acute tonsillitis or it may apparently arise *de novo* with no preceding tonsillitis. There are several interesting and unanswered questions regarding peritonsillar abscess, one being why does it mainly occur in young adults and rarely in children when acute tonsillitis is a disease of childhood? Although a patient with a peritonsillar abscess may have a previous history of recurrent episodes of acute tonsillitis, on occasions, there is no such history and it remains to be explained why the patient should suddenly develop a quinsy.

Bacteriology

The bacteriology of acute tonsillitis and peritonsillar abscess is different – and although one is a complication of the other, it may be that the complication only occurs in the presence of certain organisms. Although beta-haemolytic streptococcus is frequently isolated, it is rarely isolated on its own. In results from the Naval Medical Center, Bethesda (1991) mixed aerobic and anaerobic flora were found in 76%. Beta-lactamase producing organisms were recovered from 52% of swabs. Jokinen *et al.* (1985) also demonstrated a large variety of different organisms in their series and it may be that the involvement of anaerobic organisms predisposes to infection spreading through the tonsillar capsule. This may explain the much more frequent occurrence of peritonsillar abscess in adults.

Clinical features

The usual patient with a quinsy is a fit young adult who may have a previous history of repeated attacks of acute tonsillitis, however, the patient may never have had tonsillitis. Usually a quinsy is preceded by a sore throat for 2 or 3 days which gradually becomes more severe and unilateral. This heralds the development of a quinsy which is almost always unilateral but occasionally can be bilateral. At this stage the patient is ill with a fever, often a headache and severe pain, made worse by swallowing. There may be referred earache and pain and swelling in the neck due to infective lymphadenopathy. The patient's voice develops a characteristic 'plummy' quality as a consequence of the oropharyngeal swelling and an accumulation of saliva in the mouth. Examination reveals an ill-looking patient with pyrexia and often with severe trismus. The classical appearance of the oropharynx is the striking asymmetry with oedema and hypcraemia of the soft palate, and enlargement, hyperaemia and displacement of the tonsil on that side. There are usually tender, enlarged lymph nodes in the jugulodigastric region on the same side.

Differential diagnosis

Any condition which produces swelling or oedema of the soft palate may be mistaken for a quinsy. An abscess related to an upper molar tooth is probably the most likely condition to be confused with a quinsy because it will also produce trismus and earache. Any of the causes of a parapharyngeal swelling (see Chapter 22) may also mimic a quinsy, although a carefully taken history and examination will usually make these conditions obvious.

Treatment

The patient should be admitted to hospital and treated with analgesics and antibiotics. In general, the antibiotic should be administered by the intravenous route and benzylpenicillin (600 mg 6-hourly) is the first choice; in those patients allergic to penicillin, erythromycin (500 mg 6-hourly) should be used. Although infection is usually with a mixture of aerobic and anaerobic organisms, most are sensitive to penicillin. In a patient with an early peritonsillar abscess which is really a peritonsillar cellulitis, incision and drainage are not to be recommended. It is difficult to be certain when a discrete abscess has formed, but marked bulging of the soft palate, rather than a diffuse oedema, usually indicates this and, at this stage, incision and drainage should be performed. Failure of an assumed peritonsillar cellulitis to respond to adequate antibiotics within 24 hours is also an indication for incision. This is undertaken at the point of maximum swelling of the soft palate above the upper pole of the tonsil. The mucosa should be anaesthetized with a lignocaine spray and incised with a no.15 blade with all but the terminal 0.5–1.0 cm guarded using zinc oxide tape. Usually pus will gush out of the incision. A pair of sinus forceps should be introduced through the incision and opened to break down any loculi.

The above procedure is the time honoured and accepted form of treatment but increasingly surgeons (Ophir *et al.*, 1988; Stringer, Schaefer and Close, 1988; T-Buturo, 1990; Snow, Campbell and Morgan 1991) have suggested that permucosal needle drainage of the abscess is equally efficacious, less distressing for the patient and, of course, cost effective. In one study none of the patients required admission to hospital (Stringer, Schaefer and Close, 1988).

The majority of otolaryngologists advise a patient who has had a quinsy to undergo tonsillectomy at a suitable interval (usually 6 weeks) to avoid a recurrence. The evidence from follow-up studies on pa-

tients who have had a quinsy shows that only about 20%, at the most, have a second peritonsillar abscess, so perhaps the policy of tonsillectomy after this condition should be revised (Beeden and Evans, 1970; Brandon, 1973; Herbild and Bonding, 1981; Holt and Tinsley, 1981; Tucker, 1982b; Harris, 1991).

The alternative method of managing a quinsy is to perform emergency abscess tonsillectomy. The advantage of this is that incision and drainage are avoided and only one hospital admission is necessary. This assumes that all patients who have a quinsy will go on to need tonsillectomy to avoid recurrence and, as stated above, this may not be necessary. The risks of abscess tonsillectomy are mainly theoretical, namely increased haemorrhage and spread of infection. None of the studies of abscess tonsillectomy showed an increased incidence of these complications (Moesgaard Nielson and Griesson, 1981), whereas cold tonsillectomy at an interval following a quinsy has been shown to have an increased incidence of primary haemorrhage (Kristenson and Tveteras, 1984). However, if the recurrence rate after quinsy is only 20% then abscess tonsillectomy means that many patients are having unnecessary surgery.

Complications

There is no doubt that a peritonsillar abscess is a potentially lethal condition. Rapidly increasing oedema and spread of infection can lead to pharyngeal and laryngeal oedema with respiratory obstruction and on occasions tracheostomy is necessary. Spread of infection through the constrictor muscles of the pharynx can lead to a parapharyngeal abscess which may involve the carotid sheath leading to jugular vein thrombosis or even fatal carotid artery haemorrhage. If a parapharyngeal abscess is suspected because of tender swelling in the neck it must be incised and drained through a neck incision. In this situation there is a real risk of a salivary fistula which again puts the carotid artery at risk. However, neglect of a parapharyngeal abscess results in spread of infection and possible mediastinitis.

Parapharyngeal abscess

The parapharyngeal space lies on either side of the superior part of the pharynx – the oropharynx and nasopharynx. It is bounded laterally by the parotid gland and parotid fascia and by the medial pterygoid muscle. Medially, this space is bounded by the pharynx and separated from it by the superior constrictor muscle. Posterior to the pharynx, the parapharyngeal space communicates with the retropharyngeal space. Superiorly, the parapharyngeal space is limited by the base of the skull and inferiorly, by the fascia surrounding the submandibular gland. The parapharyngeal space contains the carotid sheath with the internal carotid artery, internal jugular vein, vagus nerve, the styloid group of muscles and last four cranial nerves. It also contains some lymph nodes. Infection can spread to the parapharyngeal space from the retropharyngeal space, the peritonsillar space and from the submaxillary space. The commonest causes of a parapharyngeal abscess are tonsillitis, peritonsillar abscess or a dental infection. Rarely mastoiditis or a pharyngeal foreign body can give rise to a parapharyngeal space abscess.

Clinical features

The symptoms and signs of a parapharyngeal abscess are very similar to those of a peritonsillar abscess except that the maximum swelling is more inferiorly placed and the soft palate is less oedematous. The other striking feature of a parapharyngeal abscess is the tender firm swelling in the upper part of the neck. This allows it to be distinguished from a peritonsillar abscess in which swelling in the neck is due to enlarged lymph nodes rather than an abscess. Of course, if a parapharyngeal abscess complicates a peritonsillar abscess the clinical features are very similar.

Treatment

The patient is treated with intravenous penicillin 600 mg 6-hourly; erythromycin is the drug of choice if the patient is allergic to penicillin. If pus is present in the neck then this must be drained. If this does not seem likely, observation for 24 hours to assess the effects of antibiotic therapy is reasonable. Drainage of a parapharyngeal abscess is not without risk as trismus and pharyngeal oedema make general anaesthesia difficult. If there is any doubt about the capability of the anaesthetist to pass an endotracheal tube then an initial tracheostomy should be performed under local anaesthesia. The abscess is drained through a collar incision in the neck at the level of the hyoid bone. The abscess is widely opened and, if it has arisen from an adjacent space, this should be opened also. Tracheostomy is performed if there is doubt about the adequacy of the patient's airway. If the infection has arisen from a dental abscess, expert advice should be sought and this should be dealt with at the same time.

Complications

A parapharyngeal abscess can lead to involvement of the carotid sheath with thrombosis of the internal jugular vein or rupture of the carotid artery. Spread of the abscess into the mediastinum can occur if treatment is not instituted rapidly. The possibility of airway obstruction has already been mentioned.

Retropharyngeal abscess

A collection of pus in the retropharyngeal space occurs in three situations. Acute suppuration in a retropharyngeal lymph node following an upper respiratory tract infection in childhood gives rise to a suppurative retropharyngeal abscess. This condition is very rare in adults because these lymph nodes atrophy in adult life; retropharyngeal abscess of this type is considered in Volume 6. Occasionally a foreign body which has perforated the posterior pharyngeal mucosa will give rise to an abscess in this situation. In adults an abscess in the retropharyngeal space is uncommon and nearly always due to tuberculous disease of the cervical spine which has spread through the anterior longitudinal ligament of the spine to reach the retropharyngeal space. This condition is virtually confined to adult patients and is nearly always due to reactivation of a dormant focus which has arisen from a previous infection of tuberculosis. The previous focus of infection which was almost certainly blood-borne has been controlled by the immune response and reactivation of the focus must be due to a change in the immune system.

Usually the infection begins as a destructive process involving the intervertebral disc and then the anterior portion of the vertebral body. Histologically, the lesion is a granuloma with caseation and with epithelioid cells, giant cells and a surrounding zone of lymphocytes and fibrous tissue.

Clinical features

In the early stages of the disease there may be few symptoms and little to be seen on examination. Pain often occurs and later the patient may have fever. As the process progresses there may be neurological signs and, occasionally, the patient may present with the signs and symptoms of spinal cord compression. The pharynx may appear normal or there may be a marked bulge of the posterior pharyngeal wall. Usually there will be nothing to feel in the neck unless the swelling is huge. Radiology usually shows evidence of bone destruction and loss of the normal curvature of the cervical spine. It must be remembered that the spine may be quite unstable and undue manipulation may precipitate a neurological event. The diagnosis is made by the radiological appearances supplemented by needle biopsy. Surgical drainage of the abscess is not normally necessary but should be carried out through a cervical incision and approach in front of and medial to the carotid sheath. Occasionally exploration of the neck is necessary to obtain biopsy material in order to make the diagnosis.

Treatment should be with chemotherapy and at all times expert advice should be sought regarding the stability of the spine. Spinal fusion is rarely necessary to stabilize the cervical spine. Occasionally, surgery is required to decompress the spinal cord if there is a progressive neurological deficit.

Acute lingual tonsillitis

This is a rare condition, although it would be surprising if some degree of infection did not occur as part of most episodes of acute pharyngitis and acute tonsillitis. It may well be that this is the case, but the infection gives little in the way of signs and is overshadowed by the more obvious infection of the tonsils or pharyngeal lymphoid tissue. Thus lingual tonsillitis is only usually recognized in patients who have had their palatine tonsils removed. The bacteriology and clinical features of the disease are similar to those of acute tonsillitis except that the sore throat tends to be made worse by speech and protrusion of the tongue and the voice has a more striking 'plummy' quality. The lingual tonsil, best visualized on indirect laryngoscopy, is hyperaemic and pus can be seen in the follicles. Treatment is as for acute tonsillitis as are the complications, except that respiratory obstruction due to swelling and oedema of the base of the tongue and supraglottic larynx is more likely to occur.

Diphtheria

Diphtheria is a specific infection caused by the Gram-positive bacillus *Corynebacterium diphtheriae*. In countries with a well-developed immunization programme it is a rare disease (200–300 cases/year in the USA), although it does still occur in epidemics in underdeveloped societies where it carries a mortality of 10%. The disease spreads rapidly in conditions of overcrowding where, in addition, medical care tends to be poor. The disease itself varies in severity depending upon the immunity of the host and also the virulence of the infecting organisms. Clinically, it can vary from an asymptomatic carrier state to a rapidly fatal toxic disease.

Clinical features

The infection remains localized to the primary site of infection, usually the pharynx, larynx and nasal cavities, although in tropical and subtropical countries it gives rise to a cutaneous infection. The systemic effects of the infection are all related to the production of an exotoxin. Spread of infection is by infected droplets of nasal, nasopharyngeal or pharyngeal secretions and the incubation period is 2–6 days. In a host with well-developed immunity to the exotoxin there may be minimal symptoms or none at all, although the organism is still capable of being transmitted. The onset of the illness is heralded by malaise, pyrexia and headache. Anterior nasal diphtheria gives rise to a mucopurulent haemorrhagic discharge with nasal obstruction due to a membrane in the nasal cavity or nasopharynx. Oropharyngeal diphtheria produces a severe sore throat with a greyish-green membrane on the tonsils, posterior pharyngeal wall and soft palate. Tender bilateral cervical lymphadenopathy occurs in the jugulodigastric region. The membrane may spread from the pharynx to the larynx causing rapidly increasing airway obstruction necessitating endotracheal intubation or tracheostomy.

Most of the deaths from diphtheria are related to the toxaemia which causes a myocarditis, cardiac conduction defect and arrhythmias producing acute circulatory failure. The exotoxin may also produce a fatal thrombocytopenia.

Neurological complications may appear 3–6 weeks after the onset of diphtheria and give rise to paralysis of the soft palate, diaphragm, external ocular muscles and occasionally a Guillain-Barré syndrome. Patients who recover from diphtheria may show severe scarring of the nasopharynx and oropharynx including the soft palate and the larynx, with fibrous bands and adhesions.

Differential diagnosis

The diagnosis of diphtheria is unlikely to be missed if the physician considers it, but it may be confused with streptococcal tonsillitis, infectious mononucleosis, the acute manifestations of leukaemia or agranulocytosis.

Treatment

The diagnosis of diphtheria must be made on clinical grounds and cannot await evidence of culture, although microscopic examination of the membrane may be helpful. Treatment involves neutralization of toxin with equine antitoxin (20 000–120 000 units depending upon the severity of the illness) together with benzylpenicillin (600–1200 mg 6-hourly). If the membrane is confined to the tonsils 20 000 units of antitoxin are usually adequate. Higher doses are required if it extends beyond the tonsil. With highly purified antitoxin anaphylactic reaction is rare, but small intramuscular doses can be given, followed in 1–2 hours by a full intravenous dose if there is no reaction.

Immunization

Active immunization against diphtheria is by injection of toxoid (produced by formalin denaturation of toxin) in three doses beginning at 3 months of age. It is this immunization which has so reduced the incidence of diphtheria.

Infectious mononucleosis

This is an acute infection caused by the Epstein-Barr virus which has been isolated from the blood, lymph nodes and saliva of patients with the disease and the latter is probably the mode of transmission. Transmission of the disease to volunteers using the virus has not been accomplished, although there is little doubt that this virus is the causative agent and individuals with antibody to the capsular antigen of the virus will not develop the disease. In general, infectious mononucleosis is a disease of young adults, being very rare in childhood.

Clinical features

The clinical manifestations of infectious mononucleosis are variable ranging from an asymptomatic state to a severe systemic illness with hepatosplenomegaly.

The incubation period is of the order of 5–7 weeks and usually there is a prodomal phase of 4–5 days with malaise, fatigue and headache. The most common manifestation of infectious mononucleosis is tender enlargement of cervical lymph nodes (hence the synonym glandular fever) which, in most patients, is accompanied by a sore throat.

The pharyngeal signs are variable. Often there is an acute follicular tonsillitis, indistinguishable from a streptococcal tonsillitis. On other occasions a limited membrane may form in the oropharynx and there may be petechiae on the soft palate. Occasionally, enlargement of pharyngeal and base of tongue lymphoid tissue together with a membranous slough may produce progressive respiratory obstruction necessitating tracheostomy.

Pyrexia usually accompanies the severe form of the disease and lymph nodes in other regions may be enlarged. Splenomegaly occurs in 50% of patients and hepatomegaly in 10%. Liver function tests are frequently abnormal in infectious mononucleosis and clinical jaundice occurs in about 10% of patients.

A rubelliform rash sometimes occurs and this is almost invariable if ampicillin is mistakenly prescribed for the condition. Ampicillin should therefore never be prescribed for a patient with a sore throat unless it is certain that this is due to acute epiglottitis.

A small proportion of patients may show periorbital oedema particularly involving the lower eyelid and occasionally this may be mistaken for sinusitis, especially in young patients. Other more rare manifestations of infectious mononucleosis include lesions such as facial palsy, Guillaine-Barré syndrome, meningo-encephalitis, myelitis, myocarditis, pericarditis, nephritis and pneumonitis. The blood picture in infectious mononucleosis usually shows a leucocytosis of which 50% are mononuclear cells and 1% are atypical with pleomorphic nuclei. Occasionally haemolytic anaemia, aplastic anaemia or thrombocytopenia will occur.

The diagnosis is made from the clinical picture together with the finding of mononucleosis in the peripheral blood. The white blood count may be normal in the first week but rises in the second. The common serological tests depend upon the development of heterophile antibodies, the most useful being agglutinins to sheep and horse red cells and these antibodies are the basis of the Paul Bunnell and monospot tests. These tests are usually positive in the first week of the disease, although around 10% of patients never develop a positive test. This proportion of negative results may be even higher in children.

Tonsillar debris and cysts

Caseous debris may accumulate in the tonsillar crypts and particularly in the supratonsillar cleft. The patient may notice the accumulation and may express it. This debris is of no significance and should be ignored.

Accumulation of debris in a crypt may form a tonsillar cyst. These appear as yellow-coloured inclusion cysts and again are of no significance and can be ignored.

Occasionally, however, patients do become extremely distressed by the nasty taste of the debris being extruded from the tonsillar crypts and in these patients it may well be reasonable to remove the offending tonsils.

Unilateral tonsillar enlargement

It is not unusual for the tonsils to be somewhat different in size but a gross difference should always be treated with suspicion, particularly if the patient feels the difference is of recent onset. If the larger tonsil appears abnormal a biopsy should be performed; if it looks normal then observation is indicated. Gross asymmetry with enlargement of the tonsil implies neoplasia, usually squamous carcinoma or lymphoma. Occasionally a peritonsillar abscess will give rise to confusion. When examining a patient with an apparent unilateral enlargement of the tonsil great care must be taken to exclude a parapharyngeal mass which is displacing the tonsil medially (see Chapter 22).

Ulceration of the tonsil

The differential diagnosis of an ulcerative lesion of the tonsil is interesting. In theory many different disorders can give rise to an ulcerative lesion of the tonsil but, in practice, most of these can be excluded on history and clinical examination. Other investigations which may be useful are blood picture, chest radiograph, specific blood serological tests and, ultimately, biopsy. Possible causes are listed below.

1 Neoplastic: squamous cell carcinoma, carcinoma of salivary gland origin (adenoid cystic, muco-epidermoid), lymphoma, rarely melanoma, myeloma.
2 Infection:
   acute – acute streptococcal tonsillitis, peritonsillar abscess, acute diphtheria, infectious mononucleosis, Vincent's angina
   chronic – syphilis, tuberculosis
3 Blood diseases: agranulocytosis, leukaemia
4 Miscellaneous: aphthous ulceration, Behçet's syndrome.

Acute pharyngitis

This is probably the most common cause of the 'sore throat' in adults. It may be associated with an upper respiratory tract infection in combination with nasal obstruction and hence mouth breathing. There is lymphoid tissue all over the posterior pharyngeal wall with particular aggregates in the lateral pharyngeal bands and of course in the tonsils (if they have not been removed). There has been a suggestion that removal of the tonsils may predispose to acute pharyngitis, but there seems to be no conclusive evidence to support this. The organisms involved are similar to those in a predominantly tonsillar infection except that viruses probably represent a much higher proportion of the infecting organisms. Because of this, definitive treatment is difficult and hence unless there is obvious bacterial involvement symptomatic relief is probably all that can be offered.

Viral pharyngitis

Many different viruses give rise to a predominantly upper respiratory tract infection which involves a rhinitis, a pharyngitis and, in some cases, a laryngitis. The possible causative organisms are shown in Table 4.1.

When nasal infection and symptoms predominate the illness is designated the common cold or coryza. When the symptoms are fever and malaise with pharyngitis, influenza is usually diagnosed. In an individual patient the signs and symptoms do not allow one to predict which virus is responsible. This can only be ascertained by serological tests showing rising antibody titres and this, of course, is rarely of practical importance. Most children

Table 4.1 Causative organisms in viral pharyngitis

Rhinoviruses
Coronaviruses
Influenza A and B viruses
Parainfluenza viruses
Adenoviruses
Enteroviruses
Respiratory syncytial virus

and adults will suffer three or four virus infections per year and these often occur in epidemics. Spread of viruses is by droplet infection and once in the upper respiratory tract the virus will enter the epithelial lining cells. It may be prevented from doing this by the presence of specific secretory antibodies in the mucociliary blanket lining the upper respiratory tract, non-specific antiviral mucoproteins or by the mechanical effect of ciliary action. Once within the epithelial cells lining the upper respiratory tract the virus divides and the cells die. The systemic effects of an acute viral illness such as fever, headache, myalgia, arthralgia, anorexia are either a result of haematogenous and systemic spread of the virus or the release of intracellular factors caused by the necrosis of epithelial cells.

Clinical features

The sore throat may be the initial symptom of an acute pharyngitis or it may be preceded by a rhinitis and/or conjunctivitis or by a day or so of malaise. It is made worse by swallowing and the pain may radiate to the ears. Cervical lymphadenopathy may occur and the clinical manifestations depend upon the nature of the virus and the resistance of the host. Thus the larynx may be involved producing hoarseness, and the lower respiratory tract may also be colonized, producing cough. It is not unusual for acute otitis media of the suppurative or non-suppurative type to be part of the illness. Secondary bacterial infection probably does occur on occasions and this will also affect the clinical picture. Examination of the patient may reveal a rhinitis, with secretions in the nasal cavities and hyperaemic congested turbinates. The nasopharynx may be hyperaemic and the mucosa covered by mucopus. The posterior pharyngeal wall also shows streams of mucopus with hyperaemic islands of lymphoid tissue which may occasionally show pustular follicles. The tonsils may be inflamed, as may the larynx. The course of the illness again depends upon host resistance and the virulence of the organism, but usually the disease is self-limiting, lasting for 3 or 4 days.

Treatment

None of these illnesses is sufficiently severe to warrant antiviral agents and so treatment must be symptomatic with bed-rest, analgesics (e.g. aspirin) and fluids by mouth. If a significant bacterial complication has occurred, antibiotics are indicated.

Complications

These are mainly local complications such as sinusitis, otitis media, laryngitis, tracheobronchitis and pneumonia. The laryngitis may occasionally result in sufficient oedema to produce a degree of respiratory obstruction, but this is much more common in children than adults. General complications are rare but include meningitis, encephalitis and myocarditis. The usual cause of death in patients with an upper respiratory virus infection is a viral pneumonia with secondary infection and this is much more likely in elderly or debilitated patients.

Herpes simplex

The herpes simplex virus occurs in two forms; type I usually affects the oral cavity and oropharynx and type II generally gives rise to genital infection. Primary infection with the type I herpes simplex virus usually affects children and causes a severe vesicular and ulcerative stomatitis affecting the lips, gums, tongue, buccal mucosa, soft palate and occasionally spreading to the oropharynx. Children with this condition are ill with pyrexia, tachycardia and cervical lymphadenopathy. Diagnosis is normally obvious, although ocasionally it can be confused with Stevens-Johnson syndrome (see below) and can be confirmed by isolation of virus from an unruptured vesicle. The virus can be identified using fluorescent antibody or can be seen as an intranuclear inclusion in the scrapings.

Usually the treatment of primary herpes is non-specific, namely analgesics and fluids, which may need to be given intravenously. Secondary herpetic infection occurs when the herpes virus resides within the posterior root ganglion following a primary stomatitis. Intercurrent illness then results in the appearance of herpetic vesicles usually on the lips or at the angles of the mouth as a typical cold sore.

Acyclovir is an active agent against herpes viruses but does not eradicate them. It is effective only if started at the onset of infection.

Uses of acyclovir include systemic treatment of zoster infections and in systemic and topical treatment of herpes simplex and infections of the skin and mucous membranes. It can be life saving in herpes simplex and zoster infections in the immunocompromised patient.

Herpes zoster

Zoster virus is the same virus as that which causes chicken-pox (varicella). Herpes zoster probably arises by the reactivation of virus particles which have remained in the cranial nerve nuclei, ganglia or spinal root ganglion following a previous attack of chicken-pox. Thus it resembles the reactivation of herpes simplex virus in cold sores. Also, however, herpes zoster can occur during an epidemic of chicken-pox. In the pharynx, eruption of zoster can occur in the distribution of the Vth, IXth and Xth cranial nerves. Thus the palate can be affected or the tonsil and posterior pharyngeal wall. This is often associated with herpes zoster oticus (see Volumes 2 and 3) and the pharyngeal manifestations are very transient and easily overlooked. They may give rise to pain on swallowing, and vesicles and shallow ulcers, which heal rapidly, may be seen on the soft palate, hard palate, tonsil or posterior pharyngeal wall.

Vesicular and bullous eruptions of the pharynx

Herpangina, herpes simplex (less commonly) and herpes zoster may give rise to vesicles in the pharynx which break down and form small ulcers which heal rapidly. Other conditions which may occur are Stevens-Johnson syndrome, pemphigus, pemphigoid and benign mucous membrane pemphigus. These conditions affect the skin and mucous membrane of the mouth and on occasions the oropharynx. Only very rarely is the pharynx involved without involvement of the oral cavity and these conditions are discussed in Chapter 3.

Other specific viral illnesses
Hand, foot and mouth syndrome

This is an illness probably caused by a coxsackie virus (an enterovirus). The disease is characterized by a vesicular eruption in both the oral cavity and the oropharynx, accompanied by vesicles on the hands and feet. There is also usually pyrexia with malaise. The illness is short-lived and self-limiting and mainly affects children.

Herpangina

This is a self-limiting vesicular eruption which occurs in the oropharynx and a number of enteroviruses have been implicated. It is distinguished from herpes simplex which is almost always restricted to the oral cavity and very rarely spreads to the pharynx.

Cytomegalovirus infections

This virus is usually transmitted by blood transfusion, although it can occur without, especially in immuno-suppressed states. It gives rise to an illness which is very similar to infectious mononucleosis. The diagnosis is made by serial antibody levels.

Other causes of acute pharyngitis

Acute gonococcal pharyngitis

This disease is acquired following orogenital sexual intercourse and the majority of patients who acquire it are asymptomatic. Some may have a transient sore throat and occasionally an exudative gonococcal tonsillitis will occur with an appearance similar to streptococcal tonsillitis or infectious mononucleosis. There will also be tender enlarged cervical lymph nodes. If the diagnosis is suspected the patient should be treated with 4.8 mega units of procaine penicillin given intramuscularly usually with probenicid. A swab should be taken for microscopy and for culture and sensitivity tests. Some gonococci produce a beta-lactamase (penicillinase) and are therefore relatively resistant to penicillin treatment. This should be suspected in patients who give a history of sexual contact in the Far East. Oral tetracycline should be used for those patients who do not improve with penicillin, and the treatment failures seem to be more frequent in patients with gonococcal pharyngitis than in those with genital infections. The dangers of gonococcal infection are those of septicaemia with septic foci in many organs, but particularly in joints and tendons. As well as septic arthritis, there occurs with gonococcal infections an arthritis which seems to be a hypersensitivity reaction and may be associated with iritis.

Oedema of the uvula

Acute oedema of the uvula (Quinke's disease) is unusual without an obvious precipitating cause. The patient complains of the onset of a tickle or irritation in the throat together with a sensation of gagging. Examination shows oedema of the uvula which on occasions may be very severe indeed. The aetiology is unknown but may be related to an inhaled or ingested allergen. The oedema usually settles down of its own accord (perhaps assisted by an intravenous injection of hydrocortisone), unless it is part of a more serious allergic reaction such as angioneurotic oedema.

Other causes which produce oedema of the uvula are numerous and include:

1 Trauma: foreign bodies, surgery, endotracheal intubation
2 Infection:

acute – peritonsillar abscess, viral pharyngitis, candidiasis
chronic – syphilis, tuberculosis
3 Tumours: squamous carcinoma
4 Radiotherapy
5 Allergic angioneurotic oedema
6 Blood diseases: agranulocytosis, acute leukaemia
7 Miscellaneous: aphthous ulceration, Behçet's syndrome.

Chronic pharyngitis

This title implies a long-standing infection or inflammation of the pharynx; classically the disease is divided into specific or non-specific types. Specific chronic infections are due to a well-defined pathological entity, although sometimes the differentiation between acute and chronic is a little blurred. Non-specific pharyngitis is a much more difficult entity to define and diagnose and therefore to treat. It is discussed first.

Chronic non-specific pharyngitis

A general practitioner sees large numbers of patients with chronic sore throats and hence the diagnosis of chronic pharyngitis is commonly made. The appearance of the pharynx shows generalized diffuse hypertrophy of the pharyngeal lymphoid tissue and particularly that of the lateral pharyngeal bands. This lymphoid tissue may or may not look inflamed and it is probably true to say that patients with no symptoms often have hypertrophy of their pharyngeal lymphoid tissue. The condition is sometimes called chronic granular pharyngitis.

The aetiology of this condition is usually obscure. Chronic sinusitis with postnasal drip should be excluded either clinically or by sinus radiographs. Bronchiectasis is said to be associated but usually the chest symptoms predominate. Severe dental caries may be the source of infection but this is now a rare finding. Irritants such as tobacco, alcohol or industrial fumes have to be inquired about and eliminated if relevant laboratory tests such as throat swabs or blood tests are of no useful value. It is always important to examine these patients carefully including their neck as very occasionally there may be an underlying pharyngeal carcinoma. Referred pain in the ear is always a dangerous sign in chronic pharyngitis.

Having said all this by far the commonest situation is the patient with a chronic sore throat and no obvious aetiological factors. Globus pharyngis (see Chapter 24) is recognized by some as a definite clinical entity and certainly the impression is often of some psychological overlay. Fear of cancer may be dominant in the patient's mind and specific denial of this is often of help in trying to reassure the patient.

A variety of somewhat non-specific remedies such as gargles, antiseptic or analgesic throat sprays have been used but it is doubtful if they do identifiable good. Surgeons have been pressed into using electrocautery or even cryosurgery to the lymphoid tissue but these produce severe discomfort and have no proven value whatsoever. Reassurance and the exclusion of malignancy are probably the two most important methods of offering the patient useful help.

Chronic specific pharyngitis

These entities are discussed below but not in order of incidence, simply in an order of convenience.

Syphilis

This is an infection by the spirochaete *Treponema pallidum* and apart from the congenital form is acquired by sexual intercourse. The disease progresses through primary, secondary and tertiary stages with the secondary most likely to give rise to pharyngeal symptoms. The disease manifests itself in a great many ways and clinical presentations, particularly in the tertiary stage where the presenting symptom may involve virtually any organ system. The lesion of primary syphilis is at the site of the initial inoculation and the organism can penetrate both normal mucosa and mucosal abrasions. The primary pathology in syphilis is an endarteritis with an increase in adventitial cells, a proliferation of endothelial cells and an inflammatory focus of lymphocytes, plasma cells and monocytes. Usually in parts of the lesion healing with fibrous tissue is taking place. In the secondary and particularly in the tertiary phase of the disease a granulomatous reaction takes place with necrosis of tissue and occasional giant cells.

Primary syphilis

The lesion is the chancre which develops after an incubation period of about 21 days. The most frequent extragenital sites for a chancre are the lips, tongue, buccal mucosa and tonsil. The lesion begins as a papule which breaks down to form a painless ulcer with indurated margins. At the same time there may be unilateral or bilateral cervical lymphadenopathy and the glands are nontender. Although the chancre is characteristically painless secondary infection can render it painful. The ulcer persists for a variable period, 2–6 weeks as a rule, and then heals. While the primary lesion is present the individual is capable of transmitting the disease.

Secondary syphilis

The secondary stage occurs several weeks (usually 4–6 weeks) after the primary lesion and about 30% of patients in the secondary stage will have evidence of a healing chancre. The features of the secondary stage are fever, headache and malaise with generalized lymphadenopathy and a mucocutaneous rash and sore throat. The pharynx and soft palate show hyperaemia and inflammation, and may show lesions which have been described as mucous patches or snail-track ulcers. These lesions are more commonly seen in the oral cavity and are ulcerated lesions covered with a greyish-white membrane which, when scraped off, has a pink base with no bleeding. The secondary stage of the disease lasts a few weeks and here again the lesions in the mouth and pharynx are infectious. About 30% of patients will go on to develop the tertiary stage of the disease.

Tertiary syphilis

This develops some years (5–25) after the initial infection and is characterized by lesions which may be widespread throughout the body or restricted to one or two organ systems. In the upper respiratory tract the manifestations are those of the gumma. This is the granulomatous necrotic lesion which begins as a nodule and then breaks down to form an ulcer. It can occur in the hard palate, the nasal septum, the tonsil, posterior pharyngeal wall or in the larynx. The gumma, whether ulcerated or not, is typically painless. There is usually no lymphadenopathy associated with these lesions unless they are secondarily infected. When treated with penicillin the gumma will rapidly heal.

Diagnosis

In the primary or secondary stage of the disease spirochaetes can be identified by dark field illumination microscopy in smears taken directly from the lesion. The spirochaetes can also be identified in biopsy specimens using silver stains or fluorescein-labelled antibody. Biopsy of a tertiary lesion gives a typical histopathological picture. Serological tests for syphilis fall into two main groups; those used to identify non-specific antibodies to cardiolipin (VDRL tests) and those to detect specific treponemal antibodies (TPI and FTA).

The VDRL (Venereal Disease Research Laboratory) tests use an antigen extracted from beef heart in a slide flocculation test. The VDRL reaction begins to become positive during the first or second week after the development of the chancre and 99% of patients with secondary syphilis give a positive reaction as do a similar proportion with tertiary syphilis. Unfortunately, a proportion of patients with other diseases also give a positive reaction. These include other infections involving non-syphilitic treponemes (yaws, bejel or pinta which are cutaneous infections) and also infections such as atypical pneumonia, malaria, smallpox and leprosy. Some patients with disordered immune systems such as those with systemic lupus erythematosus or rheumatoid arthritis will give a positive reaction and occasionally elderly patients who have never been exposed to syphilis will show a positive reaction.

Of the tests for specific antibody, the TPI (*Treponema pallidum* immobilization) is the most specific but also the most expensive. It depends upon the ability of an antibody in the patient's serum to immobilize spirochaetes which are observed by dark ground illumination. The TPI test is 100% positive in patients with established secondary and tertiary syphilis and, if carried out correctly, is entirely specific. The FTA (fluorescent treponemal antibody) test involves the absorption from the patient's serum of cross-reacting antibodies using non-pathogenic treponemes and then absorption of specific antibody by dried *Treponema pallidum* preparations. The absorbed antibody is identified by a fluorescein-labelled antihuman gamma globulin. The FTA test is positive in 100% of patients with secondary and tertiary syphilis and the false positive rate is not as high as in the VDRL reaction, but occasionally patients with systemic lupus erythematosus or rheumatoid arthritis will be positive.

Treatment

In primary and secondary syphilis a dose of 2.4 mega units of benzathine penicillin in a single or two intramuscular injections is satisfactory. In tertiary syphilis a total of 7.2 mega units of benzathine penicillin is given usually as 2.4 mega unit injections at around 7- and 14-day intervals.

Tuberculosis

The pharynx is not a common site for clinically manifest tuberculosis. However, it is the site of primary infection which nearly always occurs in children and results in an asymptomatic primary focus in the pharynx (usually the tonsil or adenoid) with cervical lymphadenopathy.

Secondary tuberculosis affects the pharynx but only in patients with massive sputum positive and usually cavitating pulmonary tuberculosis. This is in contrast with laryngeal tuberculosis when lesions do occur with low grade or inactive pulmonary disease. The pharyngeal lesions are secondary to coughing up heavily infected sputum and consist of multiple very painful shallow ulcers in the pharynx or oral cavity. Occasionally the pharynx is involved in patients with widespread miliary tuberculosis and here the lesions may be from blood-borne as well as sputum-borne dissemination of the disease. Lupus

vulgaris is a low grade cutaneous infection of tuberculosis and has been described in the nasal cavities and in the pharynx. Tuberculous otitis media is probably a blood-borne dissemination of the disease but occasionally it can arise from pharyngeal disease by spread from the eustachian tube.

Diagnosis

There is little difficulty in making the diagnosis of pharyngeal tuberculosis because of the association with pulmonary disease which is obvious clinically and radiologically.

Treatment

Pharyngeal tuberculosis needs no special treatment; it will be treated at the same time as the pulmonary disease, namely with triple therapy usually using isoniazid, rifampicin and pyrazinamide as first line drugs.

Toxoplasmosis

Toxoplasmosis is a common disease of birds and mammals caused by the protozoan *Toxoplasma gondii*. The infection can be transmitted to humans by the ingestion of cysts in uncooked meat or food contaminated with animal faeces. In immunocompetent humans acquired toxoplasmosis usually gives rise to no symptoms. Some will have a sore throat with malaise and fever and cervical lymphadenopathy and, on occasions, the patient will simply present with an enlarged cervical lymph node. The fever and malaise may last for several weeks and many organ systems may be involved, e.g. lungs, myocardium, pericardium, liver, brain and skeletal muscles. The disease is usually self-limiting and death is most unusual.

In immunodeficient individuals the disease may be much more serious with multisystem failure and death.

The diagnosis of the disease can be made by a serological test which is an indirect dye or fluorescent antibody test. On occasions lymph nodes will be removed for purposes of biopsy and the histology is typical with follicular hyperplasia and typical epithelioid cells.

Treatment

Usually no treatment is necessary but in those individuals with a severe systemic upset or in immunodeficient patients a combination of pyrimethamine and sulphadiazine is indicated.

Leprosy

Isolated leprosy of the pharynx does not occur; it spreads to the nasopharynx and occasionally to the oropharynx from the nasal cavities. Leprosy is an infection caused by *Mycobacterium leprae* which produces a chronic disease with a spectrum of clinical manifestations. Tuberculoid leprosy is a low grade lesion affecting an area of skin and its nerve supply. Lepromatous leprosy is a more florid form of the disease with massive infection of the dermis of the skin; it can affect the nasal cavities, nasopharynx and also the testes and lymphoreticular system. Disease in the pharynx spreads from the nasal cavities and gives rise to a combination of granulomatous lesions, ulcerating and healing with fibrosis. The diagnosis is usually made by biopsy and the treatment is by chemotherapy with sulphones.

Scleroma

This is a chronic infective condition caused by *Klebsiella rhinoscleromatis*. The disease begins in the nose and only secondarily spreads to involve the pharynx where it produces granulomatous lesions and scarring.

Fungal infections

Candidiasis (moniliasis)

Candida albicans is a fungus which is part of the flora of the oral cavity or oropharynx in 30–40% of normal individuals. For the organism to become pathogenic and give rise to symptoms there must be a local or systemic change in the host. It has been called a 'disease of the diseased'.

Local changes which predispose to infection by candida may be caused by local diseases such as lichen planus and leukoplakia. Systemic antibiotic administration may change the oral flora sufficiently to disturb the local balance and allow overgrowth of candida. Radiotherapy to the oral cavity and pharynx is often complicated by candida.

In patients with chronic ill health, and particularly immunocompromised individuals, candidiasis of the oral cavity or pharynx may occur. Thus diabetes mellitus, lymphoma and treatment with immunosuppressive agents predispose to candidiasis. It is a common feature in patients with acquired immune deficiency syndrome (AIDS).

Infection with candida in the oral cavity or pharynx may be asymptomatic or may give rise to severe pain with dysphagia. Clinically it gives rise to small white patches which when removed leave an erythematous ulcer.

Candidiasis can be treated by local or systemic therapy or a combination of the two. Attention must be paid to the predisposing condition if this is possible. Local antifungal agents are usually effective: nystatin 100 000 units 6-hourly, amphotericin 100 000 units 6-hourly, miconazole 125 mg 6-hourly; occasionally systemic therapy (ketoconazole 100 mg twice daily) will be more effective.

Pharyngeal symptoms of blood disease

Certain blood diseases, because of their effect on the immune system, often present with lesions in the mouth or pharynx.

Agranulocytosis

Diseases which result in a severe decrease in the number of polymorphonuclear leucocytes are unusual but often present with oral and pharyngeal symptoms. Occasionally agranulocytosis will be idiopathic, but most of these disorders are hypersensitivity reactions to drugs which only affect a small proportion of patients. Some are dose related, others are not. A large variety of different drugs is likely to produce these reactions, e.g. chloramphenicol, sulphonamides, phenylbutazone, thiouracil, carbimazole and chlorpromazine. Chemotherapeutic cytotoxic agents have a direct effect on bone marrow and result in marrow aplasia and this is dose related. The first symptoms associated with agranulocytosis are fever and headache with severe pain on swallowing. The lesions in the pharynx are necrotic ulcers with a slough and may be single but are usually multiple and coalescent. There is usually no cervical lymphadenopathy. There is often severe halitosis and the patient becomes very ill. Culture of the ulcers rarely gives any information usually only yielding normal commensal organisms. The diagnosis of agranulocytic pharyngitis is made on a blood count and film which should always be performed on any patient with a sore throat. Treatment involves withdrawal of the precipitating agent, high dose steroids and systemic antibiotics. Blood transfusions are often necessary.

Acute leukaemia

Acute leukaemia may be of three types (lymphoblastic, myeloblastic and monoblastic), although the clinical presentation is indistinguishable. The lymphatic type is most common in children, myeloid most common in young adults and the monocytic can occur at any age. These diseases present with fever, anaemia and bleeding disorders. Often the oral or pharyngeal manifestations are the first symptoms. Ulceration with slough and membrane formation occurs on the gums, in the oral cavity and in the pharynx. There is nothing specific about these lesions except for their severe extent and the fact that they are often associated with haemorrhage. Often there is an associated bilateral cervical lymphadenopathy. The diagnosis is made by a blood picture and bone marrow examination.

Vincent's angina

Vincent's angina (trench mouth) is an infection with a spirochaete, *Borellia vincentii* and an anaerobic organism *Bacillus fusiformis*. In general, Vincent's angina occurs in patients with very poor dental hygiene and a generally debilitated condition. It can occur, however, without these predisposing factors. It is essentially a necrotizing gingivitis with ulceration and bleeding of the gums which are covered with a necrotic membrane. The lesions are painful and associated with marked fetor and the patient may be pyrexial and often has tender enlarged cervical glands. The lesions may spread to involve the tonsils but, on occasions, the tonsil may be involved without a gingivitis or stomatitis. The lesion of the tonsil is a deep ulcer with a grey slough in its base. The diagnosis is made by taking scrapings from the ulcer or gingiva on a slide, staining with gentian violet and identifying both the spirochaete and the fusiform bacillus. Treatment of Vincent's angina is usually local with peroxide mouthwashes, care from a dental hygienist, together with benzylpenicillin. In addition, metronidazole (500 mg 8-hourly intravenously) should be given.

Pharyngeal stenosis

Stenosis of the pharynx is not common. When it occurs there is fibrous tissue formation with adhesions and fibrous strands covered by mucous membrane. It can occur in the nasopharynx involving the posterior choanae or the eustachian openings. It may also arise in the oropharynx and the soft palate may be firmly fixed to the posterior pharyngeal wall. Stenosis in the nasopharynx and oropharynx may affect nasal respiration, speech and eustachian tube function. Swallowing is usually affected by hypopharyngeal stenosis. Involvement of the larynx by the same pathological process which caused stenosis of the pharynx is much more serious and results in dysphonia and airway difficulty. The causes of stenosis are varied (Table 4.2) and usually stenosis is the end result of an inflammatory process. Occasionally the stenosis may occur at the same time as the active pathological process (e.g. scleroma, leprosy, Wegener's granuloma).

Treatment of established stenosis of the nasopharynx or oropharynx is rarely necessary or successful. Hypopharyngeal stenosis can be treated by repeated dilatation.

Pharyngeal manifestations of human immunodeficiency virus infection

Between 40 and 60% of patients with acquired immunodeficiency syndrome (AIDS) secondary to

Table 4.2 Causes of pharyngeal stenosis

1   Trauma
     Surgical, adenoidectomy, tonsillectomy, cleft palate repair, pharyngoplasty, laryngectomy, pharyngolaryngectomy; inhalation of corrosives, burns with smoke inhalation, radiation therapy
2   Acute infection
     Acute streptococcal tonsillitis, acute diphtheria
3   Chronic infection
     Syphilis, tuberculosis, leprosy, scleroma
4   Miscellaneous
     Wegener's granuloma, Behçet's syndrome, aphthous ulceration, pemphigus, pemphigoid

human immunodeficiency virus (HIV) infection manifest symptoms referable to the head and neck region (Sooy, 1987). During the initial seroconversion to HIV-infection patients may develop a glandular-fever-like illness. In the HIV-infected patient hairy leukoplakia, opportunistic infections, lymphoid tissue hyperplasia/hypertrophy and HIV-related neoplasia frequently involve the pharynx.

Hairy leukoplakia

Hairy leukoplakia occurs in 5–25% of patients with AIDS. Typically it affects the oral cavity, particularly the lateral and dorsal surfaces of the tongue (Greenspan *et al.*, 1984). It has also been reported to involve the oropharyngeal mucosa, usually on the soft palate (Eversole, 1989).

Opportunistic infections

Candidiasis

Oral candidiasis is common in patients infected with HIV (Greenspan *et al.*, 1990). A large number of these patients will go on to develop diffuse pharyngeal and oesophageal candidiasis. This infection may cause severe dysphagia and odynophagia. Treatment of upper aerodigestive tract candidiasis in HIV-infected patients often involves repeated courses of topical and systemic antifungal medications (De Wit *et al.*, 1989; Dull *et al.*, 1991).

Viruses

Opportunistic viral infections affect the upper aerodigestive tract. Cytomegalovirus, herpes simplex virus and the human immunodeficiency virus infection can result in pharyngeal mucosal ulceration with associated pain and dysphagia (Kansas *et al.*, 1987). These opportunistic viral infections are frequently prolonged and recurrent. Treatment with systemic acyclovir and analgesics is effective.

Lymphoid tissue hyperplasia

In the HIV-infected population lymphoid tissue hyperplasia and hypertrophy commonly occurs in the head and neck region. It may involve both nodal and extranodal lymphoid tissue. This results in cervical lymphadenopathy, adenoid hypertrophy and both lingual and palatine tonsillar hypertrophy (Olsen, Jeffery and Sooy, 1988; Barzan *et al.*, 1989). The cause of this lymphoid tissue hyperplasia is unclear. Polyclonal B-cell activation facilitated by infection with HIV, Epstein-Barr virus or cytomegalovirus has been implicated.

Nasal obstruction is a common presenting complaint and otitis media with effusion is a frequent finding. Occasionally massive adenotonsillar hypertrophy may occur and cause airway obstruction (Kraus *et al.*, 1990). Although the nasopharyngeal mass is often benign in lymphoid tissue hyperplasia, it is important that adenoidectomy is performed to rule out extranodal lymphomas, Kaposi's sarcoma and nasopharyngeal carcinoma (Lanser, Klein and Marvin, 1985; Lees, Kessler and Michael, 1987; Ergeter and Beckstead, 1988; Stern, Lin and Lucente, 1990). Extensive surgical resection of the nasopharyngeal lymphoid tissue is not indicated. Medical treatment with antibiotics and topical aqueous nasal steroid sprays will often provide symptomatic relief of the nasal obstruction. Middle ear effusions are managed with myringotomy and ventilation tube insertion. Similarly, it is important to biopsy unilateral hypertrophic palatine or lingual tonsils to rule out neoplasia in HIV-infected individuals (Sooy, 1987). In patients where massive lymphoid hypertrophy leads to airway obstruction then a more extensive procedure may be required to secure a safe airway.

Neoplasia

Benign tumours

Human papilloma virus is associated with papillomas, verruca vulgaris and condyloma acuminata. These lesions are commonly found in the oral cavity and oropharynx of HIV-infected patients and have an appearance similar to genital warts. The lesions should be excised if they are symptomatic, anogenital lesions should be treated particularly in the HIV-infected male homosexual group (Greenspan *et al.*, 1990).

Malignant tumours

Lymphoma

Lymphoma is common in patients with advanced HIV disease. Non-Hodgkin's lymphoma is the most common AIDS-associated tumour of the pharynx. The tumours are usually extranodal and typically high grade B-cell lymphomas. They occur most frequently in the nasopharynx and palatine tonsil. Treatment with systemic chemotherapy results in complete response in about 50% of patients, but survival averages less than 6 months (Kaplan *et al.*, 1989).

Kaposi's sarcoma

HIV-related Kaposi's sarcoma commonly affects the pharyngeal mucosa. It has been reported in the nasopharynx, tonsillar fossa, posterior oropharyngeal wall and the hypopharynx (Patow *et al.*, 1984a). Tumour enlargement may result in a globus pharyngis sensation, dysphagia and airway obstruction (Patow *et al.*, 1984b). Tumour ulceration may lead to considerable pain and odynophagia. Treatment of these lesions, although controversial, is with radiotherapy alone or in combination with chemotherapy. Concomitant additional treatment for antifungal and antiherpetic prophylaxis is of benefit in reducing the florid radiation-induced mucositis (Ficarra *et al.*, 1989). Surgical resection, cryotherapy and laser ablation may provide successful local treatment.

Squamous cell carcinoma

The incidence of squamous cell carcinoma of the oral cavity is increased in patients with AIDS (Silverman, 1987). The incidence of pharyngeal squamous cell carcinomas in HIV-infected patients is unknown.

Obstructive sleep apnoea

This is a subject which is incompletely understood at the present time and there are many questions which remain unanswered about apnoea during sleep. There is no doubt that normal individuals have apnoeic episodes when asleep and that these episodes are completely harmless. On the other hand, there are examples of patients who have developed right-sided heart failure and pulmonary hypertension secondary to upper airway obstruction with apnoea. The difficulty lies in the area between these two extremes and how one should define it. Apnoea during sleep has been divided into obstructive, central and mixed; obstructive apnoea being preceded by upper respiratory obstruction with increasing respiratory effort. Central apnoea occurs without this increasing respiratory effort but the mechanism could still be obstructive; it is simply that the drive to respiration is lacking. Purely central apnoea with no obstructive element does occur but is probably very rare. Mixed apnoea is a combination of failure of central control and upper airway obstruction.

The mechanism of the upper airway obstruction is unknown, but it has certainly been demonstrated that in sleep there is reduced activity in the muscles of the tongue, soft palate and pharynx and this reduced activity may have a central component (Remmers *et al.*, 1978). The loss of tone in the muscles of the tongue, soft palate and pharynx results in a collapse of the airway due to a suction effect and, as respiratory effort increases, the suction and therefore the obstruction increases. As the patient becomes hypoxic there is an arousal response which increases muscle tone and improves the airway. This loss of tone in upper airway musclature during sleep has been demonstrated in normal asymptomatic individuals and the factors which lead to the development of the full-blown obstructive sleep apnoea syndrome are probably multiple. It has arbitrarily been accepted that obstructive sleep apnoea occurs when a patient has 30 apnoeic episodes each lasting 10 seconds or more during 7 hours of sleep. This is reinforced if it can be demonstrated that during these apnoeic episodes the oxygen saturation levels in arterial blood fall. This standard for sleep apnoea is by no means universally accepted and much more investigation remains to be done.

A number of studies casts doubt upon the validity of this standard. For example an investigation of normal individuals by Black *et al.* (1979) has shown that up to 50% of these would fit the above criteria for sleep apnoea, with oxygen desaturation falling as low as 60%. The relationship between snoring and sleep apnoea is also ill-defined. Snoring is more common in elderly men and occurs in a surprisingly high proportion of the population (Lugaresi *et al.*, 1980). Snoring is associated with a high incidence of systemic hypertension and simple snorers can develop obstructive sleep apnoea after alcohol excess (Remmers *et al.*, 1978). Thus, the supposition has been raised that a proportion of patients who snore may go on to develop obstructive sleep apnoea.

Clinical features

The classical features of the pickwickian syndrome, which is the first described example of sleep apnoea syndrome, occur only rarely (Gastaut, Tassinari and Duron, 1966). The classical description is of a squat, obese individual with a short fat neck who snores heavily with increasing respiratory effort until prolonged apnoeic episodes occur with cyanosis. The patient then begins to breathe again with semi-arousal only to drift back into sleep and a further apnoeic episode. This disturbed sleep with oxygen desaturation leads to daytime somnolence such that the individual is falling off to sleep during the daytime and it may be difficult to distinguish the condition from narcolepsy.

Obstructive sleep apnoea can and does occur in non-obese individuals, although it seems to be more prevalent in elderly obese males. The reported incidence in the USA is considerably higher than that in the UK and Europe. This may be a real difference between the populations or may be an apparent one generated by the fact that many more sleep laboratories exist in the USA for the investigation of such disorders. Examination of the oropharynx of patients with obstructive sleep apnoea may reveal no abnormality, although a proportion has a rather elongated soft palate and uvula. Examination may also show a cause for nasal obstruction such as a deviated nasal septum or nasal polyps. It should be remembered that patients with asthma and those with obstructive lung disease may show sleep disturbance and nocturnal oxygen desaturation. After full clinical examination, investigation of patients with obstructive sleep apnoea requires sinus and chest radiography, full blood picture and pulmonary function tests. Polysomnography is essential but the facilities for this are sparse in the UK at present. Thus monitoring during sleep with ECG, EEG, EOG (electro-oculogram), oximetry, oral and nasal thermisters and thoracoabdominal strain gauges is necessary. Patients with obstructive sleep apnoea will show apnoeic episodes preceded by increasing respiratory effort but reduced air flow. Oxygen desaturation is often accompanied by bradycardia and cardiac arrhythmias eventually leading to right ventricular failure and hypertension.

Treatment

This is a controversial subject and even more so if one considers the treatment of snoring as well. Patients with severe obstructive sleep apnoea with oxygen desaturation certainly should be treated and the options are as follows.

In patients who are obese, weight loss may help and also may make other treatment more successful. Medical treatment of obstructive sleep apnoea includes the continuous administration of oxygen at increased pressure (CPAP), although this is not comfortable and not well tolerated by patients. Protriptyline has been shown to decrease the number of apnoeic episodes.

The most successful surgery for obstructive sleep apnoea is tracheostomy, although this has major disadvantages. Correction of obvious upper airway defects such as a severely deviated nasal septum or removal of nasal polyps may help some patients and should be carried out before more drastic measures are undertaken. Excision of part of the soft palate and uvula (palatopharyngoplasty) has been described (Blair-Simmons, Guilleminault and Silvestri, 1983) and the results documented. The surgery involves resection of the tonsils if they are still present together with a portion of the free edge of the soft palate and uvula. It is yet to be determined how much tissue should be resected and depends upon the amount which it is thought is redundant (in some patients as has already been said the soft palate looks normal and yet resection of some soft palate will improve the symptoms of obstructive sleep apnoea). In general, 10–15 mm of soft palate should be resected more medially than laterally. If the tonsils are removed at the same time, suturing the anterior to the posterior pillar has been advised. If the tonsil is not present but the pillars seem excessively flaccid a portion should be resected. The bare surface of the soft palate remaining after resection is sutured so that the mucosa of the posterior surface is brought into contact with the anterior surface.

The results of palatopharyngoplasty are variable. Some patients are cured of sleep apnoea and oxygen saturation levels of 60% before surgery may return to normal after surgery. Some patients are helped only to a marginal extent and some not at all. The implication in these patients is that the obstruction is at another level and mandibular osteotomies, hyoid bone expansion or wedge resection of parts of the base of the tongue have on occasions been helpful (Guilleminault, 1984).

In patients with very severe apnoea and desaturation levels down to 50% tracheostomy is probably the treatment of choice. The complications of palatopharyngoplasty are similar to those of tonsillectomy with the addition of palatal incompetence in some. Postoperatively, approximately 30% of patients will have regurgitation of fluid but this proportion improves until only a small percentage remains. However, in these patients nasal regurgitation of fluids and speech with nasal escape is permanent.

Tonsillectomy

Tonsillectomy in children and adults has always been a controversial topic and has promoted endless discussion for many years. For a while in the 1950s and 1960s the operation was performed when the indications for surgery were at the very least doubtful. The pendulum then swung and patients were denied the operation despite repeated periods of time off work and considerable morbidity. There is no doubt that there are indications for adult tonsillectomy, but the surgeon must be clear in his mind that he is confident that he is going to help the patient by removing the tonsils. The indications should therefore be stringent and loose indications such as halitosis, globus hystericus and others are to be condemned (Tucker, 1982a). Such indications simply expose the patient to needless trauma and risk and serve to damage the reputation of otolaryngology as a surgical specialty. Nevertheless, when performed for the correct indications adult tonsillectomy is a very worthwhile procedure.

Indications

Recurrent tonsillitis

Tonsillitis does occur in adults, usually young adults, but it is not common. Although there is no recognized association it not infrequently becomes a problem in young adults who have had infectious mononucleosis. Repeated attacks (three to four per year for 2–3 years) of true acute tonsillitis are a definite indication. Acute tonsillitis is a significant identifiable illness with severe sore throat, pyrexia, often dysphagia, and generalized systemic upset. This must be distinguished from the more vague minor or chronic sore throat and in fact like chronic appendicitis, there is no such condition as chronic tonsillitis. Chronic pharyngitis, which has already been discussed, is not helped by tonsillectomy. The general practitioner has to be relied upon to supply the information as to whether the patient has been having genuine attacks of acute tonsillitis as simple inspection of the tonsils when not infected does not help as a useful guide to the need for surgery. There is absolutely no place for a policy of performing the surgery because the patient desires it or because the surgeon cannot think what to advise for a particular symptom.

Peritonsillar abscess

There is no doubt that peritonsillar abscess is a serious illness with a definite mortality. There is also no doubt that a patient who has had one quinsy is liable to have a second or third. However, this liability to recurrence is closer to 20% than 100% and a quinsy is not an absolute indication for tonsillectomy. Each patient must be judged individually; one who has repeated episodes of acute tonsillitis who then develops a quinsy is perhaps in need of tonsillectomy more than a patient who has a quinsy with no previous tonsillitis. A second quinsy is probably the point at which to decide absolutely on tonsillectomy. Abscess tonsillectomy is discussed earlier in this chapter but in the authors' opinion has little to recommend it.

Tonsillectomy for biopsy purposes

When a tonsil is thought to be the site of a neoplasm, biopsy is essential. Thus the patient with a unilateral enlarged and abnormal looking or ulcerated tonsil should be advised to have a biopsy. This can be undertaken as an incisional biopsy and is the method of choice when a squamous carcinoma is suspected. When the swelling is thought to be a lymphoma (a large hyperaemic, fleshy looking tonsil), the approach may either be incisional biopsy or tonsillectomy. Certainly tonsillectomy provides more tissue for the histopathologist to study but is more hazardous than incisional biopsy. If the patient has obvious lymph nodes in the neck, biopsy of these may be preferable

Other indications

It is usual to perform tonsillectomy for sleep apnoea syndrome when the patient is undergoing palatopharyngoplasty.

When the glossopharyngeal nerve in treatment of glossopharyngeal neuralgia or the styloid process for Eagle's syndrome are being approached through the pharynx the tonsils must be removed to give access.

Contraindications to tonsillectomy

Bleeding disorders

Tonsillectomy should not be performed when the patient has a bleeding tendency. This bleeding disorder must be investigated, diagnosed and treated prior to tonsillectomy. Patients with a vague history of bleeding easily or with a family history of bleeding disorder must be thoroughly screened and usually their clotting mechanism will be found to be normal. In patients with a known bleeding disorder the advisability of surgery must be discussed with the patient and haematologist and the risks discussed and estimated. If it is still felt that surgery is indicated then the patient's deficiency must be corrected prior to surgery.

Recent infection

A recent attack of acute tonsillitis is normally considered as a contraindication to surgery because of the potential increased risk of haemorrhage. Most people who have acute tonsillitis have been on appropriate antibiotics and it is the authors' opinion that so long as the pyrexia has settled and the tonsils are not obviously acutely inflamed then there is no contraindication to surgery.

Another commonly stated fact is that anyone with an upper respiratory tract infection should have the tonsillectomy postponed for several weeks due to the potential danger of developing pulmonary complications from the anaesthetic. Again it is the authors' opinion that so long as there are no positive chest findings on preoperative assessment then progressing to tonsillectomy offers no additional risks.

Oral contraceptives

The risks of deep vein thrombosis after tonsillectomy are extremely low indeed and it is unproven whether this risk is increased in patients who are taking an oestrogen-containing oral contraceptive. As postoperative mobilization is so fast it is not the policy in the authors' units to take any special precautions with patients taking an oral contraceptive.

Preoperative considerations

A patient undergoing tonsillectomy must have a carefully taken history and full clinical examination prior to surgery. In particular, recent upper respiratory tract infection, bleeding tendencies, coincidental anaemia or heart murmur must all be ruled out. The state of the patient's dentition must be assessed and in particular carious or loose front teeth or capped teeth must be looked for and the patient suitably informed of the risks. Urinalysis is the minimum in the way of preoperative investigations, some surgeons require also a haemoglobin estimation, blood grouping and a chest radiograph.

The operation of tonsillectomy

Premedication should be determined by the anaesthetist, but Omnopon (papaveretum) 20 mg and scopolamine (hyoscine) 0.4 mg are suitable for the average adult. General anaesthesia is the routine for tonsillectomy in the UK and a nasotracheal tube is the usual method of maintaining the airway. A detailed description of a particular surgical technique for tonsillectomy is not desirable as this is a procedure which must be taught practically and because many different variations of technique are used. It is up to each surgeon to develop his own method under close instruction and supervision. It is worthwhile, however, making some general points which are common to most techniques.

1 Most surgeons use a technique of dissection because it allows a more careful and thorough removal of all lymphoid tissue (Figure 4.1). Guillotine tonsillectomy is a dying art and perhaps this is a good thing.

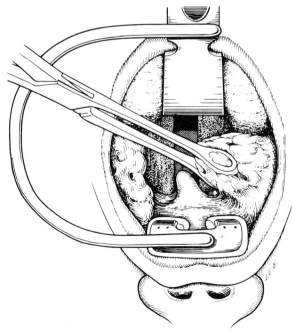

Figure 4.1 The tonsil is grasped and pulled medially. As in all surgery dissection of tissues under tension is the easiest and least traumatic

2 A Boyle-Davis gag (which is not hot) should be
positioned with care not to damage the lips, teeth
or posterior pharyngeal wall and so that the
tongue blade lies centrally along the dorsum of the
tongue.

3 The mucosa of the anterior and posterior tonsillar
pillars should be incised in such a way as to
preserve as much mucosa as possible (Figure
4.2).

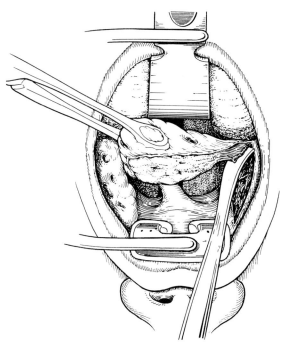

Figure 4.3 The areolar tissue between the tonsillar capsule
and the superior constrictor muscle has been dissected. The
dissection is almost complete but should be continued just
onto the base of the tongue. After removal of the tonsils
absolute haemostasis must be achieved, either using
ligatures or diathermy

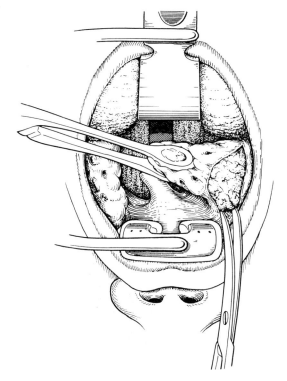

Figure 4.2 The mucosa of the anterior pillar has been
incised, the upper pole of the tonsil is being dissected prior
to incision of the posterior pillar

4 The plane of dissection of the tonsils is in the loose
areolar tissue between the capsule of the tonsil
and the superior constrictor muscle of the pharynx
(Figure 4.3). It is essential that the dissection is
performed in this plane, if too deep a plane is
dissected the muscle will be damaged and bleeding
will be increased, and if the plane is not deep
enough then lymphoid tissue will remain. It is
usual to begin this dissection at the upper pole of
the tonsil, but if difficulty is encountered the plane
should be found more inferiorly and then followed
superiorly. Most of the difficulty in tonsillectomy is
because this plane is not identified and, in some
situations, particularly after a quinsy, this identification is quite difficult. Some muscle fibres of the
superior constrictor insert into the fibrous tissue of
the tonsillar capsule and they must be gently dissected away. The dissection is carried inferiorly to
the junction of the tonsil and the base of the
tongue and the final attachment of the tonsil is
severed often using a snare.

5 The most essential part of tonsillectomy is the
control of haemorrhage and the operation is not
complete until all bleeding has ceased. The fossa
should be absolutely dry at the end of the procedure. It is usual to pack the fossa with gauze
immediately following removal of the tonsil while
the other tonsil is removed or, in the case of the
second tonsil, while bleeding from the first fossa is
dealt with. Much of the bleeding will have subsided
by the time the gauze pack is removed. Bleeding
points are identified and either ligated or diathermized depending on the surgeon's preference. Diathermy is quicker (Haase and Noguera, 1962), but
great care must be taken not to inflict an unwanted diathermy burn on the patient. The incidence of secondary haemorrhage may be greater
after diathermy (Carmody, Vamadenan and
Cooper, 1982; Siodlak, Gleeson and Wengraf,
1985).

6 When all haemorrhage has been controlled the blood clot must be aspirated from the nasopharynx where it will have accumulated and all swabs removed and counted.

The recovery of the patient from anaesthesia must be as gentle as possible, coughing and retching are liable to cause haemorrhage. The patient is recovered in the tonsil position, that is on the side with the head down so that if haemorrhage does begin the blood will flow out of the nose and mouth and not downwards to the larynx. The airway must be maintained at all times and noisy respiration may mean that there is blood in the airway. This should be inspected and the blood and secretions aspirated. At the same time the tonsillar fossae should be inspected for signs of haemorrhage.

Laser tonsillectomy

With the increased use of the laser there have been suggestions that the KTP-532 laser should be used for tonsillectomy to reduce intraoperative bleeding. A paper from Texas University Medical Branch (Strunk and Nichols, 1990) concluded that the disadvantages of laser tonsillectomy included increased cost, increased total operating time as a result of increased set up time and laser malfunction, delayed healing and no statistically significant improvement in the level of pain. The sole advantage associated with laser usage was decreased blood loss and hence this method might well be worth considering in patients with a coagulopathy.

Postoperative care

The postoperative care of a patient following tonsillectomy is directed towards early detection of haemorrhage. Thus regular observation of pulse is necessary (every 15 minutes for 4 hours, every 30 minutes for a further 4 hours and then hourly). Haemorrhage in an adult is less likely to be concealed than in a child, but a rapidly increasing pulse with increase in pallor and vomiting of blood must all be treated seriously and careful inspection of the tonsillar fossae carried out by an experienced surgeon. Should there be doubt then return to theatre to ligate the bleeding point should be carried out sooner rather than later.

Postoperative analgesia presents a problem. Some anaesthetists favour injecting local anaesthetic into the tonsil bed just prior to surgery and certainly immediately postoperatively, intramuscular Omnopon or diamorphine can be used to good effect. Problems however do arise in the maintenance of analgesia throughout the 6–8 day postoperative period. A study from Copenhagen (Stage, Jensen and Bonding, 1988) demonstrated that in 832 post-tonsillectomy patients secondary bleeding occurred in 0.5% of those receiving paracetamol in comparison with 3.1% of those receiving acetylsalicylic acid. No mention was however made with regard to the degree or otherwise of the pain control obtained.

In the authors' experience there is no available analgesia that is appropriate and sufficiently powerful to relieve post-tonsillectomy pain totally over a 7-day period.

Complications of tonsillectomy

These may be conveniently divided into perioperative and postoperative and the latter subdivided into immediate, intermediate and late, but this is a somewhat artificial classification. The most significant complication is haemorrhage and most of the deaths associated with tonsillectomy are directly or indirectly associated with this complication.

Perioperative

Haemorrhage

The amount of bleeding during tonsillectomy varies with individual patients and surgeons. Recent infection, previous peritonsillar abscess, and severe scarring are the factors which increase the haemorrhage in any one patient. The surgeon can minimize the haemorrhage by a careful, gentle dissection technique. Excessive haemorrhage from both fossae raises the question of a coagulation defect which was previously unsuspected and this must be excluded. When haemorrhage is excessive and cannot be controlled by the usual means (ligation, diathermy), other methods are available. A single difficult bleeding point may need undersewing and ligating. If excessive haemorrhage occurs throughout the fossa it can be controlled by leaving a pack in the fossa and oversewing the pillars. This is hazardous because of the risk of dislodgement of the pack in the immediate recovery period. A pack of absorbable material, e.g. Calgitex or Gelfoam, can be used or, alternatively, a gauze pack can be left in the fossa and removed the following day by dividing the sutures. If the latter is chosen a tie can be brought out of the mouth and taped to the cheek. Occasionally an aberrant internal carotid artery will be encountered in the tonsillar fossa and this leads to massive haemorrhage which can only be controlled by a ligation of the internal carotid artery in the neck. Occasionally uncontrollable haemorrhage during tonsillectomy, possibly due to a large tonsillar branch of the facial artery, requires external carotid artery ligation and this should be performed inferior to the origin of the facial artery.

Trauma

As has been said already, capped or carious teeth are at risk during tonsillectomy and the patient should be warned of this. Dental advice may be necessary before and after surgery. Gentle insertion of the gag minimizes the risk of damage to the teeth and also damage to the posterior pharyngeal wall by a hurried or careless insertion of the tongue blade. Badly placed mucosal incisions can lead to excessive loss of mucosa of the soft palate and occasional damage to the arterial supply of the uvula bilaterally may lead to loss of the uvula. Insertion of the gag can sometimes lead to dislocation of the temperomandibular joint or pain due to joint dysfunction in the postoperative period. Fire has occurred in the mouth secondary to the use of diathermy in the presence of high oxygen concentrations.

Postoperative

Immediate complications

Haemorrhage

The most significant immediate complication of tonsillectomy is so-called reactionary haemorrhage. By definition this occurs up to 24 hours postoperatively, but the vast majority of reactionary or primary haemorrhages occur within the first 8 hours.

Reactionary haemorrhage is dangerous in two ways: first, in the phase during which the patient is recovering from anaesthesia before the cough reflex is fully established, blood in the airway can result in laryngeal spasm or can asphyxiate the patient by mechanically occluding the airway. Second, haemorrhage results in hypovolaemia which, if not corrected, results in peripheral circulatory failure (shock) and eventually death.

Reactionary haemorrhage after tonsillectomy is unusual, occurring in about 0.5–1% of operations (Nesbitt, 1934; Williams, 1967). The cause is unknown but it must represent bleeding from an artery or vein which had stopped bleeding at the time of surgery. The possible causes of renewed bleeding may be dislodgement of blood clot from the lumen of the vessel or vasodilatation of a vessel which was in spasm at the time of surgery. This is probably a local problem but it is possible that changes in blood pressure or the state of vessels by anaesthetic agents may play a part. Bleeding from a vein postoperatively may be due to excessive venous pressure induced by coughing or retching. However much one speculates on the causes of reactionary haemorrhage, it must be admitted that the precise cause in the vast majority of patients is unknown.

In order to avoid disaster, any bleeding following tonsillectomy must be taken very seriously. Blood must be cross-matched at the first sign of haemorrhage. The tonsillar fossae must be inspected with great care, the clot removed if possible and a bleeding point may be seen. If the bleeding is minor it may cease once the clot has been removed or it may stop with a little pressure with a swab, possibly soaked in 1:1000 adrenaline. Even if all haemorrhage then ceases the fossae should be inspected from time to time over the next few hours as bleeding can start again. If there is any doubt, the patient must be prepared for a second anaesthetic and the bleeding point ligated under general anaesthesia. This second anaesthetic is hazardous and carries a significant mortality (Davies, 1964) because the patient has already had one anaesthetic, has blood in his airway, is hypovolaemic from blood loss and also may have a stomach full of blood.

Anaesthesia

The anaesthetic complications in the immediate postoperative period relate to the maintenance of an adequate airway, free of secretions and particularly of blood. A swab left in the airway may obviously lead to asphyxiation and it is the surgeon's responsibility to be certain that no such oversight occurs.

Intermediate complications

Haemorrhage

The most significant intermediate complication is secondary haemorrhage which by definition, is any haemorrhage which occurs more than 24 hours after surgery and classically occurs at 6–8 days. This time course implies that the most likely cause is infection. Secondary haemorrhage after tonsillectomy is not common, occurring in about 1% of patients. It is not usually as severe as primary haemorrhage but, nevertheless, must be taken very seriously as it does have a definite mortality.

The patient should be treated with systemic antibiotics (intravenous penicillin or erythromycin), a haemoglobin estimation should be performed and blood should be cross-matched.

It is usual to remove blood clot from the tonsillar fossa and perhaps hold a swab soaked in 1:1000 adrenaline in the fossa. How much these measures influence the course of events is not known.

It is most unusual for secondary haemorrhage to be severe enough or sufficiently prolonged to require formal ligation under anaesthesia. If this is contemplated a coagulation screen should be performed because a minor coagulation defect, which did not cause problems at initial surgery, can still cause problems at the secondary stage. In a tonsillar fossa which is infected and friable it is difficult to find and ligate a bleeding point. Occasionally this will be possible but more usually diathermy or suturing of a bleeding point will be necessary.

Haematoma and oedema of the uvula

Excessive surgical trauma can produce marked bruising and oedema of the uvula and, although alarming to look at, this settles down without a problem. Damage to the arterial supply to the uvula bilaterally is very rare but when it occurs the uvula may necrose. Loss of the uvula does not result in any functional disability.

Infection

Postoperatively the tonsillar fossae contain whitish slough which one would expect to be an ideal culture medium for bacteria. In fact the fossae rarely become seriously infected. When this does occur it can be recognized by increasing, rather than decreasing pain around the end of the first postoperative week and earache seems to be particularly common. The fossae look surprisingly normal but the combination of pyrexia with increasing pain leaves little doubt that there is infection. Untreated this may lead to secondary haemorrhage but usually haemorrhage is the first sign that infection has occurred. The prophylactic use of antibiotics postoperatively has not been shown to prevent secondary haemorrhage.

Pulmonary complications

Pulmonary atelectasis postoperatively leading to pneumonia is very rare. It is more likely to occur if the patient has an upper respiratory tract infection at the time of surgery and inhalation of blood or fragments of tonsil tissue may precipitate it. Very rarely a lung abscess will supervene.

Subacute bacterial endocarditis

Tonsillectomy leads to a transient bacteraemia at the time of surgery. If the patient has an abnormal heart valve or rarely, a septal defect, subacute bacterial endocarditis may complicate the operation. For this reason all patients with a heart murmur found at the preoperative investigation should have been examined by a cardiologist and, if necessary, the surgery and immediate postoperative period should be covered by systemic penicillin.

Pain

Tonsillectomy in adults and older children is typically accompanied by 7–10 days of moderate to severe local pain with or without referred otalgia. The standard management of pain has commonly been based on the use of opiates for the first 24 hours followed by the ongoing use of oral analgesics. Because of the possible interference with clotting, acetylsalicylic acid is normally avoided and paracetamol or co-proxamol most commonly recommended. None of these give totally acceptable analgesia.

Injection of bupivacaine and adrenaline into the peritonsillar tissues has not resulted in a substantial difference in pain relief (Nigam and Robin, 1991) and attempts at using Difflam oral spray or benzocaine lozenges locally have been no more successful.

More recently it has been suggested that non-steroidal anti-inflammatory drugs which have been shown to be effective against a variety of postoperative pains should be used for post-tonsillectomy pain relief. Kotecha *et al.* (1991) have shown that diclofenac (intramuscularly or by suppository) produced a statistically significant reduction in pain when compared with papaveretum on a double blind basis.

More studies are required to find the ideal analgesia for postoperative tonsillectomy pain relief.

Earache

Postoperative earache is fairly common after tonsillectomy and is usually referred pain from the tonsillar fossa, although occasionally this will herald the onset of a secondary infection. Acute otitis media has been described as a complication of tonsillectomy and the ears should always be examined in any patient who complains of otalgia.

Late complications

Postoperative scarring

Careless, traumatic surgery with loss of mucosa, particularly on the soft palate, can result in scar tissue in the palate which limits mobility. In an extreme case it is conceivable that this could affect the voice of the patient, producing nasal escape. The latter is of course much more common after a combined tonsillectomy and adenoidectomy.

Tonsillar remnants

Incomplete dissection can leave behind small islands of lymphoid tissue. Failure to remove the lower pole of the tonsil right down to the base of the tongue can result in an appearance which looks as though the tonsils have not been removed. Usually small tonsillar remnants are asymptomatic and discomfort in the throat or minor sore throats should not readily be ascribed to tonsillar remnants. Large masses of tonsil tissue remaining after tonsillectomy can result in acute tonsillitis and peritonsillar abscess has been described in a patient whose tonsils had been removed. If it is felt that tonsillar remnants are the site of recurrent acute infection then they should be removed.

Malignancy following tonsillectomy

A report by Vianna, Greenwald and Davies in 1971 suggested that patients whose tonsils had been removed were almost three times more likely to develop Hodgkin's disease when compared with patients who still had their tonsils. In fact the statistics of the study were felt to be subject to bias and further studies since have shown no difference in the occurrence of Hodgkin's disease after tonsillectomy (Ruuskanen, Vanha-Pertula and Kavalainen, 1971; Johnson and Johnson, 1972).

Acknowledgement

The section on pharyngeal manifestations of human immunodeficiency virus infection was written by Mr David W. Sim.

References

ALMADORI, G., BASTIANINI, L., BISTONI, F., PALUDETTI, G. and ROSIGNOLI, M. (1988) Microbial flora of surface versus core tonsillar cultures in recurrent tonsillitis in children. *International Journal of Pediatric Otorhinolaryngology*, **15**, 157–162

BARZAN, L., CARBONE, A., SARACHINNI, S., VACHER, G., TIRELLI, U. and COMORETTO, R. (1989) Nasopharyngeal lymphatic tissue hypertrophy in HIV infected patients. *Lancet*, i, 42–43

BEEDEN, A. C. and EVANS, J. N. (1970) Quinsy tonsillectomy – a further report. *Journal of Laryngology and Otology*, **84**, 443–448

BLACK, A. J., BOYSEN, P. G., WYNNE, J. W. and HUNT, L. A. (1979) Sleep apnoea, hypopnoea and oxygen desaturation in normal subjects. *New England Journal of Medicine*, **300**, 513–517

BLAIR-SIMMONS, M. F., GUILLEMINAULT, C. and SILVESTRI, R. (1983) Palatopharyngoplasty. *Archives of Otolaryngology*, **109**, 503–507

BOX, Q. T., CLEVELAND, R. T. and WILLARD, C. Y. (1961) Bacterial flora of the upper respiratory tract. *American Journal of Diseses of Children*, **102**, 293–301

BRANDON, E. C. (1973) Immediate tonsillectomy for peritonsillary abscess. *Transactions of the American Academy for Ophthalmology and Otolaryngology*, **77**, 412–416

CARMODY, D., VAMADENAN, T. and COOPER, S. M. (1982) Post-tonsillectomy haemorrhage. *Journal of Laryngology and Otology*, **96**, 635–638

DAVIES, D. D. (1964) Re-anaesthetising cases of tonsillectomy and adenoidectomy because of persistent postoperative haemorrhage. *British Journal of Anaesthesia*, **36**, 244–249

DE WIT, S., WEERTS, D., GOOSENS, H. and CLUMECK, N. (1989) Comparison of fluconazole and ketaconazole for oropharyngeal candidiasis in AIDS. *Lancet*, i, 746–748

DULL, J. S., SEN, P., RAFFANTI, S. and MIDDLETON, J. R. (1991) Oral candidiasis as a marker of acute retroviral illness. *Southern Medical Journal*, **84**, 733–735

ERGETER, D. A. and BECKSTEAD, J. H. (1988) Malignant lymphomas in the acquired immunodeficiency syndrome. *Archives of Pathology and Laboratory Medicine*, **112**, 602–606

EVERETT, M. T. (1979) The cause of tonsillitis. *Practitioner*, **223**, 253–259

EVERSOLE, L. R. (1989) Oral hairy leukoplakia: diagnosis and management. *Oral Surgery, Oral Medicine and Oral Pathology*, **67**, 396–403

FICARRA, G., BERSON, A. M., SILVERMAN, S. JR, QUIVEY, J. M.,

LOZADA-NUR., F. SOOY, D. D. *et al.* (1989) Kaposi's sarcoma of the oral cavity: a study of 134 patients with a review of the pathogenesis, epidemiology, clinical aspects and treatment. *Oral Surgery, Oral Medicine and Oral Pathology*, **66**, 543–550

GAFFNEY, R. J., FREEMAN, D. J., WALSH, M. A. and CAFFERKEY, M. T. (1991) Differences in tonsil core bacteriology in adults and children: a prospective study of 262 patients. *Respiratory Medicine*, **85**, 383–388

GASTAUT, H., TASSINARI, C. and DURON, B. (1966) Polygraphic study of the episodic diurnal and nocturnal (hypnic and respiratory) manifestations of the Pickwickian syndrome. *Brain Research*, **2**, 167–186

GREENSPAN, D., GREENSPAN, J. S., CONANT, M., SILVERMAN, S. and DE SOUZA, Y. (1984) Oral hairy leukoplakia in male homosexuals, evidence of association with both papilloma virus and a herpes group virus. *Lancet*, ii, 831–834

GREENSPAN, D., SCHIODT, M., GREENSPAN, J. S. and PINDBORG, J. (1990) *AIDS and the Mouth: Diagnosis and Management of Oral Lesions*. Copenhagen: Munksgaard

GUILLEMINAULT, C. (1984) New surgical approaches for obstructive sleep apnoea syndrome. *Sleep*, **7**, 1–2

HAASE, F. R. and NOGUERA, J. T. (1962) Hemostasis in tonsillectomy by electrocautery. *Archives of Otolaryngology*, **75**, 125–126

HARRIS, W. E. (1991) Is a single quinsy an indication for tonsillectomy? *Clinical Otolaryngology*, **16**, 271–273

HERBILD, O. and BONDING, P. (1981) Peritonsillar abscess: recurrence rate and treatment. *Archives of Otolaryngology*, **107**, 540–542

HOLT, G. R. and TINSLEY, P. P. (1981) Peritonsillar abscesses in children. *Laryngoscope*, **91**, 1226–1230

JOHNSON, S. K. and JOHNSON, R. E. (1972) Tonsillectomy history in Hodgkin's disease. *New England Journal of Medicine*, **287**, 1122–1125

JOKINEN, K., SIPILA, P., JOKIPII, A. M. M., JOKIPII, L. and SORRI, M. (1985) Peritonsillar abscess; bacteriological investigation. *Clinical Otolaryngology*, **10**, 27–30

KANSAS, F. J., JENSEN, J. L., ABRAMS, A. H. and WUERKER, R. B. (1987) Oral mucosa cytomegalovirus as a manifestation of the acquired immunodeficiency syndrome. *Oral Surgery, Oral Medicine and Oral Pathology*, **64**, 183–189

KAPLAN, L. D., ABRAMS, D. I., PIEGAL, E., MCGRATH, M., KAHN, J., PADRAIC, N. *et al.* (1989) AIDS-associated non-Hodgkin's lymphoma in San Francisco. *Journal of the American Medical Association*, **261**, 719–724

KOTECHA, B., O'LEARY, G., BRADBURN, J., DAROWSKI, M. and GWINNUTT, G. L. (1991) Pain relief after tonsillectomy in adults: intramuscular diclofenac and papaveretum compared. *Clinical Otolaryngology*, **16**, 345–349

KRAUS, D. H., REHM, S. J., ORLOWSKI, J. P., TUBBS, R. R. and LEVINE, H. L. (1990) Upper airway obstruction due to tonsillar lymphadenopathy in human immunodeficiency virus infection. *Archives of Otolaryngology – Head and Neck Surgery*, **116**, 738–740

KRISTENSON, S. and TVETERAS, K. (1984) Post-tonsillectomy haemorrhage and retrospective study of 1150 operations. *Clinical Otolaryngology*, **9**, 347–350

LANSER, M. J., KLEIN, H. Z. and MARVIN, A. (1985) Kaposi's sarcoma in patients with AIDS. *Archives of Otolaryngology*, **111**, 486–489

LEES, F. R., KESSLER, K. J. and MICHAEL, R. A. (1987) Non-Hodgkin's lymphoma of the head and neck in patients with AIDS. *Archives of Otolaryngology – Head and Neck Surgery*, **113**, 1104–1106

LUGARESI, E., CIRGNOTTA, F., COCCAGNA, G. and PIANNA, C. (1980) Some epidemiological data on snoring and cardio-circulatory disturbances, *Sleep*, **3**, 221–224

MOESGAARD NIELSON, V. and GRIESSON, I. (1981) Peritonsillar abscess. Cases treated with tonsillectomy a chaud. *Journal of Laryngology and Otology*, **95**, 801–807

NAVAL MEDICAL CENTER (1991) Aerobic and anaerobic microbiology of peritonsillar abscess. *Laryngoscope*, **101**, 289–292

NESBITT, B. E. (1934) Results of tonsil and adenoid operations. *British Medical Journal*, **2**, 509–513

NIGAM, A. and ROBIN, P. E. (1991) The role of bupivacaine in post-tonsillectomy pain. *Clinical Otolaryngology*, **16**, 278–279

OLSEN, W. L., JEFFREY, R. B. and SOOY, C. D. (1988) Lesions of the head and neck in patients with AIDS: CT and MR findings. *American Journal of Radiology*, **151**, 785–790

OPHIR, D., BAWNIK, J., PORIA, Y., PORAT, M. and MARSHAK, G. (1988) Peritonsillar abscess. A prospective evaluation of outpatient management by needle aspiration. *Archives of Otolaryngology – Head and Neck Surgery*, **114**, 661–663

PATOW, C. A., STEIS, R., LONGO, D. L., REICHERT FINDLAY, P. A., POTTER, D. *et al.* (1984a) Kaposi's sarcoma of the head and neck in the acquired immunodeficiency syndrome. *Otolaryngology – Head and Neck Surgery*, **92**, 255–260

PATOW, C. A., STARK, T. W., PINDLAY, P. A., STEIS, R., LONGO, D. L. and MASER, I. F. (1984b) Pharyngeal obstruction by Kaposi's sarcoma in a homosexual male with acquired immunodeficiency syndrome. *Otolaryngology, Head and Neck Surgery*, **92**, 713–716

REILLY S., TIMMIS, P., BEEDEN, A. G. and WILLIS, A. T. (1981) Possible role of the anaerobes in tonsillitis. *Journal of Clinical Pathology*, **34**, 542–547

REMMERS, J. C., DE GROOT, W. J., SAUERLAND, E. K. and ARCH, A. M. (1978) Pathogenesis of upper airway occlusion during sleep. *Journal of Applied Physiology*, **44**, 931–938

RUUSKANEN, O., VANHA-PERTULA, T. and KAVALAINEN, K. (1971) Tonsillectomy, appendicectomy and Hodgkin's disease. *Lancet*, i, 1127–1128

SILVERMAN, S. JR, (1987) Aids update: oral findings, diagnosis and precautions. *Journal of the American Dental Association*, **115**, 559–563

SIODLAK, M. Z., GLEESON, M. J. and WENGRAF, C. L. (1985) Post-tonsillectomy secondary haemorrhage. *Annals of the Royal College of Surgeons of England*, **67**, 167–168

SNOW, D. G., CAMPBELL, J. B. and MORGAN, D. W. (1991) The management of peritonsillar sepsis by needle aspiration. *Clinical Otolaryngology*, **16**, 245–247

SOOY, C. D. (1987) The impact of AIDS in otolaryngology, head and neck surgery. *Advances in Otolaryngology and Head and Neck Surgery*, **1**, 1–28

STAGE, J., JENSEN, J. H. and BONDING, P. (1988) Post-tonsillectomy haemorrhage and analgesics. A comparative study of acetylsalicylic acid and paracetamol. *Clinical Otolaryngology*, **13** 201–204

STERN, J. C., LIN, P. and LUCENTE, F. E. (1990) Benign nasopharyngeal masses and human immunodeficiency virus infection. *Archives of Otolaryngology – Head and Neck Surgery*, **1161**, 206–208

STRINGER, S. P., SCHAEFER, S. D. and CLOSE, L. G. (1988) A randomised trial for outpatient management of peritonsillar abscess. *Archives of Otolaryngology – Head and Neck Surgery*, **114**, 296–298

STRUNK, C. L. and NICHOLS, M. L. (1990) A comparison of the KTP/532 laser tonsillectomy vs traditional dissection/snare tonsillectomy. *Otolaryngology, Head and Neck Surgery*, **103**, 966–971

SUROW, J. B., HANDLER, S. D., TELIAN, S. A., FLEISHER, G. R. and BARANAK C. C. (1989) Bacteriology of tonsil surface and core in children. *Laryngoscope*, **99**, 261–266

T-BUTURO, C. G. (1990) Management of peritonsillary abscess (quinsy) at Harare Central Hospital. *Central African Medicine*, **36**, 187–190

TONER, J. G., STEWART, T. J. CAMPBELL, J. B. and HUNTER, J. (1986) Tonsil flora in the very young tonsillectomy patient. *Clinical Otolaryngology*, **11**, 171–174

TUCKER, A. G. (1982a) The current status of tonsillectomy – a survey of otolaryngologists. *Clinical Otolaryngology*, **7**, 367–372

TUCKER, A. G. (1982b) Peritonsillar abscess – a retrospective study of medical treatment. *Journal of Laryngology and Otology*, **96**, 639–643

VIANNA, N. J., GREENWALD, P. and DAVIES, J. N. P. (1971) Tonsillectomy and Hodgkin's disease: the lymphoid tissue barrier. *Lancet*, i, 431–432

WEIR, N. F. (1972) Clinical interpretation of tonsillar size. *Journal of Laryngology and Otology*, **86**, 1137–1144

WILLIAMS, A. J. (1967) Hemorrhage following tonsillectomy and adenoidectomy. *Journal of Laryngology and Otology*, **81**, 805–808

YLIKOSKI, J. and KARJALAINEN, J. (1989) Acute tonsillitis in young men: etiological agents and their differentiation. *Scandinavian Journal of Infectious Diseases*, **21**, 169–174

5

Acute and chronic laryngitis

Paul van den Broek

Acute laryngitis

Acute laryngitis is usually of infectious origin, either viral or bacterial, but can also be due to exogenous agents. In some instances autoimmune processes can manifest themselves in the larynx, simulating an acute inflammatory reaction. Swelling of the laryngeal mucosa and the underlying tissue is the common factor in all these conditions. They can be divided into several well-defined clinical entities which are discussed in this chapter.

Acute (simple) laryngitis

Aetiology

This is the most usual form of laryngitis and occurs as a symptom of a common cold. The disease is often associated with and secondary to an acute inflammation of the nose, throat or paranasal sinuses. It is an airborne infection usually caused by adenoviruses and influenza viruses. These can damage the respiratory mucosa to such an extent that secondary bacterial infection supervenes. The bacteria involved most commonly are *Moraxella catarrhalis*, *Streptococcus pneumoniae* and *Haemophilus influenzae*, which are common inhabitants of the aerodigestive tract in some patients. Unfavourable climate and diminished resistance through undue physical and psychological strain may be predisposing factors.

Pathology

The laryngeal mucosa shows all the signs of acute inflammation. There is extravasation of fluid. In the early phase infiltration by polymorphonuclear leucocytes is present and later lymphocytes and plasma cells predominate. The underlying muscles and even the perichondrium and the cricoarytenoid joints may be affected by the process.

Areas of epithelium may be destroyed and exfoliated. Full recovery is usual but, in some instances, fibrosis will result and there can be permanent damage to the laryngeal mucosa with loss of its original structure. This can be the beginning of a chronic laryngitis.

Symptoms

The main symptoms are hoarseness, discomfort and pain in the larynx. Usually there is also an irritant paroxysmal cough. The voice is hardly ever completely lost, but speaking causes discomfort and phonation often results in a high-pitched husky voice. The voice varies in strength and pitch. The irritating cough may persist after the voice has returned. The degree of pyrexia and general symptoms depends very much on concomitant infections in the other parts of the respiratory tract. The infection is often limited to the larynx with very few general symptoms.

Clinical diagnosis

The diagnosis is made by a careful history and examination of the upper and lower respiratory tracts. The presence of a generalized infection is usually apparent. It may be necessary to substantiate this further by radiographs of the sinuses and chest. The larynx is investigated by indirect laryngoscopy, which can be difficult in the presence of acute infection as a result of hypersensitivity of the mucosa. A local anaesthetic consisting of 4–10% xylocaine spray may be helpful.

When the larynx can be seen, a red and swollen mucosa is found which may prevent a deeper view into the larynx. The true vocal cords lose their whitish and contrasting colour and are also swollen, sometimes partly obstructing the laryngeal lumen. In adults this hardly ever results in impaired breathing with stridor; in children, however, the clinical course can be rapidly progressive. The presence of inspissated mucus, or sometimes a true purulent discharge, is pathognomonic of a bacterial infection which needs more aggressive treatment.

Treatment

The treatment of acute laryngitis depends on the presence of concomitant infection in the upper respiratory tract and the degree of local changes in the larynx. The treatment in all cases consists of simple supportive measures such as voice rest, medicated steam inhalations and the avoidance of cold, draught, tobacco and alcohol. Expectoration of mucus can be assisted by the administration of mucolytic agents.

With these measures most patients with viral laryngitis improve within a few days. After a viral laryngitis, it may sometimes be necessary to suppress a persisting cough with codeine.

The presence of bacterial infection, apparent by the presence of pus and general symptoms, is usually an indication for antibiotics. These should be broad spectrum whenever they are given without prior culture and sensitivity testing. The most appropriate antibiotics are broad-spectrum penicillins 500 mg four times daily, doxycycline 200 mg/day or erythromycin 500 mg twice daily.

Local application by sprays with astringent agents should be avoided. When professional activities occasionally prevent taking full vocal rest, the discomfort of speaking can be overcome by a local anaesthetic spray. This should, however, always be restricted to one or two applications to prevent further irritation.

Acute laryngitis is mostly a disease with a short and benign course. Adequate treatment along the lines described above is mandatory to prevent permanent damage of the laryngeal mucosa which can be the beginning of a chronic laryngitis.

In children the symptoms and signs of acute laryngitis may be much more alarming because the laryngeal lumen is much smaller and the laryngeal tissues are more prone to oedematous swelling. This applies especially to the separate entities known as acute laryngotracheobronchitis and acute epiglottitis.

Recently much attention has been given to the possible role of gastro-oesophageal reflux especially in children as a cause of recurring upper respiratory infections (Koufman, 1991; Contencin and Narcy, 1992).

Acute (fibrinous) laryngotracheobronchitis

Aetiology

In children, an acute respiratory infection may rarely run a fulminant course spreading to the entire respiratory system. Small children up to the age of 7 years are most often affected. The infection can be caused by any of the microorganisms commonly involved in respiratory infections, but the haemolytic streptococcus is predominant. It usually superinfects on an infection by the influenza virus.

Pathology

Acute laryngotracheobronchitis affects the entire respiratory tract. The production of tenacious mucus which can hardly be expectorated, thus adding to the respiratory distress, is characteristic. The formation of pseudomembranes is also common which, unlike diphtherial membranes, can be wiped off without causing bleeding. The inspissated secretions may cause total obstruction of the small bronchi leading to atelectasis.

Clinical features

Any mild common respiratory infection can lead to the complete picture of an acute laryngotracheobronchitis with its sometimes fulminant course. This generalization of a limited infection complicated by a bacterial superinfection must be recognized early to allow adequate treatment. The patient's temperature sometimes rises to 41°C and toxaemia may develop rapidly.

Most commonly, during or after a common cold, the child's temperature rises further and this is combined with a dry and harsh cough, hoarseness and stridor. The production of tenacious secretions which can be hardly expectorated, and the mucosal swelling are the main causes of obstruction of the airway, which is most prominent at the narrow laryngeal inlet. It is at this stage that painstaking observation is necessary to prevent the child from developing respiratory failure which can be rapidly fatal. The increased muscular energy consumption required for breathing and coughing, together with the retention of carbon dioxide, leads to a combination of metabolic and respiratory acidosis which paralyses the central regulation of respiration. During the initial phase the child is restless and sometimes cyanotic; in the later stages there may be an apparent improvement when the child becomes tired and calm. The retention of carbon dioxide causes a change of colour from cyanotic to pale and these are the first and often only signs of imminent disaster.

A small child with a temperature higher than 38.5°C and stridor should be admitted to hospital for observation. The clinical picture is usually dominated by the laryngeal stridor, the degree of which can scarcely be investigated objectively. The sequelae of rapidly developing or continuing stridor can only be properly judged by objective blood gas analysis which gives information on the degree of oxygenation, carbon dioxide retention and acidosis. It must be realized that any value can change within a very short time. Mirror examination in these children is impossible. Nowadays, the use of a 3mm flexible endoscope can give a good impression of the degree of obstruction. Auscultation of the lungs is often difficult to interpret because of the stridor and massive secretions. A chest radiograph is required to investigate the degree of involvement of the lower respiratory system. First and most important remains sound clinical judgement based on clinical examination and laboratory investigations.

Treatment

Acute laryngotracheobronchitis should be treated vigorously. Treatment should start immediately with antibiotics, preferably a broad-spectrum penicillin; this can be given orally or by injection depending on the general condition of the child. The value of corticosteroids in reducing the inflammatory reaction is debatable. However, when children are in distress the use of intravenous steroids will certainly do no harm and is probably beneficial. They should not be used for longer than is required to relieve the most acute symptoms; this is usually a few days.

The child should be isolated in a room or tent with moist air. Mucolytic agents can be added by mouth or in aerosols to facilitate expectoration of the tenacious mucus. If feeding by mouth is difficult, a nasogastric tube should be introduced. The child must be adequately hydrated and should be carefully monitored for cardiac or respiratory failure. Any sign of deterioration should lead to consultation about the necessity of airway assistance either by endotracheal intubation or tracheostomy and, if necessary, by assisted respiration. It is outside the scope of this chapter to discuss the merits of intubation versus tracheostomy. Neither method is safer than the other. They both require good instrumentation and technique but, above all, well-trained personnel to observe and nurse a child with a tracheostomy or endotracheal tube.

Subglottic laryngitis (pseudocroup, spasmodic cough)

Aetiology

Acute laryngotracheobronchitis should not be confused with the condition generally known as subglottic laryngitis (pseudocroup). Subglottic laryngitis is common in young children below the age of 3 years.

The symptoms are usually alarming. The exact aetiology is unknown, but the disease is often associated with an infection by one of the influenza viruses.

The main intralaryngeal changes, consisting of substantial swelling of the mucosa, are found on or near the undersurface of the true vocal cords and in the subglottic region.

Clinical features

An attack of pseudocroup starts abruptly in a child, who might have a mild respiratory infection with some cough. Usually after the child has gone to bed and has fallen asleep, he or she wakes up again with a dry cough and rapidly increasing stridor. The complete clinical picture develops in a very short time and seems alarming. There is usually no pyrexia or only mild fever, the voice is raw and the sound resembles the barking of seals. The cough is dry. Secretions may be present but are not marked. The child becomes restless, nervous and tends to cry. The anxiety of the parents is usually projected onto the child and the clinical signs then worsen. The child may have a red appearance from exertion and perspiration. There are no further diagnostic aids to ensure the diagnosis of this generally benign and self-limiting condition.

Treatment

The child and sometimes the parents need treatment. The child should be comforted as much as possible because further exertion during crying and coughing stimulates intralaryngeal swelling. Sedatives should never be given to the child because they suppress respiratory reflexes essential for maintaining oxygen and carbon dioxide levels within normal limits. Sedatives are probably best given to the parents! The value of corticosteroids for the treatment of the child is still debated. There is no objection to parenteral administration of corticosteroids but the effect is doubtful and injection can distress the child.

If possible the child should be taken to a room with moist air which helps to ease coughing and irritation. A bathroom with running hot water to produce steam is probably the best place. The child should be observed carefully until the worst symptoms settle. If any doubt is present about the child's breathing capabilities he or she should be admitted to hospital. Only rarely will there be a real emergency. Occasionally there may be progression to complete acute laryngotracheobronchitis, requiring more aggressive treatment.

In an emergency the treatment of choice is endotracheal intubation which can usually be limited to 1 or 2 days. Whenever this is necessary, it is of paramount importance that the correct diameter of tube should be used to prevent local damage to the mucosa which may otherwise lead to permanent stenosis: it is better to use too small than too large a tube. Siliconized tubes have the advantage of a very low friction coefficient and therefore have a less traumatic effect on the mucosa.

Although the progress of the stridor should be carefully monitored, it is hardly ever necessary to proceed to aggressive treatment. The stridor usually subsides within a few hours and the next day the child may be entirely normal. There is a tendency towards recurrence and it seems that some children have a predisposition for this condition. Possibly an allergic reaction in the subglottic region is a contributing factor.

Membranous laryngitis

Aetiology

Another rare form of laryngitis, probably closely linked with acute laryngotracheobronchitis, is known as membranous laryngitis, sometimes also called croup or pseudomembranous croup. It is not caused by *Corynebacterium diphtheriae* (Klebs-Loeffler bacillus) but by various microorganisms including streptococci, *Pseudomonas aeruginosa* or Vincent's microorganisms.

Pathology

The presence of a confluent membrane covering the surface of the larynx is the most characteristic sign. No bleeding occurs when this is removed and no ulceration remains. The main site is the supraglottis or the laryngeal vestibule. Only rarely does it spread to the vocal cords. It can descend from above as part of Vincent's infection of the pharynx.

Clinical features

The clinical picture is similar to that of other forms of laryngitis. The constitutional disturbance is often accompanied by anorexia and thirst; there is moderate fever; swallowing is painful and coughing is usually present. Later there may be stridor due to laryngeal spasm and obstruction by oedema or obstructing membranes. The disease should be differentiated from classical diphtheria which it resembles. A bacteriological investigation will establish the diagnosis and differentiate it from other forms of laryngitis.

Treatment

Antibiotics or sulphonamides are given depending on the sensitivity of the microorganism. Modern chemotherapy has altered the outlook of most forms of acute laryngitis.

Acute epiglottitis

Acute epiglottitis is a distinct form of acute inflammation of the larynx. As the name implies the epiglottis is the main site of involvement. The inflammation of the epiglottis leads to extensive swelling of the laryngeal inlet.

The disease affects both children and adults. The incidence is about 1:17 000 children and 1:100 000 adults. As vaccination against haemophilus B is becoming more common, it is likely that the incidence will diminish (Wurtele, 1990).

Aetiology

Acute epiglottitis has been shown to be caused by infection with *Haemophilus influenzae* type B.

Clinical features

The history is usually short and starts with an upper respiratory tract infection. There is a rapid rise in the patient's temperature sometimes exceeding 40°C, with signs of severe illness. The patient is quiet, and has pain in the throat which inhibits swallowing and appetite. There is often a rapid and potentially fatal increase of stridor which is most marked in children. Unlike pseudocroup the child prefers the sitting position (the tripod sign) and usually drools.

The epiglottis is often directly visible on inspection of the oropharynx as a rounded swollen red mass. Care should be taken when depressing the tongue as this can cause fatal glottic spasm.

Treatment

Acute epiglottitis should be considered an emergency and the patient should be admitted to hospital. The possibility of rapid deterioration requires careful and skilled observation in order to be able to take adequate measures when necessary. When the airway is sufficient the main treatment consists of inhalation of moist air, and antibiotics, preferably amoxycillin, should be given. Airway obstruction may develop very rapidly and some experienced surgeons advocate direct establishment of an airway.

This can be achieved by a tracheostomy or by nasotracheal intubation. Although both methods give good results there is a growing consensus that nasotracheal intubation should be the first choice (Andreassen *et al.*, 1992; Kessler, Wetmore and Marsh, 1993).

In general, the monitoring of patients, especially children, with airway obstruction due to laryngeal infection or other causes has become a separate specialty. The otolaryngologist should be a regular observer in intensive care wards where endoscopic and surgical skills may be needed when the airway becomes obstructed. The observation of a stridulous patient should include constant monitoring of heart and respiratory function, temperature, and regular analyses of the blood gases.

A child has a relatively small respiratory reserve compared with an adult; the oxygen consumption per unit of bodyweight is twice as high. Furthermore, the smaller diameter of the airways results in a higher peripheral airway resistance and a greater risk of obstruction.

The relief of life-threatening obstruction of the airways can usually be effected by passing an endotracheal tube. Except in cases of a foreign body in the airway, the laryngeal opening can be found and a tube inserted. This procedure requires a laryngoscope with good light and tubes of different sizes. After the airway has been re-established a decision should be taken as to whether an indwelling tube should be left or a tracheostomy performed. Siliconized tubes cause very little local irritation if they are of the correct size. Many paediatricians and otolaryngologists have accepted prolonged intubation as the method of choice for the first 10–14 days, provided that adequate monitoring facilities are available.

Successful results with prolonged intubation have led to less frequent use of tracheostomy for short-term airway relief in many centres. Whenever long periods of assisted ventilation are foreseen, tracheostomy should still be considered as a good and probably preferable alternative. Modern synthetic semirigid materials reduce the chance of complications which were common when metal tracheostomy tubes were used.

Nowadays, tracheostomy is rarely performed as an emergency procedure, because endotracheal intubation has usually been carried out first.

The differential diagnosis of different types of acute laryngitis in children is very important for the institution of adequate treatment in cases where this is necessary. Some conditions need rapid and aggressive treatment, others can be observed without danger.

The main features of the different forms of laryngitis are summarized in Table 5.1.

Oedema of the larynx

Oedema of the mucosa can accompany any inflammatory reaction of the larynx and is, therefore, not a specific disease but rather a sign. It may be a solitary reaction to different types of exogenous stimuli or to unknown factors. Trauma, infection and tobacco are the most important contributors. Another important cause of oedema is the physical trauma of radiation treatment. Most forms of laryngeal oedema persist over a prolonged period of time with only a limited tendency to spontaneous resolution. Several clinical entities require special mention.

Reinke's oedema

The accumulation of fluid under the epithelium of the true vocal cords is generally known as Reinke's oedema, named after the German anatomist, Reinke, who first described the loose areolar tissue in this region. The attachment of the vocal ligament along the medial edge and underneath the vocal cord by the lamellar fibres extending into the conus elasticus restricts the oedema to the superior surface of the cords (Mayet, 1961).

Aetiology

The precise cause of Reinke's oedema is not known. Allergy, infection and especially local irritants probably play a major role. Tobacco is one of the major culprits and it has been shown that an important percentage of patients are heavy smokers (Myerson, 1950). Chronic sinusitis has also been implicated, but most studies fail to mention this.

Clinical features

The condition is fairly common and comprises about 10% of benign laryngeal lesions. The disease is commoner in men but the percentage may vary greatly. The patients are mostly aged between 30 and 60 years old. The oedematous swelling of the vocal cords can easily be recognized on indirect laryngoscopy. The vocal cords are red and swollen and have a slightly translucent appearance (see Plate 5/5/I). Sometimes the mucosa becomes redundant and polypoid projections are visible. Rarely these may be so voluminous as to cause stridor. The oedema prevents

Table 5.1 Acute laryngitis in children

	Simple laryngitis	*Subglottic laryngitis*	*Laryngotracheobronchitis*	*Epiglottitis*
Age	Any	1–4 years	1–8 years	3–6 years
Onset	Gradual	Rapid	Gradual (after common cold)	Rapid
Aetiology	Viral	?	Bacterial (secondary)	*H. influenzae*
Temperature °C	< 39	< 38	< 38	> 39
Voice	Hoarse	Harsh	Hoarse	Normal
Posture	Indifferent	Restless	Lying	Sitting, drooling
Treatment	Supportive	Moist air, supportive	Antibiotics, rarely intubation	Antibiotics, intubation
Monitoring	No	No	Yes	Yes

normal vocal cord vibrations causing hoarseness often with deepening of the voice. The vocal range diminishes and the voice becomes monotonous. There is frequently a dry cough and clearing of the throat.

Treatment

The treatment of Reinke's oedema should consist of a combination of surgery and vocal rehabilitation. Naturally all known causative factors, especially smoking, should first be eliminated. If smoking is not stopped the results of any treatment will be very disappointing (Hojslet, Moesgaard-Nielsen and Karlsmose, 1990).

Surgery consists of microsurgical removal of strips of vocal cord mucosa by microlaryngoscopy (Kleinsasser, 1990). First the mucosa is incised in a sagittal direction and the fluid, which may be either thin or mucoid, is sucked out. A strip of vocal cord mucosa is then removed with microforceps and scissors.

There is some controversy whether both vocal cords should be stripped at the same session or whether an interval should be allowed. The present author agrees with Kleinsasser that it is perfectly safe to treat both cords during the same operation, but that care should be taken not to extend the incisions into the anterior commissure. After the procedure absolute vocal rest is advocated for 1 week. Healing is usually rapid and new epithelium develops with a firmer attachment to the vocal cord muscle which prevents recurrence. Speech therapy is instituted after 2–3 weeks and is continued for as long as it is felt to be beneficial. Recurrences are generally uncommon.

Some patients only come for treatment after a long history, often of many months. Delay of treatment for too long can result in the development of chronic laryngitis.

Angioneurotic oedema (angio-oedema)

This condition is characterized by recurring attacks of local swelling in various parts of the body particularly the face, larynx, extremities and buttocks. Death may result from life-threatening oedema of the larynx. Gastrointestinal disturbances presenting as colic and nausea and vomiting, are almost invariably associated with the oedema.

Generally, angio-oedema can be divided into an allergic and a non-allergic form which can be either hereditary or non-hereditary.

Angioneurotic oedema of allergic origin

This form is usually accompanied by urticaria. It presents as an acute allergic reaction to food, medicines or inhaled allergens. The diagnosis is based on the history and typical concomitant symptoms. The oedema rarely leads to laryngeal obstruction. The allergic reaction can be alleviated with antihistamines and corticosteroids. In severe cases, a subcutaneous injection of adrenalin (1:1000) 1 mg can be life saving (Frank, 1976). It is very important that the allergens are identified in order to prevent future attacks.

Recently several cases of life-threatening angio-oedema have been described which were due to medication with angiotensin converting enzyme inhibitors (ACE-inh.) used against essential hypertension. The oedema usually involves the face and lips and occasionally also the larynx.

Hereditary angio-oedema

Less frequently, angioneurotic oedema is of non-allergic origin: it can be both hereditary and non-hereditary. The hereditary form with all its clinical manifestations was described by Sir William Osler in 1888. He recognized the life-threatening character of the condition. The underlying mechanism of the disease has been recognized to be a serum deficiency of the C1-esterase inhibitor protein (C1-iNH). This enzyme is one of a series of naturally occurring inhibitors of complement activation, kinin formation and fibrinolysis.

The complement system is composed of nine serum components which are activated by each other in a strict sequence leading to the release of polypeptides which enhance vascular permeability. When C1-iNH is not present as in hereditary angio-oedema, minor events such as trauma or emotional strain, can elicit a chain of serious reactions resulting in the release of complement. The mortality from concomitant laryngeal oedema is high if treatment is not rapidly instituted.

Blok and Baarsma (1984) described a family in which 35 members over three generations were traced, 14 (40%) of whom appeared to be affected; this indicates an autosomal dominant inheritance with a high penetrance. The typical triad (abdominal pain, peripheral non-pitting oedema and laryngeal oedema) was present in four patients, laryngeal oedema being the least common symptom.

The treatment can be divided into that of the acute attack and short- or long-term prophylaxis. The acute attack is treated with an intravenous injection of 36 000 units of C1-iNH. Patients should keep this at home for use in an emergency. This preparation can also be used as short-term prophylaxis in these patients before operations such as dental extractions.

Patients suffering from frequent attacks should have long-term prophylaxis which is best effected by the fibrinolytic inhibitor epsilon aminocaproic acid (EACA) and its derivative tranexamic acid, or by the androgen methyltestosterone and its derivative danazol. These stimulate the production of C1-iNH.

Laryngeal perichondritis

Perichondritis is an inflammatory reaction in the tissues covering the laryngeal cartilages. A primary form, usually developing as a blood-borne infection, used to be quite common when typhus, typhoid and smallpox were prevalent. Immunization programmes have eliminated these diseases from many areas of the world. Perichondritis can also be secondary to a superficial infection in the larynx spreading to the deeper tissues. In the presence of abscesses or cellulitis the cartilage may also be involved.

At present, one of the major causes of perichondritis is radiotherapy. Although the improved dosage schedules and the introduction of megavoltage radiation sources have greatly diminished the chances of serious complications, perichondritis remains a potentially dangerous hazard of this form of treatment. Perichondrium and cartilage can be affected by the radiation beam resulting in a sterile inflammatory reaction with very little tendency to spontaneous resolution. When the cartilage is uncovered after the tumour resolves, the cartilage with its inherent avascularity is liable to serious infection with little healing tendency.

Clinical features

Perichondritis usually develops slowly. The characteristic sign is dull pain over the entire laryngeal skeleton. The thyroid and cricoid cartilage are thickened and tender on palpation. The swollen red laryngeal mucosa can be seen on indirect laryngoscopy. The swelling may be so pronounced as to impair vocal cord function or obstruct the airway. Sometimes the cartilage is exposed. A foul smell indicates tissue necrosis. Occasionally pieces of necrotic cartilage are expectorated.

The clinical course is usually slow and protracted but, occasionally, the clinical signs of perichondritis develop very quickly, especially during radiotherapy, necessitating emergency treatment.

Treatment

Medical treatment, consisting of high doses of broad-spectrum antibiotics effective against anaerobes, should be instituted immediately. Furthermore, corticosteroids should be given in high doses for 1 week with gradual withdrawal (prednisone 30mg/day). Whenever airway problems predominate, tracheal intubation or a tracheostomy should be performed.

Although acute perichondritis can resolve quickly, especially with regard to airway obstruction, the laryngeal oedema may last for weeks to months. Laryngeal abscesses should be drained.

Separate mention should be made of the treatment of laryngeal perichondritis after radiotherapy (Stell and Morrison, 1973). This condition is generally serious and may be very slow to resolve. It may be necessary to maintain a tracheostomy for weeks, months, or even years. Resolution is usually slow and often leaves a gradually progressive narrowing of the larynx from scar formation.

Relapsing polychondritis

Relapsing polychondritis is a rare condition which was first described in 1923 by Jaksch-Wartenhorst. There is a recurrent inflammation of cartilage especially of the auricle, nose and trachea. The aetiology is unknown, but it is thought to be an autoimmune disease linked with the collagen-vascular group of diseases. Occasionally, patients with relapsing polychondritis suffer from rheumatoid arthritis, systemic lupus erythematosus or ankylosing spondylitis.

The recurrent inflammation in the cartilages of the head and neck region such as the pinna, nasal cartilages, larynx or trachea, is the most prominent manifestation, but inflammatory lesions such as scleritis, conjunctivitis, keratitis, arthropathy and vasculitis can be found in other supporting tissues (Dolan, Lemmon and Teitelbaum, 1966). The erythrocyte sedimentation rate is raised except in the very early stages.

The laryngeal and tracheal lesions manifest themselves with signs of laryngitis and tracheitis. The mucosa is swollen especially around the epiglottis and aryepiglottic folds and descending down into the trachea. In the later stages the cartilage disappears and the epiglottis may be shrunken. The other laryngeal cartilages may also be soft and tender. Loss of cartilage of the larynx and the trachea can lead to segmental narrowing because of collapse and fibrosis.

Histologically there is degeneration of the cartilage due to invasion by inflammatory tissue. Several authors have described the microscopy of these lesions. It seems that the process is preceded by a degeneration of the marginal chondrocytes (Valenzuela *et al.*, 1980). The ground substance of the cartilage becomes acidophilic. Erosion by inflammatory tissue takes place around the cartilage and compression of lacunae can be found. Initially, the exudate is mainly composed of neutrophils but later lymphocytes, plasma cells and sometimes histiocytes can be found. In the end stages progressive fibrosis is found. Histochemical staining has shown a deficiency of matrix acid polysaccharide (Verity, 1963).

Although anticartilage antibodies have been found in the serum of patients with relapsing polychondritis, the exact meaning of these immunological findings in relation to the cause of the disease is not known (Michaels, 1984). This also applies to the finding of autoantibodies to type II collagen, a constituent of both ocular and cartilaginous tissue, which have been found in cases of relapsing polychondritis. Although there is growing evidence that relapsing polychondritis is an autoimmune disease, definite proof is still lacking.

The presenting symptoms of laryngeal involvement are hoarseness and dyspnoea due to oedema of the mucosa. Usually there are signs of acute inflammation with fever and pain. Without treatment there is progression to serious stenosis of the larynx. The course can be very slow and relatively benign but can also be rapid and fatal. The mean survival of 27 patients described in the literature who died before 1971 was 5.25 years, but varied from one month to 23 years (Hughes *et al.*, 1972).

The treatment of choice is still considered to be the administration of corticosteroids; initially high dosages are required, prednisone 30–60 mg/day. After the acute symptoms have subsided a maintenance dose (e.g. prednisone 5–10 mg/day) is necessary to prevent exacerbation. The therapy can rarely be withdrawn entirely. When exacerbations occur the dose must be increased. Gaffney, Harrison and Blayney (1992) advocated the use of racemic ephedrine for the acute laryngeal oedema. The use of other drugs such as antimetabolites and immunosuppressive drugs seems logical if the autoimmune cause is accepted but, at present, not enough evidence of their usefulness is available.

Chronic laryngitis

Any chronic non-specific inflammatory reaction of the laryngeal mucosa may be called a chronic laryngitis. The patient suffering from chronic laryngitis complains of hoarseness over a long period of time and, on inspection of the laryngeal surface, changes in the laryngeal mucosa are always visible. The clinical picture may show variations so that over the years many descriptions have been given to clinical entities which were thought to be different. These were given separate names referring to the macroscopic or microscopic appearance, and date back to the time of Virchow, the German pathologist of the second half of the nineteenth century. He introduced the term 'pachydermia' to designate local changes in the vocal cord which, on microscopic appearance, showed thickening of the epithelial layers (Virchow, 1887). Depending on the history and the site of the lesions he further divided this entity into 'pachydermia verrucosa' and 'contact pachydermia'. Although these names are not much used today the condition is still well known to every laryngologist.

Since Virchow's time many other names have been used such as *hyperplastic laryngitis, leucoplakia, keratosis, hyperkeratosis* and others meant to describe chronic laryngeal disease with certain clinical and histomorphological features. However, most are so ill-defined that they are of limited value for a clinician, although they may be informative with regard to aetiology, natural history and treatment. Furthermore, the microscopic appearance of the laryngeal mucosa and the surrounding tissues may show some differences, however these are not pathognomonic for any clinical entity. On the contrary, in most of these non-specific laryngeal conditions the microscopic picture is rather uniform, being characterized by hyperplasia of the squamous epithelium with differences only at the cellular level. The mucosa of the true vocal cords is normally covered by squamous epithelium, whereas the remainder of the larynx is normally covered by respiratory epithelium. During life this respiratory epithelium is subject to progressive metaplasia towards squamous epithelium. It has been known for a long time that the epithelial changes in the laryngeal mucosa are enhanced by tobacco and environmental pollution and can result in the development of an infiltrating carcinoma. In 1923 the American laryngologist Chevalier Jackson stated that chronic laryngitis and what he called 'keratosis' could be precancerous. These lesions should be detected early and eradicated. Several authors (Putney and O'Keefe, 1953; McGavran, Bauer and Ogura, 1960; Gabriel and Jones, 1962; Norris and Peale, 1963; Crissman, 1979; Sllamniku *et al.*, 1989; Hojslet, Moesgaard-Nielsen and Palvio, 1989) have carried out studies to investigate the chance of malignant degeneration, and it has been recognized that certain microscopic changes, especially at cellular level, can be regarded to be predictive for later malignant transformation.

Kleinsasser (1963) first stressed the importance of a classification system of histological grades which would help to alert the clinician to those lesions which have a higher chance of malignant degeneration and thus would need more aggressive treatment or closer follow up. The introduction of microlaryngoscopy by the same author around 1961 allowed well delineated and representative biopsies to be taken from the suspicious lesions in the laryngeal mucosa and was an important step towards accurate clinical assessment of these lesions. Over the past 20 years the value of this method has been repeatedly confirmed.

However, a uniform grading system has not yet been adopted and subjective interpretations of the degrees of change found in the laryngeal mucosa under pathological circumstances are an obstacle to a reliable and reproducible grading system. Perhaps more objective means of quantification of the changes at the cellular level, for instance morphometric or photometric evaluation (Hellquist and Oloffson, 1984; Hellquist *et al.*, 1984), and DNA-measurements (Cooke *et al.*, 1991; Munck-Wickland *et al.*, 1991) will enhance the reliability of such a system and make it more acceptable.

Aetiology

Chronic laryngitis primarily affects middle-aged men but the variation in age is wide. The median age is approximately 57 years, that is about 5 years less than the average age of patients with laryngeal carcinoma.

Many factors, both endogenous and exogenous,

have been incriminated as causative. The exogenous stimuli may be physical, chemical or infective, the most important being inhaled irritants and, notably, cigarette smoke. In many studies it has been shown that metaplastic changes in the surface epithelium of the airways in heavy smokers is more marked than in non-smokers. This also explains the sex differences observed.

The changes in the mucosa are most marked on the ventricular bands and the true vocal cords. Auerbach, Hammond and Garfinkel (1970), in a study of larynges at post-mortem found epithelial changes in 6% of non-smokers, 22% of smokers of 20 cigarettes and 44% of smokers of 40 cigarettes a day. The degree of cellular atypia is also strongly related to smoking habits. The presence of cellular atypia is observed in 85% of heavy smokers. After smoking has been stopped the hyperplasia remains, but the cellular atypia gradually diminishes.

In series of patients with chronic laryngitis the percentage of smokers is usually high (Putney and O'Keefe, 1953, 89.8%; Norris and Peale, 1963, 94%). Alcohol is also often mentioned as a causative factor (Hinds, Thomas and O'Reilly 1979), but much less solid evidence is available. In the author's own data on smoking and drinking habits in a large number of patients with head and neck cancer, the alcohol consumption among the laryngeal cancer patients is much lower than among patients with carcinoma of the oral cavity and pharynx. This could point towards a direct surface effect. In a study by Stevens (1979), hamsters exposed to benzopyrene and alcohol were affected more frequently by laryngeal carcinoma than those not receiving alcohol.

Chronic laryngitis is more frequently found in patients suffering from chronic infection of the upper or lower respiratory tract. Stell and McLoughlin (1976), studying a group of 58 patients with chronic laryngitis, found a history of infection in 53%. It is not clear whether this association is due to the increased incidence of coughing in these patients resulting in mechanical trauma, or whether a more generalized involvement of the respiratory mucosa including that of the larynx is the main reason. Probably both factors play a role. The stubborn nature of chronic respiratory tract infections means their elimination should play an important role in the treatment of chronic laryngitis.

Besides coughing, vocal abuse is an important physical factor which contributes to the development of inflammatory lesions of the larynx due to mechanical irritation. Muscular strain, venous congestion and forced vocal attack are probably involved. Virchow recognized the factor of vocal abuse when describing the picture of pachydermia verrucosa in a Prussian army officer. It is certain that abnormal vocal strain especially in those who use their voice professionally can be a source of tissue changes which have a disastrous effect on the voice. These are discussed in Chapter 6.

Finally endogenous factors must also be taken into account. These may be constitutional or metabolic. Short, heavily-built people are more prone to chronic laryngitis. Diabetes, hypothyroidism and vitamin A deficiency can also be contributory.

History and clinical signs

Chronic laryngitis is usually of insidious onset and rarely develops after an acute laryngitis, although this may be the trigger in a larynx which has already been affected by asymptomatic epithelial changes. When no acute infection has been present it is difficult for the patient to pinpoint the exact time of onset.

Hoarseness is the most frequent and often the only symptom. This complaint tends to vary with the time of day and with the intensity with which the voice is used. Typically the patient complains that the voice is worse in the morning. Drying of the laryngeal mucosa during the night through mouth breathing and a decreased frequency of swallowing is probably the reason for this. Inspissated mucus which has to be cleared causes dryness and the feeling of a foreign body in the throat. When the throat has been cleared and the mucosa is moistened again the voice gradually improves. However, it remains harsh with varying pitch and volume. There can be periods of complete aphonia, although these are rare. The vocal range is reduced, especially in the higher frequencies. There may be a cough caused by local irritation as a result of mucus, dryness or intraepithelial changes, which can worsen the other symptoms. Pain is rarely present unless undue strain by coughing has damaged the mucosa.

The complaints of a patient with chronic laryngitis tend to develop slowly and then become stationary. There may be variations over short periods but, in general, chronic laryngitis remains constant over a long period.

Clinical picture

Chronic laryngitis is diagnosed from the history and by indirect laryngoscopy. Direct inspection of the larynx is the cornerstone of any diagnosis. Furthermore, histopathological examination of tissue removed from the laryngeal lesions is indispensable. Without these investigations a diagnosis cannot be made.

Chronic laryngitis can be divided into several clinical conditions.

Simple diffuse chronic laryngitis

The patient complains of hoarseness and sometimes a slight cough over a long period of time. These complaints start insidiously, occasionally during an upper respiratory tract infection, and persist although they are not always present.

Examination shows a reddened hyperaemic laryngeal mucosa. The true vocal cords lose their white colour and become pink or red, sometimes with a glossy appearance or with submucosal oedema. The diagnosis is made on the findings at indirect laryngoscopy. If the laryngeal mucosa is smooth and regular, a biopsy should be avoided in the early stages to prevent damage to the laryngeal mucosa.

Simple chronic laryngitis can best be treated by vocal rest, inhalations with mentholated air and, if the slightest signs of infection are present, an appropriate antibiotic should be given. Furthermore, all possible noxious agents should be avoided especially tobacco and alcohol.

This form of laryngitis is reversible within a few weeks with adequate measures.

Chronic diffuse hyperplastic laryngitis

The most important contributing factors are chronic infection of the sinuses and lower airway; tobacco and alcohol; occupational, chemical or physical irritants; and mouth breathing. The onset is insidious and these patients often have a history of coughing.

The laryngeal picture is determined by more conspicuous changes of the laryngeal mucosa, especially the true vocal cords, which lose their normal appearance. The mucosa is clearly swollen and its normal white appearance is replaced by a red, deep red or sometimes grey colour. The surface of the mucosa is hardly ever completely smooth. Patches of epithelial thickening and broad-based polypoid lesions can be found. The picture is much more alarming than that of simple laryngitis and it may be difficult to differentiate it from carcinoma or specific laryngitis (see Plate 5/5/II).

This form of laryngitis is usually associated with chronic respiratory infections such as sinusitis and bronchitis.

Keratosis, leucoplakia, pachydermia, squamous cell hyperplasia

These terms are based partly on clinical appearance and partly on histological features. They are still often used for local or more diffuse lesions of the larynx, primarily of the vocal cords. Many clinicians would like to see these terms abandoned because they are ill-defined and confusing. Furthermore, the inter and even intra observer variation when interpreting laryngeal lesions plays an important role (Dikkers and Schutte, 1991).

The lesions are often well circumscribed and well demarcated from the surrounding tissue. One or both cords can be affected as well as the anterior commissure. Very often the surface of the lesion is white in colour as a consequence of thickening of the squamous epithelium covered by excess keratin. The elevation of the lesion from the surrounding tissue can be seen clearly with the operating microscope. The surrounding mucosa may be normal or may resemble simple chronic laryngitis. The keratinization may be so abundant that the picture may simulate a benign tumour, a squamous papilloma or a verrucous carcinoma. When the lesion lies in the posterior part of the glottis where the mucosa is redundant to allow movement of the cords, it has also been named 'posterior laryngitis'. Its possible relation with nocturnal regurgitation of gastric acid has led to the name 'acid laryngitis'. At this site the epithelium is already normally slightly thickened and the transition towards abnormal is very gradual, so that care should be taken not to overdiagnose this condition. The presence of symptoms including gastro-oesophageal reflux usually helps to make a diagnosis.

Contact ulcers – contact pachydermia

These terms were coined by Jackson (1928) and Virchow (1887) respectively and are still in use today. Although Jackson later included vocal cord granuloma, this should be considered as a separate entity.

Contact ulcers are saucer-like lesions on the medial edge of the vocal cord exactly at the vocal process (see Plate 5/5/III). They can be bilateral and symmetrical, often with a small projection on one cord which fits the saucer of the other side. There is no epithelial defect, thus the word 'ulcer' is not correct. The lesions are made up of thickened epithelium with a central indentation exactly at the site of the mucoperichondrial covering of the vocal process. Patients with a contact ulcer may complain of pain. This disease usually occurs in those with tense personalities and it is agreed that vocal overuse and abuse are important aetiological factors.

Histology of chronic laryngitis

The importance of an accurate histological diagnosis in cases of chronic laryngitis cannot be overestimated. The relation between benign-epithelial changes and carcinoma has been repeatedly demonstrated (Crissman, 1979).

The chances of malignant degeneration are related to certain histomorphological characteristics which can help to divide the lesions into high and low risk groups (Oldekalter, 1986). A reliable diagnosis demands two criteria to be fulfilled. The first is that the biopsy is taken from a representative part of the lesion. If the lesion is small, total removal will allow examination of the entire specimen. When the lesion is extensive, biopsies are taken from the most aggressive looking part. Epithelial changes such as carcinoma *in situ* are often found in the vicinity of a squamous cell carcinoma and care should be taken not to overlook the site where an infiltration of carcinoma may be present, for instance in the subglottic larynx or in the ventricle (McGavran, Bauer and Ogura, 1960). The second requirement regards the way the specimen is sent to the pathologist. If possible the removed undamaged piece of mucosa should be orientated to allow the pathologist to make sections vertically through the mucosa to avoid tangential sectioning which may simulate infiltration of tumour tissue into the underlying tissue.

Although it is recognized that squamous epithelium can undergo changes which may eventually lead to squamous cell carcinoma and that certain histological and cellular features indicate a higher chance of malignant transformation, a uniform and internationally accepted classification of these lesions is still lacking, mainly because each classification depends on a subjective interpretation. The results of objective methods such as morphometry (Oldekalter *et al.*, 1985), photometry (Hellquist and Oloffson, 1984) and others have not yet found widespread clinical application.

In Europe the most accepted classification is that originally proposed by Kleinsasser (1963), who introduced a histological grading system in which the lesions are divided into three grades. In the USA a more descriptive classification is in use based on keratosis with or without atypia. The normal squamous epithelium of the larynx is non-keratinizing in several layers. Adjacent to the subcutaneous tissue lies the basal layer (stratum germinativum), consisting of cylindrical cells with ovoid nuclei. Mitoses are frequent in this germinal layer of the epithelium. From this layer the cells move to the surface, gradually changing from round to flat cells which are shed from the surface. Although the more superficial cells contain intracellular keratohyaline granules, there is no full development towards keratin. Under normal circumstances this maturation process follows a regular pattern with normal cells grouped in layers. A disturbance of this normal maturation underlies the pathological changes found in chronic laryngitis. The degree of disturbance of this maturation process, also called *dysplasia*, forms the basis of Kleinsasser's classification. In the USA the term keratosis is preferred.

Grade I: simple squamous cell hyperplasia or keratosis

There is thickening of the entire epithelium. The basal cell layer becomes undulated, sometimes with deep projections into the stroma (acanthosis). There is further differentiation of cells towards intracellular keratin formation. The nuclei extend into the keratin layer (parakeratosis) and keratin covers the lesion to a varying degree (hyperkeratosis), but the regular maturation pattern is retained (Figure 5.1).

Grade II: squamous cell hyperplasia or keratosis with atypia

In this second stage there is early disorganization of the maturation process, but this is not very extensive; the loss of the normal organization is limited and never

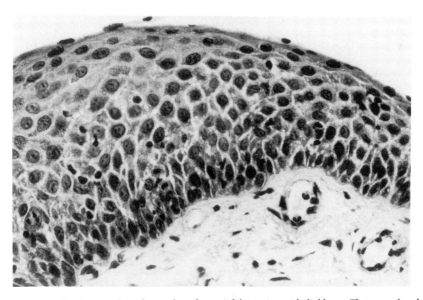

Figure 5.1 Squamous cell hyperplasia grade I. There is broadening of the entire epithelial layer. The normal architecture of the epithelium is retained. There is no atypia (× 378). (Courtesy of Dr J. F. M. Delemarre, Consultant Pathologist of the Netherlands Cancer Institute)

affects all layers at the same time. There is atypia at the cellular level, including altered nuclear/cytoplasmic ratio, abnormal DNA content, abnormal mitoses and other aberrations. Acanthosis, dyskeratosis and parakeratosis are also present (Figure 5.2 and see Plate 5/5/IV).

Grade III: carcinoma *in situ*

This third stage shows the most serious disorganization of the squamous epithelium identical to that of severe dysplasia. Frequent mitoses and cellular anomalies are found. The entire epithelium shows all cellular changes compatible with squamous cell carcinoma, but without infiltration through the basal membrane (Figure 5.3 and see Plate 5/5/V).

Malignant transformation

The chance that epithelial changes as found in cases of chronic laryngitis may develop into infiltrating carcinoma has been the subject of several studies.

Although most carcinomas of the larynx are diagnosed at the first biopsy, about 3–6% of them occur in cases which have previously been diagnosed as laryngeal keratosis.

In a retrospective analysis of 1019 patients with keratosis Sllamniku *et al.* (1989) divided the patients into four groups, depending on the degree of keratosis with or without atypia. All patients had been followed for 5–25 years. Invasive carcinoma of the larynx developed in 3% of cases of simple keratosis, 7.4% of cases with mild atypia, 17.4% with moderate atypia and 27.8% of cases with severe atypia. More than 90% showed the malignant transformation within

10 years. Similar findings were reported by Hojslet, Moesgaard-Nielsen and Palvio (1989).

Treatment

It is important to make an early diagnosis and classify the lesion in order to institute adequate treatment. Squamous cell hyperplasia should be removed locally. Microlaryngoscopy as introduced by Kleinsasser is the most appropriate method. The lesion can usually be peeled off the underlying muscular tissue and vocal ligaments adequately and accurately. Both cords can be treated in the same session if the anterior commissure is left untouched. Occasionally the lesion may be so diffuse that total removal is not possible. In these cases removal is performed as far as possible (Kleinsasser, 1990). The laser can be a very helpful tool in these cases.

Histological examination should always be performed. Grade I and II lesions normally need no further treatment. For grade III lesions opinions differ. The increased chance that an infiltrating carcinoma will develop from such a lesion means that less risk can be taken. If possible, total removal by microlaryngoscopy is the method of choice and should be performed as soon as possible. A laryngofissure is rarely indicated. Furthermore, a good inspection of the surrounding mucosa is mandatory, especially in the subglottic region, in order not to overlook an infiltrating carcinoma.

Radiotherapy is only indicated when removal must be repeated for recurring or diffusely spreading lesions. Although some authors prefer radiotherapy as the

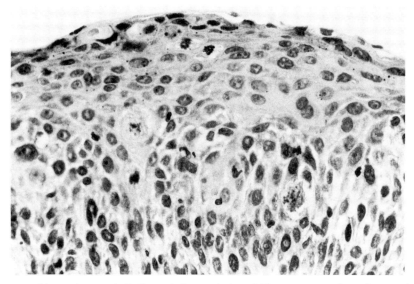

Figure 5.2 Squamous cell hyperplasia grade II. The epithelium is thickened. There is an irregular architectural pattern in the basal and adjacent layers. Occasional mitoses are found. Cell and nuclear polymorphism are present (× 378). (Courtesy of Dr J. F. M. Delemarre, Consultant Pathologist of the Netherlands Cancer Institute)

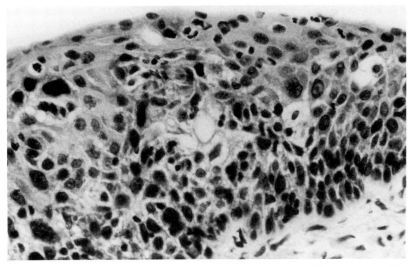

Figure 5.3 Squamous cell hyperplasia grade III: carcinoma *in situ*. The cellular pattern of the squamous epithelium shows all the features of a true squamous cell carcinoma. There is no invasion (× 378). (Courtesy of Dr J. F. M. Delemarre, Consultant Pathologist of the Netherlands Cancer Institute)

primary treatment of choice, others feel that the recurrence rate after radiotherapy is too high and therefore advocate surgical removal or laser treatment.

Patients suffering from squamous cell hyperplasia of the larynx need careful follow up because of the increased risk of squamous cell carcinoma (Hellquist, Lundgren and Oloffson, 1982).

Atrophic laryngitis

This rare entity is also called laryngitis sicca. It is characterized by atrophic changes in the respiratory mucosa with loss of the mucus-producing glands. It is usually part of an atrophic rhinitis caused by *Klebsiella ozaenae*, but is much rarer.

Pathology

Fibrosis of the corium of the mucosa leads to anaemia and glandular atrophy. The respiratory epithelium shows squamous metaplasia with loss of cilia. Inspissated mucus adheres to the epithelium, dries and forms thick crusts. The most common sites are the false cords, the posterior region and the subglottic region.

Clinical features

An irritable cough and hoarseness are the most important signs. Crusts which are sometimes blood stained are expectorated. The crusts can readily be seen in the larynx and are the most important diagnostic feature. If the nose and sinuses show similar abnormality the diagnosis is easily made.

In far advanced stages, when repeated crusting has led to total atrophy, there may be reactive inflammation of the cartilage with progressive fibrosis and eventually serious stenosis of the larynx.

Treatment

Treatment is directed at underlying causes such as generalized infections, poor nutrition or, rarely, syphilis. Local treatment consists of the stimulation of secretions and the removal of crusts. Secretions can be encouraged by small doses of ammonium chloride or iodide. The mucus so produced is less viscid, it softens the crusts and facilitates expectoration. The larynx can be sprayed with solutions of mucolytic agents. Local irritation especially by smoking should be strictly forbidden.

Contact granuloma (intubation granuloma)

A separate entity is formed by localized granulomas, nearly always unilateral, situated medially or superiorly on the vocal process of the arytenoid cartilage.

These lesions are often confused with contact ulcers. Jackson (1923) made no mention of granuloma when he first presented the clinical and pathological features of contact ulcers. Later he added the description of granulomas and considered them as part of the healing process. Benjamin and Croxson (1985) considered granulomas as a separate clinical entity. The granuloma has a typical polypoid appearance which is a local reaction to trauma. Granulation tissue can develop if the perichondrium is damaged either by vocal trauma or through trauma from an endotracheal tube. The granuloma may develop a long time after intubation.

Clinical features and diagnosis

Slight hoarseness is the most important symptom; the diagnosis is readily made by indirect laryngoscopy. The lesion is usually small but can become quite large and sometimes partially obstructs the laryngeal lumen. It is mostly restricted to one side and is usually attached on the superior edge. The granuloma can be pedunculated and move up and down between the cords. The colour is red, sometimes stained with dark areas due to haemorrhage (see Plate 5/5/VI).

Treatment

These granulomas are not easy to treat. Simple removal by microlaryngoscopy seems the method of choice but local recurrences are common. The carbon dioxide laser advocated in recent years for treatment of this condition has not really improved matters; repeated treatment is often necessary. A conservative approach of 'wait and see' is sometimes as effective and should be considered in every case in view of the very resistant nature of this condition in spite of surgical removal.

Amyloidosis

Amyloid is an eosinophilic hyalin material with a strong affinity to certain dyes such as Congo red. Amyloidosis is a disease which has been known for over 140 years in which infiltration of different organs may occur.

Laryngeal amyloidosis is rare. It may be part of a generalized amyloidosis with involvement of many organs, in particular the heart, kidneys, gastrointestinal tract, blood vessels, and liver. There are two main forms. Type A is the secondary type which is found in patients with long-standing inflammatory diseases; type B is the primary type which is sporadically found in the larynx. This latter form may also be found in patients with multiple myeloma or macroglobulinaemia. With modern immunohistochemical methods it is possible to differentiate further the different types of amyloid which, morphologically, are all the same. Laryngeal amyloidosis is characterized by monoclonal light chain deposition, primarily of the λ-type (Lewis *et al.*, 1992).

The clinical presentation of amyloid in the larynx is not characteristic. It may present as a solitary polyp on the vocal cord or as a more diffuse swelling in any region of the larynx or even trachea. Ulceration is not present. A biopsy of the lesion will lead to a diagnosis. A biopsy of the rectal mucosa is necessary to exclude a generalized form.

In rare instances there can be extensive infiltration from the larynx into the trachea, with progressive obstruction of the airway.

Treatment is directed towards any underlying disease. The local lesion can be removed by microlaryngoscopy with sharp instruments or with the laser. The disease usually only progresses very slowly and repeated removal may be necessary.

Granulomatous conditions

Both specific and non-specific granulomatous diseases can be found in the larynx. Sometimes the exact nature of the disease may be evident especially when a diagnosis has already been made at another site. It may be very difficult to make a diagnosis if only the larynx is involved. History, histopathological investigations and blood chemistry are essential for a correct diagnosis.

Tuberculosis

Laryngeal tuberculosis used to be commonly associated with pulmonary tuberculosis. In the western world, improved socioeconomic circumstances and the advent of chemotherapy have resulted in a marked decline in tuberculosis, which is now rare in these areas. However, in developing countries the situation is quite different (Manni, 1982; Ramadan, Tarazi and Baroudy, 1993).

Laryngeal tuberculosis is almost exclusively found in patients suffering from open pulmonary tuberculosis and, in most cases, is a result of contamination by sputum containing acid-fast bacilli. The increased incidence of pulmonary tuberculosis in patients suffering from AIDS will certainly result in an increase of laryngeal tuberculosis.

Laryngeal tuberculosis only rarely develops by a blood-borne infection which causes diffuse involvement of the laryngeal mucosa with extensive ulceration. The frequency of the involvement of the larynx is difficult to estimate and varies in the different series published. Auerbach (1946) in his historic publication found laryngeal involvement in 37.5% of patients with pulmonary tuberculosis at autopsy, but today the percentage of involvement is probably much lower. There is no sex predominance. The age of patients with laryngeal tuberculosis used to be between 20 and 40, but is now generally higher.

Pathology

The pathway of infection is not known exactly, it is believed that contact with sputum containing tubercle bacilli plays an important role. The possibility of haematogenous or lymphogenous infection has also been suggested (Ormerod, 1939). The infection starts in the subepithelial space with exudation and hyperaemia followed by round cell infiltration. There is an inflammatory reaction of the mucosa and tubercles are found consisting of a granulomatous reaction with Langhans' giant cells, caseation and necrosis. The covering mucosa has an irregular appearance. Eventually confluence of these tubercles leads to necrosis of the overlying epithelium which sloughs and ulcerates. The ulcers are shallow with undermined edges, but there may be infiltration of cartilages, especially that of the epiglottis and the arytenoids. Acid-fast bacilli may be found with special stains, but are not always present.

Tuberculosis is to some extent self-limiting and heals with fibrosis which may result in serious stenosis of the larynx. Sometimes tumour-like swellings are found with reparative processes called tuberculomas. Occasionally, there may be a diffuse oedematous reaction consistent with an allergic response to the tubercle bacillus.

Clinical features

Laryngeal tuberculosis should be suspected in any patient with pulmonary tuberculosis, especially in countries where tuberculosis is still endemic. Pain in the throat and referred earache are common. Cough, often productive, and hoarseness are nearly always present.

In advanced cases with extensive ulceration, the symptoms are very severe. The voice may be reduced to a harsh whisper. The pain and dysphagia can become unbearable. Only rarely is oedema so severe as to cause dyspnoea.

Laryngeal tuberculosis presents in many different forms. Mucosal hyperaemia and oedema are common first signs, often with irregularities of the mucosal surface. When tubercles are formed, granulomatous masses can be seen, ulceration appears later although it is relatively rare (15%, Manni, 1982). All regions of the larynx can be affected but there is a certain predilection for the posterior commissure, the arytenoids and the vocal cords (Plate 5/5/VII).

Diagnosis

Patients with pulmonary tuberculosis should undergo laryngoscopic examination. A chest radiograph is performed to assess pulmonary lesions and a sputum smear for acid-fast bacilli will usually be sufficient to confirm the diagnosis.

Other forms of non-specific laryngitis and scleroma may resemble laryngeal tuberculosis as well as the ulcerative lesions found in lupus vulgaris, syphilis and carcinoma. If there is any doubt a biopsy should be performed. Tuberculosis and a malignant tumour may present simultaneously.

Treatment

As a result of improved socioeconomic standards and the discovery of several very effective drugs, laryngeal tuberculosis is now rare. The drugs include streptomycin, para-aminosalicylic acid and rifampicin. Usually a combination of these drugs is used for maximum effect. Toxicity is still a problem, and all otologists are aware of the serious side effects of streptomycin on the auditory and vestibular organs. As well as these drugs, vocal rest should be advocated. Previously, application of local preparations containing local anaesthetic and astringents such as formaldehyde were advised, but these seem to be of limited benefit compared to chemotherapy.

Historically, galvanocautery was applied and even nerve blocks were performed of the superior laryngeal nerves for intractable pain. The recurrent nerve used to be injected with alcohol to immobilize the cord to promote better healing. These measures have now been abandoned.

The prognosis has altered entirely since the introduction of antituberculous drugs and nowadays with adequate treatment a laryngeal infection will subside within a few weeks, but treatment must be continued over a long period.

Sarcoidosis

Sarcoidosis is a chronic idiopathic granulomatous disease, also known as Besnier-Boeck disease. It may affect several organs and the mediastinal lymph nodes are usually involved. Head and neck manifestations are found in 10% of patients of whom only a minor proportion have laryngeal disease (Neel and McDonald, 1982). The symptoms are generally mild notwithstanding extensive tissue involvement. The disease is usually self-limiting. Laryngeal sarcoidosis may be the sole site of involvement in 50% of all patients whose disease affects the larynx.

Pathology

The pathology of the laryngeal lesions resembles a non-specific granuloma similar to the lesions in other organs. The granulomas are composed of epithelioid cells with a varying number of lymphocytes and plasma cells. Giant cells with inclusion bodies are few and necrosis or caseation are not found. Later fibrosis and hyalinization and possibly encapsulation by fibrous tissue are more apparent.

Clinical features and diagnosis

Usually the patient has a history of hoarseness, dysphagia and dyspnoea. In most patients the main site is the supraglottis. The epiglottis and the false cords are swollen, oedematous and pale, and the rim of the epiglottis is full and rounded. The true cords and the subglottis are only rarely affected. The lesion can progress rapidly and lead to life-threatening airway obstruction. The diagnosis is made by biopsy which reveals the granulomatous nature. Further suspicion is raised by systemic manifestations. When the diagnosis is suspected, confirmation should be obtained by a full physical and laboratory investigation. This may be very difficult, especially if no other organs are involved. In rare instances sarcoidosis can present with a neuritis of the recurrent laryngeal nerve through involvement of cervical or mediastinal nodes. A positive Kveim skin test is highly suggestive but a negative reaction does not exclude the diagnosis. An elevated serum angiotensin converting enzyme (SACE) is found in about 60% of patients. A gallium-67 scan can be very helpful in localizing enlarged lymph nodes.

Treatment

Opinions still differ as to whether sarcoidosis should always be treated. In general, sarcoid is very sensitive to high doses of corticosteroids, however, the recurrence rate is high and many lesions will regress spontaneously. The main indication for treatment in laryngeal sarcoidosis is airway obstruction and, to a lesser degree, severe dysphagia or hoarseness. Steroids may be given systemically or by local application, but their effect remains difficult to estimate. If the airway is seriously compromised a tracheostomy may be necessary and may have to remain in place for many months.

Syphilis

With the improvement in the treatment of syphilis, laryngeal syphilis is now rare. Involvement of the larynx is present in about 5% of patients and syphilitic infection of the larynx should always be considered whenever an unexplained infection is present.

All stages of this disease can be manifest in the larynx. A primary lesion has been described very rarely. A small mucosal erosion develops into a typical primary chancre. The secondary stage is also rare and multiple vesicles and papular lesions extend into the larynx from the pharyngeal mucosa. The third stage appears after a symptom-free period, sometimes of many years, and is the most important. Granulomas are found in the mucosa and form a gumma. These are characterized by a centre of necrotic amorphous tissue surrounded by an infiltrate of plasma cells and lymphocytes, sometimes with eosinophils and giant cells. There is periarterial infiltration and obliterative endarteritis.

The lesions have a predilection for the anterior parts of the larynx – the epiglottis and the aryepiglottic folds – compared to tuberculosis, which more often affects the posterior part of the larynx. The mucosa is swollen and infiltrated and later undergoes deep ulceration with central sloughing. Abundant tenacious necrotic tissue reaches and penetrates the cartilage. The vallecula and the lateral pharyngeal wall are also involved. Considerable destruction can be found which, after healing, leaves a bizarre deformation of the larynx and often stenosis.

Clinical features

The presentation of syphilis in the larynx is very similar to other granulomatous laryngeal diseases. Hoarseness and sometimes dysphagia are the primary symptoms. Pain is rare and indicates very rapid destruction of deeper structures. Swelling of the mucosa causes some degree of stridor.

The laryngeal appearances vary widely. Laryngeal syphilis can easily be confused with a malignant tumour or with other chronic granulomatous infections, such as tuberculosis. At one time, the simultaneous occurrence of laryngeal syphilis and a malignant tumour was not rare. Nowadays laryngeal syphilis has become so rare that the diagnosis is usually only suspected after a biopsy has excluded carcinoma, which is so much more frequent.

Very rarely congenital syphilis can affect the larynx in the infant.

Treatment

The treatment of laryngeal syphilis should conform to the normal treatment of syphilis. This usually means prolonged treatment with high doses of penicillin. Local treatment by inhalations may be beneficial. Removal of necrotic tissue must sometimes be done endoscopically to ensure an adequate airway. Local irritants such as tobacco and alcohol should be avoided.

Scleroma of the larynx

Scleroma, better known as rhinoscleroma, is a chronic granulomatous infection caused by *Klebsiella rhinoscleromatis*. The disease was recognized as an inflammatory process by Mikulicz in 1877 who described the characteristic foamy cells which carry his name. Initially it was considered as a lesion of the nose alone, but later, other sites of this infection were described. The disease occurs worldwide with a low incidence but it is endemic in certain parts of central Europe, North East Africa and Central America. In a fully developed infection the histological appearance is characterized by Mikulicz cells, Russell bodies and Gram-negative bacteria but, in the initial stages especially, the inflammatory reaction is non-specific and can be difficult to diagnose. Repeated biopsies may be necessary before the diagnosis is made. Other granulomatous infections including tuberculosis, leprosy and granuloma inguinale can give a similar picture with the presence of macrophages resembling Mikulicz cells.

The symptoms and signs are non-specific and, as in many other chronic laryngeal infections, the diagnosis is usually first suspected after the discovery of the characteristic findings in a biopsy specimen. The presence of nasal lesions, which are found in 95% of patients will help to make a diagnosis. Laryngeal involvement is found in 14–80% of patients. Laryngeal scleroma is rarely isolated (Jay, Green and Lucente, 1985).

Treatment consists of prolonged administration of bactericidal drugs. The spore forming properties of the organism necessitate the combination of an aminoglycoside, such as gentamicin, with an antimetabolite, such as tetracycline. Occasionally, endoscopic removal of granulomatous tissue is necessary to prevent obstruction. Relapse is common and makes close observation for long periods necessary.

Wegener's granulomatosis

Wegener's granulomatosis is a diffuse systemic disease of unknown cause. It includes a triad of necrotizing granulomatous lesions in the upper and lower respiratory tracts manifesting themselves as a sinusitis or rhinitis, a pulmonary infiltration generalized vasculitis involving arteries and veins, and a necrotizing glomerulonephritis (MacKinnon, 1970). Probably about 25% of the patients also develop laryngeal manifestations during the course of the disease. The larynx is rarely the source of primary manifestation (Terent *et al.*, 1980).

The lesion usually lies in the subglottis and may cause laryngeal obstruction. The mucosa is swollen, has a granular appearance, bleeds easily and is sometimes ulcerated.

If untreated Wegener's granulomatosis can be rapidly fatal. Corticosteroids can change the course of the disease if given early. Nowadays there is strong evidence that immunosuppressive drugs, especially cyclophosphamide, are very active against this disease and they are the treatment of first choice. In view of the toxicity of these drugs they should be used with proper precautions and only under medical supervision. Cures lasting up to 10 years have been reported.

Leprosy

Lepromatous lesions can be found in the larynx and these resemble the tuberculous and syphilitic granulomas (Soni, 1992). The disease, caused by *Mycobacterium leprae* (Hansen's acid-fast bacillus), still holds many secrets with regard to the mode of infection.

There are two forms – lepromatous and tuberculoid – both of which can arise in the larynx.

The epiglottis and aryepiglottic folds are most often affected. There is granulomatous swelling, and often ulceration and destruction, primarily in the supraglottic region. The epiglottis may be curled into a hollow rod. The mucosa may be studded with tiny nodules which may also occur in the trachea. Microscopically, the mucosa is thickened and foamy histiocytes are found (Virchow cells).

Modern chemotherapy can alter the otherwise fatal outcome to a certain extent. Dapsone, clofazimine and rifampicin are commonly used. The treatment should be prolonged over many years.

Mycosis of the larynx

Fungal infections have become much more common, partly through the widespread use of antibiotics and cytotoxic agents, which may influence the bioequilibrium allowing fungi, some of which are normal saprophytes, to spread. Also, generalized diseases such as diabetes, hypovitaminosis, malnutrition, hepatic disease and disseminated malignant disease predispose to fungal infections. It is likely that these infections will become increasingly important with the increasing incidence of AIDS.

Other mycoses have become more common as a result of the increase in worldwide travel, which has spread fungal infections from regions where they are endemic (Lyons, 1966).

Isolated involvement of the larynx is very rare. Contamination of the larynx is usually part of a fungal infection of the aerodigestive tract or of a systemic infection. These infections may be either superficial and limited to the mucosa, or spreading deeply into all tissues.

The following mycoses can affect the larynx.

Candidiasis (moniliasis)

Laryngeal involvement by *Candida albicans* is usually secondary to candidal infection of the oropharynx or of the lower airways. *Candida albicans* is essentially a saprophyte commonly found in the mouth and pharynx which can assume pathogenic properties under altered circumstances.

Manifestations of candidiasis in the larynx include oedema and erythema of the mucosa, a whitish-grey adherent fibrinous pseudomembrane and superficial ulceration surrounded by squamous cell hyperplasia. Microscopically the yeast, with its hyphae and pseudohyphae, is easily recognized.

Treatment is primarily directed towards correction of the underlying cause. Drugs containing nystatin or miconazole are given by topical application, as lozenges or as an aerosol.

Coccidioidomycosis

This infection, caused by *Coccidioides immitis*, is endemic in certain parts of California, especially the San Joaquin Valley. Primary infections are common and present as mixed respiratory infections. The disseminated form is very rare.

There have been incidental reports of involvement of the larynx presenting as a granulomatous lesion clinically identical with other granulomas such as tuberculosis. The fungus can usually be seen in biopsy specimens. Amphotericin B is the treatment of choice.

Paracoccidioidomycosis (*South American blastomycosis*)

Paracoccidioides brasiliensis is the causative organism of this fungal infection, also called South American blastomycosis. It is endemic in Central and South America.

The disease manifests itself with oropharyngeal or skin lesions and bronchopulmonary infections. Laryngeal involvement is quite common.

Ulceration of the larynx can sometimes lead to strictures. The organism can be identified in a smear or in sputum and amphotericin B is the treatment of choice.

Histoplasmosis

Histoplasmosis is caused by *Histoplasma capsulatum*: it is worldwide and is endemic in certain regions of the USA such as in the valleys of the Ohio and Mississippi rivers. Many people have been infected with *Histoplasma* during a previous respiratory infection leaving pulmonary calcification which can be seen on a chest radiograph. There is also a disseminated form attacking organs such as the liver, spleen and bone marrow. Mucosal lesions are being seen with increasing frequency.

In the larynx the characteristic lesions of a chronic granulomatous infection are indistinguishable from tuberculosis. Oedema, erythema and granulomas are present, but the lesions lie more anteriorly.

It is not always easy to identify *Histoplasma*, especially in the chronic form. Special staining tests with methenamine-silver or culture in Sabouraud's medium can be helpful. Further confirmation can be obtained by skin tests or complement fixation tests. The clinical course is variable and characterized by exacerbations and remissions.

The most important drug is amphotericin B 30–50 mg, four to six times a day. Careful monitoring is necessary as serious nephrotoxicity may occur. A newer drug, ketoconazole, is less toxic but needs further investigation as to its efficacy.

Other mycotic infections

Other fungal infections which have been described in the larynx include: North American blastomycosis (*Blastomyces dermatitidis*), cryptococcosis (*Cryptococcus neoformans*), rhinosporidiosis (*Rhinosporidium seeberi*), and aspergillosis (*Aspergillus niger*). The diagnosis can be made by using fungal staining techniques.

Actinomycosis

Actinomyces israelii is the causative agent of actinomycosis. It is not a true fungus and, according to most pathologists, should be classified in the group of the higher bacteria (Michaels, 1984). Involvement of the larynx is rare (Brandenburg, Frisch and Kirkham, 1978) and is usually secondary to a suppurative cervical lymph node. The characteristic yellow 'sulphur granules' are seen and under the microscope *Actinomyces* are identified as long slender Gram-positive branching filaments.

Parasitic infections

Parasitic diseases in the larynx are very rare. Leishmaniasis, trichinosis, schistosomiasis and ascariasis are all parasitic infections which can be found in the larynx. The diagnosis is suspected by the general manifestations of the disease, the lesions in the larynx being of the granulomatous type. Detailed descriptions can be found in textbooks of tropical diseases.

References

ANDREASSEN, U. K., BAER, S., NIELSEN, T. G., DAHM, S. L. and ARNDAL, H. (1992) Acute epiglottitis – 25 years experience with nasotracheal intubation, current management policy and future trends. *Journal of Laryngology and Otology*, **106**, 1072–1075

AUERBACH, O. (1946) Laryngeal tuberculosis. *Archives of Otolaryngology*, **44**, 191–201

AUERBACH, O., HAMMOND, E. C. and GARFINKEL, L. (1970) Histologic change in the larynx in relation to smoking habits. *Cancer*, **25**, 92–104

BENJAMIN, B. and CROXSON, G. (1985) Vocal cord granulomas. *Annals of Otology, Rhinology and Laryngology*, **94**, 538–541

BLOK, P. H. H. M. and BAARSMA, E. A. (1984) Hereditary angio-edema. *Journal of Laryngology and Otology*, **98**, 59–63

BRANDENBURG, J. H., FRISCH, W. W. and KIRKHAM, W. R. (1978) Actinomycosis of the larynx and pharynx. *Otolaryngology – Head and Neck Surgery*, **86**, 739–742

CONTENCIN, P. and NARCY, P. (1992) Gastropharyngeal reflux in infants and children. A pharyngeal pH monitoring study. *Archives of Otolaryngology – Head and Neck Surgery*, **118**, 1028–1030

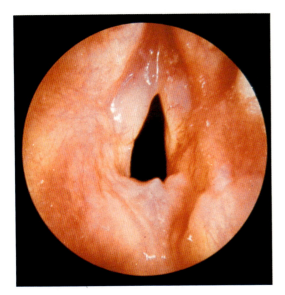

Plate 5/5/I Reinke's oedema on both vocal cords

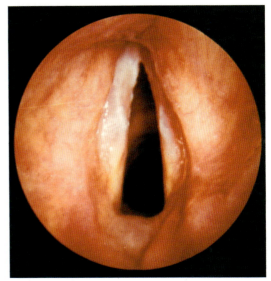

Plate 5/5/III Contact ulcer, saucer-like lesion on left vocal cord

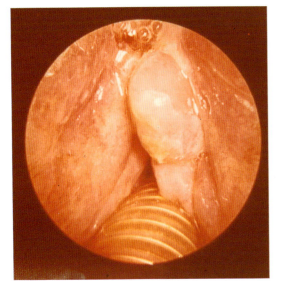

Plate 5/5/II Chronic hyperplastic laryngitis with polypoid projections. Microscopically this was a grade I squamous cell hyperplasia

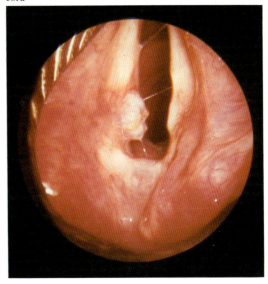

Plate 5/5/IV Chronic laryngitis with local squamous cell hyperplasia grade II

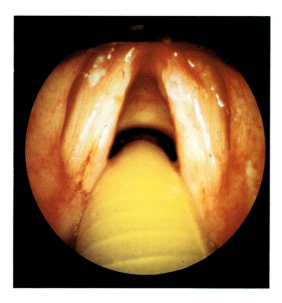

Plate 5/5/V Small lesion on right vocal cord. Microscopically a carcinoma *in situ*

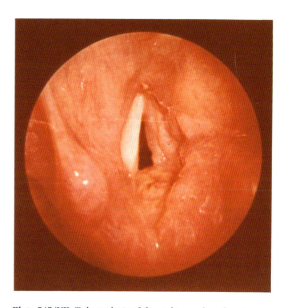

Plate 5/5/VII Tuberculosis of the right vocal cord and posterior commissure

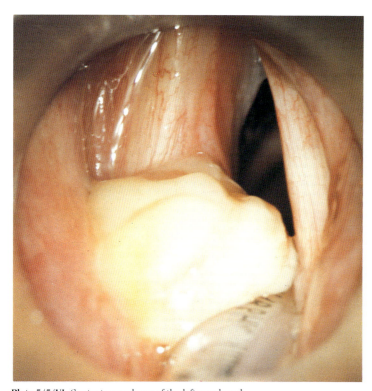

Plate 5/5/VI Contact granuloma of the left vocal cord

COOKE, C.D., COOKE, T.G., FORSTER, G., HELIWELL, T.R. and STELL, P.M. (1991) Cellular DNA content and prognosis in surgically treated squamous carcinoma of the larynx. *British Journal of Cancer*, **63**, 1018–1020

CRISSMAN, J. (1979) Laryngeal keratosis and subsequent carcinoma. *Head and Neck Surgery*, **1**, 386–391

DIKKERS, F.G. and SCHUTTE, H.K. (1991) Benign lesions of the vocal cords: uniformity of assessment of clinical diagnosis. *Clinical Otolaryngology*, **16**, 8 – 11

DOLAN, D. L., LEMMON, G. B. and TEITELBAUM, S. L. (1966) Relapsing polychondritis, analytical literature review. *American Journal of Medicine*, **41**, 285–299

FRANK, M. (1976) Hereditary angio-oedema, the clinical syndrome and its management. *Annals of Internal Medicine*, **84**, 580–593

GABRIEL, C. E. and JONES, D. G. (1962) Hyperkeratosis of the larynx. *Journal of Laryngology and Otology*, **76**, 947–957

GAFFNEY, R. J., HARRISON, M. and BLAYNEY, A. W. (1992) Nebulized racemic ephedrine in the treatment of acute exacerbations of laryngeal relapsing polychondritis. *Journal of Laryngology and Otology*, **106**, 63–64

HELLQUIST, H., LUNDGREN, J. and OLOFFSON, J. (1982) Hyperplasia, keratosis, dysplasia and carcinoma *in situ* of the vocal cords, a follow-up study. *Clinical Otolaryngology*, **7**, 11–27

HELLQUIST, H. and OLOFFSON, J. (1984) Photometric evaluation of laryngeal epithelium exhibiting hyperplasia, keratosis and moderate dysplasia. *Acta Otolaryngologica*, **92**, 157–165

HELLQUIST, H., OLOFFSON, J., LUNDGREN, J. and GRÖNTOFT, O. (1984) Photometric studies on nuclear DNA content and area in different laryngeal epithelia. *Cancer Detection and Prevention*, **7**, 275–277

HINDS, M. W., THOMAS, D. B. and O'REILLY, H. P. (1979) Asbestos, dental X-rays, tobacco and alcohol in the epidemiology of laryngeal cancer. *Cancer*, **8**, 25–30

HOJSLET, P. E., MOESGAARD-NIELSEN, V. and PALVIO, D. (1989) Premalignant lesions of the larynx. A follow up study. *Acta Otolaryngologica*, **107**, 150–155

HOJSLET, P. E., MOESGAARD-NIELSEN, V. and KARLSMOSE, M. (1990) Smoking cessation in chronic Reinke's oedema. *Journal of Laryngology and Otology*, **104**, 626–628

HUGHES, R. A., BERRY, C. L., SEIFERT, M. and LESSOF, M.H. (1972) Relapsing polychondritis. *Quarterly Journal of Medicine*, **41**, 363–380

JACKSON, C. (1923) Cancer of the larynx. Is it preceded by a recognizable precancerous condition? *Annals of Surgery*, **77**, 1–14

JACKSON, C. (1928) Contact ulcer of the larynx. *Annals of Otology, Rhinology and Laryngology*, **37**, 227–230

JAKSCH-WARTENHORST (1923) cited by Dolan *et al.* (1966)

JAY, J., GREEN, R. P. and LUCENTE, F. (1985) Isolated laryngeal rhinoscleroma. *Otolaryngology – Head and Neck Surgery*, **93**, 669–673

KESSLER, A., WETMORE, R. F. and MARSH, R. R. (1993) Childhood epiglottitis in recent years. *International Journal of Pediatric Otorhinolaryngology*, **25**, 155–162

KLEINSASSER, O. (1963) Die Klassification und Differential Diagnose der Epithelhyperplasien der Kehlkopfschleimhaut auf Grund histomorphologischer Merkmale. *Zeitschrift für Laryngologie und Rhinologie*, **42**, 339–362

KLEINSASSER, O. (1990) *Microlaryngoscopy and Endolaryngeal Microsurgery*. Philadelphia: W. B. Saunders

KOUFMAN, J. A. (1991) The otolaryngologic manifestations of gastro-esophageal reflux disease (GERD). *Laryngoscope*, **101** (suppl. 53), 1–78

LEWIS, J. E., OLSENK, D., KURTIN, P. J. and KYLE, R. A. (1992) Laryngeal amyloidosis: a clinicopathologic and immuno-histochemical review. *Otolaryngology – Head and Neck Surgery*, **106**, 372–377

LYONS, G. D. (1966) Mycotic lesions of the larynx. *Annals of Otology, Rhinology and Otology*, **75**, 162–175

MCGAVRAN, M., BAUER, W. C. and OGURA, J. H. (1960) Isolated laryngeal keratosis. Its relation to carcinoma of the larynx. *Laryngoscope*, **70**, 932–951

MACKINNON, D. M. (1970) Lethal midline granuloma of the face and larynx. *Journal of Laryngology and Otology*, **84**, 1193–1203

MANNI, J. J. (1982) The prevalence of tuberculous laryngitis in pulmonary tuberculosis in Tanzanians. *Tropical Geographic Medicine*, **34**, 159–162

MAYET, J. J. (1961) Die morphologische Grundlagen des Reinkeschen Stimmband Ödems. *Archiv für Ohren-Nasen-and Kehlkopfheilkunde*, **177**, 160–173

MICHAELS, L. (1984) *Pathology of the Larynx*. Berlin: Springer Verlag

MIKULICZ, J. (1877) Uber das Rhinoscleroma. *Archiv für klinische Chirurgie*, **20**, 485–534

MUNCK-WICKLAND, E., KUYLENSTIENNA, R., LINDHOLM, J. and AUER, G. (1991) Image cytometry DNA-analysis of dysplastic squamous epithelial lesions in the larynx. *Anticancer Research*, **11**, 587–600

MYERSON, M. C., (1950) Smokers' larynx, a clinical pathological entity. *Annals of Otology, Rhinology and Laryngology*, **59**, 541–546

NEEL, H. B. and MCDONALD, T. J. (1982) Laryngeal sarcoidosis. *Annals of Otology, Rhinology and Laryngology*, **91**, 359–362

NORRIS, C. M. and PEALE, A. R. (1963) Keratosis of the larynx. *Journal of Laryngology and Otology*, **77**, 635–647

OLDEKALTER, P. H. M. T. (1986) Morphometry and squamous cell hyperplasia of the larynx. *Thesis*, Amsterdam

OLDEKALTER, P., HULSEN, H., DELEMARRE, J. F. M., ALONS, C. L., VELDHUIZEN, R. W., MEIJER, C. J. L. M. *et al.* (1985) Morphometry of squamous cell hyperplasia of the larynx. *Journal of Clinical Pathology*, **38**, 489–495

ORMEROD, F. C. (1939) *Tuberculosis of the Upper Respiratory Tract*. London: Stapler Press Ltd

PUTNEY, F. J. and O'KEEFE, J. J. (1953) The clinical significance of keratosis of the larynx as a premalignant lesion. *Annals of Otology*, **62**, 348–357

RAMADAN, H. H., TARAZI, A. E. and BAROUDY, F. M. (1993) Laryngeal tuberculosis: presentation of 16 cases and review of the literature. *Journal of Otolaryngology*, **22**, 39–41

SLLAMNIKU, B., BAUER, W., PAINTER, C. and SESSIONS, D. (1989) The transformation of laryngeal keratosis into invasive carcinoma. *American Journal of Otolaryngology*, **10**, 45–54

SONI, N. K. (1992) Leprosy of the larynx. *Journal of Laryngology and Otology*, **106**, 518–520

STELL, P. M. and MCLOUGHLIN, M. P. (1976) The etiology of chronic laryngitis. *Clinical Otolaryngology*, **1**, 265–269

STELL, P. M. and MORRISON, M. (1973) Radiation necrosis of the larynx. *Archives of Otolaryngology*, **98**, 111–113

STEVENS, M. H. (1979) Synergistic effect of alcohol on epidermoid carcinogenesis in the larynx. *Otolaryngology – Head and Neck Surgery*, **87**, 751–756

TERENT, A., WIBBELL, L., LINDHOLM, C. E. and WILBRAND, H. (1980) Laryngeal granuloma in the early stages of Wegener granulomatosis. *Journal for Oto-Rhino-Laryngology*, **42**, 258–265

VALENZUELA, R., COOPERICHEN, P. A., GOGATE, P., DEODHAR, S. D. and BERGFELD, W. F. (1980) Relapsing polychondritis, immunomicroscopic findings in cartilage of ear biopsy specimens. *Human Pathology*, **11**, 19–22

VERITY (1963) cited by L. Michaels (1984)

VIRCHOW, R. (1887) Ueber pachydermia laryngis. *Berlin klinische Wochenschrift*, **24**, 585–595

WURTELE, P. (1990) Acute epiglottitis in adults and children: a large scale incidence study. *Otolaryngology – Head and Neck Surgery*, **103**, 902–908

6

Disorders of the voice

P. H. Damsté

The relationship of voice, speech and language

The human voice serves a number of communicative functions, some associated with spoken language and others unrelated to speech and language: voice alone can communicate several non-verbal messages.

Non-language use of the voice

Many examples of the non-verbal use of the voice can be observed in daily life. The cry of a baby attracts attention and invites care from its mother and from a very early age a baby and its mother recognize each others' voices. The voice remains an attention attracting device for people of all ages and all through life vocal characteristics are part of one's personal identity. A boy confirms his identity in the playground and shows himself off to family and play-mates, dancing and shouting at the top of his voice. In much the same way a radio or television appear-ance of a popular celebrity may carry impact more because people 'hear his voice' rather than because of what he has to say. In singing the tone of the voice always carries more meaning than the words. More than words the tone of the voice expresses attitudes such as intimacy, authority, submission, dominance towards the person to whom the message is directed. The quality of the voice gives the back-ground against which the contents of the message must be interpreted. A call of 'be careful' can convey different attitudes: genuine solicitude, a reproach or a threat. The voice, even without words, can express emotions such as grief (weeping), frustration or anger (crying). When a person cries out in anger, pain, indignation or astonishment, the tone of the voice carries most of the message.

The quality of the voice is related to other psycho-motor means of communication, such as posture, gait, gestures and facial expressions. A person is characterized by all these psychomotor manifesta-tions which are permanent personality traits. More-over, they can express transient emotional states. Voice, like the other non-verbal means of expression, is partly under voluntary control. It is also part of the involuntary 'body language'. The messages conveyed in an unintended way by body posture, movements, facial expression and voice have a significant role in human interactions. The amount of non-verbal com-munication is grossly underestimated compared to the importance of verbal language, which is usually overrated. *C'est le ton qui fait la musique* (the tone makes the music) is a French expression meaning that the contents of a message depend on the way it is delivered.

Throat and voice complaints are often non-verbal messages of emotional (psychological) disturbance and the specialist must be able to identify them as such. If loss of voice, a sore throat or the feeling of a lump are not detected as a sign of worry or distress, the patient and the doctor both start off on the wrong foot. When both are reluctant to face the true origin of the discomfort, a psychological game devel-ops. The patient avoids the issue by describing only his 'cold', 'feeling a lump', or 'having no voice'. The doctor avoids the danger zone by statements about 'red mucosa', 'laryngitis' and by prescribing medicine. This is more likely to happen if an adequate assess-ment of the emotional turmoil will cost too much time or is simply out of the range of the specialist's abilities.

Thus, even when the voice is almost absent, it is eloquent in its non-verbal language. Some people unfortunately are deaf to its meaning or pretend not to hear it. This is probably the most frequent cause of error in diagnosis and of failure in the treatment of voice disorders.

Use of the voice in language

The linguistic significance of the voice is obvious. Pairs of speech sounds such as p–b, s–z are characterized by the discriminative feature voiceless – voiced. The meaningful coding of language makes use of 'voicing' as one of the distinctive features of speech sounds (phonemes). 'Tie' differs from 'die' only with respect to voicing of the initial apicoalveolar plosive. In whispered speech the distinction is therefore harder to make.

Besides being a contributing feature to articulated speech the voice adds intonation to spoken language. This is the pattern of voice pitch in the flow of a sentence or phrase. The code for producing meaningful intonation differs in various languages and dialects. Obviously the listener must attach the same meaning to a code as the speaker has intended to convey. The intonation or prosody aspect suffers when a voice is very weak or is out of control in any other way. Monotonous speech or unusual intonation of accents is prevalent in neurological voice and speech disorders such as Parkinson's disease and suprabulbar paralysis.

The emotional expression of the voice can sometimes be understood across language barriers, just like the meaning of certain gestures is understood by all mankind. Speech, on the other hand, is only understood by those who are familiar with the particular language environment in which the speaker has grown up. Summing up, it can be said that voice is a natural medium well adapted to communicate emotional content, whereas speech is a cultural medium that is suitable to convey intellectual content. Speech may be used to express feelings but also to hide, disguise or deny them.

Anatomy and physiology of voice control

For the sake of clarity, the phonatory system can be divided into three levels and a control function:

1 The voice activating air-stream (the respiratory system)
2 The voice generator (the larynx with its vocal folds) which causes the air to vibrate and thus produces the tone
3 The voice resonator (the pharyngeal and oral cavity) which selectively transmits some frequency bands (called formants) and weakens others (antiresonances)
4 The coordinating and controlling function (the central and peripheral nervous system).

The voice activating air-stream

During phonation there is a difference in air pressure above and below the glottis. This pressure difference provides the energy that overcomes the resistance of the adducted cords, and causes them to vibrate. In efficient use of the speaking voice the pressure drop from below to above the vocal folds is small (the equivalent of 5–10 cm of water pressure) and the airflow is also low (less than 200 ml/s). A speaker or singer can learn to exert control over the subglottic pressure, the degree of glottal closure, and the flow of air. Too weak closure of the glottis causes a high flow, sometimes audible as a breathy voice with a rush of air. Too strong glottic closure accompanies a high pressure or a low flow, or both. This is audible as a hyperkinetic or croaking voice.

Patterns of breathing

At the end of expiration when the muscles of the thorax and the abdomen relax, there is a short pause before the onset of inspiration. This is called the expiratory pause. It occurs only when the body and the mind are completely at rest. Under this condition the organism has a low rate of oxygen and carbon dioxide exchange and is not expecting an approaching effort or excitement. The respiratory frequency is low and the displaced volume of air small. Slight contractions of the diaphragm suffice to meet the demand for air. The only respiratory movements that can be seen are movements of the abdominal wall as it is displaced outwards by the descent of the diaphragm.

The respiration at rest as just described can change into a more active form as a consequence of:

1 Physiological adjustment to increased CO_2 production in the tissues when muscle activity increases
2 Emotional anticipation preparing the organism for action. The latter can also occur as a poorly adapted conditioned anxiety response. When it is not followed by increased activity it can lead to neurotic hyperventilation.

Normally the first visible sign of deeper breathing is outward movement of the flanks that is added to the forward movement of the abdomen (Figure 6.1). When the large pillars of the diaphragm contract, the dome of the diaphragm is flattened and the lower ribs are pushed outwards. The flanks can also be expanded by active contraction of the external intercostal muscles. This happens when the need for air increases and breathing becomes deeper. Elevation of the ribs widens the lower thoracic aperture increasing the diameter of the thorax; it also assists the movement of the diaphragm to displace more air.

Another effective inspiratory movement is stretching the curved vertebral column: when a cervical and lumbar lordosis and a thoracic kyphosis are

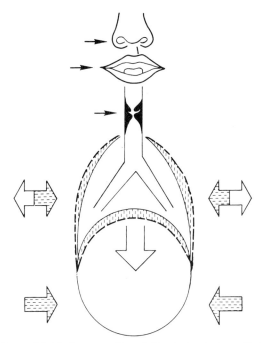

Figure 6.1 The lungs are distended by the inspiratory effort of the diaphragm and thoracic muscles. The elasticity of the lungs supplies the force to overcome the resistance of the glottis and articulatory organs during phonation. → Valve-like controls of the air resistance; ⇦ inspiratory movement; ⇨ expiratory movement

straightened out, the volume of both the abdomen and the thorax is increased. Part of the voice therapy repertoire is correction of body posture: establishing contact with the ground by planting the feet firmly and cancelling a lumbar lordosis by tilting the pelvis backwards. This increases the distance between the insertions of the diaphragm and increases the range of contraction of that powerful muscle.

Generally speaking, the respiratory pattern increases from abdominal to thoracic and accessory respiratory musculature with increasing alertness or arousal. Strong emotions can give rise to overbreathing. They prepare the body for action by autonomic and endocrine changes, and when the anticipated action is put off (e.g. by fear of its consequences) and the hyperventilation continues, too much CO_2 will be washed out of the system. A low CO_2 level in the blood and the tissues thwarts the availability of calcium ions and this can cause various problems. In its acute form it can lead to a regulatory deficit of the circulation and to fainting (collapsing is in itself an extreme withdrawal and flight response; see Voice reactions to stress). In a less acute form nervous overbreathing can cause symptoms of the so-called hyperventilation syndrome: lightness in the head, dizziness, headache, irritability, paraesthesia (a tin-

gling feeling in the extremities), muscular spasm of the hands and the face. Hyperventilation is a regular occurrence in voice abnormality, e.g. in functional dysphonia, when the patient speaks all day long with a great waste of air, and in organic paralytic dysphonia, when the patient is unable to close the glottis as a result of a vocal cord paralysis on both sides.

Effect on the voice of insufficient control of the airflow

A well-controlled voice is produced by relaxed and supple vocal folds caused to vibrate by a moderate stream of air under low pressure. In vocal dysfunction the air pressure and the air-stream are not well controlled during phonation; the vocal cords will not be closed fully during phonation and will allow passage of a large airflow. This is observed on indirect laryngoscopy as an oval or triangular glottic opening. It is incorrect to interpret such an image when seen with a mirror as a paresis of the internal arytenoid muscles; after some instruction and improved voice production the cords are seen to close perfectly, which proves that the paresis has no organic origin. Incomplete closure of the glottis is also seen when the intrinsic laryngeal musculature is in a state of excessive tension that is inappropriate for effective function. Under laryngostroboscopic observation the vocal folds do not vibrate over their full width; the resulting sound lacks resonance as a consequence of a lack of overtones.

When vocal dysfunction is caused by vocal fold closure not being in tune with breath control, it is customary to speak of hyperfunction in the case of excessive closure of the glottis and of hypofunction in the case of insufficient closure. In both conditions there is a lack of breath support. This notion is important for voice therapy, it explains how excessive airflow is kept in check during phonation.

Breath support

In respiration at complete rest the expiratory phase is caused entirely by the elastic force of lung tissue that has been stretched during inspiration and which resumes its neutral position. No additional muscular force is needed to drive the air out so long as the neutral starting point is not reached. After a deep inspiration (when preparing to speak or to sing a long phrase) the elastic expiratory force is rather large as a result of the strongly distended condition of the lungs. If this force was allowed to drive the air out through the adducted vocal folds the air pressure would be greatly in excess of that required for good phonation. Therefore the excess pressure and flow are checked by a counter/inspiratory force:

1 The weight of the abdominal contents, when the individual is standing upright

2 A certain tone of the inspiratory musculature, the diaphragm and the external intercostal muscles. The controlling activity is strongest at the beginning of phonation and can diminish gradually as the expiration progresses and the stretched tissues approach their neutral starting position. When all complementary air has been spent the expiratory muscles may enter into play to drive out the reserve volume of air (Mead, Bouhuys and Proctor, 1968).

The inspiratory control during phonatory exhalation is called breath support. Most professional speakers and singers are well aware of some form of indirect control of the resonant properties of their voice. Some feel it in the abdomen, others in the sides or the back. Some report that the back of the neck feels like a powerful control centre for the quality of their voice. The following paragraphs explain how the curvature of the neck affects the length and tension of the vocal cords.

The vibrating glottis: the voice generator

The expiratory air-stream brings the vocal folds into vibration. The impressive range of intensities, tonal qualities and pitch of the human voice is the result of:

1 The movements in the cricothyroid articulations which stretch or shorten the vocal ligaments
2 The movements of the arytenoid cartilages, each of which is in the centre of the intrinsic laryngeal muscles which cause them to rotate and glide over the articulatory surfaces of the cricoid cartilage
3 The tendinous membrane that covers the inner surface of the intrinsic musculature of the vocal folds. It inserts on the inner side of the cricoid and ends on the free margin of the vocal ligament. This membrane has also been called the conus elasticus or the cricovocal membrane.

The coordinated activity of the intrinsic laryngeal muscles causes the vocal folds to take on a certain firmness, a certain length and a degree of closure (firmly or loosely adducted folds during the production of voice sound). When close together the vocal folds narrow the airway – the site is called the glottis. The folds act like a flutter valve: they are alternately pushed apart by air pressure and sucked together by air-stream. The vibratory cycle (consisting of an open and a closed phase) repeats itself in rapid succession, 80–800 cycles (or more) per second (Figure 6.2). The closing phase is caused in part by the Bernouilli effect: when the air speed in the narrowing between the folds is at its highest, the pressure exerted on the walls of the glottis is minimal, giving rise to abrupt closure. It is this shock wave which, in the frequency of the glottal tone, excites the resonating cavity in

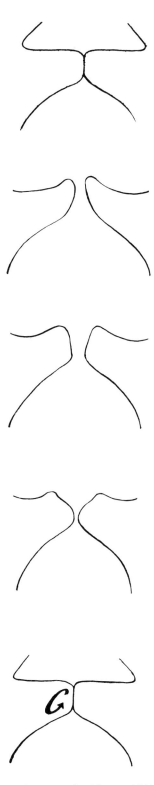

Figure 6.2 One vibratory cycle of the vocal folds

rapid succession. The more abrupt or steep the sound-wave, the more harmonic overtones are generated.

In contrast with the chest register, which is the normal mode of vibration for the male speaking voice, the production of a falsetto voice is entirely different. Here the vocal ligaments are stretched to their full length. The thyroarytenoid muscles in the vocal folds are fully relaxed and do not resist the stretching of the vocal folds. The vibrating mass is reduced to the medial rim of the vocal folds because of the tension in the ligaments. Also the folds are not completely closed as a rule; consequently the flow of air is interrupted in a less abrupt way than was the case in chest voice. The resulting pressure wave is smoother and gives rise to only one or two harmonic overtones, which gives the voice a flute-like character.

The suspension of the larynx

The way in which people use their voice is largely governed by habit. Although phonatory behaviour is in principle a voluntary activity, it is in part automatic and therefore hard to change. Most of the voice disorders that are seen in the clinic stem from faulty use of the voice. Changing voice habits is therefore the most important therapy in this chapter on voice disorders. In order to understand how a patient can, with the guidance of a therapist, attain better control of his voice technique and how this is achieved, the inside of the larynx, and its suspension system must be described (Figure 6.3). This leads to understanding of how the voice generator is linked to the respiratory system. Also the properties of the generator in relation to the volume and shape of the resonating cavities are important.

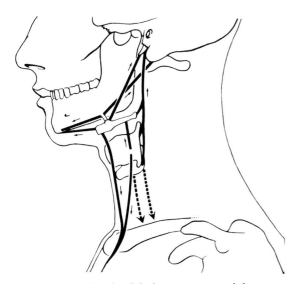

Figure 6.3 The hyoid and the larynx are suspended between the bones of the skull and the thorax

Because of the firm connection of the larynx to the hyoid bone these structures can be considered as one complex suspended between the base of the skull and the thoracic inlet. This complex can be moved up and down in front of the cervical vertebrae by long muscles such as the stylohyoid, omohyoid and geniohyoid. From the highest position, as in swallowing, to the lowest as in yawning, the larynx remains securely fastened to the vertebral column, by an ingenious suspension system by which it glides like a sledge over the vertebrae. The carriage consists of a tendinous centre that is held by the constrictor muscles. It extends from the hyoid to the cricoid, and slides over the periosteum in front of the vertebral column. Short muscles – the middle and lower pharyngeal constrictor muscles, the most caudal part of these is the cricopharyngeus muscle – connect the larynx and hyoid to the tendinous sheet. The cricopharyngeus has a particular significance in voice control. When the larynx is in a low position it tilts the cricoid forward, thus shortening the vocal folds. Together with its antagonist, the cricothyroid muscle, it controls the delicate balance of vocal cord tension. If the larynx-hyoid complex is held in an elevated position, the direction in which the contracting cricopharyngeus pulls is changed, it will pull in a horizontal or even caudal (downward) direction, and tilt the cricoid backwards. Combined with the forward pull of the pretracheal muscles this results in stretching of the vocal ligament (Sonninen, 1968). This effect of elevating the larynx is observed in people without vocal training who try to reach high notes when singing or crying. The result is a shrill and thin high tone, because the manoeuvre, apart from stretching the vocal cords, reduces the length of the vocal tract and diminishes the volume of the resonator.

Influence of the respiratory tract on the voice generator

How the muscles immediately related to the larynx and the hyoid affect the length and tension of the vocal folds has been described previously (Figure 6.4). More distant forces also influence the shape of the glottis and the consistency of the folds and the effect of the contracting diaphragm on the length of the vocal folds is significant. When the diaphragm contracts during inspiration, it moves downwards and pulls the bronchial tree with it. The caudally directed force of the trachea (which, according to Zenker and Zenker (1960) can be of the order of 1000 g) pulls the anterior part of the cricoid downwards. The anterior part is moved because the main force is applied anterior to the cricothyroid joint, situated on the posterior half of the cricoid. The cricoid is thus tilted forward by the inspiratory force of the diaphragm, and the vocal folds are shortened.

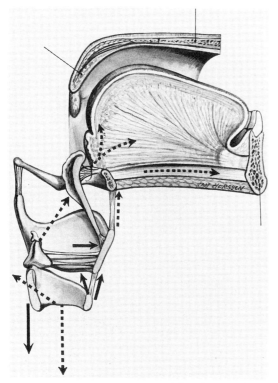

Figure 6.4 The suspended larynx and the effect of pulling forces on the length and stretching of the vocal cords. Full arrows: lengthening forces; interrupted arrows: forces that shorten the cords

The tracheal pull is maximal when the diaphragm is in the full inspiratory position and when the thorax is wide with expanded and elevated ribs. In this ready-for-phonation position the external frame in which the larynx is suspended provides complete freedom for the finest adjustment by the intrinsic laryngeal musculature. Messchaert, a great Dutch baritone, described the singer beginning a tone with his trunk full of inspired air feeling that he is, like the tone, light and floating on air.

Understanding the control of the glottis by muscle forces near and far is important for the diagnosis of vocal dysfunction. It has yet another application. Patients who have a bilateral recurrent laryngeal nerve paralysis with the cords in a paramedian position suffer from dyspnoea due to the high resistance of the glottis during inspiration. When they protrude the tongue they elevate the hyoid–larynx complex. If, at the same time, they apply abdominal breathing with a well descended diaphragm the vocal folds will be passively abducted (Zenker and Zenker, 1960). Even though the widening of the glottis may be slight, it has been sufficient to help some patients through a difficult period without having to resort to tracheostomy.

The voice-resonator

When tracheal pull is applied during the inspiratory activity of the diaphragm, it can be combined with contraction of the pretracheal muscles. The effect is one of widening and lengthening the lower pharynx and this has a considerable effect on the sound of the voice. When the volume of the pharyngeal cavity increases, lower harmonics are selected from the sound spectrum generated by the vocal fold vibrations. The transmission of lower harmonics is perceived as a full and dark sound. This is called covering of the voice, as contrasted with the open voice.

In producing an open voice the larynx is held in an elevated position (short resonator) and the vowels have a clear ai-like quality as opposed to the dark o-like quality in covered voice.

Untrained singers have a habit of moving the larynx upwards when they attempt to reach high notes. Trained singers maintain the larynx at practically the same level throughout the entire range of their voice. The covering mechanism is as it were contained within the mechanism for higher pitch. By gradually mixing the colours of the voice registers they avoid any gap or sudden transition between registers. This is attained by keeping the volume of the resonator fairly constant and by allowing the vibrating mass of the folds to decrease gradually, not suddenly as in transition to the falsetto mode.

Three parts of the oropharyngeal resonator are of special interest: the laryngeal entrance immediately above the glottis; the middle part with the velopharyngeal valve; and the outermost part between the lips (Figure 6.5). The steep waves of air pressure that emanate from the glottis do not flow out in a wide pharynx immediately, but have to pass through the narrowing between the ventricular folds. A rather strong approximation of the ventricular folds has been observed especially during the production of clear ringing tones. The situation is not unlike what happens in the bell-shaped cup of a trombone or other brass instrument. The shock waves are funnelled in a narrow enclosure and thereby reach higher pressures than if they had not met this resistance. The ventricles and the interventricular space act as a transformer or a filter of the primary glottic sound which can be modified, e.g. by raising or lowering the larynx.

The consistency of the walls of the resonator is important. Firm walls transmit the sound without loss of high frequency components, whereas soft walls absorb parts of the sound energy spectrum. The soft palate or velar valve is a 'soft spot' that can be varied at will. When the velum is firmly closed and the velar musculature firmly contracted, transmission is complete and the sound issuing from the mouth is clear. When the musculature is relaxed or thin (in the case of a congenital insufficiency) a part of the spectrum is filtered out and absorbed by the soft spot.

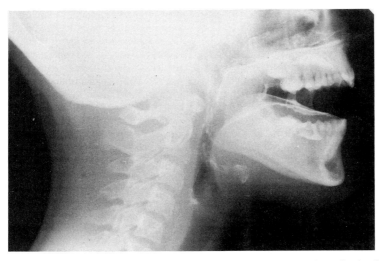

Figure 6.5 Lateral radiograph of the neck and the low facial part of the skull, showing an elevated soft palate, the resonating pharyngeal and oral cavity, the ventricle between the true and false vocal cords

It is not even necessary for the velar porch to be open; when an area as large as that of the soft palate is soft, it works as a filter: low frequencies are comparatively unaffected, frequencies above 1200 Hz disappear from the spectrum. The result is perceived as a hypernasal sound that lacks lustre.

The voice sound generated at the glottal source and transmitted through the resonating tube is finally imparted to the ambient air through the mouth. The vocal intensity (as measured) or the loudness (as perceived) is roughly proportional to the area of the mouth opening. This explains the importance of practising mandibular opening in singing and speaking.

Integration and control by the central nervous system

When a person is actively engaged in oral communication, be it in song or speech, the entire body participates in the activity. Not only the intrinsic laryngeal musculature, but also the soft palate, the tongue, the floor of the mouth, the muscles of the neck, the diaphragm, the trunk and the pelvis (for breath support) take part in expressive phonation. All this is controlled by the central nervous system. Signals arrive at the central nervous system carrying information about the condition of stretch of muscles and ligaments, the position of joints (static signals) and the changes that take place during movement (dynamic signals). Other afferent signals arrive from internal organs such as the mucosal surfaces of the respiratory tract. The central nervous system integrates the information and sends out signals for the necessary adjustment of muscular tone.

The key to voice therapy is to teach a patient to make good use of his possibilities, even if the quality of the voice is limited by organic damage. It implies intensive practice at all levels of nervous system organization. The patient will be guided in finding the best possible adjustment to the changed condition. In the case of habitual or psychogenic dysphonia, the patient is taught to become aware of emotional tension and its effect on breathing and phonation. He then practises ways to free himself from involuntary tension that blocks the free flow of air and interferes with free phonation. Awareness of emotional influences on muscle tone, on respiratory and voice control is significant in the diagnosis and therapy of voice disorders. This aspect is often neglected by those whose attention is narrowly focused on the physical aspects of the voice. A patient can normally be held responsible for his use of the voice. If he has temporarily lost control of his voice it is usually as a consequence of some form of stress. Stress is usually not a consequence of a vocal disorder, but the cause of it. Stress is translated into psychomotor disturbances that affect posture, respiration and voice control. This in turn gives rise to organic changes of the folds due to faulty use or overloading of the vocal folds.

Examination of patients with voice disorders

History

When taking the history from a patient with a voice disorder, the principal complaint is elicited first, in the patient's own words. It is supplemented by questions on the following points: the date of onset (gradual or abrupt), the course, previous treatment;

what was the voice like before the trouble began; earlier similar troubles; which activities in the patient's job or free time put demands on the voice? In a complete history all the remaining relevant data required for the diagnosis are assembled. At the very least the following are enquired about: general health and life-appreciation, respiratory and digestive tracts, cranial nerves (swallowing, hypernasality) and, most important, relationships in the family, at school or in the patient's job. Sataloff (1991) has summed up the points of relevance in the history and examination of professional singers.

The examination begins during the history taking. An impression is gained of the patient as a communicator by his conduct, facial expressions and eye contact. The opportunity is taken to listen to the sound of the voice and to note its peculiarities. For comparison at a later visit the qualities of the voice should be recorded in writing. A language has to be developed for this purpose, the following terms are more or less descriptive. Is the voice:

low	or	high
loud		soft
powerful		weak
clear		breathy, hoarse
sharp		dull
sonorous		thin
resonant		falsetto
periodic		raw, harsh
relaxed		tense, strained

It is usual to include in the description an interpretation of the manner of voice production, e.g.

hyperkinetic, i.e. a tense voice with forceful closure of the glottis and high subglottic air-pressure

hypokinetic, i.e. a voice with little energy, and with air waste.

The posture of the body is noted – tense, relaxed or slouched – and the breathing habit – quiet movements of the abdominal wall or high thoracic breathing, using the accessory muscles of respiration.

Functional assessment

Assessing the function of the voice by eliciting various kinds of voice production is important. Often the crucial point in phoniatric diagnosis is deciding how far the functional capabilities of the voice go, and to what degree they are limited by an organic factor. Taking a phonetogram (see below) is a thorough way of eliciting a large variation of voice sounds. As a preliminary examination the way in which the patient's voice alters in response to the following

instructions is observed: coughing, phonating while yawning (check whether the larynx is held in a really low position), voice production successively with a relaxed sigh, with a falsetto voice and, in the case of hypofunction, during an attempt to produce a sharp, piercing voice. Masking the patient's hearing by applying a source of noise close to the ears may result in a loud and clear voice in the case of hypofunction. In glottic insufficiency due to recurrent nerve paralysis or other causes, manual pressure on one side of the thyroid or on both sides (approximating the thyroid alae) should be tried. The effect on the quality of the voice gives a more accurate prognosis of subsequent voice therapy or phonosurgery (see below). In this way the functional potential of the larynx, the extent to which the patient can control his voice, and his readiness or resistance to change his voice can be quickly assessed.

The function of the voice is also evaluated during the examination of the ears, nose and throat when the patient's attention is distracted from the performance of his own voice. The oral cavity and the pharynx are inspected, and the length of the velum is noted in relation to the depth of the pharyngeal isthmus. The airway on both sides of the nose is tested by alternately closing off one of the nostrils, and observing if air can pass with ease through the other nasal cavity. The neck is inspected and palpated and indirect laryngoscopy performed.

Indirect laryngoscopy

During indirect laryngoscopy the vocal cords are observed in quiet and deep breathing and while performing the following manoeuvres: producing a low voice, coughing with a short dry cough, producing a high falsetto and a sharp, loud voice. Thus, an impression is gained of the motor capabilities of the larynx, and the value of an isolated abnormal phenomenon is reduced to its proper proportion. For example, if the vocal cords do not close completely during phonation, but do close completely on coughing and phonating in a harsh voice, one can conclude that closure of the glottis is possible and that the incomplete closure is of functional (habitual) origin. The result of the inspection is described and illustrated with a simple drawing. Also the estimated length is noted (long, short, or cords of average length).

The observed findings are now summarized in a conclusion which relates them to each other and ascribes them to their probable cause(s) – the diagnosis. A phoniatric diagnosis has to account for:

1 The condition of the vocal folds
2 Capabilities and limitations of voice function
3 Contributing factors of constitution and temperament
4 Factors maintaining the dysfunction: psychological, habitual and environmental.

Finally, the diagnosis is discussed with the patient and advice given. Whether the choice of therapy be medical, surgical or behavioural, the patient should be enabled to make a decision for himself based on the available information. The motivation to begin the treatment determines whether the outcome will be successful, particularly when the patient is referred for psychotherapy or voice-therapy. The referring specialist can influence that motivation.

In most patients it will be possible to arrive at a decision with the method of examination just described. Further instrumental techniques can only supply superfluous information in most cases. They should be omitted from the routine examination, lest they should give the patient a wrong impression that he has a more serious disorder than is actually the case. If the examiner wishes to collect data for scientific reasons, he should tell the patient, and ask his permission. It is ethically wrong to subject the unknowing patient to all sorts of recordings that benefit science and industry more than the patient. With this restriction, some further methods of examination can be used in particular cases.

Special methods of examination

Magnetic tape recording of the voice

Recording the voice has several advantages (Gould, 1983):

1 It provides a document for later comparison
2 When the recording is replayed the examiner can focus all his attention on features of the voice and articulation and on characteristics in the use of language, without having his attention distracted by conducting conversation
3 When replaying the recording in the presence of the patient some features can be discussed which make the patient aware of the nature of the dys-

function and motivate him to accept treatment. At the same time the examiner can obtain an idea about the patient's ability to discriminate between the abnormal and desirable qualities of the voice, which is important in prognosis
4 The recording allows various forms of acoustic analysis without further involvement of the patient.

The phonetogram or pitch-intensity profile

The examiner's subjective assessment of the loudness, pitch and quality of the voice can be supplemented by objective measurements. There are user-friendly but costly apparatus on the market that combine a number of acoustic measurements and calculations. A simple sound-intensity meter and a musical instrument which can produce a series of tones in the range between 60 and 1400 Hz will suffice for the examiner with a musical ear. The sound intensity and the pitch can be plotted against each other in a graph, which then shows clearly the range of the voice and its intensity span for all frequencies that have been tested (Figure 6.6).

The voice quality or timbre is harder to quantify. Attempts to derive a representative index for voice quality from the acoustic signal will yield results in the near future.

In the clinical judgment of voice dysfunction data from many sources are combined. One of these sources is laryngostroboscopy.

Stroboscopy

Mirror examination of the vocal folds under intermittent light is an excellent clinical tool to observe details of the epithelium and the deeper structures during phonation. The vibratory motion itself and the different phases of opening and closure of the vocal folds can be seen.

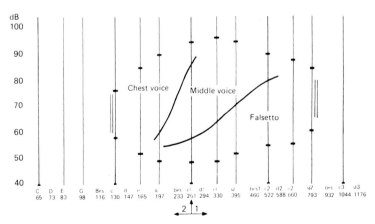

Figure 6.6 In a phonetogram both the softest and the loudest intensities are recorded on the vertical scale, at various pitches. Their frequencies are plotted on the horizontal axis (Damsté and Lerman, 1975)

The action of the laryngostroboscope rests on the fact that the vibrations of the vocal cords are periodic, so that the vocal cords return at regular intervals to the same position. If the vocal cords are illuminated in exactly the same phase of vibration by a short burst of light they appear to be standing still. Because of the speed with which the flashes of light follow each other, and because of the after image effect of the eyes the vocal cords appear to be stationary. A microphone signal ensures synchronization of the flashes of light with the vibrations of the vocal cord. A delayed image of the vibrations is produced by slightly reducing the frequency of the flashes of light compared with the vibrations of the vocal cord. The vocal cords are then illuminated in a successively later and later phase of movement by the pulses of light. This results in an apparent slow forward movement of the vibrating cord. For a description of the technique the reader is refered to Kitzing (1985).

Stroboscopic examination of the vocal folds is carried out in the same manner as conventional laryngoscopy, using a head mirror and a laryngeal mirror. However, the normal light source is replaced by the flashing xenon-tube. The stroboscopic light source can also be linked to a Hopkins rod or fibrescope. Both can be used for video display and recording of the image. The light from the stroboscope is transmitted to the larynx by a quartz fibre bundle. Mainly the upper surface of the vocal cords is seen, whereas the lower surface remains out of sight. However, the medial surfaces which are directed towards each other are easily seen, at least during the open phase of the vocal folds. This is an advantage over conventional laryngoscopy when during phonation the fast vibrations only permit a blurred view of the medial edges. Small irregularities can then escape the examiner. In stroboscopy it is possible to see accurately where an epithelial abnormality is situated and how it participates in, or impedes, phonation. In stroboscopic laryngoscopy one sees the vibrating part of the vocal folds sharply defined, and everything which protrudes from their medial surfaces is distinctly observed.

With the help of a well adjusted stroboscope the extremely fast vibratory movement appears as a gentle waving motion.

The pattern of the wave motion

In the chest or modal register the vocal folds have a soft or elastic consistency. A wave edge appears from the underside, moving the medial surfaces apart. It ebbs away when it reaches the upper surface of the folds. At the same moment the glottic chink has already begun to close from the underside. In the lower tones of the vocal range the folds are soft, and the amplitude of vibration is large. As the pitch is increased the substance of the folds becomes gradually firmer, and the amplitude of the vibration smaller. In untrained voices there is a sudden transition towards the falsetto register.

Electromyography (EMG)

The intrinsic laryngeal muscles can be approached in two ways for insertion of electrodes. Via the mouth and pharynx wire electrodes can be placed in the vocalis muscle. Through the skin of the neck concentric needle electrodes can be inserted in the various layers of the laryngeal musculature. The procedure should be reserved for research purposes. The author is of the opinion that in individual cases the results are mostly not relevant enough to warrant the use of laryngeal EMG as a clinical diagnostic tool.

Recording the airflow during phonation

Efficient use of the voice is characterized by low airflow, resulting in a clear voice of high intensity, hence the importance of measuring and recording the flow of air simultaneously with recording the sound pressure level (SPL). A mask in which a pressure gradient microphone is integrated is fitted over the face. The tracks of the flow mask and the SPL are made visible on an oscilloscope.

Electroglottogram (EGG)

EGG is the recorded change in electrical impedance over the glottis which follows the cyclical changes of the area of contact between the two vocal folds. It gives an impression of the ratio of closure of the glottis in relation to the full vibration period.

Diagnosis and treatment

Table 6.1 displays the various voice disorders. It is divided into four columns: the right column shows the disorders of primarily organic origin, such as laryngeal paralysis and papilloma. The columns on the left show the psychogenic and habitual voice disorders; there is no laryngeal disease and, from an organic point of view, the phonatory system is capable of function. The cause of dysfunction is either emotional or habitual. In the former case the voice is inhibited by psychological stress, in the latter case faulty use or overloading of the voice causes the dysfunction.

Functional dysphonia of long standing may give rise to organic adaptations to the misuse. These secondary organic affections of the vocal cords are displayed in the middle column. They are the consequences of temporary or chronic abuse of the vocal folds and, as long as they have not progressed too far, are still reversible. For this reason they belong to the large class of functional dysphonias, and not to the primary organic dysphonias.

Table 6.1 Overview of voice disorders

Functional		Organic	
Psychogenic (phononeurosis)	*Habitual*	*Secondary organic (phonoponosis)*	*Primary organic*
Emotional or psychotraumatic interference with voice control Anxiety neurosis	Improper use of the voice leads to ⟶ (habitual dysphonia)	Overloading, leading to abnormal adaptations of the cords such as:	Congenital web or asymmetry Neuromotor disorders (peripheral or central)
Compensation neurosis (reinforced by the effect)	Habitual dysphonia ⟶	Irritation of the mucosa, recurrent laryngitis	Trauma (also surgical and intubation granuloma)
Psychogenic aphonia or dysphonia	Hypofunction ⟶	Oedema, nodules (chronic nodular laryngitis)	Cysts, polyps, infections: common cold, tracheobronchitis, syphilis, systemic diseases
Spastic dysphonia	Hyperfunction ⟶	Chronic laryngitis with hyperplasia of epithelium: leucoplakia, pachydermia (contact ulcer)	
Disorders related to adolescence Prolonged mutation Mutation falsetto Incomplete mutation ⟶		Hypoplasia of muscular and connective tissue	Tumours benign/malignant Endocrine disorders Congenital weakness (sulcus glottidis)

Psychogenic voice disorders

Emotionally-conditioned voice disorders are by no means rare and they require skilful professional assistance before the patient can resume control over his voice. The voice is the mirror of the soul and in these cases the loss of control of the voice shows the soul to be in disarray. A questionable form of therapy still often used by otolaryngologists consists of suggestive laryngological actions executed with magic and/or authority. If the loss of voice has allowed the patient sufficient time to re-establish mental composure, a suggestive treatment may be appropriate. However, the chances of recurrence are high if the causes of the stress and the resulting disarray are left untreated. In such cases the needs of the patient are best answered by an appropriate form of counselling, for which the patient can be referred to the family physician, a knowledgeable speech therapist, a psychotherapist or, if applicable a priest. Every specialist should be aware of his limitations; if a laryngologist feels that he is inexperienced in counselling patients in emotional turmoil, he should help the patient to find a suitable source of moral support.

In a number of cases the pseudoparalysis is the consequence of a lack of assertiveness. A person who knows how to hold his own in difficult circumstances is less vulnerable to psychogenic dysfunction than a person who lacks self-reliance. A course in assertiveness training can provide support in episodes of aphonia and prevent recurrences.

Voice reactions to stress

A common reaction to frustration and grief is crying. In ethological terms this behaviour can be described as 'agonistic', i.e. is a response to a situation that the individual is incapable of coping with in a more adult way. He or she then resorts to a primitive behavioural pattern of withdrawal or flight: crying solicits pity and help from bystanders, appeases a threatening dominant person and is one way to solve an unbearable situation.

Even more common than crying is responding to frustration and anger by shouting. Both weeping and anger belong to the same family of agonistic behaviour. In contrast to crying, which is linked to flight and submission, shouting in anger is linked to fight and aggression.

Shouting and crying are generally felt to be socially undesirable or even unacceptable. Many people have been so conditioned by their upbringing that they consistently reject any show of emotion. Such an attitude can easily lead to repression of emotions and inhibition of vocal expression of feelings.

In this vicious circle of bottled up feelings and

unsolved displeasures, conversion symptoms may develop. The whispering voice of psychogenic aphonia is one example. It is of the submissive 'flight' type; hypokinesia prevails and it is prevalent in women. Another form more prevalent in men is vocal stuttering, also called spastic dysphonia. It is a sometimes querulous, sometimes aggressively protesting form of speech with hyperkinetic characteristics. It can have a gradual onset in which the patient feels slight irritation or involuntary contractions in the throat. These eventually give rise to scarcely perceptible interruptions of the voice in the middle of a word, or to an irregular tremor during voiced sounds. As the situational stress does not improve and the voice disorder only makes it worse, the patient starts a new vicious circle of his own design and sometimes with the help of his therapist or consultant. This is the secondary stage of the developing dyskinesia, and is more difficult to treat than the initial stage.

In his forceful attempts to cope with the vocal inhibitions and interruptions, the patient will strain to push the sound out. New symptoms are added, and the disorder may worsen, as can happen in developmental stuttering: the inadequate attempts to avoid or to overcome the difficulties cause ever more secondary symptoms.

The diagnosis is difficult (Stoicheff, 1983). The early stage of spastic dysphonia can be similar to dysarthric voice complaints as seen in degenerative disease of the motor system (amyotrophic lateral sclerosis, multiple sclerosis). The course of these two disorders is different. The voice dysfunction will persist if the communicative stress is not solved and the patient's coping abilities are not improved. However, a neurological degenerative disease will show deterioration over months or years. When there is doubt brain-stem evoked response audiometry may show an abnormality indicative of an organic process. In the author's cases of spastic dysphonia of psychogenic origin the brain-stem evoked response audiometry has always been normal. A better name would be pseudospastic dysphonia, in order to distinguish the psychogenic dysfunction from the spastic dysarthric vocal dysfunction due to brain stem disease.

Behaviour therapy for voice stuttering is, like other dyskinesias, an arduous task. Many patients prefer the immediate but temporary relief of symptoms provided by phonosurgery (see below).

Guidelines for the treatment of psychogenic dysphonia

1 Help the patient find out what may have caused him to lose control of his voice
2 Assist him to clear up misinterpretations of the complaint in the home and family environment. It is better to admit emotional stress as the cause of the voice suffering than to continue the game of 'laryngitis' or 'neurological disorder'
3 Prevent unnecessary diagnostic examination, which draws attention to the conversion symptom, promotes somatic fixation, and leads the attention away from the emotional inadequacies which have caused it
4 If the events and circumstances that caused the emotional stress have been discovered, the patient should receive support and instruction on how to cope with similar stressful events in the future
5 If the patient cannot summon up the courage to look into the emotional causes of the failure of his voice function, he needs a strengthening of his self-reliance and training of his personal resilience.

When the person's coping ability is improved, rather than treating the symptom, the symptom will disappear by itself.

Habitual dysphonia

When a person in normal circumstances nearly always uses a poor voice, this is called habitual dysphonia. The quality of the voice has no relation to stressful events and seems to be a habit. Just like an emotionally-conditioned dysphonia it is a learned behaviour which can be changed. However, there are differences. For the correct diagnosis the consultant should obtain answers to several questions. If the following series is answered in the affirmative, the complaint is probably habitual dysphonia:

1 Has the quality of the voice always been poor?
2 Has the voice problem had a very gradual onset?
3 Is the quality of the voice nearly constant?
4 Has the voice failed repeatedly after prolonged speaking?

When the following questions are answered with 'yes' the diagnosis is more likely to be psychogenic dysphonia:

1 Before the voice problem began was the voice quality good?
2 Has the change in voice quality arisen abruptly?
3 Is the quality of the voice inconstant, changing with the circumstances?
4 Has the voice failed repeatedly in situations of emotional stress?

There is no sharp division between habitual and psychogenic voice disorders. Anyone can suffer a temporary loss of control of the voice due to stressful circumstances, and people with poor vocal habits are probably more vulnerable than others. Perello (1962) has expressed this idea by assigning patients with functional voice disorders a place on the following scale:

phononeurosis and phonoponosis
←――――――――――――――――――――――――→
emotional problem misuse and overloading

Diagnostic analysis can determine to what extent emotional factors and to what extent voice use and voice load are responsible in an individual case. A combination of these factors was known by an old term 'phonasthenia'. A typical example was the teacher with a poor vocal technique, who loses his voice in the course of the day owing to emotional stress in his occupation. Instead of abiding by this ill-defined term, the therapist should see clearly whether he is working on improving the patient's voice technique and, when he is, bracing weaknesses of personality and improving the patient's skill in communicating with the environment. The two approaches can be applied in combination by one and the same therapist.

Some patients need excercises and very little counselling. Others are cured by a few counselling sessions and no voice practice at all.

Disorders of the voice in relation to adolescence

The voice changes at the start of adolescence, when a boy is between 12 and 15 years of age. A low voice, divided into a chest and a falsetto register is one of the sexual characteristics of the human male. It is the result of growth of the larynx and the vocal folds under the influence of testosterone. Increased production of testosterone is in turn initiated by decrease of gonadotrophins, secreted by the hypophysis. The voice change begins a short time before the growth of the larynx becomes noticeable. After about a year the speaking voice has fallen on average by eight semitones (from around 268 Hz to 173 Hz). These are average values but there are great individual variations. The mutation is not only a change of the tonal range but especially a change of the sound quality: the light boy's voice gives way to the heavy man's voice.

The popular association of functional mutational disorders with femininity or sexual immaturity is incorrect: cases of intersex and eunuchoidism are extremely rare. They will be mentioned in the paragraph on primarily organic voice disorders. In order to ascertain that a patient is developing normally, the first question can be if he has started to shave yet. Some hair under the nose and on the chin and the presence of acne are reliable indications of androgenic hormonal activity. A prominent junction of the thyroid alae (the Adam's apple) indicates sexual maturation of the larynx. If laryngoscopy shows vocal cords of normal length this is another sign that the voice disorder under investigation is not of hypogonadal origin.

The above applies to all three of the common mutational disorders: mutation falsetto voice, prolonged mutation and incomplete mutation. All three are abnormal functional adjustments to the change in size of the vocal folds. The audible characteristics in each are different. In prolonged mutation the heavy and the light registers alternate. For every part of a sentence that is spoken in falsetto voice, there are a few syllables or words spoken in the chest voice. Sometimes the young man is not aware of the inconsistency in timbre and pitch of his voice which may be one reason why he has not achieved control over his new voice. Inconstancy of the voice also occurs in normal cases of mutation; it is only when the duration extends over half a year or so and does not show a tendency to decrease, that it is termed a prolonged mutation.

A person with a mutational falsetto voice speaks continuously in a falsetto voice. There may be brief periods, e.g. during laughing or coughing when the voice drops into a heavy register. This event greatly facilitates the diagnosis because only a mature male larynx can generate separate registers. Hearing the heavy register, even for one short moment, confirms that a normal chest voice can be produced by the larynx and that hypogonadism is out of the question.

The diagnosis is more difficult in cases of incomplete mutation. An important fact drawn from the voice history is that the mutation has proceeded imperceptibly. The sound of the voice is less characteristic than in the previous two conditions. There is no question of split registers, the pitch of the voice is too high, the tone is dull, it lacks the low resounding quality of the modal or heavy register and the origin of the poor voice quality goes back to the time of the mutation.

Abnormal use of the voice during puberty is found in the history of some cases of incomplete mutation. Patients who have continued to sing in a boys' choir long after the pubertal change of the larynx has set in, may have impeded a normal transition of the vocal fold tissues to the post-adolescent state. Also patients who have suffered from chronic non-specific respiratory diseases, such as asthma, often have a dysphonia similar to incomplete mutation. Tense breathing habits may have prevented these individuals from establishing a pattern of relaxed and well controlled phonation.

The treatment of incomplete mutation is very different from that of prolonged mutation and mutational falsetto voice. In the latter it is always possible to elicit a voice sound in the normal register, by lowering the larynx and pressure on the Adam's apple. The change to a normal voice should be abrupt, not gradual. The duration of treatment can usually be short. In patients with incompletely mutated voices the treatment is aimed at achieving more supple cords: the structure of connective tissue and muscles in the folds must change. This requires intense work on the part of the patient over a period of months or years.

Hypo- and hyperkinetic forms of habitual dysphonia and the resulting organic laryngeal abnormality

In many cases of poor vocal habits the delicate balance between subglottic pressure, breath flow and glottal resistance (firmness of closure) is neglected. When the vocal folds are not sufficiently closed and too much air is used, the voice sounds breathy. This is called hypokinetic dysphonia. When the glottis is closed too firmly, the resulting voice sound is harsh or croaking and is called hyperkinetic dysphonia. Sometimes it is hard to distinguish hypokinesis at the level of the glottis, hyperkinesis at the ventricular and pharyngeal level (constriction) and high thoracic breathing. In that case the issue is left undecided and termed 'dyskinesis'.

Prolonged use of improper vocal habits may cause the vocal folds to adapt to the strain by forming nodules, oedema and various forms of hyperplasia. The former are seen more in children and women, the latter in men.

Vocal nodules

Vocal cord nodules are a frequent disorder in both children and adults. In children and adolescents they consist of spindle-shaped thickenings of the edges of the vocal cords, whereas in adults they constitute more localized thickenings, varying from small points to nodules, typically at the junction of the anterior and middle thirds of the vocal cords and always symmetrically on both cords.

Vocal nodules originate from a combination of overtaxing and incorrect use of the voice (habitual dysphonia). They can be prevented or cured by voice rest or by learning to use the voice properly. So strong is the influence of function on the form of the vocal cords, that the nodules can come and go in a matter of weeks, as has been observed many times in salesmen during a busy season or in housewives in a period of emotional stress. If the factors which lead to the nodules persist for a long time the nodules become permanent. A preliminary phase of submucous transudation is followed by ingrowth of vessels, then by fibrous organization. At this stage resumption of normal function leads more slowly to a return to normal.

The consistency of the nodules can be observed by laryngoscopy under stroboscopic light. Local oedematous swelling of recent onset vibrates in phase with the whole vocal fold, whereas an older and more fibrous swelling can so impede the vibrations that only a part of the cord vibrates. The improvement in the vibratory pattern during restoration of the voice can be seen well by stroboscopy.

The treatment of choice is re-education of the voice by a suitable training programme that motivates the patient to practise in his home and work environment (Boone and MacFarlane, 1988). Voice rest can be used in varying degrees. Complete voice rest, intended to be carried out literally, is too difficult for most patients to adhere to, because they would need to take sick leave and seclude themselves. The nodules will improve or disappear if this treatment is followed, but the question is what will happen as soon as talking is resumed. The patient is then exposed again to the full burden of daily life and work, still with his incorrect vocal habits. If these habits have not been changed in the interim, there is a high chance that the disorder will recur. There are two indications for voice rest: when the cause of the trouble has been a short-lived overtaxing of the voice; and as a preliminary to voice therapy. The patient who must learn new vocal habits is more likely to succeed if he is encouraged to give up his old habits. This is the case if he is freed from any vocal use apart from his exercises at the start of the retraining period. It has the best chance of success in a residential setting where all aspects of personal change, resistance to stress and voice training are taken into account.

Vocal fold oedema and laryngeal polyps

A thin layer of loose connective tissue separates the epithelium of the folds from the underlying ligament and muscles. The potential space under the epithelium is called the subepithelial space of Reinke. Accumulation of fluid in this space is called vocal fold oedema; if the accumulation is concentrated at one point and balloons the epithelium out in front of it, this is known as a vocal fold polyp.

Polyps can occur along the whole membranous part of the vocal folds, but are most common near the anterior commissure. A polyp at this point can be easily overlooked because it is out of sight behind the epiglottis. It can be brought into view by having the patient lower his larynx during the mirror examination by yawning and falsetto phonation. In most cases the cause is unknown; some polyps may have originated from phonating with excessive subglottic air pressure and incompletely closed cords, so that the mucous membrane at the anterior commissure is sucked on and ballooned out. The accumulation of fluid in the subepithelial layer is later followed by the ingrowth of new connective tissue, so that the polyp eventually becomes firm in consistency.

Oedema of the vocal cords usually affects both sides symmetrically. It can be an after effect of acute laryngitis, particularly when the voice has not been spared during the inflammatory phase. In many patients it is the consequence of heavy smoking.

The pale appearance of swollen, oedematous vocal folds is unmistakable. It is more difficult to recognize a slight degree of vocal cord oedema. Listening to the voice may give a hint when the range is a semitone deeper than usual and high tones and falsetto tones become almost impossible. Stroboscopic examination shows a floppy wave edge and an enlarged vertical component of the vibratory pattern. Slight oedema will resolve in time; when there is a large colloidal mass beneath the epithelium, resorption may take a long time and the patient may prefer to have the swollen mucosa incised, after which the excess oedema fluid can be aspirated. Voice therapy to control the breath flow and ensure sufficient glottal closure is indicated to prevent recurrence.

A vocal fold polyp never resolves and should be removed. The author has seen a few spontaneous cures in a very early stage of a polyp, by rupture of the epithelium and escape of the contents which were not yet organized by connective tissue.

Hyperplasia of the epithelium

Improper use of the voice can play an important role in the inception of a series of epithelial changes, particularly when it coincides with smoking, alcohol intake or reflux of gastric contents. These three causes of chronic irritation combine to produce adaptation reactions that are rather damaging to the voice: inflammation, acanthosis, hyperkeratosis. These conditions are discussed at length in a separate chapter and only the voice aspect will be mentioned here.

When examining the voice field (phonetogram) and listening to the voice it is observed that the patient cannot phonate at a low level of intensity. Because of the thickening of the epithelium a higher than normal airflow is needed to start vocal fold vibration. The threshold of quiet phonation may be as high as 60 dB on the phonetogram. The intensity range and the tonal range are limited. The hoarseness improves but does not disappear when posture and breath control are corrected.

Laryngostroboscopic examination is useful to determine the degree and the extent of the thickening and above all to check for malignancy. In the latter case there is absence of vibration of the infiltrated cord. In this way, follow up with stroboscopic laryngoscopy can prevent unnecessary biopsies, a fact which is naturally important to preserve the voice function.

In principle, all secondary organic affections of the vocal cords, even those with epithelial hyperplasia are reversible if all causative factors are removed. Examples of complete regression of severe forms of hyperplastic laryngitis have been observed when patients were admitted to the author's clinic, when they stopped smoking and drinking and learned new voice habits. Such a regimen is rarely practised and most patients prefer phonosurgery combined with voice correction.

Voice disorders of primarily organic origin

In the voice problems discussed hitherto the primary source of the trouble is always incorrect use of the voice. In the diagnoses discussed here misuse of the voice has not necessarily been a causal factor. A summary of these diagnoses is found in Table 6.1 under the title Primary organic voice disorders.

Vocal cord paralysis

The causes of vocal cord paralysis are dealt with in Chapter 9.

An experienced examiner can suspect a vocal cord paralysis from the sound of the voice. Even if there is no clearly audible air waste, the voice sounds weak and thin, the lower register is lost and chest resonance is absent. This is explained by the difference in levels between the two cords: when the arytenoid of the normal cord adducts it also tilts forward, bringing the cord into a more caudal position than its paralysed counterpart. Thus the vibrating folds do not touch over the whole of their medial surfaces.

During laryngostroboscopic examination hypotonia of the paralysed cord can be seen: the amplitude of vibration of the affected cord is greater during phonation than that of the healthy side. When the glottis is not fully closed, the paralysed cord flutters like a flag in the wind.

Breathing is often impaired in a bilateral paralysis with the cords in the paramedian position. The increased airway resistance is most noticeable on inspiration. Particularly rapid inspiration results in inspiratory stridor. In the opposite situation, with the cords fixed in an intermediate position, the glottis cannot be closed and offers too little resistance to the respiratory air, also during phonation. If the patient speaks a good deal, the excessive displacement of respiratory air can result in hyperventilation. A decreased tension of carbon dioxide in the blood and tissues leads to peculiar complaints, which the patient seldom connects with his voice problem. These complaints include tingling in the fingers and feet (paraesthesia), feeling light-headed or dizzy, headache, irritability and emotional lability. It is wise to enquire about symptoms of the hyperventilation syndrome before beginning voice exercises.

Treatment

In a unilateral paralysis in the intermediate position the aim of treatment is better glottic closure which can be achieved with exercises that make use of the remaining innervation and that stimulate compensation by adjoining muscles. The exercises consist of short and well controlled expiratory thrusts that bring the vocal folds into vibration. The Bernouilli (suction) effect narrows the glottis. External pressure by two fingers to the side of the larynx can improve the sound. Progress is measured by the duration of phonation. When proper care is taken development of a false vocal cord voice can be prevented.

Surgical methods for improving the voice when exercises have not had the desired effect are discussed below.

A bilateral paralysis in the paramedian position can develop into a situation in which the vocal cords lie closer together, in the median position. The voice improves, but the patient now has shortness of breath on inspiration and audible stridor. When stridor and shortness of breath become serious there comes a point at which relief must be provided, either by a tracheostomy or by an operation to widen the glottis, in other words, lateral fixation of an arytenoid. In borderline cases exercises for the improvement of breath control can forestall the need for an operation. When the glottic resistance is abnormally high, improvement of the posture can provide just that little extra widening of the glottis which makes satisfactory breathing possible. Straightening the vertebral column and increasing the tracheal pull (see Figure 6.4) by full diaphragmatic breathing are especially helpful.

After an operation to widen the glottis one should not expect too much of the vocal function, because of the air escape during speaking. Voice exercises now serve to provide clear articulation and to reduce air waste to a minimum to prevent the symptoms of hyperventilation.

Voice disturbances caused by endocrine dysfunction

A child's voice, the voice of an adult woman and that of a man sound different mainly because of the different sizes of the vocal folds and because the resonant tubes are small, medium and large respectively. The differences between the sexes (sexual dimorphism) are induced by genetic influence in early embryonic development and are later elaborated by hormonal action during the period of rapid growth of puberty and adolescence. At a more mature age the effect of the sex hormones is more limited. Oestrogens administered to a grown man change the texture of the skin and hair and increase subcutaneous fat deposits on the breasts and the hips but do not change the timbre and pitch of the voice to a perceptible degree. Androgens administered to a grown woman have a more marked effect. They cause extra nitrogen uptake and protein synthesis in the organs that change with the male secondary sex characteristics: the size of the vocal folds increases changing the voice in timbre and range, hair starts to grow in unusual places and there may be enlargement of the clitoris. The effects of oestrogens on men and of androgens on women are different in another respect. In the former, feminization effects rapidly disappear after the intake of hormones is discontinued. In the latter the virilization effect on the voice persists.

Intersexuality

Aberrant sexual development may be caused by chromosomal abnormalities. XO and XXY are the most frequent abnormal chromosome sets. In the presence of only one X-chromosome the individual develops into a girl with recognizable physical characteristics and decreased fertility (Turner's syndrome). The XXY constitution leads to individuals of male appearance who are infertile (Klinefelter's syndrome). During puberty they acquire fat deposits on the breasts and hips, the mutation of the voice is absent or incomplete, and there is little growth of facial hair. In this respect they resemble the eunuchoid syndrome. Implantation of depot-testosterone stimulates development in a more male direction. The XYY constitution (an extra Y chromosome) contrasts with Klinefelter's syndrome by creating male individuals who are mostly mentally handicapped, and sometimes over-aggressive and infertile.

Chromosomal abnormalities are comparatively rare and they are not the only cause of aberrant sexual development. The embryo's endocrine glands start to function during intrauterine life. The hormones thus produced play a role in the further development of the reproductive organs. The delicate balance of growth and differentiation can be disturbed by the relatively large amounts of oestrogens produced by the placenta. It is assumed that a male embryo in a very early stage may be affected by placental oestrogens which prevent full masculinization from taking place. The tissues do not respond to androgenic stimulation; this leads to pseudo-hermaphroditism (the non-virilizing testes syndrome). The baby is born with testes hidden in the labia or in the pelvis, the genitalia resembling those of the female. The child is often brought up as a girl until adolescence, when testosterone production by the hidden testes becomes strong enough to induce male sex characteristics. The voice changes, facial hair starts to grow and interest in girls appears. At this point it has to be admitted that at birth he had been registered with the wrong sex. In these cases a request to change the birth certificate is usually granted.

Eunuchoidism

In 1863 the Italian composer Rossini not long before his death wrote a 'Petite Messe Solennelle'. More than a century later it is impossible to comply with his advice for the performance: 'Twelve singers of three sexes will suffice: men, women and castratos'. The third sex is no longer trained in our schools of music. In order to have a career as a castrato singer, boys under the age of puberty underwent an operation which deprived them of their testes. Thus, when at puberty the hypophyseal gonadotrophic and growth hormones were disinhibited and released into the circulation, the gonadotrophic hormones did not find target organs that could start the production of testosterone. The growth hormone however induced a growth spurt. As a consequence no secondary male sex characteristics developed, but the limbs increased in length by growth uninhibited by the action of testosterone. Hence the tall stature of castratos or eunuchs; others of the third sex amassed large amounts of body fat and grew to extremely heavy proportions. The sexless, unearthly and heavenly quality of their voices appealed to audiences, as at present many are enchanted by the extraordinary musical possibilities of the male alto voice. This is the well developed falsetto register or head voice of a baritone singer.

The few castrations that still occur are usually caused by accidents. Other causes of testicular hypogonadism are infectious diseases that lead to atrophy of the testes. When this is recognized in time the hormonal defect can be replaced by the administration of testosterone.

In addition to the testicular form of hypogonadism, there is the (rare) condition of hypophyseal hypogonadism. Klinefelter's syndrome has already been mentioned as a genetic aberration with a deficient output of gonadotrophins, and subsequent hypogonadism and eunuchoidism.

Sexual orientation and gender identity

In some conditions of abnormal sexual behaviour there is no evidence of genetic or hormonal abnormality. It is very likely at the least that environmental factors have conditioned the abnormality, possibly interacting with internal predisposing factors.

Homosexuality does not give rise to any problems about the characteristics of the voice, because homosexuals, men and women alike, accept their gender and they feel no need to change their appearance. The popular conception that male homosexuals would like to have high-pitched voices was disproved by Lerman and Damsté (1969) who compared the mean fundamental frequency of the speaking voice of 13 homosexuals and 13 heterosexuals.

In trans-sexuals there is a discrepancy between the somatic gender and the gender as subjectively experienced. Some trans-sexuals feel a strong urge to live as a person of the opposite sex, others have the firm conviction that they belong to the sex opposite to that indicated by their bodies. Trans-sexuals may wish to change their physical sexual characteristics by surgical and hormonal treatment. In women the transformation proceeds by surgical and hormonal treatment. In men treatment by oestrogens produces breast enlargement but will have little influence on the voice. Two courses of action are available to change the male timbre of the voice: surgery, with the hazard of a limited voice range and a poor quality of the voice, and training in the habitual use of a light mid-register instead of a low chest-voice.

This can lead to a satisfactory result if the individual has the required auditory discriminatory ability and the motivation to practise intensively.

Virilization of the voice in women

Masculinization can occur in women of all ages. In girls before or at puberty it is called perverse mutation. It is extremely rare and the cause is endogenous – a tumour of the ovaries or the adrenal glands that produce testosterone.

A critical period for a woman's voice begins at the menopause, when ovulation and menstruation end. The hormonal balance shifts and with it come alterations inducing changes in elastic and collagenous fibres. These physiological ageing processes can be compensated for by good use of the voice. If the woman is a singer, she can take precautions that the chest register does not take control of her voice. If she practises her middle register daily in a mezza-voice, she can continue to use her feminine voice into old age.

A large number of women are prescribed testosterone at this time of their lives, because it relieves certain disagreeable symptoms related to the climacteric. This treatment always affects the voice sooner or later. The individual sensitivity to androgens varies and so does the individual's sensitivity to notice changes in the voice. Some notice a difference after one or two injections or a few weeks of oral administration; others do not complain even though they suffer gross alterations of the voice.

The anabolic steroids are related to the androgenic hormones. They are prescribed in chronic debilitating diseases and in the presence of metastases of ovarian cancer. Virilization by drugs such as these is marked by voice change before other symptoms of virilization appear. These other symptoms, especially hirsutism are usually prominent and early signs when the virilization is due to an endogenous cause (the Stein–Leventhal ovarian dysfunction, or ovarian tumours).

It is important that the initial symptoms of voice virilization are recognized, because only then can the drug be stopped in time to prevent more severe damage to the voice. The early signs are so inconspicuous that the patient is often more impressed by a slight change of her voice than the doctor, to whom the voice still seems within the normal range of pitch and quality. Only by careful questioning and listening to the patient can the doctor discriminate between this incipient organic disorder and other more passing organic or functional disorders. One listens to unsteadiness of the timbre: repeated changes between a full resonant and a thin falsetto-like voice sound within one spoken sentence. The difference between the two qualities of the timbre are very slight in the beginning. When virilization progresses a split in normal and falsetto register will become evident. When there is doubt the reaction of the patient to the almost imperceptible change of her voice is decisive: the voice sounds strange to her, it is not under control as it used to be, especially in the high tones. People who sing, professionally or as amateurs, will of course perceive this at an earlier stage than others.

In an advanced stage of voice virilization the lower part of the voice range has a distinctly heavy quality like the chest register that is normal for men. Some patients with virilization feel extremely self-conscious about this chest voice and try to avoid the low tones, even during the examination of the voice range.

Most clinicians agree that the structural change in the vocal folds caused by the virilizing agent cannot be reversed, even over a long period. The organic structure is irreversibly changed and demands a functional compensation. Blending the registers is an important goal of practice. The prognosis depends on the stage to which masculinization has progressed, the age of the patient, and her ability to compensate the damaged function, based on a good musical ear and phonatory control.

Other hormonally-induced voice disorders

Laryngopathia gravidarum is a disorder of pregnancy during which time oestrogens are produced in great quantities. These may cause mild oedema of the vocal folds, as in premenstrual hoarseness. The voice is somewhat lower and gruffer than normal. In predisposed women the disorder can assume a more serious form, with redness and oedematous swelling of the epithelium of the vocal folds, the ventricular bands and the aryepiglottic folds, sometimes with haemorrhage and loss of the epithelium. In another form, crust formation is the most prominent symptom.

The voice disorder can proceed to complete aphonia with stridor and shortness of breath. The inflammatory appearance has a hormonal cause: once the pregnancy is over the disorder usually resolves completely.

Hypothyroidism

This disorder in early childhood leads to dwarfism and mental retardation – cretinism. In later life it causes myxoedema, i.e. a thickening of the subcutaneous tissue; the voice is monotonous, low and dull; speech is slow with laborious articulation. All this is often incorrectly interpreted as the normal symptoms of old age. If correctly interpreted, replacement therapy brings a marked improvement.

Hyperthyroidism

This produces the opposite symptoms: the voice is clear, high and animated, but tends to instability and is quick to tire. Poor coordination between respiratory and laryngeal control may produce hoarseness.

Thyroid enlargement without toxic symptoms can also cause voice complaints as a result of displacement of the pretracheal muscles, and in serious cases by compression of the trachea. The dysphonia after thyroidectomy, described in the section on vocal cord paralysis, is well-known.

Congenital abnormalities of the larynx

When the voice has been abnormal since early childhood a congenital cause should be suspected, particularly when functional examination shows that the intensity and the range of the voice are limited. Indirect or direct laryngoscopy may be necessary to confirm a suspected congenital disorder, but this can be too invasive especially in a very young child, if nothing more is gained than a confirmed diagnosis of a condition that cannot be corrected. The author recommends this investigation only if there is a reasonable expectation that laryngoscopy will lead to corrective surgery, as in the case of a laryngeal web.

Webbing of the anterior commissure considerably reduces the freedom of the vocal folds to vibrate. The voice sounds unusually high and breathy and cannot produce a powerful tone. The treatment is surgery, followed by re-education of the voice.

Another congenital condition is asymmetry of the vocal folds as a result of:

1 Unequal length of the cords
2 Unequal mobility of the cords, which can be due to a congenital paresis
3 A difference in the level of the cords which can result from either of the above.

Finally two rare conditions which may lead to a mild form of voice handicap should be mentioned. One is the 'sulcus glottidis', a groove along the length of one or both vocal folds, perhaps due to hypoplasia of the connective tissue (Itoh *et al.*, 1983). The other is over-elasticity of the vocal cord ligament that is sometimes observed in boys and girls with hyperextensible joints in Ehler–Danlos syndrome. It results in a peculiar low and monotonous voice. These disorders do not usually require surgical treatment. Injection of Teflon suspension may be considered.

Other primary organic voice disorders

Senile atrophy

Women of advanced age may speak in a voice with a lower than normal pitch because of vocal fold oedema or hypothyroidism. In some older men the voice may assume a light timbre and a high pitch. At the same time they lose the ability to phonate in the chest register. The cause of this is probably shrinking of the muscle mass of the cords or stiffening of the vocal membrane and the vocal fold ligaments, so that the suppleness required for the production of the chest register is lost. It is certainly not a general symptom of old age.

Cysts of the vocal folds

Two cysts of importance in phoniatrics are the mucous retention cyst and the epithelial inclusion cyst. Both can result from laryngitis and they can interfere with the function of the voice to a greater or lesser degree, depending on their site. As this is usually halfway along the membranous part of the folds the symptoms can be considerable. They may be visually inconspicuous and may appear as a unilateral nodule or hide under 'monochorditis'. Small cysts near the edge of a vocal fold can cause a diplophonia; that is a double or interrupted tone, caused by the inequality of the vibrating masses of the two folds. Cysts are removed assuming that the underlying connective tissue is not damaged. After the operation a period of voice therapy is usually necessary to correct habits formed while the cyst was still present.

Inflammation

Specific inflammations of the larynx, such as tuberculosis and syphilis and granulomas are discussed in Chapter 5.

Papillomatosis of the larynx

When dysphonia has been present for some time and shows a gradual progression, laryngoscopy may reveal a warty epithelial mass on one of the cords. The diagnosis of a papilloma is confirmed by histological examination of the specimen, which shows a characteristic arrangement of the cells in this benign epithelial tumour. In adults, surgical removal of the growth is unlikely to be followed by a recurrence. However, in children, these tumours are apt to recur, and multiple papillomas may occur on both vocal cords and the false cords, sometimes extending to the epiglottis and the trachea.

The prognosis improves with age, the chance of extension and recurrence becomes much less with the attainment of adulthood. The quality of the voice should then be reasonable provided that multiple operations have not caused permanent scarring and stenosis. Treatment must therefore ensure that damage to the growing larynx is avoided and that the subepithelial layers are not damaged. Training in non-traumatic use of the voice makes sense because continuous trauma due to incorrect voice use might stimulate the growth of papillomatous tissue.

Trauma of the larynx

Direct trauma to the larynx can be caused by road traffic accidents: e.g. the neck can be struck by a projecting part of a car or motor cycle. A cartilaginous fracture, a ligamentous tear or a rupture of the trachea may occur. After the life-threatening condition has resolved the effects on the function of the vocal fold are important. Mucosal adhesions can impede the movement and vibration of the vocal folds. In addition the slightest interference with the cricothyroid or cricoarytenoid joints can influence the regulation of tension of the cords unfavourably, resulting in huskiness of the voice.

The examination presents certain difficulties. Since there are numerous other causes of dysphonia, it may not be easy in a particular case to decide if the symptoms are connected with an accident, especially if this occurred a long time ago. This problem is particularly difficult if there is a question of financial compensation.

In testing vocal function it is important to determine the margin between the available function on the one hand and to what extent it is being used on the other. The margin can be reduced by retraining the vocal function.

The prognosis for the voice depends on the findings at indirect laryngoscopy with respect to the position and mobility of the arytenoids, the aperture and closure of the glottis and difference in the levels of both vocal cords. Adhesions can be removed or a cord moved to a more favourable position by injection of a suspension of Teflon to improve the voice. On the other hand, unexpected results have been obtained by continued voice exercises. Experience has shown that once one has succeeded in getting a vocal fold to vibrate in the air-stream, regular voice use will bring about further improvement. The form of the vocal fold is undoubtedly modified by the use of the voice. Some feel that this can be ascribed to the Bernouilli effect, the medially directed sucking force of the air-stream by its modelling action, progressively broadening a narrow fold. To produce a tolerable voice with a somewhat rudimentary instrument is a greater art than when normal cords are present. Re-education of the voice requires considerable skill on the part of the therapist and tenacity and optimism on the part of the patient.

Stenosis of the larynx in children before the onset of speech gives rise to compensatory voice mechanisms. In the absence of laryngeal voice, these children develop a form of buccal voice, a 'frog's speech'. With the help of movements of the tongue and the bottom of the mouth air is pressed along the pharyngeal arch which is thus made to vibrate. The sound so produced is only capable of abnormal articulation, but it can nevertheless be understood by persons closely associated with the child.

In a number of cases of laryngeal stenosis, a satisfactory lumen can be obtained by plastic reconstruction. Where this has not been possible the remaining lumen has been fitted with an acrylic tube which allowed sufficient air to be forced through the larynx to produce voice. In that case the patient remains dependent on a tracheostomy for respiration.

Cancer of the vocal cords

Hoarseness is so common that despite this early symptom, vocal cord cancer is often neglected for a long time. Also, this disease usually has an insidious onset and affects mainly smokers for whom a morning cough and a break in the voice from collected mucus is nothing unusual. The hoarseness must then have reached a certain degree of severity and persistence before it becomes a reason for the patient to see his doctor. It is therefore a good rule that if a patient has been hoarse for 6 weeks he should be examined by a throat specialist. Typically this form of hoarseness is constant (not intermittent as in functional dysphonia), and does not improve but rather progressively worsens. Stroboscopic laryngoscopy may aid in the differential diagnosis from hyperplastic laryngitis: malignant infiltration must be suspected when the affected vocal cord is seen not to vibrate in stroboscopic light. Stroboscopic examination can also be used for follow up after radiotherapy: if the hoarseness has not resolved and the vibrations of the vocal fold have not returned to normal, it is justifiable to suspect that the tumour has not completely resolved.

Phonosurgery

Phonosurgery can be defined as surgery designed to improve or restore the voice (Ford and Bless, 1991). Procedures under this name have come into existence since the microscope has been used to view the vocal cords, and suspension laryngoscopy has allowed a stable view of the operative field leaving both hands free. General anaesthesia is required. Of course it is still possible to obtain good results using topical anaesthesia when using a laryngeal mirror, good lighting, and instruments with the appropriate curvature. However, the risk of recurrence of the lesion or of some form of iatrogenic damage is greater and nowadays, modern phonosurgical techniques have preference.

Phonosurgery includes internal laryngeal surgery by endoscopy, injection techniques, laser incisions, and external thyroplasty, also called laryngeal framework surgery. Surgery in connection with the voice after laryngectomy will be discussed in the paragraph on rehabilitation after laryngectomy.

Indications and aims

Vocal nodules require surgical removal only in rare instances: when indurated by fibrosis or covered by hyperkeratosis (Bouchayer and Cornut, 1992). Mucous retention cysts should be removed whenever they give rise to serious voice complaints. They may

hide under the appearance of a nodule, under a stretched mucosa the yellow contents become visible. The cyst wall should be removed in its entirety, care being taken that the underlying ligament is not damaged.

In surgery for congenital defects, such as atrophic patches and sulcus vocalis, the aim is to restore a mucosa that is free to glide over the underlying connective tissue. An inherent risk of surgery on vocal folds is adhesion of the mucosa onto the ligament, which makes normal vibration impossible. Sometimes steroid injections into the subepithelial space are used to prevent inflammation and subsequent fibrosis.

In removing multiple papillomas that obstruct the airway care is taken that healthy epithelium is saved in order to preserve the voice. Cryosurgery has the advantage of selectively treating the diseased tissue.

The use of the CO_2 laser for endolaryngeal surgery cannot be generally advocated. It requires stringent extra precautions to prevent accidents, extra courses for all personnel involved, and the results have not been shown to be better than those obtained by the use of normal microsurgical instruments. Recovery of the voice after laser surgery on the vocal fold is often slow, due to scarring and destruction of nervous tissue in the mucosa.

Chronic adductor paralysis can remain a severe voice disorder when voice training has failed to achieve compensatory glottic closure by the healthy cord. Nerve and muscle grafts have not given consistent results, the usual treatment now is injection of Teflon suspension to displace the paralysed cord towards the midline, or thyroplasty (discussed under External surgery). Since the Teflon suspension is a viscous paste a special Brünings syringe is needed equipped with a wide bore needle. The surgery is best done under topical anaesthesia. Two or three small deposits of Teflon are injected into the lateral part of the vocal fold, not more than is needed for a slight displacement. It is important that the fold should approach the opposite fold at the correct vertical level.

Surgery for improvement of the voice in (pseudo) spastic dysphonia is an issue under debate. Its aim is to paralyse one of the cords so as to replace voice stuttering by a paralytic dysphonia. This is attained by injecting the cord with botulinum toxin, or by severing the recurrent nerve. With the first method the treatment has to be repeated every 2 or 3 months. The effect of the second method lasts from between 3 and 30 months (Fritzell *et al.*, 1993). Since patients with spastic dysphonia, especially those at an early stage have been reported to be amenable to cognitive and behavioural therapy, this should be recommended and attempted before surgery is proposed.

External surgery of the larynx

Insertion of grafts, rotation of the arytenoid by suturing it to the thyroid cartilage and a variety of other procedures have a long history. At the present time procedures developed and described by Isshiki (1980) are popular. Most frequent is thyroplasty type I for medial positioning of the cord, type II produces lateralization, type III is for shortening and type IV for lengthening the vocal fold. The external approach has the advantage that the delicate interior of the larynx is not touched and that in principle the procedure is reversible, should the result be disappointing. This is a definite advantage over, for instance, the injection of a Teflon deposit, which cannot be removed if too much is inserted.

Combined surgical and re-educative approach

It is a requirement for every phonosurgeon to be a good diagnostician of voice disorders and to have experience in training and therapy for modification of vocal behaviour. In the absence of re-educational experience absurd mistakes can be made in selecting patients for surgery. It is, for example, a necessity to have command of such diagnostic tests as manual depression of the cricoid cartilage, manual compression of the thyroid alae, as described under Functional assessment. Medial compression, if it results in a clearer voice and longer phonation time, means two things:

1 The patient can learn to improve his voice by intensive practice, by addressing hypofunctional lateral parts of the intrinsic laryngeal musculature and compensating for insufficient closure by using the laryngeal suspension system
2 Chances of improvement by phonosurgery (injection, arytenoid adduction, or thyroplasty) are good.

Which of the two ways will be chosen depends on the size of the glottic gap, the possibilities and inclinations of the voice care centre which is consulted, and the motivation and readiness of the patient to engage in regular practice sessions.

During post-surgical voice therapy the patients will explore and discover how to use the new anatomical situation to best advantage. Already in the presurgical stage it may be of advantage to work on faulty habits of breath control and voice use. Close cooperation between the phonosurgeon, the voice therapist and the patient can give the latter a more solid understanding of what he can expect from surgery.

Rehabilitation of the voice after laryngectomy

Since the prognosis for cancer of the larynx is better than many forms of carcinoma, successful rehabilitation is especially rewarding. Through all the remaining years the patient enjoys an improved quality of life if he has learnt to use a good substitute voice.

There are three options: oesophageal speech, electrical or pneumatic voice substitute, and speech using a valve prosthesis connecting the trachea and oesophagus.

Informing the patient and his spouse is an essential part of the rehabilitation programme. Usually the nature and the consequences of the operation have been discussed before the operation. The spouse should always be present; the partners can discuss matters between them and what one has missed will have been heard and understood by the other. In the stress of the preoperative period much of what has been said is not remembered. It is good to repeat the information in the more quiet period after the patient has recovered from the surgery. Among the points to be discussed are:

1 The altered anatomy (Figure 6.7)
2 Moisturizing and cleaning the stoma
3 The various types of substitute voice
4 Useful aids and appliances
5 The address of the Association of Laryngectomized Patients
6 Other questions brought up by the patient and his spouse.

Depending on the organization of the clinic, most of the informative sessions will be held by a doctor, a nurse or a speech therapist. The person responsible should be aware that these sessions do more than furnish matter-of-fact information. Counselling after radical surgery includes guiding a person through phases of recovery. The counseller will have to cope with periods of depression, anxiety or protest. With her help and the cooperation of an understanding partner or relative, the patient will ultimately accept his handicapped condition. Only then will he be ready to concentrate on assignments and exercises for rehabilitation.

The appropriate time to begin speech training after surgery depends on the local condition of the wound and on the general condition of the patient. The wound should be healed and mirror examination should show no trace of fibrin in the pharynx. For his general condition the patient is encouraged to take walks and other forms of exercise. The condition of his teeth is checked. An audiogram is recorded as a preliminary to voice and speech training.

Oesophageal speech

Surgeons who performed laryngectomies early in the 20th century reported that, to their surprise, several of their patients sooner or later developed intelligible speech but only in patients with no external pharyngeal fistula. In the early days of the operation a pharyngostome was a frequent complication which interfered with food intake and with the development of substitute speech. The mysteries of speech without

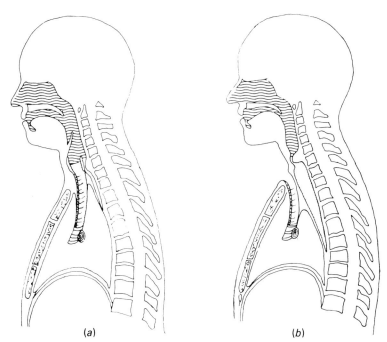

Figure 6.7 The voice organs (*a*) before and (*b*) after laryngectomy. The oesophagus takes over the bellows function of the lungs for the purpose of speaking

a larynx have been solved in subsequent years (Keith and Darley, 1993). At the present time every laryngectomized patient should have access to voice rehabilitation immediately after the surgical wound has healed and the feeding tube has been removed.

When a patient is left to his own devices after laryngectomy and he attempts to speak, the result initially is poor. His lips move, but no sounds come out of his mouth: no vowels because there is no voice, and no consonants because there is no airstream with which they can be articulated. After some practice the patient can learn to move the floor of the mouth and the root of the tongue in such a way that some air is displaced, enough to produce short sibilant and plosive sounds. This can lead to pseudo-whispered speech which is not a real whisper because it lacks the sighing sound of the glottis. It is produced with effort and lacks some indispensible voice sounds, so that it is difficult to understand. As has been mentioned under stenosis of the larynx there are people who learned to vibrate the pharyngeal arch with such a mechanism, producing buccal speech. It is a type of speech which can only be understood by the initiated and there is no reason to encourage its use by laryngectomees. On the contrary, as a sequel to pseudo-whispered speech the patient may develop so-called pharyngeal voice, which is equally unsatisfactory and is a blind alley on the road to oesophageal voice. It is produced by contractions of the pharynx, which is just the thing

to be avoided when learning to produce oesophageal speech. The correct manner in which the patient can generate a properly understandable substitute voice, is by taking air into the oesophagus. When, immediately after the intake, the air is returned, it makes the opening of the oesophagus vibrate resulting in a vowel-like sound, resounding in a wide pharyngeal and oral cavity (Figure 6.8).

The initial stage

When attempting to make his first oesophageal sounds, any manner or manoeuvre by which the patient succeeds is correct for that particular patient. There is no single method that will be suitable for all. There are several possibilities.

1 Drawing air into the oesophagus by inhalation; the entrance of the oesophagus should be opened during an inspiration
2 Pumping air into the oesophagus by injection; the tongue and the floor of the mouth compress the air, while the entrance to the oesophagus is relaxed
3 Carbonated water is used to help the patient form his first recognizable words using his 'second voice'.

A patient who is well instructed by the person in charge of his rehabilitation will soon find out which method of air intake suits him best. A few experienced

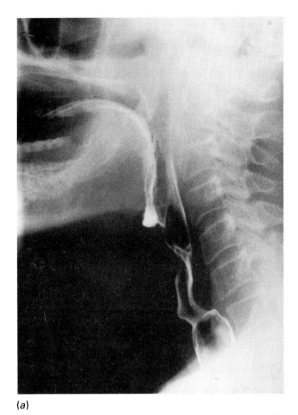
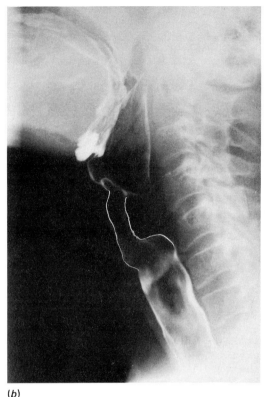

(a)   *(b)*

Figure 6.8 The pharyngo–oesophageal segment generates the oesophageal voice. (*a*) Soft phonation; (*b*) loud phonation. Lateral radiographs after swallowing bismuth paste (partly retouched with white ink)

laryngectomized speakers take air in by inhalation, most use injection or a combination of inhalation and injection. Most experienced patients can speak two to five syllables on one intake. Eventually, replenishing the air in the oesophagus is achieved so unobtrusively that it is hardly noticed. The basic sound is usually learned within 1 or 2 days. It takes 2–10 weeks before the patient can use his newly acquired voice outside his own home and the quality further improves over the next year.

Difficulties encountered in acquiring oesophageal voice

The most frequent problem for beginners is that the oesophageal opening does not relax at the moment that the air must pass through it on the way in or out. When the air does not get further than the pharynx, the sound produced is a tense, high pitched sound and of short duration, and is unsuitable as a substitute voice. Sometimes a patient succeeds in injecting air into the oesophagus but is unable to return it at will. When more than a fraction of a second elapses between injection of air and phonation, the air is passed down into the stomach and is

lost for phonation. The problem is sometimes solved by active relaxation training of the muscles of the neck and jaw: an indirect approach to relax the oesophageal sphincter. When there is great difficulty, dilation by an oesophageal bougie and insufflation of air by a catheter can help to overcome the sphincteric contraction reflex.

A diverticulum of the pharyngeal wall can have an adverse influence on the sound of the voice which may be moist and bubbling. Such a diverticulum is best prevented by stitching the pharyngeal wall with the greatest care and ensuring that the patient does not swallow in the first days after operation.

A distracting symptom in some oesophageal speakers is a hissing sound made by air passing through the stoma or the tracheostomy tube. It can be improved by teaching the patient a more controlled method of breathing during speech.

Some patients complain that their voice is too weak to be of any use in other than the quietest environments. This can be caused by flaccidity of the pharyngeal wall at the level of the vibrating structures. If light finger pressure on the skin above the tracheostome improves the quality of the voice a special neckband that applies permanent pressure can be fitted.

The artificial larynx

During the period that oesophageal speech is practised the patient is offered the option of using an artificial larynx for speech situations in which oesophageal speech cannot yet meet the demands. The artificial voice generators are essentially of two types: the pneumatic, activated by the respiratory air from the tracheostome, and the electric, driven by batteries. The first has several advantages. It can be used the day after the operation, providing it can be connected to the tracheal cannula. By carefully choosing the material for the vibrating membrane a suitable pitch and quality of the voice can be selected and because the pitch varies with the breath pressure, the fundamental frequency approaches normal speech intonation. It has no battery that can run out and is cheap. Some patients dislike the polyethylene or metal tube that transmits the sound from the vibrator at the stoma to the mouth, and see this as a disadvantage. Typical examples of pneumatic voice prostheses are the Tokyo artificial larynx and the Memacon DSP 8.

Of the many electrical external vibrators that are available most have an adjustable pitch and intensity level. Servox has the option of a manually operated tonal accent device, the use of which requires linguistic as well as other skills. All voice prostheses have the disadvantage that one hand is occupied when speaking. Every year new developments are reported so that hope for further improvements is entirely justified. Details about training in the use of artificial larynges can be found in the publication by Keith and Darley (1993).

Surgical methods to restore the voice after laryngectomy

A disadvantage of oesophageal voice is that the small supply of air that is available for phonation necessitates repeated interruptions of the speech flow for the intake of air. This drawback has been met by a procedure originally described by Singer and Blom (1980) and recently evaluated by Hilgers, Schouwenburg and Scholtens (1989). The wall between the trachea and the upper oesophagus is punctured during endoscopy. A tube of about 4 mm diameter ending in a valve is inserted into the opening. It has a dual function: it keeps the fistula open and it allows air from the trachea to pass into the oesophagus when the patient closes off his stoma and breathes out. The voice that is produced is generated at the pharyngo-oesophageal junction as is oesophageal voice. The difference is that more air is available for speech and that sustained speech is produced with a fluent quality. Another advantage is that speech is immediately available after operation. Disadvantages are that one hand is occupied during speech and the patient remains dependent on the hospital for replacement of the prosthesis every few months. The tracheo-oesophageal puncture can be performed during surgery for laryngectomy or at a later stage during the period of rehabilitation (secondary puncture). The introduction of this method has been followed by various improvements in the design of the prostheses and of the surgery of the pharyngo-oesophageal junction. As a result tracheo-oesophageal shunt surgery combined with a valve prosthesis is an important advance in speech rehabilitation after laryngectomy.

Measures for restoring other functions

The sense of smell, that is often absent in laryngectomees, can be restored. The patient learns to ventilate the nose by making the same tongue-pumping movements as he uses during oesophageal speech, this time with the soft palate lowered. The root of the tongue is moved up and down and one nostril is closed off by a finger. A hissing noise through the other nasal opening shows that air is passing. Mastery of this skill ensures that the patient can detect noxious gases in his home, can enjoy agreeable smells in the countryside and can enjoy the taste of his food better.

Swimming is not necessarily impossible for laryngectomees who were keen on this sport before the operation. A cannula with an inflatable cuff is inserted into the trachea. An air-hose connected to the cannula at one end leads to a snorkel at the other end fixed to the head by an elastic band. After the cuff has been inflated a thorough check is made that no air escapes past the cannula when the swimmer breathes out with the neck under water. The patient will have to get used to the larger dead space, which requires him to breathe more deeply, by practice sessions on dry land before actually entering the water. Being able to swim again means much for many laryngectomees: it reduces the sense of being handicapped and enables those for whom many other sports have become impossible to stay in good health.

References

BOONE, D. and MACFARLANE, S. C. (1988) *The Voice and Voice Therapy*. Englewood Cliffs: Prentice Hall

BOUCHAYER, M. and CORNUT, G. (1992) Microsurgical treatment of benign vocal fold lesions: indications, technique, results. *Folia Phoniatrica*, **44**, 101–184

DAMSTÉ, P. H. and LERMAN, J. W. (1975) *An Introduction to Voice Pathology*. Springfield; Charles C. Thomas

FORD, C. N. and BLESS, D. M. (1991) *Phonosurgery. Assessment and Surgical Management of Voice Disorders*. New York: Raven Press

FRITZELL, B., HAMMARBERG, B., SCHIRATZKI, H., HAGLUND, S., KNUTTSON, E. and MARTENSSON, A. (1993) Long term results of recurrent laryngeal nerve resection for adductor spastic dysphonia. *Journal of Voice*, **71**, 172–178

GOULD, W. J. (1983) Voice recording and vocal fold photography in the ENT office setting. *Journal of Otolaryngology*, **12**, 282–284

HILGERS, F. J. M., SCHOUWENBURG, P. F. and SCHOLTENS, B. (1989) Long term results of prosthetic voice rehabilitation after total laryngectomy. *Clinical Otolaryngology*, **14**, 365

ISSHIKI, N. (1980) Recent advances in phonosurgery. *Folia Phoniatrica*, **32**, 119–154

ITOH, T., KAWASAKI, H., MORIKAWA, I. and HIRANO, M. (1983) Vocal fold furrows. A 10 year review of 240 patients. *Auris, Nasus, Larynx*, **10** (suppl.), 17–26

KEITH, R. L. and DARLEY, F. L. (1993) *Laryngectomee Rehabilitation*, 3rd edn. Austin, Texas: Pro-Ed

KITZING, P. (1985) Stroboscopy: a pertinent laryngeal examination. *Journal of Otolaryngology*, **14**, 151–157

LERMAN, J. W. and DAMSTÉ, P. H. (1969) Voice pitch of homosexuals. *Folia Phoniatrica*, **21**, 257–265

MEAD, J., BOUHUYS, A. and PROCTOR, D. F. (1968) Mechanisms generating subglottic pressure. *Annals of the New York Academy of Sciences*, **155**, 177–181

PERELLO, J. (1962) Dysphonies fonctionelles: phonoponose et phononeurose. *Folia Phoniatrica*, **14**, 150–205

SATALOFF, R. T. (ed.) (1991) *Professional Voice*. New York: Raven Press

SINGER, M. I. and BLOM, E. D. (1980) An endoscopic technique for restoration of voice after laryngectomy. *Annals of Otology, Rhinology and Laryngology*, **89**, 529–533

SONNINEN, A. (1968) The external frame function in the control of pitch in the human voice. *Annals of the New York Academy of Sciences*, **155**, 68–90

STOICHEFF, M. L. (1983) The present status of adductor spastic dysphonia. *Journal of Otolaryngology*, **12**, 311–314

ZENKER, W. and ZENKER, A. (1960) Ueber die Regelung de Stimmlippenspannung durch von aussen eingreifenden Mechanismen. *Folia Phoniatrica*, **12**, 1–36

7

Management of the obstructed airway and tracheostomy

Patrick James Bradley

The obstructed airway

Definitions

Complete: there is no air flow.
Partial: the patient has stridor or respiratory difficulty due to narrowing of the major airway.
Potential: the patient, because of a known anatomical or physical condition, may develop airway compromise if the respiratory physiology or conscious level is altered.

Aims of management

The aims of management are to protect a jeopardized airway and to establish an airway when none is available (ATLS Manual, 1989) and to maintain the patient's oxygenation. A definitive airway is established when a cuffed tube is safely secured in the trachea.

The clinical situation may present itself in one of three environments:

1 The community
2 The hospital environment
3 The operating room.

The site of the obstruction or narrowing may be located in:

1 The mouth, oropharynx or supraglottis
2 The glottis or subglottis
3 The trachea and lower respiratory tract.

Management

The problem should be approached as follows:

1 The simplest adequate form of control should be selected

2 The lowest level of airway obstruction should be ascertained and an airway established below this level
3 Acute airway problems often evolve in association with other medical problems.

The majority of obstructed airways encountered in clinical practice can be stabilized by endotracheal intubation.

Intubation of the larynx

Certain basic equipment and instruments are required for successful laryngeal intubation (Figure 7.1). The equipment should always be checked in advance if time and the needs of the patient allow. A source of 100% oxygen and a bag-valve assembly should also be available to ventilate the patient. Tightly fitting anaesthetic face masks of a variety of sizes should be to hand to help gain initial control of the airway. Suction is essential and a large bore Yankauer type suction head is ideal to clear the airway of mucus, blood or vomit. The Macintosh laryngoscope must be available – the handle should be checked for a functional battery – with a variety of blades. A selection of different endotracheal tubes should also be available with a metal malleable stylet which occasionally is needed to aid with the insertion of the tube. The Magill forceps is often invaluable in directing the endotracheal tube if difficulties are encountered in finding or exposing the laryngeal inlet. The selection of the appropriate size of endotracheal tube is based roughly on the patient's age. An adult woman will usually need a tube of internal diameter of 8.5 mm and a man, one of 9.5 mm. It is a mistake to select a small bore tube in the belief that it will be easier to

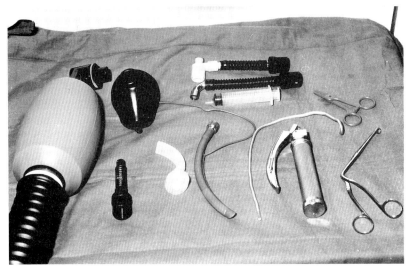

Figure 7.1 Instrumentation for laryngeal intubation

insert. Not only is this usually incorrect but there will be a large air leak past the tube, together with an increase in the resistance to spontaneous respiration, should the latter be desired. On the other hand, an over-large tube inserted with force will damage the vocal cords with possible serious long-term results. The correct length of the endotracheal tube which will be required can be estimated by measuring the distance from the lobe of the ear to the angle of the mouth and doubling it.

Indications

Absolute

1 Protection of the trachea from contamination in:
  a Non-anaesthetized patients with a depressed cough reflex, e.g. head injury, cerebrovascular accident, drug overdose and some central nervous system diseases
  b Anaesthetized patients who are likely to vomit and soil the lower airway, e.g. obstetric patients or patients with intestinal obstruction
  c Patients at risk of soiling or contamination of the trachea or lower airway from an operation site, e.g. head and neck or dental procedures
2 Severe upper airway obstruction.

Relative

1 To facilitate controlled ventilation
2 To facilitate tracheobronchial toilet
3 To maintain a clear airway under difficult circumstances, e.g. in the prone position, as required for neurosurgery

4 For diagnostic procedures, e.g. angiography or bronchoscopy.

Technique

Careful but rapid preparation of the patient will aid intubation unless the situation dictates immediate action. The occiput is elevated about 4–6 cm off the table with a pad or pillow providing that a cervical spine injury is not suspected. The neck should be flexed on the trunk and the head extended on the neck in the 'sniffing position'. Pre-oxygenation of the patient should be performed with a tightly fitting anaesthetic mask and ventilation assisted as necessary by the bag-valve-mask assembly. Sedation or topical anaesthetic or both can be used at this stage to decrease patient discomfort.

The head is placed so that the angle between the mouth and the trachea is reduced, until it forms, as near as possible, a straight line. It is a mistake to hyperextend both the head and the neck, as this produces misalignment of the mouth and the tracheal axes, so making intubation more difficult (Figure 7.2).

To achieve the correct degree of extension at the atlanto-occipital joint, the forefinger of the right hand is applied to the patient's hard palate and the upper jaw is pulled towards the operator. The lips can then be pushed away from the teeth by the middle finger and thumb.

Endotracheal intubation in the hands of experts takes less than 10 s, however, the inexperienced may take much longer. Oxygen uptake continues during the period of attempted intubation and the arterial oxygen tension declines. The lungs should therefore

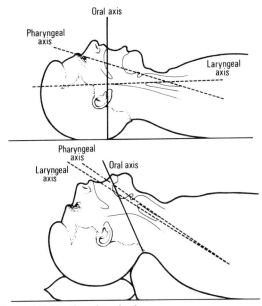

Pharyngeal axis

Oral axis

Laryngeal axis

Pharyngeal axis

Laryngeal axis

Oral axis

Figure 7.2 Mouth and tracheal axes

be inflated if possible with oxygen up to the moment when the laryngoscope is inserted into the mouth. Similarly, prolonged attempts at intubation should always be interrupted and the patient oxygenated, to prevent hypoxia.

The handle of the laryngoscope is lifted in the direction to which it points. It must not be rotated, as this movement will damage the teeth, gums and the mucous membrane of the pharynx. The uvula is seen at the tip of the blade which is advanced in the midline while elevation of the soft tissues is maintained. The tip will eventually come to lie in the vallecula between the tongue and the epiglottis. Elevation of the root of the tongue will indirectly elevate the posteriorly placed epiglottis, and the laryngeal opening will come into view, ready for intubation.

The endotracheal tube is passed between the vocal cords. If the patient is making respiratory movements, the tube should be passed during inspiration when the cords are separated maximally. If the larynx is difficult to see anteriorly, it may be brought into view by an assistant gently pressing on the thyroid cartilage.

Once the tube has been inserted the cuff should be inflated until the tracheal leak is just eliminated. The endotracheal tube is attached, as the situation demands, to an Ambu bag, ventilator or anaesthetic circuit.

The tube should be fixed to the head with a bandage or tape to prevent displacement.

Oral intubation is the most direct route, requires less time and is indicated in the moribund or apnoeic patient. An awake patient must be cooperative or adequately sedated to allow oral intubation because of the profound stimulation of the throat by the laryngoscope.

The introduction of a tracheal tube may be achieved using methods which involve manoeuvres above or below the cords.

Methods from above the cords

Blind nasotracheal intubation

This is useful when the patient is uncooperative or if manipulation of the neck is considered unsafe (Danzl and Thomas, 1980). This technique can be used if the patient has trismus, severe mandibular injuries, cervical spine rigidity, and distortion or masses in the oral cavity. The nasotracheal approach has disadvantages in that it demands greater technical expertise, and the patient must have good spontaneous respirations because the tube is guided by the breath sounds. The complication rate of this procedure is less than 3%, but includes epistaxis, sinusitis, nasal necrosis, retropharyngeal lacerations and otitis media (Tintinalli and Claffey, 1981).

Use of a firm elastic bougie

At laryngoscopy, the intubator may only be able to visualize the back ends of the vocal cords or even no part of the cords. It is frequently possible to pass a bougie blindly through the larynx into the trachea. This procedure may be helped if the bougie is hollow and a capnograph is attached to confirm its position. Either way an endotracheal tube may be passed over the bougie into the trachea. Associated with this method is trauma to the vocal cords or misplacement into the oesophagus.

Fibreoptic techniques

These can be used to aid oral and nasal intubation but are usually reserved for elective intubations because they require more expertise and time as the larynx can be easily obscured. The tracheal tube can be 'rail-roaded' over the endoscope when it has been positioned in the trachea.

Use of the rigid bronchoscope

This can frequently achieve a view of the vocal cords when no view has been possible with the laryngoscope. This is because of the angle of the approach and there frequently being missing teeth in the molar area of the upper alveolus allowing the rigid scope to pass. When the glottis is seen an elastic bougie can be passed into the trachea and the tracheal tube can be 'rail-roaded' into the correct position.

Use of the laryngeal mask airway

In the emergency situation this may be helpful as the mask covers the rima glottidis. A tracheal tube may be passed through, or a flexible endoscope may be used when the patient is stabilized and a tracheal tube may be 'rail-roaded' into position.

Methods from below the cords

Tracheostomy

This subject is dealt with in detail later in the chapter.

Retrograde intubation

This technique involves the passage of a catheter through a needle into the lumen of the trachea, once the position of the catheter is established the catheter can be advanced through the glottis in a proximal direction and the catheter can be retrieved from the mouth or the nasal cavity. Once the catheter is secured the tracheal tube can be advanced either over the tube, or a flexible endoscope can follow the catheter down and be used to 'rail-road' the tracheal tube into position.

Transtracheal ventilation

This is the method of placing a tracheal tube into the trachea after a cricothyroidotomy has been made.

Successful translaryngeal intubation is achieved if the clinician is flexible, comfortable with multiple techniques and is aware of the possible complications and difficulties that may be encountered with each technique. Emphasis is placed on the expeditious control of the airway in a rapidly deteriorating patient. If the initial approach to intubate is unsuccessful, alternative approaches must be promptly instituted (Salem, Mathrubhutham and Bennett, 1976).

Intubation difficulties

Difficulties in intubation arise from three sources:

1 Errors of technique (Table 7.1)
2 Anatomical variations
3 Transient physiological and structural abnormalities.

The incidence of difficult intubation is approximately 1:750 cases in experienced hands (Edems and Sia, 1981). Of these airways with difficulties, 90% can be anticipated and in the remaining 10% the problem is encountered unexpectedly. Any test that can predict difficult intubation may save lives, as a

Table 7.1 Common errors of orotracheal intubation

Step	Error
Positioning	Axes not aligned
Opening of mouth	Mouth not wide enough
Insertion of blade	Wrong size or type of blade
	Blade badly positioned
Exposure of cords	Leverage rather than traction
Introduction of tube	Obscured line of vision
	Failure to maintain natural curve
	Trachea angulated by traction

result of the planned use of local or regional anaesthetic techniques, or by allowing time to organize special procedures such as fibreoptic laryngoscopy. Many tests and asssessments have been recommended but have a high false positive rate (Combley and Vaughan, 1992). A modified Mallampali test (Mallampati *et al.*, 1985) and measurements of the thyromental distance have been suggested (Frerk, 1991). Patients in whom the posterior pharyngeal wall cannot be visualized below the soft palate, who also have a distance of less than 7 cm between the prominence of the thyroid cartilage and the bony prominence of the chin have proven to be significantly more likely to present difficulties with intubation.

Preintubation assessment can often identify high risk patients. Patients with head and neck problems sometimes have a number of factors which would suggest possible intubation problems. A mass can alter the normal anatomy of the pharynx and larynx, so that the glottis is impossible or extremely difficult to expose by direct laryngoscopy. Oedema and scarring of the airway secondary to radiotherapy or previous surgery may interfere with the ability to expose the glottis. The presence of temporomandibular joint ankylosis, tumour, masseteric spasm or a small mouth with a large tongue will compromise adequate exposure. Lesions that limit neck mobility such as cervical spondylosis, Klippel-Feil syndrome, as well as congenital abnormalities which produce an anteriorly placed larynx (micrognathia, Treacher-Collins and Goldenhaar's syndromes) will make alignment of the laryngeal and oropharyngeal axes difficult (White and Kander, 1975).

Temporary abnormalities often present a problem in an emergency. These abnormalities include blood, vomit and foreign bodies that interfere with the view of the airway; trismus secondary to head injuries, seizures or drug ingestion; trauma of the mouth or face; a neck injury; and hypoxia caused by shock or drugs in a conscious but uncooperative patient.

Physicians who are likely to encounter emergency situations which require rapid control of the patient's airway should be able to use techniques other than the standard oro- or nasotracheal intubation. Many techniques and devices have been used to aid blind intubation including forceps, hooks, catheters, guides, and drugs to increase the respiratory flow, and agents to sedate or paralyse the patients. The most frequently used device to facilitate the positioning of the tube during orotracheal intubation is the malleable guide wire. In its most common form a blunt ended wire is used to mould and hold the tube in a pronounced curve. However, this technique has the potential of lacerating the vocal cords or trachea.

More recently, to the above techniques has been added the flex-end tube or trigger tube. This tube is of a standard design; the wall contains a wire that allows anterior flexion of the tip by means of a trigger at the proximal end. While internal guides are generally used in orotracheal intubation, external guides are most often employed in nasotracheal intubation. The most common external guide is the Magill forceps, an instrument that allows the distal end to be grasped and be positioned between the vocal cords under direct vision.

However, at times oral and nasal intubation are difficult to achieve even with the techniques described. The flexible laryngoscope has been used for difficult intubations since first described by Davis (1973), who reported it as an alternative to blind nasal intubation. The flexible fibreoptic laryngoscope is small enough to allow the adult endotracheal tube to be passed over it. The laryngoscope acts as an introducer and allows direct exposure of the larynx. The distal 5 cm of the scope can be manoeuvred in an anterior and posterior direction. Neither neck movement nor spontaneous respiration is required. The use of the suction fibreoptic endoscopes has greatly aided the ability to remove secretions that may obscure the view (Davidson, Bone and Nahum, 1975).

Incorrect positioning of the endotracheal tube

In an emergency, and sometimes in difficult elective intubations, the endotracheal tube is occasionally placed into the oesophagus. If this situation is not recognized quickly the patient will die. There are very few absolute signs that the tube is in the trachea; in most cases reliance is placed on a good view of the larynx during intubation, the 'feel' of the lungs during bag compression, the presence of reasonable breath sounds, and the appropriate thoracic movements. The restarting of spontaneous respiration with the appearance of bag movements is reassuring. Bronchospasm or pneumothorax can confuse the picture, but the presence of these diagnoses should be accepted only on good evidence. Difficulty in ventilating is more likely to be a consequence of a tube in the oesophagus than because of bronchospasm. The detection of breath sounds is notoriously misleading, as these may be mistaken for the sound of air passing into the oesophagus (Scott, 1986). If a blue patient goes pink the tube is unlikely to be anywhere but in

the trachea. Patients do not die from 'failure to intubate', they die either from failure to stop trying to intubate or from undiagnosed oesophageal intubation. If difficulty is encountered during intubation the airway can nearly always be maintained by an oral airway and a ventilating mask and bag.

Preventing complications

The design of the current plastic disposable endotracheal tubes has greatly reduced the risks of complications compared with the old cuffed reusable, red-rubber tubes. The types of injury following endotracheal intubation have been well described (Blanc and Tremblay, 1974). The incidence and severity of mucosal damage correlates with the duration of the intubation. Minimal damage is reported in patients intubated for less than 48 hours. With longer intubation periods, the incidence of mucosal damage increases especially in the glottic and subglottic areas. Severe late complications of endotracheal intubation include glottic granulomas, laryngotracheal synechiae, vocal cord paralysis and, in severe cases, tracheal stenosis. Tracheal stenosis, although uncommon has been reported in at least one in 342 long-term intubated patients (Hawkins and Luxford, 1980).

The risk of complications greatly increases after intubation for more than 48 hours (Johnsen, 1973; Kane *et al.*, 1982). Major recent improvements which have reduced the complications of endotracheal intubation are the improved understanding of the pathogenesis of intubation injuries and advances in mechanical ventilation, respiratory therapy and endotracheal tube design and care. Prevention of airway injury from prolonged intubation depends on preventing excessive movement of the tube, avoiding excessive pressure on the airway structures by the cuff, and the preshaped endotracheal tubes which conform to the airway anatomy. Laryngeal injury from long-term nasotracheal intubation is lower than that of oral intubation, probably as a result of the smaller sized tubes and the greater stability which reduces the frictional forces of the tube in the larynx during positive pressure ventilation.

The incidence of tracheal stenosis due to cuff-induced lesions has diminished significantly with the development of the high residual volume cuff (high volume, low pressure, high compliance or 'floppy' cuff) (Arola, Inberg and Puhakka, 1981). Problems reported with the high residual volume cuff include aspiration around the endotracheal tube, a higher incidence of sore throats as a result of the greater mucosal contact, increased difficulty of intubation because the cuff obstructs the view of the larynx during insertion, obstruction of the larynx during insertion, obstruction of the endotracheal tube lumen on account of overinflation of the cuff and high peak pressure during coughing and increased incidence of post-intubation stridor after prolonged intubation. Animal studies have shown that ventilation with an endotracheal tube with a low pressure, high volume cuff causes different but significant tracheal damage when compared to the old tubes with high pressure, low volume cuffs (Sanada, Kojiwa and Fowkalsrud, 1982).

Hoarseness after an operation is relatively common and has been reported in as many as 70% of patients after intubation (Stauffer, Olson and Petty, 1981; Gleeson and Fourcin, 1983). Typically the hoarseness disappears after a few days and neither the patient nor the surgeon remains concerned about the quality of the voice. However, in some cases hoarseness or even aphonia persists associated with pain on swallowing. The following factors contribute to the development of postoperative hoarseness (Jaffe, 1972):

1 The act of intubation
2 The endotracheal tube during surgery
3 The indwelling endotracheal tube after surgery
4 Intubation and concomitant bronchitis or bronchopneumonia
5 An allergic reaction involving the larynx
6 Any operation on the neck or upper thorax.

Other symptoms may include sore throat, cough, sputum production, and haemoptysis, in descending frequency ranging from 40% to 10% of patients studied. The incidence of granuloma varies from 1:800 to 1:30 as reported in the literature, but most complications resolve spontaneously (Stauffer, Olson and Petty, 1981).

One-quarter of patients ventilated and intubated in intensive care units require ventilatory support for more than 1 week, and 10% require it for more than 2 weeks. Any inflatable cuff, no matter how soft, is potentially hazardous when confined within the tracheal lumen without a safety mechanism. Pressure control is essential, preferably by some means that does not require repeated attention. Nasotracheal intubation is generally better tolerated than orotracheal and can usually be maintained for 3–4 weeks.

Management of acute airway obstruction

A clinical history prior to the acute airway obstruction may be helpful if there is time. In the previously normal and asymptomatic patient the possibility of foreign body aspiration is real and must be excluded. In other situations patients with hoarseness may have a tumour of the larynx. The age of the patient may also be helpful to exclude coronary disease or cerebral haemorrhage with vascular arrest compounding the clinical situation. Therapy for a patient with evolving upper airway obstruction relies on clinical judgement. In the patient who is moderately stable, indirect mirror examination or flexible fibreoptic examination of the upper airway can contribute a significant amount of information regarding the

degree of airway compromise and the neuromuscular function of the larynx. Radiographs and blood gases should be performed if time permits.

At times, patients who present with respiratory distress because of injury, infective processes or even with neoplastic conditions are considered chronic but stable. The clinical situation can be either treated medically, expectantly observed, or may be electively investigated. However, the decision not to intervene needs to be reviewed should information or the clinical state of the patient change. Medical management may include the administration of oxygen, steroids or antibiotics. Oxygen may be given using a humidifier via a face mask. This method will provide only approximately 50% inspired oxygen. The addition of humidification will provide liquefaction of secretions and make the clearance of partially obstructing secretions easier for the patient. Steroids may be helpful in the presence of mild to moderate trauma or inflammatory and infectious processes. Hydrocortisone should be given; the recommended dosage is 100 mg initally and 50 mg every 8 hours for 24–48 hours. No significant data exist to show that steroids have a detrimental effect on infectious processes on a short-term basis (Hawkins and Crockett, 1983). Antibiotics should also be considered if there is any suggestion of infection or transmucosal injury is contributing to the obstructing process. A short course of antibiotics may reverse the inflammatory process. The recommended dosage is 1 million units of penicillin every 6 hours intravenously for 3–5 days.

Options for intervention

The Heimlich manoeuvre

Acute airway obstruction by a food bolus or any foreign body should be managed by the Heimlich manoeuvre. This uses the residual air in the lungs to expel a foreign body. Pressure should be exerted by a rapid squeezing motion applied against the xiphoid region of the sternum (Heimlich, 1974).

Nasopharyngeal/oral airway

This form of airway can overcome problems related to prolapse or relaxation of the palate and the base of tongue and may provide a well tolerated and fully adequate airway. The nasal airway is better tolerated in the conscious or semiconscious patient than the oral airway.

Assessment of the upper airway

Endotracheal intubation can only be performed if the correct instrumentation is available, i.e. as on a cardiac arrest trolley or in an operating theatre environment. Using a laryngoscope, the tongue and supraglottic anatomy can be inspected to exclude a local cause such as a foreign body or a cyst or haematoma. With the use of suction this area can be cleaned. The glottis can be inspected. It may be possible to insert an endotracheal tube if available. If the obstruction is considered to be lower down then a rigid bronchoscope can be passed to inspect the subglottis and the trachea down to the level of the carina. If a foreign body is found it should be removed and the patient intubated and oxygenated.

Blind nasal intubation

This procedure may be indicated when disturbance of the patient should be minimized or when orotracheal intubation is contraindicated or impossible due to trauma in the oral cavity or anatomical distortion of the upper airway or due to problems with the cervical spine.

Transtracheal needle ventilation

This method can be used to great advantage in the emergency situation. It provides rapid control while the patient is being stabilized before more definitive measures can be introduced. The following equipment is necessary: a delivery system for oxygen under pressure (50 pounds per square inch, 450 kPa), connecting hose with Leur-Lok connectors and a 16-gauge or bigger plastic sheathed needle. The needle is directed through the cricothyroid membrane and attached to the oxygen line with an interrupter in place. The patient can be fully ventilated by this technique for at least 30 minutes.

Complications of this method can occur especially in the struggling patient. The catheter or the needle may become dislodged with resultant surgical emphysema or catheters may become kinked. One should be aware that there should be adequate expiratory flow available and it may be necessary to insert a second needle or create a minitrach or even proceed to a cricothyroidotomy.

Minitracheostomy

This should not be used as this procedure offers only temporary and suboptimal airway access.

Percutaneous tracheostomy

This should not be used in the emergency situation when an airway is at risk. The current role of percutaneous tracheostomy is elective in the intubated patient in the operating room or in the intensive care environment when this procedure may be preferred to a formal tracheostomy.

Cricothyroidotomy

This operation can be performed rapidly with a minimum amount of equipment. It is usually performed

under less than optimal conditions, and the potential for laryngeal injury is high. Once the patient is stabilized, the wound should be examined in the operating room and the larynx also examined endoscopically. If there is any sign of injury or if long-term ventilation is considered necessary the cricothyroidotomy should be converted to a formal tracheostomy.

Tracheostomy

Urgent tracheostomy in a life and death situation may be very bloody and difficult. This procedure should be performed through a vertical incision and by the most experienced surgeon available.

Modified retrograde intubation

In a situation where the upper airway is soiled by blood or saliva in the partial obstructed airway, it is possible to stabilize the airway by passing an epidural catheter into the trachea and in a retrograde fashion through the glottis and out through the mouth. Then by following the catheter downward with a flexible laryngoscope the glottis can be found and the endoscope can be safely introduced into the upper trachea. The endotracheal tube can then be advanced over the endoscope and the clinical situation can be stabilized.

Tracheostomy

The term *tracheotomy* is used to refer to the creation of a surgical opening into the trachea. *Tracheostomy* is used when a formal opening or stoma is made. In common use the terms are interchangeable and in the present chapter, for the sake of consistency, *tracheostomy* will be used.

History of tracheostomy

Tracheostomy was performed in ancient times and the recordings of such events have been documented by Asclepiades, the Greek physician in 100 BC. It was only towards the end of the 19th century that peroral intubation was reintroduced and became increasingly more possible with the invention and subsequent modifications of the laryngoscope. Techniques improved, many lives were saved, and inhalational anaesthesia became routine. The development of tracheostomy has been divided into five periods: the 'period of legend' dating from 2000 BC to AD 1546; the 'period of fear' from 1546 to 1833 during which the operation was performed only by a brave few, often at the risk of their reputation; the 'period of drama' from 1833 to 1932 during which the procedure was generally performed only in emergency situations on acutely obstructed patients; the 'period of enthusiasm' from 1932 to 1965 during which the adage, 'if you think tracheostomy ... do it' became popular; and the 'period of rationalization' from 1965 to the present during which the relative merits of intubation versus tracheostomy were debated (McClelland, 1972).

Indications for tracheostomy

The four basic reasons for tracheostomy are:

1 *Upper airway obstruction*: real risk. Although still common in practice, upper airway obstruction is now the least common indication for tracheostomy. In general, once the procedure is performed, the underlying disease is no longer an immediate threat to compromise of the airway.
2 *Mechanical respiratory insufficiency*: acute respiratory failure requiring tracheostomy may occur in a a variety of diseases, including drug intoxication, head and chest injuries, elective surgery, neurological disorders and diseases, chronic obstructive airways disease, as well as pneumonia in a previously healthy patient. In these situations, there is a need for intermittent or continuous positive pressure ventilation. In prolonged cases tracheostomy provides the easiest and safest means of providing ventilatory assistance, eliminating upper respiratory 'dead-space' and allowing frequent and accurate pulmonary aspiration.
3 *Respiratory difficulties due to secretions*: this clinical situation may present with infections, congestive heart failure, pulmonary oedema, chronic lung disease, or bulbar disease secondary to cerebrovascular ischaemia or stroke. The presence of accumulated secretions in the lower respiratory tract leads to inability to allow gas diffusion at the alveoli. The presence of a tracheostomy allows secretions to be aspirated as required with minimal interference to the patient.
4 *Elective*: to effect a patent airway when the upper airway is potentially at risk. Any major operation on the mouth, pharynx and the larynx always constitutes a danger to the airway, both as a direct result of the surgical trauma and by the physiological disturbance of the swallowing mechanism. In many of these patients with uncertain general condition, particularly cardiovascular or pulmonary deficiency and advanced age, elective tracheostomy should be considered. Generally there is nothing to lose by its use – better too often than too late (Shaw, Stylis and Rosen, 1974).

Surgical technique

Tracheostomy should be performed in the operating room if possible and the procedure should be carried out under sterile conditions. If the tracheostomy is carried out with adequate preparation, meticulous surgical technique and excellent postoperative care, it is safe and reliable. It can be performed under local anaesthetic in a situation such as a patient with a large supraglottic cancer, but if the patient's condition does not preclude an endotracheal intubation the procedure should be performed in an orderly controlled environment.

Exposing the trachea requires a skin incision between the lower border of the cricoid cartilage and the suprasternal notch (Figure 7.3). Excellent rapid exposure is obtained through a vertical midline incision. In the elective situation, a horizontal incision gives a better cosmetic result. Under emergency circumstances, cosmesis becomes a lesser consideration when rapid control of the airway is required.

After the skin has been opened horizontally the strap muscles, i.e. the sternohyoid and sternothyroid, are separated vertically by blunt dissection in the midline through the linea alba. Dissection through this area should be relatively bloodless, although communicating venous channels may be encountered (Figure 7.4). The cricoid cartilage is identified

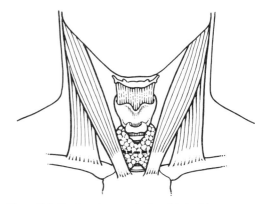

Figure 7.3 Tracheostomy – elective skin incisions

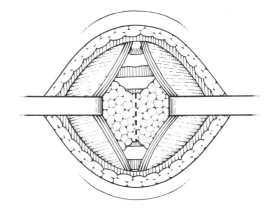

Figure 7.4 Tracheostomy – midline dissection

by palpation and the thyroid isthmus lying over the trachea is easily seen. All bleeding should be controlled during each surgical step down to the level of the trachea as identification of bleeding points may be impossible once the tracheostomy tube is placed in position. The isthmus of the thyroid gland should be clamped with artery forceps, transected in the midline, and transfixed, exposing the trachea (Figure 7.5). The thyroid gland must be divided in the midline, as deviation from this can result in profuse haemorrhage and the recurrent laryngeal nerve could be damaged. The technique of retracting the thyroid isthmus superiorly or inferiorly may be quicker, but the risk of airway obstruction during early tube change is real and this procedure of not dividing the thyroid isthmus should be condemned unless the surgeon who performed the tracheostomy performs the first tube change himself.

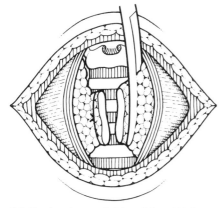

Figure 7.5 Tracheostomy – division of thyroid isthmus

The opening into the trachea should lie at the level of the second to the fourth tracheal ring to avoid damage to the cricoid cartilage which can result in subglottic stenosis. One exception to this is the patient admitted with stridor secondary to a laryngeal tumour. In this situation the incision in the trachea should be high even if this involves going through the tumour (Stell, 1973). This is so that when laryngectomy is performed the tracheostomy can be excised with the specimen. The tracheal incision should be of the type that disturbs the tracheal anatomy the least (Bryant *et al.*, 1978). A vertical incision is most suitable for this purpose. Some surgeons recommend a superiorly or inferiorly based flap (Bjork, 1960) or even the removal of a segment of cartilage; these procedures have been recommended to facilitate retention and changing of the tracheostomy tube. However, disadvantages include tracheal stenosis and delayed healing after removal of the tube with the formation of a tracheocutaneous fistula which frequently requires formal surgical closure. In the patient with a short fat neck the use of the cricoid hook

to elevate and stabilize the trachea can be invaluable when making the tracheal incision (Friedman and Venkatesan, 1990). If the trachea is soft and malleable as in the young, the insertion of laterally based sutures at the tracheal opening can be helpful and aid with tube changes later. In the elderly, it may occasionally be necessary to use Mayo scissors or even bone cutting shears to open into the tracheal lumen. If the tracheal cartilages are found to be calcified it is better to remove an adequate amount of the anterior wall to allow easy entry of the tracheostomy tube rather than outfracture the tracheal rings.

The tracheostomy tube should have been previously selected and the cuff checked for leaks before insertion. In general, tubes of size 7.5 mm or 8 mm are suitable for women and the larger tube size 8.5 mm or 9 mm for men. Once the tube has been inserted into the trachea the obturator is removed immediately, and blood and mucus are aspirated from the tracheal lumen. The wound should be checked for haemorrhage as there will not be another time to inspect the wound in these ideal circumstances. The wound must not be closed too tightly at the completion of the operation, as this may lead to the rapid development of alarming surgical emphysema of the neck. The flanges of the tracheostomy tube should be sutured to the skin to prevent dislodgement of the tube by the patient coughing or moving. The wings or flanges of the plastic tracheostomy tube can be shortened so that tapes cannot be used during the initial recovery period. The practice of tying in the tracheostomy tube with a surrounding gauze pad should be discouraged for the first 24 hours, at least, as the pad may obscure signs of bleeding and may even encourage surgical emphysema as the neck tissues become swollen.

Emergency tracheostomy

Anoxia results in death in about 4–5 minutes. Creation of an airway by tracheostomy must therefore be performed within 2 or 3 minutes. In general, this situation is to be avoided if at all possible and only usually becomes necessary because of the ill-advised conservative management of a patient with a compromised and barely adequate airway. In this situation tracheostomy is best performed using local anaesthetic since intubation in a distressed or stridulous patient with a known mass or tumour in the upper airway may be impossible. This situation frequently can be anticipated if the patient has been evaluated by indirect laryngoscopy prior to making the decision to operate. If there is any doubt of rapidly securing an airway by orotracheal intubation a tracheostomy should be performed under local anaesthetic.

Performing a tracheostomy under local anaesthetic can be harrowing both for the patient and the inexperienced surgeon. The patient should be placed in the usual position, if possible with the neck extended and the shoulders supported to give maximum exposure of the neck and trachea. The patient should be breathing 100% oxygen at this time and the surgical situation explained to him throughout the procedure. Local anaesthetic (lignocaine 1%) should be injected into the incision area and into the strap muscles. Care should be taken that the local anaesthetic is not injected into the trachea otherwise paroxysmal coughing may turn a semi-emergency into an absolute emergency. Also care should be taken not to infiltrate local anaesthetic into the paratracheal gutter as the recurrent laryngeal nerves may be paralysed, increasing respiratory distress. When the trachea has been exposed the thyroid must be divided and transfixed. Once this situation has been reached, local anaesthetic should be instilled into the trachea to suppress cough. The patient should be warned at this stage that he will no longer be able to speak. This warning can help to minimize the panic that often accompanies this type of operation. If the patient becomes distressed or the airway is lost at this stage the surgeon must act quickly and secure the airway with speed otherwise the patient could die.

If presented with a patient whose airway suddenly obstructs, obviously no time should be wasted with preparation of the patient as life is clearly at risk unless an airway is secured. The incision best suited to this situation is a vertical incision beginning from the cricoid cartilage extending inferiorly 2.5–5 cm (1–2 inches). The larynx should be stabilized by the non-dominant hand and the neck extended. Using the dominant hand a vertical incision is created through the skin, platysma, and subcutaneous tissues. Structures such as the strap muscles and thyroid isthmus are rarely identified. The index finger of the non-dominant hand is used as a retractor and a blunt dissector. It should be possible to avoid incising the cricoid cartilage and to position the actual vertical incision in the trachea at about the level of the second and third tracheal rings. So long as the dissection is in the midline in the anatomically normal neck, little irreversible damage can be done. Using an artery forceps the trachea can be opened to allow insertion of a tracheostomy tube or possibly an endotracheal tube into the tracheal lumen. The cuff is then inflated to protect and control the lower airway.

During an urgent or life and death tracheostomy the bleeding can be profuse and even terrifying to the observers as well as the inexperienced surgeon. The surgeon must not waste time attempting to stop bleeding; the priority is to secure the airway with speed. The bleeding dramatically subsides once the trachea is opened. It cannot be emphasized enough that it is the surgeon's responsibility to ensure that the assistants do not retract the trachea off the midline during this type of surgery. If the dissection is off midline then the trachea will be difficult to find and profuse haemorrhage will result.

The tracheostomy tube

The selection of a tracheostomy tube is usually governed by the requirements of the operation and the postoperative care. Usually a plastic tube with an inner cannula and a cuff is preferred if the patient requires protection of the lungs from aspiration or haemorrhage. If the patient requires controlled ventilation, a cuffed Shiley or Portex tube with a high volume low pressure cuff system is satisfactory. A fenestrated tube permits the passage of air upwards through the glottis thereby allowing the patient to speak.

There are two main type of tracheostomy tube available.

Metal tubes

Metal tubes, whatever their design, have several basic common principles: an obturator, an outer tube, and an inner tube. The inner tube is always slightly longer than the outer tube so that crusts can collect on the protruding end. Cleaning of the inner tube can be performed because the outer tube maintains the patency of the airway. Newer tracheostomy tubes have a flange which is not rigidly attached, allowing free movement of the neck. In unusual situations special tubes are available – Koenig's tube for extensive and low narrowing of the trachea, and Durham's tube in which the position of the flange is adjustable, so that it can be used for patients with either a thin or very fat neck. The main disadvantage of metal tubes is that they do not have a cuff, and cannot therefore produce an airtight seal. If the metal tubes do not fit properly, the end of the tube can erode the anterior tracheal wall. It must be remembered that metal tracheostomy tubes are manufactured and supplied as a 'set'. Therefore only complete sets should be used otherwise complications may result.

Non-metal tubes

Non-metal tubes are made of silastic. Their main advantage is that they can be made with an inflatable cuff and can be connected to an anaesthetic machine or respirator. They are also available in a cuffless model. They do not produce the same degree of mechanical damage to the trachea as metal tubes. Paradoxically the main disadvantage of these tubes is the inflatable cuff; it should be blown up to the point where there is a slight air leak past it when being used with the ventilator or the cuff pressure should be monitored and recorded to prevent ischaemia of the mucosa of the wall of the trachea, and routinely the cuff should be deflated for 5 minutes in every hour. If it is absolutely essential to maintain a permanent airtight seal, this can be achieved by the use of the Salpeker tube, which has two cuffs, one above the other, allowing alternate deflation and inflation of each cuff.

Postoperative management

Much morbidity and some of the mortality attributed to tracheostomy can be prevented by meticulous postoperative care by the surgeon and the nurse in charge of the patient, as well as the patient himself and his family. After the insertion of the tracheostomy tube the air the patient breathes must be humidified to keep the tracheal mucosa moist and thereby maintain mucociliary transport of secretions and prevent crusting and eventual obstruction of the airway. This can be done by forcing oxygen or compressed air at a rate of 5–7 l/min through a reservoir containing sterile water and delivering this air to the tracheostomy via a tracheostomy mask. The temperature of the humidified gas should be monitored to prevent overheating and consequent irritation of the tracheal mucosa. Once the patient is up-and-about, the mist may be applied three to four times a day and continuously at night. Care must be taken to remove the condensation, which may be inoculated with the patient's bacterial flora, so as not to contaminate others. The use of saline or sodium bicarbonate instilled into the trachea, 1–2 ml/h, helps to reduce the likelihood of crusting and aids with suction clearance of the secretions (Schild, 1970).

Initially, frequent suction is necessary because the tracheostomy reduces the efficiency of coughing and the patient cannot clear secretions from the tracheobronchial lumen. The secretions are profuse for the first few days and may require a full-time special nurse to perform suction very frequently if lower respiratory tract infection is to be avoided. The secretions result from the trachea being exposed to the cooler and drier air than it has been used to. The trachea therefore needs to be sucked out at frequent intervals. No specific time interval can be set and suction is required when indicated. The attending staff must obey the usual aseptic ritual: wash, wear gloves, and the suction tube should be sterile and preferably disposable. Changing the tracheostomy tube should not be necessary for at least 36–48 hours. At this time the tract will have become established and the opening in the trachea will usually be readily found. However, even in experienced hands the trachea may occasionally be difficult to find, and therefore it is important that the surgeon who has performed the tracheostomy should perform the first tube change. When the nursing staff are expected to perform tube changes medical staff should be readily available.

Patients who are having their tube changed are placed in the tracheostomy position, that is lying flat and with the neck extended. When the tube is withdrawn many patients experience paroxysmal coughing and the patient needs to be instructed and encouraged to inhale deeply, so that on removal of the tube all the secretions and debris lying in the tracheal lumen are blown out rather than aspirated.

Patients who have undergone tracheostomy must be monitored constantly. The patient's blood pressure, pulse and respiratory rate should be monitored every 15 minutes until the patient is awake, alert and aware of the situation and then every hour for the first 24 hours. Regardless of the ward type receiving the patient on admission, the patient and bed position should be within sight and sound of nursing personnel at all times. When the patient is transferred from this clinical area it must be remembered that the patient is usually unable to speak and a method of calling for assistance should be provided. All unit staff should be skilled in meeting the special needs of the tracheostomy patient, including the handling of respiratory emergencies.

Changes in vital signs or status should be reported to the medical staff. When there are other symptoms of distress including intercostal recession, restlessness or chest pain the patency of the airway must immediately be re-evaluated. Suction is performed as necessary. Dressings if used, should be sterile and must be changed at least once every shift or more often if secretions are copious, as a soiled dressing is a bacterial reservoir and could cause the wound to become infected. When sutures are used to stabilize the tracheostomy tube, these need to be cared for like the wound; the crusts need to be removed with hydrogen peroxide or saline soaks. The tapes if used should be changed when they become soiled. Routine culture of the tracheostomy wound is unnecessary and is only indicated when the secretions change in colour, odour, quantity or viscosity.

Emergency situations

Obstruction

Obstruction of a tracheostomy will lead to respiratory distress within a very short time, therefore any signs of distress should be looked for and investigated with speed. The most common cause of such airway obstruction is narrowing of the lumen of the tube by crusted secretions. Occasionally these crusts may dislodge or be dislodged leading to complete obstruction of the lumen of the tube. Instillation of saline and frequent suction should clear this problem and also prevent the situation occurring.

Acute total obstruction

Total obstruction may be encountered when trying to pass a suction catheter. The lumen may be obstructed by a mucous plug, displaced tube, or displaced cuff. If total obstruction is present, respiratory arrest will occur if it is not relieved immediately. Thus, when a suction catheter cannot be passed, the nurse must remain with the patient and attempt to relieve the obstruction while another nurse places the patient's neck in an extended position and calls for medical assistance. If a cuffed tube is in position the cuff must be deflated. Normal saline solution should be instilled into the tracheostomy tube and suctioning attempted again. If these measures fail to relieve the obstruction, it is necessary to remove the tube and reinsert a tracheostomy tube or consideration be given to orotracheal intubation if possible. At all times, because this emergency may occur at any time of night or day a second tracheostomy tube of the same size and one of the next size smaller should be at the bedside at all times, as well as a Trousseau dilator or Kelly haemostat to maintain the opening into the trachea. Oxygen may need to be administered as well and should always be available.

Accidental decannulation

Accidental displacement of the tracheostomy tube in the early postoperative period can produce an emergency. Accidental displacement of the tube or even decannulation may occur with a severe bout of coughing, chest physiotherapy, suctioning or during change of tracheostomy tube tapes. A confused or uncooperative patient may pull out his own tube. Since it takes some time for the surgical tract to mature in the early postoperative period the tissues around the tracheostomy site are oedematous and soft, and it may be very difficult to locate the opening in the anterior tracheal wall. A tracheostomy tube should not be inserted until the tracheal opening has been identified with certainty. Difficulty with locating the tracheal wall may be because at the time of the tracheostomy there was mobilization of the soft tissues lateral to the trachea leaving the tissues less rigid and more mobile. This may occur because of the type of surgical exploration undertaken or difficulty with surgical creation of the tracheostomy. This is why it is to be recommended that the surgeon who created the tracheostomy should perform the first tube change. Unintentional removal of the tracheostomy tube in the early postoperative period can be prevented by suturing the tube in place until a tract has developed rather than using cotton tapes. Occasionally the positioning of long silk ligatures fixed to the walls of the trachea at the time of surgery will be helpful. These may be pulled upwards and outwards at a 60° angle to reopen the trachea for reinsertion of the tube. Unfortunately in the experience of the author these sutures pull out in such emergencies and are therefore unreliable. In any event a Trousseau dilator or a large Kelly haemostat should be at the patient's bedside at all times so that the tracheos-

tomy can be held open after accidental decannulation until a new tube can be inserted. When a tracheostomy tube has been reinserted, the ventilation and provision of an adequate airway must be checked, since the tube may have been inserted into the soft tissues adjacent to the trachea. Should this be the case, respiratory distress, subcutaneous emphysema, or a pneumomediastinum could develop. The first step is to listen for movement of air through the tracheostomy tube and listen to the patient's respiration. If the patient is asked to cough the expiratory flow of air may be felt on the back of the hand or may be heard. Pulsation of the tube may indicate that the tube is resting against a major vessel, and erosion of the vessel wall, with subsequent bleeding may result. If there is any doubt about the correct position of the tube within the lumen of the trachea consideration must be given to orotracheal intubation if possible.

Haemorrhage

Some bleeding from a tracheostomy site is common and occurs within the first 24 hours postoperatively. Bleeding in this period should be reported to the surgeon who performed the tracheostomy, who should attend and inspect the area. Bleeding may be from the wound edge and can be dealt with easily. However, bleeding from deeper sites usually requires return to theatre for formal inspection. If the patient can easily be intubated via the orotracheal route then this should be done as this manoeuvre facilitates identification of the bleeding point. If this cannot be performed because of upper airway problems or surgery then the wound needs to be opened widely to expose all the anterior neck structures. The bleeding is frequently found from the thyroid isthmus or the thyroid itself, other areas include the divided or retracted strap muscles. If bleeding occurs after this period then the cuff of the tracheostomy tube should be inflated, the patient sedated and taken back to theatre as a major artery such as the brachiocephalic may be eroded.

Tracheostomy self-care

Patients who have a long-term need for a tracheostomy or those who have undergone a laryngectomy are often depressed. This can be manifest as an inability to perform adequate tracheostomy self-care at home. A system has been developed in Nottingham (Mason *et al.*, 1992) to teach self-care in a step-wise fashion enabling both the patient and the medical attenders to assess progress and to identify those patients who will require continuing close support if they are to self-care for their tracheostomy at home.

This system consists of 10 elements of tracheostomy care each subdivided into five teaching elements.

The elements are:

- Recognizing the need to clean and change the tracheostomy tube
- Removing the inner tube
- Cleaning the inner tube
- Inserting the inner tube
- Preparation of the equipment to change the outer tube
- Applying the tapes
- Removing the outer tube
- Cleaning the outer tube
- Inserting the outer tube
- Skin care.

The phases are:

1 Acting – the medical attendant performs the task.
2 Teaching – the medical attendant shows the patient how to perform the task.
3 Guiding – the patient and the medical attendant perform the task together.
4 Supporting – the patient performs the task while the medical attendant supervises and encourages the patient.
5 Self-care – the patient performs the task without the medical attendant.

The date on which each phase is completed is recorded.

Prior to teaching, the physical health of the patient is reviewed, and the patient and medical attendant agree on the number of days expected to be required to achieve competence in tracheostomy self-care. Upon completion a competence ratio is calculated as:

Number of days originally expected
Number of days actually required

The merits of this system are:

1 Medical staff, nursing staff, patients and relatives can readily monitor progress prior to discharge.
2 The learning process for the patient is established and not interrupted by shift changes of staff or holidays.
3 Patients struggling are identified rapidly, and the relevant care and help provided.
4 Patients with psychological problems with tracheostomy self-care can be identified and the appropriate extra support provided when they go home.

In patients with a competence ratio of < 0.6, it is now the policy to inform the general practitioner personally of our concern regarding the patients' ability to self-care for their tracheostomy. Extra support may be required and such patients will also require an earlier outpatient appointment than is routine.

Complications

Emergency situations arising after tracheostomy have already been discussed above but are included here for completeness. As with any other operation the complications of tracheostomy may be divided into immediate, that is during or immediately after the operation; intermediate, happening during the rest of the patient's stay in hospital; or late, occurring when the patient has gone home (Conley, 1979). Table 7.2 lists some of the more common of these complications. The complications of tracheostomy frequently result from improper execution of the procedure or inadequate postoperative care. Most retrospective studies have assessed the incidence of overall complications and these range from 5% to 40% (Miller and Knapp, 1984; Waldron, Padgham and Hurley, 1990). Agreed risk is approximately 15% with the most common being haemorrhage (3.7%), tube obstruction (2.7%) or tube displacement (1.5%). The incidence of pneumothorax, atelectasis, aspiration, tracheal stenosis or tracheo-oesophageal fistula is less than 1%. Death occurs in 0.5% to 1.6% of patients and is most often caused by haemorrhage or tube displacement. Moreover emergency tracheostomy carries a two- to fivefold increase in the incidence of complications over an elective procedure (Reilly and Sasaki, 1993).

Table 7.2 Complications of tracheostomy

Immediate
Haemorrhage
   thyroid veins
   jugular veins
   arteries
Air embolism
Apnoea
Cardiac arrest
Local damage
   thyroid cartilage
   cricoid cartilage
   recurrent laryngeal nerve

Intermediate
Dislodgement/displacement of the tube
Surgical emphysema of the neck
Pneumothorax/pneumomediastinum
Scabs and crusts
Infection
Tracheal necrosis
Tracheoarterial fistula
Tracheo-oesophageal fistula
Dysphagia

Late
Stenosis of the trachea
Difficulty with decannulation
Tracheocutaneous fistula/scars

Immediate

Haemorrhage

Haemorrhage during the operation is frequent, arising from the anterior jugular veins or the thyroid gland. Bleeding should be controlled at once by diathermy or by ligation. If the bleeding is profuse and difficult to control, digital pressure should be applied and the wound extended to allow better visualization of the area to identify the bleeding point. Blind groping and grasping in a small hole is to be condemned as further bleeding and other tissue damage can result (Stemmer *et al.*, 1976).

Air embolism

Air embolism is a serious complication but fortunately is uncommon. During surgery large neck veins can be inadvertently opened with large volumes of air sucked in and passing rapidly into the right atrium. If not recognized this situation can produce a crisis with tamponade and death. It should be avoided by meticulous attention to controlling bleeding by good access and visibility.

Apnoea

Apnoea is thought to be the result of the sudden discharge of the pent-up carbon dioxide from within the lungs once the airway obstruction has been suddenly bypassed. A quick way of avoiding this situation is to allow the patient to breathe a mixture of 95% oxygen and 5% carbon dioxide during the procedure if performing the tracheostomy under local anaesthetic.

Cardiac arrest

Cardiac arrest may occur during tracheostomy. The three most important factors appear to be excessive adrenaline production in the anxious patient; a rapid rise of the pH, consequent upon washing out of retained CO_2; and hyperkalaemia consequent upon respiratory alkalosis.

Local damage

In a short chubby neck great difficulty can be experienced with placing the tracheal incision in the correct position. It is better that the incision be placed too low rather than too high through the cricoid or the first tracheal ring as there is an increased risk of subsequent tracheal stenosis. Unilateral or bilateral vocal cord paralysis may arise from inadvertent injury to the recurrent laryngeal nerves during an emergency tracheostomy, particularly if the dissection deviates from the midline.

Intermediate

Dislodgement/displacement of the tube

The length of the tracheostomy tube and the thickness of the neck are clearly the most important factors, however, modern tubes are of sufficient length to prevent accidental withdrawal of the tube. Nevertheless, the silver tubes of Negus and Chevalier-Jackson are shorter and should be used only in patients with thin necks. Postoperative oedema, haematoma and emphysema will cause a broadening of the distance between the skin surface and the anterior wall of the trachea, the process of expansion dragging the tube out of the trachea. The technique of suturing the flanges to the skin will help to minimize this possibility during the early period. In the later period the tracheostomy tapes should be tied with the neck in flexion, in which the girth of the neck is at its smallest; if tied in extension the tapes will become loose once the head comes forward.

Surgical emphysema

Subcutaneous emphysema can be alarming but is seldom fatal. Many factors may contribute to this complication – a too large incision in the trachea, depression of the superior flap of the trachea above the incision, obstruction to the egress of air by the glottic or pharyngeal obstruction, a tube that is partially obstructed or diverts air into the soft tissues of the neck, too tight closure of the subcutaneous tissues and skin about the tracheostomy tube causing a ball-valve effect, and excessive coughing which may also cause a pneumothorax. The emphysema is most often confined to the neck but can extend to the face and the chest wall. It usually presents within the first day and is self-limiting by the seventh day, unless the precipitating factors persist. The patient may develop a low grade pyrexia with localized cellulitis and a feeling of discomfort caused by stretching of the skin. The most frequent causes are tight skin closure and an improperly fitting tracheostomy tube; they should be rectified at once. In this situation the risk of the tracheostomy tube being dislodged is increased because of the local increase in neck swelling.

Pneumothorax/pneumomediastinum

These conditions may arise after any operation in the root of the neck. Usually this complication occurs in patients who are having surgery under local anaesthetic and are struggling, gasping and coughing. Occasionally the apex of the lung can be high in the neck and may be punctured by accident. The diagnosis should be considered in all patients after creation of a tracheostomy if the dyspnoea has not improved. A chest radiograph will confirm the diagnosis. Under severe circumstances, i.e. if there is a tension pneumothorax, immediate needle aspiration with a 14–

16 gauge needle into the upper anterior thorax will confirm the diagnosis and improve the patient's condition. The patient almost always requires aspiration of the air and drainage for a few days.

Scabs and crusts

A tracheostomy alters the basic physiology of the inspired air from filtered, warm and humidified to dry, cold air coming into direct contact with the trachea. This alteration dries the tracheal and pulmonary secretions and this interferes with the ciliary capacity to move the mucous blanket, and thus causes production of thick, tenacious mucous scabs and crusts. This basic interference with the movement of the ciliary blanket and the perpetuation of the drying process, is one of the most important aspects in the postoperative care. If not corrected, this sequence of events leads to infection, obstruction, atelectasis and pneumonia. If the situation is not controlled the scabs will increase in size, with the result that they are difficult or impossible to cough out or even remove by suction. Therefore the air supplied to the patient needs to be humidified. Air saturated with water vapour may be supplied by an old fashioned but cheap and reliable steam tent. Commercial humidifiers are available in most hospitals nowadays. A simple method of droplet infusion is to introduce, in an adult, 15 drops per minute of saline via a fine bore plastic catheter or to instil 5 ml/h via a syringe directly into the trachea. Suction is applied as necessary with a sterile, disposable, smooth-tipped catheter; the nurse must wear sterile gloves. Many of these patients aspirate their oropharyngeal secretions and thus have an excessively wet trachea. There is a constant slow adaptation process over weeks, and ultimately the trachea adapts to its new dry environment. The patient should be encouraged to regulate and adjust his own humidification before discharge from hospital. In some instances it may be necessary to insert a bronchoscope to clear out the trachea and bronchi.

Infection

All tracheostomy wounds become locally infected within hours of their creation. However, all tracheostomy wounds should be attended with the strictest of local hygiene. Local dressings applied around the tracheostomy tube help to reduce the pressure on the neck skin and may avoid necrosis. However, during the early period these dressings need to be changed frequently as secretions and blood accumulate. Barrier creams applied to the skin help to reduce the risk of local skin infections. Some patients develop *Pseudomonas* infections locally which may progress to fatal septicaemia. Prophylaxis is the best way of avoiding this type of infection. Fortunately infections in the neck wound are usually local, indolent and produce local cellulitis with some granulations. As the wound is open drainage is adequate and seldom are antibiotics necessary.

Tracheal necrosis

This complication most frequently follows focal pressure secondary to infection. The pressure is derived from over-sized tracheostomy tubes, an improper curve of the tube, impingement of the tip of the tube or pressure of the cuff on the trachea. The effect of this pressure begins as an ulcer on the wall of the mid or low cervical trachea. Previous irradiation, low grade infection and poor physiological status exaggerate the condition. This may lead to necrosis of the trachea with subsequent stenosis, tracheo-oesophageal or tracheoarterial fistula. It is therefore essential that the regulation of the pressure of the tracheostomy cuff in the intensive care unit and on the ward receives due care and attention. Any sign of bleeding, pain or obstruction should attract immediate investigation and remedial action by elimination of the pressure factors, careful inspection of the ulcer, with a decision to allow the ulcer to heal by secondary intent or to excise the ulcer and attempt primary closure. Occasionally in large ulcers, the great vessels are at risk and need to be protected with a muscle flap with withdrawal or change in position of the ventilatory apparatus.

Tracheoarterial fistula

This tragic complication occurs in about 0.4% of tracheostomies. It carries a mortality of 80–90%. It may be heralded by the so-called 'sentinel' bleed which should prompt a thorough fibreoptic tracheal inspection (Jones *et al.*, 1976). It is associated with an improper position of the tracheostomy tube against the vessel, improper curve and length of the tube, or is secondary to pressure from the cuff. One of the essential prophylactic measures in tracheostomy is to evaluate the position of the brachiocephalic artery by digital pressure during the surgical procedure. A significant warning sign before exsanguinating haemorrhage is slight bleeding from the trachea at any time from 3 days to 3 weeks before the catastrophe (Cooper, 1977).

Tracheo-oesophageal fistula

There are two significant factors contributing to the production of a tracheo-oesophageal fistula. A combination of these factors causes necrosis of the posterior wall of the trachea and the anterior wall of the oesophagus, thus creating a fistula. These factors are an overinflated or improperly fitting cuffed tube, causing pressure on the posterior tracheal wall and, usually, an indwelling nasogastric tube in the oesophagus. Positive pressure ventilation is a significant contributing factor. The diagnosis is suspected clinically by violent coughing during eating, chronic coughing associated with swallowing of saliva and occasionally air escaping into the hypopharynx. Endoscopic examination is the best method to confirm the presence and site of the fistula. The use of contrast medium for diagnosis is often confusing because it is difficult to differentiate between aspiration of the contrast through the fistula and aspiration of the contrast material into the larynx as a result of loss of the swallowing reflex. Once the diagnosis is confirmed the best treatment is surgical closure.

Dysphagia

Difficulty in swallowing is often encountered for the first few days after the creation of a tracheostomy. This situation can be managed by feeding the patient through a Ryles tube or by inflating the cuff of the tracheostomy tube during feeds. This difficulty with swallowing may be related to the original indication for tracheostomy but other factors may contribute: tethering of the larynx so that it cannot move upwards during swallowing; the pressure of the inflated cuff on the oesophagus; or very rarely, as a result of ulceration of the tracheo-oesophageal wall producing a fistula (Bonanno, 1971).

Late complications

Stenosis of the trachea

Tracheal stenosis occurs at three distinct levels – the stoma, the cuff site or the tip of the tube. The majority of cases results from the inflatable cuff of the orotracheal or tracheostomy tube, others result from scar contracture caused by improperly placed incisions, repetitive incisions, tracheal resections and trauma, tracheal infections or organic disease of the trachea.

Difficulty with decannulation

Most tracheostomies are temporary; the patient is ultimately decannulated and the tracheocutaneous fistula is closed. In the early phase of the tracheostomy the tube can be withdrawn without much difficulty because the wound edge is clean, no granulations have formed and the skin edges are still raw which leads to rapid closure. When the tube has been in place for weeks, months or even years, removal may be difficult – granulations may have formed developing into fibrous masses resulting in tracheal strictures. Patients with a long-standing tracheostomy should be carefully examined before the tube is removed. Lateral neck radiographs or xerograms with or without tomography can show granulations or fibrous masses at the entrance of the tracheostomy. Sometimes the trachea needs to be inspected directly to assess the lumen. Some tracheal narrowing can be

demonstrated in more than 90% of patients after tracheostomy, and is most often seen near the site of the stoma (Lulenski, 1981). Functional impairment is rare unless the trachea has been narrowed by more than 50% as measured on biplane radiographs. If the airway appears adequate, tube sizes can be decreased until the patient is breathing through the glottis. The smaller tube may be closed over with tape, or a plug can be inserted for several days before final removal of the tube. If the wound is recent it will close in 1–2 days, but if it is of longer duration it may be necessary to close it surgically.

Tracheocutaneous fistula and scars

The tracheal wound and skin incision usually close by secondary intent, but occasionally fistulae persist, particularly if the tracheostomy has been present for a long time. A persistent fistula causes continual tracheal secretions with skin irritation, disturbed phonation, frequent infections and poor cosmesis. The scar after secondary closure is usually cosmetically unacceptable to the patient and her family. The skin is usually thin and frequently becomes attached to the trachea by fibrous tissue so that the scar moves up and down when the patient swallows and causes a tug on the trachea. Most fistulae heal spontaneously if they have been present for less than 16 weeks, but if they have been there longer most will need surgical closure. Surgery is best performed under general anaesthetic with endotracheal intubation; the old scar is excised and the strap muscles mobilized and approximated by sutures. The wound should be closed in layers over a small corrugated drain to avoid the risk of haematoma formation or surgical emphysema (Kulber and Passey, 1972).

The long-term tracheostomy

Long-term tracheostomies are recommended for patients who will require prolonged or permanent control (Maisel and Goding, 1991). If tracheostomies performed in the standard way are maintained for months or years, they frequently result in serious damage to the laryngotracheal complex. The difference is essentially one in which the stoma is designed for long-term patency (Eliachar *et al.*, 1984). Measures must be taken to prevent contracture or collapse of the stomal edge, and minimize or avoid rough surfaces, granulation tissue, infection or pain. The gap between the surface of the anterior cervical skin and trachea should be circumferentially lined by either skin or mucous membrane. This gap should be short and stable, obviating the need for a permanently placed tube to maintain an airway. The majority of patients with a long-term tracheostomy prefer the use of a stoma stent to cover the tracheostomal orifice, maintain its patency, and promote speech and an effective cough. An introducible, self-retaining prosthesis is preferred for patients who can breathe and speak through the larynx. The indications for long-term tracheostomy are conditions such as chronic obstructive airway disease requiring long-term ventilation, severe obstructive sleep apnoea, bilateral vocal cord paralysis, laryngeal or tracheal stenosis, and neurological or neuromuscular disorders where the airway is at risk. The technique described by Eliachar and Oringher (1990) undermines the neck tissues widely and makes a large cartilaginous opening into the trachea. After the fat and subcutaneous tissue have been removed the skin is sutured to the mucosal edge of the trachea. They advocate further additional support and protection of the anterior tracheal wall by a fibromuscular sling derived from the tendon of the sternomastoid muscle. The tendon is slung over the tracheal flap, then sutured to its counterpart on the other side.

Minitracheostomy

The innovation of a vertical stab incision made through the cricothyroid membrane under local anaesthetic allows the insertion of a 4 mm cannula to provide ready access and delivery of oxygen. This technique was described by Matthews and Hopkinson (1984) to aid with retained mucus in patients who had undergone a thorocotomy and in whom there was the need to treat their respiratory distress. The prime indication for the minitracheostomy is to remove chest secretions, but it has also been used in the treatment of respiratory failure with a high frequency jet ventilator, in obstructive sleep apnoea. It has also been described in the management of an obstructed airway before laryngectomy. Many of the complications associated with the creation of a formal tracheostomy have been reported (Ryan, 1990).

Percutaneous tracheostomy

Percutaneous tracheostomy, a minimally invasive alternative to conventional tracheostomy was first described by Toye and Weinstein (1969) but it is only recently that kits to create a full-sized percutaneous tracheostomy have become available.

There are two methods.

1 The trachea is punctured at a chosen level with a needle and cannula and a guide wire is then passed into the trachea using the Seldinger technique. This system uses graded dilators, 12–36 Fr, which are passed over the guidewire into the trachea. Passage of the dilators and the tracheostomy tube is facilitated by the liberal use of lubricating gel (Cook and Callanan, 1989; Schachner *et al.*, 1989).

2 In the Schachner (Rapitrac) system a dilator, the tracheostome, is passed over the guidewire into the trachea to dilate the tract fully in one step. The tracheostome has a bevelled metal core with a hole through its centre to accommodate the guidewire. Once inserted into the trachea, the handles of the tracheostome are squeezed together causing the metal cone to split into two halves, thus dilating the opening in the trachea. A conventional tracheostomy tube, with a specially designed obturator is passed through the tracheal opening. The dilator and obturator are then removed leaving the tracheostomy tube in place.

In an appraisal of percutaneous tracheostomy there was a significantly higher number of patients in the Rapitrac group who had complications compared with that of the Cook method and a conventional tracheostomy group (Leinhardt *et al.*, 1992). The technique is not difficult to learn but it has been repeatedly reported that there is a distinct 'learning curve', with proficiency developing after several supervised procedures (Hazard, Jones and Benitane, 1991). It has also been stated that percutaneous tracheostomy is associated with a lower rate of associated adverse events in critically ill patients. It can be conveniently performed in intensive care units at the patient's bedside, eliminating the risk and expense involved in transport to and from the operating room. All patients having a percutaneous tracheostomy require an oral or nasal endotracheal tube in position to aid with the procedure and to minimize complications. A recent report on percutaneous tracheostomy lists a number of complications (Wang *et al.*, 1992). The possibility of a false passage is a significant hazard, especially in patients with calcified rings, blind passage of the dilators and tube may also result in puncture through the side or back wall of the trachea.

Cricothyroidotomy

In an emergency, failure to clear or secure the airway with an endotracheal tube may result in the death of the patient. Entry into the airway can be achieved rapidly through the cricothyroid membrane because it is superficial and an easily identifiable landmark (Roven and Clapham, 1983).

Indications

Emergency

An emergency arises when an obstructed airway cannot be secured through the laryngeal route for whatever reason (Milner and Bennett, 1991).

Elective

Cricothyroidotomy has been condemned because of the high incidence of subglottic stenosis. In the presence of laryngeal disease and/or prolonged intubation the incidence of subglottic stenosis is high and cricothyroidotomy as an elective procedure should not be performed (Brantigan and Grow, 1982) though this statement has been questioned by others (Sisi *et al.*, 1984).

Techniques

Three ways have been described to perform a cricothyroidotomy:

1 Using an intravenous catheter
2 Using a cricothyrotome or the disposable Nu-Trake cricothyroidotomy device
3 As a formal surgical procedure.

The patient's head and neck are extended, by placing a pillow beneath the shoulders, to provide better exposure. In an emergency, a 14-gauge intravenous needle can be inserted, through the cricothyroid membrane, into the lumen of the trachea and aspirated until air is returned to signify the correct position. A catheter is then directed 45° caudally and advanced over the needle into the trachea. The cricothyrotome is used in a similar fashion. Emergency cricothyroidotomy instruments or commercial sets are available and have been found in experienced hands to achieve an airway with speed; the technique is similar to the Schachner technique (Ravlo *et al.*, 1987).

In the formal surgical procedure, the instruments needed are a scalpel, an artery forceps and an endotracheal or tracheostomy tube. The operator fixes the thyroid cartilage with the thumb and middle finger using the non-dominant hand and the cricothyroid space is identified. The scalpel should be inserted perpendicularly through the cricothyroid membrane. A stab and twist movement without reaching the posterior wall gains access to the airway. With the non-dominant hand the artery forceps is slightly opened and passed around the scalpel blade into the airway to widen the opening. The scalpel is exchanged for an endotracheal tube or a tracheostomy tube. If the cricothyroid membrane is cut transversely and parallel to the tracheal rings more bleeding can be expected because of the veins crossing this area.

After a surgical cricothyroidotomy when an endotracheal tube has been placed, ventilation can be managed in the normal way using an Ambu-bag and an adaptor. Using the intravenous catheter or the cricothyrotome with a Leur connection two immediate problems arise – connection to an inflation device, and producing adequate gas flow through a small bore tube with high resistance. In the casualty or resuscitation environment several methods are available: a 3 mm endotracheal tube using a 3 ml Luer lock; a syringe with a 7 mm endotracheal tube adaptor inserted into the barrel; a 10 ml syringe with the endotracheal tube inserted into the barrel with the cuff inflated. Enough oxygen is then supplied for tissue oxygenation but CO_2 removal is inefficient. If the minute ventilation is inadequate, the surgeon can at least 'buy-time' for the performance of a surgical cricothyroidotomy or tracheostomy. The resistance to flow through the small bore cannula can be overcome by a high pressure oxygen source (at least 400 kPa). Flow must be intermittent and allow adequate time for expiration. The jet-vent or a high pressure flow system is needed to overcome these problems. An obvious hazard is hyperventilation with high intrathoracic pressures, possibly leading to cardiac decompensation or pneumothorax. High-frequency jet ventilation is the safest way to solve the problems of hyperventilation and cardiac decompensation.

Once the emergency has been controlled, the clinician can convert to a translaryngeal tube or to a tracheostomy. The long-term management plan should be specific to the patient's needs (Weymuller and Cummings, 1982). Severe laryngeal injury will require a tracheostomy, whereas with an obstructed laryngeal lesion the blockage may be removed endoscopically.

Complications

Complications may occur during catheter insertion or during ventilation. Haemorrhage may occur from an artery or vein (Mcgill, Clinton and Ruiz, 1982). The main problems with ventilation are subcutaneous emphysema, if the catheter slips out of the trachea, and hyperinflation. Hyperinflation occurs when laryngeal obstruction limits expiration so that the lungs become more expanded with each inflation. Subglottic stenosis may follow cricothyroidotomy, although its true incidence is difficult to assess. The association of voice change has been noted following cricothyroidotomy (Gleeson *et al.*, 1984).

References

AROLA, M. K., INBERG, M. V. and PUHAKKA, H. (1981) Tracheal stenosis after tracheostomy and after oro-tracheal cuffed intubation. *Acta Chirurgica Scandinavica*, **147**, 183–192

ATLS (1989) *Manual Advanced Trauma Life Support*. Chicago: American College of Surgeons

BJÖRK, V. O. (1960) Partial resection of the only remaining lung with the aid of respiratory treatment. *Journal of Thoracic and Cardiovascular Surgery*, **39**, 179–188

BLANC, V. F. and TREMBLAY, N. A. G. (1974) The complications of tracheal intubation. *Anaesthesia and Analgesia*, **153**, 202–213

BONANNO, P. C. (1971) Swallowing function after tracheostomy. *Annals of Surgery*, **174**, 29–33

BRANTIGAN, P. C. and GROW, J. B. (1982) Subglottic stenosis after cricothyroidotomy. *Surgery*, **91**, 217–221

BRYANT, L. R., MUIJA, D., GREENBERG, S., HUEY, J. M., SCHECHTER, F. G. and ALBER, H. M. (1978) Evaluation of tracheal incisions for tracheostomy. *Archives of Otolaryngology*, **135**, 675–679

COMBLEY, M. and VAUGHAN, R. S. (1992) Recognition and management of difficult airway problems. *British Journal of Anaesthesia*, **68**, 90–97

CONLEY, J. J. (ed.) (1979) Tracheostomy complications. In: *Complications of Head and Neck Surgery*. Philadelphia: W. B. Saunders. pp. 274–292

COOK, P. D. and CALLANAN, V. I. (1989) Percutaneous dilatational tracheostomy technique and experience. *Anaesthesia and Intensive Care*, **17**, 456–457

COOPER, J. D. (1977) Tracheo–innominate artery fistula. *Annals of Thoracic Surgery*, **24**, 439–447

DANZL, D. F. and THOMAS, D. M. (1980) Nasotracheal intubation in the emergency department. *Critical Care Medicine*, **10**, 142–144

DAVIDSON, T. M., BONE, R. C. and NAHUM, A. M. (1975) Endotracheal intubation with the flexible fibreoptic bronchoscope. *Ear, Nose and Throat Monthly*, **54**, 346–349

DAVIS, N. J. (1973) A new fibreoptic laryngoscope for nasal intubation. *Anaesthesia and Analgesia*, **52**, 807–808

EDEMS, E. T. and SIA, R. L. (1981) Flexible fibreoptic endoscopy in difficult intubation. *Annals of Otolaryngology*, **90**, 307–309

ELIACHAR, I. and ORINGHER, S. F. (1990) Performance and management of long-term tracheostomy. *Operative Techniques in Otorhinolaryngology, Head and Neck Surgery*, **1**, 56–63

ELIACHAR, I., ZOHAR, S., GOLZ, A., JOACHIMS, H-Z. and GOLDSHER, M. (1984) Permanent tracheostomy. *Head and Neck Surgery*, **7**, 99–103

FRERK, C. M. (1991) Predicting difficult intubation. *Anaesthesia*, **46**, 1005–1008

FRIEDMAN, M. and VENKATESAN, T. K. (1990) The difficult tracheostomy simplified. *Operative Techniques in Otorhinolaryngology, Head and Neck Surgery*, **1**, 71–72

GLEESON, M. J. and FOURCIN, A. J. (1983) Clinical analysis of laryngeal trauma secondary to intubation. *Journal of the Royal Society of Medicine*, **76**, 928–932

GLEESON, M. J., PEARSON, R. C., ARMISTEAD, S. and YATES A. S. (1984) Voice changes following cricothyroidotomy. *Journal of Laryngology and Otology*, **98**, 1015–1019

HAWKINS, D. B. and CROCKETT, D. M. (1983) Corticosteroids in airway management. *Otolaryngology–Head and Neck Surgery*, **91**, 593–597

HAWKINS, D. B. and LUXFORD, W. M. (1980) Laryngeal stenosis from endotracheal intubation. *Annals of Otology*, **89**, 454–458

HAZARD, P., JONES, C. and BENITANE, J. (1991) Comparative clinical trial of standard operative tracheostomy with percutaneous tracheostomy. *Critical Care Medicine*, **19**, 1018–1024

HEIMLICH, H. J. (1974) Pop goes the cafe coronary. *Emergency Medicine*, **6**, 154–160

JAFFE, B. F. (1972) Post-operative hoarseness. *American Journal of Surgery*, **123**, 432–437

JOHNSEN, S. (1973) What is prolonged intubation? *Acta Otolaryngologica*, **75**, 377–378

JONES, J. W., REYNOLDS, M., HEWITT, R. L. and DRAPANAS J. (1976) Tracheo-innominate artery erosion. *Annals of Surgery*, **184**, 194–204

KANE, W. M., DENNENY, J. C., ROWE, L. D. and ATKINS, J. P. (1982) Complications of intubation. *Annals of Otolaryngology, Rhinology and Laryngology*, **91**, 584–587

KULBER, H. and PASSEY, V. (1972) Tracheostomy closure and scar revisions. *Archives of Otology and Laryngology*, **96**, 22–26

LEINHARDT, D. J., MUGHAL, M., BOWLES, B., GLEW, B., KISHEN, R., MACBEATH, J. *et al.* (1992) Appraisal of percutaneous tracheostomy. *British Journal of Surgery*, **79**, 255–258

LULENSKI, G. C. (1981) Long term tracheal dimensions after flap tracheostomy. *Archives of Otolaryngology*, **107**, 114–119

MCCLELLAND, M. A. (1972) Tracheostomy; its management and alternatives. *Proceedings of the Royal Society of Medicine*, **65**, 401–403

MCGILL, J., CLINTON, E. and RUIZ, E. (1982) Cricothyrotomy in the emergency department. *Annals of Emergency Medicine*, **11**, 361–364

MAISEL, R. H. and GODING, G. S. (1991) Tracheostomy for obstructive sleep apnoea; indications, techniques and selection of tubes. *Operative Techniques in Otorhinolaryngology, Head and Neck Surgery*, **2**, 107–111

MALLAMPATI, S. R., GATT, S. P., GUGINO, L. D., DESAI, S. P., WARAKSA, B., FREIBERGER, D. *et al.* (1985), A clinical sign to predict difficult tracheal intubation; a prospective study. *Canadian Anaesthetists Society Journal*, **32**, 429–434

MASON, J., MURTY, G. E., FOSTER, H. and BRADLEY, P. J. (1992) Tracheostomy; self–care; the Nottingham system. *Journal of Laryngology and Otology*, **106**, 723–724

MATTHEWS, H. R. and HOPKINSON, R. B. (1984) Treatment of sputum retention by mini-tracheostomy. *British Journal of Surgery*, **71**, 147–150

MILLER, J. D. and KNAPP, J. P. (1984) Complications of tracheostomies in neurosurgical patients. *Surgery and Neurology*, **22**, 186–188

MILNER, S. M. and BENNETT, J. D. C. (1991) Emergency cricothyrotomy. *Journal of Laryngology and Otology*, **105**, 883–885

RAVLO, O., BALA, V., LYBECKER, H., MOLLER, J. T., WERNER, M. and WEILSEN, H. K. (1987) A comparison between two emergency cricothyroidotomy instruments. *Acta Anaesthesiologica Scandinavica*, **31**, 317–319

REILLY, H. and SASAKI, C. T. (1993) Tracheotomy complications. In: *Complications in Head and Neck Surgery*, edited by Y. P. Krespi and R. H. Ossoff. Philadelphia: W. B. Saunders. pp. 257–274

ROVEN, A. N. and CLAPHAM, M. C. C. (1983) Cricothyroidotomy. *Ear, Nose and Throat Journal*, **62**, 488–493

RYAN, D. W. (1990) Mini-tracheotomy. *British Medical Journal*, **300**, 958–959

SALEM, M. R., MATHRUBHUTHAM, M. and BENNETT, E. J. (1976) Difficult intubation. *New England Journal of Medicine*, **295**, 879–881

SANADA, Y., KOJIMA, Y. and FOWKALSRUD, E. W., (1982) Injury of cilia induced by tracheal tube cuffs. *Surgery, Gynecology and Ostetrics*, **154**, 648–654

SCHACHNER, A., OVIL, Y., SIDI, J., ROREV, M., HEILBRONIN, Y. and LEVY, M. J. (1989) Percutaneous tracheostomy – a new method. *Critical Care Medicine*, **17**, 1052–1056

SCHILD, J. A. (1970) Tracheostomy care. *International Anaesthetic Clinics*, **8**, 649–654

SCOTT, D. R. (1986) Endotracheal intubation; friend or foe! *British Medical Journal*, **292**, 157–158

SHAW, H. J., STYLIS, S. C. and ROSEN, G. (1974) Elective tracheostomy in head and neck surgery. *Journal of Laryngology and Otology*, **88**, 599–614

SISI, M. J., SHACKFORD, S. R., CRUICKSHANK, J. C., MURPHY, G. and FRIDLUND, P. H. (1984) Cricothyroidotomy for long-term tracheal access. *Annals of Surgery,* **200**, 13–17

STAUFFER, J. L., OLSON D. E. and PETTY, T. L. (1981) Complications and consequences of orotracheal intubation and tracheostomy. *American Journal of Medicine,* **70**, 65–76

STELL, P. M. (1973) Tracheotomy and tracheostomy. In: *Recent Advances in Otolaryngology,* edited by J. Ransome, H. Holden and T. R. Bull. Edinburgh: Churchill Livingstone. pp. 275–294

STEMMER, E. A., OLIVER, C., CAREY, J. P. and CONNOLLY, J. E. (1976) Fatal complications of tracheostomy. *American Journal of Surgery,* **131**, 288–290

TINTINALLI, J. E. and CLAFFEY, J. (1981) Complications of nasotracheal intubation. *Annals of Emergency Medicine,* **10**, 142–144

TOYE, F. J. and WEINSTEIN, J. D. (1969) A percutaneous tracheostomy device. *Surgery,* **65**, 384–389

WALDRON, J., PADGHAM, N. W. and HURLEY, S. E. (1990) Complications of emergency and elective tracheostomy. *Annals of the Royal College of Surgeons England,* **72**, 218–220

WANG, M. B., BERKE, G. S., WARD, P. H., CALCATERRA, T. C. and WATTS, D. (1992) Early experience with percutaneous tracheotomy. *Laryngoscope,* **102**, 157–162

WEYMULLER, E. A. and CUMMINGS, C. W. (1982) Cricothyroidotomy; the impact of antecedent endotracheal intubation. *Annals of Otology, Rhinology and Laryngology,* **91**, 437–439

WHITE, A. and KANDER, P. L. (1975) Anatomical factors in difficult direct laryngoscopy. *British Journal of Anaesthesia,* **47**, 468–473

8

Trauma and stenosis of the larynx

A. G. D. Maran

Acute laryngeal trauma

Epidemiology

There are basically two types of laryngeal trauma – penetrating wounds and blunt injuries. The blunt injuries can be high velocity or low velocity. Penetrating wounds are caused by knives, bullets, wires and agricultural implements. High velocity blunt injuries are usually caused by road traffic accidents or injuries at work. The velocity, however, may be so high that the wound becomes compound. Low velocity blunt injuries rarely become compound and are due to blows with fists and as a result of sports injuries. The sports that are particularly associated with laryngeal injury are snowmobile racing, motor cycle racing, basketball, karate and injuries have even been reported due to contact with golf balls and cricket balls. Reports have also come from the sport of ice hockey where garrotting with the hockey stick is a hazard of the professional game.

The type of individual who suffers from laryngeal trauma is usually a young male who indulges in sport, is involved in fights, or who drives cars fast and dangerously.

In North America and Western Europe, the condition of laryngeal trauma was first associated with road traffic accidents. This was when no seat belts were used or lap-type seat belts were in vogue. Nowadays, the incidence in these countries of laryngeal damage from road traffic accidents is only a fraction of what it was. This is due to the crossover seat belt and the institution of speed limits and other safety features in cars, such as collapsible steering wheels, air cushions, etc. In developing countries, however, when driving by a large number of people is a relatively new feature, laryngeal injuries as a result of road traffic accidents present a significant problem.

Furthermore, in these countries there is an improving delivery of medical care and more patients are rescued from road traffic accidents and removed from the site of the accident to the hospital, where previously they may have died at the roadside.

Biomechanics

Any classification of types of laryngeal injury is an unhelpful exercise unless it is confined to injuries to the supraglottis, the glottis, the subglottis or mixed injuries. Basically, one must consider injuries to the surrounding skeleton of the larynx, that is the hyoid, thyroid, cricoid and tracheal rings, and injuries to the internal soft tissues. Damage to either the skeleton and the soft tissues creates different problems and requires different modes of management.

Penetrating wounds tend to bounce off the more solid pieces of the larynx, that is the supporting skeleton. It would be usual for a penetrating instrument to slide off the thyroid cartilage and penetrate the thyrohyoid membrane superiorly or go between the cricoid and the thyroid inferiorly to penetrate the cricothyroid membrane. Each of these presents different functional problems.

Penetration of the thyrohyoid membrane causes bleeding in the paraglottic space and thus airway obstruction. It does not affect the voice in any way. A little bleeding or oedema will resolve with the normal scavenging macrophage process of the body but, if there is any significant amount of bleeding, then it will not all resorb and will be organized to cause some degree of stenosis of the supraglottis.

This does not happen to such an extent if the cricothyroid membrane is penetrated. The most immediate effect of this will be that air will leave the respiratory tract and will cause some surgical emphysema in the neck. The penetrating wound, however, may be covered with thyroid tissue which may act as a valve. The bleeding may fill the subglottic space causing respiratory obstruction, but it is more likely to run down the trachea through a clean cut and cause coughing.

Low velocity blunt injuries are unlikely to fracture the thyroid or the cricoid, but fractured hyoids are not uncommon in karate and basket-ball, but the main problem is soft tissue injury. Again there will be bleeding into the soft tissues of the paraglottic space and, if the ends of the fractured hyoid are in close apposition, then movement during swallowing will cause pain which may require treatment. The patient may also have swelling of the base of the tongue and some dysphagia.

Even though the thyroid and cricoid are not fractured, there may well be bleeding within the paraglottic space and bleeding within Reinke's space on the vocal cords. The interarytenoid space, which must be present to allow gliding and separation of the arytenoids, can fill with blood ultimately causing stenosis, but the problem is usually one of oedema and minimal bleeding rather than obliterative bleeding causing airway damage or later stenosis.

High velocity blunt injuries will fracture the skeleton of the larynx. The fate of the thyroid cartilage depends on its degree of calcification and, thus, on the age of the patient. If the thyroid cartilage is pushed backwards over the cervical spine, then it splays apart (Figure 8.1). A minimal injury like this with an elastic thyroid cartilage will result in no fracture, but if there is any rigidity in the thyroid cartilage or if the force is great enough, then the cartilage will usually split down the front or down the thyroid prominence. The inherent elasticity of the uncalcified cartilage will allow it to spring back into place, and there may be little damage or there may be disruption of the anterior commissure. The

classically described situation of detachment of the tendon of the anterior commissure and the petiole of the epiglottis is hardly ever seen, but is so dramatic that it demands inclusion in any text on laryngeal injury. In this case, the epiglottis falls backwards and the vocal cords literally roll up on themselves towards the arytenoid. Usually in an elastic thyroid with a linear fracture down the prominence, however, there is little in the way of disruption of the anterior commissure, but there will be bleeding into the pre-epiglottic space and posterior displacement of the epiglottis. More important is the fate of the arytenoids. As the thyroid becomes compressed against the cervical spine, the arytenoids are sandwiched. This can result in them being displaced at worst, but at best there will be bleeding into the interarytenoid space and subsequent swelling.

If the thyroid is calcified and is then compressed against the cervical spine, it is unlikely to have enough inherent elasticity to return to its original position (Figure 8.2). It will, therefore, shatter rather like an egg and there will be loss of the thyroid prominence. There will be similar arytenoid injury as described above.

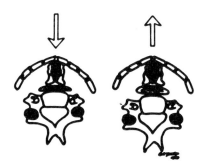

Figure 8.2 When a calcified thyroid cartilage is compressed against the cervical spine, it may well shatter with resultant bleeding into the paraglottic space

The cricoid is the most important part of the laryngeal skeleton. It is the only complete ring in the upper or lower respiratory tract. The thyroid, the hyoid and tracheal rings are all U-shaped with soft tissue attachments posteriorly. If the cricoid is disrupted then it will stenose. Even a linear fracture in the cricoid will cause some resorption of cartilage and reduction of the calibre of the airway at the level of the cricoid. This has severe effects on airflow as a consequence of Poiseuille's law relating the airflow to the fourth power of the radius of the airway. This is probably why high tracheostomies have such a damaging effect on the airway. There is nothing magic about the first ring, but a tracheostomy tube put through an opening made by excision of the first ring will be contiguous with the cricoid cartilage and may result in enough resorption of that cartilage for the cricoid to stenose. It is rare that acute injuries damage the soft tissue within the cricoid but, if a high velocity acute

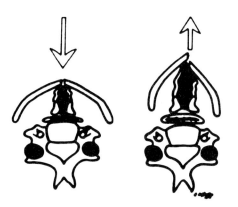

Figure 8.1 The effect of compression on the cervical spine of an uncalcified thyroid cartilage is shown. The maximum damage will be a vertical fracture down the thyroid prominence

injury damages the integrity of the cricoid cartilage, then there will be a very difficult defect to repair.

The final soft tissue injury from high velocity blunt injuries takes the form of separation of the trachea from the cricoid. This usually results in death at the roadside, but it is quite possible for enough lumen to remain for the patient to breathe long enough to come into hospital. Several tracheal rings can be damaged with this sort of injury and the cricotracheal membrane sheared off.

Pathological consequences of injury

Soft tissue

Any injury to the larynx will result in some oedema of soft tissue. This usually has no permanent effects other than in Reinke's space, where permanent oedema of the vocal cord can result or resolve into a laryngeal polyp.

Far more important is the effect of organized haematoma. This is most marked in the supraglottic space where there is the most scope for expansion of soft tissue and obliteration of the airway.

The interarytenoid area is also a very large potential space with debilitating consequences if organization occurs within the area.

The anterior parts of the vocal cords at the anterior commissure may be detached, but more commonly abrasions of the mucosa here can result in anterior web formation.

The subglottic space in children is very much more important than it is in the adult, in whom subglottic space obliteration narrowing the airway is rare. It is usually the result of disorganization of the surrounding skeleton, especially the cricoid.

Glottic competence can be lost for several reasons. The most common cause is fixation of an arytenoid in an unsatisfactory position, but it can also be made incompetent by resorption of the thyroarytenoid muscle and atrophy of the cord, and also by vocal cord paralysis due to damage to the recurrent laryngeal nerve in subglottic trauma.

Skeletal injuries

The hyoid, the only bone in the respiratory tract, may be fractured and may well heal without the patient knowing anything has happened apart from a few days of discomfort. On rare occasions, the fractured ends form a bursa which results in continual movement of the fractured edges together and this requires excision.

The thyroid cartilage, if fractured, will heal by fibrous union and, provided it is in a good position, this is just as satisfactory as wiring or stitching it together. If, however, it is compressed, as in a calcified thyroid cartilage, then it has to be reconstituted and held outwards with a stent.

The effects of disruption of the cricoid cartilage have already been described, and any rehabilitation of this area must involve widening the cricoid cartilage and keeping the edges apart with some material which does not resorb.

At this point, it is pertinent to point out the effect of blood on cartilage. If cartilage is allowed to stay in contact with blood for any length of time, then the cartilage is absorbed by the blood. This is especially important in the trachea where loss of the U-shaped rings perhaps causes no observable abnormality in the airway until the patient takes exercise or a deep breath. The increased velocity of airflow pulls in the weakened tracheal walls and the patient will have dyspnoea on exercise due to tracheomalacia.

If cartilage is left denuded of mucosa and is in contact with secretions, then the surface of the cartilage will become inflamed. This will result in the formation of granulations and is most frequently seen in intubation injuries where the vocal process of the arytenoid is sometimes damaged and an intubation granuloma results (Figure 8.3). Similarly, if too large an intubation tube is used, then the anterior commissure is split and cartilage becomes bared in that area resulting in an anterior intubation granuloma.

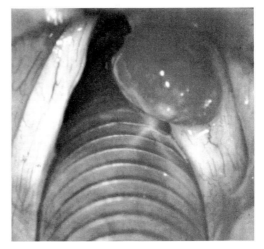

Figure 8.3 Intubation granuloma due to granulations on exposed cartilage; these injuries tend to recur unless the underlying chondritic cartilage is removed

Treatment principles

Protection of the airway

This is obviously the most important feature and is probably the reason that most victims of road traffic accidents are now saved. If there is merely oedema present, with no suggestion of intraluminal bleeding or tracheal damage, then the patient can be kept on bed rest with or without steroids or steam inhalations until the situation resolves.

More likely, however, the airway will be at risk and, rather than performing an immediate tracheostomy, the patient should be intubated. In any review of chronic laryngeal stensoses, there is always a hint of criticism in publications that anaesthetists at this point missed an acute laryngeal injury. If anyone has had a neck injury, there will be confusion and perhaps bleeding in the throat and it is quite impossible with the equipment available to an anaesthetist, in the time available to him, to recognize intraluminal or skeletal damage to the larynx. Even though an endotracheal tube is not much smaller than many of the stents that are used in the later reconstruction of a larynx, neither they nor stents do anything to stop intraluminal bleeding, especially in the supraglottic area, nor to prevent webs in either the posterior or anterior glottis.

In the first aid situation, a tracheostomy may be needed. Nowadays immediate intubation or a minitrach is the preferred alternative.

Protection of laryngeal function

Although the larynx has functions related to swallowing closure and effort closure, by far its most important functions are in relation to breathing and speaking. It is these functions that should be protected as far as possible in the management of laryngeal injury. In the assessment of results of treatment, a success with regard to breathing is a patient who does not have to wear a permanent tracheostomy tube and who is able to lead a normal life with no or minimal dyspnoea. On the other hand, if the vocal cord has been damaged, a normal speaking voice is unlikely. Success in this function, therefore, can range from normal voice to audible phonation as opposed to a whisper.

Emphasis has been laid on the importance of preventing bleeding in the laryngeal spaces in the treatment of acute injury to the larynx. In this regard it is apposite to mention the use of stents. Many stents have been described for use in laryngeal injury, but their role should be isolated to the scaffolding of a reconstituted skeletal structure. They have no part to play in stopping swelling and the subsequent organization of laryngeal spaces. A much better technique for this is to open the spaces and obliterate them with quilting sutures. If there is any significant degree of bleeding within the larynx, then it should be opened by way of a midline approach (laryngofissure) and the spaces evacuated and quilted with 3–0 Vicryl sutures. Inserting drains into the spaces is quite useless.

If there has been damage to the skeletal structure then a principle of minimal debridement should be practised. There is not very much cartilage in the larynx and excision of any tracheal rings, and certainly of the cricoid cartilage, carries with it grave consequences. Although much of this cartilage may resorb, it is better to cover it with mucosa and see if it forms a scaffold for firm fibrous tissue. The worst that can happen is what one would achieve with debridement.

In general terms, the arytenoid will be swollen in nearly every moderately severe laryngeal injury and so the patient should be fed with a nasogastric tube both to stop inhalation from glottic incompetence and to bypass the dysphagia secondary to arytenoid oedema.

Assessment

History

The most important step in diagnosing an acute laryngeal injury is to be aware of the possibility in every patient who has had trauma to the upper half of his body. Dyspnoea and dysphonia are the main features leading to suspicion, with dysphagia and pain as lesser indicators.

Examination

Marks on the neck may or may not be present and their absence does not rule out a fractured larynx, but it makes such a diagnosis unlikely (Figure 8.4).

Surgical emphysema confined to the neck is almost pathognomonic of a breach in the airway. Loss of landmarks such as the thyroid prominence is also diagnostic. It should be borne in mind that any neck wound carries with it the associated possibilities of damage to the great vessels and to the cervical spine.

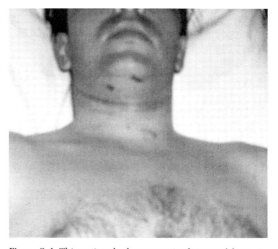

Figure 8.4 This patient had an extensive laryngeal fracture after an automobile accident, but only had minimal chest and neck bruising

Radiology

Plain radiographs of the neck are helpful in confirming the presence or absence of air in the soft tissues (Figure 8.5.). Tomography and laryngography are usually impractical in acute injuries. A CT scan in the axial plane should be done as soon as practical.

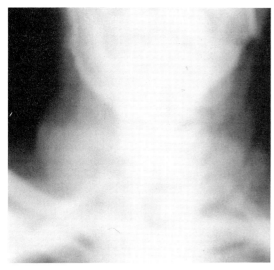

Figure 8.5 Radiograph showing surgical emphysema in a laryngeal fracture

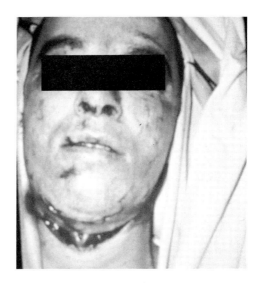

Figure 8.6 Sharp penetrating wound of larynx due to riding a motor bike into a wire fence

Laryngoscopy

This should be performed in all patients. If ordinary mirror examination is impossible, flexible laryngoscopy may yield valuable information.

Treatment

Penetrating injuries

Injuries such as those due to knife wounds, wire wounds and wounds from agricultural or industrial implements will only require treatment if there is bleeding into the supraglottic area. Nearly every such case will require to have the larynx opened and the supraglottic area drained and quilted (Figure 8.6).

Bullet wounds most certainly require exploration with debridement of cartilage, which will probably also be fractured, and exploration of the neck vessels and nerves. Reconstruction will follow the same principles as outlined previously. On occasion the injuries from bullet wounds are so severe that total laryngectomy is necessary (Figure 8.7).

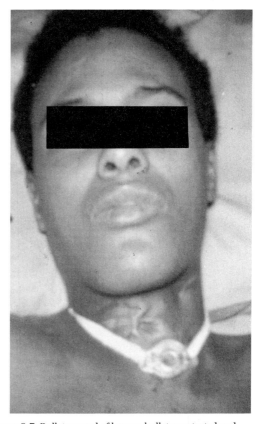

Figure 8.7 Bullet wound of larynx: bullet penetrated and exited from the neck leaving the larynx so damaged that a total laryngectomy was necessary

It is usual for patients with supraglottic injury to end up with a reasonably good voice and no permanent tracheostomy.

Low velocity blunt injuries

The majority of these patients do not require open exploration of the larynx, but most will require observation in hospital at least overnight in case of laryngeal oedema and airway obstruction. As well as sports injuries, similar pathological consequences can follow attempted strangulation and the inhalation of fumes during a conflagration (Figure 8.8). Provided both the airway and the voice are reasonable then these patients can be observed. If either of these functions is disturbed, however, then the larynx should be intubated and perhaps later explored and reconstructed.

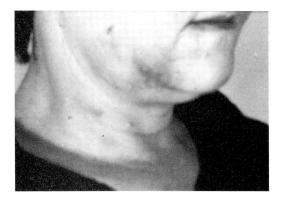

Figure 8.8 After attempted strangulation the larynx may be severely oedematous

Many of these patients will end up with a poor voice if the glottis has been damaged, because there may well be later minor web formation or arthrodesis of an arytenoid, but it is unusual for these patients to require a permanent tracheostomy.

High velocity blunt injuries

About half the patients who have laryngeal injuries as a result of road traffic accidents will require laryngeal exploration and reconstruction. Skeletal damage is repaired by reconstitution usually using stents, and soft tissue injuries are dealt with by reducing bleeding, evacuating spaces and using quilting sutures.

If the cricoid is injured, then primary repair should be attempted. Only when primary repair has failed should one of the many techniques applied to chronic cricoid stenosis be used.

Separation of the cricotracheal membrane is an unusual injury and one which is dealt with fairly reasonably by dropping the larynx in the neck and freeing the trachea down to the carina, and pulling it upwards for an end-to-end anastomosis, excising any damaged tracheal rings.

Most high velocity blunt injuries will result in combined injuries to the glottis and subglottis. If only the glottis is involved then the results with regard to breathing should be good, but if the subglottis is involved, then the patient faces certain future surgery for chronic subglottic stenosis.

Chronic laryngeal stenosis
Epidemiology

This section will be confined to chronic laryngeal stenosis in the adult. The condition, if it manifests itself in childhood, is quite different and is considered in Volume 6.

Common causes of chronic laryngeal stenosis in Western Europe and the USA are failed treatment or non-recognition of acute trauma, but stenosis is also seen as a complication of tracheostomy, intubation and partial laryngectomy (Dankle, Schuller and Mc-Clead, 1987; Cole and Aguilar, 1988). In Egypt, and other parts of the Middle East, scleroma is probably the most common cause of laryngeal stenosis. Tracheostomy is an operation performed well by nearly every medical practitioner involved in the care of trauma patients in Western Europe and North America, but there are still places in the world where tracheostomies can be performed badly, leading to laryngotracheal stenosis. Other systemic diseases, such as Wegener's granuloma, polychondritis, and various types of autoimmune thyroiditis, can also damage the subglottic area resulting in stenosis, but they are rare.

While supraglottic and glottic stenosis do occur, the most common site is the subglottic area. The main cause of this is, therefore, disruption of the supporting skeleton of the cricoid and the tracheal rings. The associated soft tissue narrowing usually reflects the lack of integrity of the supporting structures.

Pathological considerations

Much the same pathological considerations apply to chronic laryngeal stenosis as to the acute injury. The soft tissue damage is due to mucosal loss and adhesions but, most importantly, to organization of haematoma within the paraglottic, the pre-epiglottic and the interarytenoid space.

Glottic competence is affected by web formation anteriorly, and posteriorly an arthrodesis of the arytenoid can result in an unsatisfactory position. Furthermore, the recurrent laryngeal nerves, if they are not injured in the initial trauma, stand a very high chance of injury in the ensuing treatment of chronic laryngeal stenosis, and arytenoidectomy or cordopexy almost always forms part of the treatment of chronic laryngeal stenosis.

A factor in chronic laryngeal stenosis that does not, however, apply in the acute injury is that of tissue memory. If a cartilaginous framework has been disrupted, it heals with fibrous tissue, the fibrocytes of which have a directional memory. Thus, merely incising and separating scar tissue will lead to the tissue attempting to replace itself in its original scarred state. Reconstruction must be more sophisticated than incision and replacement. As much scarred tissue as possible should be excised, but the danger of repositioning will be ever present. This is most important in the cricoid where the interruption of the ring causes narrowing. The forces within the cricoid are altered, probably permanently, from this narrowing, and excision of the scarred area and separation of the cricoid ends with support from intervening tissue is probably the single most difficult problem in the management of chronic stenosis (Freeland, 1981; Eliachar *et al.*, 1987).

Excision of scarred soft tissue is not nearly so difficult. Wide excision of scarred tissue is, of course, necessary but grafting with split skin or mucosa usually gives good results. It must be re-emphasized, however, that no amount of satisfactory soft tissue healing will take place if the skeletal framework is disrupted or resumes its scarred altered position.

Stents are useful in supporting a reconstituted laryngeal framework and, to an extent, in separating mucosal surfaces that have been adherent. It bears repetition that stents are of little value in curing haematoma formation within soft tissue.

Treatment principles

Most patients presenting for treatment for chronic laryngeal stenosis will already have a tracheostomy. They should be warned that the results of treatment of chronic laryngeal stenosis are at best unrewarding and their tracheostomy may be permanent. In the postoperative period with resultant swelling, the patient will almost certainly have to be fed with a nasogastric tube at least for some days. They should also be warned that it is unlikely that they will regain a normal voice especially if the glottis has been damaged.

There is almost universal dissatisfaction with the surgical treatment of the systemic conditions that cause laryngotracheal stenosis, such as a scleroma, Wegener's granuloma and polychondritis. It is debatable whether these patients should be treated with any surgery other than occasional dilatations.

Assessment

History

The cause of the chronic stenosis is obviously important. If it is a result of an excessively zealous partial laryngectomy, then it is unlikely that enough tissue will be found to augment the lumen of the larynx. Again, if it is a systemic disease that has caused the laryngeal stenosis, it is unlikely that surgery has any place to play in the management. Exceptions to this might be confined segments of scleroma in the advanced fibrotic stage, but this would be a very rare occurrence.

Perhaps the most important communication to establish between the surgeon and the patient is a mutual sense of realism. Both should realize what is and what is not possible with surgery. Both should realize that the dynamics of tissue healing can alter any result and this should be taken into account in timing the operation. No attempts should be made to increase the laryngeal lumen until 18 months have passed from the time of the initial injury. Finally, the patient must be quite clear as to what his objectives from surgery will be. He must evaluate how much a good voice means to him and similarly whether he wants to be rid of the tracheostomy tube so much that he is willing to undergo surgery. More minor cases should also realize that the additional scarring of surgery could, in rare instances, result in the patient having a tracheostomy for the rest of his life.

Examination

The surgeon should establish with mirror or flexible endoscopy the extent of the laryngeal, glottic or subglottic stenosis, but this is not always possible and is probably the least important part of the examination. Perhaps the most important part of the physical examination is in the assessment of the length of the neck and, therefore, how much trachea is available for mobilization in the neck without having to go into the mediastinum.

Radiography

The first and probably the only investigation should be a CT scan (Figure 8.9). Only in cases where the subglottis cannot be evaluated, should laryngography be used. This is perhaps the only place that laryngography now has to play in the investigation of laryngeal disease.

Endoscopy

This is necessary to establish, as accurately as possible, the extent of laryngeal damage, but it is also useful to ascertain the lower extent of subglottic stenosis and to test for the state of the tracheal cartilages (Figure 8.10). These have to be examined

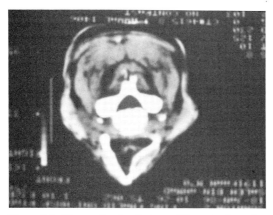

Figure 8.9 CT scan showing fracture of the anterolateral part of the thyroid cartilage

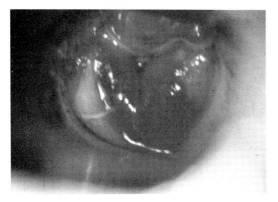

Figure 8.10 Endoscopic view of a supraglottic stenosis

serial excisions of the soft tissue with the laser and the laryngeal widening operation. Laser excision allows the patient to keep the tracheostomy tube and to evaluate the effect of serial excisions. An alternative is the laryngeal widening procedure where the larynx is opened in the midline and as much as possible of the submucosal scarred tissue removed. The remaining mucosa is stitched back against the laryngeal framework with quilting sutures or areas of scarred tissue are grafted either with skin or buccal mucosa (Figure 8.11).

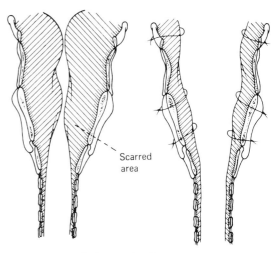

Figure 8.11 In the laryngeal widening operation, a laryngofissure gives access to the laryngeal interior. The scarred submucosal tissue is removed and the mucosa quilted

from as high as possible without creating any splinting and with the anesthetist blowing high airflows into the lungs using a Venturi system. In this way, tracheomalacia can be assessed.

The state of the arytenoids must be ascertained to see if they are fixed or not and oesophagoscopy should be carried out in every patient.

Treatment

Supraglottic stenosis

There are three choices in the treatment of this condition: first, there is supraglottic laryngectomy; second, a laryngeal widening procedure; and third, laser excision. The author does not think there is any place now for supraglottic laryngectomy in the treatment of this condition. It defies all the basic tenets of the surgery of laryngeal trauma, namely minimal excision. There is usually nothing wrong with the supraglottic skeletal framework and the lesion is nearly always of soft tissue. The choice lies between

Glottic stenosis

The anterior glottic web can be dealt with either by laser excision, by repeated endoscopic excision or by external excision and separation of the anterior glottis with a silastic or tantalum keel (McNaught keel). If an external approach is used, then the keel is kept in place for at least 5 weeks. It can then be removed with minimal reopening of the neck wound. The external approach is probably the preferred one when there is also a stenosis of the anterior parts of the false cord but, if the webbing is limited to the glottis, then laser excision or endoscopic removal is probably best in the first instance.

Posterior stenosis of the glottis is more difficult to treat. The glottis consists of roughly 50% cartilage from the medial face and vocal processes of the arytenoids and 50% membranous vocal cord from the vocal ligament and the attached mucosa and thyroarytenoid muscle. Posterior glottic stenosis lies between the arytenoids. This is usually accompanied by fixation of at least one arytenoid. The stenosis may be excised and the arytenoid separated with a modified keel with silastic stenting on the end of it to keep the posterior glottis open (Figure 8.12). For this to succeed, both arytenoids must be mobile and capable of achieving glottic competence when the keel is removed. If the arytenoids are not mobile then one should be removed via a laryngofissure and the cord stitched laterally with stenting applied to stop further adhesions.

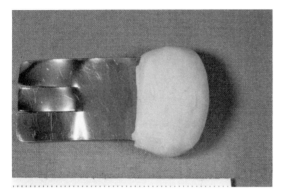

Figure 8.12 Modified keel for posterior glottic stenosis

Subglottic stenosis

Cricoid stenosis

Enough has already been written about the biomechanics of cricoid stenosis to make it clear how a free graft in this area must work. It must keep the cricoid ring open and, to do this on a permanent basis, it must adhere to the cartilaginous ends. It is unlikely that free bone or cartilage grafts, taken from ribs, can ever achieve this objective in a satisfactory and regulated manner. Furthermore, it is certain that allografts have no place.

Perhaps the best method is to swing down the body of the hyoid bone on a muscle pedicle of sternohyoid and hope that this, wired into the arch of the cricoid, can keep it open. When this is done, the soft tissue scarring must also be removed and replaced with a skin graft and a stent applied either in the form of rolled up silastic above a tracheostomy tube, or in a modified tracheostomy tube. If a Montgomery T-tube is used for this, then the greatest care must be taken to see that it does not crust.

For greater degrees of cricoid stenosis, where the ring cannot realistically be reconstituted, then it is best to remove the cricoid leaving part of the posterior lamina on which sit the arytenoids. The larynx is then dropped and the trachea pulled up and joined to the lower end of the thyroid lamina anteriorly and to the arch of the cricoid posteriorly (Gerwat and Bryce, 1974). This tends to give something of a lump in the back of the immediate subglottic space, but it is a fairly reliable procedure and can usually allow the patient to be extubated.

Tracheal stenosis

The more minor degrees of tracheal stenosis are best treated with dilatations. Very often the problem is one of tracheomalacia, rather than true stenosis, and the true stenosis cannot be seen on endoscopy or radiographs. Very often these patients are frustrated by the lack of a medical diagnosis when they know full well that they are dyspnoeic on exertion. If they are only dyspnoeic on exertion, however, they must consider very carefully whether or not to have surgery just because an operation exists to excise the weak area of trachea. This operation may well damage one or both of the recurrent laryngeal nerves and result in further surgery for vocal cord paralysis. Attempts to strengthen the tracheal wall with marlex mesh or other external devices, although intuitively attractive, are not often successful.

If a tracheal stenosis is severe enough to warrant the wearing of a tracheostomy tube, then it is a relatively easy matter to excise up to 4–5 cm of trachea and to join the trachea on to the cricoid or first tracheal ring (Wiatrak and Cotton, 1992).

Freeing the trachea into the mediastinum presents little problem, provided the operator keeps close to the wall of the trachea and does not stray outside the plane of the peritracheal fascia. Pulling the trachea up is easy because it acts as a concertina. The surgeon must remember, however, that the same pull is then applied downwards after the anastomosis. The most important part of this operation is dropping the larynx in the neck. This is done by cutting off the superior cornu of the thyroid cartilage on both sides. This releases the pull of the stylopharyngeus, salpingopharyngeus and palatopharyngeus muscles. The pre-epiglottic space should be entered by dividing the thyrohyoid membrane and the thyroid cartilage distracted from the hyoid. The middle constrictor should also be removed from the posterior lamina of the thyroid cartilage. There is enough slack in the false cords on the interior part of the larynx to allow several centimetres of displacement.

During this procedure, attempts should be made to find the recurrent laryngeal nerve on either side. If a damaged nerve is found, then it is best to perform a Woodman's operation at the time of the initial anastomosis but, if both laryngeal nerves are intact, then it can be expected that any subsequent vocal cord paralysis is due to a neuropraxia and will recover.

If this manoeuvre is not enough to close the gap of an extensive stenosis, then a procedure, described over 30 years ago by Dr Grillo of Boston, can be utilized. In the UK, it is often called Barclay's procedure and consists of carrying out a right thoracotomy and removing the right main-stem bronchus from the carina, closing the defect at the carina and joining the right main-stem bronchus on to the left main-stem bronchus at a lower level. This gives several more centimetres of length to the trachea and does not result in stenosis further down (Figure 8.13).

Results

The results from supraglottic stenoses are usually good. It is usually possible to remove the tracheostomy tube and leave the patient with a reasonable voice. Similarly the results from the treatment of glottic stenosis should also be good and it would be a rare event for the patient to have a permanent tracheostomy.

The results of the treatment of subglottic stenosis, however, are universally poor. Although isolated claims of remarkably good results in the treatment of this lesion are made by the occasional surgeon, they cannot be reproduced consistently by experienced laryngologists of long-standing merit. The key to the subglottis is the cricoid, and it does appear that we have not yet found a satisfactory solution to restoring the dynamic elastic forces necessary to preserve the integrity of the only complete ring in the respiratory tract.

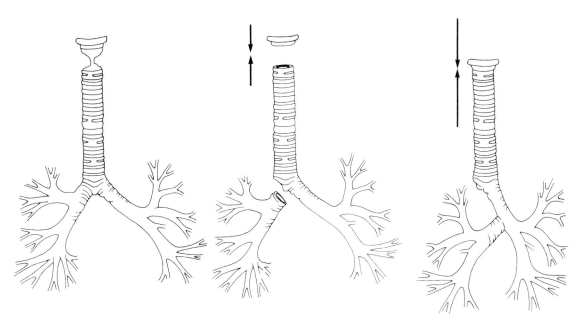

Figure 8.13 Grillo procedure where the right main-stem bronchus is detached from the bifurcation and attached lower down the left main-stem bronchus

References

COLE, R. R. and AGUILAR, E. A. (1988) Crycothyroidotomy versus tracheotomy: an otolaryngologists perspective. *Laryngoscope*, **98**, 131–135

DANKLE, S. K., SCHULLER, D. E. and MCCLEAD, R. E. (1987) Prolonged intubation of neonates. *Archives of Otolaryngology, – Head and Neck Surgery*, **113**, 841–843

ELIACHAR, I., ROBERTS, J. K., HAYES, J. D., LEVIN, H. L. and TUCKER, H. M. (1987) Laryngotracheal reconstruction: sternohyoid myocutaneous rotary door flap. *Archives of Otolaryngology – Head and Neck Surgery*, **113**, 1094–1097

FREELAND, A. P. (1981) Composite hyoid–sternohyoid graft in the correction of established subglottic stenosis. *Journal of the Royal Society of Medicine*, **74**, 729–735

GERWAT, J. and BRYCE, D. P. (1974) The management of subglottic laryngeal stenosis by resection and direct anastomosis. *Laryngoscope*, **84**, 940–957

LYONS, G. D., OWENS, R., LOUSTEAU, R. J. and TRAIL, M. L. (1980) Carbon dioxide laser treatment of laryngeal stenosis. *Archives of Otolaryngology*, **106**, 255–256

WIATRAK, B. J. and COTTON, R. T. (1992) Anastomosis of the cervical trachea in children. *Archives of Otolaryngology – Head and Neck Surgery*, **118**, 58–62

Further reading

BRYCE, D. P., BRIANT, T. D. R. and PEARSON, F. G. (1969) Laryngeal and tracheal complications of intubation. *Annals of Otology, Rhinology and Laryngology*, **77**, 442–461

COTTON, R. (1978) Management of subglottic stenosis in

infancy and childhood. *Annals of Otology, Rhinology and Laryngology*, **87**, 649–657

MCCAFFREY, T. V. (1992) Classification of laryngotracheal stenosis. *Laryngoscope*, **102**, 1335–1340

MCDONALD, T. J., NEEL, H. B. and DEREMEE, R. A. (1982) Wegener's granulomatosis of the subglottis and the upper portion of the trachea. *Annals of Otology, Rhinology and Laryngology*, **91**, 588–598

MCNAUGHT, R. D. (1950) Surgical correction of anterior web of larynx. *Laryngoscope*, **60**, 264–272

MARAN, A. G. D., STELL, P. M., MURRAY, J. A. M. and TUCKER, A. (1981) Early management of laryngeal injuries. *Journal of the Royal Society of Medicine*, **74**, 656–660

MILES, W. K., OLSON, N. R. and RODRIGUEZ, A. (1971) Acute treatment of experimental laryngeal fractures. *Annals of Otology, Rhinology and Laryngology*, **80**, 710–720

MONTGOMERY, W. W. (1968) The surgical management of supraglottic and subglottic stenosis. *Annals of Otology, Rhinology and Laryngology*, **77**, 534–546

SCHAEFER, S. D. (1992) The treatment of acute external laryngeal injuries. *Archives of Otolaryngology – Head and Neck Surgery*, **117**, 35–39

STELL, P. M., STANLEY, R. E., MARAN, A. G. D. and MURRAY, J. A. M. (1985) Chronic laryngeal stenosis. *Annals of Otology, Rhinology and Laryngology*, **94**, 108–113

WOODMAN, D. (1946) Modification of extralaryngeal approach to arytenoidectomy for bilateral abductor paralysis. *Archives of Otolaryngology*, **43**, 63–65

9

Neurological affections of the pharynx and larynx

David Howard

Anatomy

Neuronal control of the pharynx and larynx begins in the cerebral cortex at the lower part of the precentral gyrus. Additional fibres also arise from some frontal and parietal areas. The majority of fibres descend in the pyramidal tracts, with subsequent partial decussation at the upper border of the medulla to reach the nucleus ambiguus. Most palsies are produced by lesions of the nucleus ambiguus or the vagus nerve trunks and their branches. Lesions can cause unilateral or bilateral paralysis of the pharynx, often associated with palatal paralysis, and/or paralysis of the larynx and cricopharyngeus.

The cranial portion of the accessory nerve contains motor fibres destined for the muscles of the soft palate (except tensor veli palatini), pharynx, and intrinsic larynx.

Glossopharyngeal nerve

The glossopharyngeal nerve is essentially sensory. The nerve is not motor to the palate (it only supplies the stylopharyngeus which cannot be tested clinically) so that when the gag reflex is tested the stimulus is carried by the IXth nerve but the resulting palatal movement is mediated by the Xth nerve.

Vagus nerve

The vagus nerve leaves the cranium in the same sheath of dura as the accessory nerve. The glossopharyngeal nerve lies in front of these. The vagus is swollen during its exit by the superior ganglion cells. Below the jugular foramen the nerve is swollen again for approximately 2.5 cm by the inferior ganglion. This latter ganglion is crossed by the cranial root of the accessory nerve which blends with the vagus below the ganglion. The cells of the ganglion are sensory only.

The vagus nerve descends in the neck within the carotid sheath, between the internal jugular vein and the internal carotid artery, as far as the superior border of the thyroid cartilage and then between the vein and the common carotid artery to the root of the neck. Its subsequent course differs on each side.

Pharyngeal branch

This arises from the upper part of the inferior ganglion and runs between the external and internal carotid arteries to the superior border of the middle constrictor muscle. Here it divides into numerous filaments and forms the pharyngeal plexus along with branches from the sympathetic trunk, glossopharyngeal and external laryngeal nerves.

Superior laryngeal nerve

This arises from the lower portion of the inferior ganglion, and descends on the side wall of the pharynx posterior and then medial to the internal carotid artery. It divides into the internal and external laryngeal nerves.

Internal laryngeal nerve

This descends to the thyrohyoid membrane piercing it above the superior laryngeal artery. It divides and supplies sensory innervation to the supraglottis, vallecula, and posterior surfaces of the arytenoid cartilages. Inferiorly it communicates with ascending branches of the recurrent laryngeal nerve. It also carries afferent fibres from neuromuscular spindles and cricoarytenoid joint receptors (Wyke and Kirschner, 1976).

There are abundant laryngeal receptors, both tactile and pain, providing a high degree of sensitivity particularly of the supraglottic mucosa. The afferent loop of the reflex initiates a bilateral laryngeal reflex. The chemoreceptors in the larynx have unknown functions. The subglottis has a similar receptor, served by the recurrent laryngeal nerve. These subglottic chemoreceptors apparently modify breathing, since some chemical stimuli applied to them initiate slow deep breathing, as does carbon dioxide applied to this part of the tract when it is isolated. The articular joint afferent fibres are particularly well developed, producing a highly sensitive and rapid monitoring response. Some reflexes which control respiration and phonation may arise from stretch receptors in the musculature of the larynx, demonstrable both histologically and by electrophysiology. Debate continues with regard to the exact role of all the sensory receptors and the reader is referred to an excellent contribution by Wyke and Kirschner (1976). Debate also remains as to whether the internal laryngeal nerve is entirely sensory: Williams (1951) described motor fibres innervating the interarytenoid muscles. Certainly no obvious interarytenoid contraction takes place on stimulation of the superior laryngeal nerve.

External laryngeal nerve

This branch descends deep to the superior thyroid artery on the inferior constrictor muscle. It then pierces the muscle, passes around the inferior thyroid tubercle and supplies the cricothyroid muscle. It also gives branches to the pharyngeal plexus and inferior constrictor muscle.

Recurrent laryngeal nerves

The nerve on the *right* side arises from the vagus in front of the first part of the subclavian artery, winds backwards around the vessel and ascends obliquely behind the common carotid artery to the side of the trachea. On the right the nerve is commonly in front of the tracheo-oesophageal groove and may even be considerably lateral to the trachea as it reaches the lower pole of the thyroid gland. Near the lower pole both recurrent nerves are always intimately related to the terminal branches of the inferior thyroid artery. Authors differ in reporting the percentage of each variation, but on the right side the nerve occurs with approximately equal incidence behind, in front of, or intermingling with, the terminal branches of the inferior thyroid artery.

On the *left* side the nerve curves around the arch of the aorta and ascends commonly in a more protected position within the tracheo-oesophageal groove. On this side it is most likely to run behind the branches of the inferior thyroid artery, and least likely to pass in front of them.

Both nerves are intimately related to the medial surface of the thyroid lobes and their fascial coverings before passing deep to the lower border of the inferior constrictor muscle to enter the larynx behind the cricothyroid joint.

As they ascend, each nerve gives branches to the mucous membrane and muscular coat of the oesophagus and trachea. The nerves may divide before entering the larynx. They supply all the muscles of the larynx, except the cricothyroid, and sensation to the mucous membrane below the vocal cords. They also give branches to the inferior constrictor muscle and communicate with the internal laryngeal nerve.

Aetiology

It is difficult to produce an exhaustive list of causes of neurological deficits in the pharynx and larynx. The causes of many neural lesions, particularly of the larynx, are unknown.

Supranuclear lesions

Cortical lesions producing laryngeal and pharyngeal palsies are rare, and little is known about the effects on the larynx. It requires a bilateral symmetrical lesion of the cortex to produce a pharyngeal or laryngeal palsy, and in such cases respiratory and reflex laryngeal movements may be unaffected. Hemiplegia does not impair vocal cord movement.

Nuclear lesions

The nucleus ambiguus may be involved in postero-inferior cerebellar artery thrombosis, tumours of the medulla, bulbar palsy, syringobulbia, motor neuron disease, encephalitis, poliomyelitis, cranial polyneuritis, tabes and rabies. The most common cause of bilateral laryngeal paralysis arising in the nucleus is progressive bulbar palsy or cranial polyneuritis. Before the advent of lead-free paint it was a rare manifestation of lead poisoning. Nuclear lesions usually cause a combined paralysis of the soft palate, pharynx and larynx, but the larynx may be spared if only the superior part of the nucleus is affected. This may produce a palatopharyngeal paralysis – the syndrome of Avellis.

Posterior fossa and jugular foramen lesions

These involve the vagus nerves as they emerge from the brain stem and leave the skull. Nerves IX, XI and XII may also be affected and a large number of laryngopharyngopalatal palsies combined with lesions of these nerves have been named. They come under the headings of posterior fossa syndrome and jugular foramen syndrome. Although the many eponyms are of historical interest their use can lead to confusion.

The commonest combinations of associated cranial nerve lesions in the region are:

1 IX, X, XI, in the jugular foramen, Vernet's syndrome
2 X, XI, Schmidt's syndrome
3 X, XI, XII, Hughlings Jackson syndrome
4 IX, X, XI, XII, Collet-Sicard syndrome
5 IX, X, XI, XII and Horner's syndrome, Villaret's syndrome.

Having established the combination of nerve palsies the presence of an additional Horner's syndrome indicates a lesion outside the skull as the cervical sympathetic ascends to the base of the skull but does not pass through the jugular foramen. Evidence of additional brain stem compression obviously indicates an intracranial lesion.

Lesions in this region may arise from a wide range of diseases. These include skull fractures, primary tumours of the temporal bone (particularly glomus tumour or meningioma), nasopharyngeal tumours, metastases, cholesteatoma, extension of infection from the middle ear, jugular bulb thrombophlebitis, tuberculosis, and syphilitic meningitis.

Extracranial lesions

In the cervical region the list of causes includes penetrating injuries; tumours of the hypopharynx, upper oesophagus, thyroid and parapharyngeal space; enlargement of/or surgery on the regional lymph nodes; and surgery of the thyroid gland.

Arising in the thorax the left recurrent laryngeal nerve has a longer course and is more exposed to damage than the right. It is vulnerable to compression by an aortic aneurysm, an enlarged left atrium in mitral stenosis, carcinoma of the bronchus, other mediastinal tumours and enlarged mediastinal glands.

The right recurrent laryngeal nerve is more vulnerable to injury during surgery on the thyroid gland because of its more anterior and lateral position at the inferior pole of the gland, rather than being protected in the tracheo-oesophageal groove.

Paralysis of the palate and pharynx
Symptoms

Unilateral palatal paralysis may not give rise to any symptoms because of compensation by the unparalysed muscles of the opposite side. Direct questioning may reveal slight changes in phonation (especially in professional voice users), snoring, postnasal drip and occasionally a unilateral hearing loss because of eustachian tube dysfunction on the affected side.

Bilateral palatal paralysis prevents the palate from closing off the oropharynx from the nasopharynx and prevents control of airflow through the nose – fluids, and sometimes solids, thus regurgitating through the nose during deglutition. The voice has a nasal quality (rhinolalia aperta), as is heard in a patient with an untreated cleft palate. There is also a tendency to mouth breathing, snoring at night, and mucoid rhinorrhoea.

The patient with a bilateral palatal paralysis can usually swallow sufficient for his needs unless the pharynx is also involved. A combined paralysis is much more serious, particularly if the pharyngeal paralysis is bilateral; the patient cannot swallow and attempts to do so result in spasms of coughing as a result of overspill into the larynx. Soft bulky foods are usually more easily swallowed than liquids and solids. Even the patient's ordinary secretions may enter the lower respiratory tract and cause inhalation pneumonia.

In unilateral pharyngeal paralysis the compensation by the opposite constrictors is often efficient, but the patient needs to swallow in a deliberate manner, has bouts of coughing to 'clear' the throat, and may find it easier to sleep on the unaffected side to prevent laryngeal irritation from pharyngeal secretions.

Signs

Unilateral palatal paralysis is detected by examination of the oropharynx. When the patient says 'ah' the palate does not rise on the affected side and the uvula is drawn to the normal side. With a bilateral palatal paralysis the palate remains immobile during phonation. Occasionally it may be difficult to decide whether there is any movement in a bilateral paralysis. The patient cannot whistle or blow up a balloon.

Sensation is tested by touching each side of the palate gently with an orange stick and asking the patient to compare the two. Pain sensation may also be tested, with care, using a long pin. The posterior pharyngeal wall is tested in the same manner. With a unilateral pharyngeal paralysis the pharyngeal reflex is lost on the affected side and the pharyngeal wall droops. In both unilateral and bilateral pharyngeal paralysis pharyngeal secretions collect in the hypopharynx and around the laryngeal inlet and may be clearly seen on indirect laryngoscopy or fibreoptic flexible nasendoscopy. The latter has the advantage of allowing the observer to view laryngopharyngeal movement during speech and swallowing. If the symptoms are strongly suggestive of bilateral pharyngeal paralysis care should be taken on indirect laryngoscopy as it may produce sudden aspiration of these pooled secretions.

Diagnosis

Rarely, palatal paralysis in children may be referred to the otorhinolaryngologist because the symptoms are believed to be caused by 'adenoids'. The history of enlarged adenoids is very different: the child has nasal obstruction but no nasal regurgitation. The thick nasal intonation caused by enlarged adenoids produces the contrasting speech defect of rhinolalia clausa.

Reduced motility, and occasionally fixation, of the palate may be produced locally by scarring following unsatisfactory cleft palate repair, adenoidectomy or tonsillectomy, syphilis, scarlet fever, and tumours.

Investigation

Paralysis of the palate is unlikely to require investigation other than for the underlying cause. Accurate recordings of the degree and type of nasopharyngeal closure with palatal movement have been studied using video recordings obtained via flexible nasoendoscopy. This evaluation is only necessary when palatal or nasopharyngeal surgery is proposed for a long-term and stable palatal paralysis.

Pharyngeal paralysis with varying degrees of dysphagia has been the subject of physical, radiological, endoscopic and electrophysiological investigations. The long established standard barium swallow procedure was introduced primarily for the study of oesophageal disease and is inappropriate for the examination of patients with pharyngeal paralysis. In addition, these patients may have paralysis of the muscles involved in the first stage of swallowing, the oral phase. The barium swallow is inappropriate in those patients with neurological diseases who are having severe problems with swallowing and are at risk of aspiration, as is also the case in many postoperative patients who have varying degrees of pharyngeal malfunction.

The modified barium swallow

This technique allows examination of the oral cavity and pharynx radiographically. In the standard barium swallow the oesophagus must be filled with barium to be viewed and the patient lies in a supine position. However, in order to view the oral cavity and pharynx, these cavities must not be filled with large amounts of barium material as this obliterates their structure and masks their function. In addition, the patient with an oral or pharyngeal swallowing disorder, at the risk of aspiration, may have great difficulty in handling a large bolus of barium. Thus, the modified technique involves the use of only small amounts of material, generally one-third to one-half of a teaspoon per swallow. A variety of materials of different consistency may be used and most commonly these are barium paste, biscuits coated with barium paste, or biscuits with barium baked into their contents. This variety of consistency allows overall evaluation as some patients may experience difficulty in swallowing liquids but not heavier food.

The modified barium swallow is best undertaken with the patient seated upright in a normal eating position. In patients with dysphagia the performance of the oral cavity and pharynx in the normal eating position must be established first and then, if desired, the patient's position can be changed and the postural effects on swallowing noted. The procedure is initially undertaken in the lateral plane with the fluoroscopy tube defining the whole oral cavity and pharynx. The anteroposterior view is taken following the lateral assessment and the overall evaluation allows definition of oral and pharyngeal motility during swallowing, the presence of aspiration, the oral and pharyngeal transit times compared with normal, and the effects of any positional changes on the overall swallowing performance. Further oesophageal assessment can be completed as necessary depending on the lower extent of the paralysis.

Patients with pharyngeal paralysis may have inadequate initiation of the pharyngeal constrictor wave, delayed soft palate elevation and inadequate velopharyngeal closure with regurgitation into the nasopharynx and nasal cavities, abnormal pharyngeal motility patterns with prolonged pharyngeal transit time, stasis in the vallecula and/or pyriform fossa and laryngeal dysfunction.

Aspiration may be the predominant symptom in patients with bilateral pharyngeal paralysis. The modified barium swallow also allows detailed evaluation of the upper oesophageal sphincter which is not only the cricopharyngeus muscle but frequently incorporates the lower inferior constrictor muscle of the pharynx and the initial oesophageal circular fibres. It varies in length from 2.5 to 6.5 cm and this is important when 'cricopharyngeal' myotomy is considered. The results of these investigations can be compared with data from normal subjects. During swallowing, relaxation of the upper oesophageal sphincter should be complete, preceding pharyngeal contraction and terminating thereafter.

Pharyngeal pressure measurements, pH monitoring, electromyographic recording and endoscopic examination, although used in research, have yet to prove their worth in most clinical situations.

Pharyngeal disorders

Globus pharyngeus (globus 'hystericus', idiopathic globus)

This functional disorder is most common in middle-aged women and is associated with a variety of sensations in the pharynx and larynx. Emotion, particularly fear, can cause a marked sensation of a lump, dryness, or 'blockage' of the throat, so it is not surprising that people who are emotionally unstable should refer symptoms to this region. However, the term globus hystericus is misleading as true hysteria is rare and hysterical dysphagia is uncommon even in these patients.

The most common feature in globus pharyngeus is the sensation of a lump in the throat. Often the patient's attention has been drawn to the throat by a previous minor throat infection, a transient incident with food 'sticking' in, or 'catching' in the throat, or a relative or friend dying of 'cancer of the throat'. The symptom is most obvious when the patient attempts to swallow his own saliva to 'see if the lump is still there', but there is no true dysphagia and the symptoms often disappear while eating a meal. Repeated attempts at swallowing saliva may lead to aerophagy, with gastric distension and discomfort. The symptoms may have been present for many months and are usually worse if the patient is under any form of stress.

Examination often reveals a notably anxious patient with a pronounced gag reflex, but the pharynx, oral cavity, larynx and neck do not show any evidence of disease.

It is advisable to investigate these patients by a blood count to exclude anaemia, and by a barium swallow which may show obvious cricopharyngeal spasm without any other abnormality, but the role of this finding in the pathogenesis of the problem remains unclear. The spasm may be associated with lesions at the lower end of the oesophagus such as hiatus hernia, carcinoma or achalasia. There is no doubt that many globus patients can be demonstrated to have a hiatus hernia and it is postulated that the lower oesophageal abnormality causes reflex vagal stimulation and subsequent alteration in the tone of the hypopharyngeal musculature, particularly the cricopharyngeus. However, many patients have hiatus hernias without globus type symptoms and research has not yet explained the cause of globus pharyngeus.

If symptoms persist direct rigid, or flexible endoscopy may be indicated as these methods are more likely than radiology to detect early organic disease, particularly of the postcricoid area.

If no organic disease is shown by adequate investigation the patients are often rendered symptom free by reassurance and explanation. Occasionally, an anxiolytic, such as diazepam, may help troublesome symptoms but this type of medication is only required for a small proportion of patients. Speech therapists may have a useful part to play, particularly if there is an associated functional dysphonia. Rarely, the more emotionally crippled patient requires psychiatric referral.

Cricopharyngeal spasm and pharyngeal pouch

These pharyngeal disorders almost certainly have a neurogenic basis and are discussed in Chapter 10.

Glossopharyngeal neuralgia

Apart from the distribution of the pain, glossopharyngeal neuralgia resembles the much commoner condition of trigeminal neuralgia. The pain occurs in brief agonizing stabs which may be of great severity. They usually start in relation to the tonsil and radiate down the side of the neck, in front of the ear and to the back of the mandible. Very rarely the pain may begin deep in the ear.

The attacks are usually precipitated by swallowing or by protruding the tongue, but when the ear is the main site external stimulation of the ear or skin may provoke an attack. Similar, but more continuous pain may be caused by cancers of the tonsil or pharynx and these must be carefully excluded.

When the throat is the main site of pain, some relief may be obtained by direct application of cocaine to the lateral pharyngeal wall and posterior third of the tongue. Carbamazepine (Tegretol), given in increasing dosage up to 200 mg four times daily, may control the attacks and additional relief may be obtained with sedatives. If these measures prove unsuccessful operation on the nerve may be necessary. It is always wise to regard the neuralgia as evidence of an underlying lesion until proved otherwise by events or by surgical exploration. The list of findings at surgical exploration includes a long styloid process, aberrant vessels coursing over the nerve, unsuspected neurofibroma and cholesteatoma. Skull base and lateral radiographs may be useful and selected patients may require CT scanning.

The nerve may be approached via the tonsillar fossa, skull base, or intracranially. Wilson approached the nerve through the tonsillar fossa where it lies on the stylopharyngeus (Wilson and McAlpine, 1946). It may be avulsed or divided, but adequate safe dissection to the base of the skull is not possible by this route and only symptoms referable to the throat are relieved. A long styloid process may be fractured or partially removed during the same procedure (after tonsillectomy) but the vogue for this procedure seems to be declining.

Approach to the nerve at the skull base is difficult owing to its relatively small size, depth and relation to other important structures. It must be avulsed to remove the jugular and petrosal ganglia otherwise the connections with the tympanic plexus remain intact and any ear symptoms continue.

Injection of the nerve with alcohol at the point of emergence from the skull base can be undertaken but this is a difficult and hazardous procedure which has not gained wide acceptance.

The most reliable results are obtained with modern neurosurgical techniques involving craniotomy and division of the nerve fibres soon after emergence from the medulla. Additional division of the upper two rootlets of the vagus nerve containing auricular and pharyngeal branches may be necessary.

Herpes zoster

Rarely, the neurotrophic varicella-zoster virus may affect the distribution of the IXth and Xth cranial nerves. The vesicular eruption usually affects the palate, the pharynx and the laryngeal inlet on one side. The pharyngeal lesions may be isolated or be accompanied by other eruptions on the auricle or the anterior pillar of the fauces such as occur in geniculate herpes (Ramsay-Hunt's syndrome).

The eruption is usually preceded by general malaise, fever and anorexia, particularly in the elderly. Herpes zoster may occur at any age, but most patients are over 50. Initially the throat is sore for a few hours before typical vesicles appear. These break down to form shallow ulcers, and they may be accompanied by severe pain. They heal without scarring but intractable pain may persist for many years in elderly patients. Local treatment with an antiseptic mouthwash keeps the pharynx clean, and local analgesics are useful before meals. Systemic steroids have been advocated but are of no proven value. Strong analgesics such as pethidine may be required in the acute stages but are contraindicated for persistent postherpetic pain. Carbamazepine (Tegretol) is rarely useful in postherpetic pain and nerve division or injection often provides only temporary relief. A combination of chlorpromazine and dihydrocodeine can be given for long periods and antidepressants may be required to treat the depression which may accompany the persistent pain.

Diphtheria

This disease is caused by the Klebs-Loeffler bacillus, *Corynebacterium diphtheriae*. It produces a membranous exudate at the initial site of infection which is later followed by distant toxic effects, of which polyneuropathy and circulatory failure are the most important.

It has a worldwide distribution but, following the introduction of active immunization only isolated outbreaks occur in the UK. Because of the rarity at the present time the first cases of recent outbreaks have been missed and the subject deserves careful consideration.

Diphtheria is most common in the 2–10-year-old age group and is spread by droplet infection from carriers and patients. Active immunization has been followed by the elimination of the carrier state.

Pathology

The organisms remain at the site of infection and do not become invasive. The powerful exotoxin initially causes epithelial necrosis, followed by an inflammatory reaction with the necrosis forming the characteristic membrane. The membrane is 'false' as it consists of invaded and necrotic layers of mucosa and is not an exudate. The membrane is adherent and is difficult to remove. The corynebacteria are present at the margin of the membrane and swabs should be taken from this area.

The neurological symptoms are associated with fatty degeneration of the myelin sheaths of involved nerves with a consequent slowing of nerve conduction. The fauces are the commonest site of diphtheritic infection and as absorption of toxins is more rapid than from other sites (nose, nasopharynx, larynx), faucial diphtheria is usually associated with most toxaemia. Palatal paralysis is attributed to the ascent of toxin from the common faucial site of infection to the medulla. (In cutaneous infection local ascent of the nerves by the toxin is responsible for the development of paralysis.) Paralysis of accommodation, generalized polyneuropathy and myocardial damage are the consequences of dissemination of the toxin via the blood stream.

Symptoms and signs

Although infection can also occur in the nose, nasopharynx and larynx, the faucial site is much the commonest and paralysis of the palate is usually the earliest neurological symptom. The onset of faucial diphtheria is usually insidious: the child becomes quiet and anorexic but rarely complains of a sore throat. Lassitude and general malaise are associated with a normal temperature or mild pyrexia seldom above 38.4°C (101°F). Initially the membrane is absent, but may become extensive within 24 hours. It usually begins on one or both tonsils and spreads onto the fauces, uvula and palate. It may vary from cream to yellow to grey, glistens, and bleeds with removal. Paradoxically it is usually thinner and less well defined in the more severe cases but covers a wider area of the pharynx. Other sites of membrane formation, notably the nasopharynx, must always be checked. Fetor is striking and characteristic and there is usually a cervical adenitis. Early signs of toxicity are marked pallor, drowsiness, vomiting and tachycardia.

Palatal paralysis, usually bilateral, may occur within a few days but is commonest during the second or third week. It leads to regurgitation of fluids through the nose and a nasal voice. The palatal reflex is absent. Paralysis of accommodation usually develops in the third or fourth week and generalized neuropathy between 5 and 7 weeks after infection. This generalized neuropathy (which is not necessarily preceded by palatal and ocular palsies) involves paralysis of the pharynx, intrinsic muscles of the larynx and the diaphragm. It is a serious complication because dysphagia may be complete and there is a risk of aspiration pneumonia and respiratory failure.

Diagnosis

Any membranous throat condition should be regarded with suspicion particularly if the membrane is difficult to remove and associated with a low grade fever but a relative tachycardia. Infectious mononucleosis can produce a grey membrane and oedema in the throat identical to diphtheria and is the commonest infection to cause real difficulty in diagnosis. However, other signs such as generalized lymphadenopathy, splenomegaly and the finding of abnormal mononuclear cells in the peripheral blood help to distinguish the condition. Agranulocytosis and acute leukaemia may produce lesions of the throat resembling diphtheria.

Quinsy, Vincent's angina, thrush and herpes zoster should be readily distinguishable.

Nose and throat swabs should be taken in every suspected case, but negative cultures do not exclude diphtheria and bacteriological confirmation of virulent diphtheria may take 3 or 4 days. Paralytic complications increase in frequency and extent with increasing delay of treatment with antitoxin, and this therapy must never be withheld while awaiting bacteriological confirmation of the suspected clinical diagnosis. Once toxin is fixed in heart muscle or peripheral nerves it is not affected by antitoxin which can only neutralize circulating toxin.

Treatment

The importance of rest in this condition cannot be overemphasized. All patients should be nursed flat in isolation, often for many weeks. They should be mobilized gradually and only when clinical and electrocardiographic evidence of myocarditis is absent. The old fashioned adage of 'a pillow a week' until the patient is sitting up remains a good regimen. As complete recovery can ensue in may cases, it is tragic when death results from too early and too great an exertion because of impatience.

The dose of antitoxin required depends on the site of the disease and the extent and duration of the membrane. It varies from 20 000 units intramuscularly to 200 000 units intravenously. A repeat dose of antitoxin is unnecessary if the correct initial assessment is made but can be given after a 2–3 day delay if the membrane continues to spread. Penicillin should be given to all patients to limit the spread of infection. It does not affect any preformed toxin and is in no way a substitute for antitoxin. Intravenous injections of hydrocortisone and 1:1000 adrenalin drawn up into syringes must be available when administering antitoxin as it is a horse-serum preparation. A history must be taken of previous injections and allergy.

Palatal paralysis usually calls for no treatment other than that dictated by the general condition of the patient, but when the pharynx is affected a nasogastric tube must be passed and left *in situ* to provide feeding and to lessen the risk of inhalation pneumonia. A sucker may be used to remove pharyngeal secretions but, in severe cases, a tracheostomy with a cuffed tube may be necessary. If both respiratory and pharyngeal muscles are affected intermittent positive pressure ventilation can be carried out via the tracheostomy.

Although paralysis recovers spontaneously, the restoration of movements is said to be hastened by exercises, such as whistling and blowing up balloons.

Prognosis

This depends on the virulence of the infecting organism, the position and extent of the membrane, and the delay in administering antitoxin. Death from diphtheria during the first week is caused by circulatory failure or laryngeal obstruction. Myocarditis may prove fatal in the second or third weeks and respiratory failure is responsible for most later deaths. Complete recovery without sequelae is usual but may take up to 6 months in severe cases. Most patients are out of danger within 10 weeks. Active immunization with triple vaccine, commencing at 4 months of age, usually prevents or modifies diphtheria but fatal attacks may still occur.

Most convalescent and long-term carriers can be treated with a 7-day course of erythromycin. Tonsillectomy is rarely required.

Acute anterior poliomyelitis

This acute viral disease is characterized by local or widespread muscular paralysis resulting from destruction of anterior horn cells in the spinal cord and corresponding cells in the nuclei of the cranial nerves. It is of particular interest to the otolaryngologist because paralysis of the pharynx and larynx occur in the bulbar type of disease, with involvement of the brain stem nuclei.

Aetiology

This disease is also known as infantile paralysis and in areas of the world where the virus is uncontrolled and sanitation poor, young children are still the main victims. However, in developed countries there has been a shift of the age of onset towards young adults. In the UK and many other countries which have had active immunization campaigns, poliomyelitis occurs only sporadically and the classical midsummer and autumn epidemics are of historical interest only.

The neurotropic virus exists in three known types which have different antigenic properties. It is transmitted by pharyngeal secretions and food contaminated by virus excreted in the faeces. The virus enters the body via the nasopharynx or gastrointestinal tract and has an incubation period of 7–14 days. Axonal spread occurs, but the virus is also bloodborne and this is the main route of transmission to the central nervous system. Aycock and Luther (1929) indicated that the virus easily gained entry via the raw tonsillar bed after tonsillectomy. There is also good evidence that physical exertion during the stage of incubation predisposes to increased paralysis, particularly in those muscle groups used in the exercise. Paralysis may also develop in limbs into which injections are given. All these factors are obviously best avoided during an epidemic. Detailed reviews of the virology and epidemiology are available (Cohen, 1969; Drouhet, Debre and Celers, 1970).

Pathology

The virus is often widespread throughout the brain and spinal cord but has a particular affinity for the motor nuclei of cranial nerves and the anterior horn motor cells. Depending on the severity of the attack these cells necrose, usually within the first few days of the disease, following which no further destruction occurs. Other cells show evidence of damage by loss of Nissl granules but these are presumably capable of recovery. Necrosed cells are removed by neurophages, and examination of the spinal cord many years after the acute episode may show almost complete loss of anterior horn cells in the affected areas. Approximately one-third of cells have to be destroyed to induce clinical signs of paralysis. Paralysed muscle undergoes severe neurogenic atrophy.

Symptoms and signs

There are three possible distinct phases of this illness. Entirely subclinical infections and trivial illnesses lasting a few days with headache, diarrhoea and sore throat occur in most patients. The illness aborts before the paralytic stage and these apparently healthy individuals greatly outnumber those with neurological involvement and probably provide the greatest source of infection. Depending on factors such as the type and virulence of the virus, a variable proportion of patients who recover from the initial mild illness enter a second stage of meningitic involvement, the so-called pre-paralytic stage, 2–3 days after recovery from the first. Headache and general malaise return, are far more severe and are accompanied by lumbar and limb pain, and cervical rigidity. In children, delirium and convulsions may occur. This group of symptoms resembles that of other forms of viral meningitis.

Finally, a small group of patients continues into the third, paralytic phase. Unfortunately, some adults who develop paralysis do not go through the two clearly defined preceding phases. Prediction of the extent of paralysis is difficult but severe limb pain and loss of tendon reflexes suggest a bad prognosis. Rest in bed at the first sign of an attack is essential.

In most patients maximum paralysis is reached within 3 days and occurs in a random manner. Spinal paralysis may affect the respiratory muscles and early recognition is important. A useful simple test is to ask the patient to count as far as possible with a single breath, a number below 15 suggests serious respiratory insufficiency.

Brain stem damage is serious, swallowing becomes impossible and pharyngeal secretions are aspirated. Combined bulbar and respiratory paralysis is still often fatal despite the best treatment.

Fortunately, except in severe cases, only some of the muscles originally affected remain paralysed. Recovery begins after about a week, and may continue for over 3 months.

Treatment

Barrier nursing is essential. Both bulbar paralysis and respiratory paralysis may require the attention of the otolaryngologist. Respiratory embarrassment caused by accumulation and aspiration of pharyngeal secretions must be distinguished from true paralysis of the muscles of respiration. Respiratory weakness requires artificial respiration. If there is no bulbar palsy a tracheostomy is not necessary if a negative pressure cuirass or cabinet respirator is used. These respirators once widely used with good results, require careful day-to-day management with a high level of skill on an appropriate unit. Nowadays they have been largely replaced by intermittent positive pressure ventilation via a nasal or oral endotracheal tube, or through a cuffed tracheostomy tube. The advantage of intermittent positive pressure ventilation is that, if bulbar paralysis is also present, the cuffed intratracheal tube prevents the aspiration of pharyngeal secretions, food and vomit. Nasogastric feeding is obviously important in patients with bulbar paralysis. These patients require detailed management of blood gases, bronchial secretions, secondary infection, nasogastric feeding, care of the skin, bladder, bowels, and satisfactory communication. These many factors are best undertaken by an experienced team on an intensive care unit.

Prevention

Salk introduced the first vaccine by killing the three virus strains with formalin and injecting the preparation systemically. The value of this preparation became well established in the 1950s but it did not prevent colonization of the gut by wild virus and an immune patient could still be a carrier. It has therefore been superseded by the oral administration of an attenuated live vaccine of the Sabin type, given as one or two drops on a sugar lump. Immunity appears to last for at least 3 years and in children and young adults booster doses are needed at intervals of a few years. There can be no doubt that in countries where a sustained vaccination programme has been pursued paralytic poliomyelitis has been virtually abolished but it is important that standards are not relaxed allowing the problem to grow again (Paul, 1971).

Rabies

This viral disease of mammals is usually transmitted to man by the bite of a dog with infected saliva. Rabies was eradicated from the UK 80 years ago but remains enzootic in foxes in mainland Europe. It has been estimated to cause 15 000 deaths a year in other parts of the world. 'Furious' rabies is characterized by intense arousal and hydrophobia associated with inspiratory and pharyngeal muscle spasm. 'Dumb' rabies presents as an ascending paralysis.

Pathology

The virus enters via a bite and is transmitted along nerve trunks in both directions to infect many organs including the salivary and lacrimal glands. The brain and spinal cord show ganglion cell degeneration and marked perineural and perivascular round cell infiltration.

Symptoms and signs

The incubation period varies widely from 10 days to years (usually 1–2 months) depending on the distance of the infected bite from the central nervous system. The first general symptoms are depression, apprehension and insomnia. Then follows hydrophobia, the classical sign of rabies: attempts to drink water produce gross spasm of the pharynx, larynx and respiratory muscles. This spreads to all the muscles of the body producing opisthotonus. At its height even the sound or thought of water will elicit the spasm. Other signs are hypersalivation, dysphagia, cranial nerve palsies, cardiac arrhythmias and severe psychiatric disturbance. Patients sink into a coma after a few days and even with intensive care only a few patients survive.

The condition must be distinguished from tetanus which has a much shorter incubation period of 2–3 weeks. Trismus is the early symptom and pharyngeal spasm is absent. In hysteria true pharyngeal spasm is absent and the problem is amenable to drugs and suggestion.

Prophylaxis and treatment

Animal bites must be thoroughly cleaned, and the wound left open. The indications for vaccine treatment are clear (WHO Committee, 1966) and it should begin as early as possible after the bite. The newer inactivated vaccine given in human diploid strain COI38 has been shown to be safe and effective (Wiktor, Plotkin and Grella, 1973; Aoki *et al.*, 1975). Hyperimmune gamma globulin is now given as a rule with vaccine.

Patients with established rabies require heavy sedation to control spasms and suffering. Total paralysis with curare and artificial respiration offer the only hope.

Myasthenia gravis

This disease occurs in all ages and races but is twice as common in women as men. It is usually seen in young adults and may present to the otorhinolaryngologist when the bulbar muscles are involved. Current evidence suggests it is an autoimmune disease with damage to the acetylcholine receptors in the motor end-plate. Any group of muscles may be affected and the disease tends to remit and relapse. There is abnormal muscle fatiguability, sometimes confined to an isolated group of muscles. The extraocular muscles are those most commonly involved. If it is restricted to the bulbar muscles there is dysarthria, dysphagia, regurgitation of fluid through the nose, and movements of the tongue, palate and pharynx are decreased. The symptoms typically appear in the evening when the patient is tired, particularly towards the end of a meal. They improve after a night's rest. If the patient is asked to count aloud the voice becomes less distinct and more nasal.

Diagnosis depends on the typical clinical picture, the evaluation of the effects of intravenous edrophonium (Tensilon test), modern electromyographic measurements, or the detection of antiacetylcholine receptor antibodies in the blood.

The standard symptomatic treatment for myasthenia gravis is still neostigmine or pyridostigmine, the dosage of which is steadily increased until the maximal effect is obtained. This does not affect the underlying natural history. Immunosuppressive treatment with prednisone, with or without azathioprine (Imuran) may be required. Plasmapheresis has been life saving.

Most remissions occur in the first few years of the disease but unfortunately relapses are common. Most deaths also occur in the early years of the disease. Neonatal myasthenia is occasionally seen in infants of affected mothers but usually recovers in a few weeks.

Thymic enlargement is often found in young patients and may be caused by a thymoma, some of which are malignant. The place of thymectomy remains debatable. The results are best in young women with a short and severe history, but both sexes may benefit and operation is indicated if there is rapid deterioration with optimum medication. If a thymoma is present radiotherapy may be used before surgery. Only one-third of patients with a thymoma survives beyond 5 years.

Myasthenia is closely related to thyrotoxicosis and less commonly to sarcoidosis, diabetes mellitus, rheumatoid arthritis and systemic lupus erythematosus. Accumulating evidence suggests that the disease has several different clinical, immunological, and genetic forms (Feltkamp *et al.*, 1974; Fritze *et al.*, 1974).

Motor neuron disease (progressive bulbar palsy)

This is a disease of middle age or later life in which degeneration affects motor neurons in the anterior horns of the spinal cord, certain somatic motor nuclei of cranial nerves, and in the cerebral cortex. Both upper and lower motor neurons are affected and symptomatology is diverse. The cause is, as yet, unknown. Pathological fasciculation can occur in any situation where some motor neurons degenerate and others persist, but it is most common in motor neuron disease.

The most common presentation is wasting of the muscles of the hand and upper girdle, but another common presentation, of interest to the otorhinolaryngologist is progressive bulbar palsy. This is more common in women, causing dysphagia and dysarthria. It is often combined with upper motor neuron signs and evidence of pseudobulbar palsy. If weakness begins with bulbar palsy it usually spreads to the shoulders and arms.

The classical sign of the bulbar presentation is fasciculation and wasting of the tongue as a result of degeneration of the hypoglossal nuclei. This sign is unreliable in a protruded tongue, and it must be elicited with the tongue on the floor of the mouth. The differential diagnosis from myasthenia gravis is rarely difficult.

Dysphagia with aspiration is the most dangerous symptom and the course of the disease is more rapid if this is the initial symptom.

No treatment has any effect on the course of this relentless and depressing disease. Cricopharyngeal myotomy has its proponents, but does not always help the dysphagia and any improvement is usually short lived. The knowledge of a fatal creeping paralysis can lead to a complete collapse of morale, and requires careful handling.

Palatal myoclonus

In this condition there are rhythmical movements of the soft palate, occurring 60–180 times per minute (palatal nystagmus). They develop insidiously, on one or both sides, and interfere with sleep, swallowing and respiration. They persist during sleep and may be inhibited initially by voluntary control. It appears to be a disorder of the olivocerebellar modulatory projection on the rostral brain stem and is seen in multiple sclerosis and brain stem infarction.

It may occur in association with myoclonus of the pharynx, larynx, eyes and diaphragm. The palatal myoclonus may be audible as a clicking sound and is sometimes abolished by anticonvulsants.

Treatment of palatal and pharyngeal paralysis

The treatment differs according to the cause and extent of the lesion. Isolated, palatal paralysis rarely requires treatment, although troublesome nasal regurgitation may be helped by holding the nose during swallowing or by an upper dental plate with a soft palate extension. Paralysis of the oropharynx and hypopharynx is not uncommonly associated with additional paralysis of the larynx and/or the tongue. The treatment necessary will depend upon the degree and complexity of the overall paralysis.

Limited and temporary *unilateral* paralysis of the oro- and hypopharynx without associated laryngeal difficulties may allow the patient to maintain adequate nutrition without aspiration, particularly if he receives accurate evaluation and swallowing instructions from the otorhinolaryngologist and speech and swallowing therapist. The latter can instruct the patient with regard to simple measures, such as turning the head towards the affected side or tilting the head in order to maximize swallowing down the normal side of the pharynx, which will improve swallowing under these circumstances. If there is limited aspiration this may be prevented by teaching the patient the method of swallowing while generating a positive intralaryngeal pressure.

Bilateral oro- and hypopharyngeal palsy, particularly when associated with other tongue and laryngeal abnormalities is frequently a life-threatening problem. Many of these patients aspirate even their own saliva and are at risk of serious chest infection. If the difficulties are short term and temporary, help might be obtained by a soft fine bore nasogastric tube for feeding and repeated pharyngeal suction to protect the airway. However, these are completely unsatisfactory in the long term, and tracheostomy and gastrostomy/jejunostomy may be necessary. A modern, light-weight cuffed tracheostomy tube is frequently used in a tracheostomy, but this frequently fails to provide adequate protection against laryngeal secretions – particularly if inappropriate oral feeding is attempted at the same time. If the neurological deficit is likely to continue beyond a few weeks without the chance of spontaneous improvement more satisfactory methods of protection of the airway are necessary and these are dealt with later under the heading of denervation of the larynx.

Laryngeal neurological lesions

Functional disorders

Many patients of a type similar to those with globus pharyngeus present with disorders of laryngeal sensation or voice production. These are related to social upsets, anxiety, smoking and vocal misuse. Following exclusion of organic disease local measures, reassurance, and advice from a speech therapist are usually successful.

Laryngeal paralysis or the 'spastic' larynx

Paralysis of the larynx may be caused by peripheral or central damage. As mentioned previously the latter is rare at a cortical level and the lesions are 'spastic'. This must not be confused with the so-called 'spastic' dysphonia which has been discussed at length in recent years.

Spasmodic dysphonia (laryngeal dystonias)

The assessment and treatment of spasmodic dysphonia has expanded considerably since the last edition of this chapter and most authors now recognize at least two disorder patterns, the adductor and abductor types. The term spasmodic dysphonia is increasingly being replaced by the term focal laryngeal dystonia and, to complicate matters even further, mixed abductor/adductor and a respiratory type of dystonia have also been described (Koufman and Blalock, 1991). In all variants of these laryngeal dystonias there is a severe movement disorder of the vocal folds characterized by inappropriate hyperadduction or hyperabduction. The dysphonia is usually associated with vocal fatigue and marked tightness of the chest and neck musculature, the voice is harsh and strained but the patient is often able to laugh, clear the throat and sometimes even sing. It can be difficult to distinguish true spasmodic dysphonia from muscle tension dysphonia, particularly when supraglottic contraction is present. These patients require detailed laryngological examination by video endoscopic means in conjunction with evaluation by an experienced speech therapist. Screening neurological examination, laryngeal electromyography and most recently spectral analysis of the voice help to clarify the situation (Koufman and Blalock, 1991).

The cause of spasmodic dysphonia remains uncertain, although many authorities feel that a faulty central neural integration is the most likely cause. Many treatments have been advocated for spasmodic dysphonia varying from conservative voice therapeutic techniques to the more radical solution of recurrent laryngeal nerve section. This latter technique was introduced by Dedo in 1976 and has remained the subject of debate ever since. Initial success rates were high with many patients relieved of their disabling voice symptoms and able to return to normal lifestyles, but the long-term success rate is not nearly as good with a recurrence rate of over 50% at 5 years and EMG studies suggest that the dystonia increases on the unoperated side. Tucker (1989) introduced anterior laryngoplasty, a technique which relaxes the vocal cords and was proposed as an option for laryngeal dystonia of the adductor type. The effect of this operation on spasmodic dysphonia is unpredictable and many patients have a marked decrease in phonatory pitch and volume.

In 1986, Blitzer *et al.* introduced the technique of botulinum toxin injection into the vocalis muscle. This technique has markedly improved the situation for these patients and, at the same time, the routine use of transnasal fibreoptic laryngoscopy, video recording, electromyography and the concentration of patients within centres has led to an increasingly improved outcome and clarification of laryngeal dystonia.

A variety of techniques for the injection of botulinum toxin has now been introduced and each has its advantages and disadvantages. Transcutaneous injection is commonly performed through the cricothyroid membrane using EMG and or fibreoptic localization. EMG monitoring has a distinct advantage in that virtually all patients can be injected and it is possible to localize the vocalis muscle. Bilateral injection may be used but dosage protocols vary. Most patients experience 1–2 weeks of rather breathy dysphonia, followed by up to 6 months of complete relief with a relatively normal voice. Most authors would agree that the abductor type and mixed dystonias are more difficult to treat and may account for the variable early results when these types are not clearly demarcated. In the case of abductor type spasmodic dysphonia, the posterior cricoarytenoid muscle is injected.

Laryngeal spasm

This rather ill-defined condition is rarely neural and in young children is usually infective in nature. In the past, poor living conditions, rickets, whooping cough, upper respiratory tract sepsis, poliomyelitis, tetanus, and rabies have all been involved. Nowadays these are all rare in the UK.

Adults may suffer from 'choking' attacks with considerable panic and functional overlay. If these episodes are severe and there is concomitant vagal activity, a frank fainting episode may occur. Laryngeal spasm may arise at night in individuals with marked oesophageal reflux and cricopharyngeal incompetence from any cause. It is presumed that a small amount of stomach content is aspirated into the larynx and the patient awakes with a 'choking' attack. This is an unusual disorder and other more common causes of nocturnal dyspnoea should be excluded.

Superior laryngeal nerve palsy

Paralysis of this nerve whether on one or both sides is often clinically unrecognized and it has been somewhat neglected in laryngeal studies.

In unilateral superior laryngeal nerve paralysis, the voice is not severely affected and compensation occurs quickly. The disability to a professional voice user, in particular a singer, may, however, be significant. This form of paralysis is more readily recognized on examination because of the asymmetrical tilt and shift of the larynx and the ipsilateral, bowed, and flabby vocal fold. Deprived of one of its tensors the affected fold also appears longer. Arytenoid movements are unimpaired. The voice sometimes fails to regain its former strength even though its quality returns.

Bilateral superior laryngeal nerve palsy is even more rarely recognized. The symmetry of the larynx at rest and during phonation makes the presence of this combined paralysis difficult to detect. The absence of anterior tilt allows the epiglottis to hang more over the endolarynx and the slightly flaccid, bowed and hyperaemic vocal folds are more difficult to see. The bowed folds allow excess leakage of air during phonation and the voice is lower, weaker, breathy and lacks inflection. With good compensation the speaking voice returns to normal but the singing voice is severely compromised.

The detection of both these paralyses has been aided by modern fibreoptic laryngeal endoscopes, stroboscopy, and video recording (Howard and Lund, 1986).

Superior laryngeal nerve palsy occurs in a significant number of patients undergoing thyroid surgery and a detailed knowledge of the variable anatomy of this nerve is essential. Dissection and division of the superior pole vessels immediately adjacent to the capsule of the upper pole of the thyroid gland will lessen the chances of damage. Trauma to the neck, particularly from road traffic accidents can cause superior laryngeal nerve palsy.

Recurrent laryngeal nerve palsy

The eventual static position and appearance of a paralysed vocal fold will depend on the degree and permanency of denervation and the degree of associated muscle and joint atrophy and fibrosis. Semon (1881) and his contemporaries, and laryngologists up to this day have failed to recognize these variables, and this has produced an unnecessary amount of disagreement and controversy. Indeed accurate re-

cording of the position of a paralysed vocal fold is difficult because only 3–6 mm separate the median, paramedian and so-called 'cadaveric' positions. Therefore, many cases are reported inaccurately and this may help to explain the apparent inconsistencies between the various theories.

The 'cadaveric' position does not always occur after death and is best replaced by the term 'lateral'. By far the most satisfactory method of describing the position of the paralysed fold is to state clearly, in millimetres, the distance it lies from the midline. If detailed follow up and evaluation is to be undertaken for research and publication, then endoscopic photographic documentation should be used to ensure accuracy of long-term measurements.

It is also best to describe the paralysis, whether unilateral or bilateral, in terms of abductor or adductor paralysis, i.e. the direction of movement which the vocal fold cannot make.

Semon's law

Semon's law is of *historical interest only*. The weight of neurohistological and neurophysiological evidence against it is now overwhelming, and it plays no part in modern laryngology. Briefly, Semon proposed that the motor fibres innervating the adductor and abductor muscles lay in separate bundles in the recurrent laryngeal nerve and that they had different susceptibilities to an advancing lesion of the nerve giving rise first to an abductor paralysis with the vocal fold in the median position, and then adductor paralysis so that the fold came to rest in the lateral (cadaveric) position. There are many clinical inconsistencies to this, in addition to neurohistological and neurophysiological evidence that this is not the case. The reader is referred to the excellent account by Wyke and Kirschner (1976) for further study.

Wagner and Grossman theory

Wagner (1890) and Grossman (1897) proposed a theory which has had more recent experimental confirmation by Arnold (1962) and Dedo (1970). In the absence of cricoarytenoid joint fixation, an immobile vocal fold in the paramedian position has a total pure unilateral recurrent nerve paralysis, and an immobile vocal fold in the lateral (cadaveric) position has a combined paralysis of superior and recurrent nerves (the adductive action of cricothyroid is lost).

However, clinically it is not uncommon to see patients with intrathoracic lesions (which should produce a pure recurrent palsy) with the paralysed fold in the lateral (cadaveric) position. Purported explanations for this are stretching of the nerve by the intrathoracic lesion thus pulling the vagus down from the skull base and injuring the superior laryngeal nerve; and possible retrograde atrophy of the vagus to the nucleus ambiguus. Damage to the laryngeal nerves produces loss of sensation as well as motility. This may produce an incompetent laryngeal sphincter and possible life-threatening aspiration.

No doubt controversy with regard to the above considerations will continue but, from a practical point of view, the management of a patient with a vocal fold palsy depends on the aetiology of the lesion and on the defect it causes. In the case of a unilateral fold palsy the patient may obtain excellent vocal compensation without treatment, only the timbre of the voice being altered. 'Idiopathic' defects may rarely recover up to 2 years after onset and traditionally it has been necessary to wait a minimum of 12 months to see if recovery occurs in a paralysed cord before undertaking any definitive treatment. With increasing use of EMG electrodes in specialist voice centres and clinics it may be possible to consider earlier treatment if the EMG confirms complete loss with no signs of recovery.

Aetiology

Stell and Maran (1978) reviewed five large series of paralysis of the recurrent laryngeal nerve in the literature. The following groups were discernible.

Malignant disease

This accounted for 25% of patients, one-half being caused by carcinoma of the lung.

Surgical trauma

This was responsible for 20% with surgical procedures on the lung, heart, oesophagus and mediastinum now outnumbering those produced by thyroidectomy.

Idiopathic

In 13% no cause could be found although virus infections such as influenza and infectious mononucleosis have been suggested as aetiological agents. In this idiopathic group all patients who are smokers should be considered to have carcinoma of the lung until proved otherwise.

Inflammatory

Another group accounting for 13% of patients with pulmonary tuberculosis still being the major cause.

Non-surgical trauma

In 11% of patients the cause was stretching of the nerve by enlargement of the left atrium, aortic aneurysm, or neck trauma.

Neurological

A proven neurological cause was found in 7%, i.e. cerebrovascular disease, Parkinson's disease, multiple sclerosis, head injury, alcoholic and diabetic neuropathies.

Miscellaneous

The remaining 11% of patients did not fit neatly into any of the above categories and they included a wide range of illnesses such as rheumatoid arthritis, haemolytic anaemia, syphilis, and collagen diseases.

Owing to its long course the left recurrent laryngeal nerve is affected in approximately three-quarters of patients and the right in about 15%, the remainder being bilateral.

Symptoms and signs

Evaluation begins with listening to the patient's voice as he gives the history. A faint whisper suggests a functional adductor paralysis, a forced whisper an organic adductor paralysis. A voice which tires with use suggests a unilateral abductor paralysis and stridor and aspiration occur with a bilateral abductor paralysis. The patient's age and occupation are of paramount importance.

Additional symptoms in the upper respiratory and gastrointestinal tracts, and the rest of the head and neck are obviously of relevance and the patient's past medical history and smoking habits are of particular importance.

Investigations

Haematological tests

A full blood count, erythrocyte sedimentation rate and serology are useful screening tests, but other indices such as viral studies and blood glucose tests are rarely useful.

Radiology

In the past a wide variety of radiological examinations has been advocated to assist with the investigation of these patients. However, in many countries the increasing availability of high quality CT scanning combined with contrast media, has now made this the investigation of choice. The scan is performed from skull base to mid-thorax and is the definitive investigation (MacGregor *et al.*, 1994). Where this technique is not available, plain radiographs, tomograms of the chest and a good submentovertical skull base view yield the best results. Further plain radiographs of the nasopharynx, neck and petrous bones are occasionally useful and a barium swallow and thyroid scan may be added if indicated.

Endoscopy

Panendoscopy with rigid and flexible instruments may be used to elucidate or confirm the diagnosis and the causative lesion. Particular points of note are the need for biopsy of the fossa of Rosenmüller and the bronchial carina even if these appear normal. This is particularly necessary in those patients whose history and radiology have not suggested a cause. The affected arytenoids must be palpated to distinguish vocal fold paralysis from cricoarytenoid fixation.

Treatment

Evaluation of these patients will show them to belong to one of the four following groups. The treatment may vary even within the same group depending on the general state of the patient and the aetiology of the lesion. Many patients will be helped by speech therapy, with or without associated surgery.

Unilateral abductor paralysis

This is an important group to consider first because speech therapy may be the only treatment necessary. The single paralysed vocal fold lies in the paramedian position and any initial hoarseness may disappear as the unaffected fold compensates. When the left fold is involved, the aetiology is commonly that of carcinoma of the lung and presentation with the vocal fold palsy means that the carcinoma is already inoperable.

For many of these patients the vocal fold palsy is part of a disordered protective mechanism and they may aspirate, particularly liquids, and have a weak cough. Under these circumstances surgical intervention may be indicated immediately, particularly in a patient who is not expected to live for a long period.

In patients with other less serious causes, the dysphonia may persist and become distressing or, if the voice becomes reasonable it may, nevertheless, tend to tire with repeated use. Professional voice users are particularly likely to request treatment.

The surgical methods available for the treatment of a unilateral abductor paralysis are: vocal fold injection; medialization (laryngoplasty); arytenoid rotation; nerve muscle pedicle reinnervation; recurrent laryngeal nerve reinnervation; or, indeed, a combination of these procedures. Teflon injection is most likely to produce a good result when the fold is in the paramedian position but the amount used is critical and the technique is more fully described later. The post-injection voice is rarely entirely 'normal', although the volume and quality are improved. It is important that the patient with a paralysed fold is advised before surgery that, although there is a good chance of improving the voice, it will not necessarily return to its previous 'normal' level.

Unilateral adductor paralysis

The flaccid paralysed fold lies in the lateral position and gives rise to a weak husky voice, sometimes no more than a whisper. In addition, as this lesion is most commonly the result of damage to the vagus or both superior and recurrent laryngeal nerves, the laryngeal sphincter is incompetent, part of the larynx insensitive, and consequently aspiration may occur.

Both the type and timing of treatment depend on the aetiology of the unilateral adductor paralysis. If the cause is a carcinoma, particularly of the bronchus, then the patients appreciate the improvement of voice and ability to cough that can be obtained with a prompt Teflon injection. Many of these patients with carcinoma will have only a few months to live and delay to await any possible laryngeal compensation is unwarranted. There is also increasing support for immediate injection of a paralysed vocal fold resulting from major thoracic operations, thus enabling the patient to cough satisfactorily during the postoperative period. Teflon injection for an adductor paralysis gives overall poorer results than for abductor lesions. This is a result of the difficulty of closing the posterior part of the glottis between the arytenoids where there will always be some air wastage. Overspill may be helped by injection or laryngeal framework surgery, but the results are more difficult to predict and require experience and care on the part of the surgeon.

Unilateral adductor paralysis not caused by carcinoma requires a waiting period of at least 2 months to allow for compensation or evidence of recovery. Speech therapy should be given during this time. If the unilateral adductor paralysis is a result of laryngeal trauma there is usually considerable scarring, particularly of the thyroarytenoid muscle and it may not be possible to displace the vocal fold medially by means of a Teflon injection. In order to alter the position of the scarred fold from lateral to medial a number of alternative procedures have been advocated. Collagen injection has been used in an attempt to augment an atrophic vocal fold by injection superficially and is said to cause scar tissue to soften. A combination of both medialization laryngoplasty and arytenoid adduction has been advocated when the posterior commissure gap is more then the usual 2–3 mm.

Bilateral abductor paralysis

This lesion is usually the result of damage to both recurrent laryngeal nerves at thyroidectomy. Other treatable causes are rare. The vocal folds lie in the paramedian position and the voice is good but the degree of stridor is very variable. In the acute situation stridor may be life threatening and a tracheostomy required. However, if the lesion develops more slowly and the patient is relatively inactive there may be little or no stridor. Nevertheless, at some point, usually associated with an upper respiratory tract infection, all these patients will develop stridor. If the lesion is diagnosed soon after thyroidectomy immediate re-exploration of the neck is indicated. This is not so much to re-anastomose sectioned nerves (which gives overall poor results), but more in the hope of finding the nerves caught in a ligature. Removal of this often allows good long-term recovery. The author advocates a positive approach to post-thyroidectomy paralysis, but re-exploration of the nerves is pointless after a delay of more than 2 months because of motor end-plate degeneration and fibrosis of laryngeal muscles.

The choice of treatment for patients with established bilateral abductor paralysis is varied and numerous operations have been described. No operation should be attempted until at least 2 months after the onset of paralysis, thus allowing for any possibility of spontaneous recovery, unless detailed EMG studies are available showing complete denervation. If there is recovery of any movement in one fold then possible operations should be undertaken only on the other fold.

When considering treatment it is important to remember the basic point that the patient has a good voice but poor airway. Any operative procedure to improve the airway will decrease the quality of voice and on occasions fail to improve the airway. Many of these patients will require or present to the laryngologist with a permanent tracheostomy. If this is fitted with a speaking valve they have the excellent situation of a good airway and a good voice. The only disadvantage to this being the actual wearing of the tube which some patients are unable to accept. A permanent speaking valve tracheostomy may be the best choice in the professional voice user. It is the author's experience that patients who have become used to wearing such a tube will decline further surgical intervention and they should not be persuaded into undergoing one of the many variants of arytenoidectomy, cordectomy or reinnervation.

Bilateral adductor paralysis

Apparent bilateral adductor paralysis may occur in patients with psychiatric disturbances. There may be a severe dysphonia but the commonly used term 'hysterical aphonia' is often inappropriate. The milder cases may be considerably helped by speech therapy particularly if the underlying problems (usually social) can be resolved. A few patients may need psychiatric referral and recurrence of symptoms is not uncommon.

Organic disease producing this bilateral lesion is fortunately rare but is usually a serious central nervous system disease or neoplastic process involving the medulla, skull base or upper neck. With both vocal folds in the lateral position these patients are not only aphonic but are unable to cough well and have incoordinated swallowing. This laryngeal incompetence results in life-threatening aspiration in a very short time. Initial management involves a tracheostomy with a cuffed tube and a nasogastric tube for feeding. Further management is usually required depending on the aetiology. Total laryngectomy is the only sure way to protect the lungs but may not be undertaken if there is a possibility of neurological improvement. Epiglottopexy (Brookes and McKelvie, 1983) is the procedure of choice in neurological problems where subsequent neurological improvement may occur.

Other methods of management have been advocated such as Teflon injection of the folds and supraglottis, closure of the glottis by suturing the cords, and cricopharyngeal myotomy. The results of these other methods are variable and often poor, particularly when adequate preoperative videofluoroscopic assessment and investigations have not been undertaken.

Phonosurgery

The term phonosurgery is increasingly used throughout the world when referring to any surgery designed primarily for the improvement or restoration of voice. It was first popularized by Hans von Leden in the late 1950s (von Leden, 1991) when there was a renewed interest in procedures for functional improvement of the larynx. More recently the terms laryngoplasty, thyroplasty and laryngoplastic phonosurgery, have all been used to describe surgical procedures on the laryngeal framework. Phonosurgery in its widest context covers all laryngeal injection techniques, microsurgery, laser surgery, laryngeal framework surgery and laryngeal re-innervation techniques.

An understanding of this developing branch of our speciality is not possible without a detailed study of the anatomy, physiology and pathology of the larynx and such is the increasing complexity of the subject that this detailed knowledge is essential before treating patients with significant voice problems. While thousands of patients with vocal fold paralysis have been treated by Teflon injection and have obtained reasonable results, the assessment of vocal function has become more critical in recent years. The limitations of a simple injection technique performed by the occasional operator with inadequate pre- and postoperative assessment have now become apparent.

The surgical correction of symptomatic unilateral vocal fold paralysis began with Brüning's attempts in 1911 to treat patients by injecting paraffin into the laterally placed vocal fold. A modification of the injection syringe he described is still widely used today. Subsequent to his description, injected paraffin in other parts of the body was found to cause embolization and paraffinoma and its use was abandoned.

Over 40 years later, Arnold (1955) revived the technique using cartilage particles as the injection material. Following this a variety of substances such as bone paste, silicon, tantalum oxide powder, tantalum and Teflon were evaluated. Teflon paste emerged as the material of choice. Its permanence, low tissue reactivity and lack of carcinogenicity in over 20 years of use are well documented. The reader is referred to the excellent review of the characteristics of Teflon paste by Montgomery (1979).

In 1915, Payr described the first laryngeal framework procedure, in which an anteriorly-based rectangular thyroid cartilage flap was used for vocal fold medialization. However, this flap did not provide definitive medialization to produce good glottic apposition and the technique did not become popular. In 1952, Meurman reported 15 patients on whom he carried out medialization by implanting rib cartilage lateral to the vocal fold. In 1968, Sawashima *et al.* improved on Meurman's technique and in 1980 Isshiki reported the use of a silastic implant for medialization. This latter development stimulated great interest and throughout the 1980s medialization laryngoplasty has steadily become the treatment of choice for many patients with vocal fold paralysis.

Laryngeal injection techniques

At the time of writing, the most common technique for correcting glottic insufficiency remains the injection of a filler substance to displace the medial edge of the involved vocal fold towards the midline. Indications for its use and the correct timing of surgery have already been considered in the previous section. Materials such as Teflon cause permanent change in the structure of the vocal fold when injected and therefore should not be used with patients whose vocal function may return. Under these circumstances gel-foam paste, fat or collagen may be used if absolutely necessary. It is important to try to preserve the integrity of the membranous vocal fold to achieve optimal vibratory function.

Teflon injection

The injection of Teflon should produce sufficient medial displacement of the affected vocal fold towards the midline to ensure glottic closure during phonation. The displacement should be in the plane of the true vocal fold and Teflon must not be injected into the membranous vocal fold itself. Injections that are not in the correct plane of the contralateral vocal fold may appear to produce glottic closure on laryngoscopic examination but produce relatively poor voice with persistent breathy dysphonia. Injection into the subglottic or supraglottic soft tissues is unhelpful and in the case of the subglottis may produce dyspnoea in its own right. Adequate glottic soft tissue is a prerequi-

site for success with Teflon injection and poor results may be expected in patients who have had previous severe laryngeal trauma with extensive scarring, those who have atrophied vocal folds for whatever reason, and those who have had a cordectomy for squamous carcinoma or previous arytenoidectomy.

When Teflon is injected the particles are walled-off by foreign body reaction and the suspending glycerol is slowly absorbed. The resulting mass is hard and will produce notable dysphonia if vocal fold mobility returns. Subsequent removal of the Teflon by means of a CO_2 laser is difficult and preservation of normal vocal fold anatomy is impossible. Inadequate exposure at laryngoscopy may make Teflon injection difficult or impossible and, in these circumstances, transcutaneous injection advocated by Ward, Hanson and Abemayeor (1985) remains an option. It is often not possible to inject enough Teflon posteriorly to displace the vocal process medially in patients who have marked posterior glottic deficiency on attempted closure.

Anaesthesia

Injection can be performed under local or general anaesthesia and each method has its advantages and disadvantages, together with surgeons who strongly advocate each method. The final choice will depend on the patient, his overall condition, and the local method of practice and facilities. It is preferable for the surgeon to be familiar with both techniques.

Method

Dedo, Urrea and Lawson (1973) gave an excellent account of the method using local anaesthesia with results in 135 patients. This technique is done with the patient in a sitting position with the larynx and pharynx anaesthetized by sprays and droplets of cocaine. The surgeon views the larynx by indirect laryngoscopy and injects Teflon from a Brünings syringe into the paralysed vocal fold. Following withdrawal of the needle the patient can be asked to phonate and the quality of the voice checked. Further injection can be undertaken if necessary. This method undoubtedly gives good results but is not tolerated well by all patients and, indeed, is refused by some. The ability to assess the right amount of Teflon paste should not be too highly regarded since oedema of the surrounding fold occurs rapidly within 2–3 minutes and unless the injections can be completed in this time the true depot size is unpredictable. Subsequent resolution and absorption also occur over several postoperative weeks.

The method is of course most useful in patients whose overall condition contraindicates general anaesthesia. Ward, Hanson and Abemayeor (1985) described a transcutaneous technique, injecting the fold via a needle placed through the anterior neck into the larynx, in a patient with severe trismus, the result was checked using a flexible fibreoptic endoscope passed into the pharynx and attached to a video camera.

The major criticism of the technique under general anaesthesia has been the likelihood of over-injection. However, this rarely occurs when the basic requirements are observed. These are that the other fold should be fully functional and the injected fold should not be pushed right up to the midline. The author's preference is for the following technique. Under general anaesthesia (via a laryngeal mask initially and then Venturi ventilation), a Dedo laryngoscope is inserted and fixed with the Loewy suspension. A Brünings syringe is loaded with Teflon paste and care is taken to ensure that the paste has filled the attached needle and passes easily. The first injection is made into the posterolateral corner of the middle third of the vocal fold just anterior to the vocal process. With each click of the syringe ratchet 0.2 ml of paste is deposited and usually 0.4–0.8 ml is required to push the cord medially to lie close to the midline. It is important to realize that paste is compressible and is not all delivered immediately the handle is squeezed. Therefore several seconds should be allowed to elapse following each click so that all the paste is extruded and the fold accurately assessed. The injection should cause a gentle fusiform enlargement and care should be taken to avoid placing the paste in Reinke's space, too far laterally into the ventricular floor, or too deeply into the subglottis. A second injection is usually required in the anterolateral corner of the middle third of the vocal fold, i.e. the midpoint of the membranous fold. Because of the firm adherence of the mucous membrane to the vocal process it is impossible to inject posteriorly to close any gap between the arytenoids.

An intramuscular injection of dexamethasone 8 mg is given at the time of the procedure to minimize oedema but routine antibiotics are unnecessary. The majority of these operations can be carried out on a day-case basis, but a postoperative overnight stay may be indicated by the general condition of the patient.

Complications

The morbidity from this procedure is small but in all large series there is an incidence of about one in 100 patients requiring tracheostomy. The patient should be warned of this possibility preoperatively. Tracheostomy may be required because of acute progressive oedema which usually responds promptly to steroids, antibiotics and humidification allowing decannulation after only a few days. Less often a hemilaryngitis will occur 7–10 days postoperatively and requires antibiotic treatment.

The minimal soreness and foreign body sensation experienced by many patients subsides in a few days

and an improvement in the voice should be obtained in over 90% of patients. As stated previously, the best results are in patients with a pure unilateral recurrent nerve lesion.

Collagen injection

The collagen is bovine dermal collagen which has been solubilized, purified and reconstituted in phosphate buffered physiological saline. The preparation has a low viscosity which allows it to be injected through a fine needle and placed precisely into an atrophied vocal fold. Following injection the collagen implant forms a cohesive mass to which connective tissue cells migrate. The implant slowly resorbs and is replaced to some extent by loose connective tissue. Because the manufacturing process removes the most highly species-specific segments of the collagen molecules, this reduces the potential for the animal collagen to cause hypersensitivity reactions and adverse problems with this preparation are rare.

The technique is different from that of Teflon injection in that the material is placed superficially in the plane of the vocal ligament and not lateral to the thyroarytenoid muscle. A specially designed, 27-gauge disposable needle is used attached to a tuberculin-type syringe. The tip of the needle is inserted directly into the posterior one-third of the membranous vocal fold and once through the epithelium the resistance of the vocal ligament is felt. Injection is started at this point and between 0.2 ml and 0.8 ml of collagen is required to augment an atrophic paralysed vocal fold. Provided there is not a serious degree of scarring the collagen will spread forwards as the injection continues, filling out the vocal fold in the midmembranous and anterior portion. It may be necessary to inject collagen at other points and softening of scar tissue may allow subsequent, somewhat easier, injections on a second or third separate occasion, to achieve the desired result. This can be a difficult procedure and the author recommends that this is undertaken under general anaesthesia with microscopic control. Over injection, producing blebs of raised epithelium on the membranous vocal fold should be avoided.

Assessment of results of injection

Transcutaneous techniques may be observed endoscopically, while transoral procedures are best evaluated with microscopic control. For the majority of patients the most important parameter of success is the subsequent quality and strength of their voice and Dedo, Urrea and Lawson (1973) judged their success rate by listening to pre- and postoperative recordings. However, in recent times laryngeal videostroboscopy has been found to be a good indicator of success and an increased amplitude of vocal fold vibration and an increased mucosal wave can be seen on comparison of pre- and postoperative videos. Acoustic measures using long-time average spectral analysis remain a research-orientated assessment, but the simple measurement of increased maximum phonation time is a clinical test which can indicate improvement after, or during an injection procedure. It is not wholly reliable however because factors such as the patient's overall condition and pulmonary function may influence the results.

Many variables affect the functional outcome in these patients and the author feels strongly that, if at all possible, they should receive both pre- and postoperative speech therapy to aid the surgical results. Both Teflon and collagen induce varying degrees of oedema and foreign body reaction over differing lengths of time and the speech therapist is able to advise on all aspects of vocal use during periods of variable function.

Commercially available Teflon contains particles ranging in diameter from 5 μm to 80 μm and the smaller particles are known to migrate into lymphatics and have been shown in the contralateral lymphatics of the larynx using routine histological sectioning (Ellis *et al.*, 1987). Recent concerns about the long-term consequences of injected Teflon, particularly in North America, cast doubt as to whether Teflon injection remains a satisfactory technique but many laryngologists have used it over the last 30 years and in the author's experience the main problems have been related to poor injection technique with over-injection into the subglottic tissues and the vocal fold itself, with further deterioration of the voice and airway. The injection must be done accurately and conservatively and little is lost by under-injecting and performing a second injection at a later date.

Steroids

Synthetic corticosteroid suspensions have been injected into the glottis to treat a variety of conditions such as inflammatory lesions, granulomas and rheumatoid arthritis of the cricoarytenoid joints. The results are variable but the collagen injector device provides the best method for injection, giving excellent control of the amount of steroid.

Medialization laryngoplasty

Unilateral vocal fold paralysis, vocal fold atrophy, and sulcus vocalis are the main indications for medialization laryngoplasty. Unilateral vocal fold paralysis is by far the most common indication. Isshiki's work in the 1970s outlined the reasons for performing this type of laryngeal framework surgery in order to improve dysphonia by indirectly altering the position, shape and tension of the vocal folds (Isshiki, 1980). Isshiki's classical type 1 thyroplasty involves displacing the paralysed vocal fold medially by means of

medial displacement of a small rectangular musculo-cartilaginous flap of thyroid cartilage with attached periosteum and thyroarytenoid muscle. The thyroid cartilage is exposed through a small transverse incision and the point midway between the superior notch and inferior border is identified and marked. A horizontal line is then drawn across the ala parallel to its inferior border beginning 5–6 mm from the midline. The window measures 5 mm by 12 mm in men and 4 mm by 10 mm in women. This window should be no closer to the midline, so as to avoid entering the larynx at the anterior commissure. The rectangular window is created in the thyroid cartilage using a fine perforating burr and completed using small periosteal elevators. Care is taken to avoid damaging the highly vascular inner perichondrium. This procedure can be difficult when the cartilage is highly calcified but once freely mobilized the window can be pressed inwards and the inner perichondrium undermined around the periphery of the window to obtain satisfactory mobilization and gain space for inserting a silastic plug. On average the cartilage is advanced inward to a distance approximately equal to the thickness of the thyroid ala and the results are monitored with a flexible fibreoptic endoscope attached to a video monitor. The mobilized window may be depressed medially in several different locations while the patient is asked to phonate.

This now classical operative procedure has been modified by many subsequent authors and a variety of silastic inserts of varying shapes and other materials have been advocated. It is to be hoped that modern methods of assessing the aerodynamics, acoustics and stroboscopic imaging dynamics of the larynx will be reported in a definitive manner, so that the various thyroplasties at present advocated can be reviewed to find which produces the optimum results.

Arytenoid adduction

Arytenoid adduction is the procedure of choice when the glottic aperture is wider as previously outlined in the unilateral adductor palsy group. The immobile vocal fold may be at a higher level posteriorly in the area of the vocal process. The condition also occurs in abductor paralysis due to rotational motion around the long axis of the cricoarytenoid joint. It is a technically more difficult procedure but involves rotating the arytenoid cartilage by pulling the muscular process in the direction of the force of the adductor muscle, bringing the tip of the vocal process towards the midline. It is also best performed under a combination of preoperative sedation and local anaesthesia in the same way as thyroplasty, but the skin incision is extended laterally several centimetres to expose the posterior edge of the thyroid ala. The thyropharyngeus component of the inferior constrictor muscle is exposed and vertically sectioned along the posterior edge of the thyroid cartilage. The cricothyroid joint is dislocated and the posterior edge of the thyroid ala is reflected anteromedially. The mucosa of the pyriform sinus is elevated upwards. The location of the muscular process is identified by palpation of the upper rim of the cricoid cartilage anterosuperiorly and the cricoarytenoid joint is opened laterally. The muscular process is pulled anteromedioinferiorly with a 3 0 nylon suture, which is then fixed to the thyroid ala through two small drilled holes. The holes are made near the junction of the anterior third and lower quarter of the thyroid ala. The necessary tension on the sutures is determined by phonation and monitored by a flexible fibreoptic endoscope.

Arytenoidectomy for bilateral abductor paralysis

This procedure was first used by veterinary surgeons in the 19th century on race horses with unilateral cord palsies. Ivanoff (1913) undertook the first human arytenoidectomy. King (1939) described an extralaryngeal approach to move the arytenoid and affected cord laterally and attach it to a severed omohyoid muscle and the thyroid ala. Woodman (1946) modified this procedure by excising the arytenoid and suturing the residual vocal process to the inferior cornua of the thyroid cartilage. This latter operation became popular during the following 30 years but is associated with variable results with respect to voice and airway and complications of infection and stenosis.

Arytenoidectomy can also be accomplished via a laryngofissure or lateral thyrotomy approach, combined with lateral cord mobilization and fixation. The thyroidotomy approach allows good access to the arytenoid and a submucosal dissection.

Endolaryngeal arytenoidectomy was first described by Thornell in 1949 and, like the other procedures, gives variable results. It can be a difficult operation to perform with microsurgical instruments but can now be carried out bloodlessly and precisely using the CO_2 laser. It may be combined with partial or complete cordectomy using the laser.

Cordectomy for bilateral abductor paralysis

Since the early part of this century various open and endoscopic methods of cordectomy have been advocated but variable results and, in particular, granulation formation have made surgeons wary of the procedure. With the advent of the CO_2 laser the endoscopic operation is precise and quick to perform and may be combined with arytenoidectomy. Removal of the posterior half of one vocal fold and the anterior two-thirds of the arytenoid gives a good compromise between voice and airway. The operation is completed in a bloodless field and is associated with minimal postoperative oedema and granulation formation. The inpatient stay is very short and more tissue can easily be removed at a second endoscopy if necessary. The operation can be undertaken in those patients who have a compromised airway but who have so far managed without a tracheostomy, and is the author's treatment of choice.

Reinnervation procedures

In 1927 Colledge and Ballance demonstrated in monkeys, baboons and a single human patient that bilateral recurrent nerve damage could be repaired by anastomosis of the phrenic nerve to the recurrent laryngeal nerve. This resulted in abduction of the vocal fold in quiet respiration with an adequate airway. Crumley (1982) has described splitting the phrenic nerve to anastomose to the recurrent nerve giving respiratory abduction of the vocal fold while preserving diaphragmatic motion. This procedure deserves further evaluation but the nerve–muscle pedicle technique first reported in humans by Tucker in 1976 has not produced good results in many other surgeons' hands. This latter technique involves transferring a portion of the sternohyoid muscle with its nerve supply from the ansa cervicalis into the posterior cricoarytenoid muscle to try to produce reinnervation and movement.

References

AOKI, F. Y., TYRELL, D. A. J., HILL, L. E. and TURNER, G. S. (1975) Immunogeniatry and acceptability of human diploid-cell culture rabies vaccine in volunteers. *Lancet*, i, 660

ARNOLD. G. E. (1955) Vocal rehabilitation of paralytic dysphonia: I. Cartilage injection into a paralyzed vocal cord. *Archives of Otolaryngology*, **62**, 1–17

ARNOLD. G. E. (1962) Vocal rehabilitation of paralytic dysphonia: VII. Paralysis of the superior laryngeal nerve. *Archives of Otolaryngology*, **75**, 549–570

AYCOCK, W. L. and LUTHER, E. H. (1929) The occurrence of poliomyelitis following tonsillectomy. *New England Journal of Medicine*, **200**, 164

BROOKES, G. B. and MCKELVIE, P. (1983) Epiglottopexy: a new surgical technique to prevent intractable aspiration. *Annals of the Royal College of Surgeons of England*, **65**, 293–296

BRÜNINGS, W. (1911) Uber eine neue Behandlungsmethode der Rekurrenslahmung. *Verhandlungender Deutschen Laryngolischen Gesellschaft*, **18**, 93–151

BLITZER, A., BRIN, M. F., FAHN, S., LANGE, D. and LOVELACE, R. E. (1986) Botulinum toxin (BOTOX) for the treatment of 'spastic dysphonia' as part of a trial of toxin injection for the treatment of other cranial dystonias. *Laryngoscope*, **96**, 1300–1301

COHEN, A. (1969) *Textbook of Medical Virology*. Philadelphia: Lippincott

COLLEDGE, L. and BALLANCE, C. (1927) Surgical treatment of paralysis of vocal cord and of paralysis of diaphragm. *British Medical Journal*, 1, 609–612

CRUMLEY, R. L. (1982) Experiments in laryngeal reinnervaton. *Laryngoscope*, 92, 530–536

DEDO, H. (1970) The paralyzed larynx. An electromyographic study in dogs and humans. *Laryngoscope*, 80, 1455–1519

DEDO, H. (1976) Recurrent laryngeal nerve section for spastic dysphonia. *Annals of Otology, Rhinology and Laryngology*, 85, 451–459

DEDO, H., URREA, R. D. and LAWSON, L. (1973) Intracordal injection of Teflon in treatment of 135 patients with dysphonia. *Annals of Otology, Rhinology and Laryngology*, 82, 661–667

DROUHET, V., DEBRE, R. and CELERS, J. (1970) Laboratory diagnosis of enterovirus infections. Poliomyelitis: pathophysiology, and poliomyelitis: prophylaxis. In: *Clinical Virology*, edited by R. Debre and J. Celers. Philadelphia: W. B. Saunders. pp. 69–79

ELLIS, J. C., MCCAFFREY, T. V., DESANTO, L. W. and REIMAN, H. V. (1987) Migration of Teflon after vocal cord injection. *Otolaryngology – Head and Neck Surgery*, 96, 63–66

FELTKAMP, T. E. W., VAN DEN BERG-LOONEN, P. M., NIJENHUIS, L. E., ENGLEFIRET, C. P., VAN ROSUN, J. J. and OOSTERHUIS, H. J. G. H. (1974) Myasthenia gravis, auto antibodies and HL-A antigens. *British Medical Journal*, 1, 131

FRITZE, D., HERMANN, C., NAIEM, F., SMITH, G. S. and WALFORD, R. L. (1974) HL-A antigens in myasthenia gravis. *Lancet*, i, 240

GROSSMAN, M. (1897) Experimentelle Beitrage zur Lehre von der 'Posticuslahmung'. *Archiv für Laryngologie und Rhinologie*, 6, 282

HOWARD, D. J. and LUND, V. J. (1986) Endoscopic surgery in otolaryngology. *British Medical Bulletin*, 42, 234–239

ISSHIKI, N. (1980) Recent advances in phonosurgery. *Folia Phoniatrica*, 32, 119–154

IVANOFF, A. (1913) Excision of the arytenoid cartilage in laryngeal stenosis. *Ushni Gorlov i Nosov Bollezn*, 5, 1067

KING, B. T. (1939) New and function restoring operation for bilateral abductor cord paralysis: preliminary report. *Journal of the American Medical Association*, 112, 814–823

KOUFMAN, J. A. and BLALOCK, P. D. (1991) Functional voice disorders. *Otolaryngologic Clinics of North America*, 24, 1059–1073

MACGREGOR, F. B., ROBERTS, D. N., HOWARD, D. J. and PHELPS, P. D. (1994) Vocal fold palsy: a reevaluation of investigations. *Journal of Laryngology and Otology*, 108, 193–196

MEURMAN, Y. (1952) Operative medio fixation of the vocal cord in complete unilateral paralysis. *Archives of Otolaryngology*, 55, 544–553

MONTGOMERY, W. W. (1979) Laryngeal paralysis Teflon injection. *Annals of Otology, Rhinology and Laryngology*, 88, 647–657

PAUL, J. R. (1971) *A History of Poliomyelitis*. New Haven: Yale University Press

PAYR, E. (1915) Plastik am schildknorpel zur behebung der folgen einseitiger stimmbandlahmung. *Deutsche medizinische Wochenschrift*, 43, 1265–1270

SAWASHINA, M., TOTSUKA, G., KOBAYASHI, T. and HIROSE, H. (1968) Reconstructive surgery for hoarseness due to unilateral vocal cord paralysis. *Archives of Otolaryngology*, 87, 289–294

SEMON, F. (1881) Clinical remarks on the proclivity of the abductor fibres of the recurrent laryngeal nerve to become affected sooner than the adductor fibres, or even exclusively, in cases of undoubted central or peripheral injury or disease of the roots or trunks of the pneumogastric, spinal accessory or recurrent nerves. *Archives of Laryngology*, 2, 197

STELL, P. M. and MARAN, A. G. D. (1978) *Head and Neck Surgery*, 2nd edn. London: William Heinemann Medical Books. pp. 194–204

THORNELL, W. C. (1949) New intralaryngeal approach in arytenoidectomy in bilateral abductor paralysis of vocal cords: a report of three cases. *Transactions of the American Academy of Ophthalmology and Otolaryngology*, 54, 631–636

TUCKER, H. M. (1976) Human laryngeal reinnervation. *Laryngoscope*, 86, 769–779

TUCKER, H. M. (1979) Laryngeal framework surgery in the management of spasmodic dysphonia. Preliminary report. *Annals of Otology, Rhinology and Laryngology*, 98, 52–54

VON LEDEN, H. (1991) The history of phonosurgery. In: *Phonosurgery: Assessment and Management of Voice Disorders*, edited by C. N. Ford and D. M. Bless. New York: Raven Press. pp. 3–24

WAGNER, R. (1890) Die Medianstellung der Stimmbander bei der Rekurrenslahmung. *Archiv für pathologische Anatomie und Physiologie*, 210, 124–127

WARD, P. H., HANSON, D. G. and ABEMAYEOR, E. (1985) Transcutaneous Teflon injection of the paralyzed vocal cord: a new technique. *Laryngoscope*, 95, 644–649

WHO EXPERT COMMITTEE ON RABIES (1966) *World Health Organization Technical Report Series no. 321*. Geneva: World Health Organization

WIKTOR, T. J., PLOTKIN, S. A. and GRELLA, D. W. (1973) Human cell culture rabies vaccine. Antibody response in man. *Journal of the American Medical Association*, 224, 1170

WILLIAMS, A. F. (1951) Nerve supply of laryngeal muscles. *Journal of Laryngology and Otology*, 65, 343–348

WILSON, C. P. and MCALPINE, D. (1946) Glossopharyngeal neuralgia treated by transtonsillar section of the nerve. *Proceedings of the Royal Society of Medicine*, 40, 81

WOODMAN, D. G. (1946) A modification of the extralaryngeal approach in arytenoidectomy for bilateral abductor paralysis. *Archives of Otolaryngology*, 48, 63–65

WYKE, B. D. and KIRSCHNER, J. A. (1976) Larynx-neurology. In: *Scientific Foundations of Otolaryngology*. London: William Heinemann Medical Books. pp. 546–574

10

Pharyngeal pouches

D. A. Bowdler

An acquired diverticulum is a circumscribed pouch caused by the protrusion of mucosa through the muscle layers of the wall of an organ. A congenital diverticulum, such as a Meckel's diverticulum, is much rarer and is covered by all the muscle layers of the wall of the viscus.

Oesophageal diverticula are well documented and are divided, according to their supposed aetiology, into traction and pulsion diverticula. However, the aetiology still remains uncertain and controversial and they have been redefined on anatomical grounds into three groups: pharyngo-oesophageal, middle or thoracic, and lower or epiphrenic diverticula.

Pharyngo-oesophageal diverticula may be congenital or acquired, multiple or single, and sited laterally, or posteriorly. The majority arise above the cricopharyngeus muscle, including the posterior pharyngeal pulsion diverticulum which is most frequently encountered, and are actually therefore pharyngeal, but a few arise below and are oesophageal in origin. They are relatively uncommon lesions, carcinoma and benign strictures being the main causes of dysphagia. While they may present at any age, most diverticula present in later life, which suggests an acquired rather than congenital origin and they may cause severe dysphagia, malnutrition and pulmonary disease but are normally curable unless complicated by carcinoma.

Embryology and anatomy

In order to understand the classification, it is necessary to review the embryology and anatomy. During development there are six branchial arches, each consisting of a cartilaginous bar surrounded by mesoderm. The skeleton of the mandible, pharynx and larynx is derived from these bars, and the muscles differentiate from the mesoderm. An artery and cranial nerve supply each arch. Depressions between the arches are lined by endoderm internally and are called pouches and, on the external surface, are lined by ectoderm and called clefts.

The fifth pouch regresses during development. The remaining four pouches, except the first, grow laterally dividing into a dorsal and ventral component, which contribute to the structures of the head, neck and mediastinum. Meanwhile the ectoderm of the second arch grows caudally, covering the lower arches and clefts, eventually joining the skin distal to the last arch. The enclosed ectoderm then disappears, though persistence of it can give rise to a cervical sinus or branchial cyst.

The three constrictor muscles develop from splanchnic mesoderm which migrates around the pharynx, but they are partially deficient anterolaterally where the neurovascular bundle to each branchial arch enters the pharynx. The constrictor muscles overlap each other like a stack of plastic cups, the superior lying innermost, and the inferior outermost, and all insert into a posterior midline raphe. The superior constrictor muscle arises from the lower two-thirds of the posterior border of the pterygoid plate to the tip of the hamulus, from where its origin continues, arising from the pterygomandibular raphe and the mandible, at a point above the mylohyoid line, level with the third molar tooth. It inserts posterosuperiorly into the pharyngeal tubercle and below into the median raphe to the level of the vocal cords. A gap lies above the superior constrictor through which the eustachian tube passes. The middle constrictor muscle arises from the greater cornu and the angle with the lesser cornu of the hyoid bone before fanning out to insert into the posterior midline raphe, superiorly as high as the pharyngeal tubercle and inferiorly to the level of the vocal cords. The neurovascular bundle of the second arch, of which the nerve is the glossopharyngeal, passes through the gap which remains between the superior and middle constrictors, and is related to the tonsil medially.

The inferior constrictor muscle is described in two parts, the thyropharyngeus and the cricopharyngeus. The thyropharyngeus arises from an oblique line on the thyroid ala and a fibrous arch between the thyroid and cricoid cartilages, its upper fibres overlapping the superior and middle constrictors as they pass postero-superiorly, its lowest fibres lying edge to edge with the cricopharyngeus. The gap between the middle and inferior constrictors, which is bounded anteriorly by the thyrohyoid muscle, lies over the pyriform fossa and is pierced by the third arch neurovascular bundle, of which the nerve is the superior laryngeal. The term Killian's dehiscence was coined following the finding that the thyropharyngeus was unsupported by the other constrictor muscles below the level of the vocal cords and above the cricopharyngeus.

The cricopharyngeus muscle is thicker and bulkier than the thyropharyngeus passing from one side of the cricoid to the other, around the back of the pharynx. The sixth neurovascular bundle, of which the nerve is the recurrent laryngeal, enters the pharynx laterally under the lower border of cricopharyngeus and above the circular fibres of the oesophagus, and is a relatively weak point described as the Killian–Jamieson area.

The circular fibres of the oesophageal musculature lie below and parallel to the cricopharyngeus, while the longitudinal muscles sweep forward to insert into the cricoid cartilage, leaving another relatively weak posterior triangle, known as the Laimer–Hackermann area. It is also of clinical importance that the oesophagus is not exactly midline at this point, tending to veer to the left, as posterior pharyngeal pulsion diverticula usually present on the left.

The motor supply to the constrictor muscles arises from the pharyngeal branch of the vagus nerve, which forms a plexus on the middle constrictor. The cricopharyngeus muscle is an exception and may be supplied by the recurrent laryngeal and external laryngeal nerves. The sensory supply of the pharynx is via the glossopharyngeal nerve, the internal laryngeal nerve and the recurrent laryngeal nerve.

In summary, several relatively weak areas exist through which mucosal bulges or diverticula may develop (Figures 10.1 and 10.2).

Lateral

1 Above the superior constrictor
2 Between the superior and middle constrictors
3 Between the middle and inferior constrictors
4 Below cricopharyngeus – Killian–Jamieson's area.

Posterior

5 Laimer–Hackermann's area
6 Killian's dehiscence.

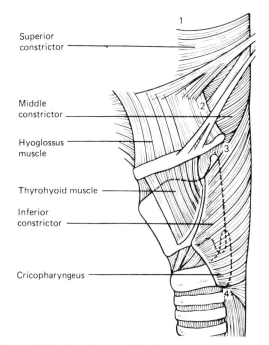

Figure 10.1 A lateral view of the pharynx demonstrating the weak areas which are indicated: (1) above the superior constrictor; (2) between the superior and middle constrictors; (3) between the middle and inferior constrictors; (4) below cricopharyngeus – Killian–Jamieson's area

Classification

Classifications have been based on developmental, anatomical and aetiological grounds (Korkis, 1958; Wilson, 1962). Hurst (1925) described an anterior pharyngeal diverticulum but later retracted his findings recognizing that it was an overdeveloped or deep vallecula. The classification given in Table 10.1 is based primarily on anatomical site, and then subdivided by aetiology.

Lateral pouches

Lateral pharyngeal diverticula are uncommon and can be divided into congenital and acquired, a distinction which is obvious when occurring at the extremes of age, but is controversial in those patients presenting in early adult life. In the literature, congenital lateral pharyngeal diverticula are reported soon after birth and present with complications early in infancy, making it unlikely that they would remain undetected until adulthood or old age, while in most patients presenting in early adult life there are clear predisposing factors. They arise from the posterior faucial pillar and the upper or lower pyriform fossae, and are

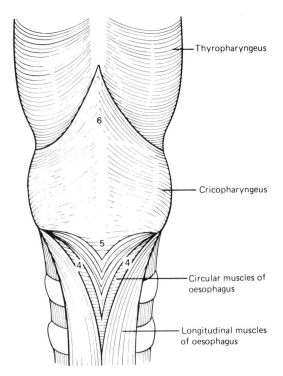

Thyropharyngeus

Cricopharyngeus

Circular muscles of
oesophagus

Longitudinal muscles
of oesophagus

Figure 10.2 A posterior view of the pharyngo-oesophageal
segment which shows: (5) Laimer–Hackermann's area; (6)
Killian's dehiscence

Table 10.1 Classification of pharyngeal diverticula

Lateral
1	Congenital		
2	Acquired	a	normal bulges
		b	traumatic
		c	raised intrapharyngeal pressure 'pharyngocoeles'

Posterior
1	Congenital		
2	Acquired	a	traumatic
		b	raised intrapharyngo-oesophageal pressure
		c	posterior pharyngeal pulsion diverticulum (Zenker's diverticulum)

normally been attributed to branchial cleft remnants
which communicate internally, usually in association
with the second cleft, though also with the third and
fourth clefts.

Burge and Middleton argued that they are
branchial pouch derivatives based on three findings.
First, all nine patients presented with a lesion on the
left side of the neck, and often the ultimobranchial
body growth on the right is diminished or absent.
Second, they suggested that the histological finding
of Hassal's corpuscles and thyroid tissue in the operative specimens indicates pouch origin, though Hassals
corpuscles are found in lymphoid tissue and the
thyroid could have been trimmed along with the
tract. Finally, in following the tract they felt that it
passed between the recurrent laryngeal and external
laryngeal nerves and therefore was of fourth pouch
origin. Whatever the true explanation, it seems certain that these rare diverticula are the result of a
developmental defect in some part of the branchial
apparatus.

All patients presented in the first two decades of
life, and in the majority there was a history of recurrent infected swellings in the neck, often having been
treated previously with antibiotics or incision and
drainage. The signs are a tender fluctuant swelling in
the anterior triangle of the neck, pyrexia, mild dysphagia and occasionally mild stridor. In one patient
the diverticulum was discovered because it was repeatedly intubated in error during an anaesthetic shortly
after birth.

Plain radiographs of the neck usually show air in
the diverticulum, but the lesion can be more effectively demonstrated by a contrast swallow using high
density barium. Once the acute episode has settled
with antibiotics or by incision and drainage, the
treatment is excision of the diverticulum and tract to
the pharynx where the neck is oversewn.

Acquired

Argument about the aetiology of acquired lateral
pharyngeal diverticula still continues. Some consider
the basic defect to be a congenital weakness and so
classify these diverticula as congenital, but the potential weak areas are present in all persons, with the
variable or precipitating factor being raised intrapharyngeal pressure, or muscular laxity in association
with ageing. These diverticula do not seem to occur
in the absence of such a predisposing factor and are
usually found in patients well into adult life, supporting the argument that they are acquired lesions.

Normal bulges

Frequent and incidental findings on routine barium
swallows are small lateral pharyngeal bulges which
can be seen either arising in the pyriform fossa or

best observed by frontal contrast enhanced cineradiography while being emphasized by raised intrapharyngeal pressure, achieved clinically by performing a
modified Valsalva manoeuvre.

Congenital

Congenital lateral pharyngeal diverticula are
extremely rare, with only a few reported in the
literature (Burge and Middleton, 1983). They have

more rarely the tonsillar fossa while performing a modified Valsalva manoeuvre (Bachman, Seaman and Macken, 1968). They are more common in the elderly, probably due to reduced muscular tone and loss of elasticity of the tissues, and they are usually asymptomatic and bilateral, which is the reason they are thought by many to be normal variants.

Those diverticula which arise through Killian–Jamieson's area can probably be included in this subdivision, though it has been suggested that these cases may account for those supposed Zenker's diverticula that present with hoarseness, due to their proximity to the recurrent laryngeal nerve. However, any large pouch will lie close to the nerve which casts doubt on this supposition. In any event it is difficult to believe that such differentiation is of any clinical significance.

Radiological contrast studies demonstrate the bulges as smooth, hemispherical prominences arising from the pyriform fossa or tonsillar fossa, the appearance lending itself to the name pharyngeal 'ears' (Figure 10.3). These are largest when a modified Valsalva manoeuvre is performed (blowing hard against pursed lips), often collapsing down to a normal pharyngeal contour under normal pressure, and most easily seen on frontal views. At this stage they require no treatment, but it has been postulated

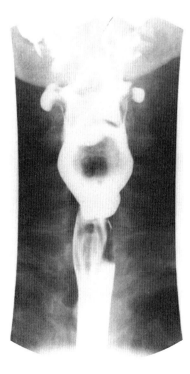

Figure 10.3 A barium swallow demonstrating prominent bulges from both the tonsillar and pyriform fossae

that they represent an early stage in the evolution of larger symptomatic diverticula.

Traumatic

Atkinson (1952) reported the findings of Colonel M. Morris (late RAMC), in certain nomadic groups of habitual criminals from the Central and United Provinces of India, who presented with self-inflicted diverticula. These were produced by the repetitive introduction of a piece of lead, the size of a pigeon's egg, into the tonsillar fossa creating a diverticulum that could be kept patent with a finger and in which coins or jewellery could be hidden, and recovered when required, by tilting the head forwards and effecting a vomiting motion. The diverticulum probably lies between the middle and superior constrictors, and if not maintained, disappears rapidly.

Raised intrapharyngeal pressure (pharyngocoeles)

These large and occasionally symptomatic diverticula may arise from precursor pharyngeal 'ears'. Their development is probably either due to frequent repetitive increase in intrapharyngeal pressure or from loss of muscular resilience associated particularly with advancing years, or perhaps both. The diverticula protrude through one of the weak areas in the lateral pharyngeal wall and develop into pouches with obvious necks that are sometimes called 'pharyngocoeles'.

A pharyngocoele was first described by Wheeler (1886), in a patient who had been in the army and took considerable pride in his ability to command a full brigade on the parade ground with his own voice. He had both a pharyngocoele and a Zenker's diverticulum, the latter causing hoarseness and so threatening his career! Pharyngocoeles were also noted in Egyptian muezzins who sang verses of the Koran from the minarets of mosques. Many developed pharyngocoeles which became so marked, that special collars or neck trusses were required to restrain them. These diverticula while usually unilateral have been found bilaterally and though usually symptomatic are not generally severely distressing. They affect men more commonly than women in a ratio of 8:1. Those occurring in younger patients normally have a predisposing factor such as playing wind instruments, or violent sneezing and coughing (Norris, 1979), but in the older age group the main reason is probably simply laxity of the musculature. In both groups there would appear to be an intrinsic weakness in the lateral wall, as suggested by the anatomy, a fact of which the nomadic criminals, described by Colonel Morris, took full advantage!

Symptoms may develop due to food entrapment in the diverticulum, and are insidious in onset, so that the patient presents with long-standing problems. The main symptom is dysphagia which is usually intermittent and mild, though occasionally it may become severe. Sometimes there is regurgitation of undigested food, with associated foul taste and foetor, which in addition may lead to nocturnal coughing and choking. Dysphonia results from the effects of spillage into the larynx, though some suggest this is due to compression of the recurrent laryngeal nerve by the pouch. Chronic pulmonary problems may be the first hint of the condition.

Signs are scarce, but just anterior to the sternomastoid muscle, there may be a palpable lump, which is soft, compressible and which may gurgle due to a mixture of air and fluid within the diverticulum. Indirect laryngoscopy shows little, though a slit-like ostium may be observed in the region of the posterior faucial pillar or the upper part of the pyriform fossa. The diverticulum can usually be inflated voluntarily by the patient blowing against closed lips in a modified Valsalva manoeuvre.

Plain radiographs may show the diverticulum as a transluscency, lateral to the pyriform fossa, however the mainstays of diagnosis are cine or videofluoroscopic techniques, using high density barium which coats the mucosa more effectively and is retained longer. The patient is asked to take a small amount of contrast medium and then to perform a modified Valsalva manoeuvre to emphasize the diverticulum. It will be seen as a rounded, contrast-lined opacity communicating with the pyriform fossa or tonsillar fossa by an isthmus or neck (Figure 10.4). Ultrasound has also been used to make the diagnosis (Hayashi *et al.*, 1984). Occasionally barium studies fail to reveal the diverticulum and direct pharyngoscopy is necessary to attempt to find the slit-like opening of the diverticulum, the search being concentrated in the areas where they are known to occur, however, it can still be very easily missed.

If the diverticulum causes no symptoms, no treatment is required except for follow up. In those who develop troublesome symptoms, the diverticulum should be excised through an external approach. The diverticulum is followed through the cervical region to its opening into the pharynx, amputated at its neck and the pharyngeal mucosa oversewn. Postoperatively it is advisable to feed the patient by nasogastric tube for 3–5 days to diminish the risk of fistula formation and ensure healing.

Posterior pouches

Posterior pharyngeal diverticula are far more common than lateral pharyngeal diverticula, with the posterior pharyngeal pulsion diverticulum or Zenker's diverticulum being the one most frequently encountered.

Congenital

Congenital posterior pharyngeal diverticula are very rare and were first described in two infants who

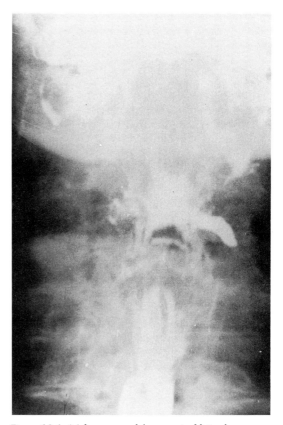

Figure 10.4 A 'pharyngocoele' or acquired lateral pharyngeal diverticulum shown by a barium swallow study (by kind permission of Dr P. Phelps)

developed symptoms similar to oesophageal atresia soon after birth (Britnall and Kridelbaugh, 1950). A further case has been reported with an almost identical history, with clinical, radiological and surgical evidence all suggesting the presence of a congenital posterior pharyngeal diverticulum (MacKellar and Kennedy, 1972). Radiological evidence of air in the stomach, in the absence of a tracheo-oesophageal fistula, confirms oesophageal patency. The diverticulum arises from above the cricopharyngeus and is lined by normal pharyngeal mucosa, distinguishing it histologically from a traumatic pseudodiverticulum. The whole diverticulum is covered with muscle, differentiating it from an acquired pulsion diverticulum. On contrast radiological studies there is an elongated smooth walled diverticulum which lies posteriorly to the oesophagus, and extends into the posterior mediastinum. The position of the diverticulum in relation to the oesophagus differentiates it from duplication when the two lumens are closely adherent. The treatment is excision of the diverticulum to restore pharyngeal continuity.

Acquired

Traumatic pharyngeal pseudodiverticulum

This very rare condition usually presents in newborn infants (Wells *et al.*, 1974), but has been reported in adults. The aetiological factor is hypopharyngeal trauma, either from damage caused by the obstetrician's finger during breech delivery or blind passage of suction tubes and endotracheal tubes, though in one of the adult patients the cause was spontaneous rupture of a retropharyngeal abscess in an immunosuppressed patient (Morton, 1983). The hypopharyngeal mucosal tear may be either transmural or submucosal, the former causing more severe symptoms, due to a false passage tracking down into the posterior mediastinum within the prevertebral space. Cricopharyngeal spasm precipitates the early symptoms of increasing dysphagia and excessive oropharyngeal secretions, though symptoms do not usually present until some hours after the trauma. Eventually attempts to feed cause coughing and choking due to overspill into the larynx, sometimes resulting in cyanotic episodes and, at worst, aspiration pneumonia. The patient becomes pyrexial and increasingly ill, developing symptoms and signs of mediastinitis. There may also be cervical subcutaneous emphysema. The symptoms and signs mimic other conditions including oesophageal atresia, oesophageal duplication, and congenital posterior pharyngeal diverticulum, though a clear antecedent history helps to distinguish it from the above conditions.

An initial plain abdominal radiograph may show air in the stomach which excludes oesophageal atresia. An attempt is then made to pass a radiolucent nasogastric tube and, if aspiration reveals gastric contents, retrograde contrast studies are performed up to the pharynx to delineate the pouch. If a nasogastric tube cannot be passed into the stomach, contrast material is injected down the tube at the pharyngeal level which should demonstrate the diverticulum, or alternatively the patient sucks a contrast material feed. However, with the two latter methods, there is a considerable risk of inhalation and worsening of the pulmonary condition.

The radiological appearance of a traumatic pharyngeal pseudodiverticulum is an irregular elongated tract originating in the pharynx and passing behind the oesophagus into the posterior mediastinum (Figure 10.5).

The treatment is not clearly defined, but whatever, it should be rapidly instituted upon diagnosis. If a nasogastric tube can be passed safely and the general condition of the patient is stable, conservative management with intravenous antibiotics and nutritional support is suggested. However, if any deterioration in the general condition of the patient develops, surgical drainage of the pseudodiverticulum either via a cervi-

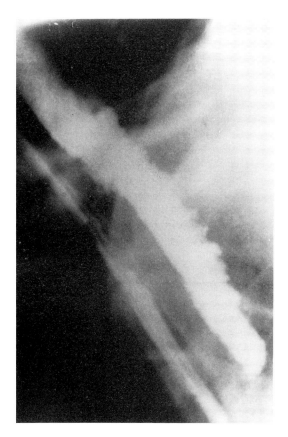

Figure 10.5 A barium study demonstrating the irregular and elongated contour of a pharyngeal pseudodiverticulum. (By kind permission of Mr R.P. Morton and the Editor, *Journal of Laryngology and Otology*, 1983, **97**, 79–83)

cal incision or a thoracotomy is indicated, at which time it is usual to perform a gastrostomy for nutritional support. Antibiotic cover is continued. The excised track shows fibrous or inflammatory tissue rather than epithelium.

Diverticulum resulting from raised intrapharyngo-oesophageal pressure

This rare diverticulum protrudes through the Laimer–Hackermann area, and presents in older people, again probably due to weakness of the musculature. It is probably more common than reported as it is always asymptomatic, requiring no treatment. Being asymptomatic such diverticula are noted endoscopically or radiologically and vary in size depending on the position of the peristaltic wave (Ekberg and Nylander, 1983). Some authors discount their existence altogether.

Posterior pharyngeal pulsion diverticulum (Zenker's diverticulum)

History

The posterior pharyngeal pulsion diverticulum is known by many names including pharyngo-oesophageal pouch or diverticulum, retropharyngeal pouch or diverticulum, posterior pharyngeal pouch or diverticulum, and Zenker's diverticulum.

The first case was described by Mr A. Ludlow, a surgeon from Bristol, in 1764 in a letter to Dr William Hunter of the Society of Physicians in London. His report was published in *Medical Observations and Inquiries* in 1769, and his description of the symptoms and morbid anatomy closely mirrors our present knowledge (Ludlow, 1769). The treatment consisted of swallowing weighted threads, attempted passage of whalebone bougies and ingesting mercury, but all failed to save the patient! The post-mortem examination was beautifully illustrated by Jan Van Rymsdyk and showed a pouch lying between the oesophagus and vertebral column originating from the posterior pharyngeal wall.

Early classifications of oesophageal diverticula by Zenker called this type 'pulsion diverticula'. Zenker and Von Ziemssen (1878) reviewed 22 cases between 1764 and 1876, in addition to five of their own, and gave an accurate account of the symptoms and also suggested the possible pathogenesis. Many early commentators thought that these diverticula arose between the upper oesophagus and the inferior constrictor via the Laimier–Hackerman area, despite Zenker's anatomical description.

Early suggestions about the aetiology included foreign body impaction. Sir Charles Bell (1817) suggested that the cause was ineffectual swallowing attempts leading to pharyngeal distension, while Killian felt that the cause was spasmodic contraction of the circular fibres at the upper end of the oesophagus. It is perhaps interesting to note that diverticula occur normally in some animals including pigs, camels and elephants.

Early treatment was palliative. The mainstay of treatment was dilatation of the cricopharyngeus with bougies and nutritional support through stomach tubes or, if there was total dysphagia, via a gastrostomy. Faradism was used to stimulate emptying of the sac and some claimed success but, in view of the lack of muscle coat, this must be viewed with scepticism.

Direct surgical intervention was suggested as early as 1864, and the first operation was performed in 1877 by incising the diverticulum and bringing it out to the skin, however the patient died 8 days postoperatively of bronchopneumnia. The first excision of a diverticulum was performed in 1884 but the patient died from a massive haemorrhage after 24 hours. The first successful excision was carried out by Wheeler in 1886 which was followed by other reports over the next decade, though the mortality rate was high and most patients developed a fistula.

In 1910 Stetten reviewed the literature and of 48 patients treated by excision of the pouch, nine had died, a mortality rate of 18.7%, furthermore, the primary healing rate was only 42%. Due to the high mortality and morbidity alternative techniques were sought. Girard (1896) invaginated the pouch into the oesophagus and this was later modified in the Sippy Bevan technique which used several purse string sutures along the length of the pouch to reduce it to a stump. In 1909 Goldmann described a two-stage technique which was modified and subsequently used by Lahey (1954) who was the staunchest advocate of this technique. Schmid (1912) described a diverticulopexy which was taken up by others, but this technique never gained wide acceptance. An endoscopic method with division of the party wall with scissors was devised by Mosher (1917) but, after a fatality from haemorrhage, he abandoned the technique, though it was later repopularized by Dohlman (1949). Since the advent of antibiotics the two-stage procedure has been largely superceded by one-stage excision of the diverticulum.

In more recent years the treatment has been focused on the suspected cause as well as the effect, and cricopharyngeal myotomy has been strongly advocated (Lichter, 1978). While the Dohlman technique divides the muscle as part and parcel of the method, it still leaves the pouch and thus the attendant risk of a carcinoma developing later. For this reason, as well as the higher recurrence rate and need for multiple procedures, it is not popular in the UK or North America.

More recently the treatment has again been modified by the use of stapling guns during excision, and the carbon dioxide laser for endoscopic treatment, as well as inversion of the pouch instead of excision. However, despite all the surgical advances in the relief of symptoms, the aetiology of the condition remains uncertain.

Mechanism of swallowing

Swallowing is a complex mechanism by which a bolus is passed from the mouth to the pharynx, and then into the oesophagus, in a quick, coordinated fashion. The shortest phase is the pharyngeal, or second stage of swallowing, lasting less than a second. The mechanism of the second stage begins as the first stage is completed with the bolus being injected into the oropharynx. The larynx is elevated with the hyoid to lie under the mandible and base of the tongue and the aryepiglottic folds contract to complete closure of the larynx, already closed at the glottic level due to adductor contraction. The epiglottis is inverted by the bolus passing down the pharynx, and the pharynx is elevated over the bolus simultaneously. A pharyngeal peristaltic or stripping wave then pushes the bolus down through the pharynx and cricopharyngeal sphincter, which is passively or reflexly relaxed as the second stage of swallowing begins. Most of the bolus has preceded this wave, which clears only the more solid particles.

Aetiology

The aetiology of the posterior pharyngeal pulsion diverticulum is still unknown, though many theories have been advanced. There is much conflicting evidence from investigations using anatomical, radiographic, manometric and electromyographic studies even when using the same method of study. The main theories fall into four main categories:

1 Tonic spasm of the cricopharyngeus (Negus, 1950)
2 Lack of inhibitory stimuli to the cricopharyngeus (Dohlman and Mattsson, 1959)
3 The second swallow (due to pharyngeal laxity) (Wilson, 1962)
4 Neuromuscular incoordination and congenital weakness (Korkis, 1958).

1 Negus believed that Killian's dehiscence was the result of man's evolution to an erect position, with the larynx and cricopharyngeus moving lower down the neck, causing the other constrictors to lie obliquely. The lack of posterolateral longitudinal muscles, found elsewhere in the alimentary tract, compounded this effect. As this was present in all humans, he proposed that the variable was cricopharyngeal incoordination, in particular spasm as a result of inflammation, stenosis or a neurological deficit. He proposed that the bolus was squeezed down by the pharyngeal stripping wave, where it met the sphincter in spasm so forcing mucosa through Killian's dehiscence, long-standing repetition leading to diverticulum formation. As the pouch increased in size he believed it would force the cricopharyngeus anteriorly so that the bolus would impinge more directly into the diverticulum.
2 Dohlman and Mattsson theorized that the sphincter failed to relax, rather than being in active spasm. They believed that the cricopharyngeus was normally tethered to the prevertebral fascia, but that this attachment was weakened with ageing so that, on deglutition, the larynx was elevated pulling the cricopharyngeus upwards with it rather than stretching the muscle, which would normally trigger off a reflex arc resulting in relaxation of the sphincter in readiness for the bolus. This failure of relaxation would result in increased intrapharyngeal pressure causing mucosal bulging posteriorly, which was further compounded by a negative pressure in the prevertebral space, sucking the mucosa backwards.

3 Wilson (1962) studied a group of patients with posterior pharyngeal pulsion diverticula and noted that there was a very high incidence of enlargement of the pharynx or a megapharynx. In addition he found that, following a barium contrast swallow, there was always a residue left in the pharynx. He speculated that due to pharyngeal muscular laxity, there was a weak pharyngeal stripping wave that was unable to clear the whole bolus from the pharynx before the cricopharyngeal sphincter contracted. Consequently, a second swallow was needed to try to clear the residue but this would occur against a closed sphincter resulting in a high pressure area between the stripping wave and cricopharyngeus leading to mucosal bulging posteriorly. If long standing this would allow diverticulum formation.
4 Korkis agreed with Negus that a neurological disorder was the most probable precipitating factor but that it occurred in the presence of a congenital weakness predisposing to diverticulum formation, usually in later life. He supported his argument by commenting on the congenital posterior pharyngeal diverticulum and on the reports of familial diverticula. Furthermore, he claimed that if the lesions were acquired as a result of obstruction at the level of the cricopharyngeus, then they should occur in patients with long-standing upper oesophageal stenosis or dysphagia of other causes. However, dysphagia is commoner in women than in men and diverticula are more common in men.

It is therefore necessary to consider the evidence derived from the various methods of study undertaken.

Anatomical

It is an established fact that there is an area of potential weakness in the inferoposterior part of the pharynx. However, there is contradictory evidence as to the exact site described by Killian. Perrott (1962) in a study of cadavers found several different patterns of fibre arrangement in the gap between the thyropharyngeus and cricopharyngeus, and in each individual muscle. He suggested that certain patterns, in particular where divarications occur in the cricopharyngeus leaving denuded portions, were more liable to mucosal herniation. He therefore called into question the exact site of weakness and consequently the validity of the so-called Killian's dehiscence. That some individuals may have an even greater chance of developing a diverticulum due to a congenital weakness is supported, as previously mentioned, by reports of familial diverticula.

However, the cadaveric findings are dependent on interpretation of fibre arrangements in a non-physiological state. Surgical findings are of a fairly clearly defined cricopharyngeal sphincter with the diverticulum arising above. Certainly at oesophagoscopy there seems to be a definite sphincter at the cricoid level with the opening of the pouch arising above and behind it.

Radiological

Contrast cine or video-fluoroscopy is the main method of examination of the mechanism of swallowing both of normal people and of patients with diverticula.

One of the features of contrast studies is the presence or absence of a cricopharyngeal sphincter bulge indenting the posterior wall of the pharyngo-oesophageal segment. Crichlow (1956) believed that its presence indicated a pathological condition, whereas Siebert, Stein and Poppel (1959) found it to be present even in normal asymptomatic patients. Lichter (1978) considered that, in the presence of a diverticulum, a prominent cricopharyngeal bulge was a definite indication for myotomy. However, interpretation of the findings in the presence of an abnormality is open to observer bias.

Ardran, Kemp and Lund (1964) argued that since most studies were performed in patients with established diverticula, which disturbed the normal physiology of swallowing, the results might be due to the disease and not reflect the cause. Using contrast cineradiography, they examined 16 patients with diverticula of differing sizes and 17 normal subjects. After the initial part of the swallow, the main bolus descended into the pharynx to be moved on by the pharyngeal stripping wave. In patients with diverticula they found this to be defective in two ways: first, the oropharyngeal contraction was weak or absent, and second, pharyngeal constrictor function below this level was disturbed, which together with premature cricopharyngeal closure, caused a residue to remain in the pharynx with a bulge or diverticulum forming as a result. Consequent upon their studies they proposed a mechanism of pouch formation. The cricopharyngeus contracts prematurely and the posterior wall bulges backwards. As the stripping wave descends to the closed sphincter, it pushes the posterior wall down and forwards to meet the back of the cricopharyngeal sphincter, which is facing upwards and forwards, and so a dimple is produced which might well go on to enlarge and become a diverticulum.

In some patients they noted failure of complete cricopharyngeal relaxation which led to a nipping between the sphincter and the stripping wave with a consequent bulge, which they suggested could also exacerbate diverticulum formation.

In their study they noted no megapharynges in normal subjects and only one out of 16 patients with known diverticula, which contradicts the findings of Wilson. Also, the cricovertebral distance was the same when comparing normal subjects with patients with diverticula, which does not support the Dolmann Mattsson theory.

Manometry

Using manometric techniques information about the intraluminal pressures, and therefore the actions of different muscle groups, can be investigated. Atkinson *et al.* (1957) showed that the pressure in the resting pharynx was atmospheric, with a band of high pressure (10–60 mmHg) at the cricoid level. The oesophagus had a negative resting pressure. On swallowing, a positive pressure wave passed through the pharynx (15–80 mmHg), and at the same time there was a sudden fall in the sphincter pressure and a rise in oesophageal pressure.

Fyke and Code (1955) felt that oesophageal closure was achieved by a state of tonic contraction in the cricopharyngeal sphincter at rest, but on swallowing the cricopharyngeus relaxed while a coordinated peristaltic wave pushed the bolus through the pharynx, sphincter and oesophagus. Winnans (1972) and Berlin *et al.* (1977) suggested that the cricopharyngeus acts as a pinchcock valve by demonstrating a greater pressure in an anteroposterior plane. In the presence of posterior pharyngeal pulsion diverticula, various deviations from normal have been described.

Kodicek and Creamer (1961), using open-tipped recording tubes attached to a capacitance manometer, were able to show that the cricopharyngeus relaxed normally and that there was no incoordination. Their results are supported by Hunt, Connell and Smiley (1970) who, while demonstrating a high resting cricopharyngeal pressure, showed normal relaxation of the cricopharyngeus in relation to the pharyngeal stripping wave in patients with diverticula.

However, Ellis *et al.* (1969) and later Lichter (1978) demonstrated, by manometric techniques, early cricopharyngeal closure, while Lichter also described premature relaxation of the sphincter, followed by early contraction leading to raised intrapharyngeal pressure. He did not demonstrate any weakness of pharyngeal contraction, but in some patients noted a repetitive swallowing pattern, probably as a result of the obstruction. In the same study he examined patients following surgery, all of whom had had cricopharyngeal myotomy, and demonstrated reduced resting pressures in the region of the sphincter, which led him to suggest that cricopharyngeal myotomy should be performed whenever the cricopharyngeus was noted to be prominent radiologically.

Smiley, Caves and Porter (1970) found that in 32 of 34 patients with Zenker's diverticulum, there was an associated oesophageal reflux or hiatus hernia. On studying patients with oesophageal reflux alone, they noted a high resting sphincter pressure though no incoordination of swallowing. They proposed that oesophageal reflux or hiatus hernia might well play a causal role in the formation of Zenker's diverticulum. Delahunty *et al.* (1971) confirmed these findings and Gage–White (1988) found the incidence of hiatus hernia was more than doubled in patients with diverticula compared with a control group.

Knuff, Benjamin and Castell (1982) using modern manometric techniques including a low compliance infusion system, studied nine patients with a known posterior pharyngeal pulsion diverticulum initially diagnosed by barium swallow studies. The result of their research showed normal relaxation of the cricopharyngeus which did not contract until the end of the pharyngeal stripping wave, though they found a low resting pressure in the sphincter or pharyngo-oesophageal segment, which seriously questions the theories of diverticulum formation. More recently Nilsson, Isberg and Schiratzki (1988), using cineradiography and manometry, demonstrated that there was a split between the fibres of the sphincter and also incoordination during swallowing. This is directly contradicted by Frieling *et al.* (1988) who found no disturbance of the sphincter, again using a combination of radiological and manometric studies.

Electromyography

The potential advantage of these studies is that direct information about individual muscles can be gathered. Basmajian and Dutta (1961) showed relaxation of the constrictors at rest, with contraction only occurring during the second stage of swallowing. Kawasaki and Ogura (1968) demonstrated in dogs that, due to inhibition of the muscle action potential coincident with laryngeal elevation, the pharyngo-oesophageal sphincter opens passively to allow the bolus to pass. The difficulties arise in that this method is invasive and may alter the patient's normal response or swallow. Furthermore, the results may reflect field effects and thus be invalidated. However, more information may be forthcoming by following this line of research.

Summary

Despite all the aforementioned studies, which so frequently contradict each other, the aetiology is no more certain than when Sir Charles Bell proposed his ideas in 1817. However, nearly all authors agree that there is abnormal pharyngeal function probably at the cricopharyngeal level, which is supported by the fact that dilatation gives temporary relief.

Incidence

It is difficult to quantify the incidence of pharyngeal diverticula in the general population, as not all cases are reported, and centres with a special interest in these diverticula attract patients from other areas, thus magnifying their figures in relation to population. The only report that gives figures in relation to population is from Juby (1969), who reported 17 patients in a population of 300 000 over a 12-year period, which is 0.47 cases per 100 000 persons per year. Most authors refer to numbers seen over a fixed period or relate them to hospital admissions, operations or radiographic studies. Shallow and Clerf (1948) stated an incidence of 1 in 1400 admissions, or 800 operations. MacMillan (1932) recorded finding 18 diverticula in 1000 contrast radiographs for patients with dysphagia, Baron (1982) 1 in 800 routine barium studies.

Age, sex and race

Figures for age and sex are more certain, although there is variation between different centres. A collection of some of the largest series gives a ratio of about 2.1 men to one woman. Patients are generally aged over 50 years at diagnosis but are occasionally younger. From a number of the American series it is suggested that blacks are rarely affected by this condition.

Symptoms

Patients present with symptoms of variable severity, not necessarily related to the size of their diverticulum. Though some patients present after only a few months of symptoms, most complain of long-standing problems (Huang, Unni and Payne, 1984), having adapted to the slowly progressive symptoms. Indeed, it is the insidious nature of the onset that causes most patients to present with a well-developed diverticulum. There have been attempts to stage symptoms in relation to the size of the diverticulum:

Stage I: small mucosal protrusions (the initial stage)
Stage II: a definite pouch but with the oesphagus and hypopharynx still in line (the intermediate stage)
Stage III: a large pouch with the hypopharynx in line with the neck of the diverticulum, and the oesophageal inlet pushed anteriorly.

Each stage was said to be associated with a symptom pattern: stage I, the sensation of food sticking in the throat; stage II, regurgitation and gurgling from the pouch; stage III, the development of severe dysphagia.

Different patients present with different symptom patterns but the symptoms are listed below roughly in order of their frequency.

Dysphagia

This symptom may be misinterpreted by the clinician, leading to prolonged delay before investigation. Initially the patient may complain of a sensation of a lump in the throat, which can frequently be misdiagnosed as globus hystericus. Other early symptoms are a feeling of food sticking in the throat, requiring repeated swallowing attempts. Generally, however, the story is of increasing difficulty in swallowing solids, requiring the patient to chew every mouthful down to small fragments. As the condition progresses it becomes impossible to enjoy a meal out with friends, due to the length of time taken to eat a meal, indeed eating becomes acutely embarrassing. Eventually difficulty with semisolid foods and then liquids develops. Occasionally a patient cannot swallow his own saliva, having to spit out the excessive secretions. It has been suggested that the pressure of the pouch on the upper oesophagus causes obstruction, but manometric studies have detected no change in oesophageal pressures, even with large pouches.

Regurgitation

Patients suffer from regurgitation of undigested food into their mouths, sometimes during a meal, though more often afterwards. It is exacerbated by positional change, especially lying down in bed at night. This symptom can wake the patient in the middle of the night, when spillage from the pouch causes coughing and choking. A few adapt to this by evacuating the pouch before going to bed, by pressing on the side of their neck over the diverticulum.

Associated with this symptom, the second most common after dysphagia, is a foul taste in the mouth due to the prolonged retention of undigested food. A gurgling sound on swallowing is sometimes noticed by the patient due to a mixture of air and fluid in the sac.

Weight loss

Due to dysphagia, which may be present for a considerable time before presentation, some patients present with severe weight loss and malnutrition complicating the treatment of this benign condition.

Hoarseness

Overflow of sac contents into the larynx causes chemical irritation and laryngitis. It is suggested that this can be due to the pressure of the sac on the recurrent laryngeal nerve, though this has not been effectively demonstrated. Vocal cord paralysis is more likely to be due to the presence of a carcinoma in the diverticulum.

Pulmonary complications

A serious sequel to the spillage of sac contents into the larynx is aspiration pneumonia. Pulmonary complications are well recorded with large pouches, including pneumonitis, lung abscesses, bronchiectasis

and collapse, which require treatment before surgical resection of the diverticulum.

Miscellaneous

There is usually no pain except in the presence of carcinoma. Occasionally other strange presentations occur. Bleeding has been reported from a diverticulum, due to ulceration. Also rare is a diverticulo-tracheal fistula which causes the patient to cough when eating, and leads to pulmonary complications. Resection of the tract and diverticulum cures this problem. An odd presentation was one patient's failure to respond to medication for another condition due to the tablets lodging in the sac (Baron, 1982). This was again cured by resection.

Signs

The signs include emaciation, which can be severe, though it is less common than in the past, as diverticula are usually diagnosed earlier. A soft swelling may be found in the neck, usually on the left side, in the lower part of the anterior triangle, and may gurgle on palpation (Boyce's sign). A spasm of coughing may be caused by palpation due to spillage of contents into the larynx. Indirect laryngoscopy may demonstrate laryngitis and pooling of saliva in the pyriform fossa in which undigested food particles may be seen. Very occasionally blood may be found in the regurgitated contents of a pouch suggesting the development of a carcinoma.

Investigations

While the history and the examination may be virtually pathognomonic, it is necessary to confirm the diagnosis with radiological evidence, generally contrast cine or video-fluoroscopy.

Radiography

Plain radiographs of the neck may reveal a triangular lucency in the prevertebral tissues with its apex at the level of the cricoid, due to air in the upper part of the pouch. The base of the triangle has a meniscus due to the fluid in the fundus of the pouch.

Contrast video-fluoroscopy allows constant monitoring of the swallowing mechanism which is valuable as single shot barium swallows may miss a small diverticulum, especially if the films are taken from the wrong angle. Video-fluoroscopy demonstrates the pouch, especially the upper and lower lips of the neck seen most clearly near the end of the second stage of swallowing. The lower lip represents the cricopharyngeal sphincter which may project anteriorly into the pharyngo-oesophageal lumen as an obvious bulge. Fluoroscopy has the additional advantage of being able to view the pouch from different angles to achieve the optimum view of the neck of the pouch. This is particularly important for larger pouches which tend to be displaced so that they overlie the oesophagus, usually to the left seen on an anteroposterior view. The pouch changes shape during different phases of the deglutition cycle, the classical pear shape appearing when the cricopharyngeus contracts at the end of the pharyngeal stripping wave (Figure 10.6). An anterior view is needed by surgeons to see in which side of the neck the pouch lies though it is usually to the left. In a large pouch a tracheogram may occur due to overspill.

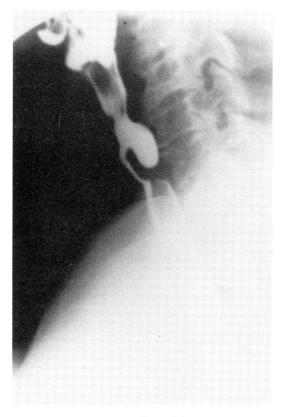

Figure 10.6 A diverticulum filled with barium posterior to the oesophagus demonstrating the diverticulo-oesophageal septum containing the cricopharyngeal sphincter

Although many long-term radiographic follow-up studies have been performed, no one as yet has seen a diverticulum develop in a patient or a transient diverticulum develop into a full-blown diverticulum. Ardran, Kemp and Lund (1964), in their series saw very little variation in the size of existing pouches during a 10-year follow up. Radiological staging has been attempted: stage I, small, i.e. less than one vertebral body; stage II, medium; stage III, large, i.e. greater than three vertebral bodies. The main value of staging is in relation to the mortality and morbidity of surgical procedures. The internal contours should be examined, as an irregularity or filling defect (Figure 10.7) within the diverticulum itself may be caused by solid food remnants or by a carcinoma. If the filling defect is constant and in the lower two-thirds of the sac, it is highly suspicious of a carcinoma, whereas in the neck, food and air bubbles causing filling defects are common findings.

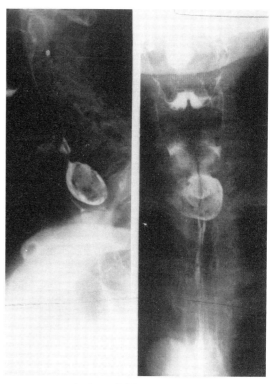

Figure 10.7 Multiple small filling defects are seen within the diverticular sac, in this case due to retained food debris

The radiographic study is incomplete if it does not include the lower oesophagus, stomach and duodenum, in order to look for other abnormalities such as hiatus hernia or peptic ulceration, with which there is a strong association (Smiley, Caves and Porter, 1970; Delahunty *et al.*, 1971).

The diagnosis can also been confirmed by ultrasound, but radiological investigations remain the primary method of diagnosis. Occasionally, diagnosis is made at oesophagoscopy, and biopsy may be necessary to confirm a suspected carcinoma of a diverticulum.

Pathogenesis

The diverticulum starts as a small bulge at Killian's dehiscence. As it enlarges it comes to lie between the oesophagus and the vertebral column and may remain static for many years or slowly increase in size until eventually it passes into the posterior mediastinum (Figure 10.8). The plane of the neck of the diverticulum alters as the size increases until it, rather than the oesophagus, lies in line with the hypopharynx, so that the food will pass into the pouch preferentially. This feature also makes identification of the oesophageal opening quite difficult at oesophagoscopy, and often prevents blind attempts to pass a nasogastric tube into the oesophagus.

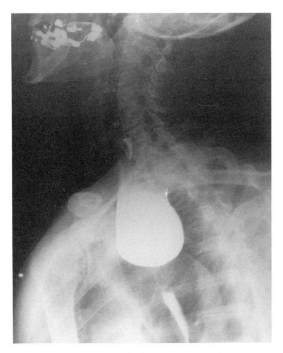

Figure 10.8 A large diverticulum passing into the posterior mediastinum

The histology shows an epithelial lining of stratified squamous epithelium and submucosa, often with fibrous tissue surrounding it. Nearer the neck of the sac scanty muscle fibres are found in the wall. Occasionally, there are variations, in particular carcinoma *in situ* and frank invasive squamous cell carcinoma. Other histological oddities have been reported, including ulceration of the pouch with underlying submucosal infiltration by plasma cells, lymphocytes and eosinophils. Harrison and Tighe (1970) reported a sac which appeared to be covered completely with a fibromuscular layer, as one might expect in a true diverticulum. The sac was lined with hyperplastic stratified squamous epithelium with some acute inflammation and ulceration, but underlying this were cysts lined with stratified columnar mucus-secreting epithelium. The only explanation that could be offered for this rather odd finding, was of a developmental abnormality similar to the congenital posterior pharyngeal diverticulum described by Britnall and Kridelbaugh (1950).

Treatment

No treatment is indicated if the patient's general condition is poor for other medical reasons, or for a patient with a diverticulum with few symptoms. The basis of treatment is to correct the cause of the pouch and the methods for achieving this aim are endoscopic or external surgery. It is agreed by most surgeons that the cricopharyngeal sphincter is probably involved in the aetiology of the posterior pharyngeal pulsion diverticulum, though its exact relationship is not yet understood and therefore a cricopharyngeal myotomy is generally recommended. It is well documented that there is a higher recurrence rate in those patients who do not have a myotomy.

Endoscopic treatment

The main endoscopic techniques for treatment of posterior pharyngeal pulsion diverticula are dilatation of the sphincter and endoscopic diathermy of the diverticulo-oesophageal septum.

Dilatation

Early treatment of diverticula was aimed at dilating the cricopharyngeal sphincter to alleviate the dysphagia and this was effective, though temporary, in relieving symptoms. There is an additional risk of perforation of the pouch and this was especially true in the early days when blind bouginage was performed. An alternative method of dilatation is extensive stretching of the sphincter using a hydrostatic bag. However, dilatation by bouginage or hydrostatic bag is rarely used nowadays except to dilate a postoperative stenosis.

Endoscopic diathermy (Dohlman's operation)

This operation has failed to gain wide acceptance in the UK or the USA, but is more popular in some European countries. It was first described by Mosher in 1917 in the USA, in a series of six patients in whom he divided the septum between the diverticulum and the oesophagus with scissors. However, despite good results in the resolution of symptoms, he abandoned this method after a fatality due to haemorrhage. The technique was modified and popularized by Dohlmann and Mattsson (1959) who used it extensively and recorded over 100 operations in which there were no deaths or serious complications, though the recurrence rate was 7%. The major theoretical risk is of mediastinitis, but this was discounted by Dohlman in 1949, who said, 'if the ledge between the pouch and the oesophagus is incised down the entire length of the diverticulum, there cannot be any increased intradiverticular pressure in the act of swallowing, because the pouch can empty unobstructed into the oesophagus. This is, presumably, the reason why the food is not pressed into the mediastinum, and that therefore there is no considerable risk of infection'.

The rationale behind this operation, in preference to an external approach, is based on the general health of these patients. The patients are generally old and unfit, due to emaciation and pulmonary complications from aspiration of the sac contents and also have a higher incidence of cardiac and pulmonary disease, therefore representing a poor anaesthetic and surgical risk. Endoscopic diathermy of the diverticulo-oesophageal septum is a short operation, lasting only 5–10 minutes, and can be performed under local anaesthetic, if a general anaesthetic is contraindicated. Recovery is rapid and the patient is normally ready for discharge 4 or 5 days after operation. Furthermore, the size of the sac does not affect the division of the septum. While the procedure does not remove the pouch, it relieves the symptoms and restores swallowing by dividing the cricopharyngeus and widening the mouth of the diverticulum. Re-operation is far easier than after external operations where scar tissue makes identification of recurrent diverticula hazardous.

Specialized instruments have been developed for the endoscopic technique (Figure 10.9). The oesophagoscope is split distally, the upper beak being longer than the lower one with a slit between them. The instruments include a toothed diathermy forceps to prevent slipping, a knife and a suction tube, all of which are insulated except at their working ends, and a pair of insulated paddles, which protect the oesophageal and pouch walls.

At operation, the long beak of the oesophagoscope is inserted into the oesophagus and the short beak into the diverticulum (Figure 10.10*a*). The wall between the diverticulum and the oesophagus lies in the slit as a horizontal spur, containing the cricopharyngeus (Figure 10.10*b*). The spur is then grasped in the midline between the jaws of the diathermy forceps and coagulation diathermy applied until a longitudinal strip of blanching occurs which is divided by a diathermy knife. Insulated paddles are used to prevent

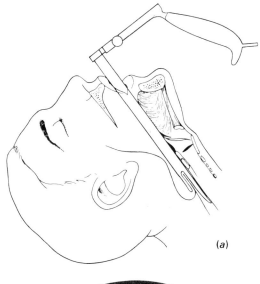

(a)

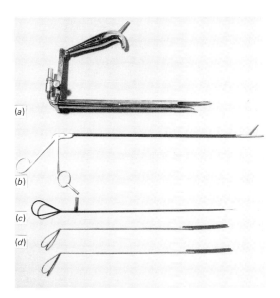

Figure 10.9 Specialized instruments for use in endoscopic diathermy division of the diverticulo-oesophageal septum: (*a*) oesophageal speculum with split beak; (*b*) diathermy forceps; (*c*) knife; (*d*) insulated paddles

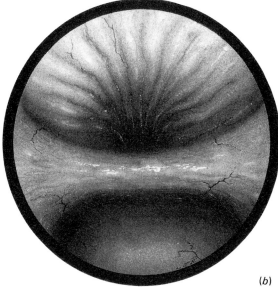

(b)

Figure 10.10 (*a*) Oesophagoscope in position, with the longer beak in the oesophagus and the shorter beak in the diverticulum. (*b*) The endoscopic view of the spur with the beaked oesophagoscope in position (by kind permission of Mr H. B. Juby and the Editor, Butterworth's *Operative Surgery*)

may be continued caudally until the fundus of the diverticulum is seen.

With large sacs the operation is often staged, being completed after one or two repeat operations, each separated by 5–6 days. The procedure is stopped before the floor of the diverticulum is reached to minimize the risk of mediastinitis. Fluids are given orally the following morning, if there are no contraindications, a soft diet being instituted on the second or third day. The success of the operation is gauged by postoperative barium studies performed at 5 days. Although some residue may be noted temporarily, the operation is deemed successful if there is only a short party wall remaining with minimal delay in the emptying, as well as an absence of symptoms. The patient is discharged after 5 days and is on a normal diet after 2 weeks.

Wouters and Van Overbeek (1990), in a series of 323 patients, claimed that 92.1% were 'highly satisfied' and 7.3% 'fairly satisfied' with their treatment. They reported only one death (0.47%) but 28 complications (8.7%), though most resolved quickly. Eight patients (3.8%) had stenosis and therefore presumably recurrent symptoms, though this was not stated.

Endoscopic division of the diverticulo-oesophageal septum provides a quick safe technique for relieving symptoms, the major risks being haemorrhage, mediastinitis, emphysema and stenosis, the latter being treated by further division or dilatation. However, there is a risk of carcinoma in a pouch being missed, as reported by Juby (1969), in a patient who had undergone six diathermy treatments, and Mackay (1976), who found one patient with carcinoma following Dohlman's procedure, a fact which has caused many to abandon its use.

Knegt, de Jong and Van der Schans (1984) reported on 28 patients in whom they had used a carbon dioxide laser to divide the diverticulo-oesophageal septum. Twenty-two patients had complete relief of symptoms and the remainder were considerably improved. One patient had postoperative mediastinitis, which responded to antiobiotics, and 21 of the 28 patients had a sharp rise in temperature for the first 24 hours, the reasons for which are unexplained. Wouters and Van Overbeek (1990) used laser surgery in 184 patients and felt that it causes less tissue necrosis and therefore less scarring. Complications have been less than 5%, but include four instances of mediastinitis.

External surgical approach

One-stage diverticulectomy

Though this was the first successful method it was not repopularized until antibiotics were in regular use. In the preoperative investigation the patient is admitted 1–2 days preoperatively to empty the sac of food and to restrict the patients to clear fluids for the last 24 hours.

The patient's general health is assessed, with particular emphasis on the treatment of any chest disease.

The operation is generally performed under general anaesthesia with the patient intubated and paralysed. Once anaesthetized, an oesophagoscope is passed and the openings to the pouch and oesophagus identified. A nasogastric tube is passed down the oesophagus after which the diverticulum is inspected to exclude carcinoma and to aspirate any residual debris from it before packing with ribbon gauze soaked in proflavin, the proximal end of the strip being brought out through the mouth to the head of the table so that the anaesthetist can remove it at the appropriate time. Attempts at passing the nasogastric tube after packing the pouch can be hampered by the proflavin in the pharynx and the bulk of the pack impinging on the oesophagus, so it should be inserted before packing.

The patient is then placed in the reverse Trendelenberg position with a sandbag under the shoulders and the head is extended and rotated away from the side of the incision. The operation area is sterilized and draped, and a collar incision, usually on the left side of the neck, is marked out on the skin at the level of the upper border of the cricoid from the midline to halfway across the sternomastoid muscle, preferably in a skin crease. The incision line is infiltrated with adrenalin to minimize bleeding and the incision made through skin, subcutaneous tissues and platysma to the strap muscles and sternomastoid. The deep cervical fascia is then incised along the anterior border of the sternomastoid muscle which is retracted laterally. The omohyoid is identified, mobilized and divided at which point the internal jugular vein comes into view (Figure 10.11a). The middle

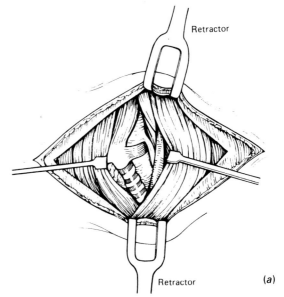

Figure 10.11 (*a*) Incision and exposure of the pharyngo-oesophageal segment. The strap muscles and thyroid gland are retracted medially to improve exposure (by kind permission of Mr H. B. Juby and the Editor Butterworth's *Operative Surgery*)

thyroid veins are divided and ligated so that the dissection may proceed medial to the carotid sheath, which is retracted laterally avoiding undue pressure on the carotid artery. The inferior thyroid artery is identified and divided as necessary and if possible the recurrent laryngeal nerve is identified at this point of the operation. The diverticulum, which is packed with proflavin, can be easily identified by colour or palpation and the fundus grasped with a pair of Babcock forceps. The diverticulum is dissected free of the oesophagus, the thyroid gland and thyroid cartilage being retracted medially, with care not to damage the recurrent laryngeal nerve. The neck of the pouch is then carefully cleaned of muscle fibres to its junction with the pharynx, which is identified by palpating the nasogastric tube (Figure 10.11*b*). Great care must be taken to avoid tearing the neck of the sac at this juncture. The proflavin pack is removed and stay sutures are inserted into the neck of the pouch inferiorly and superiorly, care being taken not to place them too medially, which would lead to a stricture.

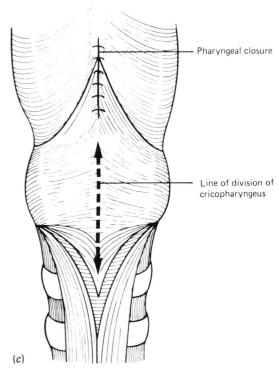

Figure 10.11 (*c*) The line of division for the cricopharyngeal myotomy. By dividing the cricopharyngeus posteriorly the recurrent laryngeal nerve is avoided (by kind permission of Mr H. B. Juby and the Editor Butterworth's *Operative Surgery*)

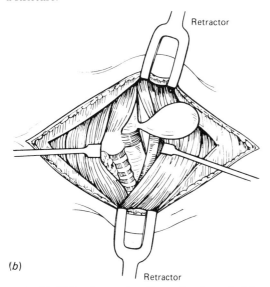

Fig. 10.11 (*b*) The diverticulum dissected to the neck of the sac and clamped prior to excision. (by kind permission of Mr H. B. Juby and the Editor Butterworth's *Operative Surgery*)

The cricopharyngeal spincter and upper circular fibres of the oesophagus are then divided posteriorly in order to avoid the recurrent laryngeal nerve (Figures 10.11*c* and *d*), after which the wound inferior to the neck of the pouch is packed with gauze to catch any debris which may discharge and the pouch is amputated. The mouth of the neck is closed with a continuous inverting suture and the stay sutures removed. A second layer of interrupted catgut or silk is used to bury the first (Figure 10.11*e*). Haemostasis is secured before wound closure, a drain is inserted inferiorly,

and the wound is closed in two layers. Antibiotics should be reserved for complications and are not routinely used. The drain is removed when there is minimal drainage, usually after 2 or 3 days. Nasogastric feeding is continued for 5–7 days, after which fluids are given. If there are no complications, the nasogastric tube is removed and a soft diet started the next day. Normal diet is given after 10 days.

The stapling gun has been in use in bowel surgery for many years and it is now becoming increasingly popular for resection of pouches. The first report was by Hoehn and Payne (1969) who used it successfully in four patients. In the 1980s it was reported more frequently and offers a real contribution to the safety and ease of surgery, the effective closure of the pouch neck being most important in preventing local infection, emphysema and mediastinitis. Westmore (1990) reported on 18 patients in whom the repair was performed using a staple gun and they had no complications as a result of the procedure.

Inversion

Inversion of the diverticulum was first described by Girard (1896). Bevan (1917) in the Sippy–Bevan

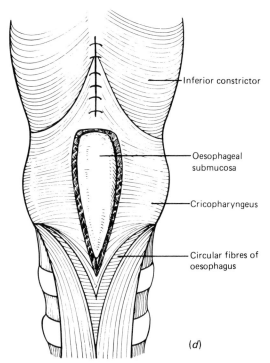

Inferior constrictor

Oesophageal submucosa

Cricopharyngeus

Circular fibres of oesophagus

(*d*)

Fig. 10.11 (*d*) The myotomy is extended inferiorly to include the upper part of the circular fibres of the oesophagus (by kind permission of Mr H. B. Juby and the Editor Butterworth's *Operative Surgery*)

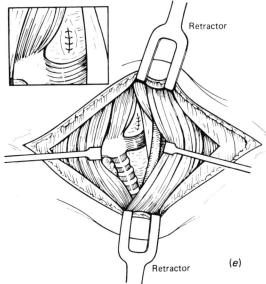

Retractor

Retractor   (*e*)

(*e*) Closure of the pharyngeal defect (by kind permission of Mr H. B. Juby and the Editor Butterworth's *Operative Surgery*)

operation, modified the inversion by placing a series of purse string sutures along the length of the sac in order to obliterate it. This technique was developed

to avoid the risk of opening the pouch. Recently, it has become more popular again as it has considerable advantages. There is a low complication rate, in particular of fistula, abscess or mediastinitis, and the patient has a short hospital stay of 2–3 days. Patients are able to drink within 24 hours of surgery, though occasionally they complain of a sensation of a lump in the throat for 2 or 3 days, but this quickly subsides.

The operation is carried out in the same way as for excision to the point of full mobilization of the pouch and cricopharyngeal myotomy, the pouch is then invaginated into the oesophagus and its neck oversewn with interrupted catgut sutures, instead of being excised (Figure 10.12). A small drain is placed in the wound which is then closed.

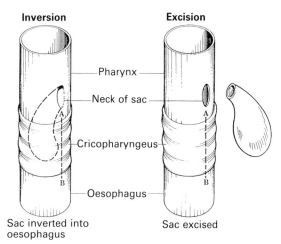

Inversion   **Excision**

Pharynx

Neck of sac

Cricopharyngeus

Oesophagus

Sac inverted into oesophagus   Sac excised

Figure 10.12 Diagrammatic representation of inversion versus excision

Escher (1984) reported on 40 patients with only one death due to cardiac failure, and one fistula, he also reported two recurrences. Although generally described for small pouches there is no reason why this operation should not be applied to large pouches. Bowdler and Stell (1987a) compared excision with inversion and found a significantly lower rate of complications in the inversion group, in addition the complications were less serious, permitting far earlier discharge from hospital.

Cricopharyngeal myotomy

While cricopharyngeal myotomy has been performed in isolation for neurological disorders, its use in patients with posterior pharyngeal pulsion diverticula, with or without diverticulectomy, remains a contentious matter. Circumstantial evidence, in particular dilatation giving temporary relief of symptoms, supports the view that it is necessary, even with the obvious lack of concrete evidence.

Many investigators have found that myotomy decreases the pharyngo-oesophageal pressure (Ellis *et* al., 1969; Berlin *et al.*, 1977; Lichter, 1978), however, Black (1981), in one patient, noticed that, despite an initial fall, the pressure had returned to normal within 4 weeks. It has been suggested that resection of a segment of the muscle may prevent this phenomenon (Gullane *et al.*, 1983). Although Hansen, Gundtoft and Sorensen (1973) questioned the value of myotomy, more recently the operation has gained many advocates (Lichter, 1978; Gullane *et al.*, 1983) who believe that it decreases the recurrence rate and adds little time or risk to the conventional operation.

Ellis *et al.* (1969) treated 18 patients with myotomy, and on follow up averaging 17 months, 14 were asymptomatic, three had occasional mild symptoms and only one had persistent symptoms. Postoperative studies showed a 50% fall in sphincter pressure.

The procedure itself is relatively simple and may be done with diverticulectomy or on its own (see Figures 10.11*c* and *d*). The muscle is divided as posteriorly as possible, to avoid damage to the recurrent laryngeal nerve, and is extended 3–4 cm caudally into the oesophageal musculature as the high pressure zone can be at least that long (Atkinson *et al*, 1957).

A bougie, catheter, or endotracheal tube may be introduced into the oesophagus to stretch the fibres to facilitate division or a microscope can be used. Myotomy is most simply achieved by creating a tunnel between the circular muscle fibres and submucosa with a curved artery forceps and dividing the muscle between the opened forceps. The mucosa then bulges through the gap.

When carried out in isolation the patient is able to drink the following day and go home within 2 or 3 days, eating normally. The dangers are those of damage to the recurrent laryngeal nerve and accidentally creating a fistula.

Complications

The mortality and morbidity of diverticulum surgery have been reduced significantly since the early days and, in particular, have been reduced by the advent of antibiotics. Large single surgeon series have better results than smaller series especially where the latter series represents the efforts of several surgeons. Complications can be divided into immediate, early and late.

Immediate

1 Haemorrhage. This usually results from poor haemostasis at surgery, or a ligature slipping from one of the vessels tied during surgery.
2 Pneumothorax. While this is uncommon it may occur during the mobilization of a large pouch particularly if adhesions are present.
3 Surgical emphysema. This may result if an unseen mucosal tear is left or the suture line is not complete.

Early

1 Secondary haemorrhage is usually due to infection.
2 Hoarseness. Endoscopic surgery avoids the recurrent laryngeal nerve but in external approaches there is always the danger of damage to the nerve (3–5%), resulting in either temporary or permanent palsy.
3 Wound infection or wound abscess. These are more likely if there has been spillage of the contents of the pouch or pharyngeal contents during surgery, although infection may result from a leak through the suture line (1.5–5%). Infection will predispose to fistula formation.
4 Fistulae are usually secondary to infection (1–8%). Saliva or food leaking from the incision is diagnostic of this condition, which may be confirmed by a gastrograffin swallow. A fistula usually closes spontaneously and until it does the patient is fed with a nasogastric tube.
5 Mediastinitis may result from a leak tracking caudally. If it is not noticed at surgery the patient develops symptoms several hours or days later, complaining of pain in the neck and back, and becoming severely distressed and dyspnoeic. Plain radiographs of the chest will show air in the mediastinum or neck. If doubt exists, a small quantity of gastrograffin is swallowed and radiographs repeated. Treatment should be with intravenous antibiotics initially, and the patient should be monitored for signs of deterioration in the vital signs. If this occurs the leak should be found and closed and a large drain inserted into the posterior mediastinum; occasionally a thoracotomy is necessary.
6 Aerocoele. This is a rare complication, a large aerocoele forming in the superior mediastinum and communicating with the pharynx.

Late

1 Persistent hoarseness occurs when the recurrent laryngeal nerve has been divided. No recovery can be expected.
2 A stricture results from taking too much mucosa when excising the pouch, or closing the pharynx. It is treated by dilatation which is generally successful, though it may need to be repeated. Occasionally surgical correction is necessary.
3 Recurrence. All methods have a recurrence rate, although it is higher for endoscopic diathermy than diverticulectomy. However, it is easy to reoperate endoscopically, whereas re-opening a neck to identify a recurrent pouch is more difficult. The recurrence rate for endoscopic diathermy is about 6–7%. Recurrence rates for diverticulectomy vary between 0.5% and 4% but some authors believe that there is a considerable difference between symptomatic and radiological recurrence rates. Bertelsen and Aasted (1976) had a 2% symptomatic

recurrence rate in his series but suggested that a 10–12% radiological recurrence rate might be present. Gullane *et al.* (1983) found an 18.6% symptomatic recurrence rate and a 55.6% radiological recurrence rate. Gammelgaard (1955) reported on 20 patients who had diverticulectomies without myotomy and when reviewed up to 8 years later, 14 had developed a radiological recurrence. If a myotomy is not done the recurrence rate of diverticulectomy is higher.

Complications using external approaches are higher when the sac is larger, being greatest in those patients falling into the stage III group. The mortality rate varies with different series but is generally between 0.5% and 3.0%.

Carcinoma of the diverticulum

Described first by Vinson (1927), it is a rare problem with only about 30 patients reported in the English literature. Huang, Unni and Payne (1984) in a series of 1249 patients, found four patients with malignancy arising from the diverticulum, which is an incidence of 0.32%. Others have reported a higher incidence of up to 3.4%, but most reports of a higher incidence are from smaller series. The true incidence is probably between 0.5 and 1.0% (Bowdler and Stell, 1987b). It affects men predominantly in a ratio of about 5:1 (Huang, Unni and Payne, 1984) and usually occurs in a long-standing diverticulum, the average duration of symptoms being greater than 7 years. The age at diagnosis is usually over 50 years. The main predisposing factor is thought to be chronic irritation and inflammation of the diverticular lining from food retention. Symptoms indicating carcinomatous change are an acceleration of dysphagia and weight loss and occasionally blood in the regurgitated food. Nodes or a mass may be found in the neck. The usual lesion is an invasive squamous cell carcinoma but four patients with carcinoma *in situ* have been reported in the literature.

Barium studies show a constant filling defect as opposed to the filling defect due to food debris which moves between films or repeat swallows. The carcinoma is usually seen in the distal two-thirds of the pouch but can easily be missed, the diagnosis frequently being made at surgery when careful examination with the oesophagoscope should be performed.

The treatment best suited to this lesion is uncertain. Radiotherapy alone has always failed to effect a cure. Most commonly a simple diverticulectomy is performed but there are only a few patients reported to be free from disease at 5 years the longest being 8 years (Huang, Unni and Payne, 1984). Following the operation, radiotherapy is often given. Some authors advocate a more radical treatment as for carcinoma of the cervical oesophagus.

References

ARDRAN, G. M., KEMP, F. H. and LUND, W. D. (1964) The aetiology of the posterior pharyngeal diverticulum. A cineradiographic study. *Journal of Laryngology and Otology*, 78, 333–349

ATKINSON, L. (1952) Pharyngeal diverticula: with particular reference to lateral protrusions of various types. *Archives of the Middlesex Hospital*, 2, 245–254

ATKINSON, M., KRAMER, P., WYMAN, S. M. and INGELFINGER, F. J. (1957) The dynamics of swallowing. I. Normal pharyngeal mechanisms. *Journal of Clinical Investigation*, 36, 581–588

BACHMAN, A. L., SEAMAN, W. B. and MACKEN, L. (1968) Lateral pharyngeal diverticula. *Radiology*, 91, 774–782

BARON, S. H. (1982) Zenkers diverticulum as a cause for loss of drug availability: a new complication. *American Journal of Gastroenterology*, 77, 152–153

BASMAJIAN, J. V. and DUTTA, C. R. (1961) Electromyography of the pharyngeal constrictors and levator palati in man. *Anatomical Record*, 139, 561–563

BELL, C. (1817) Preternatural bag, formed by the membrane of the pharynx. *Surgical Observations*, 1, 64–72

BERLIN, B. P., FIERSTEIN, J. T., TEDESCO, F. and OGURA, J. H. (1977) Manometric studies of the upper oesophageal sphincter. *Annals of Otology, Rhinology and Laryngology*, 86, 598–602

BERTELSEN, S. and AASTED, A. (1976) Results of operative treatment of hypopharyngeal diverticulum. *Thorax*, 31, 544–547

BEVAN, A. D. (1917) Pulsion diverticulum of the oesophagus – cure by the Sippy-Bevan operation. *Surgical Clinics of Chicago*, 1, 449–457

BLACK, R. J. (1981) Cricopharyngeal myotomy. *Journal of Otolaryngology*, 10, 145–148

BOWDLER, D. A. and STELL, P. M. (1987a) Surgical management of posterior pharyngeal pulsion diverticula: inversion versus one-stage excision. *British Journal of Surgery*, 74, 988–990

BOWDLER, D. A. and STELL, P. M. (1987b) Carcinoma arisng in posterior pharyngeal pulsion diverticulum (Zenker's diverticulum). *British Journal of Surgery*, 74, 561–563

BRITNALL, E. S. and KRIDELBAUGH, W. W. (1950) Congenital diverticulum of the posterior hypopharynx simulating atresia of the oesophagus. *Annals of Surgery*, 131, 565–574

BURGE, D. and MIDDLETON, A. (1983) Persistent pharyngeal pouch derivatives in the neonate. *Journal of Pediatric Surgery*, 18, 230–234

CRICHLOW, T. V. L. (1956) The cricopharyngeus in radiography and cineradiography *British Journal of Radiology*, 29, 546–556

DELAHUNTY, J. E., MARGULIES, S. I., ALONSON, W. A. and KNUDSON, D. H. (1971) The relationship of reflux esophagitis to pharyngeal pouch (Zenker's diverticulum) formation. *Laryngoscope*, 81, 570–577

DOHLMAN, G. (1949) Endoscopic operations for hypopharyngeal diverticula. *Proceedings of the Fourth International Congress of Otolaryngology (London)*, 2, 715–717

DOHLMAN, G. and MATTSSON, O. (1959) The role of the cricopharyngeus muscle in cases of hypopharyngeal diverticula. *American Journal of Roentgenology*, 81, 561–569

EKBERG, O. and NYLANDER, G. (1983) Lateral diverticula from the pharyngo-esophageal junction area. *Radiology*, 146, 117–122

ELLIS, G. H., SCHLEGEL, J. F., LYNCH, V. P. and PAYNE, S. W.

(1969) Cricopharyngeal myotomy for pharyngo-esophageal diverticulum. *Annals of Surgery*, **170**, 340–349

ESCHER, F. (1984) Zur Therapie des Zenkershen Divetikels. *Schweiz Med. Wochenschrift*, **114**, 1428–1433

FRIELING, T., BERGES, W., LUBKE, H. J., ENCK, P. and WIENBECK, M. (1988) Upper esophageal sphincter function in patients with Zenker's diverticulum. *Dysphagia*, **3**, 90–92

FYKE, F. E. and CODE, C. F. (1955) Resting and deglutition pressures in the pharyngo-oesophageal region. *Gastroenterology*, **29**, 24–34

GAGE-WHITE, L. (1988) Incidence of Zenker's diverticulum with hiatus hernia. *Laryngoscope*, **98**, 527–530

GAMMELGAARD, A. (1955) Esophageal diverticula. *Acta Chirurgica* Scandinavica, **109**, 181–183

GIRARD, C. (1896) Du traitement des diverticules de l'oesophage. *Congres Français de Chirurgie*, **10**, 392–407

GOLDMANN, E. E. (1909) Die zwiezerfge operation von Pulsiondivertikeln de Speiserohre. *Berl. Klin Chir*, **61**, 741–749

GULLANE, P. J., WILLETT, J. M., HEENEMAN, H., GREENWAY, R. E. and RUBY, R. R. F. (1983) Zenker's diverticulum. *Journal of Otolaryngology*, **12**, 53–57

HANSEN, J. B., GUNDTOFT, J. P. and SORENSEN, H. R. (1973) Pharyngo-esophageal diverticula. *Scandinavian Journal of Thoracic and Cardiovascular Surgery*, **7**, 81–86

HARRISON, K. and TIGHE, J. R. (1970) Glandular inclusions in a pharyngeal pouch. *Journal of Laryngology and Otology*, **84**, 225–227

HAYASHI, N., TAMAKI, N., KONISH, J., ENDO, K., HISAKA, T., TORIZUKA, K. *et al.* (1984) Lateral pharyngoesophageal diverticulum simulating thyroid adenoma on sonography. *Journal of Clinical Ultrasound*, **12**, 592–594

HOEHN, J. G. and PAYNE, W. S. (1969) Resection of pharyngoesophageal diverticulum using stapling device. *Mayo Clinic Proceedings*, **44**, 738–744

HUANG, B., UNNI, K. K. and PAYNE, W. A. (1984) Long-term survival following diverticulectomy for cancer in pharyngoesophageal (Zenker's) diverticulum. *Annals of Thoracic Surgery*, **38**, 207–210

HUNT, P. S., CONNELL, A. M. and SMILEY, T. B. (1970) The cricopharyngeal sphincter in gastric reflux. *Gut*, **11**, 303–306

HURST, A. F. (1925) Anterior pharyngo-oesophageal pouch as a cause of dysphagia. *Guy's Hospital Reports*, **5**, 367–372

JUBY, H. B. (1969) The treatment of pharyngeal pouch. *Journal of Laryngology and Otology*, **83**, 1067–1071

KAWASAKI, H. and OGURA, J. H. (1968) Interdependence of deglutition with respiration. *Annals of Otology, Rhinology and Laryngology*, **77**, 906–913

KORKIS, F. B. (1958) The aetiology, diagnosis and surgical treatment of pharyngeal diverticula. *Journal of Laryngology and Otology*, **72**, 509–521

KNEGT, P. P., DE JONG, P. C. and VAN DER SCHANS, E. J. (1984) Endoscopic laser surgery for hypopharyngeal diverticula – a preliminary report. *Clinical Otolaryngology*, **9**, 277–279

KNUFF, T. E., BENJAMIN, S. B. and CASTELL, D. O. (1982) Pharyngoesophageal (Zenker's) diverticulum: a reappraisal. *Gastroenterology*, **82**, 734–736

KODICEK, J. and CREAMER, B. (1961) A study of pharyngeal pouches. *Journal of Laryngology and Otology*, **75**, 406–411

LAHEY, F. H. (1954) Esophageal diverticula. *Surgery, Gynecology and Obstetrics*, **98**, 1–28

LICHTER, I. (1978) Motor disorder in pharyngoesophageal

pouch *Journal of Thoracic and Cardiovascular Surgery*, **76**, 272–275

LUDLOW, A. (1769) A case of obstructed deglutition, from a preternatural dilatation of, and bag formed in the pharynx. *Medical Observations and Inquiries*, **3**, 85–101

MACKELLAR, A. and KENNEDY, J. C. (1972) Congenital diverticulum of the pharynx simulating esophageal atresia. *Journal of Pediatric Surgery*, **7**, 408–411

MACKAY, I. S. (1976) The treatment of pharyngeal pouch. *Journal of Laryngology and Otology*, **90**, 183–190

MACMILLAN, A. S. (1932) Pouches of the pharynx and esophagus. *Journal of the American Medical Association*, **98**, 964–969

MORTON, R. P. (1983) Pharyngeal pseudodiverticulum in an adult. *Journal of Laryngology and Otology*, **97**, 79–83

MOSHER, H. P. (1917) Webs and pouches of the oesophagus, their diagnosis and treatment. *Surgery, Gynecology and Obstetrics*, **25**, 175–187

NEGUS, V. E. (1950) Pharyngeal diverticula. Observations on their evolution and treatment. *British Journal of Surgery*, **38**, 129–146

NILSSON, M. E., ISBERG, A. and SCHIRATZKI, H. (1988) The hypopharyngeal diverticulum. *Acta Otolaryngologica*, **106**, 314–320

NORRIS, C. W. (1979) Pharyngoceles of the hypopharynx. *Laryngoscope*, **89**, 1788–1807

PERROTT, J. W. (1962) Anatomical aspects of hypopharyngeal diverticula. *Australian and New Zealand Journal of Surgery*, **31**, 307–317

SCHMID, H. H. (1912) Vorschlag eineseinfachen operations – verfahrens zur Behandlung des oesophagus-divertikels. *Weiner Klinische Wochenschrift*, **25**, 487–488

SHALLOW, T. A. and CLERF, L. H. (1948) One stage pharyngeal diverticulectomy. *Surgery, Gynecology and Obstetrics*, **86**, 317–322

SIEBERT, T. I., STEIN, J. and POPPEL, M. H. (1959) Variations in the roentgen appearance of the 'esophageal lip'. *American Journal of Roentgenology*, **81**, 570–575

SMILEY, T. B., CAVES, P. K. and PORTER, D. C. (1970) Relationship between posterior pharyngeal pouch and hiatus hernia. *Thorax*, **25**, 725–731

STETTEN, D. (1910) The radical extirpation of pharyngoesophageal pressure diverticula. *Annals of Surgery*, **51**, 300–319

VINSON, P. P. (1927) Simultaneous occurrence of multiple lesions in the esophagus: a report of three cases. *Archives of Otolaryngology*, **5**, 502

WELLS, S. D., LEONIDAS, J. C., CONKLE, D., HOLDER, T. H., AMOURY, R. A. and ACHCRAFT, K. W. (1974) Traumatic prevertebral pharyngoesophageal pseudodiverticulum in the newborn infant. *Journal of Pediatric Surgery*, **9**, 217–222

WESTMORE, G. A. (1990) Staple gun in the surgery of hypopharyngeal diverticula. *Journal of Laryngology and Otology*, **104**, 553–556

WHEELER, W. I. (1886) Pharyngocoele and dilation of pharynx, with existing diverticulum at lower portion of pharynx lying posterior to the oesophagus, cured by pharyngotomy, being the first case of the kind recorded. *Dublin Journal of Medical Science*, **82**, 349–356

WILSON, C. P. (1962) Pharyngeal diverticula, their cause and treatment. *Journal of Laryngology and Otology*, **76**, 151–180

WINNANS, C. S. (1972) The pharyngoesophageal closure mechanism: a manometric study. *Gastroenterology*, **63**, 768–777

WOUTERS, B. and VAN OVERBEEK, J. J. M. (1990) Pathogenesis and endoscopic treatment of the hypopharyngeal (Zenker's) diverticulum. *Acta Gastro-Enterologica Belgica*, **53**, 323–329

ZENKER, F. A. and VON ZIEMSSEN, H. (1878) *Cyclopedia of the Practice of Medicine*. Baltimore: W. Wood & Company

11

Tumours of the larynx

P. E. Robin and Jan Olofsson

In their broadest sense the terms tumour, swelling or space-occupying lesion have a significance in the larynx beyond that in most other sites, not only because of the early prejudice of the airway, but also because of interference with function in some patients, even when the lesion is miniscule. It is for this latter reason that many lesions are identified which are tumours but not true neoplasms.

Pseudotumours

Cysts

Cysts of the larynx may be congenital or acquired. They may arise in the vocal cords (55%), ventricular bands (25%) or in the epiglottis (20%) (Kleinsasser, 1978). They may be lined by squamous or columnar epithelium.

Congenital cysts

Congenital cysts are rare and are most common in the ventricular bands or aryepiglottic folds. They may be diagnosed in the neonatal period as a consequence of breathing difficulties. They may originate from sequestration of embryonic cells in the saccule or laryngeal ventricle or arise from the seromucinous glands.

Incision of the cysts may be sufficient or excision can be performed if possible. If the airway is secured the intubation tube may be removed, otherwise it has to be left in place to allow repeat laryngoscopies. However, if the clinical course is prolonged, a tracheostomy is necessary.

Retention cysts

Retention cysts of the larynx are squamous or columnar; both forms may originate from obstructed sero-mucinous salivary glands. The squamous variant is common on the lingual surface of the epiglottis, in the vallecula and on the aryepiglottic folds (Figure 11.1). These cysts may reach a considerable size before being diagnosed but minor cysts are often incidental findings at a routine otolaryngological examination. If possible these cysts should be excised entirely.

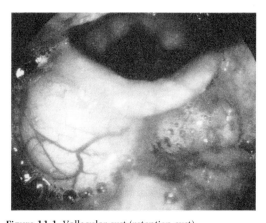

Figure 11.1 Vallecular cyst (retention cyst)

Squamous cysts also present on the squamous-lined portion of the vocal cords. They are most common on the undersurface of the anterior part of the cords. Minor cysts on the vocal cords are filled with clear mucus. Larger cysts contain yellowish, thick fluid, which sometimes includes cholesterol crystals.

The laryngoscopic appearance of vocal cord cysts and vocal cord polyps may be very similar and it is microscopic examination that reveals the true nature of the lesion. Larger cysts are easier to recognize with their yellow colour and location under a thin translucent epithelium.

The treatment consists of excision of minor vocal cord cysts and marsupialization of larger ones.

Cysts of the ventricular band or cavity may be misinterpreted as neoplasms (Figure 11.2) – a differential

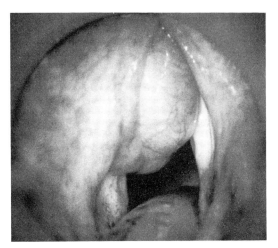

Figure 11.2 Ventricular cyst (retention cyst)

diagnosis which must be ruled out. Cysts are most common above the age of 60 years and are lined by columnar or sometimes oncocytic cells (Figure 11.3).

Under light microscopy oncocytes are large cells with an abundant pale, dark, or 'colloid' cytoplasm which is more or less acidophilic, and a small dense darkly staining nucleus. Electron microscopic studies show that the cytoplasm of the oncocytes contains large numbers of tightly packed mitochondria accounting for the granular or homogeneous appearance of the cells (Hamperl, 1962). Histochemically the oncocytes are characterized by the abundance of oxidative enzymes (Balogh and Roth, 1965; Johns, Regezi and Batsakis, 1977). The oncocytes tend to appear with increasing frequency in ageing individuals and occasionally form the predominant component of cysts and tumours. Such oncocytic lesions have most commonly been reported in the parotid glands. In the larynx a variety of names such as oncocytic cysts, oncocytic papillary cystadenomas, oncocytic adenomatous hyperplasia, oxyphilic granular cell adenoma, oncocytoma, and oxyphilic adenoma, has been given to these lesions. Nohteri (1946) found oncocytes in eight out of 37 (22%) laryngeal autopsy specimens. De Santo, Devine and Weiland (1970) in an analysis of material at the Mayo Clinic over 20 years found that 11% (33% of the saccular and 4% of the ductal cysts) were lined with oncocytes or contained such cells.

Granulomas

Non-specific granulomas are nearly always caused by trauma. Postoperative granulomas may occur after laryngeal endoscopic procedures or partial laryngectomies. Sometimes a stitch is found in the

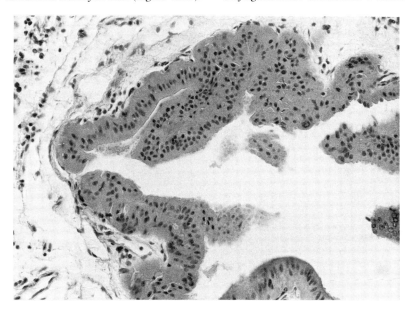

Figure 11.3 Oncocytic ventricular cyst. Photomicrograph showing the cyst lined with a single layer of typical oxyphilic cells (haematoxylin and eosin, × 320)

granuloma. Microlaryngoscopy should be performed to rule out recurrence in patients treated for malignant disease. The more commonly used laser surgery sometimes shows a tendency to excessive granulomatous tissue formation during the healing period.

Intubation granulomas are often caused by long-term intubation with prolonged pulmonary ventilation (Figure 11.4). The granulomas are caused by ulceration of the mucosa overlying the vocal process. The duration of intubation, as well as the size and type of the tube, and the degree of relaxation of the patients, are all causative factors. Prolonged intubation in adults is frequently discussed in the literature. Most intubation granulomas are diagnosed within a few weeks of extubation. Hoarseness, irritation and sometimes pain may occur. Microlaryngoscopy and excision should be performed, however, recurrences may occur. Intubation ulceration and granulomas are certainly more common than is realized, but most of these granulomas may be coughed up and the base heals spontaneously.

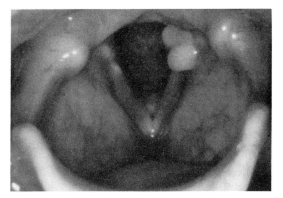

Figure 11.5 Contact granuloma of the left vocal cord. Telescopic view

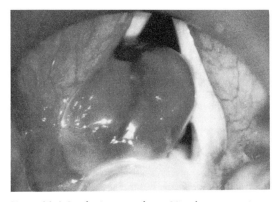

Figure 11.4 Intubation granuloma. Microlaryngoscopic view with the intubation tube in the posterior commissure

Contact ulcers and granulomas located over the vocal processes (Figures 11.5 and 11.6) and often on both sides, probably have a multifactorial aetiology and the patients should be considered from several different aspects. They are nearly exclusively seen in men over the age of 30 years (Kleinsasser, 1978; Ohman *et al.*, 1983). Vocal abuse has been considered to be the most important aetiological factor as suggested by Jackson (1928), who first described this lesion. He recommended treatment consisting of vocal rest for a long period of time and, in some cases, vocal rest combined with surgical excision (Jackson and Jackson, 1935). Peacher and Holinger (1947) reported good results with voice therapy, which have been confirmed in many reports. Patients with contact ulcers or granulomas have a low pitch quality of voice as their most pronounced feature. They often

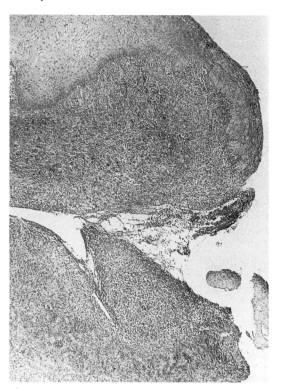

Figure 11.6 Contact ulcer – granuloma. Photomicrograph showing the ulceration and the granulomatous tissue partially with an overlying epithelium (haematoxylin and eosin, × 70)

have irritation and pain localized to the larynx, cough frequently and need to clear the throat. Emotional stress is considered another aetiological factor (Peacher, 1961). Other factors, such as hiatus hernia and gastro-oesophageal reflux have been discussed (Cherry and Margulies, 1968; Goldberg, Noyek and Pritzler, 1978; Ward *et al.*, 1980). In an oesophageal manometric study, 74% of the patients examined with contact ulcers or granulomas were found to have oesophageal dysfunction such as hiatus hernia, gastro-oesophageal reflux, dysmotility, etc. About 30% of the general population of the corresponding age have oesophageal dysfunction (Öhman *et al.*, 1983). It is difficult to know whether oesophageal dysfunction is an aetiological or concomitant factor of contact granulomas. Ward *et al.* (1980) reported good results with antireflux therapy. Biopsy should be performed to rule out cancer which rarely occurs at this site. No difference in healing could be seen when voice therapy combined with surgery was compared to voice therapy alone (Öhman *et al.*, 1983). Excessive granulomas should be excised to facilitate voice therapy.

Amyloidosis

The pathogenesis of amyloidosis is unknown but it is characterized by extracellular deposits of a proteinaceous substance. The disease was first described by Rokitansky in 1842, and the term 'amyloidosis' was introduced by Virchow in 1851. Burow and Neumann reported the first patient with laryngeal amyloidosis in 1875. Many hundreds of cases of laryngeal amyloidosis have been reported since that time.

Amyloidosis can be either generalized – primary or secondary – or localized. The larynx is rarely involved in generalized primary amyloidosis. It is, however, the usual site for amyloidosis of the respiratory tract (Figure 11.7). However, the real nature of amyloidosis is still an enigma. Amyloidosis makes up 1% of all benign laryngeal 'tumours'. It is slightly more common in men than in women and usually occurs between the ages of 40 and 60 years (Stark and New, 1949; McAlpine and Fuller, 1964). The sites of

occurrence are, in descending order of frequency, the false vocal cords, aryepiglottic folds and the subglottis (Leroux–Robert, 1962; d'Arcy, 1972), but Ryan, Pearson and Weiland (1977) cited the vocal cords as the prime site.

Amyloidosis within the larynx occurs in two forms: one tumour-like and the other displaying diffuse infiltration. The symptomatology will of course, depend on the site of involvement. Hoarseness will occur if the vocal cords are involved, and increasing inspiratory problems are typical of subglottic deposits; patients with supraglottic amyloidosis have uncharacteristic and more diffuse symptoms.

Histopathology

Congo red is the most commonly used staining reaction for amyloid and gives a bright red colour (Figure 11.8). In polarizing light apple-green birefringence is obtained. Low-angle X-ray diffraction is the third principal method, after light and electron microscopy, for identifying the amyloid substance (Kyle and Bayrd, 1975). The congo red reaction is sensitive, and false positives and negatives are rare. However, Phorwhite BBU is more sensitive with even fewer false staining reactions (Waldrop, Puchtler and Valentine, 1973).

The following differential diagnoses have to be ruled out: hyalinized myxomatous polyps, benign and malignant tumours beneath an intact mucosa, retention cysts and laryngocoele. Plasmacytoma with amyloid deposits is another differential diagnosis.

Treatment

The treatment for laryngeal amyloidosis is surgery, which can be performed microlaryngoscopically. Localized lesions may be removed entirely. In diffuse submucosal deposits repeated excision may be necessary to restore the airway and to preserve the voice. Extra care should be taken when removing amyloid tissue at the level of the cricoid ring to avoid subglottic stenosis. A laryngofissure approach may be indicated for extensive lesions. The use of the carbon dioxide laser should not be overlooked. In amyloidosis of immunoglobulin origin the use of immunosuppressive or cytostatic agents has been suggested (Jones *et al.*, 1972).

Benign mesodermal tumours
Vascular neoplasms

Vascular neoplasms arise from blood or lymphatic vessels. The tumours arising solely from lymph vessels are extremely rare within the larynx. Combined lymphangiomas and haemangiomas may be present. The blood vessel neoplasms may be benign (haemangioma) or malignant (haemangiosarcoma). In addition

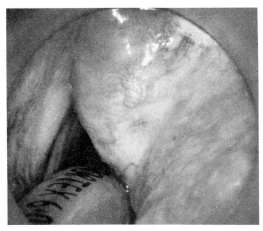

Figure 11.7 Amyloidosis of the right ventricular band. Bulging of the false vocal cord is seen at microlaryngoscopy

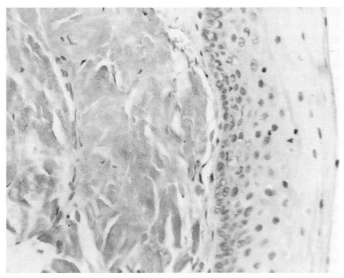

Figure 11.8 Amyloidosis. Photomicrograph showing infiltration of an amorphous substance, staining positively with Congo red, lying in the submucosa with intact overlying epithelium (× 370)

haemangiopericytomas and Kaposi's sarcoma also occur.

Haemangioma

Haemangiomas are rare in adults. Vascular but non-neoplastic lesions occur such as the 'telangiectatic' vocal cord polyp, which is filled with thin-walled blood vessels. Some of these vessels may be filled with old or recently formed thrombi. Around such polyps older submucous haemorrhage may be seen at microlaryngoscopy.

Another differential diagnosis is the pyogenic granuloma, often located on the posterior part of the vocal cord and related to a previous intubation.

Infantile haemangioma

This is discussed in Volume 6, Chapter 22.

Chondroma

Since 1816, when a cartilaginous tumour of the larynx was first described by Travers (van de Catsijne, 1965), more than 200 such tumours have been reported and approximately 20% of these have been chondrosarcomas (Fombeur *et al.*, 1974; Zismor, Noyek and Lewis, 1975). These tumours tend to occur between the ages of 40 and 70 years and are more frequent in men than in women, with a ratio of four to one. Most of the tumours originate in the cricoid cartilage (70%) and most often from the posterior cricoid plate (Figure 11.9) (van de Catsijne, 1965; Neis, McMahon and Norris, 1989).

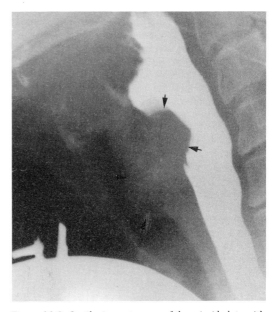

Figure 11.9 Cartilaginous tumour of the cricoid plate with marked narrowing of the airway necessitating a tracheostomy. The tumour is bulging into the hypopharynx as seen in this barium swallow

Symptomatology

The symptomatology of laryngeal cartilaginous tumours is generally non-specific, with hoarseness and dyspnoea as prominent features, their degree depending on the site and size of the tumour. Tumours arising from the cricoid cartilage often extend into the subglottic space and thereby cause progressive inspiratory stridor. Hoarseness may occur if vocal cord mobility is impaired. Extension of the tumour posteriorly into the hypopharynx may result in dysphagia. A swelling may be noted externally if the tumour is located in the cricoid ring or in the thyroid cartilage.

Clinical findings

Indirect laryngoscopy usually reveals a smooth mass covered by an intact mucosa. While radiological examination may disclose peripheral or central calcific stippling, coarse irregular calcification is the rule. This feature is considered to be pathognomonic of cartilaginous tumours and is found in about 75% (Zismor, Noyek and Lewis, 1975). Because the tumour may be so hard and difficult to penetrate, biopsy specimens may be unrepresentative often consisting of the overlying mucosa only.

Histopathology

The histopathological evaluation of cartilaginous tumours often presents considerable difficulties as regards both classification and grading of malignancy (Figure 11.10). Difficulty in distinguishing between chondroma and highly differentiated chondrosarcoma lies in the fact that pronounced cellularity and polymorphism often occur only in small foci (Lichten-

stein, 1965). DNA measurements may assist in a correct diagnosis (Kreicbergs, 1981) but are not available in all laboratories.

Treatment

Surgery is the treatment of choice, radiotherapy being of little value (van de Catsijne, 1965; Ackerman and del Regato, 1970). The operation of choice has generated much discussion (Goethals, Dahlin and Devine, 1963; Al-Saleem *et al.*, 1970; Hyams and Rabuzzi, 1970; Lawson, Bryce and Briant, 1972). Conservative surgery, whenever possible, has been recommended for both chondromas and chondrosarcomas on account of the slow growth rate of these tumours and the low incidence of metastases of the latter.

Myogenic tumours

Leiomyoma

Leiomyomas comprise three different types – common, vascular and 'bizarre'. The latter has not been described in the larynx (Kleinsasser and Glanz, 1979). The leiomyoma is one of the most common benign tumours in the human being.

Leiomyomas have been reported in children but they occur more often in adults of all ages. They seem to be most common in the supraglottic region,

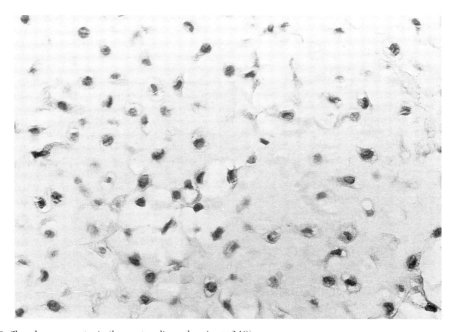

Figure 11.10 Chondroma, no atypia (haematoxylin and eosin. × 340)

have been of pea to pigeon-egg size and have been removed endoscopically or by an external approach.

Rhabdomyoma

Rhabdomyomas of the true adult type are extremely rare tumours. Kleinsasser and Glanz (1979) found only eight descriptions of confirmed cases of rhabdomyoma in the larynx and added one of their own. Most rhabdomyomas in the larynx originate in the vocal cord region and appear as a polypoid mass but may extend above and below the cords.

Microscopic examination shows a tumour composed of round to oval cells with a pale, faintly granular cytoplasm. There are many large vacuoles in the cytoplasm, mainly placed in the periphery. The nuclei are round to oval and vesicular with prominent nucleoli, also located in the periphery. Cross-striations are usually visible in some cells with ordinary haematoxylin-eosin staining, but are accentuated by phosphotungstic acid-haematoxylin (PTAH) staining. Electron microscopic examination may be useful especially in uncertain cases. The differential diagnosis is primarily granular cell tumour.

Fetal rhabdomyoma is extremely rare in the larynx. The precise nature of this tumour is unknown. The lesion may be a hamartoma and not a true neoplasm. It usually presents shortly after birth but may occur in adults and present as a vocal cord polyp (Michaels, 1984).

The treatment for these lesions is surgery and endoscopic measures may be sufficient.

Granular cell tumours

In the past, benign granular cell tumours have been considered to be of mesenchymal origin. Abrikossoff (1926) suspected a myogenic origin and suggested the term 'myoblastic myoma'. The exact histogenesis of this tumour, however, still remains uncertain. A Schwann cell origin has been suggested (Azzopardi, 1956). Ackerman and Rosai (1974) concluded that the multiplicity of current aetiological data suggests that a granular cell tumour is the consequence of degradation and that it is not a specific neoplastic entity.

The most common location for granular cell tumours of the larynx is the true vocal cords and they may be managed endoscopically.

Fibroma

Fibromas are composed of fibrillar connective tissue. In the large series of benign laryngeal tumours presented by New and Erich (1938) only six of their 722 tumours were fibromas. Eight of the miscellaneous tumours listed in Table 11.1 are fibromas (Shaw, 1979). The appearance may vary. New and Erich (1938) described them as soft and pedunculated and Shaw (1979) as round, firm, smooth and sessile.

The treatment is endoscopic removal in most cases.

Lipoma

Neoplasms may arise from the adipose tissue present, especially in the false cords. Many of the reported lipomas arose in the hypopharynx and extended into the larynx (Michaels, 1984).

Macroscopically, lipomas are light-coloured, encapsulated and lobulated tumours. Microscopically they are composed of fat cells of varying size and a fibroreticular stroma.

The treatment is endoscopic removal or by an external approach depending on the size and location.

Table 11.1 **Benign tumours of the larynx seen at the Institute of Laryngology and Otology, London 1948–1969 (Shaw, 1979)**

Non-neoplastic		*Neoplastic*	
Vocal cord polyps	1122	Papilloma*	170*
Retention cysts	72	Adenoma	16
Tuberculous granuloma	44	Chondroma	3
Intubation granuloma	18	Miscellaneous	16
Contact ulcer granuloma	14	(includes fibroma, haemangioma,	
Amyloid deposit	13	lipoma, and neurofibroma)	
Wegener's granuloma	8		
Granular cell myoblastoma	6		
Miscellaneous	3		
Total	1300 (86%)		205 (14%)

* Approximately 25% were multiple juvenile papillomas

Benign ectodermal tumours

Adenoma

Benign tumours arising from the seromucinous glands of the larynx are rare. The statistics given by Friedmann (1975) from the Institute of Laryngology and Otology, London, reported 16 cases seen during a 21-year period (see Table 11.1). Sabri and Hajjar (1967) reported on 37 neoplasms of the larynx of which 19 were mixed tumours. Most of these occurred in the subglottic larynx (Som *et al.*, 1979).

Symptoms may be few until the tumour obstructs the breathing. The differential diagnoses should be limited to those lesions that are expansile masses with smooth overlying mucosa – a retention cyst, internal laryngocoele, angioma or adenoid cystic carcinoma.

The treatment is by surgery and the approach depends on the size and location of the adenoma within the larynx.

Neurogenic tumours

Along with the other benign tumours, neurilemmoma of the larynx is not common. New and Erich (1938), in their major review of 722 benign laryngeal tumours, reported one neurilemmoma. Holinger and Johnston (1951) reported one in a series of 1197 benign laryngeal tumours. Nanson (1978) found 87 reported in the literature.

Neurilemmoma is a benign tumour arising from the Schwann cells of the axon sheath. The term was coined by Stout (1935). It is usually a well-encapsulated, slowly growing tumour which can be fairly large. A neurilemmoma with a diameter of a few centimetres is obviously more serious in the larynx than when subcutaneous. Symptoms develop insidiously but can be prominent if degeneration and haemorrhage occur into the tumour causing a life-threatening situation.

Treatment

Treatment is by surgery. Small tumours may be removed endoscopically, others via a laryngofissure or a lateral laryngotomy, depending on the size and location.

Paraganglioma

More than 30 paragangliomas of the larynx have been reported in the literature with an equal sex incidence and with a peak in the fifth decade of life (Olofsson *et al.*, 1984). Most of these tumours arise from the supraglottic paraganglia and less frequently from the inferior ones. The location of the tumours

means that they often do not give symptoms until they have reached an advanced stage. Haemoptysis may occur. Angiography can provide information about the vascularity of these tumours. Computerized tomography or magnetic resonance imaging are the best radiological methods to determine the extent of these tumours. Paraganglioma arising from the inferior paraganglia may present as thyroid tumours depending on the close relationship to the thyroid capsule (Figure 11.11). The diagnosis is made entirely on the microscopic examination. Strikingly few of the laryngeal paragangliomas have been diagnosed pre-operatively, which to some extent may be the result of too superficial biopsies but also of the rarity of this entity.

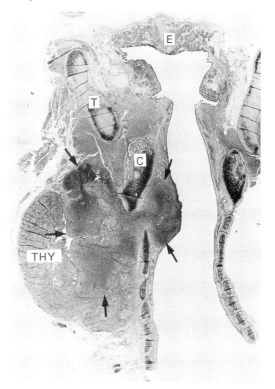

Figure 11.11 Paraganglioma probably arising from the inferior paraganglia and with involvement of the thyroid gland and the subglottic larynx. The tumour extends through the cricotracheal space and has a dumb-bell shape (coronal section through a laryngectomy specimen). C: cricoid cartilage; E: epiglottis; T: thyroid cartilage; THY: thyroid lobe

Histopathology

Important criteria for making the diagnosis of paraganglioma include the typical 'Zellballen' pattern on light microscopy, which is best demonstrated by reticulin staining (Figure 11.12). The presence of argyrophilic granules is revealed by Grimelius' stain. Ultrastructural examination shows neurosecretory granules. The main differential diagnoses are haemangiopericytoma, carcinoid tumour, granular cell tumour, salivary gland tumours, haemangiomas and thyroid carcinoma, which may invade the larynx and trachea. A relatively high percentage of laryngeal paragangliomas shows malignant behaviour with regional and distant metastases (Wetmore *et al.*, 1981).

Treatment

The treatment for paragangliomas varies considerably because of the rarity of the tumour and the often incorrect diagnosis. Conservative surgery should be performed whenever possible.

Table 11.2 Incidence of malignancy of head and neck

	Males (%)	*Females* (%)
Skin	8.2	7.0
Oral cavity	0.6	0.3
Oropharynx	0.4	0.1
Nasopharynx	0.1	0.1
Hypopharynx	0.3	0.2
Nasal cavity and sinuses	0.2	0.2
Larynx	1.3	0.2
Thyroid	0.2	0.6
Lymphoma	0.3	0.3
Sarcoma	0.1	0.1
All head and neck	11.7	9.1
All sites: total number	9177	8585

(from Powell and Robin, 1983, courtesy of Castle House Publications)

Malignant tumours

Cancer of the larynx is a particularly important malignancy. In the UK it represents approximately 1% of all malignancies (Powell and Robin, 1983) in men, although somewhat less in women (Table 11.2). It has, in common with many other head and neck cancers, a predominantly squamous pathology as well as early interference with both function and emotion. It shares with only a few other types of cancer (such as cervical, skin, lymphoma, perhaps colonic) a high rate of cure which, in certain subsites, may reach over 85% (Table 11.3) and overall exceeds 50% (Powell and Robin, 1983). Carcinoma of the larynx, therefore, places upon the clinician a much greater responsibility than usual, for careful evaluation and treatment offer a probability of cure while, in common with a number of other head and neck neoplasms, failure may be followed by a relatively uncomfortable death. Even further demands are made at the present time, for not only the survival of the patient but rehabilitation is becoming of even greater importance than formerly. Thus the selection of treatment and types of surgery must be made with more insight than previously into its behaviour and response to treatment. Because of the differences in prognosis, not only between laryngeal tumours and

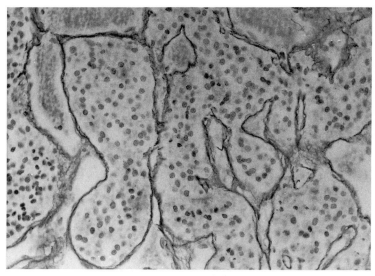

Figure 11.12 Paraganglioma. Photomicrograph demonstrating the reticulin fibres that enclose groups of cells creating the 'Zellballen' appearance so typical for paraganglioma (Laidlaw reticulin stain, × 375)

Table 11.3 Histological differentiation: 5-year survival, age-adjusted, males only 1957–1976

Squamous carcinoma	Supraglottis		Glottis		Subglottis	
	Total	5-year survival (%)	Total	5-year survival (%)	Total	5-year survival (%)
In situ	3	0.0	89	88.5	2	59.2
Well differentiated	128	38.8	531	71.1	15	29.8
Moderately differentiated	120	33.8	215	67.2	17	13.6
Poorly differentiated	197	29.3	195	54.7	26	44.8
Not specified	99	37.4	276	71.4	11	72.3
Total number	547	33.8	1306	69.3	71	38.8

Source: Birmingham and West Midlands Regional Cancer Registry, 1986

those of neighbouring sites, but also of the various sites within the larynx, a greater than usual attention must be paid to the accurate assessment of each tumour, so that the appropriate management may be instituted.

Incidence

Carcinoma of the larynx is not common, nor is it rare. Incidence world-wide varies (Waterhouse *et al.*, 1982), and a number of areas of relative high (> 10/100 000) incidence can be identified, for example Brazil (Sao Paulo), the black populations in parts of the USA, Hong Kong, India (Bombay, Poona), France (Bas Rhins, Doubs), Italy (Varesa), Poland (Katowice), Spain, and Switzerland (Geneva), while low incidence areas (< 2/100 000) include Japan, Norway, Sweden, New Guinea, and Senegal (Dakir). The UK suffers from an intermediate to low incidence (4/100 000). Incidence, it must be remembered, is as reliable as the statistical infrastructure, and a number of less developed countries may suffer from underreporting. It is clear, nevertheless, that significant differences do occur between and within various countries. In Hawaii the Caucasians suffer an incidence (8.1/100 000), more than five times that of the Chinese (1.4), four times the Filipino (2.0) and nearly three times that of the Japanese (3.3), who live in the same place (these figures are for men, those for women are proportionately less). Where the urban population can be identified separately from the rural population the incidence is almost always higher in the former. Where racial groups can be identified, the respective incidence appears to follow that of the country of origin, e.g. in Hawaii the Japanese incidence is similar to that of the Japanese in Japan, the Caucasians to that in the USA. The racial characteristic extends between countries, e.g. the in-

cidence in the Chinese in Shanghai and the USA generally is similar. Black populations in the USA have a higher incidence of carcinoma of the larynx than Caucasians in the same area. One invariable characteristic of carcinoma of the larynx is its greater predominance in men, compared with women, 6:1 at its lowest in Canada (Mannitoba) and 32:1 at its maximum in Italy (Varesa). Indeed, it is in the higher incidence areas that the male/female disparity is greatest.

It is difficult to draw firm conclusions from observations of incidence beyond remarking that the social and racial differences probably reflect different habits, and in the case of cancer of the larynx along with those of the mouth and pharynx, tend to reflect the already recognized effects of tobacco and alcohol (Newhouse, Gregory and Shannon, 1980). Of interest is the relatively low rate of laryngeal cancer in the UK compared with the definitively high rates of (smoking-related) lung cancer. A small rise in incidence of laryngeal cancer has been observed in England and Wales 1960–1968 and 1972–1978, a rise proportionately greater in females (McMichael, 1978; Robin *et al.*, 1991a) attributed to the rise in smoking during the 1939–1945 war. This rise is not apparent when only glottic tumours are considered. The already high and increasing levels of mortality from laryngeal cancer in France, Italy and Spain contrast with the rest of Europe, and examination of birth cohorts in France have led to the suggestion that alcohol plays a promoting role, particularly in the supraglottis (Tuyns and Audigier, 1976).

Presentation (Figure 11.13)

The *incidence* (as opposed to mortality) of cancer of the larynx, in common with most head and neck cancers, increases with increasing age, but because of the reducing numbers of persons surviving as age progresses, the actual number of cases *presenting* for

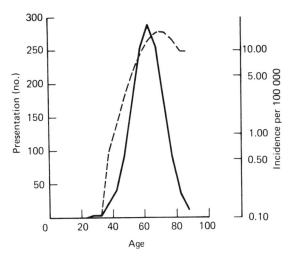

Figure 11.13 Presentation (——) compared with incidence per 100 000 (– – –) of carcinoma of the larynx (glottis) in males. (Source: Birmingham and West Midlands Regional Cancer Registry, 1957–1976)

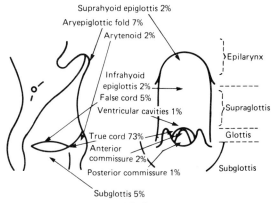

Figure 11.14 Carcinoma of the larynx in men – percentage distribution (Powell and Robin, 1983, reproduced by courtesy of Castle House Publications)

treatment falls with age (Ramadan *et al.*, 1982). The peak age of presentation is therefore younger than that of maximum incidence (that of the glottis in the UK being approximately 62 years). Supraglottic lesions present at an earlier age than those of the glottis. The trend of increasing incidence with age is not universal and does not apply, e.g. in Spain (Zaragoza) (Waterhouse *et al.*, 1982) and Finland (Taskinen, 1969) where the cancer is more often supraglottic. These observations suggest that there may be a significant difference in the aetiology and behaviour of these cancers compared with the glottic tumours which predominate in the UK.

Classification

Laryngeal lesions are diverse in their behaviour and prognosis and thus classification is particularly important. Attempts at classification were begun as long ago as 1876 (Isambert). Over a period of years (since 1954) the International Union against Cancer (UICC) has undertaken the task of establishing a classification of a number of cancers, the larynx being one of the first, and now agreement has been reached generally with the American Joint Committee (AJC) and other similar bodies (UICC) about what may become a definite classification, at least for a decade. The basis of the UICC classification is anatomical (Figure 11.14).

It is important to understand the purpose of classification. The original intention of classification was to enable different sources to standardize their material in order that numbers and extent of tumours could be compared. The various sites were selected because of both their anatomical ease of identification and also

their behavioural homogeneity. The definitions of the original UICC proposals have changed slightly to achieve the original intent. There was never any primary intention to use the classification to promote any treatment, although clinicians have found it useful to use the UICC terminology for this purpose. Classification is fundamental in studies of epidemiology.

Tumours were originally designated 'intrinsic' and 'extrinsic' laryngeal tumours. The latter, and also the term 'laryngopharynx' have been discarded for they represent the present day hypopharynx (sometimes oropharynx). Even now there is some difficulty in definition, and the term 'marginal zone' has been selected to designate the area of difficulty. The TNM (UICC, 1987) classification of larynx (International Classification of Diseases for Oncology, 1987) is given in Appendix 11.1.

There is a lack of a precise definition of the 'vocal cord'. Several interpretations are permissible: the free edge; the point where the vestibule meets the upper surface to a point or line 1 cm below; the free edge to 1 cm below; that area of the cord beneath which lies Reinke's space, that is the upper surface and free edge of the membranous cord. The lack of definition of the cord may undermine the credibility of the TNM system, yet in practice the use of the last interpretation seems to create little real difficulty. This was the agreed definition at the Centennial Conference on Laryngeal Cancer in Toronto (1974).

Of all the sites of cancer the larynx not only has one of the more detailed and precise TNM classifications, but it is also one of the most well tried and useful. It is for this reason it justifies some degree of study.

Staging

Staging is the grouping together of (TNM) features which may share a level of prognosis or a certain treatment. Staging has not been utilized in this and subsequent discussion.

Aetiology

The cause of cancer of the larynx is not known. A number of possibly related factors (male predominance, some racial predilection, a greater incidence among urban dwellers) have been designated, and there is an indisputable relationship between tobacco and alcohol (US Surgeon General, 1979; Hinds, Thomas and O'Reilly, 1979). Radiation (Sakamoto, Sakamoto and Sugano, 1979), asbestos (Parnes, 1990), and a number of occupational factors have been cited (Elwood *et al.*, 1984), but none can be regarded as conclusive in the manner of those causing, for instance, lung cancer. Laryngeal keratosis and leucoplakia (see Plates 5/11/I(*a*), (*b*) (Hellquist, Olofsson and Gröntoft, 1981; Crissman, 1982) are related to carcinoma of the larynx, but metaplasia (although smoking-related) has not satisfied the criteria for designation as a clear aetiological factor (Auerbach, Hammond and Garfinkel, 1970). One of the highest alcohol-consuming populations in Europe – the French – also shows the highest laryngeal carcinoma incidence in that continent. Contrary to common belief, the perceived consumption of spirits (Scotland, UK) does not have a similarly matching laryngeal cancer incidence (Waterhouse *et al.*, 1982). There is almost invariably an associated social relationship between alcohol and tobacco, and thus a distinction between the two factors is difficult to make, and cohort studies in France (Tuyns and Audigier, 1976) seem to postulate a reduction of laryngeal cancer as a result of deprivation (during World War II) of both alcohol and tobacco (the opposite of the features of the apparent rise in incidence, particularly in women (UK), as a result of their increase in smoking and alcohol consumption during the same war period).

It is reasonable to accept that although no close and irrefutable aetiological factor can be designated, there are several often related environmental factors which are clearly associated with an increased incidence of cancer, i.e. tobacco, alcohol, environmental (urban) pollution, asbestos, therapeutic radiation (thyroid), as yet unidentified social and possibly genetic factors which affect racial groups, and certain uncommon occupational influences (Maier, de Vries and Snow, 1991).

Symptoms of carcinoma

The symptoms of carcinoma of the larynx are not greatly different from those of any space-occupying lesion of the larynx, but certain features make a carcinoma more distinguishable.

Progressive and unremitting dysphonia. The feature of a malignant tumour is its relentless advance, although in the early stages, in particular, the dysphonia may be intermittent. A further consideration is the cancer which develops in one who suffers from chronic laryngitis, and these individuals are particularly at risk from delay in diagnosis.

Dyspnoea and *stridor* are less frequent but, as a sequel to neglected dysphonia, almost invariably indicate an advanced tumour. Subglottic carcinoma may present with these as the only symptoms.

Pain is a relatively uncommon and late symptom and more typical of supraglottic lesions. Pain referred to the ear is particularly sinister and should always promote a high suspicion of cancer.

Dysphagia is relatively rare but carries a worse prognosis because it almost invariably indicates invasion of the pharynx.

Swelling of the neck or larynx may reflect the direct penetration of a tumour outside the larynx and as such its origin, without other symptoms, may initially be difficult to distinguish conclusively. Secondary malignant deposits in the lymph nodes of the neck have few distinctive features other than their predominantly ipsilateral situation, usually in the upper/middle deep cervical chain. A prelaryngeal or tracheal lymph node must be distinguished from thyroid disease.

Cough and *irritation* in the throat may be early nondescript symptoms; *haemoptysis* is rare and is most often seen in a lesion of the (margin of the) epiglottis; while *anorexia*, *cachexia* or *fetor* are usually late symptoms.

Examination and diagnosis

Diagnosis will be made after consideration of:

1 History
2 Examination of the larynx
3 Examination of the neck
4 General examination of the patient
5 Radiology
6 Clinical investigations
7 Histological examination.

History

The history follows from the symptoms already discussed. Of no small importance is the temporal factor, unfortunately not considered in the UICC classification. The rate of advance of a cancer is important in its progress and prognosis – thus a small lesion with a long history of symptoms suggests a slowly growing lesion, whereas a massive cancer with a short history inevitably has a correspondingly poor outlook. Cancer can coexist with or supervene in leucoplakia, chronic laryngitis, tuberculosis, etc., and the symptoms of cancer or of any of the other disorders are not necessarily distinguishable from each other.

Examination of the larynx

This is generally, initially performed with a mirror (see Chapter 1). Any focal abnormality of the larynx can be a tumour, but typically a vocal cord lesion may appear as a warty enlargement on one cord, but variation from a nodule or thickening of a vocal cord through extensive hyperkeratotic sheets of epithelium to gross ulceration may be seen. In the supraglottis there is focal swelling, redness or ulceration, while a mass may be visible in the subglottis. The subglottis is often difficult to see, but a tumour may appear, most usually as an asymmetrical swelling often masked by mucoid debris. A second difficult area may be the posterior surface of the epiglottis hidden by the backward curve of the tip. The laryngeal ventricle is a third area that it is difficult to assess, where the initial or only clue to the presence of cancer may be a slight fullness. A feature associated with ulceration of these hidden areas can be pain, referred to the (ipsilateral) ear. It cannot be too strongly emphasized that any focal abnormality may prove to be malignant.

A most important feature to be assessed is the *mobility* of the larynx. Mobility of any moving part of the larynx can be impaired by invasion of the tumour into muscle layers and it carries a much more sinister prognosis. Mobility may occasionally be impaired by the sheer bulk of a large tumour, but as distinct from deeper invasion, this is uncommon and often uncertain. Subglottic lesions often limit vocal cord movement by invasion of either the muscles or the cricoarytenoid joint, and both indicate an advanced tumour.

Indirect laryngoscopy is satisfactory for most patients, and provides added information about mobility. However, *flexible endoscopes* allow examination of almost every patient without general anaesthesia (which may prejudice the assessment of mobility). Furthermore, the subglottis can sometimes be examined.

Direct laryngoscopy is necessary for most patients for biopsy purposes; microlaryngoscopy is desirable in many.

Examination of the neck

This must be carried out carefully to identify the possible spread of tumour beyond the larynx either directly or by metastasis to the regional lymph nodes. The most frequent site of secondary deposits is the ipsilateral deep cervical chain, usually in the upper/middle region. Glottic tumours rarely metastasize (Table 11.4), while deposits in the lymph nodes are more frequent from subglottic and particularly supraglottic lesions. Nodes invaded by subglottic lesions are often found in the upper mediastinum, an added reason for the relatively poor prognosis of these lesions. The frequency of ipsi-, and indeed, bilateral deposits derived from supraglottic cancer is also reflected in the prognosis. Occasionally deposits can be identified in the prelaryngeal nodes and,

Table 11.4 Incidence of nodal metastases of carcinoma of the larynx (males) 1957–1976

	Number with known node status	Node positive (%)
Supraglottis	598	38.8
Glottis	1394	4.8
Subglottis	77	13.0

Source: Birmingham and West Midlands Regional Cancer Registry, 1986

even more infrequently, beyond the cervical region. Examination must include an assessment of the number, mobility and level of the lymph nodes.

Some swelling of the larynx, whether widening or as a result of penetration of tumour through the cricoarytenoid membrane, may be felt. An enlarged thyroid lobe should suggest invasion by tumour.

General examination

A general physical examination is required to identify metastases, e.g. to the liver, and to assess the overall physical status of the individual who is likely to need an anaesthetic and biopsy, possibly surgery, radiotherapy or chemotherapy. This examination applies to any patient with a malignancy and need not be detailed here.

Radiological investigations

Chest

In many respects this is the most important investigation at this stage, for assessment of the chest not only indicates the presence or likely absence of distant metastases (and the chest is undoubtedly the most common site of such metastases in cancer of the larynx); but may also indicate the presence of other disorders. It is indeed, nowadays, an integral part, together with a clinical examination, of the assessment of the general physical status of the older adult.

Larynx

Radiological examination of the larynx is undertaken in order to attempt to delineate the extent of the tumour. It is described in detail in Chapter 2.

Clinical investigation

It is appropriate at an early stage to undertake laboratory investigations, i.e. a full haematological screen and biochemical profile including liver functions and serum proteins; in the past, serological tests for syphilis were regarded as essential, although in the UK the yield is unrewarding. A (urine) screen for diabetes, and electrocardiography are also indicated.

Histological examination

Currently it is normal to acquire a specimen (biopsy) of the tumour by direct laryngoscopy, and this is usually carried out under general anaesthesia allowing a careful and thorough direct examination of the tumour. Direct examination should include the use of a microscope in most circumstances. Biopsy material should include an adequate amount of tissue both from ulcerated areas and elsewhere if practicable. If the tumour is very small, care must be taken, first to obtain sufficient material, and second, not to damage normal tissue.

It is essential in the climate of medical practice today to obtain a biopsy of all cases, unless by so doing the patient's well-being will be prejudiced – this latter situation is rare (Table 11.5). Biopsy of the primary tumour is most advantageous although on occasions a biopsy of the secondary deposit is enough and occasionally even more appropriate. Sometimes both are required. The general principle should be firmly adopted not to make incisional biopsies in the neck except at definitive surgery unless this is unavoidable. Fine needle aspiration biopsy is used increasingly (Cusumano *et al.*, 1989).

Table 11.5 Histological confirmation of cancer of the larynx 1957–1976

	Histologically confirmed (%)
Supraglottis	90.9
Glottis	94.1
Subglottis	89.0

Source: Birmingham and West Midlands Regional Cancer Registry, 1986

The biopsy material is important on three grounds:

1 Definite diagnosis of malignancy is required. It is not possible in every case either to diagnose or to exclude the presence of malignancy purely by inspection, and all experienced surgeons have found this. Even the most benign-looking polyp or nodule has occasionally been found to be malignant. Conversely, some quite active looking keratoses may not be malignant. Tuberculosis in former times was a diagnostic complication (Hautant, 1937).
2 Identification of the type of tumour. While squamous carcinoma is undoubtedly the most common, other rare forms of malignancy are found and need individual consideration.
3 Differentiation. Often neglected, the degree of differentiation may be significant. Biopsy material may, unless representative, be misleading, and thus where possible several biopsies should be taken. The degree of differentiation may scarcely be worthy of consideration when a prognosis is to be made (see Table 11.3).

Difficulties in diagnosis

Negative biopsy

If a biopsy of a malignant-looking lesion is found to be negative, the biopsy should be repeated, but on some occasions reliance is placed on clinical diagnosis alone (usually advanced cases).

Keratosis

Sometimes a keratotic lesion yields a non-malignant histopathological diagnosis. It is often difficult to decide just when such a lesion becomes malignant (Silamniku *et al.*, 1989).

Previous radiation

Previous radiation is a common source of dilemma. A low-grade perichondritis may prevent a larynx from returning to normal. Careful observation is required. If a larynx does return to normal after radiation treatment and changes later, recurrent cancer is the most likely cause.

Miscellaneous conditions

Various conditions such as chronic laryngitis, tuberculosis, syphilis and benign tumours may give rise to diagnostic confusion or difficulty (Hautant, 1937).

Pathology

The vast majority of malignant tumours arising in the larynx are squamous cell carcinomas. All other types of malignancy arising in the larynx are rare. The histopathological classification can be performed according to Broders (1920, 1932) (Figures 11.15,

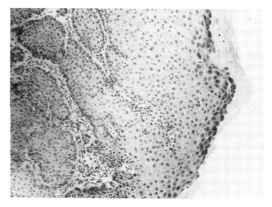

Figure 11.15 Well-differentiated microinvasive squamous cell carcinoma of the vocal cord (haematoxylin and eosin, × 80)

11.16 and 11.17). To determine whether the initial biopsy specimen yielded prognostic information, Jakobsson *et al.* (1973) introduced an eight-factor malignancy grading system and applied it to glottic carcino- mas. Nuclear polymorphism, mode of invasion and the total malignancy score were the factors that were most important in predicting the outcome for the patients (Jakobsson, 1973).

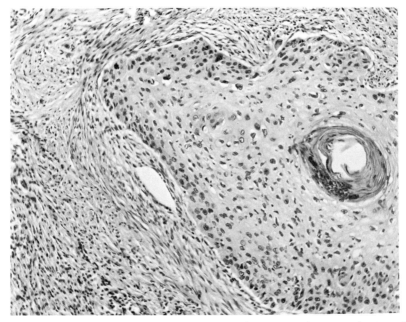

Figure 11.16 Well-differentiated squamous cell carcinoma of the supraglottic region, showing nuclear irregularity, cell mitosis and keratin pearl formation (× 120)

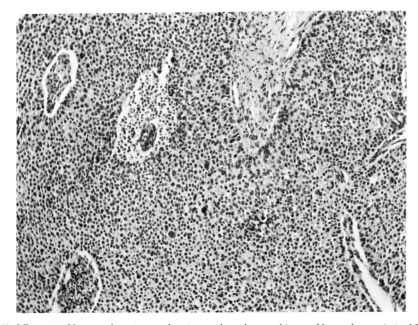

Figure 11.17 Undifferentiated laryngeal carcinoma showing nuclear pleomorphism and hyperchromasia (× 120)

A distinct variant of well-differentiated squamous cell carcinoma is the verrucous carcinoma (Figures 11.18 and 11.19) (Ackerman's tumour), which is most frequently reported arising in the oral cavity, but makes up a small proportion of all laryngeal carcinomas (van Nostrand and Olofsson, 1972; Ferlito and Recher, 1980; Michaels, 1987).

Spread of laryngeal carcinoma

The growth and spread of laryngeal carcinoma is determined to a great extent by the site of origin of the primary tumour. Important factors in determining the directions and extent of tumour growth are the anatomical barriers produced by the laryngeal compartments described by Pressman (1956), Tucker and Smith (1962) and Pressman, Simon and Monell (1969). The growth and spread of laryngeal carcinoma is described by Olofsson and van Nostrand (1973).

Glottic carcinoma

Most of the tumours arising in the glottic region originate on the free margins of the vocal cords which are covered by squamous epithelium (Figures 11.20, 11.21, 11.22 and 11.23). According to the agreements reached at the Centennial Conference on Laryngeal Cancer in Toronto (1974), the glottic region comprises the free margins and the horizontal surfaces of the vocal cords and the commissures. The anterior commissure is defined as a line between the vocal cords measuring a few millimetres in height. The subsurfaces of the vocal cords belong to the subglottic region.

Figure 11.18 Microlaryngoscopy. Verrucous carcinoma involving the anterior part of the right vocal cord and the anterior commissure. This patient was treated by endoscopic excision and laser evaporation of the surface. The patient has been followed for 4 years and there is no sign of recurrence, the vocal cords look normal and his voice is excellent

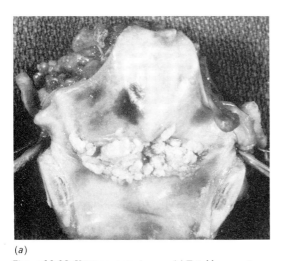

(a)

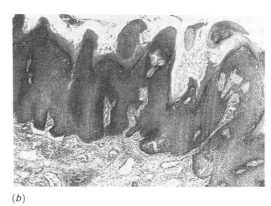

(b)

Figure 11.19 Verrucous carcinoma. (a) Total laryngectomy specimen showing a fungating cauliflower-like tumour involving the true and false vocal cords on both sides. (b) Photomicrograph showing the marked acanthosis with formation of broad, blunt rete ridges extending into the submucosa (haematoxylin and eosin, × 50) (Reproduced by permission from *Cancer* (1972) 30, 691–702)

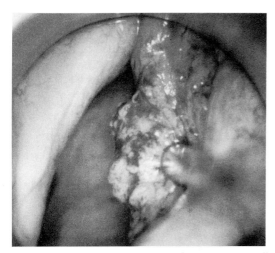

Figure 11.20 Microlaryngoscopy. Exophytic squamous cell carcinoma of the right vocal cord

Glottic carcinomas may arise in, or extend to, the anterior commissure area (see Plate 5/11/IIa), where there is only a thin layer of submucosa and a fibrous cord, 'the anterior commissure tendon', that separates the mucosa from the underlying cartilage. This explains the increased risk of cartilage invasion in the anterior commissure area compared with that for tumours involving other parts of the vocal cords where muscle and perichondrium intervene.

The anterior midline is the most frequent location for invasion of the laryngeal framework (Figure 11.24) (Olofsson and van Nostrand, 1973). When the framework is invaded this occurs most frequently in the ossified parts of the cartilage. Local bone destruction by osteoclasts active at the margins of the tumour precedes the tumour invasion. The vascularization of the cartilage is of great importance too. Unvascularized cartilage has a great resistance to tumour invasion (Olszewski, 1976).

Tumours involving or crossing the anterior commissure often extend below the cords and they may then escape outside the larynx through the cricothyroid membrane anteriorly, sometimes using the preformed vascular channels (see Figure 11.24). Tumours may also extend laterally to the conus elasticus and can then escape through the cricothyroid triangle – bounded by the cricothyroid membrane, the thyroid cartilage and the medial edge of the cricothyroid muscle.

When the vocal cord muscles are invaded the tumour may extend along the muscle bundles anteriorly or posteriorly and may then reach lateral to the arytenoid cartilage where the tumour comes close to the mucosa of the pyriform sinus. Invasion of the posterior cricoarytenoid muscle may occur. Tumour extension lateral to the arytenoid cartilage is difficult to assess by conventional laryngoscopic and radiological means, but may be assessed by computerized tomography. Widening of the thyroarytenoid space indicates such tumour spread. The mucosa of the pyriform sinus on the affected side should be included

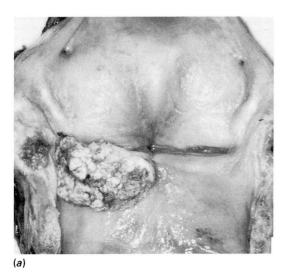

(a)

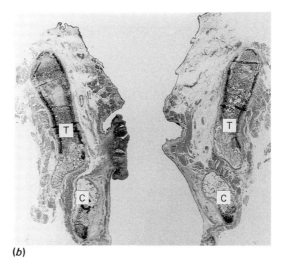

(b)

Figure 11.21 Glottic carcinoma with subglottic extension. (*a*) Total laryngectomy specimen showing a tumour involving the full length of the left vocal cord and with subglottic extension. (*b*) Coronal section of the laryngectomy specimen through the middle third of the vocal cords. The tumour extends to the subsurface of the vocal cord but there is only slight invasion of the thyroarytenoid muscle. C: cricoid cartilage; T: thyroid cartilage

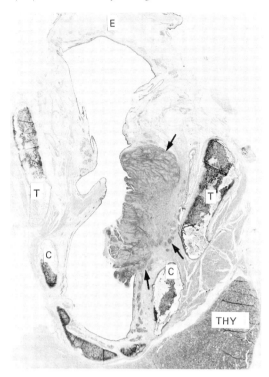

Figure 11.22 Glottic, sub- and supraglottic carcinoma. Coronal section through the middle third of the vocal cords of the laryngectomy specimen. The exophytic 'transglottic' carcinoma has a tendency to spread through the cricothyroid space. C: cricoid cartilage; E: epiglottis; T: thyroid cartilage; THY: thyroid lobe

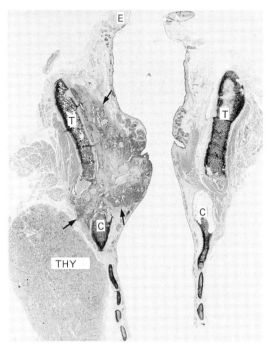

Figure 11.23 'Transglottic' carcinoma of the left hemilarynx. The tumour is growing mainly beneath intact mucosa and invading the ossified portions of the thyroid ala (T) and the cricoid cartilage (C) and spreading outside the larynx through the cricothyroid space, which is typical for these tumours. Note the close relationship between the tumour and the thyroid lobe (THY), which has been (and should be) included in the laryngectomy specimen when dealing with such a tumour. E: epiglottis

in the laryngectomy specimen in these cases to avoid a recurrence above the stoma.

Vertical extension of a glottic carcinoma to the subglottis and/or supraglottis seems to occur more frequently than extension to the opposite side (see Plate 5/11/II(*b*); Figures 11.21, 11.22 and 11.25) (Olofsson and van Nostrand, 1973).

Fixation of the vocal cord indicates deep invasion with involvement at least of the thyroarytenoid muscle (see Figure 11.22). When the posterior part of the vocal cord is involved, fixation of the cord may be the result of invasion of the arytenoid or cricoid cartilages or the cricoarytenoid joint. Perineural invasion may be another aetiological factor but is seen mainly in large carcinomas. Fixation of the vocal cord indicates that the laryngeal framework is invaded and/or that the tumour has spread outside the larynx through cartilage and/or through the cricothyroid membrane or space as in about 50% of the cases (see Figure 11.23) (Olofsson and van Nostrand, 1973; Olofsson, Lord and van Nostrand, 1973). This means that fixation in many cases is a contraindication

to partial surgery. Impaired mobility indicates more superficial invasion of the thyroarytenoid muscle and is often not a contraindication to conservative surgery.

With previously used diagnostic methods, more than 50% of patients with vocal cord fixation in glottic carcinoma were under-assessed, as methods were lacking to determine cartilage invasion and spread outside the laryngeal framework. Computerized tomography and magnetic resonance imaging have become valuable complements in the radiological diagnosis of laryngeal carcinoma and add important information about deep tumour invasion, cartilage destruction and extension of tumour outside the larynx (Gregor, Lloyd and Michaels, 1981; Sökjer and Olofsson, 1981; Werber and Lucente, 1989; Castelijns *et al.*, 1987).

Several reports have stressed the risk of cartilage invasion for tumours which traverse the laryngeal ventricle to occupy at least the glottic and supraglottic regions and often also the subglottis causing a fixed hemilarynx. These tumours extend within the paraglottic space and spread outside the larynx

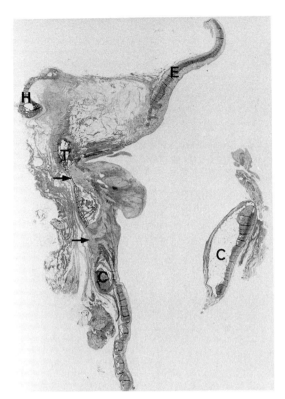

Figure 11.24 Anterior glottic-subglottic carcinoma. Sagittal section of the laryngectomy specimen close to the midline. The tumour invades the ossified part of the thyroid cartilage (T), extends subglottically with spread through the cricothyroid membrane. C: cricoid cartilage; E: epiglottis; H: hyoid bone

through the cartilage and the cricothyroid space (see Figure 11.23).

Supraglottic carcinoma

The growth and spread of supraglottic carcinoma (see Plate 5/11/II(c); Figures 11.26, 11.27 and 11.28) is well studied by the use of whole organ (specimen) serial sections (Olofsson and van Nostrand, 1973).

McGavran, Bauer and Ogura (1961) noted that supraglottic carcinomas often had 'pushing margins' (see Figure 11.28) often involving both sides of the supraglottic larynx. Bocca, Pignataro and Masciario (1968) stressed that supraglottic carcinomas seldom extend to the glottic region because 'the larynx consists of two distinct parts, an upper and a lower part, whose line of demarcation runs at the level of the vocal cords'. The different embryological derivations and the various lymphatic supplies were also stressed. Supraglottic carcinomas do not always respect the glottic region, but the various opinions in reported series depend to a certain extent on the selection of the material examined

(Olofsson and van Nostrand, 1973). Exophytic supraglottic lesions do not often extend to the glottic region and seldom invade the thyroid cartilage. Ulcerative lesions may extend down below the anterior commissure, and when doing so they have a great tendency to invade the thyroid cartilage. Invasion of the cartilage does not seem to occur unless the tumours can be seen macroscopically extending below the anterior commissure. This observation is certainly important in selecting patients for horizontal supraglottic laryngectomy.

Invasion of the pre-epiglottic space is a prominent feature of supraglottic carcinoma and especially those that involve the posterior (laryngeal) surface of the epiglottis (see Figures 11.27 and 11.28). The tumours may extend into the pre-epiglottic space through the fenestrations in the epiglottic cartilage or by destruction of the cartilage. The lateral parts of this space are in direct continuity with the paraglottic space (Tucker and Smith, 1962) and this is another, but not so common, pathway for tumours to reach the pre-epiglottic space. Nearly all tumours that invade the pre-epiglottic space involve the laryngeal surface of the epiglottis, which in most cases can be assessed at laryngoscopy (see Plate 5/11/II(c); Figures 11.26 and 11.27) (Olofsson and van Nostrand, 1973). Invasion of the pre-epiglottic space occurs in 40% of all supraglottic carcinomas and in 70% of all epiglottic tumours (Olofsson and van Nostrand, 1973).

Supraglottic carcinomas may extend cranially to the vallecula and to the base of the tongue. Posteriorly, the tumours may extend to the arytenoid cartilage, invasion of which seems to occur only when the arytenoids are grossly involved by tumour (Kirchner and Som, 1971). The pyriform sinus can be involved by tumours riding over the aryepiglottic folds. The pyriform sinus may also be reached by deep invasion.

Subglottic carcinoma

Primary subglottic carcinomas are rare and are characterized by a tendency to grow circumferentially and to be extensive before symptoms, such as inspiratory stridor, occur. Invasion of the vocal cords may cause impairment of their mobility and thereby hoarseness for which the patient may seek medical advice.

Subglottic carcinomas can spread through the cricothyroid membrane (Figure 11.29) anteriorly or through the cricotracheal space, e.g. posteriorly, or invade the trachea caudally.

Lymph node involvement

The lymphatics within the larynx can be divided into a supraglottic and a subglottic network, separated by the free margin of the vocal cords, which has minimal lymphatic drainage (Rouvière, 1931). This explains

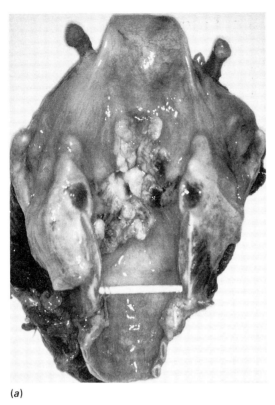

(a)

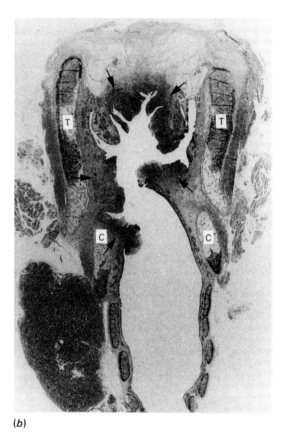

(b)

Figure 11.25 Extensive anterior glottic, sub- and supraglottic carcinoma. (*a*) Total laryngectomy specimen showing the exophytic tumour. (*b*) Coronal section through the anterior third of the vocal cords. The exophytic tumour (arrows) involves the vocal and false vocal cords and extends subglottically but has no deeper invasion. C: cricoid cartilage; T: thyroid cartilage

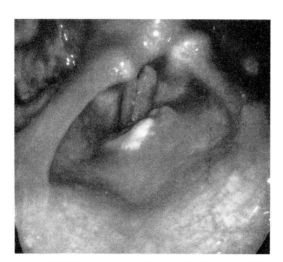

Figure 11.26 Telescopic view. Ulcerated limited supraglottic squamous cell carcinoma involving the lower laryngeal surface of the epiglottis

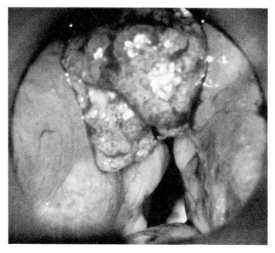

Figure 11.27 Microlaryngoscopy. Exophytic supraglottic squamous cell carcinoma occupying the lower laryngeal surface of the epiglottis and the anterior parts of the false vocal cords

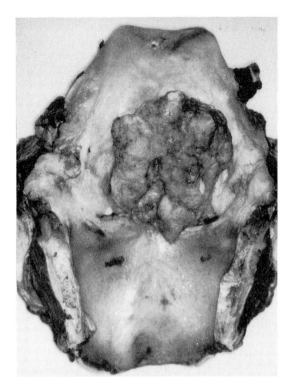 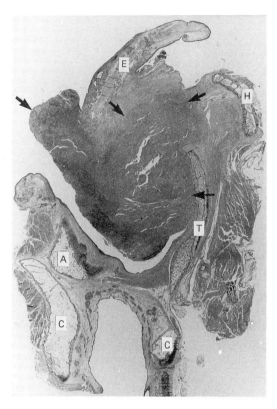

Figure 11.28 Supraglottic carcinoma with invasion of the pre-epiglottic space. (*a*) Total laryngectomy specimen showing the ulcerofungating tumour on the laryngeal surface of the epiglottis. (*b*) Sagittal section through the specimen lateral to the midline showing the extensive invasion of the pre-epiglottic space. The tumour is growing with 'pushing' margins – typical for supraglottic carcinomas. The epiglottic cartilage (E) is destroyed but the thyroid cartilage (T) is not invaded and the tumour does not extend down to the glottic region. A: arytenoid cartilage; C: cricoid cartilage; H: hyoid bone

the low incidence of lymph node metastases in tumours confined to the vocal cords.

The supraglottis is rich in lymphatics, which accounts for the high incidence of lymph node metastases in supraglottic carcinoma, 32% as reported by Som (1970) and 73% as reported by Baclesse (1949). Sand Hansen (1975) found that 44% of the patients with a supraglottic carcinoma but only 5% of those with primary glottic carcinoma and 6% of those with subglottic carcinoma, had palpable cervical lymph nodes at the time of initial diagnosis. In total, 18% of patients with laryngeal cancer had lymph node metastases at the time of referral.

The incidence of palpable lymph nodes increases with the extent of the primary tumour. Of patients with T1 supraglottic carcinoma, 17% had lymph node metastases compared with 47% for the T2–T4 tumours. For glottic carcinoma the highest incidence of lymph node metastases was found when the sub- and supraglottic regions were involved (17%) (Sand Hansen, 1975).

Distant metastases

Few patients present with distant metastases at the time of diagnosis of their laryngeal carcinoma. Secondary distant metastases are more common. Sand Hansen (1975) reported 11% with distant metastases, most of which occurred in the lung (6.8%). The occurrence of pulmonary metastases seemed to some extent to be influenced by the presence of lymph node metastases, the macroscopic appearance and histology of the tumour. Poorly differentiated, necrotic tumours and tumours with lymph node metastases had the highest incidence of pulmonary metastases.

Multiple primary tumours

A number of papers stress the occurrence of synchronous and metachronous second and third primary tumours in patients with head and neck cancer. Wagenfeld *et al.* (1980, 1981) found 6.5% of second

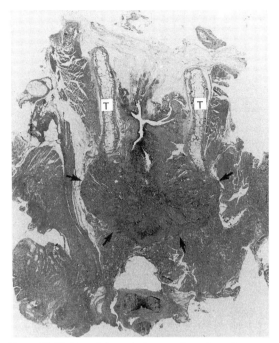

Figure 11.29 Spread through the cricothyroid membrane. Coronal section close to the anterior commissure. Anterior glottic-subglottic carcinoma with spread through the cricothyroid membrane (arrows). T: thyroid cartilage

primary carcinomas within the respiratory tract in patients with glottic carcinoma and 12.3% in those with supraglottic carcinoma; more than half of these tumours were located in the lungs and have to be separated from metastases.

Prospective panendoscopic examinations in patients with neoplasms arising in the upper respiratory tract have yielded a high percentage of synchronous multiple primary carcinomas (McGuirt, Matthews and Kourman, 1982) and introduce interesting aspects in the clinical management of patients with upper aerodigestive tract malignancies. The value of such procedures, especially in the follow-up of patients has been discussed by Olofsson (1993).

Treatment

Almost all carcinomas of the larynx are treated (Table 11.6). Like most head and neck tumours, the therapeutic problem is local, not merely because in the majority of patients there is no evidence of spread beyond the local tissue or regional nodes, but also because even in those patients where dissemination is evident, the local lesion is the one causing symptoms that require some form of management. Even temporary control of the local and regional disease may require energetic treatment.

Most cancers of the head and neck show a reduced or uncertain response to second treatments (the separate treatment of regional nodes which appear after the treatment of the primary tumour is excepted from this statement), but the larynx is, in this respect, rather different. The so-called 'salvage' surgery of the primary lesion is thus a legitimate approach and must be considered in the treatment planning (Lederman and Dalley, 1965; Bryce, 1972; Stell *et al.*, 1982).

Treatment may fall into the following categories:

1 No treatment
2 Palliation
    a pain relief
    b tracheostomy
    c other surgery
    d radiotherapy
    e chemotherapy
3 Curative (radical)
    a radiotherapy
        radioactive implants
        megavoltage
        neutrons
    b surgery
    c chemotherapy
4 Rehabilitation

Since squamous carcinoma makes up the overwhelming proportion of malignancies of the larynx, the discussion will refer almost exclusively to this disorder. Rare forms of malignancy of the larynx will be dealt with separately.

No treatment (see Table 11.6)

A few patients require no treatment, including those presenting *in extremis*, who are no longer conscious of pain or distress, or in whom disseminated tumours cause their death without the primary tumour or regional disease causing symptoms. In a retrospective sense this category also includes those who do have cancer of the larynx but who die of other disorders, the laryngeal cancer unrecognized. The fact that cancer of the glottis, especially the small lesion of the vocal cord, has a relatively long natural history may occasionally raise the question of the necessity of any treatment in those who have another debilitating or lethal disorder, and careful judgement is required before instituting treatment at all. Approximately 7–8% of patients presenting clinically with a carcinoma of the larynx receive no treatment (Stell, Morton and Singh, 1983) (see Table 11.6).

Palliation

It is appropriate to consider palliation of cancer of the larynx at an early stage, not because of its importance

Table 11.6 Treatment of cancer of larynx (males only), radical, palliative or none, 1957–1976

	Radical		Palliative		None		Total	
	No.	*%*	*No.*	*%*	*No.*	*%*	*No.*	*%*
Tis	59	95.2	1	1.6	2	3.2	62	100.0
T1a	671	95.7	9	1.3	21	3.0	701	100.0
T1b	208	95.0	9	4.1	2	0.9	219	100.0
T2	392	93.6	8	1.9	19	4.5	419	100.0
T3	409	88.5	28	6.1	25	5.4	462	100.0
T4	172	75.1	32	14.0	25	10.9	229	100.0
NK	42	64.6	2	3.1	21	32.3	65	100.0
NA	80	48.8	14	8.5	70	42.7	164	100.0
Total	2033	87.6	103	4.4	185	8.0	2321	100.0

Source: Birmingham and West Midlands Regional Cancer Registry, 1986
NK: details insufficient to stage
NA: cancer of type not applicable to staging

numerically (see Table 11.6), but because it is necessary to consider carefully the purpose of the treatment and the means used. Palliation indicates the attempt to suppress the carcinoma and its symptoms but without expectation or intent to cure. It may be of little value if the result is short term, and allows the disease to recur in a more distressing or painful form. Palliation which, for instance, suppressed the disseminated disease but not the troublesome primary lesion could be unwelcome. Palliation is commonly used in the later stages of disease.

Pain relief

Pain is not particularly common in laryngeal cancer. Paradoxically it is the slowly growing, sometimes underestimated and thus undertreated, lesion which can be the most intractable. A carcinoma with a long previous history, often of recurrences, is likely to take a long time to destroy the sufferer, and once pain develops a long period of control may be required. Such patients need the benefit of pain control specialists and the various adjuvant psychological, electrical and pharmaceutical methods. Such patients, too, may be subjects for treatment by a combination of methods including radiation, surgery and chemotherapy.

Tracheostomy

The relief of airway obstruction in a patient with incurable cancer often provides a dilemma. Dyspnoea is indeed distressing and its relief in such patients may merely delay for a very short period the inevitable death and on some occasions preserve a life temporarily only for other suffering and pain. These patients often provide problems, not only because a decision may be required rapidly, but also because the individual may be unable to indicate his wishes. Discussion with relatives is important, and often the time gained by tracheostomy is required for the relatives and the patient to come to terms with the unpleasant reality. It is this situation which requires the most informed and sympathetic management by the surgeon.

Tracheostomy may well be required as a preliminary before the possibility or practicability of treatment has been assessed. Tracheostomy in these patients also requires considerable thought and judgement, but is more appropriately discussed in relation to curative management.

The third instance where tracheostomy may be considered as a palliative procedure is in conjunction with other palliative procedures. Certain lesions are incurable – examples are all those with disseminated metastases, or those already treated where the airway becomes prejudiced and recurrence(s) are identified which may be temporarily controlled by chemotherapeutic agents, allowing a period of relative well-being. Each case must be considered upon its own merits.

Other surgery

Too often surgery, otherwise regarded as 'radical', is neglected as a palliative procedure. On occasions a total laryngectomy is the most reliable method of pain control, and a radical neck dissection, even in those with disseminated metastases, may remove a fungating or painful local lesion which is otherwise difficult to control and which is the source of the current symptoms. Such treatment, permitting sometimes months of relative well-being, may be a simple substitute for debilitating and time-consuming radiotherapy or chemotherapy, the modes of treatment usually invoked for palliation but which often impose more discomfort than the cancer itself.

Radiotherapy

Radiation therapy is commonly used for palliation. Radiation is of particular value under these circumstances because it can be applied locally and selectively, focusing on the area or cause of symptoms; thus patients in whom the primary lesion is obtrusive, or those where local (or even distant) metastatic lesions are the major problem, may be treated sufficiently to suppress those symptoms.

Usually the approach to palliation is simpler than for curative therapy. A complicating factor may be larger volumes requiring treatment (the larger the volume the less radiation per unit volume can be given) and less likelihood of complete control – often the original reason for the palliative nature of treatment. Sometimes the detailed planning and preparation is waived since these exercises are designed to promote maximum dosage to an accurately limited volume, the need for accuracy being heightened by the desire to treat to tolerance, while tolerance is not sought when palliation is required. Radioactive implants of gold are useful for local treatment, especially of secondary deposits. Palliative courses of radiation can be delivered in fractions, but over a shorter period, since extension of the period is desirable only where treatment to tolerance is sought. Even so, there are limitations to the value of palliative radiotherapy and, as a general rule, only one course to a particular area is offered, the patient, like any other, being at risk from the destructive effects of radiation if the appropriate dosage is exceeded.

Chemotherapy

As yet (with a few anecdotal exceptions) no carcinoma of the larynx has been cured by drugs. Nevertheless, chemotherapy has become an integral component of the armamentarium used to manage cancer, although in realistic terms it is predominantly a palliative therapy. Its use as an adjuvant will be discussed in the section on radical treatment.

Response to chemotherapy may be measured by partial or complete regression of tumours (as in phase II trials) or by the survival of the patient (phase III). Complete regression is rare while partial response, even then in only one patient in five, can demonstrate the effect of the chemical treatment, but is, in effect, a complete failure. Chemotherapy can in no way be compared with radiation or surgery, for survival has not yet been shown to be improved; rather it is an alternative to analgesics.

Chemotherapy has two other major disadvantages. First it is a 'blunt instrument' influencing cancer wherever it may be, that is both local and distant (where the local lesion is the one causing symptoms); indeed it may be negatively selective, being more effective against the metastases (perhaps better perfused) than the local lesion. The second objection is the tendency towards significant side effects and the associated malaise, rather than a promotion of well-being, in a significant proportion of patients. It is as well to consider that suffering induced by non-curative treatment is hard to justify.

Curative treatment (see Table 11.6)

Curative or radical treatment may involve radiotherapy, surgery, or chemotherapy, of which the last is not used alone. The first two, may be used either separately or together.

Radiotherapy

At the present time a radiotherapist is a specialist in his own right, skilled in the application of all forms of radiation treatment, trained in medical physics and internal medicine at least to the extent of appreciating the interaction of disease with the treatment proposed and the variety of complications both early and late. The radiotherapist is also, essentially, an oncologist with experience of a very wide range of cancers. It is thus the radiotherapist who has a major role in the assessment and selection of treatment for most cancers, as well as cancer of the larynx. Joint clinics are now regarded as almost indispensable in the management of cancer of the larynx, particularly because most patients are treated by radiation.

Radiation is biologically most effective where the tissues are well oxygenated. This would seem to imply that it is most valuable in small lesions and where the vascular supply is undamaged, for example where it has not been preceded by surgery. (There is no real evidence to suggest that surgery is actually prejudicial.) Attempts to use hyperbaric oxygen have not borne fruit (Hurley, Richter and Torrens, 1972). Conversely, the less attractive cases for radiotherapy are those where the tumour is large or widespread, not only because the volume is large and a tumoricidal dose more difficult to achieve without unacceptable side effects, but also because the centre of larger tumours is often avascular and tends to be necrotic. In addition, the characteristics, even of megavoltage radiation, are such that tumours in bone are less responsive, and the cure of lymph nodes is uncertain. Radiation is thus *theoretically* more applicable on the oxygenated periphery of the tumour, while surgery could deal with the mass.

Selection of cases

Radiation is chosen in those patients where cure is likely with preservation of function. It may be used in a few circumstances where surgery is contraindicated or refused. Preliminary radiation of unresectable tumours is only rarely helpful. Radiation may be chosen, even if cure is uncertain, but with surgery in reserve. Radiation may be used for a majority of patients with cancer of the larynx.

The combination of radiation with chemotherapy may be considered, although the results of such treatments are not yet fully validated (Coker *et al.*, 1981). Chemotherapy before radiation may increase the response but not survival.

Few circumstances contraindicate radiotherapy: these include active perichondritis, where cartilage is invaded, and where radiation has been used previously.

Interstitial radiation

Historically, radium-226 needles were implanted (Finzi and Harmer, 1928) by surgically removing part of the thyroid ala. This has now been superseded by external radiation.

Radioactive gold-198 grains can be inserted using a special gun in a pattern which can give a very high dose (100 Gy) localized to nodes or nodules in the neck, with little damage to normal structures.

Radiation reactions

Radiation reactions are frequent but usually not severe. They may be minimized by the avoidance of smoking, alcohol and careful attention to the skin and to nutrition. It is usual for the patients to develop mucositis, or painful erythematous reactions in the larynx and pharynx. In many cases, it is sufficient to require hospitalization for a week or so towards and after the end of treatment. Local and systemic analgesic mixtures are generally sufficient to control the symptoms. Rarely antibiotics and steroids are required. Similarly, erythema or moist desquamation of the skin may develop, and patients are discouraged from washing or abrading the skin until a little time after treatment is complete. Severe reactions may progress to necrosis of the skin, although this is very rare except where the tumour originally involved the skin.

Perichondritis is a deeper inflammatory reaction of the laryngeal skeleton. Whether true necrosis of cartilage occurs is uncertain. The symptoms are persistent pain, earache, more severe dysphagia and, where sepsis supervenes, severe illness. Perichondritis may require the suspension of radiation treatment. Mild symptoms during or after the treatment usually respond to steroids and antibiotics. If perichondritis is severe, urgent removal of the larynx is required. Mild symptoms may occur some years after radiation, provoked usually by a respiratory tract infection. When laryngeal oedema follows radiation, it can be hard to establish whether perichondritis or local residual disease is the cause, and it can be immensely difficult to reach a decision. It is essential, however, to monitor such patients carefully, for if residual tumour is present but allowed to extend beyond the larynx, the prognosis is poor.

Generally, a patient who undergoes radiotherapy for carcinoma of the larynx must undergo a relatively strenuous treatment, because of hospitalization or travelling and the almost invariable interference with nutrition, together with general side effects of malaise, weakness, anorexia, insomnia, followed by dryness of the mouth and throat, loss of taste, and sometimes pigmentation of the skin and telangiectasia with some subcutaneous fibrosis.

Radiation is not an easy course or 'soft option', and many patients who have been subjected to both surgery and radiation will readily volunteer that radiation was by far the most miserable form of treatment. On the other hand, treatment for many small glottic tumours is relatively easy.

Most patients who have undergone successful radiation therapy retain a good or useful voice. A number are subject to dysphonic episodes with respiratory tract infections. Treatment of larger tumours, particularly if the reaction was severe, may be followed by some change in the voice, but this is preferable to its loss by surgery.

Neutrons

Fast neutron radiotherapy (Catterall, 1977) has shown a capacity for local control of malignancy apparently in excess of the success of photons in some sites. Its value has yet to be the subject of closely supervised trials and it is not generally available.

Surgery

Microendolaryngeal and laser surgery

The advent of the carbon dioxide laser used with the surgical microscope has added further impetus to the treatment of the smaller cancers of the larynx. Carcinoma *in situ* can be treated by microsurgical excision (Hellquist, Olofsson and Gröntoft, 1981) and laser surgery makes this even easier. Ideal cases are uncommon and require long and careful follow up. There is an attraction to avoid radiation in younger persons where a sufficient length of life remains during which the risk of radiation-induced or other cancers is significant. Certain localized supraglottic lesions may be excised using a laser (Schechter and El Mahdi, 1984). The real value of this method is still being fully evaluated (Epstein *et al.*, 1990).

Excisional surgery

Surgical treatment of carcinoma of the larynx historically precedes radiation treatment (Gussenbauer, 1874). Almost invariably there is some risk, if not some prejudice to, or loss of, the voice – and in supraglottic laryngectomy risk to the protection of the airway. In contrast with this, radiation generally preserves function. Today surgery is not associated with the major risks of former years, and physical fitness or age are not often the limiting factors. Most patients are fit for treatment and all may generally be offered surgery or radiation, the choice being made according to the likely effective control of the cancer and the relative consequences of the treatment.

Surgery is effective in almost all cases where the lesion can be encompassed. As a primary or sole treatment it is more effective than radiation in larger tumours (Table 11.7) and where there are secondary deposits of carcinoma in the lymph nodes of the neck. Rehabilitative procedures do much to minimize the disability after surgery. Surgery, however, may be used in combination with, or as a sequel to radiation therapy, especially in its role as 'salvage' or secondary surgery for recurrence, in many cases without detriment to the expectation of cure (Bryce, 1972; Stell *et al.*, 1982). Partial resection of the larynx may also maintain near normal function with high rates of cure (Ogura, Sessions and Spector, 1975). After radiation failure, surgery is the appropriate course for most potentially curable cancers.

Table 11.7 Recurrence-free rates (%) for T3 glottis, males and females (N0 M0) for radical radiotherapy and surgery as the primary treatment, 1957–1976

Years	1	2	3	4	5	No. cases
Radiotherapy	54	43	38	38	38	84
Surgery	77	64	60	60	58	49

Source: Birmingham and West Midlands Regional Cancer Registry, 1986

Selection of treatment

With the principles outlined above, the selection of treatment of cancer of the larynx can be outlined.

Those cases of doubtful malignancy, keratosis and those with carcinoma *in situ* in the glottis and supraglottis may be treated by microendoscopic removal (Kleinsasser, 1978) and with the help of lasers (Strong, 1974, 1975). Small tumours of the marginal zones (suprahyoid epiglottis, aryepiglottic fold, sometimes false cord) may also be candidates for such surgery. Once the need arises to remove tissue which may interfere with function (e.g. the vocal cord), alternatives should be considered.

Smaller tumours of the supraglottis and glottis (especially Tla and Tlb lesions) are usually treated by radiation with good results, although some regard many such lesions of the supraglottis, especially those arising from the base of the epiglottis and the false cords, as most appropriately treated by conservative (horizontal partial) laryngectomy (Schechter and El Mahdi, 1984) with good results (Ogura and Mallen, 1967; Bocca, Pignataro and Masciaro, 1968). The relative values of radiation versus surgery are not clear. T2 lesions are treated by radiation – the alternative being total laryngectomy. Larger T3 and T4 lesions may best be excised if surgery is the only mode of treatment to be used. T3 glottic lesions may be treated by radiation with salvage surgery without a reduction in cure (Robin *et al.*, 1991b). Subglottic lesions too may be irradiated (Lederman, 1970) with possible secondary surgery if required, but follow up with endoscopy is a necessary part of management. Where there are secondary nodal deposits the use of primary surgery is much more appropriate, particularly if conservative surgery is possible for, although small or subclinical nodes are effectively controlled by radiation (Fletcher, 1972), the expansion of the field may make cure more difficult, and conservative surgery after radiation is less attractive (Radcliffe and Shaw, 1978).

Other less common forms of malignancy of the larynx are almost invariably treated by laryngectomy; these include adenocarcinoma (Whicker *et al.*, 1974), verrucous carcinoma (van Nostrand and Olofsson, 1972), salivary adenocarcinoma (Spiro *et al.*, 1976), fibrosarcoma (Flanagan, Cross and Libcke, 1965), melanoma (Moore and Martin, 1955), chondrosarcoma (Swerdlow, Som and Biller, 1974) and chemodectoma (Adlington and Woodhouse, 1972).

Emergency laryngectomy

This controversial issue was proposed by Kiem, Shapiro and Rosin (1965) as a result of their studies of 116 laryngectomy patients of whom 17 developed peristomal recurrence. Peristomal recurrence occurred without particular reference to the original site (supra/subglottic) but more frequently in those who had tracheostomy as a preliminary procedure at the time of laryngectomy (13.9%) and even more frequently (40.9%) in those whose tracheostomy preceded laryngectomy by 2 days or more. Peristomal recurrence was uniformly fatal. Baluyot, Shumrick and Everts (1971) described the policy, and also the role of radiotherapy.

The difficulties in achieving the proposed ideal management are, naturally, the possible lack of availability of frozen section histology, and the doubt whether a patient with a compromised airway can give rational consent to a laryngectomy. Nor has the effectiveness of the policy been demonstrated either in terms of reduced peristomal recurrence or mortality.

Surgical techniques

Many different techniques for the treatment of laryngeal cancer have been devised since Buck in 1853 first performed a successful partial laryngectomy by laryngofissure in the USA, and Billroth of Vienna carried out the first total laryngectomy for cancer in 1873 (Gussenbauer, 1874). All the subsequent techniques have derived from the work of these early pioneers, and later modifications have concerned mainly such details as anaesthesia, skin incisions, succession of stages and methods of closure.

In the early years of the present century, although these operations were increasingly used, serious complications were the rule and operative mortality caused by haemorrhage, wound infection and bronchopneumonia was at times as high as 25% for the smaller procedures and 50% or more after complete removal of the larynx.

From about 1910 onwards this toll was gradually reduced through the work of pioneers such as Gluck (1922), and Thomson and Colledge (1930). Their achievements were obtained not merely by technical skill, but by a realization of the importance of adequate preparation of the patient before surgery and careful postoperative nursing to combat the dangers of infection.

After 1940, with the advent of surgical aids such as antibiotics, safer anaesthetics and blood transfusion, the whole scene changed. There are now few definite contraindications to laryngeal surgery and serious complications are rare. Operative mortality for major laryngeal operations is no more than about 1%.

The following types of procedure are now used:

1 Vertical partial resection
   a cordectomy
   b frontal partial laryngectomy
   c lateral partial laryngectomy ⎫
   d frontolateral partial laryngectomy ⎬ hemilaryngectomy
   e extended frontolateral partial laryngectomy ⎭
2 Horizontal partial resection
   a epiglottectomy
   b supraglottic partial laryngectomy
   c extended supraglottic partial laryngectomy
3 Total resection
   a total laryngectomy alone

b total laryngectomy with partial pharyngectomy or partial glossectomy.

The operation of radical block dissection of cervical lymphatics on one or both sides may need to be combined with any of these procedures. It is seldom required in the first group owing to the paucity of lymphatics in the true cords and therefore the improbability of metastatic spread. In addition, partial or total thyroidectomy may be obligatory in the major resections.

Lateral or vertical partial laryngectomy (Figure 11.30a, b), often termed 'laryngofissure', is today performed less frequently owing to the equally effective results achieved by radiation in suitable cases. However, it still has a very definite place in situations where good radiation is not available, in some cases of radiation failure, possibly for limited cordal tumours in young adults, where radiation may provoke future neoplastic changes, and perhaps also in a few older patients unsuitable for prolonged radiation. Primarily it is indicated for T1a lesions of one vocal cord which should not extend into the anterior commissure or on to the arytenoid cartilage. It is also a suitable operation for the removal of many large benign laryngeal tumours.

Frontolateral partial laryngectomy may be useful where a glottic tumour crosses the anterior commissure to involve the anterior third of the opposite cord and without any reduction of mobility ('horseshoe tumour') (Figure 11.30c, d) (Som and Silver, 1968).

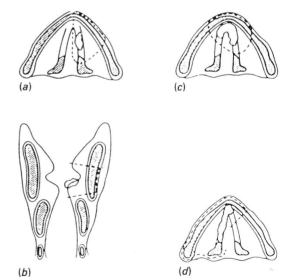

(a)   *(c)*

(b)   *(d)*

Figure 11.30 Diagram to show in (*a*) transverse and (*b*) coronal section, the extent of resection by vertical partial laryngectomy, and (*c*) the frontolateral and (*d*) extended frontolateral operations

The older more anatomical hemilaryngectomy is no longer employed, but provided that there is no evidence of deep infiltration, an extension of the lateral partial laryngectomy technique to include the whole ventricular band and arytenoid cartilage may on occasion be used in highly selected cases (Ogura and Mallen, 1967), and is often termed 'hemilaryngectomy'. This term is also rather loosely applied to other types of partial resection.

Pharyngotomy, either by the anterior transverse approach or by the lateral route (Trotter, 1926), provides a satisfactory access to limited T1 or T2 supraglottic tumours. The anterior pharyngotomy approach is also useful in excising small tumours of the tip of the epiglottis and marginal aryepiglottic folds (Martin, 1957). The larger operation of supraglottic horizontal partial laryngectomy for T1a and T1b lesions of the epiglottis and laryngeal vestibule is more modern in concept. Although popular in Europe and centres in the USA it is still not widely practised in the UK partly because of the relative rarity of suitable cases. However, it deserves greater acceptance in view of the consistently good results published compared with those of radiation. Primarily it is indicated for T1a or T1b lesions confined to the supraglottis. Transglottic extension or involvement of the tongue base usually contraindicates the procedure. It is also inadvisable in some patients much over 65 years and those with reduced pulmonary function (Som, 1970), for these accommodate relatively poorly to the changed swallowing and compromised laryngeal sphincters.

Consent for total laryngectomy must always be obtained before attempting any type of partial resection and prudence indicates that the operation should start with a direct endoscopy. Previous full-dosage radiation is certainly no bar to lateral partial laryngectomy but greatly increases the hazards of the horizontal supraglottic operations. Nor should surgery be performed without a precise knowledge of the extent of the lesion before radiation (Radcliffe and Shaw, 1978; Stell and Ranger, 1974).

Preparation for surgery It is a most important preoperative measure in this type of surgery to ensure the health of the mouth as far as possible. Unhealthy teeth should be treated and particular attention must be paid to the periodontal tissues. Operation ought not to be undertaken until the mouth has healed. Nasal sepsis should be eliminated as far as is practicable. Attention must be given to general health, haemoglobin level, chest, and the control of other medical conditions. A systemic antibiotic should be given commencing at the beginning of operation (e.g. ampicillin).

From a psychological point of view the surgeon will naturally assess each case individually. It is highly desirable that the patient is informed in some detail as to what the procedure is and what to expect, for thus is obtained not only the necessary informed consent but the better cooperation of the patient during the postoperative period.

Anaesthesia The operations can be performed under local anaesthesia, but general anaesthesia is preferable, and essential for the more exacting supraglottic (horizontal) partial laryngectomy.

Where the resting airway is seriously reduced by the tumour, there should be no hesitation in carrying out a preliminary tracheostomy under local anaesthesia with insertion of an angled cuffed anaesthetic tube. As soon as the trachea is exposed, the cuffed tube is inserted and general anaesthesia is induced.

Position of the patient This should be similar to that used for tracheostomy; the head is extended by placing a roll or a sandbag beneath the shoulders. It is important that the pillow or sandbag be evenly placed in order to ensure that the larynx and trachea are strictly in the midline.

Lateral (vertical) partial laryngectomy

Using this technique it is possible to remove completely many tumours confined to the vocal cord, with an adequate margin of healthy tissue and without removal of the arytenoid cartilage. The principles of operative surgery for malignant disease elsewhere apply, with the exception that it is unnecessary to remove the associated cervical lymph nodes for reasons already given.

The tumour must be removed in one piece with as wide a margin of apparently healthy tissue as is practicable. It has been suggested that this margin should be at least 0.5 cm and, although this suggestion is of some practical value, the tissue removed must be as much as is possible and prudent. Even in the earliest case it should consist of the whole of the side of the larynx anterior to the arytenoid cartilage, including its tip, and from the upper border of the cricoid cartilage below to the upper border of the thyroid ala above. It may be more than 1 cm above, but may be less anteriorly if the tumour approaches the commissure, or less posteriorly if it approaches the tip of the arytenoid cartilage.

Naturally, the smaller the margin of healthy tissue removed, the less satisfactory are the results likely to be.

If, on histological examination of the specimen removed at operation, any doubt exists as to the complete removal of the lesion with an adequate margin of healthy tissue, a full course of radiation should at once be given if the larynx has not previously been irradiated. However, in the latter event, vigilant follow up alone is permissible with recourse to total laryngectomy at the first sign of recurrent disease.

Incision A transverse incision over the upper border of the cricoid cartilage gives adequate exposure (Figure 11.31) with a separate lower one for the tracheostomy.

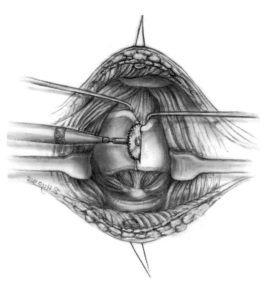

Figure 11.32 Vertical partial laryngectomy. Thyrotomy saw-cut

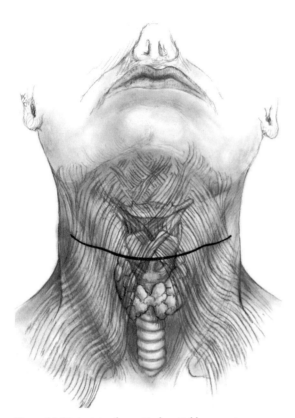

Figure 11.31 Incision for vertical partial laryngectomy

The strap muscles are separated and retained for later use. The thyroid isthmus is divided. The tracheostomy is prepared by excising a disc of the anterior tracheal wall or by a midline incision only.

Excision of the thyroid ala (Figures 11.32 and 11.33) is achieved by first separating the outer perichondrium as far as the oblique line, and sectioning the cartilage (with a saw) in the midline and laterally.

Excision of tumour The midline (or just to the contralateral side if the tumour reaches the commissure) is incised, and the growth excised, above through the ventricular band, below just above the cricoid, and posteriorly including the tip of the vocal process of the arytenoid (Figure 11.34).

Closure After haemostasis, and using the sternohyoid muscle placed inside the preserved outer perichondrium to reduce the dead space, the perichondrium is

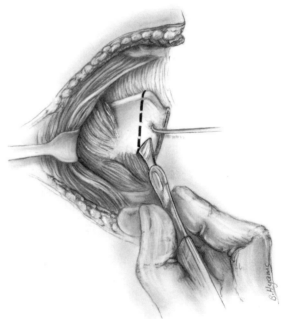

Figure 11.33 Vertical partial laryngectomy. Second thyrotomy saw-cut

sutured in the midline and the wound closed in layers. A nasogastric tube is inserted.

Postoperative care The main complications of haemorrhage and chest infections are avoidable, the former by meticulous haemostasis, the latter by care of the tracheostomy (see Chapter 9). Early activity should be encouraged. Swallowing is painful at first, and

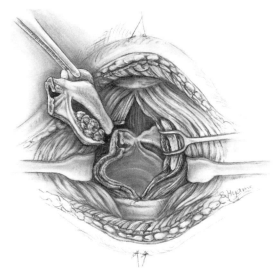

Figure 11.34 Excision of specimen in vertical partial laryngectomy

nutrition is by nasogastric tube for a few days. The tracheostomy may be closed when the airway is demonstrably adequate. Antibiotics should be continued for some weeks, especially if there has been previous radiation. Granulations may form over unepithelialized cartilage and will need to be removed.

Late results of operation The larynx heals by slow fibrosis and epithelialization, and this rarely results in stenosis, especially if the thyroid ala has been removed. Usually, however, a fibrous replica of the cord is produced which, after a year, may become a very passable substitute for the true cord. Conley (1961) claimed better healing and an improved voice by fashioning a new cord from an inturned flap of cervical skin used to line the raw side of the larynx. Other reconstructive techniques have been tried.

There is no satisfactory movement of this band of scar tissue and, although the voice will be useful, it is husky, variable in strength and usually cannot be said to approach the normal. Singing is impossible. There is often some stenosis of the anterior part if the opposite cord has been removed as in the frontolateral operation. Marked stenosis may limit the airway, and in these cases the tracheostomy is retained using a valve to permit phonation.

Local recurrence either in the scar or in adjacent tissue is uncommon. If a growth later occurs on the opposite cord it is difficult to decide whether it is a recurrence or a second primary growth. Metastasis is rare but may become evident in the cervical or medias-

tinal lymph nodes months or years after operation and with no evidence of local recurrence in the larynx.

Supraglottic partial laryngectomy

Incision The T-shaped incision (Figure 11.35) described by Som (1970) or a simple transverse incision is adequate. A tracheostomy is performed.

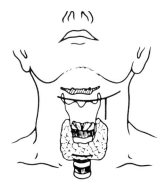

Figure 11.35 Incision for horizontal partial (supraglottic) laryngectomy

Approach to supraglottis After elevation of skin flaps, the strap muscles are divided from the hyoid bone and the superior laryngeal vascular bundles ligated, defining the hyoid, superior cornua, and posterior borders of the thyroid cartilage. If a neck dissection is required, or is indicated, it is performed at this stage. The external perichondrium is dissected (Figure 11.36) and the cartilage sectioned horizontally (Figure 11.37).

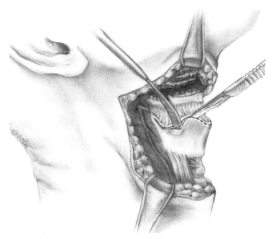

Figure 11.36 Incision of perichondrium in supraglottic laryngectomy

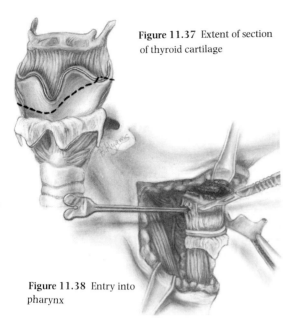

Figure 11.37 Extent of section of thyroid cartilage

Figure 11.38 Entry into pharynx

Excision of the tumour Working from above, the tumour is excised with scissors (Figures 11.40 and 11.41) with a blade each side of the aryepiglottic fold, preserving the arytenoid. Extended operations (Ogura, Sessions and Spector, 1975) are described (Figure 11.42).

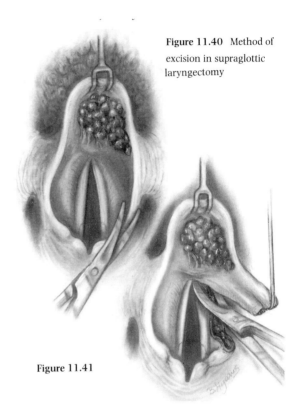

Figure 11.40 Method of excision in supraglottic laryngectomy

Figure 11.41

Exposure of the tumour The pharynx is entered laterally just below the greater cornu of the hyoid (Figure 11.38). The hyoid bone is removed. The incision is carried across the base of the tongue, maintaining an adequate margin until the tumour can be viewed from above (Figure 11.39).

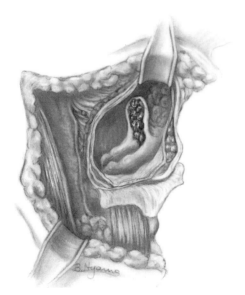

Figure 11.39 Pharyngotomy and exposure of larynx

Cricopharyngeal myotomy A myotomy is performed, and a nasogastric tube inserted.

Closure After haemostasis, closure is of the raw surfaces first by suturing the cut edges of mucosa (Figure 11.43) and then of the pharynx in layers (Figure 11.44) by approximating the base of the tongue to the cut edge of the thyroid cartilage, and the infrahyoid muscles to the cut suprahyoid muscles, and finally of the skin.

Postoperative care A routine similar to that for partial laryngectomy and tracheostomy is followed, but even with particular care, spillover and aspiration are almost inevitable.

Rehabilitation Gradual use of the voice is begun after about 7–10 days. Once spillover is reduced, oral food, initially semisolids, is begun. This aspect of care is

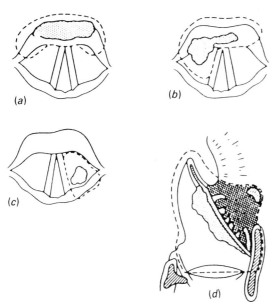

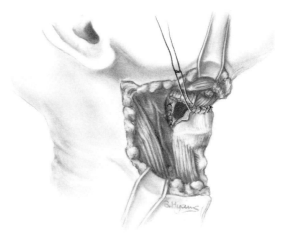

Figure 11.44 Closure of the pharynx after supraglottic laryngectomy

Figure 11.42 Extent of excision in lesions of (*a*) epiglottis, (*b*) epiglottis and false cord, (*c*) false cord, and (*d*) sagittal section to indicate plane of section above arytenoid and vocal cord

over 65 years; previous radiation may also be a contraindication (Radcliffe and Shaw, 1978).

Subtotal laryngectomy

In all parts of the world partial laryngectomy has been developed into various forms of *subtotal laryngectomy*, including *vertical subtotal laryngectomy* (see Figure 11.30*d*) removing up to 90% of the larynx (Wang and Zhu, 1990) or extending to *horizontal subtotal laryngectomy* and removing one arytenoid leaving only part of one cord, the larynx being reconstructed by crico-hyoid-epiglottidopexy. A review and description of this procedure, applicable to up to T3 (occasionally T4!) glottic tumours and used relatively widely in those countries where supraglottic tumours are more common, is given by Piquet and Chevalier (1991).

Total laryngectomy

Billroth of Vienna first removed the larynx as a treatment for cancer in 1873 (Gussenbauer, 1874).

At first, the results of operation were bad and not a single patient survived for one year in the first 25 cases recorded. Postoperative complications were frequent and severe, the most common causes of death being general septicaemia, spreading cellulitis or mediastinitis, septic pulmonary complications, haemorrhage and shock.

An attempt to improve on these poor results was made by performing the operation in two stages, the first consisting of the establishment of a tracheostomy, the larynx being removed a few weeks later.

Single-stage laryngectomy was suggested in 1921 by Moure and Portmann and, since that time, most

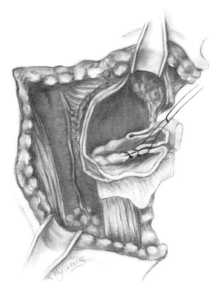

Figure 11.43 Closure of raw surfaces in the larynx in supraglottic laryngectomy

paramount for patients after horizontal partial laryngectomy, and it is because of this difficulty that the operation may not be appropriate in those with reduced pulmonary function and who are aged much

surgeons have practised a one-stage operation with increasing safety.

Incisions A commonly used incision was first recommended by Gluck (1922) and modified by Sœrenson (1930). The incision commences on the anterior border of the sternomastoid muscle about the level of the hyoid bone, passes down along the anterior border of the muscle for about 6–7 cm and then curves across the midline at the level of the second or third ring of the trachea (Figure 11.45).

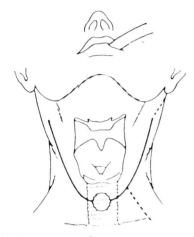

Figure 11.45 Sœrensen U-flap

Other incisions (Figure 11.46) are used, especially for combined total laryngectomy and radical neck dissection, and all have advantages. Jackson's single vertical incision is not now used. A single horizontal incision midway between the hyoid bone and the sternum with a separate one for the tracheostomy, is adequate and can be adapted for neck dissection (see Figure 11.31).

Exposure of the larynx (Figure 11.47) The larynx is dissected from the sternomastoid and carotid sheaths on each side, tying the vascular bundles. The strap muscles are sectioned low in the neck, and usually the contralateral lobe of the thyroid freed from the specimen.

Tracheostomy The trachea is divided below the tumour and a tracheostome fashioned now or later (Figures 11.48 and 11.49).

Removal of the larynx This is easier from above downwards, sectioning the constrictor muscles from the thyroid cartilage, and preserving mucosa as far as appropriate. Care should be taken to ensure adequate margins, especially over the cricoarytenoid joints.

Closure (Figure 11.50) Closure of the pharynx is in layers in the shape of either an I or a Y, ideally with a Connell suture. A long posterior myotomy (Singer and Blom, 1981) may avoid segments of spasm. The skin is closed in layers over suction drains.

Postoperative care This is as before, and much as for tracheostomy (see Chapter 9). Feeding is by nasogastric tube. Antibiotic cover (e.g. ampicillin) may be continued for a few days.

Complications The most frequent complication (apart from those associated with any surgery) is pharyngocutaneous fistula. This may develop at 4–10 days with a collection under the skin which requires drainage. Most fistulae close spontaneously after some days or weeks, assisted by frequent dressing, adequate nutrition and maintenance of the haemoglobin level. They are prevented by good technique, haemostasis, antisepsis, and a well-prepared patient. Rarely, extensive sloughing and large fistulae need repair by full thickness distant flaps.

Other complications include haemorrhage, wound infection, pulmonary and cerebral embolism, cardiac infarction, tracheal crusting and stomal recurrence, and the chest complications associated with any laryngeal operation and tracheostomy.

Thyroid insufficiency In some cases a total thyroidectomy is necessary as part of the surgical procedure. In such cases, thyroid replacement in the form of L-thyroxine is required, 0.1–0.3 mg daily. Replacement therapy is not necessary immediately but can await the resumption of swallowing in 1–2 weeks.

Rather more insidious is the hypothyroidism which may follow surgery and radiotherapy. While the patient may have retained one lobe of the thyroid, previous or later radiotherapy may on occasions impair the function, and hypothyroidism may supervene even after several years. Treatment is straightforward once the condition is recognized.

Parathyroid insufficiency This usually, but not invariably, follows total thyroidectomy. The problem may be acute in the immediate postoperative period. It may be delayed, or it may be temporary and may occur even after partial thyroidectomy.

In cases where it is anticipated, pretreatment with a vitamin D preparation may reduce the postoperative problem; otherwise intravenous calcium maintenance is necessary until either control is achieved by vitamin D medication or the condition resolves.

Respiration Most surgical procedures on the larynx require a tracheostomy to maintain the airway during and often after the surgical procedures. Total laryngectomy requires a permanent end-tracheostomy, and the maintenance of respiration depends on a good formation of the tracheostome and good healing without crusting. Most patients require no special care afterwards but, not infrequently, a respiratory tract infection is followed by tracheitis and

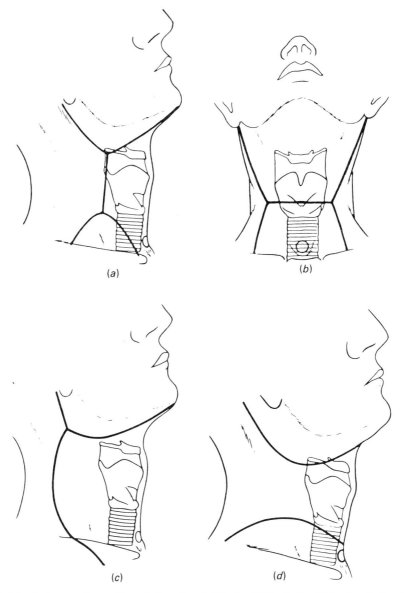

Figure 11.46 Incision for laryngectomy with neck dissection: (*a*) Martin, (*b*) Martin (for bilateral neck dissection), (*c*) Schobinger-Conley, (d) McFee

crusting, and a short period of treatment may be required to control it.

A partial laryngectomy ideally does not require a permanent tracheostomy, and the tube may be withdrawn once the natural airway can be shown, by occluding the tube, to be adequate. However, the benefits of retaining part of the natural larynx in respect of phonation are so great that the retention of the temporary tracheostomy should not be regarded as of overriding concern and should be infinitely preferable to a total laryngectomy if the control of the cancer permits it. However, the retention of a

tracheostomy in a horizontal partial laryngectomy may in itself be prejudicial to the recovery of the effective protective function of the glottic sphincter. Fine judgement may be required.

Swallowing after total laryngectomy As a rule this presents no difficulty. Even while a nasal feeding tube is in position a patient can swallow his saliva and drink fluids quite satisfactorily, although the act of swallowing is painful for the first few days. If healing has proceeded well and a fistula is not anticipated, it should be possible to remove the feeding

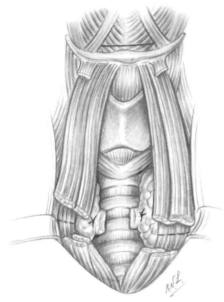

Figure 11.47 Exposure of thyroid, thyroid section at isthmus, and section strap muscles

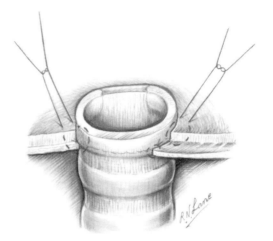

Figure 11.49 Formation of tracheostome

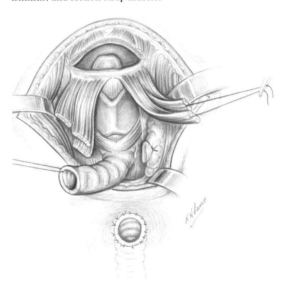

Figure 11.48 Incision above hyoid bone. Section of trachea and preparation of the tracheostome

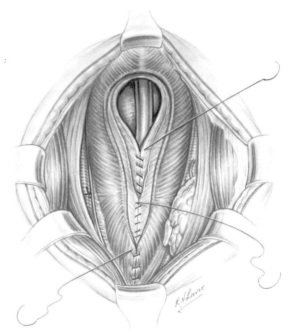

Figure 11.50 Closure of the pharynx in layers

tube after about 6 days, but if there has been previous radiation it would be much wiser to leave the tube in position for about 10 days since it is often not until the tenth day or later that the pharyngeal wound tends to break down. If the wound does break down, the tube should be left in position until the full extent and size of the fistula is revealed.

Functional rehabilitation of the voice Because the voice is impaired by operations on the larynx, the cooperation of a speech therapist is essential in maximizing its recovery.

Partial vertical and horizontal laryngectomy are operations designed to retain at least part of the glottis. The benefit of this is quite clear in that it utilizes the remains of the glottic vibrator in order to phonate, and the pulmonary reservoir to permit the production of a flow which can be modulated, and sufficient to produce sentences rather than a few words. The cords are often intact after horizontal partial laryngectomy and the voice is relatively little impaired, while vertical partial laryngectomy rarely allows a normal voice. In both cases a speech therapist can improve the production and efficiency of voice production.

Oesophageal voice Many patients who have undergone a total laryngectomy have been able to develop abnormal but functionally satisfactory oesophageal speech. This mechanism relies upon the subject charging the oesophagus with air and utilizing the vibrations, at either the cricopharyngeal sphincter level or another level, to phonate (Dworkin and Banton, 1982). The preoperative and postoperative assistance of a speech therapist is essential in most cases, not only to teach the mechanism of voice production, but also to improve and teach other normally subsidiary communication methods. While it is optimistically said that 60% of laryngectomees develop satisfactory phonation, it is evident that a significant minority does not. Often the elderly do not have the capacity or even the will to phonate adequately, and even those who do so are restricted, because of the limitation of the oesophageal air reservoir, in the length of word sequences they can achieve. It is not surprising therefore that much ingenuity has been applied to assist laryngectomees to improve upon the relatively poor outlook (for speech) after total laryngectomy. Conservative surgery has developed because of its capacity to preserve speech (Bocca, Pignataro and Masciario, 1968; Ogura *et al.*, 1969; Som, 1970) and has been applied in vertical partial laryngectomy since inception.

An early method of improving speech or voice production has been to develop a small tracheo-oesophageal fistula (Conley, de Amnesti and Pierce, 1958) which allows the oesophagus to be charged with air more continuously from the trachea (i.e. the pulmonary 'bellows' is brought back into play). Such a procedure relies upon the development of the oesophageal or pharyngeal vibrator, which is not developed by all patients.

Neoglottis More definite attempts at laryngeal voice replacements are represented by the method of Staffieri (1974). This procedure also develops a tracheo-oesophageal fistula. One method uses the fistularized redundant mucosa derived from the postcricoid region positioned over the cut end of the trachea, and the second prepares a fistula through the posterior wall of the trachea. In each case the tracheostomy is made through the anterior wall of the trachea lower down and no end-tracheostome is fashioned. Both these methods are intended to provide a form of neoglottis which itself generates a voice, but the second method, particularly, may act as a recharging mechanism for the oesophagus, utilizing a phonatory vibration in the pharynx.

The construction of such a neoglottis is more appropriately described in a textbook of operative surgery.

Many of these techniques are attractive but have the same problems. Their attraction is that, in the majority of cases, speech at least as good as oesophageal speech is obtained, and often it is better because the reservoir (the lungs) of air is large. In addition, it is easy to ensure that phonation is achieved rapidly just as a patient with a tracheostomy but retaining the larynx is quickly returned to speaking normally. However, the disadvantages are those associated with a tracheo-oesophageal fistula, and no method has so far been described where aspiration has not been experienced – if the neoglottis is too wide, aspiration may occur; if too narrow, phonation is impaired.

Valves In order to improve upon the achievements associated with the construction of a neoglottis, Singer and Blom (1980) and Panje (1981) devised replaceable valves which, when inserted, behave in a manner which is an advance on the quality of phonation usually produced by a neoglottis. The low resistance indwelling, Provox, is used quite frequently, especially in Europe (Hilgers and Balm, 1993). Since they are one-way valves, aspiration is prevented. Their disadvantage is the need to replace the valve regularly and the associated cost; nor are these methods entirely free of the risk of aspiration. However, both the Blom-Singer and the Panje valves can be inserted as a secondary procedure (Singer and Blom, 1980) after a standard laryngectomy and end-tracheostomy have been performed. An essential part of the procedure is the prevention of muscular spasm of segments of the pharynx, and Singer and Blom (1981) emphasized the need for a (posterior) myotomy of the pharyngeal wall at laryngectomy or as a secondary procedure. Hamaker *et al.* (1985) have summarized the results.

A reasonable approach to voice rehabilitation may be as follows. A total laryngectomy with an end-tracheostomy is carried out and healing allowed to be completed. A myotomy of the pharyngeal musculature from the level of the tongue to the upper oesophagus is performed. This minimizes the operative risk and allows any adjuvant radiotherapy and chemotherapy to take place. Voice rehabilitation should be pursued and will be achieved by a proportion of patients. A later reassessment will permit the identification of those whose rehabilitation is inadequate, and a neoglottis or valve preparation can be provided as a secondary procedure. A practical compromise may be to construct a tracheostomy in the anterior wall of the trachea, leaving the end prepared with a pharyngeal wall cover, but not fistularized, in order to be able to construct the neoglottis more satisfactorily at a second stage if a Staffieri type is preferred to a replaceable valve; or alternatively to prepare the puncture for later valve insertion.

Disability after total laryngectomy The main disability from which the patient will suffer after operation is naturally the loss of the normal voice. The sense of smell is also impaired because there is no regular air current through the nose, and taste and the appreciation of flavours are reduced.

The patient must take care that water does not enter the tracheostome when bathing or washing, and swimming must be prohibited.

Heavy lifting or strenuous digging are not possible as these actions entail fixation of the chest wall by closure of the larynx, but light physical work is possible and, occasionally, the patient can partially close the tracheostome by contracting any muscle remnants surrounding it. Some young women who have undergone this operation have subsequently married and borne children without difficulty (Shaw, 1965; Albrechtsen *et al.*, 1994).

If radical neck dissection has been necessary, some reduction in the usefulness of the arm at the shoulder level may be expected, especially in the older age groups, together with a variable amount of persistent discomfort more evident in those whose range of movement is most impaired (Ewing and Martin, 1952).

Apart from these disadvantages, patients generally come to terms with their disabilities, adaptation being usually good in age groups up to 65 years. Unfortunately, many patients are older and less adaptable but, with instruction and encouragement from surgeons, speech therapists, laryngectomee clubs and associations, the majority lead happy and useful lives although they are often socially limited.

Other malignant ectodermal tumours

Verrucous carcinoma (see Figures 11.18 and 11.19)

This rare carcinoma (approximately 1% of laryngeal malignancies) (Ryan *et al.*, 1977) has a male predominance, causes the usual laryngeal symptoms, frequently has an extensive warty papillomatous appearance, and its site is glottic more often than supraglottic. Lymphatic spread is rare (Biller, Ogura and Bauer, 1971). Traditionally treatment is surgical by partial or total laryngectomy. Radiotherapy has been employed, but anaplastic change and death have been reported after this (Burns, van Nostrand and Bryce, 1976), while uniformly good results follow surgery (and this may include local or biopsy excision) (Maw, Cullen and Bradfield, 1982).

Carcinosarcoma

An equally rare lesion (less than 1% of laryngeal malignancies) (Goellner, Devine and Weiland, 1973), carcinosarcoma presents with typical symptoms and usually a polypoid or pedunculated appearance (Brodsky, 1984). Treatment is by excision, with either partial or total laryngectomy. Radiation has rarely been used and is difficult to evaluate (Hyams and Rabuzzi, 1970).

Adenoid cystic carcinoma

Adenoid cystic carcinoma of the larynx is also very rare (Olofsson and van Nostrand, 1977) (Figure 11.51) with the typical rather long history of laryngeal symptoms. The subglottis, in contrast with other laryngeal malignancies, is the commoner site. Local or wide-field surgery is the generally favoured treatment, although radiotherapy is used on some occasions. The slow and relentless course of this tumour makes 5-year 'cures' meaningless and the vast majority of patients eventually succumb.

Other rarities include *anaplastic small cell carcinoma* (Figure 11.52) (Olofsson and van Nostrand, 1972), *acinous cell carcinoma* (Kallis and Stevens, 1989), *spindle cell carcinoma* (Hellquist and Olofsson, 1989) and *mucoepidermoid carcinoma* (Cumberworth *et al.*, 1989). These tumours are treated with primary radiotherapy and adjuvant chemotherapy (Baugh *et al.*, 1986) and/or surgery.

Malignant mesodermal tumours

Chondrosarcoma is exceedingly rare, and usually occurs in the posterior segment of the cricoid. Surgery, inevitably in the form of total laryngectomy, is the only useful treatment in most cases, although tumours in certain locations could be excised conservatively (Hellquist, Olofsson and Grontöft, 1979).

Non-Hodgkin's lymphoma is rare (Figure 11.53), but once diagnosed is treated, as other extranodal lymphomas, by radiotherapy and/or chemotherapy. *Melanoma* (Conley, 1967) (Figure 11.54) and *fibrosarcoma* are equally rare, and are treated by excision. *Neuroendocrine carcinomas* are rare.

Summary and selection of treatment

Assessment of the relative value of differing treatment methods for laryngeal cancer is not easy. Despite the gradual international adoption of the TNM classification system, confirmed in 1978, and revised in 1987 for the larynx, and greater uniformity in end-result reporting, most accounts are still based on retrospective studies. Adequate conclusions by randomized controlled prospective studies are still lacking, in part as a consequence of difficulty of application in cancer therapy. Despite this, much knowledge has been gained in recent years by extensive clinical experience using increasingly refined methods of surgery and radiation and also by the histological study of serially-sectioned laryngeal specimens (Olofsson and van Nostrand, 1973). Important knowledge of lymphatic pathways within the larynx (Pressman and Simon, 1961) and patterns of local spread and cervical lymph node involvement has also been gained (Olofsson and van Nostrand, 1973; Kirchner, 1974).

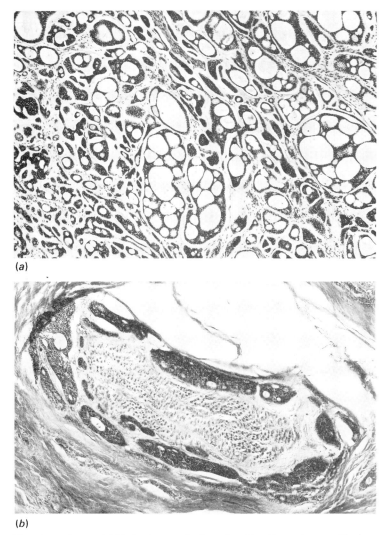

Figure 11.51 Adenoid cystic carcinoma. (*a*) Photomicrograph of an adenoid cystic carcinoma of the larynx illustrating the typical cribriform pattern of this tumour. Uniform double rows of cells surround long tubular cylinders of mucinous stromal material (haematoxylin and eosin, × 150). (*b*) Photomicrograph illustrating the great tendency for perineural invasion of adenoid cystic carcinoma (haematoxylin and eosin, × 275)

Over 50 years ago radiotherapy was condemned even for limited cordal cancer (Colledge, 1940). Today it is established as the treatment of choice in such lesions. In early glottic cancer (T1 and T2), modern radiation techniques still allow the surgeon to perform partial or total laryngectomy for failures with good salvage rates (Lederman, 1970; Bryce, 1972). In support of radiation for early glottic lesions, Lederman (1970) reported 5-year survival rates of at least 77% in his large series. Recurrence of glottic cancer after radiation and still treatable by lateral partial laryngectomy, can give a salvage for 3-year survivals of about 60% with preservation of voice and natural airway (Radcliffe and Shaw, 1978). In

more advanced recurrent glottic or transglottic cancer after radiation, a 5-year survival rate of 47% by total laryngectomy can still be otained (Robin *et al.*, 1992b) (Table 11.8).

On the other hand, 5-year survival results for initial treatment by radiation of smaller supraglottic and epilaryngeal cancer without nodal spread are very satisfactory (Lederman, 1970; Fletcher *et al.*, 1970; Fletcher and Goepfert, 1977), but salvage for failures will generally require total laryngectomy. Such cases treated by supraglottic partial laryngectomy may give a 5-year survival of 70% with voice preservation and equally good chances of salvage by total laryngectomy for the failures (Som, 1970;

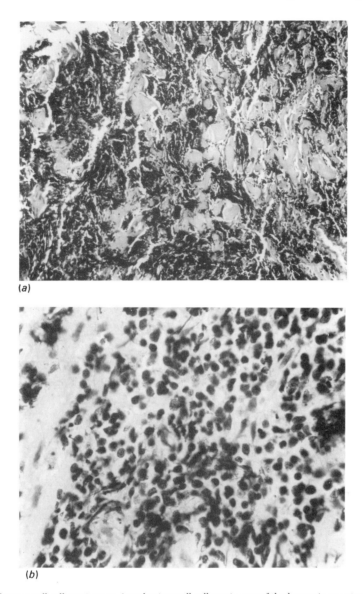

Figure 11.52 Anaplastic small cell carcinoma. Anaplastic small cell carcinoma of the larynx is an extremely rare tumour. The tumour cells most probably arise from Kultschitzky type cells and contain neurosecretory granules. These photomicrographs derive from the first described case of 'oat-cell carcinoma' of the larynx reported by Olofsson and van Nostrand (1972). (*a*) Biopsy specimen showing a tumour composed of irregular clumps and cords of tumour cells separated by a mucoid stroma (haematoxylin and eosin, × 100). (*b*) Higher magnification showing small tumour cells with round, dark-staining nuclei and scanty cytoplasm (haematoxylin and eosin, × 400). (Reproduced by permission from *Annals of Otology, Rhinology and Laryngology* (1972), **81**, 284–287)

Shumrick, 1971; Leroux–Robert, 1975; Ogura, Marks and Freeman, 1980). Primary conservation surgery therefore compares favourably with primary radiation treatment (de Santo, Willie and Devine, 1976). Supraglottic laryngectomy may be preferable in those cancers which include the false cord and base of epiglottis and those with metastatic nodes (Ogura, Sessions and Spector, 1975).

T3 glottic lesions, once automatically recommended for primary surgery or planned combined radiotherapy and surgery (Lederman, 1970; Sisson, 1974), should now be considered for primary radiation treatment with 'salvage' surgery if there is recurrence (Bryce, 1972; Stell *et al.*, 1982). Larger T4 lesions are still much more appropriately treated by surgery, although some clinicians would challenge this.

The rare cases of true subglottic cancer are generally advanced when diagnosed and planned combined treatment by radical surgery with postoperative radiation to the lower neck and mediastinum probably gives the best chance of a cure (Harrison, 1971; Bryce, 1972). However, Lederman (1970) has shown that where the disease is limited to the anterior half of the subglottic space with no palpable neck nodes and no vocal cord fixation, a 5-year survival rate of 60% can be obtained by radiation, particularly in women.

A more recently emerging treatment, apparently of value when used as an adjuvant method in advanced lesions (T3 and T4), is cytotoxic chemotherapy. Since 1974, the use of a kinetically based multidrug protocol has been on trial either before or after conventional therapy or integrated with radiation. Results are beginning to emerge from both techniques with

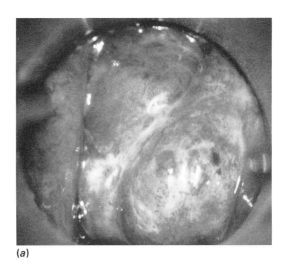

(a)

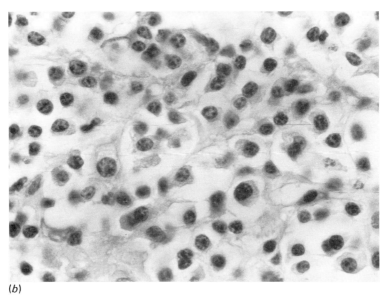

(b)

Figure 11.53 Plasmacytoma of the larynx. Extramedullary plasmacytomas are relatively rare tumours which are most frequently located in the upper airways. (*a*) This patient had a plasmacytoma involving the right false vocal cord as shown by microlaryngoscopy. The bulging, rather firm, reddish tumour obliterates the airway and is covered by intact mucosa. (*b*) The photomicrograph of the tumour shows densely packed neoplastic plasma cells upon a fine reticular stroma (haematoxylin and eosin, × 100). (Reproduced by permission from the *Journal of Otolaryngology* (1981), **10**, 28–34)

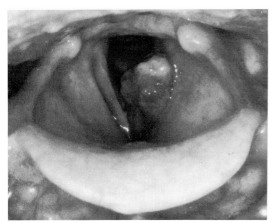

Figure 11.54 Metastasis of a malignant melanoma. Telescopic view showing the tumour that involves the laryngeal ventricle on the left side

minimal side effects (O'Connor *et al.*, 1979; Department of Veterans Affairs, 1991).

These results illustrate certain definite trends in the management of laryngeal cancer. First, that radiation gives excellent results in the early glottic lesions with absolute preservation of function. Second, that the balance of judgement between conservative and radical surgery of the larynx is becoming more refined, with the results of the former approximating to the latter for supraglottic tumours and at least equalling the results of radiation. Third, that the attack on cancer at the molecular level through cytotoxic drugs is now being applied to the larynx as an aid to conventional methods or combined treatment, again with cure and functional conservation as the objectives.

Perhaps in contrast with the foregoing has been the development of endolaryngeal procedures with the laser, permitting more accurate excision and, combined with careful follow up, an even more conservative approach to non-malignant lesions, to carcinoma *in situ* and to a few very small invasive malignancies. The development of a more positive attitude to rehabilitation, including the neoglottis and valve techniques, should encourage a more definitive and constructive approach to laryngeal cancer in general. Whether still further advances can be made by prevention (that is alcohol reduction and a non-smoking generation) and by further therapeutic developments, remains to be seen.

Table 11.8 5-year survival, males only, age-adjusted by extent (T) and nodes (N) 1957–1976

	N0		*N1a*		*N1b*		*N2a*		*N2b*		*N3*	
	Total	*5-year survival (%)*	*Total*	*5-year survival (%)*	*Total*	*5-year survival (%)*	*Total*	*5-year survival (%)*	*Total*	*5-year survival (%)*	*Total*	*5-year survival (%)*
Tis	58	86.1	0	0.0	—	—	—	—	—	—	—	—
T1a	580	84.1	2	55.1	1	0.0	1	0.0	0	0.0	1	0.0
T1b	115	66.9	1	117.4*	2	0.0	0	0.0	1	0.0	0	0.0
T2	262	69.1	2	0.0	9	0.0	0	0.0	0	0.0	0	0.0
T3	275	48.0	3	46.2	20	29.5	2	58.7	0	0.0	6	0.0
T4	33	31.7	3	35.5	7	32.8	0	0.0	0	0.0	1	0.0

Of 10 M1 cases there were no survivors
Source: Birmingham and West Midlands Regional Cancer Registry, 1986
*Refers to one case and is age-adjusted

Appendix 11.1 Larynx (ICD-O 161) (revised, 1987)
Rules for classification

The classification applies only to carcinoma. There should be histological confirmation of the disease.

The following are the procedures for assessment of the T, N and M categories:

T *categories* Physical examination, laryngoscopy and imaging
N *categories* Physical examination and imaging
M *categories* Physical examination and imaging

Anatomical sites and subsites

1 Supraglottis (161.1)
  Epilarynx (including marginal zone)
  i   Suprahyoid epiglottis (including the tip)
  ii   Aryepiglottic fold
  iii Arytenoid
  Supraglottis excluding epilarynx
  iv   Infrahyoid epiglottis
  v   Ventricular bands (false cords)
  vi   Ventricular cavities
2 Glottis (161.0)
  i   Vocal cords
  ii   Anterior commissure
  iii Posterior commissure
3 Subglottis (161.2)

Regional lymph nodes

The regional lymph nodes are the cervical nodes.

TNM clinical classification

T – *primary tumour*

TX Primary tumour cannot be assessed
T0 No evidence of primary tumour
Tis Carcinoma in situ

Supraglottis

T1 Tumour limited to one subsite of supraglottis, with normal vocal cord mobility
T2 Tumour invades more than one subsite of supraglottis or glottis, with normal vocal cord mobility
T3 Tumour limited to larynx with vocal cord fixation and/or invades postcricoid area, medial wall of pyriform sinus or pre-epiglottic tissues
T4 Tumour invades through thyroid cartilage and/or extends to other tissues beyond the larynx, e.g. to oropharynx, soft tissues of neck

Glottis

T1 Tumour limited to vocal cord(s) (may involve anterior or posterior commissures) with normal mobility
    T1a Tumour limited to one vocal cord
    T1b Tumour involves both vocal cords
T2 Tumour extends to supraglottis and/or subglottis, and/or with impaired vocal cord mobility
T3 Tumour limited to the larynx with vocal cord fixation
T4 Tumour invades through thyroid cartilage and/or extends to other tissues beyond the larynx, e.g. to oropharynx, soft tissues of the neck

Subglottis

T1 Tumour limited to the subglottis
T2 Tumour extends to vocal cord(s) with normal or impaired mobility
T3 Tumour limited to the larynx with vocal cord fixation
T4 Tumour invades through cricoid or thyroid cartilage and/or extends to other tissues beyond the larynx, e.g. to oropharynx, soft tissues of the neck

N – *regional lymph nodes*

See definitions

M – *distant metastasis*

See definitions

pTNM pathological classification

The pT, pN and pM categories correspond to the T, N and M categories.

Histopathological grading

See definitions

Stage grouping

Stage 0	Tis	N0	M0
Stage I	T1	N0	M0
Stage II	T2	N0	M0
Stage III	T3	N0	M0
	T1	N1	M0
	T2	N1	M0
	T3	N1	M0
Stage IV	T4	N0, N1	M0
	Any T	N2, N3	M0
	Any T	Any N	M1

Summary

Larynx

Tl	*Glottis*
T1	Limited/mobile
T1a	One cord
T1b	Both cords
T2	Extends to supra- or subglottis/impaired mobility
T3	Cord fixation
T4	Extends beyond larynx

Supra- and subglottis

T1	Limited/mobile
T2	Extends to glottis/mobile
T3	Cord fixation
T4	Extends beyond larynx

All Regions

N1	Ipsilateral single $\leqslant$ 3 cm
N2	Ipsilateral single > 3 to 6 cm
	Ipsilateral multiple $\leqslant$ 6 cm
	Bilateral, contralateral $\leqslant$ 6 cm
N3	> 6 cm

References

ABRIKOSSOFF, A. (1926) Über Myome ausgehend von der quergestreiften willkürlichen Muskulatur. *Virchows Archiv für Pathologische Anatomie und Physiologie und für klinische Medizin*, **260**, 215–233

ACKERMAN, L. V. and DEL REGATO, J. A. (1970) Endolarynx. In: *Cancer. Diagnosis, Treatment and Prognosis*, 4th edn. St Louis: C. V. Mosby Co. p. 323

ACKERMAN, L. V. and ROSAI, J. (1974) *Surgical Pathology*, 5th edn. St Louis: C. V. Mosby Co

ADLINGTON, P. and WOODHOUSE, M. A. (1972) The ultrastructure of chemodectoma of the larynx. *Journal of Laryngology and Otology*, **86**, 1219–1232

ALBRECHTSEN, S., JULSETH, E., OLOFSSON, J. and DALAKER, K. (1994) Outcome of pregnancy and childbirth following laryngectomy. *Acta Obstetricia et Gynecologica Scandinavica*, **73**, 83–84

AL-SALEEM, T., TUCKER, G. F., PEALE, A. R. and NORRIS, C. M. (1970) Cartilaginous tumours of the larynx. Clinical pathologic study of ten cases. *Annals of Otology, Rhinology and Laryngology*, **79**, 33–41

AUERBACH, O., HAMMOND, E. C. and GARFINKEL, L. (1970) Histologic changes in the larynx in relation to smoking habits. *Cancer*, **25**, 92–104

AZZOPARDI, J. G. (1956) Histogenesis of the granular cell 'myoblastoma'. *Journal of Pathology*, **71**, 85–94

BACLESSE, F. (1949) Carcinoma of the larynx. Radiotherapy of laryngeal cancer. Clinical, radiological and therapeutic study. Follow-up of 341 cases treated at the Foundation Curie, from 1919 to 1940. *British Journal of Radiology*, **3** (suppl.), 1–62

BALOGH, K. and ROTH, S. I. (1965) Histochemical and electron microscopic studies of eosinophilic granular cells (oncocytes) in tumors of the parotid gland. *Laboratory Investigation*, **14**, 310–320

BALUYOT, S. T., SHUMRICK, D. A. and EVERTS, E. C. (1971) Emergency laryngectomy. *Archives of Otolaryngology*, **94**, 414–417

BAUGH, R. F., WOLF, G. T., BEALS, T. F., KRAUSE, C. J. and FORASTIERE, A. (1986) Small cell carcinoma of the larynx: results of therapy. *Laryngoscope*, **96**, 1283–1290

BILLER, H. F., OGURA, J. H. and BAUER, W. C. (1971) Verrucous carcinoma of the larynx. *Laryngoscope*, **81**, 1323–1329

BOCCA, E., PIGNATARO, O. and MOSCIARIO, O. (1968) Supraglottic surgery of the larynx. *Annals of Otology, Rhinology and Laryngology*, **77**, 1005–1026

BRODERS, A. C. (1920) Squamous cell epithelioma of the lip. *Journal of the American Medical Association*, **74**, 656–664

BRODERS, A. C. (1932) Practical points on the microscopic grading of carcinoma. *New York State Journal of Medicine*, **32**, 667–671

BRODSKY, A. (1984) Carcino (pseudo) sarcoma of the larynx – the controversy continues. *Otolaryngologic Clinics of North America*, **17**, 185–197

BRYCE, D. P. (1972) The role of surgery in the management of carcinoma of the larynx. *Journal of Laryngology and Otology*, **86**, 669–683

BUCK, G. (1853) On the surgical treatment of morbid growths within the larynx, illustrated by an original case and statistical observations, elucidating their nature and forms. *Transactions of the American Medical Association*, **6**, 509–535

BURNS, H. P., VAN NOSTRAND, A. W. P. and BRYCE, D. P. (1976) Verrucous carcinoma of the larynx – management by radiotherapy and surgery. *Annals of Otology, Rhinology and Laryngology*, **85**, 538–543

BUROW, A. and NEUMANN, L. (1875) Amyloide Degeneration von Larynxtumoren, Canüle Sieben Jahre lang getragen. *Archiv für klinische Chirurgie*, **18**, 242–246

CASTELIJNS, J. A., KAISER, M. C., VALK, J., GERRITSEN, G. J., VAN HATTUM, A. H. and SNON, G. B. (1987) MR imaging of laryngeal cancer. *Journal of Computer Assisted Tomography*, **1**, 134–140

CATTERALL, M. (1977) First randomised trial of fast neutrons compared with photons in advanced carcinoma of the head and neck. *Clinical Otolaryngology*, **4**, 359–372

CENTENNIAL CONFERENCE ON LARYNGEAL CANCER, TORONTO (1974) Workshop No. 1. Classification, anatomy, growth, and spread of laryngeal cancer (Chairmen: D. F. N. Harrison and A. W. P. van Nostrand). *Canadian Journal of Otolaryngology*, **3**, 407–511

CHERRY, J. and MARGULIES, S. I. (1968) Contact ulcer of the larynx. *Laryngoscope*, **78**, 1937–1940

COKER, D. D., ELIAS, G. E., CHRETIEN, P. M., GRAY, W. C., COLEMAN, J. J., ZENTAI, T. A. *et al.* (1981) Combination therapy for advanced squamous cell carcinoma of the head and neck. *Head and Neck Surgery*, **4**, 111–117

COLLEDGE, L. (1940) Radiotherapy and surgery in carcinoma in the head and neck. *Journal of Laryngology and Otology*, **55**, 433–436

CONLEY, J. J. (1961) Glottic reconstruction and wound rehabilitation. Procedures in partial laryngectomy. *Archives of Otolaryngology*, **74**, 239–242

CONLEY, J. (Ed.) (1967) Melanoma of the head and neck. In: *Cancer of the Head and Neck*, Washington: Butterworths. pp. 106–113

CONLEY, J. J., de AMNESTI, F. and PIERCE, N. K. (1958) A new surgical technique for the vocal rehabilitation of the laryngectomized patient. *Annals of Otology, Rhinology and Laryngology*, **67**, 655–664

CRISSMAN, J. D. (1982) Laryngeal keratosis preceding laryngeal carcinoma. *Archives of Otolaryngology*, **108**, 445–448

CUMBERWORTH, V. L., NARULA, A., MCCLENNAN, K. A. and BRADLEY, P. J. (1989) Mucoepidermoid carcinoma of the larynx. *Journal of Laryngology and Otology*, **103**, 420–423

CUSUMANO, R. J., KAUFMAN, D., WEISS, M., GALLO, L., REEDE, D. and MYSSORIEK, D. (1989) Needle aspiration of the pre-epiglottic space. *Head and Neck*, **11**, 41–45

D'ARCY, F. (1972) Localized amyloidosis of the larynx. *Journal of Laryngology and Otology*, **94**, 494–497

DEPARTMENT OF VETERANS AFFAIRS LARYNGEAL CANCER STUDY GROUP (1991) Induction chemotherapy plus radiation compared with surgery plus radiation in patients with advanced laryngeal cancer.*New England Journal of Medicine*, **324**, 1685–1690

DE SANTO, L. W., DEVINE, K. D. and WEILAND, L. H. (1970) Cysts of the larynx – classification. *Laryngoscope*, **80**, 145–176

DE SANTO, L. W., WILLIE, J. D. and DEVINE, K. D. (1976) Surgical salvage after radiation for laryngeal cancer. *Laryngoscope*, **86**, 649–657

DWORKIN, J. P. and BANTON, A. (1982) Review: oesophageal and mechanical instrument speech rehabilitation for the laryngectomee. *Clinical Otolaryngology*, **7**, 269–277

ELWOOD, J. M., PEARSON, J. C., SKIPPEN, D. H. and JACKSON, S. M. (1984) Alcohol, smoking, social and occupational factors in the aetiology of cancer of the oral cavity, pharynx, and larynx. *International Journal of Cancer*, **34**, 603–612

EPSTEIN, B. E., LEE, D. J., KASHIMA, H. and JOHNS, M. E. (1990) Stage T1, glottic carcinoma: results of radiation therapy or laser excision. *Radiology*, **175**, 567–570

EWING, M. R. and MARTIN, H. (1952) Disability following radical neck dissection. *Cancer*, **5**, 873–883

FERLITO, A. and RECHER, G. (1980) Ackerman's tumour (verrucous carcinoma) of the larynx. A clinicopathologic study of 77 cases. *Cancer*, **46**, 1617–1630

FINZI, N. S. and HARMER, D. (1928) Radium treatment of intrinsic carcinoma of the larynx. *British Medical Journal*, **2**, 886–889

FLANAGAN, P., CROSS, R. MCP. and LIBCKE, J. H. (1965) Fibrosarcoma of the larynx. *Journal of Laryngology and Otology*, **79**, 1049–1056

FLETCHER, G. H. (1972) Elective irradiation of subclinical disease in cancers of the head and neck. *Cancer*, **29**, 1450–1454

FLETCHER, G. H., JESSE, R. H., LINDBURG, R. D. and KOONS, C. R. (1970) The place of radiotherapy in the management of squamous cell carcinoma of the supraglottic larynx. *American Journal of Roentgenology*, **108**, 19–26

FLETCHER, G. N. and GOEPFERT, H. (1977) Irradiation in the management of squamous cell carcinoma of the larynx. In: *Otolaryngology*, edited by A. M. English, vol. 5 Hagerstown: Harper and Row. pp. 1–45

FOMBEUR, J. P., SEGUIN, D., DESPRÈS, P. H. and GENNEVIÈVE, J. P. (1974) Chondrome du cricoïde chez une femme de 78 ans. *Annales d'Otolaryngologie et de Chirurgie Cervicofaciale*, **91**, 485–490

FRIEDMANN, I. (1975) Sarcomas of the larynx. *Canadian Journal of Otolaryngology*, **4**, 297–302

GLUCK, T. (1922) Operationen für Kehlkopfkrebs. In: *Handbuch der speziellen Chirurgie des Ohres und der oberen Luftwege*, edited by L. Katz and F. Blumenfeld, vol. IV, Leipzig: Kabitash. p. 15

GOELLNER, J. R., DEVINE, K. D. and WEILAND, L. H. (1973) Pseudosarcoma of the larynx. *American Journal of Clinical Pathology*, **59**, 312–326

GOETHALS, P. L., DAHLIN, D. C. and DEVINE, K. D. (1963) Cartilaginous tumors of the larynx. *Surgery, Gynecology and Obstetrics*, **117**, 77–82

GOLDBERG, M., NOYEK, A. M. and PRITZLER, K. P. H. (1978) Laryngeal granuloma secondary to gastro-oesophageal reflux. *Journal of Otolaryngology*, **7**, 196–202

GREGOR, R. T., LLOYD, G. A. S. and MICHAELS, L. (1981) Computed tomography of the larynx: a clinical and pathologic study. *Head and Neck Surgery*, **3**, 284–296

GUSSENBAUER, C. (1874) Ueber die erst durch Th. Billroth am Menschen ausgeführte Kehlkopfextirpation und die Anwendung eines künstlichen Kehlkopfes-Langenbeck. *Archiv für klinische Chirurgie*, **17**, 343–356

HAMAKER, R. C., SINGER, M. I., BLOM, E. D. and DANIELS, H. A. (1985) Primary voice reconstruction and laryngectomy. *Archives of Otolaryngology*, **111**, 182–186

HAMPERL, H. (1962) Benign and malignant oncocytoma. *Cancer*, **15**, 1019–1027

HARRISON, D. F. N. (1971) The pathology and management of subglottic cancer. *Annals of Otology, Rhinology and Laryngology*, **80**, 6–12

HAUTANT, A. (1937) Abnormal forms of tuberculosis simulating cancer of the larynx and the converse. *Journal of Laryngology and Otology*, **52**, 65–74

HELLQUIST, H. and OLOFSSON, J. (1989) Spindle cell carcinoma of the larynx. *Acta Pathologica Microbiologica et Immunologica Scandinavica* **97**, 1103–1113

HELLQUIST, H., OLOFSSON, J. and GRÖNTOFT, O. (1979) Chondrosarcoma of the larynx. *Journal of Laryngology and Otology*, **93**, 1037–1047

HELLQUIST, H., OLOFSSON, J. and GRÖNTOFT, O. (1981) Carcinoma *in situ* and severe dysplasia of the vocal cords. A clinicopathological and photometric investigation. *Acta Otolaryngologica*, **92**, 543–555

HILGERS, F. J. M. and BALM, A. J. M. (1993) Long-term results of vocal rehabilitation after total laryngectomy with the low resistance indwelling Provox^TM voice prosthesis system. *Clinical Otolaryngology*, **18**, 517–523

HINDS, M. W., THOMAS, D. D. and O'REILLY, H. P. (1979) Asbestos, dental X-rays, tobacco and alcohol in the epidemiology of laryngeal cancer. *Cancer*, **44**, 1114–1120

HOLINGER, P. H. and JOHNSTON, K. C. (1951) Benign tumors of the larynx. *Annals of Otology, Rhinology and Laryngology*, **60**, 496–509

HURLEY, R. A., RICHTER, W. and TORRENS, L. (1972) The results of radiotherapy with high pressure oxygen in carcinoma of the pharynx, larynx and oral cavity. *British Journal of Radiology*, **45**, 98–109

HYAMS, V. J. and RABUZZI, D. D. (1970) Cartilaginous tumors of the larynx. *Laryngoscope*, **80**, 755–767

INTERNATIONAL CLASSIFICATION OF DISEASES FOR ONCOLOGY (ICD-O) (1977) In: *Manual of the International Statistical Classification of Diseases, Injuries and Cause of Death*, vol. 1. Geneva: World Health Organisation

ISAMBERT, A. (1876) Contribution à l'étude du cancer larynge. *Annales des Maladies de l'Oreille du Larynx*, **2**, 1–23

JACKSON, C. (1928) Contact ulcer of the larynx. *Annals of Otology, Rhinology and Laryngology*, **37**, 227–230

JACKSON, C. and JACKSON, C. L. (1935) Contact ulcer of the larynx. *Archives of Otolaryngology*, **22**, 1–15

JAKOBSSON, P. Å. (1973) *Glottic carcinoma of the larynx.*

Factors influencing prognosis following radiotherapy. Thesis. Stockholm: Printab AB

JAKOBSSON, P. Å., ENEROTH, C. M., KILLANDER, D., MOBERGER, G. and MÅRTENSSON, B. (1973) Histologic classification and grading of malignancy in carcinoma of the larynx. *Acta Radiologica Therapy Physics Biology*, **12**, 1–8

JOHNS, M. E., REGEZI, J. A. and BATSAKIS, J. G. (1977) Oncocytic neoplasms of salivary glands: an ultrastructural study. *Laryngoscope*, **87**, 862–871

JONES, N. F., HILTON, P. J., TIGHE, J. R. and HOBBS, J. R. (1972) Treatment of 'primary' renal amyloidosis with melphalan. *Lancet*, ii, 616

KALLIS, S. and STEVENS, D. J. (1989) Acinous cell carcinoma of the larynx. *Journal of Laryngology and Otology*, **103**, 638–641

KIEM, W. F., SHAPIRO, M. J. and ROSIN, H. D. (1965) Study of postlaryngectomy stomal recurrence. *Archives of Otolaryngology*, **81**, 183–186

KIRCHNER, J. A. (1974) *Centennial Conference on Laryngeal Cancer.* Workshop No. 10, edited by P. W. Alberti, D. P. Bryce. Toronto

KIRCHNER, J. A. and SOM, M. L. (1971) Clinical and histological observations on supraglottic cancer. *Annals of Otology, Rhinology and Laryngology*, **80**, 638–645

KLEINSASSER, O. (1978) *Microlaryngoscopy and Endolaryngeal Microsurgery – Techniques and Typical Cases.* Baltimore: University Park Press

KLEINSASSER, O. and GLANZ, H. (1979) Myogenic tumours of the larynx. *Archives of Oto–Rhino–Laryngology*, **225**, 107–119

KREICBERGS, A. (1981) *Malignancy grading of chondrosarcoma. A cytochemical, morphological and clinical study.* Thesis. Stockholm: Kollegietryck

KYLE, R. A. and BAYRD, E. D. (1975) Amyloidosis: review of 236 cases. *Medicine*, **54**, 271–299

LAWSON, V. G., BRYCE, D. P. and BRIANT, T. D. R. (1972) Chondroma and chondrosarcoma of the larynx. *Canadian Journal of Otolaryngology*, **1**, 213–218

LEDERMAN, M. (1970) Radiotherapy of cancer of the larynx. *Journal of Laryngology and Otology*, **84**, 867–896

LEDERMAN, M. and DALLEY, V. M. (1965) The treatment of glottic cancer. The importance of radiotherapy to the patient. *Journal of Laryngology and Otology*, **79**, 767–770

LEROUX–ROBERT, J. (1962) 'Tumeurs amyloïdes' du larynx. *Annales d'Oto–Laryngologie et de Chirurgie Cervico-faciale*, **79**, 249–270

LEROUX–ROBERT, J. (1975) Statistical study of 620 laryngeal carcinomas of the glottic region personally operated upon more than 5 years ago. *Laryngoscope*, **85**, 1440–1452

LICHTENSTEIN, L. (1965) Chondrosarcoma of bone. In: *Bone Tumours*, 3rd edn. St Louis: C. V. Mosby Co. pp. 180–201

MCALPINE, J. C. and FULLER, A. P. (1964) Localized laryngeal amyloidosis, a report of a case with a review of the literature. *Journal of Laryngology and Otology*, **78**, 296–314

MCGAVRAN, M. H., BAUER, W. C. and OGURA, J. H. (1961) The incidence of cervical lymph node metastases from epidermoid carcinoma of the larynx and their relationship to certain characteristics of the primary tumor. A study based on the clinical and pathological findings for 96 patients treated by primary *en bloc* laryngectomy and radical neck dissection. *Cancer*, **14**, 55–66

MCGUIRT, W. F., MATTHEWS, B. and KOURMAN, J. A. (1982) Multiple simultaneous tumours in patients with head and neck cancer. A prospective, sequential panendoscopic study. *Cancer*, **50**, 1195–1199

MCMICHAEL, A. J. (1978) Increases in laryngeal cancer in Britain and Australia in relation to tobacco and alcohol trends. *Lancet*, i, 1244–1247

MAIER, H., DE VRIES, N. and SNOW, G. B. (1991) Occupational factors in the aetiology of head and neck cancers. *Clinical Otolaryngology*, **16**, 406–412

MARTIN, H. (1957) Cancer of the larynx. In: *Surgery of Head and Neck Tumours.* New York: Hoeber Harper, Cassell & Co. Ltd. ch. 8, pp. 337–389

MAW, A. R., CULLEN, R. J. and BRADFIELD, J. W. B. (1982) Verrucous carcinoma of the larynx. *Clinical Otolaryngology*, **7**, 305–311

MICHAELS, L. (1984) *Pathology of the Larynx.* Berlin, Heidelberg: Springer Verlag

MICHAELS, L. (1987) *Ear, Nose and Throat Histopathology*, Springer-Verlag, pp. 409–415

MOORE, E. S. and MARTIN, H. (1955) Melanoma of the upper respiratory tract and oral cavity. *Cancer*, **8**, 1167–1176

MOURE, E. J. and PORTMANN, A. (1921) De la laryngectomie totale – technique operatoire. *Presse Medicale*, **29**, 561–563

NANSON, E. M. (1978) Neurilemmoma of the larynx: a case study. *Head and Neck Surgery*, **1**, 69–74

NEIS, P. R., MCMAHON, M. F. and NORRIS, C. W. (1989) Cartilaginous tumours of the trachea and larynx. *Annals of Otology, Rhinology and Laryngoloy*, **98**, 31–36

NEW, G. B. and ERICH, J. B. (1938) Benign tumours of the larynx. A study of 722 cases. *Archives of Otolaryngology*, **28**, 841–910

NEWHOUSE, M. L., GREGORY, M. M. and SHANNON, H. (1980) Etiology of carcinoma of the larynx. *International Agency for Research on Cancer.* (IARC) Scientific Publications, **30**, 687–695

NOHTERI, H. (1946) A case of laryngeal cyst composed of oncocytes and the appearance of oncocytes in the mucous membrane of the nose and larynx. *Acta Pathologica et Microbiologica Scandinavica*, **23**, 473–483

O'CONNOR, A. D., CLIFFORD, P., DALLEY, V. M., DURDEN–SMITH, D. J., EDWARDS, W. G. and HOLLIS, B. A. (1979) Advanced head and neck cancer treated by combined radiotherapy and VBM cytotoxic regimes – 4-year results. *Clinical Otolaryngology*, **4**, 329–337

OGURA, J. H. and MALLEN, R. W. (1967) Conservation surgery for cancer of the epiglottis and hypopharynx. In: *Cancer of the Head and Neck*, edited by J. Conley, Washington: Butterworths. p. 407

OGURA, J. H., BILLER, H. F., CALCATERRA, T. C. and DAVID, W. H. (1969) Surgical treatment of carcinoma of the larynx, pharynx, base of tongue and cervical oesophagus *International Surgery*, **52**, 29–40

OGURA, J. H., MARKS, J. E. and FREEMAN, R. B. (1980) Results of conservation surgery for cancers of the supraglottis and pyriform sinus. *Laryngoscope*, **90**, 591–600

OGURA, J. H., SESSIONS, D. G. and SPECTOR, G. J. (1975) Conservation surgery for epidermoid carcinoma of the supraglottic larynx. *Laryngoscope*, **85**, 1808–1815

ÖHMAN, L., OLOFSSON, J., TIBBLING, L. and ERICSSON, G. (1983) Esophageal dysfunction in patients with contact ulcer of the larynx. *Annals of Otology, Rhinology and Laryngology*, **92**, 228–230

OLOFSSON, J. (1993) Routines for follow-up and the risk of multiple primaris. In *Neoplasms of the Larynx*, edited by Ferlito, pp. 591–598

OLOFSSON, J., GRÖNTOFT, O., SÖKJER, H. and RISBERG, B. (1984)

Paraganglioma involving the larynx. *Otorhinolaryngology*, **46**, 57–65

OLOFSSON, J., LORD, I. J. and VAN NOSTRAND, A. W. P. (1973) Vocal cord fixation in laryngeal carcinoma. *Acta Otolaryngologica*, **75**, 496–510

OLOFSSON, J. and VAN NOSTRAND, A. W. P. (1972) Anaplastic small-cell carcinoma of the larynx. *Annuals of Otology, Rhinology and Laryngology*, **81**, 284–287

OLFOSSON, J. and VAN NOSTRAND, A. W. P. (1973) Growth and spread of laryngeal and hypopharyngeal carcinoma with reflections on the effect of pre-operative irradiation. *Acta Otolaryngologica Supplementum*, **308**

OLOFSSON, J. and VAN NOSTRAND, A. W. P. (1977) Adenoid cystic carcinoma of the larynx. A report of four cases and a review of the literature. *Cancer*, **40**, 1307–1313

OLSZEWSKI, E. (1976) Vascularization of ossified cartilage and the spread of cancer in the larynx. *Archives of Otolaryngology*, **102**, 200–203

PANJE, W. R. (1981) Prosthetic vocal rehabilitation following laryngectomy. The voice button. *Annals of Otology, Rhinology and Laryngology*, **90**, 116–120

PARNES, S. M. (1990) Asbestos and cancer of the larynx: is there a relationship? *Laryngoscope*, **100**, 254–261

PEACHER, G. M. (1961) Vocal therapy for contact ulcer of the larynx. A follow-up of 70 patients. *Laryngoscope*, **71**, 37–47

PEACHER, G. and HOLINGER, P. (1947) Contact ulcer of the larynx: II. The role of vocal re-education. *Archives of Otolaryngology*, **46**, 617–623

PIQUET, J. J. and CHEVALIER, D. (1991) Subtotal laryngectomy with crico-hyoid-epiglottidopexy for the treatment of extended glottic carcinomas. *American Journal of Surgery*, **162**, 357–361

POWELL, J. and ROBIN P. E. (1983) Cancer of the head and neck: the present state. In: *Head and Neck Cancer*, edited by P. Rhys Evans, P. E. Robin and J. W. L. Fielding. Tunbridge Wells: Castle House Publications. pp. 3–16

PRESSMAN, J. J. (1956) Submucosal compartmentation of the larynx. *Transactions of the American Laryngological Association*, **77**, 165–172

PRESSMAN, J. J. and SIMON, M. B. (1961) Evaluation of subtotal laryngectomy based upon studies of the lymphatics of the larynx and neck. *Laryngoscope*, **71**, 1019–1027

PRESSMAN, J. J., SIMON, M. B. and MONELL, C. (1969) Anatomical studies related to the dissemination of cancer of the larynx. *Transactions of the American Academy of Ophthalmology and Otolaryngology*, **64**, 628–638

RADCLIFFE, G. and SHAW, H. J. (1978) Partial laryngectomy for recurrent cancer after irradiation. *Clinical Otolaryngology*, **3**, 49–62

RAMADAN, M. F., MORTON, R. P., STELL, P. M. and PHAROAH, P. O. D. (1982) Review: epidemiology of laryngeal cancer. *Clinical Otolaryngology*, **7**, 417–428

ROBIN, P. E., REID, A., POWELL, D. J. and MCCONKEY, C. J. (1991a) The incidence of cancer of the larynx. *Clinical Otolaryngology*, **16**, 198–201

ROBIN, P. E., ROCKLEY, T. POWELL, D. J. and REID, A. (1991b) The survival of cancer of the larynx related to treatment. *Clinical Otolaryngology*, **16**, 193–197

ROKITANSKY, K. F. V. (1842) In: *Handbuch der Pathologischen Anatomie*, vol. 3. Vienna: Braunmüller & Siedel

ROUVIÈRE, H. (1931) *Anatomie des Lymphatiques de l'Homme*. Paris: Mason et Cie

RYAN, R. E., PEARSON, B. W. and WEILAND, L. H. (1977)

Laryngeal amyloidosis. *Transactions of the American Academy of Ophthalmology and Otolaryngology*, **84**, 872–877

RYAN, R. E. JR DE SANTO, L. W., DEVINE, K. D. and WEILAND, L. H. (1977) Verrucous carcinoma of the larynx. *Laryngoscope*, **87**, 1989–1994

SABRI, J. A. and HAJJAR, M. A. (1967) Malignant mixed tumor of the vocal cord. *Archives of Otolaryngology*, **85**, 118–120

SAKAMOTO, A., SAKAMOTO, G. and SUGANO, H. (1979) History of cervical radiation and incidence of carcinoma of the pharynx, larynx and thyroid. *Cancer*, **44**, 718–723

SAND HANSEN, H. (1975) *Neoplasma Malignum Laryngis*. Thesis. Copenhagen: Polyteknisk Forlag

SCHECHTER, G. L. and EL MAHDI, A. M. (1984) Conservation surgery of the larynx – when? *Otolaryngologic Clinics of North America*, **17**, 215–225

SHAW, H. J. (1965) Glottic cancer of the larynx 1947–56. *Journal of Laryngology and Otology*, **79**, 1–14

SHAW, H. (1979) Tumours of the larynx. In: *Scott–Brown's Diseases of the Ear, Nose and Throat*, 4th edn. edited by J. Ballantyne and J. Groves. London: Butterworths. pp. 421–508

SHUMRICK, D. A. (1971) Partial laryngectomy. *American Journal of Surgery*, **122**, 440–444

SILAMNIKU, B., BAUER, W., PAINTER, C. and SESSIONS, D. (1989) The transformation of laryngeal keratosis into invasive carcinoma. *American Journal of Otolaryngology*, **10**, 42–54

SINGER, M. I. and BLOM, E. D. (1980) An endoscopic technique for restoration of voice after laryngectomy. *Annals of Otology, Rhinology and Laryngology*, **89**, 529–533

SINGER, M. I. and BLOM, E. D. (1981) Selective myotomy for voice restoration after total laryngectomy. *Archives of Otolaryngology*, **107**, 670–673

SISSON, G. A. (1974) *Centennial Conference on Laryngeal Cancer*. Workshop No. 5., edited by P. W. Alberti and D. P. Bryce. New York: Appleton Century Crofts

SÖKJER, H. and OLOFSSON, J. (1981) Computed tomography in carcinoma of the larynx and piriform sinus. *Clinical Otolaryngology*, **6**, 335–343

SOM, M. L. (1970) Conservation surgery for carcinoma of the supraglottis. *Journal of Laryngology and Otology*, **84**, 655–678

SOM, M. L. and SILVER, C. E. (1968) The anterior commissure technique of partial laryngectomy. *Archives of Otolaryngology*, **87**, 138–145

SOM, P. M., NAGEL, B. D., FUERSTEIN, S. S. and STRAUSS, L. (1979) Benign pleomorphic adenoma of the larynx. A case report. *Annals of Otology, Rhinology and Laryngology*, **88**, 112 114

SOERENSEN, J. (1930) Quoted by St. Clair Thompson and L. Colledge in *Cancer of the Larynx*, p. 61. London: Kegan Paul, Trench, Trubner and Co. Ltd

SPIRO, R. H., LEWIS, J. S., HAJDU, S. I. and STRONG, E. W. (1976) Mucous gland tumours of larynx and laryngopharynx. *Annals of Otology, Rhinology and Laryngology*, **85**, 498–503

STAFFIERI, M. (1974) Laryngectomie totale avec reconstitution de la glotte phonaire. *Revue Laryngologie, Otologie, Rhinologie (Bordeaux)*, **95**, 63–83

STARK, D. B. and NEW, G. B. (1949) Amyloid tumors of the larynx, trachea or bronchi. A report of 15 cases. *Annals of Otology, Rhinology and Laryngology*, **58**, 117–134

STELL, P. M., DALBY, J. E., SINGH, S. D., RAMADAN, M. F. and BAINTON, R. (1982) The management of glottic T3 carcinoma. *Clinical Otolaryngology*, **7**, 175–180

STELL, P. M., MORTON, R. P. and SINGH, S. D. (1983) Squamous carcinoma of the head and neck – the untreated patient. *Clinical Otolaryngology*, **8**, 7–13

STELL, P. M. and RANGER, D. (1974) *Centennial Conference on Laryngeal Cancer*, Workshop No. 6., edited by P. W. Alberti and D. P. Bryce. New York: Appleton Century Crofts

STOUT, A. P. (1935) Peripheral manifestations of specific nerve sheath tumor (neurilemmoma). *American Journal of Cancer*, **24**, 751–796

STRONG, M. S. (1974) Laser management of premalignant lesions of the larynx. *Canadian Journal of Otolaryngology*, **3**, 560–563

STRONG, M. S. (1975) Laser excision of carcinoma of larynx. *Laryngoscope*, **85**, 1286–1289

SWERDLOW, R. S., SOM, M. L. and BILLER, H. F. (1974) Cartilaginous tumours of the larynx. *Archives of Otolaryngology*, **100**, 269–272

TASKINEN, P. J. (1969) Radiotherapy and TNM-classification of the larynx. A study based on 1447 cases seen at the radiotherapy clinic of Helsinki during 1936–1961. *Acta Radiologica*, Suppl. 287

THOMSON, ST. CLAIR and COLLEDGE, L. (1930) Operations of the larynx. In: *Cancer of the Larynx*. London: Routledge Kegan Paul. p. 161

TROTTER, W. (1926) The surgery of malignant disease of the larynx. *British Medical Journal*, **1**, 269–273

TUCKER, G. F. and SMITH, H. R. (1962) A histological demonstration of the development of laryngeal connective tissue compartments. *Transactions of the American Academy of Ophthalmology and Otolaryngology*, **66**, 308–318

TUYNS, A. J. and AUDIGIER, J. C. (1976) Double-wave cohort increase for oesophageal and laryngeal cancer in France in relation to reduced alcohol consumption during the second world war. *Digestion*, **14**, 197–208

UICC (1978) *TNM Classification of Malignant Tumours*, 3rd edn, edited by M. H. Harmer. Geneva: Union Internationale Contre le Cancer

UICC (1987) *TNM Classification of Malignant Tumours*, 4th edn. edited by P. Hermanek and L. H. Sobin. Berlin: Springer–Verlag

US SURGEON GENERAL (1979) In *Smoking and Health: a report of the Advisory Committee to the Surgeon General of the Public Health Service*, 1:16 and 5:32–4. Washington, DC: US Department of Health, Education and Welfare. Publication PHS 79–50066

VAN DE CATSIJNE, L. (1965) Les tumeurs cartilagineuses du larynx. *Acta Oto-Rhino-Laryngologica*, **19**, 875–912

VAN NOSTRAND, A. W. P. and OLOFSSON, J. (1972) Verrucous carcinoma of the larynx. A clinical and pathologic study of 10 cases. *Cancer*, **30**, 691–702

VIRCHOW, R. (1851) Bau und Zuzammensetzung der Corpora amylacea des Menschen. *Verhandlung phys. Med. Ges.*, Würzburg, **2**, 51

WAGENFELD, D. J. H., HARWOOD, A. R., BRYCE, D. P., VAN NOSTRAND, A. W. P. and DE BOER, G. (1980) Second primary respiratory tract malignancies in glottic carcinoma. *Cancer*, **46**, 1883–1886

WAGENFELD, D. J. H., HARWOOD, A. R., BRYCE, D. P., VAN NOSTRAND, A. W. P. and DE BOER, G. (1981) Second primary respiratory tract malignant neoplasms in supraglottic carcinoma. *Archives of Otolaryngology*, **107**, 135–137

WALDROP, F. S., PUCHTLER, H. and VALENTINE, L. S. (1973) Fluorescence microscopy of amyloid using mixed illumination. *Archives of Pathology*, **95**, 37–41

WANG, T. D. and ZHU, P. (1990) Vertical frontal subtotal laryngectomy and immediate reconstruction of the larynx with cervical skin flap. *Chinese Medical Journal*, **103**, 921–924

WARD, P. H., ZWITMAN, D., HANSON, D. and BERCI, G. (1980) Contact ulcers and granulomas of the larynx: new insights into their etiology as a basis for more rational treatment. *Otolaryngology – Head and Neck Surgery*, **88**, 262–269

WATERHOUSE, J., MUIR, C., SHANMUGARATNAM, K. and POWELL, J. (eds) (1982) In: *Cancer Incidence in Five Continents*, vol. IV. IARC Scientific Publication No. 42. Lyon: International Agency for Research on Cancer

WERBER, J. L. and LUCENTE, F. E. (1989) Computed tomography in patients with laryngeal carcinoma: a clinical perspective. *Annals of Otology, Rhinology and Laryngoloy*, **98**, 55–58

WETMORE, R. F., TRONZO, R. D., LANE, R. J. and LOWRY, L. D. (1981) Non-functional paraganglioma of the larynx: clinical and pathological considerations. *Cancer*, **48**, 2717–2723

WHICKER, J. H., NEEL, H. B., WEILAND, L. H. and DEVINE, K. D. (1974) Adenocarcinoma of the larynx. *Annals of Otology, Rhinology and Laryngology*, **83**, 487–490

ZISMOR, J., NOYEK, A. M. and LEWIS, J. S. (1975) Radiologic diagnosis of chondroma and chondrosarcoma of the larynx. *Archives of Otolaryngology*, **101**, 232–234

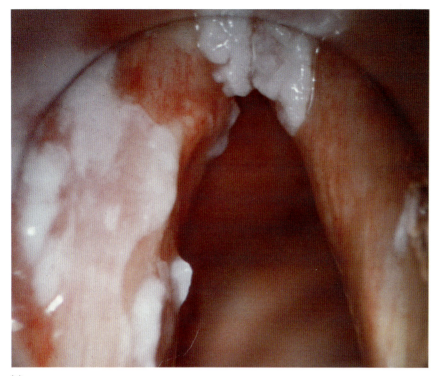

(a)

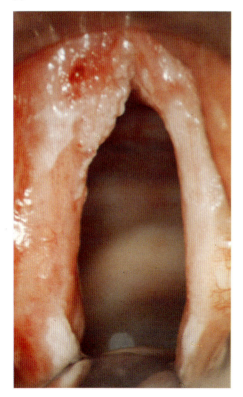

(b)

Plate 5/11/I (*a*) Keratosis. Extensive hyperplasia and keratosis (leucoplakia) of the left vocal cord and anterior commissure area; (*b*) severe dysplasia. The mucosa of the left vocal cord is red and somewhat oedematous and there is a papillomatous lesion anteriorly. Histological examination showed severe dysplasia

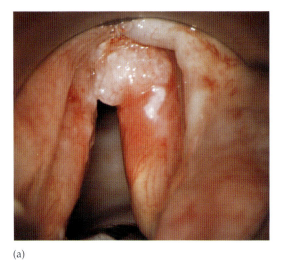

(a)

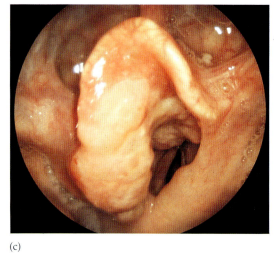

(c)

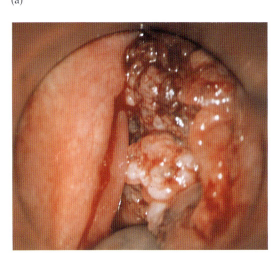

(b)

Plate 5/11/II (*a*) 'Anterior commissure carcinoma'. Squamous cell carcinoma involving the anterior part of the right vocal cord and the anterior commissure: (*b*) exophytic squamous cell carcinoma of the right hemilarynx with a fixed vocal cord: (*c*) supraglottic squamous cell carcinoma involving the epiglottis and left aryepiglottic fold (telescopic view)

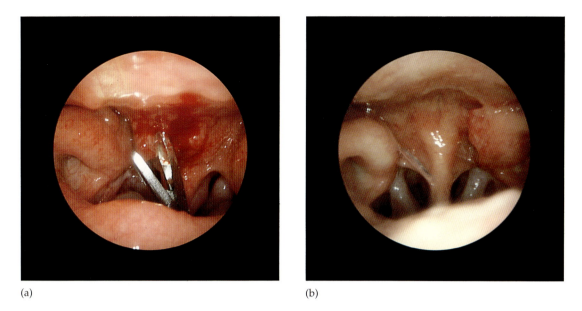

(a) (b)

Plate 5/13/I   (*a*) Endoscopic view of Henckel's biopsy forceps sampling the tissue in a typical undifferentiated carcinoma with ulcerative polypoidal appearance. (*b*) Posterior rhinoscopic picture of a very early carcinoma arising from the left torus and tubal recess depicting the most common site of tumour origin with minimal anatomical distortion. Such early detection is not common and the tumour can easily be missed without a proper endoscopic inspection

12

Angiofibroma

O. H. Shaheen

Angiofibroma is a vascular swelling arising in the nasopharynx of prepubertal and adolescent males and exhibiting a strong tendency to bleed. Alternative titles such as juvenile angiofibroma, nasopharyngeal fibroma, bleeding fibroma of adolescence and fibroangioma have largely been superseded by the simpler label of angiofibroma.

Much of the previous literature concerning aetiology and treatment was speculative and controversial, but a clearer picture of the nature of these swellings, their site of origin, behaviour and safer management has emerged in recent years.

Background

At one time, the impression existed that the incidence of angiofibromas was higher in certain parts of the world, e.g the Middle East and the Americas. It is probable that such an assumption was arrived at by equating large reported series from specific centres with a high geographical incidence. The series reported by Shaheen (1930), Figi (1940) and Handousa, Farid and Elwi (1954) are classical examples of major centres drawing patients from far and wide and suggesting a disproportionately high incidence of angiofibroma for the areas in question.

The ratio of angiofibromas to other ear, nose and throat conditions, as recorded in diagnostic registers, is likely to show wide variations, even between hospitals within a single large conurbation, and is therefore valueless as a guide to the prevalence of the condition. Martin, Ehrlich and Abels (1948) reported an annual admission rate of one or two patients for the 2000 or so patients treated in the Head and Neck service of the Memorial Hospital, New York. In an institution with a formidable reputation such as that of the Memorial Hospital, it would not be surprising if it received a far larger number of referrals than a lesser institution of comparable size within the same city.

In London, Harrison (1976) recorded the figure of one per 15 000 patients at the Royal National Throat, Nose and Ear Hospital which might prompt one to conclude that there are fewer angiofibromas in London than in New York. However, the two situations are not comparable and, in any case, the large number of London teaching hospitals existing in parallel with the Royal National Hospital is more likely to result in a fairer distribution of cases, so that even if the influx of tumours per hospital is small, the collective total might match that of any large metropolis.

Some doubt has been cast about the authenticity of certain of the series reported in the past, the main objections being questionable histology, and the inclusion of females and patients of extreme age.

There is now general agreement that this is exclusively a disease of males and that the mean age at presentation is around 14 years (Harrison, 1976). The range, however, is wide and varies between 7 and 19 years (Martin, Ehrlich and Abels, 1948) with isolated patients presenting earlier or later.

Many of the older reports implied that patients suffering from the condition displayed signs of delayed maturity as judged by secondary sexual characteristics, and that tumour pathogenesis was somehow linked to this. The regression which was observed with age or supposedly under the influence of hormones, was cited as evidence of hormonal aetiology, but was never supported by objective biochemical signs of hormonal insufficiency.

The suggestion that total regression occurs in the late teens or early twenties has never been convincingly demonstrated, although most authorities concede that some shrinkage, hardening and loss of vascularity of the tumour may occur with age.

The lack of complete regression could well explain the inclusion of older patients in some of the earlier reports, and would exonerate their authors of the charge of having misdiagnosed such cases.

Pathology

Grossly, angiofibromas appear as firm, slightly spongy lobulated swellings, the nodularity of which increases with age. Their colour varies from pink to white. That part which is seen in the nasopharynx and therefore covered by mucous membrane is invariably pink, whereas those parts which have escaped to adjacent extrapharyngeal areas are often white or grey. On section the tumour has a reticulated, whorled or spongy appearance, and lacks a true capsule. The edge, however, is sharply demarcated and easily distinguishable from the surrounding tissues.

Microscopically, the picture is of vascular spaces of varying shape and size abounding in a stroma of fibrous tissue, the relative proportions of which alter with the age of the swelling. In the earlier lesion, the vascular component stands out as an all-pervasive feature, whereas in the more long-standing tumours collagen predominates. It would seem that, as one strays from the heart of the tumour, the fibrous tissue element overshadows the vascular.

The vascular pattern consists of large thin-walled sinusoidal vessels lined by flattened epithelium, unsupported by a muscular coat, and the closer the vessels are to the surface of the swelling, the smaller they become.

In more long-standing tumours, there is a tendency towards gradual compression of the sinusoids so that the lining endothelial cells are pushed against each other like cords, while in others intravascular thrombosis occurs (Hubbard, 1958).

The stroma is composed of coarse parallel wavy or interlacing bundles of collagen in which stromal cells are seen to radiate outwards from the vessels (Steinberg, 1954) and in which localized areas of myxomatous degeneration may be observed.

Pathogenesis

A number of theories have been propounded over the years to explain the origin of angiofibromas and, although one or two are seemingly plausible, none is entirely convincing.

Ringertz (1938) suggested that the tumour arose from the periosteum of the nasopharyngeal vault, while Som and Neffson (1940) believed that inequalities in the growth of the bones forming the skull base resulted in hypertrophy of the underlying periosteum in response to a hormonal influence. Bensch and Ewing (1941) thought that the tumour probably arose from embryonic fibrocartilage between the basi-occiput and basisphenoid, whereas Brunner (1942) suggested an origin from the conjoined pharyngobasilar and buccopharyngeal fascia.

More plausibly, Osborn (1959) considered two alternatives, namely the possibility that the swellings were either hamartomas, or residues of fetal erectile tissue which were subject to hormonal influences.

Girgis and Fahmy (1973) noted cell nests of undifferentiated epithelioid cells or 'zellballen' at the growing edge of angiofibromas, an appearance which they likened to that of paragangliomas. They also commented on the existence of paragangliomatous tissue around the terminal part of the maxillary artery in the pterygopalatine fossa of stillborn infants and put forward the view that these might be the forerunners of angiofibromas.

With the possibility of vascular malformations still in mind, it would not be too far fetched to suggest that angiofibromas might arise from vestiges of the atrophied stapedial artery, although clearly it is not possible to validate such an assertion.

Site of origin and behaviour of angiofibromas

It was previously assumed that the vault of the nasopharynx was the most likely site of origin because of the broad-based attachment to the skull base which is so typical of the majority of tumours. Others considered the choana to be a more probable site in view of the frequency with which both the nasopharynx and the nasal fossa are involved, but failed to specify the precise point of origin.

Modern methods of investigation and ambitious surgical procedures have focused attention on the region of the sphenopalatine foramen as the site of origin and this would most reasonably explain the subsequent behaviour of angiofibromas. This is based on the observation that larger tumours present as bilobed dumb-bell swellings straddling the sphenopalatine foramen, with one component filling the nasopharynx and the other extending out into the pterygopalatine and infratemporal fossae. The central stalk joining the two portions occupies the sphenopalatine foramen at the upper end of the vertical plate of the palatine bone, without appearing to enlarge it very much. In the absence of any significant degree of erosion of the sphenopalatine foramen, the only logical way that such a dumb-bell arrangement can come about is if the rudiment of the swelling were to be either in or very close to the foramen.

The seedling swelling arising from such a site would migrate medially beneath the mucous membrane of the nasopharynx, displacing it downwards in the process, and eventually growing to fill the postnasal space. As the process of growth continues, the anterior face of the sphenoidal sinus is encroached upon and eroded, and the sinus is invaded. The swelling then follows the line of least resistance and grows forwards into the nasal fossa where it may acquire secondary attachments. Having filled the nasal fossa it will displace the nasal septum over to the opposite side, so that the healthy side of the nose also becomes blocked.

Growth in a lateral direction may take place in some cases, and the starting point is once again the sphenopalatine foramen. The pterygopalatine fossa is thus invaded and, once filled, causes forward bowing of the posterior wall of the antrum. Eventually, the swelling comes to occupy the infratemporal fossa and when insufficient room remains for further expansion, it will encroach on the orbital fissures.

However, this is not to say that every angiofibroma behaves in this way; indeed, some remain confined to the nasopharynx but usually with a bias towards one side.

That portion of a bilobed angiofibroma which lies outside the nasopharynx eventually becomes very hard and nodular, and in the course of its spread into the pterygopalatine and infratemporal fossae may well erode the anterior face of the greater wing of the sphenoid so as to make contact with the dura of the middle fossa. It may displace the maxillary nerve upwards, and less commonly the optic nerve, and if it invades the orbit through the inferiorly placed fissure of that cavity, will eventually cause proptosis.

The main blood supply to angiofibromas comes by way of an enlarged maxillary artery, but other arteries, such as the ascending pharyngeal, vidian, unnamed branches of the internal carotid and rarely the vertebral, may contribute to their vascularization.

Symptoms and signs

The two cardinal symptoms of angiofibromas are nasal obstruction and intermittent epistaxis. The latter may vary in severity from the occasional show to an alarming and sometimes life-threatening torrent. Chronic anaemia is thus a common feature of the established condition.

It should be stressed that the bleeding which is so characteristic of much of the surgery of angiofibromas is caused by breaking into the parenchyma of the swelling or by disrupting the feeding vessels, whereas the bleeding which occurs prior to operation is entirely spontaneous and usually unconnected with trauma.

The completeness of nasal obstruction is such that stasis of secretions and sepsis are virtually inevitable, followed by hyposmia or anosmia.

The voice acquires a nasal intonation and, if the swelling is large enough to force the soft palate down, there may be an added plummy quality to it. Blockage of the eustachian tube is not uncommon in such a situation and leads to deafness and otalgia.

Anterior rhinoscopy is likely to confirm the presence of abundant mucopurulent secretions together with bowing of the nasal septum to the uninvolved side. Posterior rhinoscopy in the cooperative relaxed patient should display a pink or red mass filling the nasopharynx, but the sheer bulk of the lesion rarely allows the examiner to determine its precise site of origin.

Gross physical signs are evident when extensive disease has involved the nose and infratemporal fossa; the nasal bones are often splayed out and there may be obvious swelling in the temple and cheek. Intraoral palpation in the interval between the ascending ramus of the mandible and the side of the maxilla may also reveal a fullness caused by a tumour which has crept around the back of the antrum.

Impaction of bulky disease in the infratemporal fossa results in extreme signs such as trismus and bulging of the parotid gland, while proptosis is a definite sign that the orbital fissures have been penetrated. The classical frog face as displayed in older publications is the ultimate picture of massive escape of disease.

Headache is not uncommon in patients with large tumours and is often attributable to chronic sinusitis. In other instances the cause is not so obvious and explanations, such as dural compression at sites of bone erosion or invasion of the sphenoidal sinus, can only be speculative.

Failing vision has been seen by the author on two occasions and indicates tenting of the optic nerve over a substantial extrapharyngeal extension of the tumour.

Investigations

Standard radiographs of the paranasal sinuses taken in the occipitofrontal or lateral projections may sometimes be misleading in that opacity of the maxillary sinus, in association with a soft tissue shadow in the postnasal space, may be mistaken for an antrochoanal polyp.

On the other hand, tomography in the fronto-occipital plane may be helpful in localizing the position of the mass, and showing areas of bone destruction or invasion of the sphenoidal sinus – findings which are inconsistent with an antrochoanal polyp. Lateral tomograms are desirable as they may reveal forward bowing of the posterior antral wall which is typical of an angiofibroma filling the pterygopalatine fossa (Figure 12.1).

The introduction of computerized tomographic scanning with enhancement, and more recently, the technique of magnetic resonance, has to a large extent pre-empted the routine use of arteriography (Levine *et al.*, 1979) (Figure 12.2).

Invasion of the sphenoidal sinus, erosion of the

greater wing of the sphenoid, and extension into the pterygopalatine and infratemporal fossae is detectable with remarkable clarity on the latest generation of scanners. When doubt exists about the accuracy of the imaging, or in cases of recurrent angiofibroma, selective arteriography should be performed and the results displayed to the best advantage using subtraction techniques.

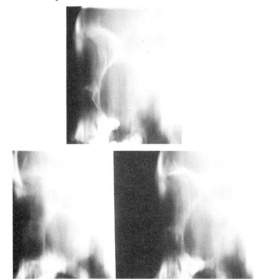

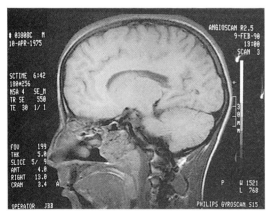

Figure 12.1 Typical bowing of the posterior wall of the antrum by an angiofibroma

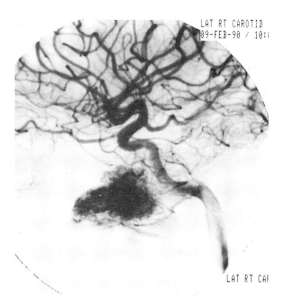

Figure 12.3 Subtraction film to show the vascular blush of an angiofibroma during arteriography

Biopsy is no longer justifiable in view of the risk of severe and protracted haemorrhage and because modern radiological techniques will establish the diagnosis with a high degree of accuracy.

Differential diagnosis

The list of possible diagnoses with which angiofibromas may be confused includes antrochoanal polyp, large adenoids, tumours of the postnasal space and chordoma. In practice there is rarely any doubt about the issue once the patient has been fully investigated.

Treatment

The treatment of angiofibroma has been subject to considerable change over the years, but appears to be coming round full circle.

In the earlier part of the century treatment was surgical because other alternatives were either not available or had not been considered. Surgical efforts were thwarted by the absence of preoperative investigations to delineate the lesion and by the amount of peroperative bleeding. Furthermore, the anaesthetics of the era were unsophisticated and poorly administered, thus adding to the problem of bleeding.

It was not universally appreciated that the severe bleeding which accompanied operations for an angiofibroma was in large measure due to the surgeons'

Figure 12.2 MRI to show a typical angiofibroma

The vascular blush, which shows up in the postnasal space and adjacent areas, is diagnostic of the condition and obviates the need for biopsy (Figure 12.3). Useful information is obtained from the arteriograms on the size and site of the lesion and the size and location of feeding vessels, some of which arise from unusual sources such as the internal carotid and vertebral arteries (Thomas and Mowat, 1970; Ward *et al.*, 1974).

failure to avoid breaching the surface of the swelling during the course of the dissection. This is hardly surprising in the light of present knowledge about its tendency to fill nooks and crannies and to invade adjacent areas. Even as late as the 1960s, the practice of grasping an angiofibroma with giant bone-holding forceps and wrenching it out was still in evidence in some centres.

The disillusionment created by the uncertainties and dangers of surgery led to a search for alternative and safer methods of treatment.

Attention was directed to hormone therapy and external beam irradiation, often as a preliminary to surgery, on the basis that such treatment promoted collagen formation and thereby reduced vascularity.

Testosterone was used on its own (Martin, Ehrlich and Abels, 1948), as were oestrogens (Patterson, 1973), and a combination of the two was advocated by Schiff (1959). There is some evidence to support the view that either type of hormone may encourage maturation of collagen while, at the same time, reducing vascularity (Arolde and Schatzle, 1971), but whether this contributes significantly to the safety of surgery is impossible to determine.

The case for using radiotherapy exclusively as a definitive treatment for angiofibromas is not without merit. Briant, Fitzpatrick and Brook (1970) advocated it on the grounds that surgery carries a high recurrence rate, but others have felt that radiotherapy should be reserved for selected patients, such as those with inoperable intracranial extensions and recurrent tumours (Ward *et al.*, 1974). The effect of ionizing radiation on angiofibromas has been studied in those patients who subsequently underwent surgery, and is judged to bring about a shrinkage and hardening of the tumours with a resultant reduction of their vascularity. Many clinicians, however, view the prospect of irradiating young adolescents with considerable diffidence and feel that it cannot be justified in the face of possible carcinogenicity.

The resurgence of interest in surgery as the definitive treatment has gathered momentum in recent years, largely because of improvements in preoperative assessment and a better understanding of the condition. There is some reason to suppose that preoperative embolization may reduce bleeding provided that the timing is right, although its hazards should not be minimized (Lasjaunias, 1980; Lang, McKellar and Lang, 1983).

The argument as to which surgical approach is best for the removal of angiofibromas implies that all swellings are identical – a notion which is nonsensical. Empiricism has no part in surgical judgement, and each case should be approached on the results of the preoperative findings. The transpalatal operation, favoured exclusively by many, would be rational if all angiofibromas were confined to the nasopharynx, a state of affairs which borders on the exceptional (English, Hemenway and Cundy, 1972).

An alternative and possibly more adaptable approach combines a transpalatal route with a gingivo-buccal incision for access to the pterygomaxillary region (Jafek *et al.*, 1973), but even this entails a degree of empiricism which is incompatible with the philosophy of tailoring the operation to the disease.

A tumour which is confined exclusively to the postnasal space should be removed transpalatally, but one which has escaped into the pterygopalatine fossa, or beyond, requires a more ambitious approach. This must entail adequate access to the extensions of the tumour and allow dissection between the swelling and surrounding structures in such a way as to ensure that the tumour parenchyma is not breached in the process (Shaheen, 1984). It should also provide the surgeon with sufficient room to ligate the principal feeding vessel to the tumour, and not compromise his ability to deal with major haemorrhage.

For tumours which encroach on the nasal fossa and just spill over into the pterygopalatine fossa, a lateral rhinotomy combined with resection of the medial antral wall may suffice to deliver the tumour and its extensions. For larger tumours which invade the infratemporal fossa access is improved by a combined transnasal/transantral approach, and this can be achieved either via a Weber Ferguson incision (Shaheen, 1982) or a facial degloving approach (Howard and Lund, 1992).

The objective of either incision is to expose the maxillary antrum sufficiently so that the anterior, lateral, posterior and medial walls of the antrum can be removed, leaving the orbital floor and upper alveolar arch as two intact shelves (Figure 12.4). By ensuring that all of the medial antral wall is removed, including the vertical plate of the palatine bone, the nasal cavity, antrum, infratemporal fossa, pterygopalatine fossa and nasopharynx are converted into

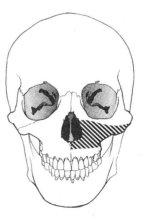

Figure 12.4 The extent of bone removal in the transantral approach to the infratemporal fossa for dumb-bell angiofibromas

one large continuous space, a state of affairs which affords access to both the components of the swelling and its central stalk.

Starting laterally, the infratemporal part of the swelling is first identified and the maxillary artery found and ligated. The tumour is then mobilized in a medial and forward direction towards the antrum and nasopharynx. Removal of the perpendicular plate of the palatine bone serves to uncap the central stalk of the dumb-bell, which previously occupied the sphenopalatine foramen, and facilitates the subsequent mobilization of the nasopharyngeal component of the swelling.

The latter is dissected free from the base of the skull and from within the sphenoidal sinus, and the mucous membrane covering its undersurface is then divided at its periphery in order to complete the removal of the tumour. No attempt is made to strip the mucous membrane off the inferior aspect of the swelling because of the intimacy of attachment between the two.

Complications

A palatal fistula may result when the transpalatal route is used, especially if the incision is sited directly over the junction of the hard and soft palate. With the Weber–Ferguson approach, anaesthesia of the cheek is inevitable, although it rarely assumes troublesome proportions in this age group. Slight ectropion of the lower lid occasionally results and crusting of the nose may occur in some patients for some time afterwards.

The frequency of recurrence is very much dependent on the adequacy of the approach, the conditions at operation, the experience of the surgeon, and the extent of the lesion in question.

References

AROLDE, R. and SCHATZLE, W. (1971) Histologisch histochemische untersuchungen juveniler nasenbachenfibrome vor und nach hormon behandlung, *HNO*, **19**, 69–74

BENSCH, H. and EWING, J. (1941) *Neoplastic Disease*, 4th edn. Philadelphia: Saunders & Co

BRIANT, T. D. R., FITZPATRICK, P. J. and BROOK, H. (1970) The radiological treatment of juvenile nasopharyngeal angiofibromas. *Annals of Otology, Rhinology and Laryngology*, **79**, 108–113

BRUNNER, H. (1942) Nasopharyngeal fibroma. *Annals of Otology, Rhinology and Laryngology*, **51**, 29–65

ENGLISH, G. M., HEMENWAY, W. G. and CUNDY, R. L. (1972) Surgical treatment of invasive angiofibroma. *Archives of Otolaryngology*, **96**, 312–318

FIGI, F. (1940) Fibromas of the nasopharynx. *Journal of the American Medical Association*, **115**, 665–671

GIRGIS, I. H. and FAHMY, S. A. (1973) Nasopharyngeal fibroma: its histopathology. *Journal of Laryngology and Otology*, **87**, 1107–1123

HANDOUSA, A. S., FARID, H. and ELWI, A. M. (1954) Nasopharyngeal angiofibroma and its treatment. *Journal of Laryngology and Otology*, **68**, 647–666

HARRISON, D. F. N. (1976) Juvenile postnasal angiofibroma – an evaluation. *Clinical Otolaryngology*, **1**, 187–197

HOWARD, D. J. and LUND, V. J. (1992) The midfacial degloving approach to sinonasal disease. *Journal of Laryngology and Otology*, **106**, 1059–1062

HUBBARD, E. M. (1958) Nasopharyngeal angiofibromas. *Archives of Pathology*, **65**, 192–204

JAFEK, B. W., NAHUM, A. M., BUTLER, R. M. and WARD, P. H. (1973) Surgical treatment of juvenile nasopharyngeal angiofibroma. *Laryngoscope*, **83**, 707–720

LANG, D. A., MCKELLAR, N. J. and LANG, W. (1983) Juvenile nasopharyngeal angiofibroma. The preferred treatment. *Scottish Medical Journal*, **28**, 64–66

LASJAUNIAS, P. (1980) Nasopharyngeal angiofibromas. Hazards of embolization. *Radiology*, **136**, 119–123

LEVINE, H. L., WEINSTEIN, M. A., TUCKER, H. M., WOOD, V. G. and DUCHESNEAU, T. M. (1979) Diagnosis of juvenile nasopharyngeal angiofibroma by computed tomography. *Otolaryngology: Head and Neck Surgery*, **87**, 304–310

MARTIN, H., EHRLICH, H. E. and ABELS, J. G. (1948) Juvenile nasopharyngeal angiofibroma. *Annals of Surgery*, **127**, 513–536

OSBORN, D. A. (1959) The so-called juvenile angiofibroma of the nasopharynx. *Journal of Laryngology and Otology*, **69**, 295–316

PATTERSON, C. N. (1973) Juvenile nasopharyngeal angiofibroma. *Otolaryngologic Clinics of North America*, **6**, 839–861

RINGERTZ, N. (1938) Pathology of malignant tumours arising in the nasal and paranasal cavities and maxilla. *Acta Oto-Laryngologica Supplementum*, **27**, 1–405

SCHIFF, M. (1959) Juvenile nasopharyngeal angiofibroma. *Laryngoscope*, **69**, 981–1016

SHAHEEN, H. (1930) Nasopharyngeal fibroma. *Journal of Laryngology and Otology*, **45**, 259–264

SHAHEEN, O.H. (1982) Swellings of the infratemporal fossa. *Journal of Laryngology and Otology*, **96**, 817–836

SHAHEEN, O.H. (1984) *Problems in Head and Neck Surgery*. London: Baillière Tindall. p. 100

SOM, M.L. and NEFFSON, A.H. (1940) Fibromas of the nasopharynx: juvenile and cellular types. *Annals of Otology, Rhinology and Laryngology*, **49**, 211–218

STEINBERG, S.S. (1954) Pathology of juvenile nasopharyngeal angiofibroma – a lesion of adolescent males. *Cancer*, **7**, 15–28

THOMAS, M.I. and MOWAT, P.D. (1970) Angiography in juvenile nasopharyngeal haemangiofibroma. *Clinical Radiology*, **21**, 403–406

WARD, P.H., THOMPSON, R., CALCATERRA, T. and KADIM, M.R. (1974) Juvenile angiofibroma, a more rational therapeutic approach based upon clinical and experimental evidence. *Laryngoscope*, **84**, 2181–2194

13

Nasopharynx (the postnasal space)

Chuan-Tieh Chew

The human nasopharynx is mainly derived from the primitive pharynx. It represents the nasal portion of the pharynx behind the nasal cavity and above the free border of the soft palate. It is a transitional zone between the nasal cavity and the oropharynx and has also been called the postnasal space or epipharynx, with debate as to the proper terminology. The concept that there is an anterior 'nasal' and a posterior 'pharyngeal' component is supported by embryological, morphological and functional considerations (Kanagasuntheram, Wong and Chan, 1969; Leela, Kanagasuntheram and Khoo, 1974). Morphological and histological studies have shown that the anterior portion proximal to the tubal orifice resembles the nasal cavity while the posterior portion resembles the oropharynx. The junctional zone is the belt along the tubal orifice where the first and third pharyngeal arches meet. The tubotympanic recess, the precursor of the eustachian tube, is formed mainly from the second pharyngeal pouch (between the first and third pharyngeal arches) while the pharyngeal muscles are derived from the third and fourth pharyngeal arches.

Innervation studies show that the portion proximal to the tubal orifice is innervated by the maxillary division of the trigeminal (Vth) nerve, and the portion posterior to the tubal orifice by the glossopharyngeal (IXth) nerve. Motor fibres are carried by the vagus (Xth) nerve with a contribution from the cranial portion of the XIth nerve. Functional studies with contrast and cinefluorography reveal structural differences between the two components. Contractility is observed only in the posterior portion.

Surgical anatomy

The average dimensions of the nasopharynx in the adult are 4 cm high, 4 cm wide and 3 cm in an anteroposterior dimension. The posterior wall is about 8 cm from the pyriform aperture along the nasal floor.

The anterior wall is formed by the choanal orifice and posterior margin of the nasal septum.

The floor is formed by the upper surface of the soft palate which occupies the anterior two-thirds and by the nasopharyngeal isthmus.

The roof and posterior wall form a continuous sloping surface bounded by the body of the sphenoid, the basiocciput and the first two cervical vertebrae to the level of the soft palate. The upper portion of the posterior wall lies in front of the anterior arch of the atlas with a mass of lymphoid tissue embedded in the mucosal membrane (nasopharyngeal tonsil or adenoid). The prevertebral fascia and muscles separate the adenoid from the vertebrae.

The lateral wall is dominated by the pharyngeal orifice of the eustachian tube. Located in the middle of the wall, it is about 1.5 cm equidistant from the roof, posterior wall, choana and the floor. The torus tubalis or tubal elevation, created by the elastic cartilage of the tube, is particularly prominent in its upper and posterior lips. Behind the posterior margin of the torus, between it and the posterior wall, lies the lateral pharyngeal recess or the fossa of Rosenmüller. Aggregates of lymphoid tissue of variable size around the tubal orifice and part of the recess are collectively called the tubal tonsil.

The fossa of Rosenmüller (Figures 13.1 and 13.2) is situated in the corner between the lateral and dorsal walls. Although not obvious in infants, the recess can measure up to 2.5 cm in depth in adults. More often than not it appears as a cleft, trabeculated at times, and recedes posterolaterally to an apex near to the edge of the carotid canal opening. It opens into the nasopharynx at a point below the foramen lacerum.

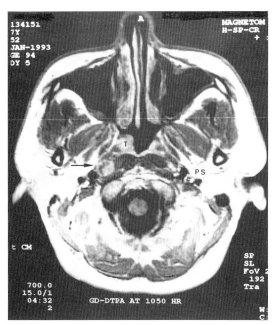

(*a*)

Figure 13.1 (*a*) Axial magnetic resonance scan with gadolinium-DTPA contrast enhanced T1 image of the nasopharynx and skull base characterizing various soft tissues showing the nasopharynx and its anatomical relations to the parapharyngeal and infratemporal region. It depicts normal anatomy on the left and a contralateral early nasopharyngeal carcinoma with a retropharyngeal node of Rouviere metastasis. T: tumour, arrow pointing to node of Rouviere, PS: Parapharyngeal space (*b*) Diagram of the anatomical relationship of the nasopharynx:

 1   Pterygoid plates
 2   Tensor palatini muscle
 3   Eustachian tube orifice and torus
 4   Levator palatini muscle
 5   Fossa of Rosenmüller
 6   Retropharyngeal node of Rouviere
 7   Lateral pterygoid muscle
 8   Medial pterygoid muscle
 9   Buccopharyngeal fascia
10   Parotid gland
11   Styloid process
12   Digastric muscle
13   Longus capitis muscle
 A   Prestyloid parapharyngeal space
 B   Retrostyloid parapharyngeal space
 C   Retropharyngeal space
 T   Tumour

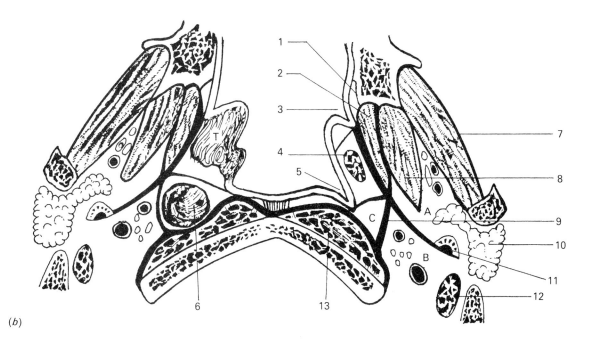

(*b*)

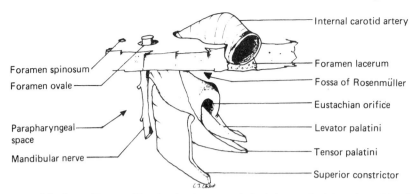

Figure 13.2 Diagram of the fossa of Rosenmüller showing its anatomical relations to the internal carotid and parapharyngeal space at the skull base

The anatomical relationships of the fossa of Rosenmüller are:

Anteriorly: eustachian tube and levator palatini
Posteriorly: pharyngeal wall mucosa overlying the pharyngobasilar fascia and retropharyngeal space, containing the lateral retropharyngeal node of Rouviere
Medially: nasopharyngeal cavity
Superiorly: foramen lacerum and floor of carotid canal
Posterolateral (apex): carotid canal opening and petrous apex posteriorly, foramen ovale and spinosum laterally
Laterally: tensor palatini and the mandibular nerve, and the prestyloid compartment of the parapharyngeal space. The fossa forms the medial border of the most superior part of the parapharyngeal space.

As the superior constrictor does not reach the base of the skull, a lateral gap (the sinus of Morgagni) is created. This gap is bridged only by the pharyngobasilar fascia. Through this, the eustachian tube with its two muscles, one on each side, enters the nasopharynx. Along the inferior border of the two muscles the fossa of Rosenmüller is separated from the parapharyngeal space by mucosa and the pharyngobasilar fascia. Tumours can easily infiltrate and breach this area to spread into the parapharyngeal space.

Epithelial lining of the nasopharynx

The nasopharyngeal mucosa is thrown into numerous folds and crypts with serous and mucous glands in the submucosal layer. The actual surface area is approximately 50 cm² in the adult. During fetal life there is a gradual transition of the respiratory ciliated epithelium to squamous type in the lower and posterior part of the nasopharynx. True squamous metaplasia occurs only in postnatal life and is completed by about 10 years of age. About 60% of the total epithelial surface is lined by stratified squamous epithelium

(Ali, 1965). The mucosa abutting the choanae and immediate nasopharyngeal roof is completely lined by ciliated epithelium. Patches of squamous and ciliated epithelium, intermingling with islets of transitional or intermediate cell types, cover the rest of the roof and lateral walls. The posterior wall is dominated by squamous epithelium. The nasopharyngeal mucosa has a distinct basement membrane and differs from the rest of the upper respiratory tract in that the subepithelial connective tissue is rich in lymphoid tissue. It consists of numerous small lymphocytes, plasmacytes, reticular cells and fibroblasts. This lymphoepithelial tissue together with aggregates of lymphoid tissue and the tonsils constitute Waldeyer's ring.

Lymphatic drainage

The nasopharynx has an extensive submucosal lymphatic plexus. The first-order drainage sites are the retropharyngeal nodes situated in the retropharyngeal space between the posterior nasopharyngeal wall, pharyngobasilar fascia and the prevertebral fascia. The node of Rouviere forms the main and constant lateral group. It lies anterior to the lateral mass of the atlas at the lateral border of the longus capitis muscle, anteromedial to the internal carotid artery. Efferent vessels then drain to the uppermost deep internal jugular chain at the skull base in the retrostyloid parapharyngeal space compartment deep to the upper end of the sternomastoid muscle. The nodes then drain downwards posteriorly to the accessory nerve group and anteriorly to the jugulodigastric group. The nasopharynx is essentially a midline structure, rich in lymphatic channels with cross-drainage hence contralateral and bilateral spread of tumour cells is not uncommon.

Adenoid and nasopharyngeal lymphoid tissue

Anatomically, the adenoid is covered by epithelium which is thrown into numerous folds separating the lymphoid follicles. There are also deep crypts similar to those in the palatine tonsil. The lymphoid tissue consists of both T and B lymphocytes, with the latter predominating. Detectable at around the fourth month of embryonic development embedded in the mucosa at the junction of the roof and posterior nasopharyngeal wall, the adenoid is poorly developed at birth. It is not visible on plain radiographs in infants under the age of 1 month but is clinically identifiable by the fourth month. It is radiologically demonstrable in only 50% of infants under 6 months, and in all infants by the age of 6 months (Capitanio and Kirkpatrick, 1970). By the age of 2 years, hypertrophy and hyperplasia of the adenoid occurs. Rapid growth occurs from 3 to 5 years with a consequent decrease in the nasopharyngeal airway. After that the adenoid size remains relatively constant while the nasopharynx increases in size (Jeans *et al.*, 1981). Involution of the adenoid occurs after puberty; however, the lymphoid tissue persists into old age.

The adenoid is of clinical importance. Any diminution in size or its absence could indicate an underlying immunodeficiency, e.g. familial hypogammaglobulinaemia and Wiskott-Aldrich syndrome. The presence of a nasopharyngeal mass in infants under the age of 1 month should raise the suspicion of a tumour such as an encephalocoele, as the adenoids are not detectable at this age.

In children, postnasal and throat infection affecting the adenoid and retropharyngeal nodes is known to cause atlantoaxial subluxation. This happens as a result of inflammatory loosening of the intervertebral ligament. Most subluxation occurs about 1–2 weeks after the onset of the infection and presents with torticollis and spasm of the posterior spinal muscles.

Pharyngeal hypophysis

The anterior pituitary gland is formed by a median ectodermal upgrowth from an invagination (Rathke's pouch) of the stomatodeum immediately in front of the buccopharyngeal membrane. This upgrowth migrates cranially through the mesenchymal tissue, which later forms the body of the sphenoid, to rest in the anlage of the sella turcica. Its original course is identified by the craniopharyngeal canal. Breaks may occur in the buccohypophyseal stalk to form accessory or aberrant endocrine tissue in the body of the sphenoid (Boyd, 1956). Remnants of the stalk persist in the nasopharyngeal roof to form the pharyngeal hypophysis which is a tiny elongated body of tissue in the mucoperiosteum underlying the posterior vomerosphenoidal articulation. Histologically the pharyngeal hypophysis contains chromophobe cells similar to those in the pituitary. Its functional role is not clear but it has been observed to undergo hypertrophy in women over the age of 50 years (McGrath, 1971). The pharyngeal and ectopic hypophyseal tissue may give rise to a chromophobe adenoma in the nasopharynx or sphenoid (without sellar enlargement or involvement).

The pharyngeal bursa – Thornwaldt's cyst

This structure is often confused with Rathke's pouch. It is a cystic notochordal remnant found inconsistently. When present, it appears as a median sac in the posterior nasopharyngeal wall just above the upper fibres of the superior constrictor (Figure 13.3). It may extend upwards to the tubercle of the occiput. Inflammation of the pharyngeal bursa is known as Thornwaldt's bursitis.

Tumours of the nasopharynx

Many types of tumour, including rare, primitive ones, have been described in the nasopharynx (Table 13.1). Tumours arising here often have a long latent period with few primary symptoms. This has often led to delayed diagnosis and treatment. Only a few nasopharyngeal tumours, e.g. hairy polyps, have a characteristic macroscopic appearance. Preliminary biopsy is often required for diagnosis before starting treatment. The histological diagnosis of some tumours can be difficult without various specific immunohistochemical staining. Of all the tumours, carcinoma is the most common. It is unique in its epidemiology and racial predisposition, with distinctive immunogenetics influencing prognosis and survival.

Nasopharyngeal cancer

Besides the 'lymphoepithelium', the nasopharyngeal wall also contains glandular and connective tissue surrounded by the bone and cartilage of the skull base. A wide variety of malignant tumours may originate in the nasopharynx from the many types of tissue elements present (Table 13.2).

The relative proportion of cancer types in the nasopharynx varies in different countries. Nasopharyngeal carcinoma is the most common form irrespective of geography and race. It constitutes 75–95% of nasopharyngeal cancers in low-risk populations and virtually all nasopharyngeal cancers in high-risk populations. In south-east Asia nasopharyngeal carcinoma predominates over other types of cancer, so much so that the ratio is approximately 99:1.

Epidemiology of nasopharyngeal carcinoma

Geography and race

Nasopharyngeal carcinoma has a distinctive epidemiological pattern. Its incidence among the Chinese and

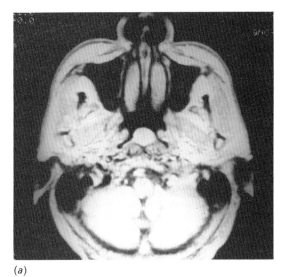
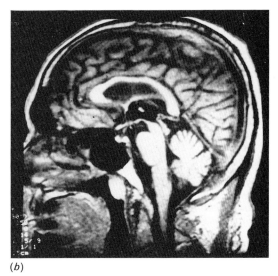

(*a*)   (*b*)

Figure 13.3 Thornwaldt's cyst in the nasopharynx of an adult – magnetic resonance T2 image in (*a*) axial and (*b*) frontal section showing the distinct anatomical outlines of the cyst

Table 13.1 WHO classification of tumours of the nasopharynx (Shanmugaratnam and Sobin, 1991)

I Epithelial tumours
a Benign
  1 Papilloma
  2 Pleomorphic adenoma
  3 Oncocytoma
  4 Basal cell adenoma
  5 Ectopic pituitary adenoma
b Malignant
  1 Nasopharyngeal carcinoma
  2 Adenocarcinoma
  3 Papillary adenocarcinoma
  4 Mucoepidermoid carcinoma
  5 Adenoid cystic carcinoma
  6 Polymorphous low-grade adenocarcinoma

II Soft tissue tumours
a Benign
  1 Angiofibroma
  2 Haemangioma
  3 Haemangiopericytoma
  4 Neurilemmoma
  5 Neurofibroma
  6 Paraganglioma
b Malignant
  1 Fibrosarcoma
  2 Rhabdomyosarcoma
  3 Angiosarcoma
  4 Kaposi's sarcoma
  5 Malignant haemangiopericytoma
  6 Malignant nerve sheath tumour
  7 Synovial sarcoma

III Tumours of bone and cartilage

IV Malignant lymphomas
  1 Non-Hodgkin's lymphoma
  2 Extramedullary plasmacytoma
  3 Midline malignant reticulosis
  4 Histocytic lymphoma
  5 Hodgkin's disease

V Miscellaneous tumours
a Benign
  1 Meningioma
  2 Craniopharyngioma
  3 Mature teratoma
b Malignant
  1 Malignant melanoma
  2 Chordoma
  3 Malignant germ cell tumours

VI Secondary tumours

VII Unclassified tumours

VIII Tumour-like lesions
  1 Cyst
  2 Heterotopic pituitary tissue
  3 Meningocoele/meningoencephalocoele
  4 Fibroinflammatory pseudotumour
  5 Infective granuloma
  6 Wegener's granulomatosis
  7 Pseudoepitheliomatous hyperplasia
  8 Oncocytic metaplasia and hyperplasia
  9 Granuloma pyogenicum
10 Lymphoid hyperplasia
11 Malakoplakia
12 Amyloid deposits

Table 13.2 Types of malignant nasopharyngeal tumours

1 *Epithelial*
   Nasopharyngeal carcinoma, adenocarcinoma, adenoid cystic carcinoma, mucoepidermoid carcinoma, others
2 *Lymphoid and haematopoietic*
   Malignant lymphomas, Hodgkin's disease, Burkitt's lymphoma, plasmacytomas, midline malignant recticulosis
3 *Bone and cartilage*
   Chondrosarcoma, osteosarcoma
4 *Soft tissue*
   Fibrosarcoma, rhabdomyosarcoma, angiosarcoma, Kaposi's sarcoma, malignant haemangiopericytoma, malignant nerve sheath tumours, others
5 *Miscellaneous*
   Malignant melanoma, chordoma, craniopharyngioma, neuro endrocrine tumour, others

Table 13.3 International comparison 1983–87. Annual age-standardized rate per 100 000 persons for nasopharyngeal cancer in different populations of the world (Parkin *et al.*, 1992)

Country	Population	Male	Female
Hong Kong	Chinese	28.5	11.2
Singapore	Chinese	18.1	7.4
USA (Hawaii)	Chinese	8.9	3.7
China (Shanghai)	Chinese	4.0	1.9
Singapore	Malay	4.3	0.4
USA (Hawaii)	Hawaiian	1.3	1.1
USA Connecticut	White	0.5	0.2
	Black	1.0	0.1
Singapore	Indian	1.0	0.2
USA (Bay Area)	Black	0.8	0.4
	White	0.7	0.2
India (Madras)		0.7	0.4
Australia (New South Wales)		0.8	0.2
Denmark		0.7	0.3
Japan (Osaka)		0.6	0.2
UK (Birmingham)		0.5	0.1
New Zealand	Maori	1.2	0.0
	Non-Maori	0.5	0.3
Columbia, Cali (South America)		0.5	0.1

other south-east Asians is about 10 to 50 times higher than that of other countries. This cancer is not strictly associated with the Mongoloid race *per se*, as the northern Chinese, Koreans and Japanese all have a low incidence.

The highest incidence (age-standardized rate (ASR) of 30–50/100 000 males) is observed in southern China in the central Guangdong province and Guangxi Autonomous Region. The high incidence ASR of 15–30/100 000 males) occurs in Hong Kong, south-east Asian Chinese and emigrant Chinese elsewhere. A moderately elevated incidence (ASR 5–15 / 100 000 males) is found among other south-east Asian races (Malays, Indonesians, Kadazans, Thais, Vietnamese and Filipinos), Eskimos (in Canada, Alaska and Greenland) and some north Africans. Populations in Malta, Tunisia, Algeria, Morocco and the Sudan have a much lower incidence than the Asian countries but are still appreciably higher than those in America and Europe. A low incidence (ASR 1 or less per 100 000 males) is present in the rest of the world (Table 13.3).

Geographical and migrant variations in Chinese nasopharyngeal carcinoma

Descriptions of neck tumours with eventual death were documented in the ancient Chinese medical literature. These descriptions were most probably those of nasopharyngeal carcinoma. In 1930 Digby, Thomas and Hsiu published in the Hong Kong *Caduceus* the comprehensive features of nasopharyngeal carcinoma with its classical massive cervical lymphadenopathy. Remarkable geographical variations in incidence are observed. It is highest in the south and declines towards the north. When and where the southern Chinese emigrate, they retain their high risk of nasopharyngeal carcinoma. Their incidence is

appreciably higher than that of the indigenous population. The incidence of nasopharyngeal carcinoma among Chinese born in the USA is about 20 times higher than that of the Caucasians, but is significantly lower – about one-half – that of Chinese born in China.

Racial differences

There is a variation of incidence of nasopharyngeal carcinoma among different ethnic groups in countries with multiracial populations, e.g. Hawaii and Singapore. In Singapore, the incidence of nasopharyngeal carcinoma is highest among the Chinese, intermediate among the Malays and lowest among the Indians. The Indians, basically a low-risk group, have not shown any increase in the incidence of nasopharyngeal cancer despite residing in a country with high incidence. This contrasts with the Eskimos in Alaska, Canada and Greenland who live in low-risk countries but have a high incidence, approximately 15–20 times that of the general population. The Greenlandic Inuit Eskimo migrants to Denmark too maintain the high risk of nasopharyngeal carcinoma (Prener *et al.*, 1987).

Even among the southern Chinese, there is a marked variation in the incidence of nasopharyngeal cancer among the dialects or specific community groups. The rate of nasopharyngeal carcinoma among the Cantonese is higher than that of other Southern Chinese dialect groups.

Sex

Nasopharyngeal carcinoma is more common in males with the age-standardized male: female ratio between 2–3:1.

Age

The plateau age distribution curve

The age-incidence rate curve of nasopharyngeal carcinoma is different from the other forms of cancer. In the Chinese it begins to rise from 15 to 19 years of life, remains the most frequent cancer in males aged 15–34 years, reaches a plateau between 35–64 years and declines thereafter (Figure 13.4). This contrasts sharply with other leading epithelial carcinomas of the aerodigestive tract and the bowel with the exception of carcinoma of the cervix. The shape of the age distribution curve suggests that events early in life are important. Exposure to external carcinogens, if involved must occur early in life to interact with susceptible genes. The absence of a progressive increase in older age suggests either the exposure is not continuous or there is reduced susceptibility with age. Alternatively the curve is consistent with a genetic hypothesis with the plateau and later decline attributed to exhaustion of the genetically susceptible members of the population.

Bimodal age distribution

In the Chinese, nasopharyngeal carcinoma is rare below the age of 15 years. However, in mid-incidence and certain low risk populations, the age incidence curve shows two separate peaks, the first peak at a postadolescent age between 10 and 20 years and a second later in life at 55–65 years. This is seen in the Maghreb Arab population in North Africa and in Tunisia where 15% of patients with nasopharyngeal carcinoma are below the age of 16 years (Ellouz *et al.*, 1978). There is also a high proportion of nasopharyngeal carcinoma in patients below the age of 20 years in other low risk countries such as India (Madras and Bombay), Uganda, Sudan, among whites and blacks in the USA and in the Kadazans (high-risk group) in East Malaysia. This bimodal distribution suggests the influence of different aetiological factors or variations in the host response.

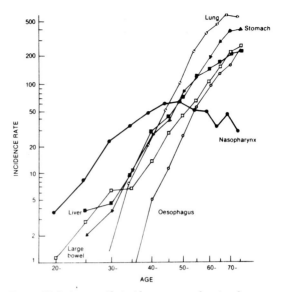

Figure 13.4 Age-specific incidence curves showing the plateau in nasopharyngeal carcinoma in comparison with the steep rise in the older age groups with lung, oesophageal, liver, stomach and large bowel cancers in Singapore Chinese males

Genetic factors

The hereditary factors related to nasopharyngeal carcinoma are discussed below.

Environmental factors

The aetiology of nasopharyngeal carcinoma remains obscure. A susceptible genetic constitution clearly plays a part and some environmental cofactors are equally important. The significance of environmental factors is supported by the following observations:

1 Epidemiological data on geographical clustering in Southern China and Chinese emigrant populations
2 The age-incidence rate curve in the high-risk population
3 Time trend: the high risks for the disease among the Chinese in Southern China, Hong Kong and Singapore have virtually remained unchanged for the past 50 years. The incidence of the disease in the second and third generation USA-born Chinese has declined when compared with that of their forefathers and relations in the East. The difference can be partly attributed to the change in the environment and life-style of the USA-born Chinese. On the other hand, the environmental

change is not profound in south-east Asia. The Chinese have retained their 'micro-environment' preserving the oriental life-style especially with regard to food and customs. It is therefore likely that any associated environmental risk factor is closely linked to the traditional rather than the modern life style of the southern Chinese. Besides the Epstein-Barr virus, a variety of inhaled and ingested agents has been proposed (Table 13.4). Some of these propositions are supported by findings from controlled studies and laboratory evidence; but most are inconclusive.

Table 13.4 Various environmental agents/factors implicated in the aetiology of nasopharyngeal carcinoma

Agents/factors	
Epstein-Barr virus	Raised antibody
	Viral genome in tumour cells
Chemical	
tobacco	Cigarette smoking
drugs	Chinese herbal medicine
plant products	EBV activating properties/ cofactors
diet	Salted fish
	Preserved vegetables, fermented food stuff
	Nitrosamines and nitro-precursors
	Tunisian preserved spice meat (*quaddid*) and stewing base (*touklia*)
Cooking habits	Household smoke and fumes
Religious practices	Incense and joss stick smoke
Occupation	Industrial fumes and chemicals
	Metal smelting
	Furnaces
	Formaldehyde
	Wood dust
Others	Socioeconomic status
	Previous otolaryngological ailments
	Weaning habits
	Nutritional deficiencies
	Metals (arsenic, chromium, nickel)

Household smoke and cigarette smoking

Exposure to smoke from cooking fires or burning incense had been suggested as a risk factor long ago following observations on indoor cooking in homes without chimneys in southern China. There appears to be no relationship between nasopharyngeal carcinoma and household smoke. The boat people of southern China who cook in the open air have a higher incidence of nasopharyngeal carcinoma. The women who are more exposed to smoke from fire-

wood used in cooking have a lower risk than men. Active and passive tobacco smoking have not been conclusively proven as risk factors in high-risk populations. The geographical distribution of nasopharyngeal carcinoma bears no relationship to the pattern of cigarette consumption or the incidence of lung cancer.

Occupation

Exposure to nickel, chromium and radioactive metals has been associated with cancer of the nose and paranasal sinuses but not with nasopharyngeal carcinoma. Inhalation of chemical fumes in certain occupations may explain the occurrence of nasopharyngeal carcinoma in industrialized countries with low incidence. A nationwide study in Sweden identified glassmakers, shoemakers, bookmakers and fireboard plant workers to be at a significantly increased risk of nasopharyngeal carcinoma (Malker *et al.*, 1990). An increased risk of nasopharyngeal cancer is noted among wood workers, loggers and foresters in New Zealand (Kawachi, Pearce and Fraser, 1989). A south China case-control study identified the high risk of nasopharyngeal carcinoma with occupations involving exposure to combustion products from welding, coal/coke and liquid fuels (Yu *et al.*, 1990) while the metal workers of Shanghai in low-risk northern China have a significantly elevated risk of nasopharyngeal carcinoma (Zheng *et al.*, 1992).

Ingestants and chemicals

Salted fish has been proposed as an important aetiological factor in the southern Chinese population. Ungutted salted marine fish contain an appreciable amount of volatile nitrosamines, principally N-nitrosodimethylamine and N-nitrosodiethylamine. They are known to induce squamous cell carcinoma and adenocarcinoma in the nasal and paranasal cavities in experimental animals. A series of controlled studies relating the incidence of nasopharyngeal carcinoma to that of diet in Hong Kong and China indicate a strong association especially with the consumption of salted fish in early childhood (Yu, 1991). Besides salted fish, high volatile nitrosamine levels are also found in many other food stuffs in Tunisia, China and Greenland; some of these preserved food substances have been shown to contain high levels of nitrosable precursors that yield volatile nitrosamine in the human stomach after ingestion (Poirier *et al.*, 1989). However, it is interesting to note that high levels of nitrosamine are consumed in Japan in dried fish and preserved vegetables and yet the Japanese incidence of nasopharyngeal carcinoma is very low. Furthermore, the bulk of human nitrosamine comes from endogenous sources in the gut. It does not also satisfactorily explain the male predominance of nasopharyngeal carcinoma.

Chemicals in Croton plants which have a geographical distribution parallel to that of the incidence of nasopharyngeal carcinoma in China, and many other traditional medicinal plants possess strong Epstein-Barr-virus-activating properties. To prove their role as cofactors in the aetiology of nasopharyngeal carcinoma would need further prospective studies. There is evidence suggesting a relationship between chemicals and activation of the Epstein-Barr virus. A remarkably high detection rate of nasopharyngeal carcinoma was reported in a chemical factory during an Epstein-Barr viral serological survey in Wuzhou City of Zangwu County, a region of high incidence in China (Zeng *et al.*, 1985).

Epstein-Barr virus

The relationship between nasopharyngeal cancer and the Epstein-Barr virus is discussed below.

Histopathology

Nasopharyngeal carcinoma arises from the crypts and squamous or respiratory epithelium lining the nasopharynx. It may be preceded by squamous metaplasia. There has been considerable disagreement over the histological classification of nasopharyngeal carcinoma and many classifications have been proposed. Terminology like lymphoepithelioma, undifferentiated carcinoma, non-keratinizing carcinoma, and anaplastic carcinoma have been used to describe the poorly differentiated carcinoma that commonly occurs in the nasopharynx. The term 'lymphoepithelioma' is used to described non-keratinizing and undifferentiated nasopharyngeal carcinoma with a heavy infiltration by lymphocytes among the tumour cells. The lymphoid elements are reactive and not neoplastic. Carcinomas of identical histological appearance have been reported in the salivary gland notably the so-called 'Eskimomas' prevalent in the Eskimos of Alaska, Canada and Greenland. According to the WHO Classification adopted since 1978 (Shanmugaratnam and Sobin, 1991) three histological types of nasopharyngeal carcinoma are recognized on the basis of their light microscopic appearances:

1 Squamous cell carcinoma
   a well differentiated
   b moderately differentiated
   c poorly differentiated
2 Non-keratinizing carcinoma
3 Undifferentiated carcinoma.

Squamous differentiation

All histological subtypes of nasopharyngeal carcinoma consistently show ultrastructural and cytokeratin immunohistochemical evidence of squamous differentiation. These include the non-keratinizing and undifferentiated carcinomas with no evidence of squamous differentiation on light microscopy. Therefore they may be considered variants of squamous carcinoma. The most common subtype seen in high-risk countries is the undifferentiated type and, with its variant including the non-keratinizing carcinoma, constitutes over 90% of all cases. In low-risk countries squamous cell carcinoma predominates in nasopharyngeal cancer and is 10–30 times more common. Generally keratinizing squamous cell carcinoma is relatively radioresistant but less aggressive in behaviour. The undifferentiated nasopharyngeal carcinoma is more radiosensitive but aggressive, frequently with advanced locoregional spread.

Immunological historeactions in nasopharyngeal carcinoma

Nasopharyngeal carcinoma is an unusual epithelial carcinoma where tumour cells have an intimate relationship with lymphocytes. Analysis of the immune cells infiltrating the tumour show that the predominant lymphocyte is the T cell and most of these are CD8 positive (Hsu and Lin, 1986; Chong *et al.*, 1988). These could be T cytotoxic or T suppressors. The presence of activated T cells and natural killer cells and antigens on tumour cells indicates immune reactions at the tumour site; what precisely these cells are reacting to is unknown.

Natural history of nasopharyngeal carcinoma

Inception ⟶	Silent period ⟶	Local invasion ⟶	Primary lymph node station ⟶	
Genetic		Blood-stained mucus	Retropharyngeal	Systemic spread
Environmental		Eustachian tube blockage	Locoregional spread ⟶	
Viral			Paranasopharyngeal/parapharyngeal	
			Skull-base erosion	

The timescale over which inception takes place and that of the silent period in nasopharyngeal carcinoma is unknown. The only available marker is the Epstein-Barr viral IgA serological marker which has been shown to be elevated months or perhaps years prior to the clinical onset of cancer.

Premalignant conditions

Nasopharyngeal carcinoma is an epithelial cancer. Even in its well differentiated form, no definitive premalignant condition can be identified macroscopically or has been shown conclusively on light-microscopy on routine biopsy specimens. Supravital staining and cytological screening has not achieved significant diagnostic accuracy. While most of the nasopharyngeal tumour cells on an exfoliation smear show positive Epstein-Barr viral nuclear antigen in contrast to other head and neck cancers, the presence of positive Epstein-Barr nuclear antigen is not diagnostic of nasopharyngeal carcinoma because normal cells may also contain the nuclear antigen.

Anatomical sites of tumour origin

Most nasopharyngeal carcinomas originate from the lateral and/or superolateral wall of the nasopharynx around the fossa of Rosenmüller (see Plate 5/13/I(a) and I(b)). This is the most complex of all walls because of its close association with the contents of the parapharyngeal space and the lymphatics. The tumour can be multicentric involving more than one site.

Early diagnosis

Over the last two decades improved methods of examination and health education have changed little in the initial clinical presentation of nasopharyngeal carcinoma. Stage I tumours still account for less than 10% of all cases. The first nodal station is the retropharyngeal node which is not clinically palpable but may be shown on cross-sectional imaging. Early diagnosis hence must precede the cervical lymphadenopathy which remains the most common presentation. Besides the fact that the tumour bed is a lymphoepithelium rich in lymphatics allowing early locoregional spread to one or both sides of the neck, there are other reasons for this aggressive tumour behaviour making early diagnosis a difficult task.

Anatomical seclusion

The nasopharynx is a clinical blind spot in the middle of the skull base. It is a difficult area to see or feel, and being situated in a relatively big and inert space where only air and mucus are in transit, nasopharyngeal carcinoma can remain silent for a long time causing few primary symptoms. The earliest primary symptom is probably occasional blood-stained mucus or eustachian tube blockage. These symptoms are not different from those of occasional colds and rhinosinusitis. It is understandable why they are conveniently disregarded. This often leads to delayed diagnosis and treatment for months.

Host–tumour response

The host reaction to nasopharyngeal carcinoma is variable and unpredictable. The nasopharyngeal primary can be inconspicuously tiny yet gives rise to marked 'downward' locoregional lymphatic spread invariably with elevated Epstein-Barr viral IgA serology. On the other hand, the primary tumour can be invasive and advance with 'upward' spread eroding the skull base with no downward spread and yet preserves an equally deceptively normal nasopharynx with normal Epstein-Barr viral serology.

It is important to keep in mind that in all painless head and neck lumps, malignancy must be suspected and a primary tumour in the nasopharynx can evade exhaustive investigations, including computerized tomographic study and biopsy. If a nasopharyngeal carcinoma is suspected continued searching is worthwhile, because very often the elusive answer may lie beneath the apparently normal mucosa. Nasopharyngeal carcinoma has remained one of the most consistently misdiagnosed diseases and is known to be a great imposter.

Clinical presentations of nasopharyngeal carcinoma

Nasopharyngeal carcinoma may appear ulcerative and be infiltrative or can be a more exuberant polypoidal type of tumour. Inflammation of the lymphoepithelium mimics tumour appearance. Very early preclinical and infiltrative carcinoma retains a relatively normal mucosal appearance. The diagnosis is based on histopathology.

Symptomatology

The marked invasive and metastatic potential of nasopharyngeal carcinoma is responsible for the symptomatology. From the primary site the tumour may spread in one or more of the following directions:

1 Anteriorly to the nasal cavity and paranasal sinuses, pterygopalatine fossa and apex of the orbit
2 Posteriorly to the retropharyngeal space and node of Rouviere, destroying the lateral mass of the atlas
3 Laterally into the parapharyngeal space (Figure 13.5)
   a prestyloid compartment: with involvement of the mandibular nerve, pterygoid muscles and infiltration of the deep lobe of the parotid
   b poststyloid compartment: vascular compression of the carotid sheath and vessels, and invasion of the last four cranial nerves and cervical sympathetic nerves

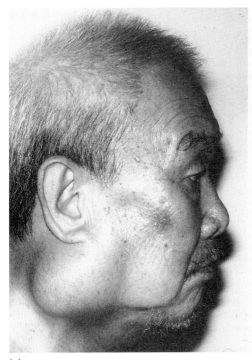

(a)

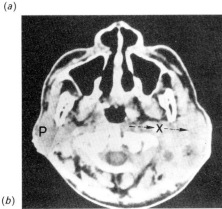

(b)

Figure 13.5 (a) Metastatic parotid lymph node mimicking primary parotid tumour in a patient with nasopharyngeal carcinoma – an uncommon occurrence but nevertheless an entity to be reckoned with. (b) Axial CT scan showing overt parotid metastasis produced by a small nasopharyngeal carcinoma breaching the buccopharyngeal fascia and parapharyngeal space infiltrating into the deep lobe of the parotid. P: Superficial lobe of parotid gland; X: deep lobe of parotid in parapharyngeal space

4 Superiorly through the sphenoid body and sinus involving the parasellar structures and optic nerve, petrous apex and foramen lacerum; along the carotid canal into the cavernous sinus involving nerves III, IV, V, and VI. The brain is affected by direct tumour extension and not haematogenous spread

5 Inferiorly to the oral cavity and retrotonsillar regions.

Clinical features

Patients with nasopharyngeal carcinoma are rarely totally asymptomatic with the exception of patients detected by screening. Most patients have multiple symptoms which are insidious in onset and are sometimes disregarded by the patients for months. The main symptoms and signs are painless cervical lymphadenopathy (60%), epistaxis and nasorespiratory symptoms (40%), audiological symptoms (tinnitus, otalgia, deafness) (30%), neurological symptoms (headache, cranial nerve palsies and Horner's syndrome) (20%), and metastases which can be locoregional (paranasal sinus, parapharyngeal space, infratemporal fossa, orbit, parotid and cervical lymphadenopathy) or distant (bone, lung and liver).

Cervical lymphadenopathy

Nasopharyngeal carcinoma has a tendency for early lymphatic spread. The lateral retropharyngeal lymph node (of Rouviere) is the first lymphatic filter but is not palpable. The common first palpable node is the jugulodigastric and/or the apical node under the sternomastoid which are second echelon nodes (Figure 13.6). Bilateral and contralateral lymph node metastases are not uncommon (Figure 13.7).

Epistaxis and nasorespiratory symptoms

Epistaxis of severe degree as a first presenting symptom is unusual; it is more commonly seen in advanced nasopharyngeal carcinoma with or without skull-base erosion. Blood-stained nasal mucus and

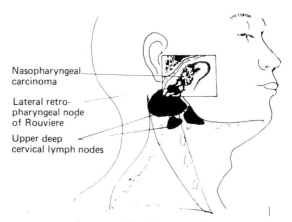

Nasopharyngeal carcinoma

Lateral retropharyngeal node of Rouviere

Upper deep cervical lymph nodes

Figure 13.6 The routes of lymphatic spread in nasopharyngeal carcinoma

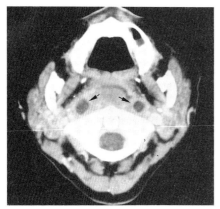

Figure 13.7 Axial CT scan at the level of the atlas showing bilateral lateral retropharyngeal nodes with low density necrotic centre and the ring-like peripheral enhancement characteristic of metastatic nodes in undifferentiated nasopharyngeal carcinoma (arrows)

saliva on clearing the throat are frequently seen. Erosion into the maxillary antrum mimics sinusitis. The blood-stained rhinorrhoea from nasopharyngeal carcinoma may masquerade as a primary maxillary cancer. Complete nasal obstruction is a late presentation; should it occur in the early stage of the disease, it is often due to superimposed infection. Ozaena occurs as a result of tumour necrosis and is typical of advanced nasopharyngeal carcinoma.

Tinnitus and aural symptoms

Otitis media with effusion causing tinnitus is not an uncommon presentation of nasopharyngeal carcinoma. It is often insidious in onset and the primary tumour can be insignificant in the peritubal region. *Adult Chinese patients with unresolving otitis media with effusion have to be presumed to have nasopharyngeal carcinoma until proven otherwise.*

Neurological palsies

All the cranial nerves, either singly or in groups can be affected by nasopharyngeal carcinoma through tumour invasion or compression. The most frequently involved cranial nerves are V, VI, IX and X accounting for 50% of all palsies (Khor *et al.*, 1975). Nerves IX and X are invariably involved together and are the most common group to be affected. The nerves to the ocular muscles (III, IV and VI) are the next group commonly affected within the cavernous sinus (Figure 13.8). Isolated single cranial nerve palsy is common with nerves V and VI.

Pain and headache

Pain is an ominous symptom in nasopharyngeal carcinoma. Severe and excruciating pain and headache is the hallmark of terminal disease. It signifies tumour erosion into the skull base and surrounding structures. Sepsis, particularly in sphenoidal sinusitis also

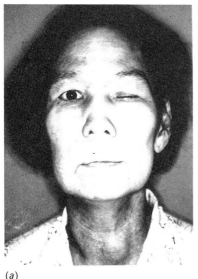

(*a*)

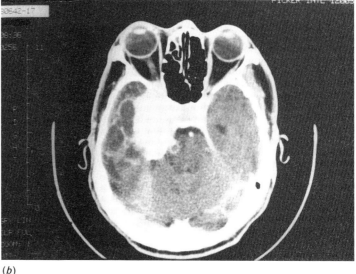

(*b*)

Figure 13.8 (*a*) Picture and (*b*) CT scan of a Chinese female patient with dermatomyositis, a condition known to associate strongly with nasopharyngeal carcinoma presenting with total ophthalmoplegia and blindness due to parasellar invasion of cranial nerves II, III, IV, V, VI by the tumour

produces severe headache. If accompanied by trismus, the disease is at an advanced stage and has involved the pterygopalatine fossa and the pterygoid muscles. Atypical facial pain or inexplicable headache may be a presenting symptom of nasopharyngeal carcinoma. Nasopharyngeal endoscopic assessment may not detect the true extent of the tumour and cross-sectional imaging of the nasopharynx and base of skull is most helpful in delineating outlying tumour extension and skull-base erosion.

Cross-sectional imaging

Computerized tomographic scanning is sensitive for detecting bone changes and hence useful for tumour staging. Nodes affected by undifferentiated carcinoma frequently have marked ring-like peripheral enhancement with contrast due to their peripheral vascularity and/or central tumour necrosis. Magnetic resonance owing to its multiplanar imaging capability is a more sensitive modality than CT scanning for detecting small tumours and soft tissue extension or invasion through the fascia (Figures 13.9 and 13.10). Gadolinium DTPA enhancement helps to delineate the lesion

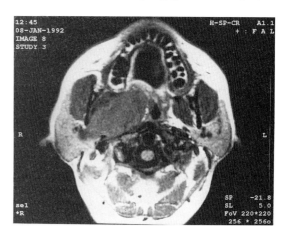

Figure 13.10 A magnetic resonance T1 image showing a right nasopharyngeal carcinoma breaching the buccopharyngeal fascia into the parapharyngeal space; invading the deep lobe of the parotid and presenting as a parapharyngeal space swelling

and the extension into the cranial cavity. It is best for evaluating central nervous system involvement and postradiation changes. Currently its role is complementary to the CT scan.

Distant metastases

Distant metastases are not uncommon in nasopharyngeal cancer and skeletal metastases account for more than half. The thoracolumbar spine is the most common site of involvement followed by the lung and liver. Distant metastases indicate a grave prognosis with a median survival of 3 months, and 90% of patients die within a year of diagnosing the first metastasis. In a study of 352 consecutive patients with nasopharyngeal carcinoma treated with radiotherapy (Khor *et al.*, 1978), 60% who manifested distant metastases had no evidence of recurrent disease in the nasopharynx or cervical nodes. This implies a significant proportion of patients probably have occult metastases at the time of initial diagnosis.

Second malignancies

The risk of developing a synchronous second primary or a metachronous malignancy in the upper aerodigestive tract is about 4%, in comparison to a 12% risk estimated for patients with other head and neck epithelial cancers (Cooper *et al.*, 1991).

Nasopharyngeal examination

Examination of the nasopharynx can be difficult. Although anatomically the width of the nasopharynx

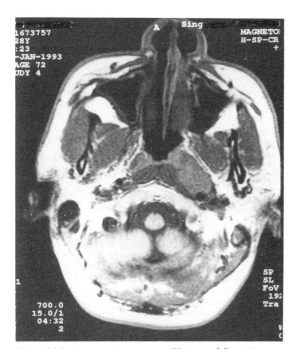

Figure 13.9 A magnetic resonance T1 image delineating a left nasopharyngeal carcinoma with marked submucosal infiltration encroaching onto the vessels in the retropharyngeal space. The tumour extends through the parapharyngeal space fascia with a fairly distinct margin of advancement. The nasopharyngeal appearance is deceptively small representing the tip of the 'tumour iceberg' which is well demonstrated here and in Figure 13.10

is 4 cm, the 'functional channel' is only about 2 cm. Posterior rhinoscopy is also restricted by the pharyngeal reflex, patient cooperation and inability to open the mouth. Furthermore, the mirror may only give an 'edge-on' view of the fossa of Rosenmüller due to the fossa's posterolateral inclination. Nevertheless, mirror examination is still the quickest way to assess the nasopharynx. It is sometimes performed under anaesthesia. In this procedure, the patient is placed in the tonsillectomy position with a Boyle-Davies gag. Two polythene tubes or catheters inserted naso-orally, retract the soft palate forward. Transoral mirror examination is then performed with a mirror that has been warmed and dipped in solution to prevent misting. Although a transoral 90° nasopharyngoscope will provide a panoramic view under magnification, it has not eliminated the limiting factors of posterior rhinoscopy.

The advent of rigid and flexible endoscopes has allowed a close-up view of the nasopharynx and its recesses. With the choice of rigid sinus endoscopes of 0°, 30° and 70° angle view and the flexible nasopharyngoscope of various diameters with or without a biopsy channel, tiny growths, especially in the tubal recess which escape detection with routine rhinoscopic mirror examination, can be identified.

Nasopharyngeal biopsy

Endoscopic transnasal biopsy is the standard procedure. The slim Hildyard postnasal biopsy forceps for routine nasopharyngeal biopsy are preferred and specimens from its 3 mm diameter cup are more than adequate for tissue histopathology. For deep biopsy and biopsy of the fossa recess, the 45° angled Henckle forceps (see Plate 5/13/I) with sharp small cups is ideal for angulating upwards and laterally to biopsy the posterolateral nasopharyngeal wall. Clinically positive nasopharyngeal carcinomas are often diagnosed at the first biopsy. About 5% of patients have a deceptively normal endoscopic appearance of the nasopharynx with submucosal disease. The cardinal rule is that a normal looking nasopharynx does not exclude microscopic disease. Experience has demonstrated that a high clinical suspicion mandates endoscopic biopsy, repeated if necessary, regardless of the fact that the nasopharynx may look normal.

Flexible fibreoptic nasopharyngoscope

This is the most useful and versatile endoscope for nasopharyngeal and upper aerodigestive system examination. Before the procedure, the nose is first anaesthetized with 5% cocaine spray (or 4% lignocaine if the patient is allergic to cocaine). Two orange sticks (one for each nostril) with cotton pledgets soaked with 5% cocaine are inserted along the floor to the nasopharynx. With this method, anaesthesia of the nasopharynx is often achieved. However, one must watch out for a common pitfall, that is the failure to hold the pledget sticks in the nasopharynx. This is due to the soft palate which propels the pledget sticks away from the nasopharyngeal wall. This reflex action usually stops once the nasopharynx is anaesthetized. An induction time of 10 minutes is allowed before the endoscopic procedure. The flexible scope is then inserted transnasally. It gives a good view of the nasal floor, the walls of the nasopharynx and the fossa of Rosenmüller.

Flexible endoscopic biopsy

The flexible nasopharyngoscope is first introduced through the nose contralateral to the side of the suspected nasopharyngeal tumour. Its tip is directed towards the tumour. As the nasopharyngoscope is rather short it can be steadied with one hand once it is in the nasopharynx. The Hildyard or 45° angled Henckel forceps is then inserted along the nasal floor on the side of the tumour into the nasopharynx. In fact, it is small enough to be introduced through the same nostril as the endoscope in most cases. The position of the biopsy forceps can be checked by the scope.

The advantage of this method is that tiny tumours in any quadrant including the difficult fossa of Rosenmüller can be seen and accurately biopsied. It is also a reliable method to detect and biopsy postradiation tumour recurrence beneath the necrotic scab that may persist long after radiotherapy.

Rigid 0° and 30° sinus endoscopes can similarly be used in the clinical setting. Generally their manipulation in the nose causes more discomfort to the patient. They are however the scopes of choice in examination and biopsy under anaesthesia should this be necessary.

Stage-classification of nasopharyngeal carcinoma

Few staging systems of head and neck cancers have generated more disagreement than that of nasopharyngeal carcinoma. To date there are no fewer than 12 different classifications.

1952 Geist and Portman
1962 UICC (Modified 1974, 1978 and 1987)
1965 Chinese Classification (Shanghai)
1970 J.H.C. Ho (Hong Kong, modified 1978)
1971 Chen and Fletcher (M.D. Anderson Hospital, Houston)
1975 German work group of clinical oncology (Cologne)
1976 American Joint Committee (modified 1978 and 1988)
1977 Kyoto symposium (Japan)
1979 Changsha conference (China)

1981 Guangzhou stage-classification
1985 Huang's stage-classification
1990s Modified Ho's (Hong Kong, Singapore)

None has gained general acceptance. Nasopharyngeal carcinoma is classically treated by radiotherapy but certain subsets of patients require neoadjuvant or adjuvant chemotherapy. The relatively simple UICC and AJC staging systems widely used in Europe and America have stages similar to other head and neck cancers. They are generally considered inadequate by centres treating nasopharyngeal carcinoma in the high-risk population. The Changsa and Guangzhou stagings are often used to report results in the People's Republic of China (Zhang *et al.*, 1989) while Huang's classification (Huang, 1980) is used in Taiwan. Ho's stage classification is adopted in Hong Kong and Singapore. A synopsis of the stage classifications currently in use is given in Appendix 13.1.

While the Ho's stage classification is reported to correlate well with the prognosis in high-risk population patient cohorts, it has drawbacks. It is unconventional with five stage-groupings instead of the usual four and neck crease for N staging ignoring the nodal size and impact of bilaterality of nodes. Tumour volume relates to radioresistance and hence has to be taken into treatment consideration.

Paradoxical T and N stage relationship

Nasopharyngeal carcinoma in the high-risk population has very different biological tumour behaviour from its well-differentiated counterpart predominant in low-risk populations, and other squamous cell cancers of the head and neck. It exhibits a paradoxical relationship between the local T and regional N disease; the most advanced T stage is often associated with N0 stage whereas the early T stage is more often associated with nodal disease.

Cross-sectional imaging and its impact on stage-classification

Sobin and Ros (1990) highlighted the future impact of radioimaging on the revised 1987 TNM classification. All staging systems for nasopharyngeal cancer currently in use were devised prior to cross-sectional radioimaging. CT and magnetic resonance scanning have revolutionized the mapping of nasopharyngeal tumours delineating paranasopharyngeal, parapharyngeal tumour extension/nodal spread and skull-base erosion with such accuracy hitherto not possible by conventional radiology. This has resulted in upstaging of the T and N disease stage in many cases. The incorporation of skull base cross-sectional imaging information into the retrospective analysis of treatment results necessitates modification of the current staging systems. Dedicated staging systems based

upon the modifications of Ho's system have been proposed in Hong Kong and Singapore (Teo *et al.*, 1991; Tsao, 1993).

Treatment

Radiotherapy

Radiotherapy is the definitive treatment for nasopharyngeal carcinoma and its regional node metastases. Tumour mapping with cross-sectional imaging has added a new dimension in therapeutic radiation oncology. It enables precise pretreatment planning and modulation of techniques. Parapharyngeal space encroachment by tumour is a conspicuous cause of local treatment failure requiring booster doses and extension of radiation target volumes. The use of facial shells is standard practice ensuring precise reproducibility of the treatment dose geometry. Prophylactic neck irradiation is advocated in patients with N0 neck disease, failure to do this results in regional relapse in one-third of the patients (Lee *et al.*, 1989).

Brachytherapy

Brachytherapy has a rapid fall off of radiation at short distances from the source thus enabling the delivery of a high tumour dose while sparing the neighbouring structures and the brain. Transnasal intracavity brachytherapy with afterloaded iridium-192 is used to treat localized residual or recurrent tumour in the nasopharynx or adjacent areas.

Complications of radiotherapy

The inevitable ablation of radiosensitive parotid glands results in alteration of quantity and quality of saliva affecting the pH of the oral cavity. Mucositis, xerostomia, dental caries and radiation otitis media with effusion are some of the long-term sequelae of the treatment. Pretreatment dental clearance and treatment of oral sepsis is mandatory and is a prophylactic measure against postradiation radionecrosis.

Lhermitte's sign of paraesthesia is an uncommon complication of radiation to the cervical spinal cord with lightning-like electrical sensation spreading into both arms, down the dorsal spine and into both legs on neck flexion. Radiation myelitis and encephalomyelitic damage, osteoradionecrosis of the skull base, brain stem damage, optic atrophy and retinitis are rare with one course of treatment. Temporal lobe necrosis usually associated with repeated radiation is a serious and potentially fatal complication. Hypopituitarism is attributed to hypothalamic–pituitary stalk damage if the radiation field is above the clinoid. In affected patients the progressive hypofunction can be demonstrated as early as 6 months to 1 year after irradiation.

Chemotherapy

In nasopharyngeal carcinoma, advanced nodal disease (> 6 cm), besides posing a treatment problem with radiation dosimetry, has a high locoregional relapse rate and risk of distant metastases. Adjunctive chemotherapy with various cytotoxic agents has been attempted to achieve control of advanced nodal disease. Neoadjuvant chemotherapy has been effective in reducing locoregional relapses (Teo *et al.*, 1987). However, the high rate of initial tumour response to chemotherapy has not been translated into improved survival or reduction of distant metastases. It is not yet known what is the most effective chemotherapeutic agent or regimen, the optimal timing with radiotherapy or the duration of cycles of chemotherapy in nasopharyngeal carcinoma.

Results

The results of treatment vary with the histological type and stage of disease, sex and the age of the patient. Well-differentiated nasopharyngeal carcinoma has poorer local control rates while advanced undifferentiated carcinoma has a higher distant metastasis rate (Sham and Choy, 1990; Ingersoll *et al.*, 1990; Lee *et al.*, 1992). Comparison of treatment results between different centres is made difficult by the lack of a generally accepted stage-classification. Generally 90% of the relapses and distant failures occur within the first 2–3 years; the main prognostic determinant is advanced nodal disease. The accepted overall 5-year survival rate is 40–50% with megavoltage radiation therapy. Women and patients below the age of 40 are reported to have better results. However, concurrent pregnancy or pregnancy within one year of treatment is associated with a very poor prognosis (Jie-hua, Caisen and Yuhua, 1984).

Surgery

Surgery plays a minor role in the treatment of nasopharyngeal carcinoma. It is limited to radical neck dissection in controlling radioresistant nodes and postradiation cervical metastases and, in selected patients, salvage surgery for recurrence in the nasopharynx.

Radical neck dissection

Neck dissection is indicated for persistent and recurrent cervical disease after a full course of radiation in the absence of primary disease proven by endoscopic biopsy. Postradiation tissue fibrosis and reaction frequently preclude an accurate assessment of the extent of the cervical nodal disease both clinically and radiologically. Fine needle aspiration cytology has not always been reliable because of tumour nests encapsulated in fibrosis. The anatomical extent and level of nodal involvement are often more extensive than expected with involvement of the apical posterior triangle and spinal accessory chain making it necessary to perform a classical radical neck dissection. Extracapsular spread and isolated clusters of tumour islands amidst the fibrosis are common features in the neck specimen histopathology. Limited neck skin involvement can also be resected en-bloc with the dissection and the tissue defect surfaced by a myocutaneous flap.

Nasopharyngectomy

There is a less definite and currently limited role of skull base resection for recurrent or residual carcinoma in the nasopharynx that has failed all treatment modalities. These are tumours often indolent but symptomatic with pain. CT and magnetic resonance imaging are essential to map the extent of disease. The internal carotid artery and the carotid canal are in such close proximity to the lateral nasopharynx where most tumours recur that this is often the key limiting factor in surgical resection. Surgical technique is impeded by the radiation fibrosis and lack of adequate surgical margins of healthy tissue. Proper extirpation of tumour requires drilling the bony margins and the clivus (Figure 13.11). It is at best a palliative procedure and limited to primary recurrent tumour with no bony skull base involvement (Tu *et al.*, 1988; Fee, Roberson and Goffinet, 1991). Postoperative trismus of varying degree is a definite problem in all patients.

Surgical approaches to the nasopharynx

Surgical access providing safe control of vessels and adequate exposure of the nasopharynx remains a challenge. Its anatomical position encased in the middle of the skull base flanked by vital structures superiorly and laterally restricts access. Dissection is very much intracavity surgery and tumour margins are often difficult to define and excise to achieve complete removal. The many surgical approaches attest to the difficulty of surgery of this region (Figure 13.12). Head and neck and maxillofacial surgeons employ anterior and inferolateral approaches while neuro-otological surgeons prefer a posterolateral approach. More than one surgical approach is often needed to provide adequate and optimal exposure.

The various extracranial approaches include:

1 Transnasal-maxillary
  a lateral rhinotomy
  b LeFort I osteotomy
  c extended subtotal maxillectomy

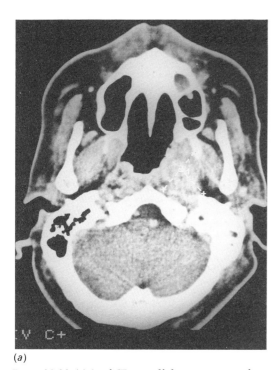

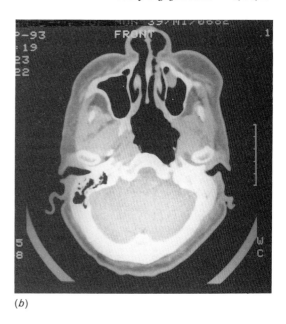

(*b*)

(*a*)

Figure 13.11 (*a*) Axial CT scan of left recurrent nasopharyngeal carcinoma after radiotherapy, brachytherapy and chemotherapy with no skull base erosion. (*b*) Post-nasopharyngectomy scan showing defect after removal of the pterygoid plates, left posterosuperior and lateral wall of the nasopharynx exposing the clivus and internal carotid canal

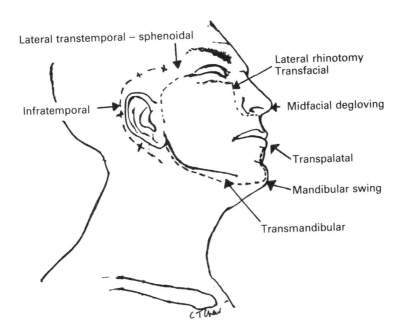

Figure 13.12 The various surgical approaches to the nasopharynx

2 Transpalatal
3 Sublabial midfacial degloving approach
4 Transfacial – maxillary swing
5 Transmandibular and mandibular swing
6 Infratemporal approach
7 Others
   a lateral transtemporal-sphenoidal
   b transpharyngeal
   c transcervical

Tumours that are limited to the nasopharynx can be removed by the standard transpalatal approach. Such tumours include minor salivary gland tumours (pleomorphic adenomas, mucoepidermoid tumours) haemangioma, inverted papilloma and melanoma. A combined intra- and extracranial approach may be required for tumours that demonstrate notable intracranial extension, e.g. craniopharyngioma and angiofibroma. The selection of an appropriate surgical approach depends upon the extent of the tumour and which structures and spaces are involved.

Postoperative haemostasis can be achieved by postnasal packing and/or a Foley catheter (inflated with 20–30 ml water) brought out through the nose. The advantage of using a Foley catheter is that should bleeding recur on removing the pressure, it can be re-inflated.

Transnasal-maxillary approach

The transnasal and transantral approaches provide good access only for removing tumours in the maxilloethmoid region. Often they are combined as a transnasal-maxillary approach (resecting the maxilla and lateral nasal wall) to provide reasonable access to the nasopharynx. Denker's extension of the Caldwell-Luc procedure is one such modification. The exposure is however limited by the soft tissue of the lip and nose. The use of lateral rhinotomy or a Weber-Ferguson incision improves the exposure but is limited by its unilaterality and midfacial scarring.

LeFort I osteotomy approach

The LeFort I osteotomy approach to the nasopharynx and central skull base is achieved by downfracturing the entire hard palate and inferior maxilla. It is basically a sublabial transverse maxillary osteotomy through the anterior and lateral walls of the maxillary sinus. Non-erupted teeth could be damaged and the osteotomy may affect facial growth.

Transpalatal approach

This is the shortest and most direct approach to expose the nasopharynx and allows extension to the sphenoid and choana. There are many variations to the palatal incision. The U-shaped incision is usually preferred as it can be extended around the maxillary tuberosity to join the sublabial incision to reach the pterygopalatine fossa (Figure 13.13). In this procedure, after the mucoperiosteal flap has been elevated (preserving the greater palatine neurovascular pedicle), removal of bone from the posterior hard palate exposes the tumour.

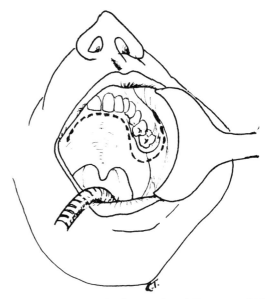

Figure 13.13 Transpalatal approach with U-incision which can be extended in an 'S' fashion around the tuberosity of the maxilla to join the sublabial incision to reach the pterygopalatine fossa

Sublabial midfacial degloving approach

This procedure is essentially a bilateral extended sublabial and transnasal-maxillary approach. It avoids visible facial scarring and allows adequate exposure of the nasal complex, nasopharynx and mid-third of the face. The initial gingivolabial incision is across the midline from one maxillary tuberosity to the other. The soft tissue on both sides of the face is then elevated subperiosteally up to the infraorbital foramina. The infraorbital nerves are exposed and preserved. Routine intracartilaginous incisions are used, separating the soft tissue of the nose from the upper lateral cartilage as in rhinoplasty. A transfixing septal incision then separates the cartilaginous septum from the medial crura of the alar cartilage. Finally, an incision along the pyriform aperture connects the circumferential septal-vestibular incisions to the sublabial incision. This allows total midfacial degloving up to the root of the nose. The necessary bone is then resected from the maxilla, antrum and the lateral nasal wall and modification such as translocating the nasal septum allows access to the nasopharynx from both sides of the face. The pterygopalatine and infratemporal fossae can also be reached by this approach. One of its postoperative complications is vestibular stenosis.

Transfacial approach

This approach combines the Weber-Ferguson-Longmire facial incision with splitting of the hard palate shelf and multiple osteotomies detaching all bony attachments of the maxillary complex. The disarticulated maxilla is attached to the cheek-masseter flap supplied by the facial and superficial temporal arteries. The lateral swing of the maxilla allows transfacial access to the nasopharynx and parapharyngeal space (Hernandez Altemir, 1986; Wei, Lam and Sham, 1991).

Transmandibular and mandibular swing approach

This approach is via an extended preauricular neck incision with mandibulotomy swinging open the mandible to reach the nasopharynx transorally or via the parapharyngeal space/stylomandibular tunnel. Various osteotomies in oblique or stepped fashion, at the angle or body of the mandible have been proposed to improve surgical access. The jaw fragments are reopposed and fixed by miniplates and screws which do not interfere with postoperative radiotherapy if required. Temporary tracheostomy is necessary to maintain the airway in the immediate postoperative period. The major disadvantage of this approach is sectioning or injury to the inferior dental and lingual nerves.

Lateral infratemporal approach

The lateral infratemporal approach (Fisch, 1983) is a radical skull-base approach transecting the auditory canal and zygoma with extended radical mastoidectomy re-routing the facial nerve, exposing and displacing the internal carotid artery to reach the nasopharynx. This approach allows good visualization and resection of the infratemporal portion of the tumour with good control of the proximal internal carotid and dural venous sinuses. The medial and inferior nasopharynx however is at a distance from this approach.

Other approaches

The lateral transtemporal approach transects the temporalis muscle and zygomatic arch to reach the infratemporal and sphenoid-nasopharyngeal region. Other approaches, e.g. transcervical (for high cervical and disc surgery) and transpharyngeal (through the floor of the pharynx above the hyoid) are seldom employed nowadays.

Immunology of nasopharyngeal carcinoma

General cell-mediated immunity

The general cell-mediated immunity of patients with nasopharyngeal cancer is impaired. Impaired T-cell functions are found in more than half of the newly diagnosed and untreated patients. This can be demonstrated *in vivo* by the Mantoux test and *in vitro* by the phytohaemagglutinin (PHA) response of lymphocytes. Similar impairment is also observed in treated patients who are in remission. Cell-mediated immunity to Epstein-Barr virus is present but impaired as demonstrable by lymphocyte stimulation assays or by T-cell cytotoxicity (Chan *et al.*, 1979). The impaired viral specific T-cell immunity and increased suppressor T-cell activity in nasopharyngeal carcinoma suggests immunosuppression. The degree of cell-mediated immunity impairment is directly proportional to the prognosis.

It is possible that the defective specific cell-mediated immunity allows the Epstein-Barr virus to be reactivated in the salivary glands. Its associated mucosal stimulation then leads to high anti-Epstein-Barr virus IgA antibodies. Tumour burden correlates inversely with cell-mediated immunity, the higher the tumour burden, the lower the cell-mediated immunity which then leads to higher Epstein-Barr virus antibody levels. Such antibodies are a measure of humoral response and not cell-mediated immunity.

Epstein-Barr virus and its association with nasopharyngeal carcinoma

This is one of the herpes viruses. Its lymphotropic action is restricted to the B lymphocytes which are found in abundance in the lymphoepithelium of the nasopharynx. The primary infection of Epstein-Barr virus takes place in childhood and is always accompanied by seroconversion and harbouring of the virus in a dormant state for life in small numbers of circulating B lymphocytes or in saliva. The virus may be reactivated with raised serological titres in immunosuppressed states. Among human cancers, only African Burkitt's lymphoma, nasopharyngeal carcinoma and some Hodgkin's lymphomas are closely associated with Epstein-Barr virus. They have different seroepidemiological backgrounds. Nasopharyngeal carcinoma is an epithelial tumour and is not related to the endemicity of the Epstein-Barr virus. Decades elapse between primary infection (> 90 % by age of 5 years in southern Chinese) and the occurrence of nasopharyngeal carcinoma (peak around fourth decade). The association of nasopharyngeal cancer with Epstein-Barr virus is supported by:

1 The presence of a humoral immune response in patients with nasopharyngeal carcinoma against Epstein-Barr virus determined antigens, including the structural antigens such as the viral capsid antigen (VCA), early antigen (EA) and nuclear antigen (EBNA)
2 The presence of Epstein-Barr viral markers, Epstein-Barr viral DNA and nuclear antigen in nasopharyngeal carcinoma tumour cells. However, Epstein-Barr viral particles have yet to be observed in nasopharyngeal carcinoma cells from biopsy samples.

Aetiological role of Epstein-Barr virus in nasopharyngeal carcinoma

More than 90% of patients with nasopharyngeal cancer have elevated antibody titres to Epstein-Barr virus-determined antigens, particularly the IgA class antibodies compared with controls of the same ethnic group and geographical location. Of the many types of nasopharyngeal carcinomas, only the undifferentiated / poorly differentiated carcinomas have a consistent immunocytological association with the Epstein-Barr virus; its viral genome is consistently found in the tumours irrespective of race or geographical location. The genome has also been reported, albeit in lesser degree, in well-differentiated nasopharyngeal carcinomas (Rabb-Traub *et al.*, 1987) but, like the normal population, this patient group does not have elevated antibody levels to Epstein-Barr viral antigens. Other aerodigestive tract carcinomas have so far failed to produce Epstein-Barr viral markers (Niedobitek *et al.*, 1991) except in undifferentiated carcinoma of the parotid and thymoma (McGuire *et al.*, 1988).

It is not clear how the viral DNA becomes associated with the epithelial carcinoma cells and when the epithelial cells are infected by the Epstein-Barr virus, whether it is before or after the malignant change (passenger virus), or as a result of impaired host immunity. The Epstein-Barr virus is capable of transforming B lymphocytes but there is no convincing evidence at present that it can transform epithelial cells, *in vitro or in vivo* even though viral receptors are present on certain normal pharyngeal epithelial cells (Young *et al.*, 1986). The Epstein-Barr virus itself is not replicating in nasopharyngeal carcinoma tumour cells and its viral antigens (VCA and EA) are not expressed in these tumours. Why only a few individuals develop nasopharyngeal carcinoma in a population that is ubiquitously infected with Epstein-Barr virus in early life remains to be explained. The aetiological role of Epstein-Barr virus in nasopharyngeal carcinoma is still very much a debate.

Epstein-Barr serological markers

In comparison to other head and neck cancers, patients with nasopharyngeal carcinoma have a broader spectrum and higher geometric mean titres of a series of antibodies directed against Epstein-Barr specific antigens. Important Epstein-Barr virus related antibodies in nasopharyngeal carcinoma are:

1 IgA and IgG to viral capsid antigen
2 IgA and IgG to early antigen
3 Antibody to nuclear antigen
4 Antibody-dependent cellular cytotoxicity antibodies.

These are of clinical importance in evaluating a patient with nasopharyngeal carcinoma for the stage of the disease at the time of diagnosis, the effect of and response to therapy, as well as the clinical course and survival.

Antibodies against viral capsid antigen, early antigen and nuclear antigen are the most useful in clinical practice and their titres correlate well with each other. The IgA response to Epstein-Barr viral antigens in nasopharyngeal carcinoma is unique and characteristic of patients with nasopharyngeal carcinoma. Antibody-dependent cellular cytotoxicity, a process known to be effective in the destruction of virus infected cells, appears to act on Epstein-Barr induced membrane antigens. It is capable of destroying the infected cells. Antibody-dependent cellular cytotoxicity antibodies may represent a functional immune response against tumour cells *in vivo*.

Seroimmunological index in the diagnosis of nasopharyngeal carcinoma

Immunoglobulin IgA/VCA, IgG/VCA, and IgA/EA IgG/EA are useful diagnostic markers of nasopharyngeal carcinoma. Their titres are related to the tumour load and geometric mean titres increase with advancing stage of the disease in untreated patients. The normal anti-Epstein-Barr viral antibody titres in adult Chinese populations are:

Anti-EBV VCA/IgG = up to 1:160
Anti-EBV EA/IgG = up to 1:160

Anti EBV VCA/IgA = 86 % below 1:5
                                10% from 1:5 to 1:10
                                4% at 1:40
Anti-EBV EA/IgA = below 1:5

Antibodies of the IgA class constitute the most frequent seroimmunological index used clinically. IgA/VCA has a sensitivity of 95% and specificity of 97% depending on the laboratory cut-off point and the stage of presentation. IgA/EA on the other hand is more specific with 99% specificity but has a sensitivity of only 90%. IgG/VCA has the least discriminatory value as a primary serological diagnostic indicator of nasopharyngeal carcinoma (Chan, 1989; Chew, 1990).

Clinical course and survival

The titres of IgA/VCA and IgA/EA are useful clinical indices for follow up of patients after treatment. Titres may decline to a low level or remain static after successful treatment. An increase of VCA, EA and EBNA antibodies would indicate clinical recurrence and/or metastasis. They may be useful to indicate the occurrence of an occult tumour and would necessitate careful evaluation of the patient.

Figure 13.14 shows the geometric mean titres of early antigen (EA), viral capsid antigen (VCA), Epstein-Barr nuclear antigen and antibody dependent cytototoxic antibodies (ADCC) in various groups of patients and controls and surviving and dead patients in various stages of the disease. The geometric mean titres of EA, VCA and EBNA (taken at the time of diagnosis) were significantly higher in the patients who died (within 4 years) of the disease compared with those who survived. ADCC antibody titre was highest in long-term survivors while VCA and EA antibody titres showed an inverse relationship to survival. The geometric mean titres of EA, VCA and EBNA increase stepwise with disease stage but decline

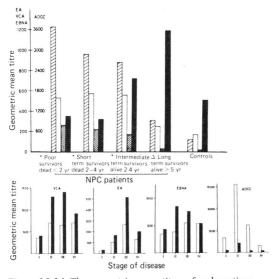

Figure 13.14 The geometric mean titres of early antigen (EA) ▨, viral capsid antigen (VCA) ☐, Epstein-Barr nuclear antigen ▥ and antibody dependent cytotoxic antibodies (ADCC) ■ in various groups of nasopharyngeal carcinoma patients and controls; and (bottom figure) surviving ☐ and dead ■ patients with nasopharyngeal carcinoma in various stages of the disease. * Sera obtained at time of diagnosis; △ sera obtained > 5 years after diagnosis

towards the end-stage. ADCC antibody clearly demonstrates its value as a biological titre in determining the survival of patients.

Prognostic serological markers

The prognostic markers of nasopharyngeal carcinoma include specific Epstein-Barr virus antibody titres. The EBV titres are dependent on histological type, the availability (load) of various Epstein-Barr viral antigens and host immune competence. The titres may not be elevated in early and end stage disease and in patients with intracranial extension without significant lymph node involvement.

1 Prognosis and survival are inversely proportional to the geometric mean titres of VCA and EA antibodies.
2 Good prognosis is indicated by high ADCC antibody titres. The titre appears to be independent of the disease stage and this suggests that a parameter independent of the tumour load is involved.

Other clinical applications

Screening for nasopharyngeal carcinoma in high risk populations

IgA/VCA is of practical value in serological screening for nasopharyngeal carcinoma in endemic regions. A large scale seroepidemiological survey has been conducted in southern China since 1978 in three different counties involving over 195 000 subjects. Cohorts surveyed included populations of rural and urban areas including ethnic minorities and of high-risk subgroups such as workers in chemical factories and boat people (Zeng *et al.*, 1983; Zeng, 1985). The percentage of IgA/VCA positive individuals ranged from 0.6% to 10%. From these, 106 patients with nasopharyngeal cancer were identified with a detection rate ranging from 1.6% to 13.6%. More than half those detected were in an early clinical stage. In Zangwu county (Guang Xi province) with a population of 450 000 of which 148 029 subjects were screened for IgA/VCA, 3 533 individuals (2.4%) were found to be positive and from this group 55 patients with nasopharyngeal carcinoma were detected, i.e. 1.6% of the IgA/VCA positive cohort. A further 32 patients were diagnosed in the second year of follow up. The period between detection of raised IgA/VCA and clinical onset of stage I nasopharyngeal carcinoma ranged from 8 to 30 months (mean 13). Of note was the prevailing high incidence of nasopharyngeal carcinoma in a chemical factory where three patients were detected out of 22 IgA/VCA positive workers among the 216 individuals screened.

The detection rate of a screened IgA/VCA positive population was estimated to be more than 80 times the annual nasopharyngeal carcinoma incidence of the general population of comparable age. This indicates the existence of subclinical and early nasopharyngeal carcinomas in the otherwise asymptomatic IgA/VCA positive individuals. The long subclinical period (months or even years) with raised IgA/VCA probably indicates the slow tumour growth with ample time for the Epstein-Barr virus antigens to stimulate the immune system. As there is no diagnostic macroscopic appearance of early nasopharyngeal carcinoma, it is likely that tumour in the early stage is indistinguishable from the normal 'lymphoepithelium' and chronically inflamed lymphoid aggregations commonly seen in the nasopharynx. A raised IgA/VCA titre identifies those high-risk individuals for further clinical and immunohistological evaluation of the nasopharynx.

Differential diagnosis of nasopharyngeal carcinoma

Morphologically nasopharyngeal carcinoma can be confused with lymphoma especially in the low-risk population.

Occult primary with cervical metastases

The nasopharynx is still the most frequent site for an occult primary in the head and neck with cervical metastases. In certain clinical situations where the primary is difficult to detect, a positive EBV/IgA serology and positive immunohistological markers on the metastatic tumour tissue serve as an adjunct to pathological identification.

Multiple nasopharyngeal biopsies under endoscopic vision are indicated if the Epstein-Barr virus serological markers are positive. Should the serology be negative and other head and neck regions are clear, an enlarged lymph node should be excised *in toto* with the capsule intact. Fresh lymph node tissue is sent for identification of nuclear antigen and DNA in the tumour cells. If nuclear antigen is demonstrated the primary tumour is most likely to be a nasopharyngeal carcinoma. Although the nuclear antigen has been identified in undifferentiated parotid gland carcinoma, one must be aware of the fact that a small primary nasopharyngeal carcinoma is known to give rise to overt tumour deposits in the parotid gland (see above).

Indiscriminate excision biopsy of lymph nodes should be discouraged. Such biopsy offers little in the clinical management if the primary is still undetected. It would further compromise the prognosis in nasopharyngeal carcinoma and increases the morbidity to radiation should the wound break down due to tumour seeding.

Immunogenetics of nasopharyngeal carcinoma

Patients with nasopharyngeal carcinoma have

shown a genetic susceptibility to this cancer. This is evident by the following observations:

1 High risk among the southern Chinese population
2 Differential high risk in emigrant Chinese in comparison to the indigenous population
3 Family clustering among first degree relatives in Chinese and other populations in Eskimos and Caucasians (Ireland *et al.*, 1988; Coffin, Rich and Dehner, 1991; Levine *et al.*, 1992)
4 Elevated risk in people having genetic admixture with Chinese
5 Low risk in other racial groups despite living in high risk countries, e.g. Indians in Singapore.

Familial nasopharyngeal carcinoma in low risk white populations is usually of the poorly differentiated type in contrast to the common well differentiated cell type in sporadic cases.

Genetic markers in nasopharyngeal carcinoma

The patients with nasopharyngeal cancer among the Chinese come from a genetically distinct subpopulation. HLA is the only genetic system so far shown to have a strong association with this cancer. The HLA loci involved with nasopharyngeal carcinoma are the HLA-A, B and DR locus situated on the short arm of chromosome 6.

Linkage disequilibrium in histocompatibility leucocyte antigen

The alleles for HLA vary in frequency and presence among different ethnic groups. The linkage pattern also differs between different human populations. In the general population, certain alleles of one locus tend to be associated with that of another, with a frequency far exceeding that expected if the two genes were to be segregated independently and separately. This is called linkage disequilibrium and is observed in Chinese patients with nasopharyngeal carcinoma (A2-B46, A33 (split of A19) – B58 (split of B17)).

HLA and nasopharyngeal carcinoma in Chinese

History of Sin 2 antigen

An oriental B antigen was discovered with high frequency among Singapore Chinese patients with nasopharyngeal cancer in a pilot study in 1974. It was designated Singapore-2 (Sin 2) (Simons and Day, 1977). Meanwhile an independent study in America also found an HLA-antigen (designated HS) occurring with high frequency among the Chinese Cantonese patients in California (Payne, Radvany and Grumet, 1975). It is now known that Sin 2 and HS are identical, and it is designated B46 by the

WHO committee on leucocyte nomenclature. The HLA association with nasopharyngeal carcinoma is haplotype (whole chromosome or large chunk of chromosome 6) in nature. Two different haplotypes are associated with newly diagnosed nasopharyngeal carcinoma – A2, Cw1, B46 and A33, Cw3, B58, DR3.

Differential HLA frequency distribution and survival

Differential frequency distributions of HLA antigen are seen among the newly diagnosed Chinese patients with regards to the age of onset of the disease. They are as follows:

1 A2, Cw1, B46 haplotype is associated with older onset patients (> 30 years old)
2 A33, Cw3, B58, DR3 haplotype is associated with both young and old patients but particularly with younger patients (< 30 years old)
3 A11 and B13 alleles are associated with a decreased risk (B13 is also associated with younger patients).

The A33, Cw3, B58, DR3 is associated with poor survival. A2, without B46 or B58 including A2, B13 appear to be associated with long-term survival (Table 13.5).

Table 13.5 Summary of HLA types and their relationship to survival pattern and clinical behaviour of nasopharyngeal carcinoma

HLA pattern	Clinical behaviour and survival
A33–B58	Short-term survival Mostly young onset < 30 years Poor CMI, PHA and Mantoux High VCA/EA titres, low ADCC titre Most die within 2 years from onset
A2–B46	Intermediate-term survivals Older onset > 30 years
A2 without B46 or B58	Long-term survivals (40% 5-year survival) Low VCA/EA titres, high ADCC titres

Haplotype distribution and relative risk

The association of a particular disease with a particular HLA antigen is quantitated by calculating the relative risk. This can be defined as the chance an individual with the disease-associated HLA-antigen has of developing the disease compared to an individual who lacks the antigens.

Relative risk

HLA	A2	1.5	Haplotype A2, Cw1, B46	3.4
	B46	1.9	A33, Cw3, B58, DR3	2.2
	B58	2.1		

Haplotype or joint occurrence of A33 – B58 and A2 – B46 are associated with a higher risk than B58 or B46 alone. This suggests that the risk is associated with haplotype rather than individual antigens. These two pairs are known to be in linkage disequilibrium in the general Chinese population. Siblings with nasopharyngeal carcinoma have been found to share the haplotypes significantly more frequently than expected and the first degree relatives have an over 20-fold increased risk of nasopharyngeal carcinoma.

Despite the occurrence of 100 or more alleles at the HLA-A and B loci, only a very limited number are associated with nasopharyngeal cancer. A11 is rarely found with B58 or B46, while the association of A2 with B46 in nasopharyngeal carcinoma is stronger than in control patients. No stronger linkage is seen than the A33-B58 association. The different HLA association with varying age of onset suggests that there is heterogenicity within the Chinese patient population. The HLA pattern suggests a genetic difference between younger and older onset patients even though there is no bimodal peak in the age incidence among Chinese patients. The same HLA locus A and B antigen are associated with Chinese patients in Singapore, Malaysia, Hong Kong and China as well as in California. Of the racial groups, there are certain similar HLA findings among Malay and Chinese patients – the association with B58 (Chan et al., 1985).

B46 origin and nasopharyngeal carcinoma

B46 has the highest frequency in South China with a gene frequency of about 12%. It appears to correlate with the population where nasopharyngeal carcinoma incidence is the highest. Its frequency decreases with distance from that region. It does not occur commonly nor is it in linkage with HLA-A2 in non-Chinese Asian populations and is absent in the Caucasian, Indian and African population. The HLA gene association is the most convincing evidence for the role of genetics in the aetiology of nasopharyngeal carcinoma.

HLA and nasopharyngeal carcinoma in non-Asian populations

HLA association among non-Asian patients has been inconsistent. A29 is associated with East African Black patients. The frequency of A3, B5 and B15 is noted to increase in northern African patient cohorts yet in the other mid-risk north African population, the Tunisians, no HLA link is noted.

Nasopharyngeal carcinoma and dermatomyositis

Dermatomyositis is an immunological systemic disorder with predominant involvement of skin and skeletal muscles. It is known to be associated with malignancy. Nasopharyngeal carcinoma is the most frequent malignancy constituting about 80% of all cancers associated with adult dermatomyositis in the southern Chinese (Chan, 1985; Hu, 1986) (see Figure 13.8).

Tumours of lymphoid and haematopoietic tissue

These tumours possess no gross characteristics which allow differentiation from the epithelial tumours of the nasopharynx. The symptomatology is similar to that of other invasive tumours occurring in this region. Epistaxis and nasal obstruction are the usual presenting symptoms. Pain may signify pressure or invasion of adjacent structures. Biopsy is needed for a definitive diagnosis. Patients with no involvment of regional lymph nodes may have disseminated disease at the time of diagnosis. Management requires a multidisciplinary approach involving the radiotherapist and medical oncologist.

Malignant lymphoma

About 25% of malignant lymphomas are of extranodal origin, with Waldeyer's ring second only to the stomach as the most common site of involvement (Freeman, Berg and Cutler, 1972). Within Waldeyer's ring, the faucial tonsil is the most frequent site of lymphomatous involvement, followed by the nasopharynx. In a review of the world literature from 1935 to 1969, Banfi *et al.* (1970) reported malignant lymphoma to account for between 1% (in South East Asia) and 43% (in Europe) of all nasopharyngeal tumours. The low incidence in the East Asian population is related to the prevalence of nasopharyngeal carcinoma. The clinical and histological distinction between undifferentiated nasopharyngeal carcinoma (particularly in low-risk populations) and malignant lymphoma can be a significant problem. Distinction can be made by immunohistochemical detection of monoclonal immunoglobulins, absence of keratin staining and epithelial features on electron microscopy in malignant lymphoma.

Diagnosis and treatment

Advances in immunopathology using tissue marker and monoclonal antisera has further classified lymphomas into various immunological types. The normal or reactive lymphocyte population is heterogeneous whereas a malignant, non-Hodgkin's lymphoma is a clone of lymphocytes carrying specific surface markers. These markers enable the non-Hodgkin's lymphoma to be identified and typed as being B or T cell. Hodgkin's disease has no monoclonal marker pattern and is a morphological diagnosis. Staging follows the definitive diagnosis. Gastrointestinal tract evaluation is needed; its involvement adversely affects the prognosis. In localized disease, radiation alone is the treatment of choice. For systemic disease, chemotherapy alone or in combination with radiation is the preferred treatment.

Plasmacytoma

Plasmacytic dyscrasia occurs in the bone marrow (medullary) and any structure containing reticuloendothelial tissues (extramedullary plasmacytoma). They are histologically similar. The extramedullary plasmacytoma occurs most commonly in the head and neck region and has a predilection for the upper aerodigestive tract, especially the nasal sinuses and the nasopharynx (Batsakis *et al.*, 1964). It can be solitary or multiple in form. It is relatively rare and the incidence compared to multiple myeloma is 1:40 (Pahor, 1977). Males predominate in the ratio 3:1 and the peak incidence is in the fifth decade.

Diagnosis and treatment

When the histological diagnosis is made, it is necessary to exclude multiple and systemic involvement. Investigations would include radiological skeletal survey, haematological evaluation, bone marrow biopsy and aspirate, and immunoglobulin electrophoresis. Solitary plasmacytomas in the head and neck are generally treated by excision (depending on the site and accessibility) or local radiotherapy. The clinical course of the nasopharyngeal or upper aerodigestive tract plasmacytomas is unpredictable. Despite treatment, they may recur or eventually evolve into the systemic form after a variable latent period. Hence long-term follow up and surveillance are necessary.

Paediatric nasopharyngeal tumours

Paediatric nasopharyngeal tumours are rare. They cause respiratory obstruction, and create problems in diagnosis and management. Besides adenoid hypertrophy (which is unusual in early infancy) and antrochoanal polyp, the differential diagnosis of a nasopharyngeal mass includes:

1 Teratoid
   dermoid, teratoma, epignathus
2 Neuroectodermal
   encephalocoele, brain heterotopia, meningioma
3 Dysontogenetic
   chordoma, craniopharyngioma
4 Miscellaneous
   cysts, haemangioma, angiofibroma, hamartoma, rhabdomyosarcoma.

Teratoid tumours

Most of the tumours arise from the midline or lateral wall of the nasopharynx and may be attached to the palate. Females outnumber males by 6:1. In contrast to dermoids, teratomas of the nasopharynx tend to be recognized later in infancy (Foxwell and Kelham, 1958).

Dermoids or hairy polyps

This is the commonest variety. They probably arise from inclusion errors during the fusion of the lateral palatine process. They are often pedunculated and covered by hairy skin containing dermal glands. Occasionally the main tumour mass is connected to an intracranial portion through a perforation in the skull base. Histologically, they are bidermal with fibroadipose tissue, bone, cartilage and fragments of striated muscle.

Teratomas

These are more complex than the dermoids in structure. Histologically they are tridermal with nervous tissue. They are frequently associated with deformities of the skull, e.g. anencephaly, hemicrania and palatal fissures. Teratomas tend to grow aggressively and, in this respect are true neoplasms. However, nasopharyngeal teratomas have not been reported to undergo malignant degeneration in contrast to teratomas elsewhere in the body.

Epignathus

This is the least common variety. It consists of the well-formed organs and limbs of a parasitic fetus. Highly developed teratoid tumours are much rarer in the head and neck, they often result in stillbirths.

Basal encephalocoeles and brain heterotopia

The human nasopharynx is closely related to the embryonic development of the neural tube. The juxtaposition of the nasopharynx and the prosencephalon may further account for the very rare nasopharyngeal neuroectodermal tumours, e.g. basal brain heterotopia. Generally encephalocoeles occur in approximately 1:4000 births and less than 10% are of the basal type (Blumenfeld and Skolnik, 1965). Among the basal encephalocoeles, the sphenopharyngeal type is the most common. Within the nose and nasopharynx it can cause obstruction and deform the upper airway. The intranasal sac may be mistaken for a nasal polyp. It must be differentiated from nasal glioma and brain heterotopia.

Chordoma and craniopharyngioma

The chordoma is a slow growing tumour of low malignancy. The craniocervical form occurs along the embryonic craniocervical axis of the notochord bar – the clivus, nasopharynx and first two cervical vertebrae. It tends to erode bone extensively with displacement of the surrounding structures, making complete surgical removal difficult. This tumour is not very sensitive to radiotherapy.

A few cases of craniopharyngioma in the nasopharynx have been described (Johnson, 1962). It is probably derived from the remnants of Rathke's pouch and the craniopharyngeal canal. Devoid of a definite capsule, the tumour proper is soft with multiple septa separating cystic spaces. Calcification may be present. Clinically, the intracranial portion of the tumour may cause increased intracranial pressure, endocrine disturbances and retarded sexual development. Surgical decompression may be required to relieve the raised intracranial pressure. Complete removal of the main cyst necessitates a subfrontal approach and is difficult (Matson and Crigler, 1969).

Nasopharyngeal cysts

Nasopharyngeal cysts occur in the roof and the lateral wall. They include Rathke's pouch cyst, Thornwaldt's cyst from the pharyngeal bursa and branchial cleft cyst (on the lateral wall).

Symptomatology

The clinical picture will depend on the size, nature and site of the tumour. Choanal obstruction may give rise to stertor and rhinorrhoea. Long pedunculated tumours may cause intermittent attacks of coughing, apnoea and dysphagia. Sessile tumours may block the nasopharyngeal airway completely and distort the palate, impeding mouth breathing and feeding. Nasopharyngeal obstruction is often dramatic in the first few months of life as infants are obligate nose breathers (Moss, 1965; Swift and Emery, 1973). The risk of asphyxia and difficulty in feeding is greater in nasopharyngeal tumours than in bilateral choanal atresia. Any intracranial communication of the tumour always predisposes the infant to the threat of cerebrospinal fluid rhinorrhoea and ascending meningitis. In such cases enlargement of the mass with crying or jugular vein compression may be elicited (Furstenberg sign).

Radiological investigations

Radiological investigations would include plain radiographs or tomograms and cross-sectional imaging with CT scans and or magnetic resonance imaging. Plain lateral skull radiographs may show a soft tissue mass obstructing the nasopharynx and displacing the soft palate anteroinferiorly. Adenoid hypertrophy in early infancy is very unusual. In older children widening of the pterygopalatine fissure (anterior bowing of the posterior wall of the maxillary antrum and posterior bowing of the pterygoid plate) is the classical sign of angiofibroma but is not pathognomonic. Similar radiological features have also been observed in other tumours; schwannomas, fibrous dysplasia and nasopharyngeal cancer (Som *et al.*, 1981).

CT scans in both axial and coronal planes are necessary to exclude intracranial extension particularly through the sella turcica and spheno-occipital synchondrosis. They also provide information on the nature of the tumour, its site of origin and both its intra- and extracranial extension. Magnetic resonance imaging delineates the soft tissue character making it possible to distinguish for example a glioma from meningeal encephalocoeles and demonstrates any intracranial connection.

Surgical management

Large teratoid masses may cause acute respiratory obstruction and need immediate surgical removal. The more common pedunculated 'hairy polyp' can be removed easily. In less urgent cases endoscopic assessment under anaesthesia and careful biopsy is required to establish the diagnosis before definitive treatment. Laryngoscopy and bronchoscopy should also be carried out to exclude other causes of upper airway obstruction. The transpalatal approach is used to remove sessile tumours. Intracranial communication is uncommon but must be excluded prior to any surgery. The existence of such a communication may necessitate a combined intra–extracranial approach.

Paediatric nasopharyngeal cancer

The common cancers affecting the nasopharynx in children are nasopharyngeal carcinoma, rhabdomyosarcoma and malignant lymphoma. Paediatric nasopharyngeal carcinoma, rare in high-risk populations, remains a common cause of nasopharyngeal cancer

in children over 10 years of age in mid- and low-risk populations (Greene, Fraumeni and Hoover, 1977). Rhabdomyosarcoma tends to occur in younger children and the nasopharynx is the second most common head and neck site after the orbit (Felman, 1982).

Diagnosis is often delayed and the tumour spreads to involve the sinuses and surrounding structures. The symptoms are not different from nasal obstruction as in adenoid hypertrophy and upper respiratory infection. The presence of rapidly increasing postnasal obstruction and pressure symptoms should suggest the possibility of a tumour.

Appendix 13.1 Stage classification of nasopharyngeal carcinoma currently in use

1 UICC TNM Classification

UICC (1987)

a Anatomical regions and sites

Posterior-superior wall: extends from the level of the junction of the hard and soft palate to the base of the skull
Lateral wall: including the fossa of Rosenmüller
Inferior wall: Consists of the surface of the soft palate
Note: The margin of the choanal orifices including the posterior margin of the nasal septum is included with the nasal fossa.

b TNM Pretreatment categories

T: primary tumour

TX primary tumour cannot be assessed
T0 no evidence of primary tumour
Tis pre-invasive carcinoma (carcinoma in situ)
T1 tumour limited to one subsite of nasopharynx
T2 tumour invades more than one subsite of nasopharynx
T3 tumour invades into nasal cavity and/or oropharynx
T4 tumour invades skull and/or cranial nerves

N: regional lymph nodes

NX Regional lymph nodes cannot be assessed
N0 No regional lymph node metastasis
N1 Metastasis in a single ipsilateral lymph node, 3 cm or less in greatest dimension
N2 Metastasis in a single ipsilateral lymph node, more than 3 cm but not more than 6 cm in greatest dimension, or in multiple ipsilateral lymph nodes, none more than 6 cm in greatest dimension, or in bilateral or contralateral lymph nodes, none more than 6 cm in greatest dimension
  N2a metastasis in a single ipsilateral lymph node, more than 3 cm but not more than 6 cm in greatest dimension

N2b metastasis in multiple ipsilateral lymph nodes, none more than 6 cm in greatest dimension

N2c Metastasis in bilateral or contralateral lymph nodes, none more than 6 cm in greatest dimension

N3 Metastasis in a lymph node more than 6 cm in greatest dimension

M: distant metastases

MX presence of distant metastasis cannot be assessed
M0 no distant metastases
M1 distant metastases

c Stage-grouping

Stage 0	Tis	N0	M0
Stage I	T1	N0	M0
Stage II	T2	N0	M0
Stage III	T3	N0	M0
	T1	N1	M0
	T2	N1	M0
	T3	N1	M0
Stage IV	T4	N0, N1	M0
	Any T	N2, N3	M0
	Any T	Any N	M1

2 The American Joint Committee on Cancer – Stage Classification

In 1988 the AJCC modified its 1983 N definitions for N2 and N3 with addition of N2c and a single N3 but the T definitions remained unchanged. The 1992 AJCC stage-classification adopted the 1988 system unchanged.

AJCC TNM Stage Classification (1988/1992)

Anatomy (1988)

Posterosuperior wall, extends from the level of the junction of the hard and soft palates to the base of the skull.
Lateral wall, includes the fossa of Rosenmüller.
Inferior (anterior) wall, consists of the superior surface of the soft palate.

Note: The margin of the choanal orifices including the posterior margin of the nasal septum is included with the nasal fossa.

TNM categories

Primary tumour (T)

TX Primary tumour cannot be assessed
T0 No evidence of primary tumour
Tis Carcinoma in situ
T1 Tumour limited to one subsite of nasopharynx
T2 Tumour invades more than one subsite of nasopharynx

T3 Tumour invades nasal cavity and/or oropharynx
T4 Tumour invades skull and/or cranial nerve(s)

N: Regional lymph nodes (midline nodes are considered as homolateral nodes)

NX Regional lymph nodes cannot be assessed
N0 No regional lymph node metastasis
N1 Metastasis in a single ipsilateral lymph node, 3 cm or less in greatest dimension
N2 Metastasis in a single ipsilateral lymph node, more than 3 cm but not more than 6 cm in greatest dimension, or in multiple ipsilateral lymph nodes, none more than 6 cm in greatest dimension, or in bilateral or contralateral lymph nodes, none more than 6 cm in greatest dimension
   N2a Metastasis in a single ipsilateral lymph node more than 3 cm but not more than 6 cm in greatest dimension
   N2b Metastasis in multiple ipsilateral lymph nodes, none more than 6 cm in greatest dimension
   N2c Metastasis in bilateral or contralateral lymph nodes, none more than 6 cm in greatest dimension
N3 Metastasis in a lymph node more than 6 cm in greatest dimension

Distant metastasis (M)

MX Presence of distant metastasis cannot be assessed
M0 No distant metastasis
M1 Distant metastasis

Stage-grouping

Stage 0	Tis	N0	M0
I	T1	N0	M0
II	T2	N0	M0
III	T3	N0	M0
	T1	N1	M0
	T2	N1	M0
	T3	N1	M0
IV	T4	N0	M0
	T4	N1	M0
	Any T	N2	M0
	Any T	N3	M0
	Any T	Any N	M1

3 Ho's Classification (Ho, 1978)

Ho's Classification (1978)

TNM categories

Primary tumour (T)

T1 tumour confined to the nasopharynx (space behind the choanal orifices and nasal septum and above the posterior margin of the soft palate in its resting position)

T2   tumour extending to the nasal fossa, oropharynx or adjacent muscles or nerves below the base of the skull

T3   tumour extending beyond T2 limits and subclassified as follows:

   T3a   bone involvement below the base of the skull (including floor of sphenoid sinus)

   T3b   involvement of base of skull (including the lateral and posterior walls of sphenoid sinus)

   T3c   involvement of cranial nerve(s)

   T3d   involvement of orbit, laryngopharynx (hypopharynx) or infratemporal fossa

N: Regional lymph nodes

N0   no palpable nodes (excluding nodes thought to be benign)

N1   node(s) wholly in the upper cervical level, bounded below by the neck crease extending laterally and backwards from or just below the thyroid notch (laryngeal prominence)

N2   palpable node(s) between the crease and the supraclavicular fossa, the upper limit being a line joining the upper margin of the sternal end of the clavicle and apex of an angle formed by the lateral surface of the neck and the superior margin of the trapezius

N3   palpable node(s) in the supraclavicular fossa and/or skin involvement in the form of carcinoma en cuirasse or satellite nodules above the clavicles

Stage-grouping

Stage I   Tumour confined to the nasopharynx (T1 N0)

   II   Tumour extending to nasal fossa, oropharynx or adjacent muscles or nerves below the base of the skull (T2) and/or N1 involvement (T1 N1, T2 N0 and T2 N1)

   III   Tumour extending beyond T2 limits or with bone involvement (T3) and/or N2 involvement (T1–2 N2, T3 N0–1)

   IV   N3 involvement, irrespective of the stage of the primary tumour (T1–3 N3)

   V   Haematogenous metastasis and/or involvement of the skin or lymph node(s) below the clavicle (T1–3 N0–3 M1)

References

ALI, M. Y. (1965) Histology of the human nasopharyngeal mucosa. *Journal of Anatomy*, **99**, 657–672

AMERICAN JOINT COMMITTEE ON CANCER (1992) *Manual for Staging of Cancer*, 4th edn, edited by O. H. Bealirs, D. E. Henson, R. V. P. Hutter and B. J. Kennedy. Philadelphia: Lippincott. pp. 33–38

BANFI, A., BONADONNA, G., CARNEVALI, C., MOLINARI, R., MONFARDINI, S. and SALVINI, E. (1970) Lymphorecticular sarcoma with primary involvement of Waldeyer's ring: clinical evaluation of 225 cases. *Cancer*, **26**, 341–351

BATSAKIS, J. G., FRIES, G. T. GOLDMAN, R. T. and KARLSBERG, R. C. (1964) Upper respiratory tract plasmacytoma: extramedullary myeloma. *Archives of Otolaryngology*, **79**, 613–618

BLUMENFELD, R. and SKOLNIK, E. M. (1965) Intranasal encephaloceles. *Archives of Otolaryngology*, **82**, 527–531

BOYD, J. D. (1956) Observation on the human pharyngeal hypophysis. *Journal of Endocrinology*, **14**, 66–77

CAPITANIO, M. A. and KIRKPATRICK, J. A. (1970) Nasopharyngeal lymphoid tissue. *Radiology*, **96**, 389–391

CHAN, H. L. (1985) Dermatomyositis and cancer in Singapore. *International Journal of Dermatology*, **24**, 447–450

CHAN, S. H. (1989) Screening for NPC. *Annals of the Academy of Medicine of Singapore*, **18**, 80–82

CHAN, S. H., LEVINE, P. H., DE-THE, G. B., MULRONEY, S. E., LAVOUE, M. F., GLEN, S. P. P. *et al.* (1979) A comparison of the prognostic value of antibody-dependent lymphocyte cytotoxicity and other EBV antibody assays in Chinese patients with nasopharyngeal carcinoma. *International Journal of Cancer*, **23**, 181–185

CHAN, S. H., CHEW, C. T., PRASAD, U., WEE, G. B., SRINIVASAN, N. and KUNARATNAM, N. (1985) HLA and nasopharyngeal carcinoma in Malays. *British Journal of Cancer*, **51**, 389–392

CHEW, C. T. (1990) Early diagnosis of nasopharyngeal carcinoma. *Annals of the Academy of Medicine of Singapore*, **19**, 270–274

CHONG, P. Y., CHEW, C. T., CHAN, K. C. and OW, C. K. (1988) Tumour infiltrating lymphocytes in nasopharyngeal carcinoma. *Annals of the Academy of Medicine of Singapore*, **17**, 238–242

COFFIN, C. M., RICH, S. S. and DEHNER, L. P. (1991) Familial aggregation of nasopharyngeal carcinoma and other malignancies. A clinicopathologic description. *Cancer*, **68**, 1332–1338

COOPER, J. S., SCOTT, C., MARCIAL, V., GRIFFIN, T., FAZEKAS, J., LARAMORE, G. *et al.* (1991) The relationship of nasopharyngeal carcinoma and second independent malignancies based on the Radiation Therapy Oncology Group experience. *Cancer*, **67**, 1673–1677

DIGBY, H. K., THOMAS, G. H. and HSIU S. T. (1930) Notes on carcinoma of nasopharynx. *Caduceus*, **9**, 45–68

ELLOUZ, R., CAMMOUN, M., BEN ATTIA, R. and BAHI, J. (1978) Nasopharyngeal carcinoma in children and adolescents in Tunisia: clinical aspects and the paraneoplastic syndrome. In: *Nasopharyngeal Carcinoma: Aetiology and Control*, edited by G. De The and Y. Ito. IARC Scientific Publ 20. Lyon: IARC, pp. 115–29

FEE, W. E., ROBERSON, J. B. and GOFFINET, D. G. (1991) Long term survival after surgical resection for recurrent nasopharyngeal carcinoma. *Archives of Otolaryngology – Head and Neck Surgery*, **117**, 1233–1236

FELMAN, B. A. (1982) Rhabdomyosarcoma of the head and neck. *Laryngoscope*, **92**, 424–440

FISCH, U. (1983) The infratemporal fossa approach for nasopharyngeal tumours. *Laryngoscope*, **93**, 36–44

FOXWELL, P. B. and KELHAM, B. H. (1958) Teratoid tumours of the nasopharynx. *Journal of Laryngology and Otolaryngology*, **72**, 647–657

FREEMAN, C., BERG, J. W. and CUTLER, S. J. (1972) Occurrences and prognosis of extranodal lymphomas. *Cancer*, **29**, 252–260

GREENE, M. H., FRAUMENI, J. F. and HOOVER, R. (1977) Nasopharyngeal cancer among young people in the United States: racial variation by cell type. *Journal of the National Cancer Institute*, 58, 1267–1270

HERNANDEZ ALTEMIR, F. (1986) Transfacial access to the retromaxillary area. *Journal of Maxillofacial surgery*, 14, 165–170

HO, J. H. C. (1978) Stage classification of nasopharyngeal carcinoma: a review. In: *Nasopharyngeal carcinoma: Etiology and Control*, edited by G. De The and Y. Ito. IARC Scientific Publ. 20. Lyon: IARC. pp. 99–113

HSU, M. M. and LIN, B. L. (1986) Characterisation of T-cell subsets using monoclonal antibodies in nasopharyngeal carcinoma patients. *Annals of Otology, Rhinology and Laryngology*, 95, 298–301

HU, W. H. (1986) Nasopharyngeal carcinoma (NPC) with dermatomysitis – an analysis of 30 cases. *Chung Hua Chung Liu Tsa Chih*, 8, 133–135

HUANG, S. C. (1980) Nasopharyngeal cancer: a review of 1605 patients treated radically with cobalt 60. *International Journal of Radiation, Oncology, Biology and Physics*, 6, 401–407

INGERSOLL, L., WOO, S. Y., DONALDSON, S., GIESLER, J., MAOR, M. H., GOFFINET, D. et al. (1990) Nasopharyngeal carcinoma in the young: a combined MD Anderson and Stanford experience. *International Journal of Radiation, Oncology, Biology and Physics*, 19, 881–887

IRELAND, B., LANIER, A. P., KNUTSON, L., CLIFT, S. E. C. and HARPSTER, A. (1988) Increased risk of cancer in siblings of Alaskan native patients with nasopharyngeal carcinoma. *International Journal of Epidermiology*, (GR6), 17, 509–511

JEANS, W. D., FERNANDO, D. C., MAW, A. R. and LEIGHTON, B. C. (1981) A longitudinal study of the growth of the nasopharynx and its contents in normal children. *British Journal of Radiology*, 54, 117–121

JIE-HUA, Y., CAISEN, L. and YUHUA, H. (1984) Pregnancy and nasopharyngeal carcinoma: a prognostic evaluation of 27 patients. *International Journal of Radiation Oncology, Biology and Physics*, 10, 851–855

JOHNSON, N. E. (1962) Craniopharyngioma – a review with a discussion of transpalatal approach. *Laryngoscope*, 72, 1731–749

KANAGASUNTHERAM, R., WONG, W. C. and CHAN, H. L. (1969) Some observations on the innervation of the human nasopharynx. *Journal of Anatomy*, 104, 361–376

KAWACHI, I., PEARCE, N. and FRASER, J. (1989) A New Zealand Cancer Registry-based study of cancer in wood workers. *Cancer*, 64, 2609–2613

KHOR, T. H., TAN B. C., CHUA, E. J. and CHIA, K. B. (1975) Tumours of the nasopharynx – Singapore 1969–1971. The presenting picture. *Singapore Medical Journal*, 16, 236–243

KHOR, T. H., TAN, B. C., CHUA, E. J. and CHIA, K. B. (1978) Distant metastases in nasopharyngeal carcinoma. *Clinical Radiology*, 29, 27–30

LEE, A. W., SHAM, J. S., POON, Y. F. and HO, J. H. (1989) Treatment of stage 1 nasopharyngeal carcinoma: analysis of patterns of relapse and results of withholding elective neck radiation. *International Journal of Radiation Oncology, Biology and Physics*, 17, 1183–1190

LEE, A. W., POON, Y. F., FOO, W., LAW, S. C., CHEUNG, F. K., CHAN, D. K. et al. (1992) Retrospective analysis of 5037 patients with nasopharyngeal carcinoma treated during 1976–1985: overall survival and patterns of failure. *International Journal of Radiation Oncology, Biology and Physics*, 23, 261–270

LEELA, K., KANAGASUNTHERAM, R. and KHOO, F. Y. (1974) Morphology of the primate nasopharynx. *Journal of Anatomy*, 117, 333–340

LEVINE, P. H., POCINKI, A. G., MADIGAN, P. and BALE, S. (1992) Familial nasopharyngeal carcinoma in patients who are not Chinese. *Cancer*, 70, 1024–1029

MCGRATH, P. (1971) The volume of the human pharyngeal hypophysis in relation to age and sex. *Journal of Anatomy*, 110, 275–282

MCGUIRE, L. J., HUANG, D. P., TEOH, R., ARNOLD, M., WONG, K. and LEE, J. C. K. (1988) Epstein-Barr virus genome in thymoma and thymic lymphoid hyperplasia. *American Journal of Pathology*, 131, 385–390

MALKER, H. S. R., MCLAUGHLIN, J. K., WEINER, J. A., SILVERMAN, D. T., BLOT, W. J., ERICSSON, J. L. et al. (1990) Occupational risk factors for nasopharyngeal cancer in Sweden. *British Journal of Industrial Medicine*, 47, 213–214

MATSON, D. D. and CRIGLER, J. F. (1969) Management of craniopharyngioma in childhood. *Journal of Neurosurgery*, 30, 377–390

MOSS, M. L. (1965) The veloepiglottic sphincter and obligate nose breathing in the neonate. *Journal of Paediatrics*, 67, 330–331

NIEDOBITEK, G., HANSMANN, M. L., HERBST, H., YOUNG, L. S., DIENEMANN, D., HARTMANN, C. A. et al. (1991) Epstein-Barr virus and carcinoma: undifferentiated carcinoma and not squamous cell carcinomas of nasopharynx are regularly associated with the virus. *Journal of Pathology*, 165, 17–24

PAHOR, A. L. (1977) Extramedullary plasmacytoma of the head and neck, parotid and submandibular salivary glands. *Journal of Laryngology and Otology*, 91, 241–258

PARKIN, D. M., MUIR, C. S., WHELAN, S. L., GAO, Y.-T., FERLAY, J. and POWELL, J. (eds) (1992) *Cancer Incidence in Five Continents*, vol VI. IARC Scientific Publ No 120, Lyon: International Agency for Research on Cancer

PAYNE, R., RADVANY, R. and GRUMET, C. (1975) A new second locus HL–A antigen in linkage disequilibrium with HL–A_2 in Cantonese Chinese. *Tissue Antigen*, 5, 69–71

POIRIER, S., BOUVIER, G., MALAVEILLE, C., OHSHIMA, H., SHAO, Y. M., HUBERT, A. et al. (1989) Volatile nitrosamine level and genotoxicity of food samples from high risk areas for nasopharyngeal carcinoma before and after nitrosation. *International Journal of Cancer*, 44, 1088–1094

PRENER, A., NIELSEN, N. H., HANSEN, J. P. H. and JENSEN, O. M. (1987) Cancer pattern among Greenlandic Inuit migrants in Denmark. *British Journal of Cancer*, 56, 679–84

RAAB-TRAUB, N., FLYNN, K., PEARSON, G., HUANGE, A., LEVINE, P., LANIER, A. et al. (1987) The differentiated form of nasopharyngeal carcinoma contains Epstein-Barr virus DNA. *International Journal of Cancer*, 39, 25–29

SHAM, J. S. and CHOY, D. (1990) Prognostic factors of nasopharyngeal carcinoma: a review of 759 cases. *British Journal of Radiology*, 63, 51–58

SHANMUGARATNAM, K. and SOBIN, L. (1991) Histological typing of tumours of the upper respiratory tract and ear. *World Health Organization International Histological Classification Of Tumours*, 2nd edn. Berlin: Springer-Verlag. pp. 7–9

SIMONS, M. J. and DAY, N. E. (1977) Histocompatibility leukocyte antigen patterns and nasopharyngeal carcinoma. *National Cancer Institute Monographs*, 47, 143–146

SOBIN, L. H. and ROS, R. R. (1990) Radiology and the new TNM classification of tumours: the future. *Radiology*, **176**, 1–4

SOM, P. M., SHUGAR, J. M., COHEN, B. A. and BILLER, H. F. (1981) The nonspecificity of the anterior bowing sign in maxillary sinus pathology. *Journal of Computer Assisted Tomography*, **5**, 350–352

SWIFT, P. F. G. and EMERY, J. L. (1973) Clinical observation on response to nasal obstruction in infancy. *Archives of Disease in Childhood*, **48**, 947–519

TAYLOR, J. N. S. and BURWELL, R. G. (1954) Branchiogenic nasopharyngeal cysts. *Journal of Laryngology and Otology*, **68**, 667–669

TEO, P., HO, J. H., CHOY, D., CHOI, P. and TSUI, K. H. (1987) Adjunctive chemotherapy to radical radiation therapy in the treatment of advanced nasopharyngeal carcinoma. *International Journal of Radiation, Oncology Biology and Physics*, **13**, 679–685

TEO, P. M. L., TSAO, S. Y., HO, J. H. C. and YU, P. (1991) A proposed modification of Ho stage-classification for nasopharyngeal carcinoma. *Radiotherapy and Oncology*, **21**, 11–23

TSAO, S. Y. (1993) A new working staging system for nasopharyngeal carcinoma (NPC). In: *The Epstein–Barr Virus and Associated Diseases*, edited by T. Tursz, J. S. Pagano, D. V. Ablashi, G. De Lenoir and G. R. Pearson. Colloque: INSERM/John Libbey Eurotest Ltd. vol 225, pp. 727–734

TU, G. Y., HU, Y. H., XU, G. Z. and YE, M. (1988) Salvage surgery for nasopharyngeal carcinoma. *Archives of Otolaryngology – Head and Neck Surgery*, **114**, 328–329

UICC (1987) *TNM Classification of Malignant tumours*, 4th edn. Berlin: Springer-Verlag. pp. 19–24

WEI, W. I., LAM, K. H. and SHAM, J. S. (1991) New approach to the nasopharynx: the maxillary swing approach. *Head and Neck*, **13**, 200–207

YOUNG, L. S., CLARK, D., SIXBEY, J. W. and RICHINSON, A. B. (1986) Epstein-barr virus receptors on human pharyngeal epithelia. *Lancet*, i, 240–242

YU, M. C. (1991) Nasopharyngeal carcinoma: epidemiology and dietary factors. *IARC-Scientific Publication*, **105**, 39–47

YU, M. C. GARABRANT, D. H., HUANG, T. B. and HENDERSON, B. E. (1990) Occupational and other non-dietary risk factors for nasopharyngeal carcinoma in Guangzhou, China. *International Journal of Cancer*, **45**, 1033–1039

ZENG, Y. (1985) Seroepidemiological studies on nasopharyngeal carcinoma in China. *Advances in Cancer Research*, **14**, 121–138

ZENG, Y., ZHONG, J. M., LI, H. Y., WANG, P. Z., TANG, MA, Y. R. *et al.* (1983) Follow-up studies on Epstein Barr virus IgA/ VCA antibody-positive persons in Zangwu country, China. *Intervirology*, **20**, 190–194

ZENG, Y., ZHANG, L. G., WU, Y. C., HUANF, Y. S., HUANG, N. Q., LI, L. Y., *et al.* (1985) Prospective studies on nasopharyngeal carcinoma in Epstein-Barr virus IgA/VCA antibody positive persons in Wuzhou City, China. *International Journal of Cancer*, **36**, 545–547

ZHANG, E. P., LIAN, P. G., CAI, K. L., CHEN, Y. F., CAI, M. D. and ZHENG, X. X. (1989) Radiation therapy of nasopharyngeal carcinoma: prognostic factors based on 10 year follow-up of 1302 patients. *International Journal of Radiation Oncology, Biology and Physics*, **16**, 301–305

ZHENG W., MCLAUGHLIN, J. K., GAO, Y. T., GAO, R. N. and BLOT, W. J. (1992) Occupational risks for nasopharyngeal cancer in Shanghai. *Journal of Occupational Medicine*, **34**, 1004–1007

14

Tumours of the oropharynx and lymphomas of the head and neck

Peter Rhys Evans

Tumours of the oropharynx are relatively rare in the UK although this is one of the commoner sites in the head and neck for carcinoma. Extranodal lymphomas of the head and neck usually arise from the lymphoid tissue of the tonsil and tongue base and for this reason are included with tumours of the oropharynx. Although the lymphoid tissue of the nasopharynx (adenoids) is also included in Waldeyer's ring, tumours arising in the nasopharynx have quite a different morphology and natural history to those arising in the oropharynx.

For descriptive purposes the oropharynx is that part of the pharynx which extends from the level of the hard palate above to the hyoid bone below (Figure 14.1). The oropharynx is further subdivided into four main sites used for the purpose of tumour classification (Table 14.1).

Table 14.1 Oropharyngeal sites

1 Anterior wall (glossoepiglottic area)
  a Tongue posterior to the vallate papillae (base of tongue or posterior third)
  b Vallecula
    (Anterior or lingual surface of the epiglottis is included in the larynx – suprahyoid epiglottis)
2 Lateral wall
  a Tonsil
  b Tonsillar fossa and faucial pillars
  c Glossotonsillar sulci
3 Posterior wall
4 Superior wall
  a Inferior surface of soft palate
  b Uvula

Tumours may arise from any site within the oropharynx but there is considerable variation in the type and behaviour of tumours in these different sites even for squamous carcinomas. It is therefore of practical importance to divide the oropharynx into the palatine arch and the oropharynx proper (Table 14.2). There is also considerable difference in the incidence of squamous carcinomas in different sites of the oropharynx due to environmental and other aetiological factors. For instance there is a high incidence of squamous carcinomas of the soft palate in women in some parts of Asia due to the habit of reverse smoking. In France and in other Mediterranean countries there is a higher incidence of oropharyngeal tumours than in the UK because of the difference in tobacco and alcohol consumption. In these areas tumours are more common in the glossotonsillar sulcus and in the pharyngoepiglottic fold. In general, squamous carcinoma of the palatine arch is less aggressive and metastasizes later than that elsewhere in the oropharynx.

Two further points of surgical anatomy require emphasis. First, some authors have included the retro-

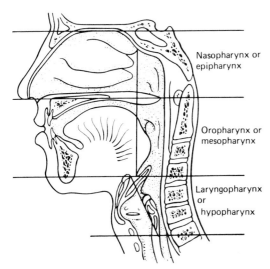

Figure 14.1 Divisions of the pharynx (by kind permission of Blackwell Scientific Publications Ltd, Oxford)

Table 14.2 Divisions of the oropharynx

Palatine arch
Soft palate and uvula
Anterior faucial pillars

Oropharynx proper
Lateral and posterior walls of oropharynx including
    pharyngoepiglottic fold
Base of tongue
Glosso-palatine sulcus
Tonsillar fossa and posterior faucial pillars
Vallecula and lingual surface of epiglottis

molar trigone as part of the oropharynx but strictly speaking this is part of the oral cavity and tumours of the trigone should not be considered as arising in the oropharynx. Second, tumours of the anterior (lingual surface of the epiglottis) are regarded as epilaryngeal tumours and are classified with laryngeal tumours (suprahyoid epiglottis). They do behave and are treated in a similar way to other supraglottic laryngeal tumours but these structures used to be part of the oropharynx in the old UICC classification.

Pathology

As with other sites in the upper aerodigestive tract tumours may arise from different epithelial elements. The lining of the oropharynx contains three structures of importance for the development of tumours:

1 A lining of squamous epithelium
2 The paired tonsils, and the collection of minor lymphoid follicles in the base of the tongue
3 Collections of minor salivary tissue within the epithelium concentrated in the soft palate, the uvula and the capsule of the tonsil.

Growth and metastatic spread of tumours of the oropharynx will be influenced by the surgical anatomy and lymphatic drainage which is described elsewhere.

Generally in the upper aerodigestive tract squamous cell carcinoma constitutes roughly 90% of all epithelial tumours. In the oropharynx the proportion is less (70%) because of the higher incidence of non-Hodgkin's lymphoma (25%) and salivary gland tumours (5%).

Epithelial tumours

Benign epithelial tumours such as papillomas arise from the squamous epithelium and are often seen as incidental findings growing from the margin of the soft palate. These are rarely of any importance. The most important epithelial tumour is squamous cell carcinoma and its variant lymphoepithelioma.

Squamous carcinoma

Approximately 500 new cases of squamous carcinoma of the oropharynx are registered annually in England and Wales. The incidence is 0.8 per 100 000 population per annum with a male to female ratio of 2.5:1. (Figure 14.2). The largest oncology centres see fewer than 30 cases per annum with most seeing fewer than 10. With these small numbers in any one centre there is a lack of published results. National survival figures are difficult to assess because cancer registries use the ICD classification system which often leads to confusion between oropharyngeal and oral cavity tumours (Henk, A'Hern and Taylor, 1993). Another effect of the rarity of this disease is that few clinicians can gain wide experience in tumours of this site and most surgical and radiotherapeutic data are largely anecdotal.

Because of its rich lymphatic drainage lymph node metastases are common and may often be the only presenting feature. For a similar reason metastatic nodes in the neck presenting with an apparent occult primary are often found to have an unsuspected

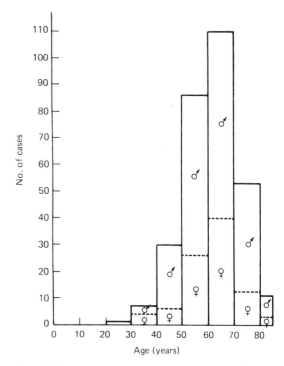

Figure 14.2 Age and sex incidence of squamous carcinoma of the oropharynx (by kind permission of Blackwell Scientific Publications Ltd, Oxford)

primary tumour in the tonsil or tongue base which is only found on histological examination of tonsillectomy or blind biopsy specimens. Table 14.3 shows the subsite distribution and incidence of site and neck node metastases (65%) in a series of 127 patients seen at The Royal Marsden Hospital between 1983 and 1991 with previously untreated squamous cell carcinoma of the oropharynx. This is not influenced by the histological type of tumour since neck metastases are as common with poorly differentiated or anaplastic tumours as with well differentiated lesions. The clinical stages of the tongue base and tonsil tumours are listed in Table 14.4. None had distant metastases at presentation. Performance status was assessed at the beginning of treatment using the WHO system; 75 were performance status 0, 29 status 1, 15 status 2 and eight unrecorded. One characteristic of oropharyngeal carcinomas, particularly those of the tonsil is that nodal metastases occur just as commonly with T1 as with T4 tumours (Table 14.4).

Table 14.3 Subsite and nodal incidence in oropharyngeal squamous carcinoma

Site	No. of patients	Node positive
Base of tongue	42	25 (60%)
Tonsil	73	53 (73%)
Soft palate	8	3
Posterior wall	4	2
Total	127	83 (65%)

The inaccuracy of clinical detection of lymph node metastases is quite high and is generally accepted to be in the region of 30% (20% false negative, 10% false positive). The use of computerized tomography (CT) and magnetic resonance imaging (MRI) has increased the accuracy of detection of neck node metastases particularly in patients with short thick necks. The majority of lymph node metastases from oropharyngeal tumours are in the jugulodigastric node (level 2) and this is also the commonest site for the so-called branchial cyst carcinoma (Figure 14.3). Several studies have shown that a true branchial cyst carcinoma is extremely rare and this diagnosis usually represents cystic degeneration in a metastatic jugulodigastric node from a small undetected primary in the tonsil or tongue base.

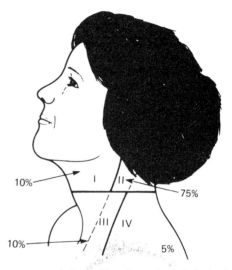

Figure 14.3 Level of palpable nodes in the neck (by kind permission of Blackwell Scientific Publications Ltd, Oxford)

The TNM classification (UICC and AJC) of the primary tumour and that of the neck nodes is given in Table 14.5 and Table 14.6 with the following provisions:

1 The classification applies only to squamous carcinoma
2 There must be histological verification of the disease. The histological features are variable: keratinization may be present or absent, and the degree of differentiation ranges from poorly differentiated or anaplastic tumours to well differentiated lesions

Table 14.4 Clinical staging of tongue base and tonsil squamous carcinomas

	Base of tongue					Tonsil				
	N0	*N1*	*N2*	*N3*	*Total*	*N0*	*N1*	*N2*	*N3*	*Total*
T1	1				1	7	7	7	2	23
T2	13	5	1	3	22	6	5	6	3	20
T3	1	5	2		8	5	4	4	5	18
T4	1	4	1	5	11	2	5	1	4	12
Total	16	14	4	8	42	20	21	18	14	73

reminiscent of normal structures. Spindle and basal cell variants are occasionally seen

3 The extent of disease must be assessed clinically, radiologically and endoscopically.

Synchronous or metachronous primary tumours in the upper aerodigestive tract or lung are found in 10% of patients with a squamous carcinoma of the mouth and oropharynx, although in some geographical areas, particularly where there is a high intake of tobacco and alcohol, this incidence is as high as 20%.

Table 14.5 Classification of primary tumour (UICC/AJC)

Tis	Pre-invasive carcinoma (carcinoma *in situ*)
T0	No evidence of primary tumour
T1	Tumour 2 cm or less in its greatest dimension
T2	Tumour more than 2 cm but not more than 4 cm in its greatest dimension
T3	Tumour more than 4 cm in its greatest dimension
T4	Tumour invades adjacent structures, e.g. through cortical bone, soft tissues of neck, deep (extrinsic) muscle of tongue
TX	The minimum requirement to assess the primary tumour cannot be met

Table 14.6 Nodal classification

N	Regional lymph nodes
N0	No evidence of regional lymph node involvement
N1	Clinically positive homolateral nodes 3 cm or less in diameter
N2	Clinically positive nodes less than 6 cm in diameter
N2a	Single clinically positive homolateral node 3–6 cm in diameter
N2b	Multiple clinically positive ipsilateral nodes less than 6 cm in diameter
N2c	Clinically positive contralateral or bilateral nodes 3–6 cm in diameter
N3	Massive homolateral bilateral or contralateral nodes more than 6 cm in diameter
N3a	Clinically positive homolateral nodes, one more than 6 cm in diameter
N3b	Bilateral clinically positive nodes or contralateral nodes one node larger than 6 cm. (In this situation each side of the neck should be staged separately, i.e. N3b right N2a left)

Lymphoepithelioma

This tumour is widely permeated by lymphocytes which are not neoplastic, though the Regaud type contains nests of non-keratinizing squamous cells and the Schmincke type exhibits isolated transitional cells (hence the alternative name of transitional cell carcinoma).

The important clinical characteristics of this tumour are its extreme radiosensitivity, its tendency to metastasize and its sites – the nasopharynx, the tonsil and the base of tongue. Quick and Cutler recognized this in 1927 as a subdivision of squamous carcinoma, and evidence for an acceptance of this view has grown since. Sometimes these tumours may be confused with lymphoma, as the squamous cell component may be extremely undifferentiated. Immunocytochemistry using the leucocyte common and cytokeratin antibodies may be helpful in doubtful cases. Surface marker studies of the lymphocytic population of lymphoepithelioma have shown these cells to be reactive, because they are composed of B cells, T helper and T suppressor cells and show no evidence of monoclonality or phenotypic restriction. Post-mortem studies on patients who died of this disease also show that the tumour is a variant of squamous cell carcinoma with a coincidental lymphocytic content, because metastases to non-lymphatic sites particularly the liver, contain tumour cells resembling the primary tumour only and do not contain lymphocytes (Stell and Nash, 1987).

Aetiology of squamous cell carcinoma

Squamous cell carcinoma is most common in the sixth and seventh decades and is more frequent in men. It used to be about five times more common in men than women but recently due to the increase in tobacco consumption in women the incidence in this group has doubled. Keratosis with dysplasia is a well recognized precancerous condition in the mouth but it seldom occurs in the oropharynx except on the palatine arch. The practice of reverse smoking in women in some parts of Asia is an important aetiological factor in squamous carcinomas of the palatine arch in this group.

As with other squamous carcinomas of the upper aerodigestive tract, tobacco and alcohol are thought to be the most important aetiological factors which are synergistic. The nitrocarbon carcinogens in tobacco are relatively insoluble in normal saliva but are more soluble in alcohol and therefore are more readily absorbed into the surface epithelium. This is most commonly seen in the sulci of the tonsils and also the glossotonsillar sulcus and the pharyngoepiglottic fold or junctional area between the oropharynx and hypopharynx where squamous carcinomas are particularly common in France.

The mucosal atrophy associated with iron deficiency anaemia might be a precursor of oropharyngeal carcinoma in women but, as seen in the dramatic fall in postcricoid carcinoma in this group, this is probably less important as are other aetiological factors such as syphilis and dental sepsis. Submucosal fibrosis of the palatine arch may also be seen in association with squamous carcinoma.

More recently an association has been found between the development of squamous carcinoma of the oropharynx and human papilloma viruses 8 and 16.

Lymphoma of the head and neck

Lymphomas of the head and neck may arise in nodal or extranodal sites. Both Hodgkin's disease and non-Hodgkin's lymphoma commonly present as lymph node deposits but, whereas Hodgkin's disease is very rare in the oropharynx, non-Hodgkin's lymphoma accounts for about 15–20% of tumours at this site, most being of the B cell type. These have features in common with other tumours of MALT (mucosa associated lymphoid tissue) sites, remaining localized to the MALT sites longer than nodal lymphomas. The commonest type of B cell lymphoma in the oropharynx is the large cell lymphoma of high grade malignancy.

Aetiology

As for most lymphomas the aetiology is largely unknown. Certain associations are recognized, such as the development of lymphoma, often of lymphocytic or immunocytic type (see below), in long-standing cases of Sjögren's disease. African Burkitt's lymphoma, a B cell high grade lymphoma of lymphoblastic type, shows a well known association with immunosuppression due to chronic malaria infection. Epstein-Barr virus is present in nearly all cases, and the lymphoma appears to favour sites of current epithelial proliferations: the odontogenic tissue in the young child, and the breast of the pregnant woman. T cell lymphoma, rare in the oropharynx, shows a well documented association with human T lymphotrophic virus type 1 (HTLV-1) especially in Japan and the Caribbean countries (Stell and Nash, 1987).

Many of the lymphomas of the oropharynx are primary in the sense that there is no demonstrable deposit elsewhere in the body at the time of diagnosis. Sometimes, however, they appear to be secondary to or coincident with deposits at other sites including the neck. These may also include the gastrointestinal tract, the lung and testis.

Classification

Until the early 1970s, the classification of lymphomas was based on morphological features only. A large variety of schemes was used, the best known being that of Rappaport (Rappaport, Winter and Hicks, 1956). When immunological data on the cellular immunoglobulins, and later surface markers, of the lymphoma cells became available, it was apparent that the morphological criteria did not always correspond with the cells' immunological functional characteristics. In particular Rappaport's histiocytic group of large cell lymphomas was found to be principally of B cell type, not of the macrophage type implied by the term. The Kiel classification (Lennert *et al.*, 1975)

is widely used in Europe, and incorporates immunological and morphological data (Table 14.7). Over the past 15 years modifications have been required and in 1982 a National Cancer Institute sponsored study of the six major classifications of non-Hodgkin's lymphoma was published in order to produce some working formulation for clinical usage (Table 14.8). The commonest types of lymphoma in the oropharynx (Table 14.9) are centroblastic (high grade) accounting for about 50% and centroblastic/centrocytic (low grade) (Figures 14.4, 14.5 and 14.6). The centroblastic lymphoma is composed predominantly of large follicle centre transformed lymphocytes with prominent nucleoli, together with variable numbers of infiltrating reactive T cells. This tumour behaves in a highly aggressive manner, but if seen at an early stage (1 and 2) may be curable by local treatment. The low grade lymphomas are less aggressive and contain mixtures of B cells of various types: follicle centre cells in centroblastic/centrocytic lymphoma, lymphocytes in lymphocytic lymphoma and immunocytes (lymphoplasmacytoid cells) in immunocytoma. All types contain T cells, presumably of reactive nature. Paradoxically these low grade tumours may be less curable than the high grade lymphomas because even though the progress is slower, they are frequently disseminated by the time of diagnosis (stages 3 and 4).

Table 14.7 Kiel classification of non-Hodgkin's lymphoma

1 Low grade malignant lymphoma
   a Lymphocytic lymphoma (B cell, T cell, hairy cell leukaemia, mycosis fungoides and Sezary's syndrome, T-zone lymphoma)
   b Immunocytoma
   c Plasmacytoma
   d Centrocytic lymphoma
   e Centroblastic/centrocytic lymphoma (follicular or diffuse)

2 High grade malignant lymphoma
   a Centroblastic lymphoma
   b Lymphoblastic lymphoma (B or T)
   c Immunoblastic lymphoma (with or without plasmablastic differentiation, B and T)

Simplified from Lennert *et al.*, 1978

The relative site incidence of non-Hodgkin's lymphoma of the head and neck and the staging system are shown in Tables 14.10 and 14.11.

Salivary gland tumours

Salivary gland tumours account for about 5% of all tumours of the oropharynx, but this is only a very small proportion of salivary gland tumours arising in the head and neck.

Table 14.8 A working formulation of non-Hodgkin's lymphoma for clinical usage (equivalent or related terms in the Kiel classification are shown)

Working formulation	Kiel equivalent or related terms
Low grade	
A Malignant lymphoma	
Small lymphocytic	
consistent with CLL	ML lymphocytic, CLL
plasmacytoid	ML lymphoplasmacytic/lymphoplasmacytoid
B Malignant lymphoma, follicular	
Predominantly small cleaved cell	
diffuse areas	
sclerosis	ML centroblastic-centrocytic (small), follicular + diffuse
C Malignant lymphoma, follicular	
Mixed, small cleaved and large cell	
diffuse areas	
sclerosis	
Intermediate grade	
D Malignant lymphoma, follicular	
Predominantly large cell	
diffuse areas	
sclerosis	ML centroblastic-centrocytic (large), follicular + diffuse
E Malignant lymphoma, diffuse	
small cleaved cell	
sclerosis	ML centrocytic (small)
F Malignant lymphoma, diffuse	
Mixed, small and large cell	ML centroblastic-centrocytic (small), diffuse
sclerosis	ML lymphoplasmacytic/-cytoid, polymorphic
epithelioid cell component	
G Malignant lymphoma, diffuse	
Large cell	ML centroblastic-centrocytic (large), diffuse
cleaved cell	ML centrocytic (large)
non-cleaved cell	ML centroblastic
sclerosis	
High grade	
H Malignant lymphoma	
Large cell, immunoblastic	ML immunoblastic
plasmacytoid	
clear cell	
polymorphous	T-zone lymphoma
epithelioid cell component	Lymphoepithelioid cell lymphoma
I Malignant lymphoma	
Lymphoblastic	
convoluted cell	ML lymphoblastic, convoluted cell type
non-convoluted cell	ML lymphoblastic, unclassified
J Malignant lymphoma	
Small, non-cleaved cell	
Burkitt's	
follicular areas	ML lymphoblastic, Burkitt type and other B-lymphoblastic
Miscellaneous	
Composite	
Mycosis fungoides	Mycosis fungoides
Histiocytic	
Extramedullary plasmacytoma	ML plasmacytic
Unclassifiable	
Other	

In contrast to the major salivary glands where the majority of tumours are benign, a far higher proportion of tumours arising in the minor salivary glands of the oropharynx are malignant. In a large series of 530 minor salivary gland tumours, 3% affected the oropharynx, almost all of them arising in the tonsillar

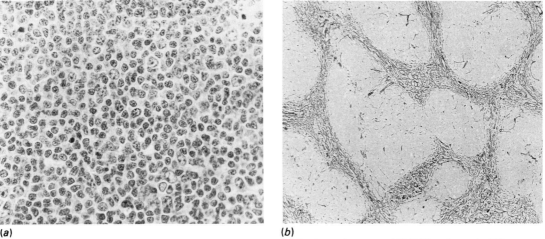

(a) *(b)*

Figure 14.4 *(a)* Cellular details of CB/CC lymphoma (× 600). *(b)* Follicular architecture of CB/CC lymphoma (× 60)

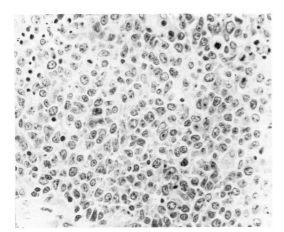

Figure 14.5 Cellular detail of centroblastic lymphoma (× 600)

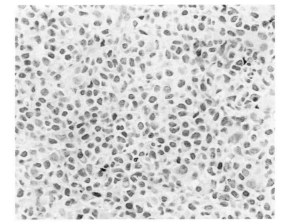

Figure 14.6 Cellular detail of immunocytoma (× 600)

area (Spiro *et al.*, 1973). The vast majority of the malignant tumours are adenoid-cystic carcinomas and most of these arise either in the tonsil or in the soft palate. As with other sites in the head and neck

these tumours behave in a similar way spreading along the nerve sheaths in the perineural lymphatics and also metastasizing to lymph nodes, bone and lung. Although the short-term prognosis with these tumours is good with 80% 5-year survival, between 60 and 80% of patients eventually die from or with metastatic disease.

Table 14.9 Histological types of non-Hodgkin's lymphoma of the oropharynx (%) (Stell and Nash, 1987)

Low grade	
Centroblastic/centrocytic B cell lymphoma	16
Immunocytoma	13
T cell low grade	7
Lymphocytic lymphoma	2
Centrocytic lymphoma	2
High grade	
Other B cell lymphomas (lymphoblastic immunoblastic)	3
Centroblastic lymphoma	53
T cell high grade	4

Table 14.10 Site incidence (%) of non-Hodgkin's lymphoma of the head and neck

Lymph nodes	25
Oropharynx	45
Nasopharynx	15
Nose and sinuses	10
Miscellaneous	5

Table 14.11 Staging classification of non-Hodgkin's lymphoma

Stage 1	Involvement of a single lymph node region (I) or of a single extralymphatic organ site (IE)
Stage 2	Involvement of two or more lymph node regions (number to be stated) on the same side of the diaphragm (stage 2); or localized involvement of an extralymphatic organ or site of one or more lymph node regions on the same side of the diaphragm (IIE)
Stage 3	Involvement of lymph node regions on both sides of the diaphragm which may also be accompanied by local involvement of extralymphatic organs or site (IIIE), by involvement of the spleen (IIIS), or both (IIIE + S)
Stage 4	Diffuse or disseminated involvement of one or more extra lymphatic organ tissues with or without associated lymph node enlargement. The reason for classifying the patient as stage 4 is identified further by specifying the site

Clinical features

Symptoms

The commonest symptoms of oropharyngeal tumours are soreness or discomfort in the throat, pain on swallowing or referred otalgia. About 60% of patients also present with lymph node metastases in the neck, and the oropharynx must be considered as one of the most common sites of origin of an apparently occult primary presenting as lymph node metastases. Large tumours of the base of the tongue give the voice a typical 'plum in the throat' quality and those obstructing the nasopharyngeal opening give a typical hyponasal quality to the voice.

Clinical examination

A full clinical examination of the upper aerodigestive tract and the neck, including fibreoptic examination where appropriate, is essential. In patients with lymphoma, other nodal areas such as the axilla, inguinal region, liver and spleen should also be examined. Two main clinical types of squamous cell carcinoma may be recognized: the exophytic (Figure 14.7) and the ulcerative (Figure 14.8). In general the exophytic type spreads superficially and may be associated with other areas of leucoplakia elsewhere and the ulcerative type infiltrates deeply, but exceptions do occur. An adenocarcinoma presents as a smooth non-ulcerated swelling (Figure 14.9) and the malignant lymphoma (Figure 14.10) as nodular enlargements in the tonsillar fossae or base of tongue. Ulceration eventually supervenes but bleeding is much more commonly associated with squamous carcinoma than with other tumour types.

Most tumours of the oropharynx can be seen easily with good lighting but those originating in the lower part of the oropharynx and tongue base are best viewed with a laryngeal mirror. Fibreoptic nasopharyngeal endoscopy under local anaesthesia has greatly enhanced the ease of examination of these tumours, particularly in assessing the lower extent of the tumour and mobility of structures at the level of the hyoid and also the superior extent if the nasopharynx is involved. Fixation of the palate or tongue should also be noted and careful palpation should be carried out to estimate the extent of infiltration, although this examination will be limited by the sensitivity of the patient.

Some carcinomas may arise deep in the tongue base and any unexplained symptom particularly persistent pain in the throat, especially if this is associated with referred otalgia or a node in the neck, should be assumed to be due to tumour until proven otherwise by thorough palpation under general anaesthetic.

Full examination of the neck must also be carried out to detect any lymph node metastases and each level must be carefully palpated, particularly the upper and middle deep cervical nodes deep to the sternomastoid, from behind the patient, using the tips of the fingers. The inaccuracy of this clinical examination has already been noted with a 20% false negative and 10% false positive error in most series. Nodal metastases from squamous cell carcinomas are typically hard and when small are generally mobile. As they enlarge, those in the deep cervical chain initially become attached to the structures in the carotid sheath and the overlying sternomastoid

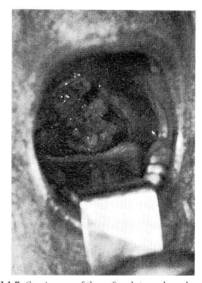

Figure 14.7 Carcinoma of the soft palate and uvula: exophytic type

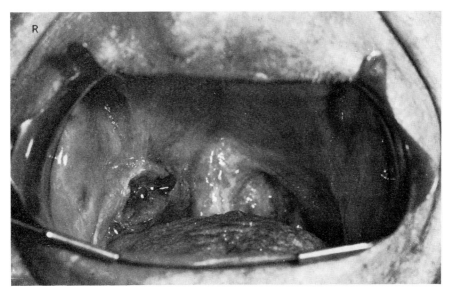

Figure 14.8 Carcinoma of the right tonsil: ulcerative type

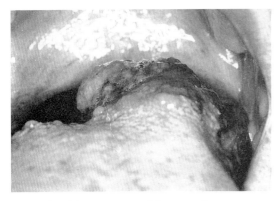

Figure 14.9 Adenocarcinoma of the tongue base

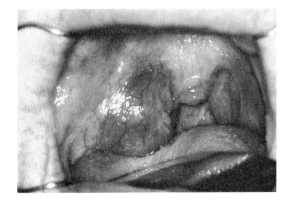

Figure 14.10 Lymphoma of the right tonsil

muscle with limitation in vertical mobility, but later become attached to deeper structures in the prevertebral region with absolute fixation. Lymphomas on the other hand have a rubbery consistency and are generally larger and multiple with matting together of adjacent nodes. Cystic degeneration in a metastatic jugulodigastric node from a squamous carcinoma of the oropharynx may have a similar presentation to a branchial cyst but the latter is a far less likely diagnosis in the older patient.

Investigations

Fine needle aspiration cytology

This should now be considered as an essential part of any examination of the head and neck where there is a suspicious swelling or node enlargement in the neck. It should allow rapid differentiation between a simple branchial cyst and cystic degeneration in a metastatic node, and also confirmation as to whether an enlarged node is simply reactive, carcinomatous or lymphomatous. This has been shown to be of great value as an additional aid in diagnosis complementing clinical examination, and is not associated with seeding deposits.

Radiological examination

Improvements in CT scans using contrast and MRI have significantly improved the assessment of oropharyngeal tumours and nodal metastases. CT scans are more useful and more widely available and will help to show deep infiltration into the tongue base and parapharyngeal space as well as the pterygoid fossa and also show up small suspicious metastatic nodes in necks that are difficult to palpate. The radiological assessment of the head and neck is described more fully elsewhere. Deposits of squamous carcinoma are characterized by peripheral enhancement, central necrosis and irregular margins whereas deposits of lymphoma are larger and more diffuse. Routine chest radiographs should be performed and if lymphoma is suspected, CT scanning of the thorax, abdomen and pelvis is essential.

Ultrasound examination

Ultrasound examination of the neck has recently been shown to be a valuable aid in the diagnosis of lymph node enlargement and recent reports have indicated that this can be as helpful as CT scans but it has the advantage of being cheaper and more accessible for clinical evaluation in the clinic. It may also be used for more accurate fine needle aspiration biopsy techniques.

More recently endoscopic ultrasound probes have been developed to assess the three-dimensional volume of tumours in the upper aerodigestive tract which do appear to correlate more accurately with prognosis than simply the two-dimensional surface area.

Biopsy

Where a tumour is accessible in the oropharynx it is often tempting to take a simple biopsy under local anaesthetic either under direct vision or using a fibreoptic endoscopic technique. It must however be emphasized that a full examination of the upper aerodigestive tract is essential under general anaesthetic to assess the full extent of tumour spread and fixation and also to examine carefully for a second primary lesion. The biopsy specimen needs to be of adequate size and ideally should include a wedge of tissue from the growing margin of the lesion.

Lymph node biopsy is not always necessary if positive histology is available from the primary site and the node is obviously metastatic from the clinical or radiological examination or from a fine needle aspirate examination. In uncertain situations a trucut biopsy may be taken, but if lymphoma is suspected or no primary site is obvious, careful excisional biopsy of the node is far more preferable to incisional biopsy, so that overall architecture is available for assessment.

Blood investigation

This should include complete blood count, erythrocyte sedimentation rate, liver function tests, plasma proteins and immunoglobulins.

Bone marrow aspiration and biopsy

A bone marrow biopsy is essential for lymphoma staging and it is important that a trephine is taken as well as an aspirate; the proportion of positives in bone marrow aspirates from patients with centroblastic/centrocytic lymphoma may be as low as 10%, while trephines give a figure of at least 50%. Decalcification of the specimen is required and immunocytochemical methods can be used as in the lymph node or oropharyngeal specimen (Nash, 1986).

Bone marrow involvement by lymphoma may take several forms (Bartl *et al.*, 1984). In involvement by lymphocytic and immunocytic lymphoma, the pattern is frequently diffuse, which makes minimal involvement difficult to detect. Some small nodules may be seen: these must not be confused with the lymphoid nodules frequently present in normal marrow, especially in elderly people. Centroblastic/centrocytic lymphoma frequently gives a nodular picture in the marrow but these are large pale nodules containing follicle centre cells and are clearly abnormal. A diffuse pattern may also occur and this does not seem closely related to the presence of nodularity in the primary lymphoma. Centroblastic lymphoma is less frequently seen in the marrow but forms clumps or sheets of large transformed follicle centre cells. Individually scattered centroblasts are less frequently seen and, if present in small numbers, might be confused with myeloid precursors (Stell and Nash, 1987).

Treatment of squamous cell carcinoma of the oropharynx

The only two curative forms of treatment for oropharyngeal carcinoma are radiotherapy and surgery, used either separately or combined for more effective treatment of larger tumours. Chemotherapy is still used in some centres as adjuvant or neoadjuvant treatment combined with radiotherapy or surgery but its role has been largely relegated to palliative treatment. Cryosurgery and laser surgery both have a small role to play in some situations. Lastly there is a number of patients where no specific treatment is appropriate.

The treatment modalities adopted in a series of 127 patients with previously untreated squamous cell carcinoma of the oropharynx at the Head and Neck Unit at The Royal Marsden Hospital between 1983 and 1991 are given in Table 14.12. Primary surgical resection was the treatment of choice in 23 patients and in 21 of these patients postoperative radiotherapy was given. The vast majority of patients received primary radical radiotherapy with 96 receiving external beam to the primary and two brachytherapy. Induction neoadjuvant chemotherapy was given in 15 patients of whom four were subsequently

Table 14.12 Treatment of oropharyngeal squamous cell carcinoma The Royal Marsden Hospital 1983–1991 (127 patients)

Primary surgery	23	(Postoperative radiotherapy 21)
Primary radiotherapy	96	(salvage surgery 13)
Primary brachytherapy	2	
Palliative treatment	4	(Died before
No treatment	2	treatment)
Total	142	

(After Henk, A'Hern and Taylor, 1993)

treated by surgery and 11 by irradiation. Four patients received only palliative treatment because of poor general condition and advanced disease, and two died before treatment could be commenced.

Radiotherapy

Radiotherapy is undoubtedly the treatment of choice for localized non-Hodgkin's lymphoma and many squamous cell carcinomas of the oropharynx, giving local disease free control rates of 73% at 3 years.

Lederman's largely historical series dating from 1933 showed an overall survival of 20% (Lederman, 1967). Fletcher and Lindberg's (1966) series from the USA, starting in 1954, showed a 5-year survival of 35% for tonsillar carcinoma and of 50% for palatal tumours.

From 1960 super voltage radiotherapy became widely available in the UK and most oropharyngeal cancer was treated by this modality. Neoadjuvant and synchronous chemotherapy came into vogue in the 1970s, and in the 1980s development of the myocutaneous and free cutaneous flap techniques led to a growing interest and enthusiasm for surgical management.

Results of the UK experience with external beam radiotherapy over the last 30 years have been published by three major centres and do show some interesting trends. The South Wales series consisted of 144 patients treated from 1960 to 1971 and was reviewed in 1978 by Henk. The median age was 67 and 32 patients were considered unsuitable for any attempt at curative treatment because of poor general condition or distant metastases. One hundred and eleven patients received radical radiotherapy of whom 57 had clinically positive nodes; neck dissection was part of the initial planned treatment in only six. The radiotherapy policy was to give a dose of 50 Gy in 15 fractions in 3 weeks to the primary tumour and clinically involved nodes. There was no attempt at elective neck irradiation. Five year crude survival was 28% overall, and 37% in the

radically treated patients. Local control of the primary tumour was 58% and 57% in the radically radiated neck nodes. Twenty two patients died under 5 years after treatment from intercurrent disease and only two from distant metastases. The series from Mount Vernon Hospital reported 86 patients with essentially similar results (Hong, Saunders and Dische, 1990).

The most recent published results from The Royal Marsden Hospital are shown in Table 14.13. The median age of patients in this group was 62 years (34–89 years) and the number of tumours at each of the four subsites in the oropharynx are listed in Table 14.3. Sixty five per cent of the total number had clinically involved nodes at presentation (see Tables 14.3 and 14.4).

Table 14.13 Patients treated by radical radiotherapy

	No. treated	Local disease-free at 3 years (%)
Base of tongue		
T2	21	78
T3	12	72
Tonsil		
T1	11	100
T2	17	58
T3	24	78

After Henk, A'Hern and Taylor, 1993

Of the 127 patients, 119 had irradiation (96 external beam primary treatment, two brachytherapy, 21 postoperative treatment). The radiotherapy policy was to irradiate the primary site and first station lymph nodes in node-negative necks, and the whole neck in node-positive patients. Most patients received a radiation dose of approximately 65 Gy in 6 weeks using daily fractionation; 20 patients in whom the irradiated volume was small, i.e. field area less than 45 cm^2, received 55 Gy in 20 fractions over 40 weeks.

Of the 98 patients who had primary radiotherapy 13 had salvage surgery, four had palliative radiotherapy and two had no treatment at all or died before treatment was instigated.

The actuarial survival of the whole group was 40% at 5 years and the relationship between survival and performance status, stage and age is given in Table 14.14. The local disease-free rate at the primary site was 73% at 3 years and all but one recurrence occurred within 2 years of treatment (Tables 14.13 and 14.14). The probability of freedom from local recurrence at 3 years is given in Table 14.15 according to performance status and stage. Univariate analysis showed that there were significant differ-

Table 14.14 5-Year actuarial survival (95% confidence limits)

All patients		40%	(29–50)	
Performance status	0	54%	(38–68)	
	1	23%	(8–42)	
	2	0		*P < 0.01
Stage	T1	49%	(9–80)	
	T2	47%	(30–62)	
	T3–4	29%	(15–44)	*P < 0.02
	N0	58%	(41–72)	
	N1	47%	(24–67)	
	N2–3	14%	(3–34)	*P < 0.02
Age	< 55	59%	(35–77)	
	55–64	50%	(28–69)	
	> 65	21%	(9–36)	*P < 0.01

* Log-rank test for trend. After Henk, A'Hern and Taylor, 1993

Table 14.15 Probability of freedom from local recurrence at 3 years (95% confidence limits)

All patients		73%	(62–81)	
Performance status	0	80%	(68–88)	
	1	62%	(39–79)	
	2	0		P < 0.001
Stage	T1	87%	(59–97)	
	T2	67%	(50–80)	
	T3–4	72%	(54–84)	n.s.

After Henk, A'Hern and Taylor, 1993

ences in survival according to the T stage, the N stage, age and especially performance status but that on multivariate analysis the overwhelming significant factor was performance status.

As with carcinoma at most sites in the head and neck, 5-year survival has not increased dramatically over the past 30 years, although local disease free control has increased by about 20%. This improvement in local control is due to several factors including the introduction of megavoltage treatment with improvement of radiotherapy techniques using larger treatment volumes and smaller fraction sizes, earlier diagnosis, possibly a more aggressive therapeutic approach, and the combination of surgery with postoperative radiotherapy in more advanced disease.

The median age of the most recent series was younger (62 versus 67 years) and although the two groups cannot strictly be compared, it does reflect an ominous trend of increasing incidence of these tumours in younger patients. The performance status in the younger group however is correspondingly better which does influence 5-year survival rates.

Although better local cure rates in oropharyngeal and other head and neck carcinomas are being achieved, the overall survival rate has not improved because of a corresponding increase in deaths from metastases, second primaries and intercurrent disease. As at other sites however the most distressing aspect is uncontrolled pharyngeal tumour and at least with improved local control and rehabilitation the quality of life in these patients is in general significantly better.

Surgery

Surgery was first described for tonsillar carcinoma at the end of the nineteenth century but until antibiotics became available in the 1940s the risk of infection was too great to attempt combined operations on the neck and the pharynx. Indeed Crile's original indications for radical neck dissection were confined to very favourable cases (Crile, 1906).

In the 1950s Hayes Martin pioneered the development of more radical en bloc resection of tumours of the oropharynx and neck with the benefit of sulphonamides and penicillin and also blood transfusion. In 1951, he described how the term 'Commando' operation came to be used for this type of operation: the technical definition of the operation was too long winded for every day use and was therefore shortened to Commando (*com*bined neck dissection, *mand*ibulectomy and resection of the *o*ropharynx). At that time the Commandos were recruited for aggressive warfare in difficult circumstances and his house staff borrowed the term and applied it to the operation (perhaps with similar analogy!). No attempt was made at reconstruction, although resection of the ascending ramus of the mandible allowed primary closure. The functional results were adequate but usually there was quite unsightly deviation of the remaining mandible across the midline with occlusion problems and also a cosmetic defect in the side of the face (Figure 14.11*a, b*).

The introduction of the deltopectoral flap by Bakamjian in 1965 allowed repair of larger defects, albeit with a two-stage procedure. The ability to close larger defects allowed the surgeon more confidence with wider resection margins with less risk of local recurrence.

During the last 15 years however there have been great strides in reconstruction which have allowed far better functional and cosmetic rehabilitation of these patients. There is however still considerable controversy about the primary management of oropharyngeal tumours and the place of surgery. In patients where there is little chance of cure they should not be offered surgery, e.g. those with trismus or bilateral fixed neck glands. Most patients with an oropharyngeal tumour without a palpable lymph node in the neck do quite well with radical radio-

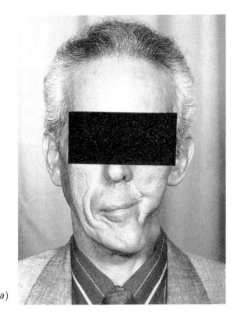

(a)

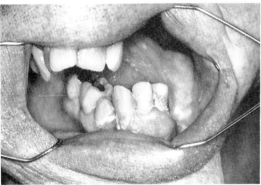

(b)

Figure 14.11 (a) Typical long-term cosmetic appearance after Commando operation with primary closure and no reconstruction of oropharynx. (b) Intraoral view showing mandibular swing

survival for patients with nodes over 3 cm in diameter was 14% (see Table 14.14).

In our experience those patients with no gland or a gland smaller than 3 cm may have a reasonable chance of responding to radiotherapy as the initial treatment but in larger nodes there is a very high incidence of capsular rupture (over 99% in nodes over 3 cm) and these patients do very poorly with radiotherapy. It has therefore been shown fairly clearly that surgery usually with postoperative radiotherapy for these larger tumours with large nodes in the neck achieves far better results than primary radiotherapy (60% compared with 0%; Calamel and Hoffmeister, 1967). It is a sad reflection that in some centres squamous cell carcinoma in the head and neck is routinely given radiotherapy irrespective of the stage or the expected results. These tumours are rare and frequently the necessary surgical expertise is not available. It is however quite wrong to opt for radiotherapy in this instance, since by the time a recurrence or persistent disease is recognized after radiotherapy, salvage surgery is often not possible. If attempted, the risks of complications are far greater and cure is seldom achieved. For advanced tumours of the pharynx, combined surgery with postoperative radiotherapy achieves much better results and if the surgery is not available locally patients should be referred to regional centres where major head and neck surgery is carried out routinely.

Of the 13 patients who had primary radiotherapy for early stage disease and salvage surgery, the 5-year survival rate after initial diagnosis and treatment is 50% and after the actual surgery is 39%.

Tumours of the lingual surface of the epiglottis are uncommon and are best treated with supraglottic laryngectomy or epiglottectomy. A small tumour at this site may be excised endoscopically and it does seem difficult to justify a course of radical radiotherapy since the defect in the epiglottis is much the same with either method but the morbidity associated with the prolonged radiotherapy course is far greater. For larger tumours of the epiglottis supraglottic laryngectomy does give very good results.

Cervical metastases

Despite overwhelming evidence that neck nodes greater than 3 cm (N2 and N3) from an oropharyngeal primary do badly with primary radiotherapy treatment this modality is still used in many centres. Radical neck dissection (or modified neck dissection with preservation of the accessory nerve in suitable cases) is the treatment of choice in these patients together with resection of the primary tumour and reconstruction. Bilateral nodes can usually be treated surgically by careful preservation of one or both internal jugular veins. Fixed nodes may be resected successfully particularly if there is a significant inflammatory element in which case the CT scan may well

therapy and should be offered this form of treatment initially.

There are therefore two groups of patients who should be offered surgery: those whose tumour has failed to respond or recurred after radiotherapy, and those with a tonsillar carcinoma and a palpable gland on one side of the neck. Although the latter patient is treated in many centres by primary radiotherapy followed by a radical neck dissection if the gland is persistent, in the author's experience the gland in the neck may become inoperable by the time the radiotherapy reaction has settled, and such a policy gives poor results. In Lederman's (1967) series the 5-year survival was 12.5% for this group and in the recent Royal Marsden experience 5-year

overestimate the extent of disease. The natural history of the disease can rarely be altered in the presence of bilateral fixed nodes.

The treatment of small nodes up to 3 cm in diameter (N1) is more controversial and there is some justification in treating a small primary with a small node with radiotherapy followed by neck dissection at 3 months since about 50% of these necks can be controlled.

The treatment of the neck in patients with no palpable nodes is also controversial since at least 60–70% of apparently N0 necks will contain nodes with microscopic tumour deposits. In a study of nasopharyngeal and oropharyngeal carcinoma, Fletcher (1972) showed a 12% recurrence rate in necks where the upper cervical nodes and the tumour were irradiated compared with a 1.7% incidence of recurrence in the neck where the whole neck and the tumour were irradiated. He also showed a 24% incidence of eventual contralateral node involvement where ipsilateral neck irradiation was given compared with 3% eventual contralateral nodes where bilateral neck radiotherapy was given. On this basis bilateral prophylactic neck irradiation seems logical where radiotherapy is given to the primary tumour. If the primary tumour is treated surgically, however, a prophylactic neck dissection is justified particularly if reconstruction is being carried out with a myocutaneous pedicled flap or a free radial forearm flap. Although prophylactic neck treatment has not been shown to improve 5-year survival rates the local control rate is significantly improved.

Combined surgery and radiotherapy

Combined surgery with postoperative radiotherapy is generally considered to give the best result in terms of survival for more advanced oropharyngeal tumours. An analysis of the failures of radiotherapy shows that the most frequent cause of failure is from local and regional recurrence. The causes of radiation failure are:

1 The central portion of the primary tumour may be relatively anoxic and hence most radioresistant. While peripheral, better oxygenated parts of the tumour might be killed, the central portion could regain its malignant potential after a period of quiescence.
2 Metastases to lymph nodes are relatively radioresistant.
3 Local or distant spread outside the treated field may have taken place before therapy, and radiation then does not encompass the lesion.
4 The tumour itself may be radioresistant, i.e. it may be able to resist ionizing radiation better than surrounding vital tissue. Preoperative radiotherapy has been promoted in the past but prospective

randomized trials, such as that carried out by Strong *et al.* (1978), have shown that preoperative radiotherapy does not increase survival. Postoperative radiotherapy has however been shown to increase survival particularly for larger oropharyngeal tumours.

Reconstruction after surgery

There have been four phases of repair of the surgical defect: using local flaps, axial flaps, myocutaneous flaps and free flaps.

Local cervical flaps (Figure 14.12 *a, b, c, d*) tend to be of poor viability; 33% of flaps are lost partially or completely because of necrosis; furthermore the use of these flaps leads to a temporary fistula in the neck and possible exposure of the carotid vessels with potentially dangerous results. This method has now been abandoned.

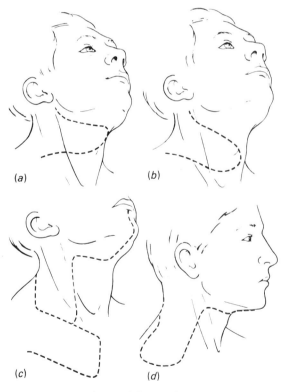

Figure 14.12 Local cervical flaps used in repair of oropharyngeal defects

Axial flaps include the temporal and deltopectoral flaps. The temporal flap (Figure 14.13) has few of the disadvantages of cervical flaps. The flap is virtually always viable provided that the external carotid

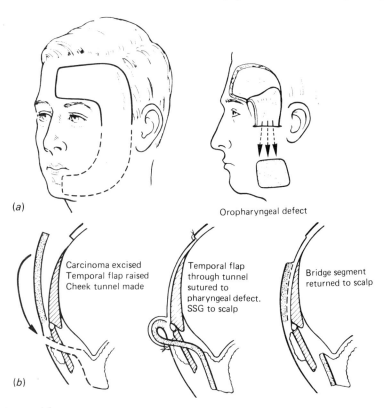

(a)

Oropharyngeal defect

Carcinoma excised
Temporal flap raised
Cheek tunnel made

Temporal flap
through tunnel
sutured to
pharyngeal defect.
SSG to scalp

Bridge segment
returned to scalp

(b)

Figure 14.13 The temporal flap

artery has not been ligated with the radical neck dissection. There is a temporary fistula below the zygomatic arch but this does not leak saliva because it is placed high in the lateral oral cavity above the saliva flow and the carotid sheath is not exposed so carotid bleeding is not necessarily a problem. The main disadvantage of this type of flap is the very obvious defect on the forehead which is covered with a split skin graft. For this reason a forehead flap is not the primary reconstructive method of choice but may be used as an alternative method where there is a high risk of arterial disease and where prolonged anaesthesia is contraindicated. It may however be a useful alternative in balding patients where the graft can be taken from the central part of the scalp and successfully camouflaged by a split skin graft.

The deltopectoral flap can also be used for repair following excision of tumours of the oropharynx. The flap is delivered into the mouth through a temporary fistula and sutured to the edges of the defect. The subcutaneous part of the pedicle may be de-epithelialized to avoid a secondary operation but alternatively, the base of the flap is divided after 3 weeks and the proximal end of the flap is returned to the chest wall and the fistula closed. It is important at the primary

operation to protect the carotid sheath with some form of flap such as the levator scapulae muscle which prevents leakage into the lower part of the neck. The necrosis rate of these flaps is less than 10% if proper precautions are taken and the functional result for speaking and swallowing and the cosmetic appearance is satisfactory.

Over the last 15 years the development of myocutaneous flaps and free flaps has superseded the use of local or regional axial flaps for reconstruction of the oropharynx. The pectoralis major myocutaneous flap (Figure 14.14 *a, b*) can be used for one stage reconstruction of oropharyngeal defects (Rhys Evans and Das Gupta, 1981) but this flap does suffer from the disadvantage of being tethered through the neck to the chest wall below the clavicle by its pedicle.

Perhaps the most important development in reconstructive surgery of the oropharynx in the last 10 years has been the use of the free vascularized flaps, the commonest being the radial free forearm flap (Figure 14.15*a, b*). The flap is designed to conform to the oropharyngeal defect on the lower forearm and raised with the radial artery and either the cephalic vein or the venae comitans of the radial artery. The flap is then transferred to the neck where the vessels are anastomosed to appropriate vessels in the upper

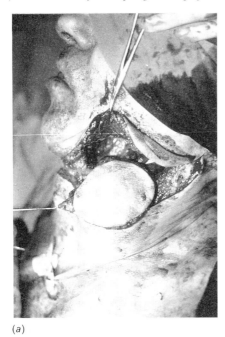

(*a*)

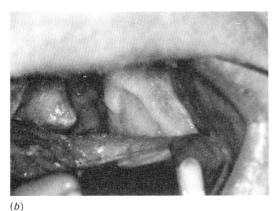

(*b*)

Figure 14.14 (*a*) The pectoralis major myocutaneous flap being delivered into the neck for reconstruction of the oropharynx. (*b*) The left tonsillar area reconstructed with a pectoralis major myocutaneous flap at 3 years

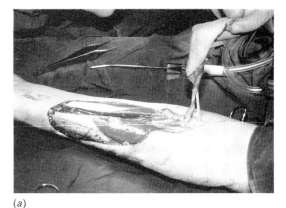

(*a*)

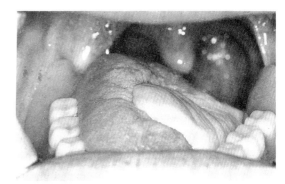

(*b*)

Figure 14.15 (*a*) A radial forearm flap being raised on the radial artery and cephalic vein before transfer to the oropharynx. (*b*) An oropharyngeal/tongue base defect repaired with a radial forearm flap at 2 years with dentures in use

Chemotherapy

The role of chemotherapy has largely been relegated to that of palliative treatment in patients with advanced or recurrent squamous carcinomas of the oropharynx. There have been numerous phase 2 trials where the response of tumours is measured, but the survival of patients has not in general been increased by more than 6 months. Only about 25% of head and neck cancers respond to chemotherapeutic regimens but the advantages of a slight increase in survival rates are heavily outweighed by the adverse effects of toxic reactions. Only rarely have phase 3 trials been carried out, i.e. with untreated controls and with measurement of patient survival. These have shown that only cisplatin is effective and that some agents actually reduce the survival because of increased toxicity. The results of phase 3 trials of adjuvant chemotherapy with radiotherapy for treatable tumours have been even more disappointing and, although a high proportion of tumours do respond temporarily, there is no increased benefit in terms of survival.

neck and the flap is sutured into the defect. In our experience the most appropriate arterial anastomosis is to the external carotid artery or main branches of that artery and venous drainage is to the internal or external jugular veins. Special reconstructive expertise is required for this microvascular anastomosis but in experienced hands the viability of these flaps is in the region of 90%. The myocutaneous flap has the advantage of bulk and is more reliable in less experienced hands but the free flap has better results in terms of speech and swallowing rehabilitation because of its relative mobility.

Cryosurgery

The destructive properties of freezing have been known for a long time, but cryosurgery has been used clinically only in the last few decades. It appears to achieve its effects by rupture of nuclear and cellular membranes, alterations in lipoprotein components of cell membranes, pH changes, toxic concentration of electrolytes, polymerization and denaturation of proteins, and vascular stasis and microthrombi leading to ischaemia. It appears that there must be rapid repeated freezing and thawing with sufficient duration of freezing to a temperature of at least $-20°C$ for a good therapeutic response to be achieved. The advantages claimed for cryosurgery are relative avascularity with little or no postoperative bleeding, minimal tissue response, pain relief mediated by destruction of nerve endings, resistance of some tissues such as bone to the effect of freezing and possibly an immunological effect due to the altered antigenicity of the tumour tissue.

Cryosurgery does have a place in the treatment of tumours of the oral cavity and oropharynx, but this is mainly for benign lesions, hyperkeratosis, haemangioma and tonsillectomy in haemophiliacs for instance. Small salivary tumours may respond well in unfit patients and small recurrences of squamous carcinoma will also sometimes resolve. But for the average large recurrence of squamous carcinomas cryosurgery can at best achieve reduction in size of the tumour and pain relief. For the vast majority of patients with squamous carcinoma this form of treatment is at best only palliative.

Laser therapy

Excision of oropharyngeal tumours with the laser may achieve useful bloodless dissection of tumours, particularly in the elderly, providing a simple technique appropriate for patients who cannot be considered for major reconstructive surgery, with minimal postoperative sequelae.

Treatment of non-Hodgkin's lymphoma

Localized lymphoma is potentially curable by radiotherapy. The use of this modality followed by chemotherapy is another approach to treatment and the available data show an advantage for patients treated by the combined approach compared with radiotherapy alone. For disseminated non-Hodgkin's lymphoma the treatment of choice is systemic chemotherapy.

Single agent chemotherapy

A wide variety of agents is active in non-Hodgkin's lymphoma. They include the alkylating agents (nitrogen mustard, cyclophosphamide and chlorambucil), the vinca alkaloids (vincristine and vinblastine), procarbazine and prednisolone, bleomycin, doxorubicin and the nitrosoureas (BCNU and CCNU). The response to single agent chemotherapy, the duration of response and the overall survival vary with histological type, results consistently being superior in patients with nodular lymphoma in contrast to those with diffuse disease. Single agent chemotherapy with an alkylating agent may be the treatment of choice in patients with advanced 'favourable' histology.

Combination chemotherapy

Combination chemotherapy is the treatment of choice in patients with unfavourable histological types which, in contrast to the favourable histological lymphomas, show a rapidly progressive and fatal course unless complete remission is achieved. Once complete remission has been maintained for 2 years, the probability of a relapse is low, suggesting that a cure is possible. A partial response in these histological types gives little survival benefit.

The first successful combination regimen for non-Hodgkin's lymphoma was cyclophosphamide, vincristine and prednisolone, forming the CVP and COP regimens. CVP consists of short pulses of chemotherapy at 21-day intervals with cyclophosphamide on days 1–5 at a dose of 400 mg/m²/day. The South West Oncology Group called their regimen COP and administered cyclophosphamide at a dose of 800 mg/m² every 2 weeks for six courses. Other modifications have included cyclophosphamide on day 1 only on a day 1–8 schedule or on a day 1–4 schedule. CVT and COP produce complete responses in 60–90% of patients with favourable histological lymphoma and may be used as an alternative to single agent therapy in this group, although the superiority of combination therapy has not been established.

In an attempt to improve results in the unfavourable histological types more aggressive regimens including MOPP and C-MOPP (cyclophosphamide replacing mustine) and regimens developed by adding bleomycin and doxorubicin to the CVP regimens to form BACOP, have been tested. Each of these regimens gave complete response rates in more than 40% of patients.

The South West Oncology Group added doxorubicin to a modified COP to produce the CHOP regimen. In a study comparing CHOP with COP, the complete remission rate achieved with CHOP was 67%, superior to the 60% remission rate on COP for patients with diffuse lymphoma. The addition of bleomycin does not appear to have improved the results of treatment.

Involvement of the central nervous system is a common problem in lymphoma, being the site of first relapse in 26% of patients in one series. It is suggested that, in parallel with acute lymphoblastic lymphoma, prophylactic intrathecal therapy should be a component of treatment in patients with advanced diffuse lymphoma (Carter, Bakowski and Hellmann, 1981).

Treatment of salivary gland tumours

Benign salivary gland tumours are almost exclusively pleomorphic adenomas, and are treated by local excision with a generous margin. Malignant tumours, generally adenoid cystic carcinomas are treated by radical surgery as for squamous carcinoma. Radiotherapy has no place in the primary treatment of these diseases but is very useful if tumour remains at the surgical margins and may be used for palliation.

References

BAKAMJIAN, J. A. (1965) A two stage method for pharyngo-esophageal reconstruction with a primary pectoral skin flap. *Plastic and Reconstructive Surgery*, **36**, 173–184

BARTL, R., FRISCH, B., BURKHARDT, R., JAGER, K., PAPPENBERGER, G. and HOFFMAN-FEZER, G. (1984) Lymphoproliferations in the bone marrow: identification and evolution, classification and staging. *Journal of Clinical Pathology*, **37**, 233–254

CALAMEL, P. M. and HOFFMEISTER, F. S. (1967) Carcinoma of the tonsil: comparison of surgical and radiation therapy. *American Journal of Surgery*, **114**, 582–586

CARTER, S. K., BAKOWSKI, M. T. and HELLMAN, K. (1981) *Chemotherapy of Cancer*, 2nd edn. New York: John Wiley and Sons

CRILE, G. (1906) Excision of cancer of the head and neck with special reference to the plan of dissection based upon 132 operations. *Journal of the American Medical Association*, **47**, 1780–1786

FLETCHER, G. H. (1972) Elective radiation of subclinical disease in cancers of the head and neck. *Cancer*, **29**, 1450–1454

FLETCHER, G. H. and LINDBERG, R. D. (1966) Squamous cell carcinoma of the tonsillar area and palatine arch. *American Journal of Roentgenology*, **96**, 574

HENK, J. M. (1978) Results of radiotherapy for carcinoma of the oropharynx. *Clinical Otolaryngology*, **3**, 137–143

HENK, J. M., A'HERN, R. P. and TAYLOR, K. (1993) *Carcinoma of the Oropharynx in the United Kingdom. Head and Neck Cancer*, vol. 3, edited by J. T. Johnson and M. S. Didolkar. London: Excerpta Medica. pp. 779–784

HONG, A., SAUNDERS, M. I., DISCHE, S., FERMONT, D., ASHFORD, R. F. and MAHER, J. (1990) An audit of head and neck cancer treatment in a regional centre for radiotherapy and oncology. *Clin. Oncol.*, **2**, 130–137

LEDERMAN, M. (1967) Cancer of the pharynx. *Journal of Laryngology and Otology*, **81**, 151

LENNERT, K., MOHRI, N., STEIN, H. and KAISERLING, E. (1975) Histopathology of malignant lymphoma. *British Journal of Haematology*, **31** (suppl.), 193–203

MARTIN, H., DELVALLE, B., EHRLICH, H. and CAHAN, W. B. (1951) Neck dissection, *Cancer*, **4**, 41–99

NASH, J. R. G. (1986) An immunohistochemical study of non-Hodgkin's lymphomas: correlation of morphological appearances and immunophenotype in 148 cases. *Histopathology*, **10**, 793–813

NATIONAL CANCER INSTITUTE SPONSORED STUDY OF CLASSIFICATIONS OF NON-HODGKINS LYMPHOMA (1982) *Cancer*, **49**, 2112–2135

QUICK, D. and CUTLER, M. (1927) Transitional cell epidermoid carcinoma: radiosensitive type of oral tumour. *Surgery, Gynecology and Obstetrics*, **45**, 320–325

RAPPAPORT, H., WINTER, W. J. and HICKS, E. B. (1956) Follicular lamphoma. A reevaluation of its position in the scheme of malignant lymphomas. *Cancer*, **9** 792–795

RHYS EVANS, P. H. and DAS GUPTA, A. (1981) The use of pectoralis major myocutaneous flap for one-stage reconstruction of the base of the tongue, *Journal of Laryngology and Otology*, **95**, 809–816

SPIRO, R. H. KOSS, L. G. HAJDU, S. I. and STRONG, M. S. (1973) Tumours of minor salivary gland origin. *Cancer*, **31**, 117–123

STELL, P. M. and NASH, J. R. G. (1987) Tumours of the oropharynx. In: *Scott Brown's Otolaryngology*, 5th edn, edited by A. G. Kerr, Vol. 5, *Laryngology*, edited by P. M. Stell, London: Butterworths. pp. 235–249

STRONG, M. S., VAUGHN, C. W., KAYNE, H. L., ARAL, I. M., UCKMAKLI, A. and FELDMAN, M. (1978) A randomised trial of preoperative radiotheraphy in cancer of the oropharynx and hypopharynx. *American Journal of Surgery*, **136**, 494–500

15

Tumours of the hypopharynx

Randall P. Morton and Nicholas P. McIvor

Surgical anatomy

The hypopharynx lies below and behind the base of the tongue, and behind and on each side of the larynx. It extends from the level of the hyoid bone superiorly to the lower border of the cricoid inferiorly. The three anatomical subsites are the pyriform fossa, the postcricoid area and the posterior pharyngeal wall (Figure 15.1; Table 15.1).

The *pyriform fossae* are channels formed on either side of the larynx and are open posteriorly. The lateral walls are continuous with the posterior pharyngeal wall, and the medial wall on each side contributes to the aryepiglottic fold and merges posteriorly with the postcricoid mucosa.

The upper part of the fossa is bounded laterally by the thyrohyoid membrane, and medially by the aryepiglottic fold. The deepest (most inferior) portion of the fossa is known as the *apex*. The apex is related laterally to the thyroid cartilage, medially to the cricoid cartilage, and inferiorly to the paraglottic space, which is the potential space bounded by the

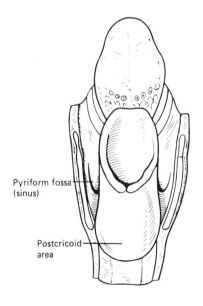

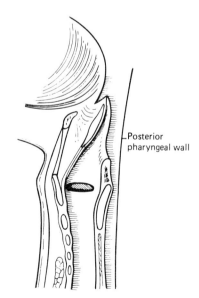

Posterior pharyngeal wall

Pyriform fossa (sinus)

Postcricoid area

Figure 15.1 Anatomical regions of the hypopharynx

Table 15.1 Definition of hypopharyngeal subsites (after UICC)

1 Pyriform fossa (sinus) extends from the pharyngoepiglottic fold to the upper end of the oesophagus. It is bounded laterally by the thyroid cartilage and medially by the surface of the aryepiglottic fold and the arytenoid and cricoid cartilages
2 Postcricoid area (pharyngo-oesophageal junction) extends from the level of the arytenoid cartilages and connecting folds to the inferior border of the cricoid cartilage
3 Posterior pharyngeal wall extends from the level of the floor of the vallecula to the level of the cricoarytenoid joints

thyroid ala laterally and the conus elasticus and the quadrangular membrane medially (Figure 15.2, see Figure 15.5). Tumours involving the medial wall and apex of the pyriform fossa easily gain entrance to the paraglottic space and then pass inferiorly lateral to the vocal cord.

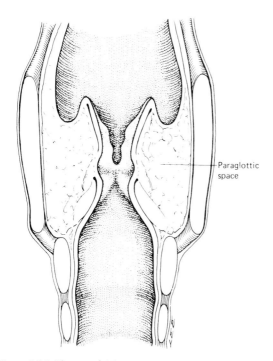

Figure 15.2 The paraglottic space

The *postcricoid* area lies behind the larynx and extends from the level of the arytenoid cartilages to the inferior border of the cricoid cartilage. It is continuous below with the upper end of the oesophagus.

The *posterior pharyngeal wall* is less well defined. It can be regarded as that part of the hypopharynx

lying between two lines projected posteriorly from the vocal cords as they lie in the cadaveric position (Figure 15.3). It begins superiorly at the level of the hyoid bone and ends inferiorly at the level of the arytenoids. It is separated from the prevertebral muscles by a fascial space.

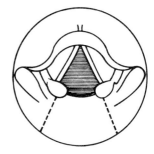

Figure 15.3 Schematic depiction of the posterior pharyngeal wall

The hypopharynx acts as a conduit for oral intake, participating in a complex neuromuscular coordinated activity involving also the oral cavity, oropharynx, larynx and cervical oesophagus. Tumours can impair this activity by virtue of a mass effect and, rarely, by invasion of the nerve supply.

The hypopharynx is lined throughout by squamous epithelium. There is a rich underlying network of lymphatics in the pyriform fossae but this is less pronounced in the other subsites. The lymphatics generally drain to the deep cervical chain. The inferior part of the pyriform fossa and the postcricoid area also drain to the paratracheal nodes; the posterior pharyngeal wall is served by the retropharyngeal nodes.

Carcinomas of the hypopharynx readily invade neighbouring structures, so that postcricoid tumours often involve the cervical oesophagus and vice-versa. Similarly it is not unusual for pyriform fossa tumours to spread to the supraglottic larynx (Figure 15.4). Tumours arising on the aryepiglottic fold may straddle the fold, making it difficult to determine whether they are primarily supraglottic or hypopharyngeal in origin.

Pathology

Tumours of the hypopharynx may be mesodermal or epithelial in origin, and benign or malignant in nature.

Benign tumours are very rare, the most common being the fibrolipoma and leiomyoma. They are polypoid tumours which usually present with dysphagia, and on videofluoroscopy or barium swallow have the typical appearance of a smooth constant mass lying in the lumen of the oesophagus. Other benign tumours usually arise from minor salivary tissue, and

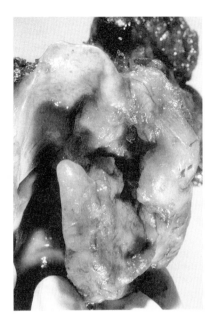

Figure 15.4 A large right pyriform fossa cancer occupies the whole of the fossa, and has destroyed the right aryepiglottic fold. The epiglottic free margin is intact. The larynx has been divided posteriorly in the midline to illustrate the normal left hemilarynx (see also Figures 15.5 and 15.7)

are either pleomorphic adenomas or cystadenomas (similar in histological appearance to Warthin's tumour) and characterized by a submucosal mass which can go unnoticed until quite large.

Malignant tumours of the hypopharynx are almost exclusively squamous cell carcinomas. Moderately and poorly differentiated tumours predominate, especially pyriform fossa tumours. Jones (1992) reported only 20% of hypopharyngeal tumours to be well differentiated. Batsakis (1979) stated that 'the great majority' of hypopharyngeal tumours are poorly differentiated. In any event, the malignant tumours of the hypopharynx carry a poor prognosis, with most series reporting less than 30% 5-year survival.

Non-squamous hypopharyngeal malignancies are generally minor salivary gland in origin (usually adenoid cystic carcinomas) or mesenchymal tumours such as plasmacytomas.

Surgical pathology

Tumours are usually classified according to the anatomical site of origin (see Table 15.1). It can be difficult to ascribe a site of origin when the tumour has spread to involve one or more anatomical sites. Even differentiation between laryngeal and hypopharyngeal tumours can be difficult when the aryepiglottic fold has been replaced or covered by tumour.

Such difficulties may explain some of the observed differences in the reported rate of relative frequency of tumours from the various subsites. Even so there is an undoubted marked variation in relative frequency of postcricoid cancers among series of hypopharyngeal cancers (see below, Epidemiology).

Tumours of the pyriform fossa which involve the lateral wall may invade through the thyrohyoid membrane and become palpable in the neck. This can be mistaken for a nodal metastasis rather than direct extension; however, a nodal metastasis generally will not move with swallowing. Tumours of the medial wall may invade the aryepiglottic fold and enter the paraglottic space. This will lead to vocal cord fixation (Figure 15.5).

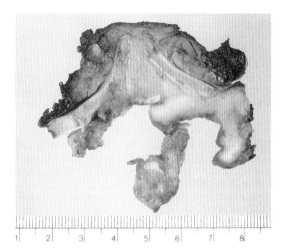

Figure 15.5 Horizontal section through the specimen shown in Figure 15.4. The tumour of the right pyriform fossa extends into the right paraglottic space, to the anterior commissure

Vocal cord paralysis will also occur if either the recurrent laryngeal nerve or the cricoarytenoid joint is invaded. This is more likely with postcricoid carcinoma than with pyriform fossa tumours.

Submucosal spread of 10 mm or more must be borne in mind when considering resection margins (Harrison, 1970). This is particularly important in the membranous tracheo-oesophageal wall where postcricoid tumours often recur.

Hypopharyngeal tumours may metastasize early to the cervical nodes. This is most likely in pyriform fossa lesions and least likely in postcricoid tumours. Typical rates of lymph node metastases evident at presentation are shown in Table 15.2.

Bilateral nodal metastases may occur, especially in tumours which cross the midline; the rich lymphatic network also crosses the midline, so late contralateral nodal metastatic recurrences are to be expected.

Many patients with clinically negative nodes will

Table 15.2 Incidence of lymph node metastases at presentation (Stell and Swift, 1987)

	N_0 (%)	$N_{1/2/3}$ (%)
Pyriform fossa	35	65
Postcricoid area	70	30
Posterior pharyngeal wall	60	40
Overall	55	45

be found to have occult metastases (see below, Management). Distant metastases (commonly liver, lung and bone) usually occur late; generally only those patients who attain locoregional control live long enough for them to become symptomatic.

Epidemiology

Reports on the descriptive epidemiology of hypopharyngeal cancer are generally unhelpful because:
1 It is not a common tumour, and numbers are small
2 The two principal subsites (pyriform fossa and postcricoid area) give rise to tumours with patterns of occurrence and behaviour which differ greatly from one another
3 Most reports amalgamate the subsites, and even include oropharyngeal, and sometimes oral carcinomas in the same group analysis.

For example, postcricoid carcinoma is the only cancer in the buccopharyngeal region more common in women than men, and with wide geographical variation in its frequency relative to other hypopharyngeal sites. Postcricoid cancer forms up to 50% of hypopharyngeal cancers in the UK and Canada, but is uncommon in North America and Australasia. Postcricoid cancer has also been linked aetiologically to dietary factors more than other hypopharyngeal sites, and this is discussed further below.

Age-specific incidence rates for pharyngeal cancer reveal an increased risk of developing the disease with increasing age, for both men and women. Even though the incidence rate is greater in people aged over 70 years, the number of people in this age group in the general population is low, and therefore, in clinical series, the peak incidence appears in people below 65 years of age. While the age-adjusted mortality rates for cancer of the hypopharynx in England and Wales this century have fallen in men, those for women have risen over the same period. In the USA, incidence and mortality rates for hypopharyngeal cancer have also increased for women from 1947 to 1984, but not for men.

These observations may suggest that different causative factors are operating for men and for women.

Alternatively, if the same aetiological agents are involved for both, then they are factors to which men are less exposed than they were, while women have experienced an increased exposure.

Alcohol and tobacco are the two principal carcinogens implicated in the upper aerodigestive tract. These factors have been examined in case-control studies in the past 40 years (Table 15.3). Most research has been conducted in men, and the evidence suggests that tobacco and alcohol are co-factors in carcinogenesis. This conclusion seems reasonable in the light of strong epidemiological evidence in favour of alcohol and tobacco being major risk factors in oral and oropharyngeal cancers, and the causal relationship demonstrated for alcohol in oesophageal cancer.

Table 15.3 Results of case-control studies which have examined the impact of tobacco and alcohol in association with the occurrence of hypopharyngeal cancer

1 *Studies supporting tobacco as a risk factor in hypopharyngeal cancer*
USA: Wynder *et al.* (1957), Hammond (1964)
Hawaii: Kato *et al.* (1992) (Japanese Hawaiians)
India: Jussawalla (1973)
Europe: England – Whitaker *et al.* (1979)
Ireland – Herity *et al.* (1981)
Italy – Barra *et al.* (1991)
Korea: Choi and Kahyo (1991)
2 *Studies showing no association between tobacco consumption and hypopharyngeal cancer*
USA: Mills and Porter (1950), Keller (1967), Weir and Dunn (1970)
England: Whitaker *et al.* (1979)
3 *Studies supporting alcohol as an independent risk factor in hypopharyngeal cancer*
Puerto
Rico: Martinez (1969)
USA: Kissen *et al.* (1973), Williams and Horn (1977)
Canada: Schmidt and Popham (1981)
Italy: Barra *et al.* (1991)
4 *Studies demonstrating synergistic effect between alcohol and tobacco consumption as risk factors in hypopharyngeal cancer*
USA: Schottenfeld (1979)
Hawaii: Hinds *et al.* (1980), Kato *et al.* (1992)
England: Herity *et al.* (1981)
Korea: Choi and Kahyo (1991)
5 *Studies which showed no increased effect of alcohol over tobacco as a risk factor in hypopharyngeal cancer*
USA: Wynder *et al.* (1957)

Even so, much more work needs to be done in this area, especially in the distinction between pyriform fossa tumours and postcricoid tumours.

Other studies of interest have examined tea consumption (La Vecchia *et al.*, 1992) and serum cholesterol (Chyou *et al.*, 1992) as risk factors. Tea consumption did not emerge as an important risk factor, but hypopharyngeal cancers were not separated from other buccopharyngeal cancers, and therefore a true association may have been obscured. An inverse association was found with serum cholesterol, in which low levels were found to be associated with emergence of pharyngeal cancer within 10 years, suggesting that nutritional or metabolic effects may be operative in the carcinogenesis. A similar inverse association has been found with oral cancer and serum vitamin A levels, and may apply to pharyngeal cancer also.

Migrant studies (e.g. Stemmermann *et al.*, 1991) demonstrate that the risk of pharyngeal cancer in a migrant population changes to that of the adopted country, suggesting that either migrants adopt the customs of their new country, or that environmental risk factors have been avoided by migration. Certainly our experience has been that postcricoid cancer (normally comprising about 40% of hypopharyngeal cancers in British series) is rare in the British emigrants to New Zealand.

A major dietary risk factor, iron-deficiency, has been reported to be associated with postcricoid carcinoma, especially in patients with Plummer-Vinson syndrome (Larsson, Sandstrom and Westling, 1975). This observation was first reported from Sweden by Ahlbom (1936). Jacobsson (1951) subsequently analysed a large number of hypopharyngeal and tongue cancers there and reported a 90% incidence of sideropenia in the women involved. Keane *et al.* (1981) have observed that the incidence of both Plummer-Vinson syndrome and hypopharyngeal cancer in Sweden has decreased with improvement in nutrition and a better health service.

Clinical presentation

Demographic characteristics have already been discussed above. The capacity of the hypopharynx allows considerable tumour growth before the passage of food is hindered, so most patients already have advanced tumours at presentation (see Figure 15.4). Important neighbouring structures, such as the larynx and prevertebral muscles are readily invaded, and the rich lymphatic drainage allows early metastatic spread to jugular, retropharyngeal, paratracheal and mediastinal nodes. A high index of suspicion is therefore needed to detect hypopharyngeal cancer before it has spread.

Patients with hypopharyngeal carcinoma usually present with dysphagia, pain or discomfort on swallowing, or a neck mass. Swallowing disorders are common 'innocent' complaints in otolaryngology, however, and the clinician therefore needs (as well as a high index of suspicion) a reliable system that enables the differentiation between neoplastic and non-neoplastic disease. Symptoms which need to be investigated for hypopharyngeal cancer to be excluded are summarized in Table 15.4.

Table 15.4 Symptoms which may reflect the presence of a tumour of the hypopharynx

Pain	usually lateralized, often radiating to, or most noticeable in, the ipsilateral ear
Dysphagia	usually constant, and progressive; if food 'sticks' on swallowing this must be viewed with extreme suspicion
Haemoptysis	this is an unusual, but important symptom which may appear particularly with pyriform fossa tumours
Hoarseness	in association with dysphagia and/or referred otalgia, this suggests extension to the larynx
Neck mass	always should be regarded as a possible nodal metastasis in adults
Weight loss	should be asked about, as it suggests serious disease in the absence of an attempt to lose weight

A patient with hypopharyngeal carcinoma must not be falsely diagnosed to have globus pharyngis which presents as a sensation of a 'lump' in the throat. This is usually midline, between the hyoid and the suprasternal notch, but generally at cricoid level. Globus pharyngis is intermittent, typically occurring between meals when swallowing saliva or during times of stress. Although uncomfortable, it is never painful.

Lateralization is more likely to reflect a tumour, as is dysphagia to solids, and progression of symptoms.

Pharyngeal pain requires investigation if it persists for more than 2 or 3 weeks. When associated with malignancy it reflects deep invasion of laryngeal structures and/or perineural infiltration. Pain is usually lateralized either within the pharynx or referred to one ear. It is typically exacerbated by eating and in particular the eating of hot or spicy foods. Initial symptoms are unlike those of globus as they occur during the swallowing of food and not between meals, are often lateralized, and are progressive.

Occasionally the initial *presenting* symptom may be hoarseness. Fixation of the hemilarynx gives a coarse, raspy voice. Less commonly a breathy and diplophonic voice is present secondary to involvement of the recurrent laryngeal nerve.

Diagnosis/investigation
Examination

Any patient presenting with throat complaints or a lateral neck mass requires a thorough head and neck examination. Because hypopharyngeal carcinoma is typically advanced at presentation, there is usually obvious abnormality either in the neck or pharynx. The pharynx must be adequately visualized either with a mirror, a rigid endoscope through the mouth, or a flexible scope through the nose. With flexible nasopharyngeal endoscopy the pyriform fossae may be distended by the patient performing Valsalva's manoeuvre with the glottis open and the nostrils pinched. Rarely, the stubborn or hypersensitive patient requires examination under general anaesthesia.

Involvement of the larynx must be assessed and a note made of vocal cord mobility and airway compromise. There may be only subtle signs of disease, such as fullness or pooling of saliva unilaterally in the case of the pyriform fossa tumours, or bilaterally in postcricoid lesions. The remainder of the upper aerodigestive tract is examined to exclude a second tumour. All regions of the neck are assessed in a systematic manner with particular importance given to the jugular chain. Any nodes are individually assessed in terms of site, size, texture, contour, tenderness, and mobility. If a node is 'fixed' then it should be noted to what, e.g. larynx, sternomastoid, carotid sheath, or prevertebral muscles, as each has different implications. Loss of laryngeal crepitus (the grating sensation of the laryngeal cartilages over the prevertebral tissues) may indicate postcricoid or posterior pharyngeal wall involvement.

Investigation

Diagnostic investigations comprise radiology, and endoscopy with biopsy.

Patients with symptoms referred to the hypopharyngeal region and no abnormality found on thorough examination, and with an apparently low risk of malignancy (i.e. no major risk factors) should proceed to barium videofluoroscopic swallow which is most useful in disorders of pharyngo-oesophageal motility. If no mucosal lesion is seen then conservative management is appropriate. If the patient does not improve and malignancy is a possibility, however remote, then endoscopy is necessary. The summary of this approach is given in Table 15.5.

Prior to endoscopy a full blood count, urea and electrolytes, and liver function tests should be performed to exclude nutritional deficiency, liver, and renal disorders. Many patients with tumours will require formal nutritional assessment.

A chest radiograph should be taken to detect a second primary or metastases in the lungs, and a plain lateral radiograph of the neck will reveal any retrolaryngeal soft-tissue mass.

At endoscopy a thorough examination of all regions of the hypopharynx is required and any tumour must be staged carefully, with any laryngeal extension being especially noted. Superior spread into the base of the tongue and tonsil, inferior spread into the apex of the pyriform fossa or down the oesophagus, and lateral extension directly into the neck should be determined. Tumours involving the posterior pharyn-

Table 15.5 Investigation plan after history and examination

1   When risk of tumour seems low:
      videofluoroscopy
      Haemoglobin/serum iron studies
      likely diagnoses
         pharyngo-oesophageal dysmotility
         reflux/stricture
         reflux/oesophagitis
         pharyngeal pouch
         pharyngeal web
2   When (a) videofluoroscopy shows a probable tumour, or
      (b) clinical suspension is high:
      Chest radiograph
      Lateral neck radiograph (soft-tissue views)
      Haematological/biochemical assessment
      Pharyngoscopy/laryngoscopy/oesophagoscopy –
      biopsy

geal wall must be evaluated for any involvement of the prevertebral muscles as this carries a poor prognosis. Furthermore, assessment of submucosal skip lesions extending beyond the apparent limit of the tumour should be made. Endoscopic examination is completed by the visualization of the oropharynx, larynx, oesophagus and bronchi to exclude further malignancy.

Before waking the patient, examine the neck in the relaxed state using bimanual palpation of the upper deep cervical region, in the same fashion employed in the submandibular area. The gloved fingers can sometimes reach down to the apex of the pyriform fossae.

Staging

The clinical stage of the tumour is determined by clinical examination (in the clinic, and at endoscopy), in conjunction with whatever organ-imaging has been employed.

A barium swallow may demonstrate the inferior limit of a lesion extending down the oesophagus (Figure 15.6). CT and MRI scanning may identify extension into the larynx, pre-epiglottic space, base of tongue, tonsil, or prevertebral muscles (Figure 15.7), but in our experience they add little to the clinical and endoscopic examination of the primary lesion. If palpable neck disease is present imaging modalities are not likely to change the management unless they are used to determine the feasibility of neck dissection, e.g. invasion of the prevertebral muscles or internal carotid artery.

In the neck, the most accurate means of staging is ultrasound-guided fine needle aspiration (USFNA) but this is very much user dependent (McIvor *et al.*, 1994). Provided that the operator is highly trained

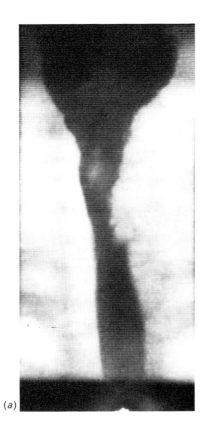

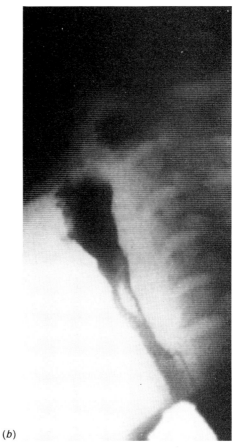

(a)

(b)

Figure 15.6 (*a*) and (*b*)   Videofluoroscopic swallow examination showing a large postcricoid carcinoma with widening of the retropharyngeal tissues and extension into the left pyriform fossa

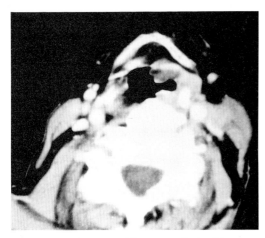

Figure 15.7 Axial CT scan of the tumour depicted in Figures 15.4 and 15.5. There is a horse-shoe shaped tumour in the right pyriform fossa, with invasion anteriorly into the pre-epiglottic space. An enlarged ipsilateral cervical node is deep to the sternomastoid muscle

and motivated then this modality can detect the majority of occult metastases (van den Brekel *et al.*, 1991). Some reports comparing CT or MRI with clinical staging, show an advantage and others not. Our own series showed no improvement with CT and we now use USFNA in the clinically N0 neck (McIvor, Morton and Dorman, 1991) because USFNA may show an otherwise (i.e. clinical and radiological) N0 neck to be N1.

The staging classification is shown in Table 15.6. Clinical stage is a useful measure, as it assists in treatment planning, and enables one to compare results between treatments and between treatment centres. It does not always correlate with the pathological stage, which is determined by histopathological review of the resected tumour and/or cervical nodes. The pathological stage is useful for prognostic purposes, and for deciding whether single modality (i.e. surgery or radiotherapy) or combination (e.g. surgery plus radiotherapy) treatment is appropriate. Often the decision to use adjuvant radiotherapy is clear from the clinical staging. Sometimes it is only

Table 15.6 Staging of hypopharyngeal cancer (UICC/AJC)

T1 Tumour limited to one subsite of hypopharynx (refer to Table 15.1)
T2 Tumour invades more than one subsite of hypopharynx, or an adjacent site, without fixation of hemilarynx
T3 Tumour invades more than one subsite of hypopharynx, or an adjacent site, with fixation of the hemilarynx
T4 Tumour invades adjacent structures, e.g. cartilage or soft tissues of the neck
NX Regional nodes cannot be assessed
N0 No regional lymph node metastasis
N1 Metastasis in a single ipsilateral lymph node, 3 cm or less in greatest dimension
N2 Metastases in a single ipsilateral lymph node, more than 3 cm but not more than 6 cm in greatest dimension; or in multiple ipsilateral lymph nodes, none more than 6 cm in greatest dimension; or in bilateral or contralateral lymph nodes, none more than 6 cm in greatest dimension
   N2a Metastases in a single ipsilateral lymph node, more than 3 cm but not more than 6 cm in greatest dimension
   N2b Metastasis in multiple ipsilateral lymph nodes, none more than 6 cm in greatest dimension
   N2c Metastasis in bilateral or contralateral lymph nodes, none more than 6 cm in greatest dimension
N3 Metastasis in a lymph node more than 6 cm in greatest dimension

Table 15.7 Important determinants involved in the treatment planning process

Tumour factors are:
   anatomical subsite of tumour origin
   clinical stage
   histological grade
Patient factors include:
   general condition
   nutritional status
   immune competence
External factors include:
   consideration of the results obtained using various modalities in any particular centre
   availability of expertise (e.g. vascularized free flap reconstruction)
   ethnic considerations
   other social factors

apparent that postoperative radiotherapy would be appropriate once pathological staging is available. Of course, if a patient receives radical radiotherapy as primary treatment, then a pathological stage cannot be established.

Treatment planning

Benign tumours

Benign tumours are treated surgically: the pedunculated lesion is exposed via a lateral pharyngotomy and removed once the pedicle has been divided. Other lesions must be treated on merit: generally some form of pharyngotomy will be necessary, even for the 'submucosal' lesions, but usually the resection of mucosa is limited and primary closure is easily obtained.

Malignant tumours

Both tumour and patient factors must be taken into account when deciding upon treatment. These are summarized in Table 15.7. It is important that the patient and family have a good understanding of the likely outcomes of the proposed treatment. They must be aware of the changes in lifestyle that can occur and the support services that are available to them. If the larynx is to be removed it is important that the patient and family understand how speech will be re-established. They must be given the opportunity to meet a laryngectomee and it is often helpful for them to view videotapes of patients who have been through similar procedures.

An important initial consideration is whether treatment is to be of palliative or curative intent. If palliative, then only troublesome symptoms such as pain, dysphagia, or airway obstruction should be treated. Treatment for treatment's sake can cause more problems from side effects than it alleviates. It is often kinder to insert a nasogastric or gastrostomy feeding tube than to treat an incurable lesion with radiotherapy that will only increase discomfort through mucositis.

Treatment philosophy

Pyriform fossa tumours

Small tumours of the pyriform fossa may be effectively treated either by radiotherapy (with or without neck dissection), or by total laryngectomy and partial pharyngectomy with or without radiotherapy (Inoue, Shigematsu and Sato, 1973; El Badawi *et al.*, 1982; Mendenhall *et al.*, 1987; Jones, 1992). Partial surgery with laryngeal preservation followed by radiotherapy gives similar results (Vandenbrouck *et al.*, 1987). Lesions that do not extend to the apex of the pyriform fossa, the postcricoid region, or the posterior wall may be resected while preserving the larynx. If the lesion involves the lateral wall of the fossa alone (a rare event), then a partial pharyngectomy with resection of the upper thyroid ala may be adequate. Extension to the medial wall without cord fixation may be manageable by partial pharyngectomy and partial laryngectomy. More extensive involvement of the medial wall and hemilarynx may be resectable by near total laryngectomy.

More advanced (T3 and T4) tumours of the pyriform fossa have higher locoregional recurrence rates and distant metastases. Loco-regional control is better with surgery, perhaps in combination with radiotherapy, than after radiotherapy alone (Mendenhall *et al.*, 1987). This does not necessarily translate to longer patient survival, however. The more recent techniques of hyperfractionated radiotherapy (smaller fractions, increased number of fractions, higher total dose) and accelerated hyperfractionation (smaller fractions, increased number of fractions, shorter duration of treatment) provide a higher biological dose to the tumour and show great promise in the treatment of advanced lesions of the head and neck but further trials are needed to identify their role in the treatment of advanced lesions (Marcial *et al.*, 1987; Johnson, Schmidt-Ullrich and Wazer, 1992).

Chemotherapy rapidly alternating with accelerated radiotherapy has also shown promise in advanced hypopharyngeal tumours, but requires further evaluation (Vikram *et al.*, 1991).

Although perhaps most advanced hypopharyngeal tumours are treated with combination surgery and radiotherapy, there is little evidence to show that combination therapy is better than surgery alone. There is also debate on the relative effectiveness of preoperative versus postoperative radiotherapy, with conflicting evidence in the literature (Kramer *et al.*, 1987).

Postcricoid tumours

Few tumours in this site are small (i.e. < 5 cm length) at presentation, but the smaller lesions can be treated quite successfully by radical radiotherapy alone. Larger (and recurrent) tumours require total laryngopharyngectomy. Extension into the oesophagus usually means that oesophagectomy is necessary. Tumour resection and pharyngo-oesophageal reconstruction is discussed below.

Posterior wall tumours

Small lesions may be treated by radiotherapy or partial pharyngectomy with laryngeal preservation (Jones and Stell, 1991). Conservation surgery requires that the pyriform fossae and oesophagus are not involved. More advanced lesions require total pharyngolaryngectomy provided that the anterior spinal ligament is not involved. If there is direct extension or skip lesions involving the oesophagus then oesophagectomy is also indicated. Close surgical margins should be treated with postoperative radiotherapy.

The neck

Approximately 60% of pyriform fossa tumours are accompanied by clinically positive nodes and a further 30–40% of clinically uninvolved necks harbour occult disease. The numbers relating to postcricoid cancer are closer to 30% and 15–20%, respectively. Therefore it is prudent to treat both the primary site and the neck in every patient. The modalities chosen to treat the primary site and the neck are determined not only by the combined stage but also independently by the stage of the primary and of the neck. For example, a T3N0 tumour may be treated by surgery to the primary and radiotherapy to the neck, whereas a T1N3 tumour may be treated by radiotherapy to the primary and combined therapy to the neck.

Radiotherapy can probably control the large majority of occult metastases. While radical neck dissection is seldom justified in the N0 neck because of its morbidity, selective neck dissections in which nodes are removed from the high risk levels II–IV carry few side effects because major structures are preserved. An elective, conservation neck dissection in an N0 neck has an advantage over radiotherapy in that it provides a pathological staging which may be used in the decision regarding postoperative radiotherapy.

Whenever nodal dissection is performed, the ipsilateral (and contralateral, in large primary tumours) paratracheal nodes should be cleared, in order to reduce the risk of peristomal recurrence, and improve prognosis (Weber *et al.*, 1993).

Radiotherapy for N1 disease may be appropriate when the primary is small (Vandenbrouck *et al.*, 1987), but the authors prefer surgery for palpable nodes. If, in the neck dissection specimen, there is extranodal spread of disease or histological evidence of multiple levels of nodal involvement, then the neck should receive postoperative radiotherapy, as well as the primary site. If radiotherapy for the primary tumour is to be given before the neck dissection, then the regional nodes should be included in the field. We prefer surgery first; the patient is unlikely to have the radiotherapy delayed because of the surgery and the radiotherapy fields can be tailored, depending on the operative and histopathological findings.

Whenever a pyriform fossa tumour crosses the midline, or where there are ipsilateral palpable nodes, we recommend bilateral neck dissection, using the selective lateral dissection technique for the N0 neck (Figure 15.8). This provides considerably more information on pathological stage, and allows more rational planning of radiotherapy, with minimal additional operative morbidity.

Advanced neck disease (N2 and N3; extracapsular invasion) is best managed with a combination of surgery and postoperative radiotherapy (see below, Radiotherapy).

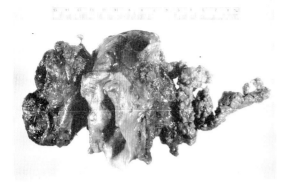

Figure 15.8 Complete surgical specimen (total laryngopharyngectomy) of the tumour shown in Figures 15.4 and 15.5. There is a large right pyriform fossa tumour with attached larynx, ipsilateral radical neck dissection and contralateral selective neck dissection (i.e. resection of nodal groups II–IV, with preservation of sternomastoid muscle, internal jugular vein and accessory nerve)

Treatment methods

Radiotherapy

Radiotherapy fields cover the primary site and both sides of the neck from the skull base to the clavicle, and to the trapezius posteriorly. If combined with surgery, radiotherapy may be given preoperatively or postoperatively. Conventional doses range from 60 to 74 Gy at 180–220 cGy per fraction. Hyperfractionation consists of two fractions per day, separated by 3 to 6 hours, to a total dose of up to 60 Gy. Fractions may vary from 120 to 180 cGy.

Preoperative radiotherapy is given to a dose of around 50 Gy with surgery 3–6 weeks later. There is conflicting information regarding complication rates associated with preoperative versus postoperative therapy. Peters *et al.* (1993) have concluded from a prospective randomized study that a minimum dose of 57.6 Gy at 180 cGy per fraction should be given to the whole tumour bed, and a boost to 63 Gy to areas of increased risk of recurrence, especially where any extranodal metastatic disease has been demonstrated. These measures will significantly reduce the risk of recurrent disease. Treatment should start as soon as possible after surgery, and certainly within 6 weeks.

Surgery

Partial pharyngectomy

If the tumour is small, and confined to the posterior pharyngeal wall or to the lateral wall of the pyriform fossa, it is possible to resect the primary via a pharyngotomy. This is normally only done if there is associated advanced nodal disease, rendering primary radiotherapy alone inappropriate.

Entering the pharynx either through the thyrohyoid membrane, or via a transhyoid approach allows adequate visualization and access, without compromising tumour margins or residual laryngeal and pharyngeal function. For the pyriform fossa tumours, the inferior constrictor must be separated from the thyroid cartilage so that a portion of the thyroid ala can be removed with the specimen. The pharynx is entered laterally in the region of the greater horn of the hyoid. The superior laryngeal nerve can usually be identified, and often preserved using this technique. Pharyngeal closure is not normally a problem with the lateral (pyriform fossa) resection. For the posterior wall tumours closure is usually a split skin graft or revascularized radial forearm graft (see below, Pharyngeal reconstruction).

Partial pharyngectomy, partial laryngectomy

There are two categories of partial laryngeal resection that can be incorporated with a partial pharyngectomy. The rationale for surgery is, as with partial pharyngectomy alone, related to the nodal status, because the primary tumour will be small. If there is fixation of the ipsilateral vocal cord, partial laryngectomy is unlikely to gain adequate resection margins, and total or near-total laryngectomy is recommended.

If the tumour involves the *superior* aspect of the medial wall of the pyriform fossa and does not extend into the apex, then a partial pharyngectomy can be extended medially to include a supraglottic laryngectomy. This usually incorporates the aryepiglottic fold, ipsilateral false cord, and epiglottis. The lateral wall of the pyriform fossa can be largely preserved. Access to the pharynx for this resection is through the lateral pharyngeal wall.

If the tumour involves the *medial* wall and apex of the pyriform fossa (with normal cord mobility), the resection can be extended medially to incorporate the vocal cord and false cord together with the aryepiglottic fold. The surgical approach is similar to that used for partial pharyngectomy alone (see above). If there is any restriction of vocal cord movement, then near-total laryngectomy and partial pharyngectomy is preferred.

Near-total laryngectomy, partial pharyngectomy

See Chapter 11.

Partial pharyngectomy, total laryngectomy

See Chapter 11.

Pharyngeal reconstruction

In deciding which form of pharyngeal reconstruction to employ, remember that most patients with hypopharyngeal carcinoma have advanced disease and a poor prognosis at presentation. Many patients will be dead within 2 years of uncontrolled disease or from second primaries. Plan a reconstruction that will offer a high probability of a short hospital stay with the patient ultimately being able to maintain his weight through per-oral feeding.

Partial pharyngeal reconstruction

Posterior pharyngeal wall resections with preservation of the larynx may be closed with skin or mucosa. Split skin can be sutured to the excision margins and to the prevertebral muscles. Similarly a pectoralis muscle or musculocutaneous flap may be used to close the defect although this may prove too bulky. The radial forearm flap provides thin skin of excellent vascularity and works well. A free jejunal 'patch' graft provides excellent mucosal tissue for reconstruction, and is favoured by some surgeons.

The deltopectoral flap requires staged operations and a temporary pharyngostome and should not be used for this reconstruction.

Total pharyngeal and pharyngo-oesophageal reconstruction

The possibilities here are skin flaps or visceral flaps. All skin flaps require tubing before insetting and therefore have a vertical suture line as well as proximal and distal anastomoses. They function as simple conduits and rely on the propulsion of food by the base of tongue and remaining pharyngeal musculature above the resection. They have a high fistula and stenosis rate. The pectoralis major flap has been a common means of pharyngeal reconstruction; it is bulky, but still a useful method in patients unfit for more extensive surgery, or where local expertise is limited. The radial forearm flap is also reliable in this location (Harii *et al.*, 1985; Takato *et al.*, 1987). A Z-plasty at the lower anastomosis helps to prevent stricture formation although this may still occur in 15% or more of patients (Takato *et al.*, 1987). The deltopectoral flap is a last resort.

The two most common forms of visceral reconstruction are gastric transposition and free jejunal transfer. These provide mucosa and therefore lubrication but, as in skin tubes, function as conduits with no useful peristaltic action.

Stell *et al.* (1983) reviewed the literature relating to hospital mortality following pharyngo-oesophageal reconstruction after surgery for hypopharyngeal cancer, and found hospital death rates of 5.5%, 19%, and 25% respectively for skin flaps, gastric transposition and jejunal transfer. By today's standards, and from our experience, these rates are excessive.

The functional impact of the different reconstructions on patients are considered further, below, under 'Rehabilitation'.

Free jejunal transfer

This is ideal when the area of resection is above the thoracic inlet. The lumen is of appropriate diameter (see Figure 15.2) and the vessels are relatively large for microvascular anastomosis. Success rates are reported in the vicinity of 90% and hospitalization is usually short (2–3 weeks). Two teams are required and harvesting of the graft carries all the risks of abdominal surgery. Perioperative mortality is reported as varying from 6% (Coleman *et al.*, 1987) to 17% (Biel and Maisel, 1987). There is also a high complication rate although generally minor; if a fistula develops it is mainly from the more difficult to perform proximal anastomosis.

Gastric transposition

This is the preferred technique when the lesion extends to the thoracic inlet because of the inherent danger of a visceral anastomosis in the mediastinum. It allows a single anastomosis that can be as high as the nasopharynx although the perfusion is reduced with anastomoses at this level. This technique also eliminates the potential for skip lesions and second primaries occurring in the oesophagus. Swallowing is restored within a few days and most patients are eating almost a normal diet (albeit in small, frequent meals) within a week or two. Also, the repair can be regarded as durable in the sense that swallowing tends to be maintained even if tumour recurs in the neck.

Gastric transposition is contraindicated in the patient with previous gastric surgery and, like the jejunal free flap, it requires a two-team effort. Mobilization of the stomach requires extensive and meticulous dissection and, in a few patients, there is some tendency to reflux and to dumping. Spiro *et al.* (1991) reported complications in 55% of 120 gastric transpositions with a perioperative mortality of 11%. Fistulae occurred in 13% of patients. Postoperative radiotherapy was associated with gastric haemorrhage.

Other visceral forms of pharyngo-oesophageal reconstruction include jejunal and colonic transposition that can be tunnelled through the mediastinum or beneath chest wall skin. These techniques are usually more appropriate for palliation of extensive oesophageal tumours.

Techniques of surgical reconstruction

Gastric transposition

At operation the two surgical teams will usually start their procedures synchronously, but if a bilateral neck dissection is included the abdominal surgeon will complete the mobilization before the neck dissection is finished.

The pharynx and larynx are mobilized from the carotid sheath on each side as described for total laryngectomy, and the superior and inferior laryngeal neurovascular pedicles are divided. One or both lobes of the thyroid gland are mobilized with preservation of the parathyroid glands and their blood supply from the inferior thyroid artery. The ipsilateral thyroid lobe, with accompanying parathyroids, is removed with the specimen whenever the primary tumour invades the larynx or pyriform apex. The trachea is divided and the tracheostome created. The upper thoracic oesophagus is mobilized by blunt finger dissection, and the paratracheal lymph nodes are mobilized en bloc with the oesophagus. Simultaneously the abdominal team opens the abdomen through an upper paramedian incision. The abdominal oesophagus is freed, followed by mobilization of both curvatures of the stomach, dividing the left gastric artery but preserving the right gastro-epiploic artery. Finally the first two parts of the duodenum are freed, and a pyloromyotomy is performed. The thoracic oesophagus is now mobilized by blunt finger dissection from above and below. Once it is free, the stomach is pulled into the neck. The pharynx is divided above the level of the hyoid, the oesophagus is divided from the stomach and this opening is oversewn. An incision is made in the fundus of the stomach which is anastomosed to the base of the tongue.

At the end of the procedure and before the patient leaves the theatre a radiograph of the chest must be taken, and if a pneumothorax is present, this must be treated appropriately by aspiration or by insertion of an intercostal drain attached to an underwater seal unless the pneumothorax is very small. In any event the chest radiograph must be repeated after a few hours.

Jejunal free flap

A two-team system is used. While the tumour and regional lymphatics are being resected, the jejunal flap is harvested from the abdomen. During the neck operation consideration is given to retaining suitable vessels for microvascular anastomosis. As jejunal vessels are quite large, the external carotid artery itself is an ideal recipient but the superior thyroid or facial arteries will suffice. Venous anastomosis may be planned to the external jugular vein or even one internal jugular vein. While the oncological resection must never be compromised by this consideration for recipient vessels, microvascular anastomosis will be facilitated if selected vessels are dissected as atraumatically as possible.

In the abdomen the jejunum is retracted on its mesentery and its vascular pedicle identified (Figure 15.9). The length of graft is determined (usually 10–12 cm) and its vascular pedicle isolated. The graft is then clamped and separated, and the remaining jejunum is reanastomosed. The graft is allowed to perfuse until the neck resection is complete and recipient

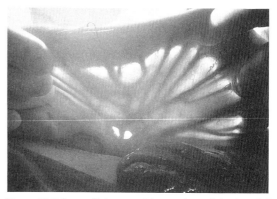

Figure 15.9 Loop of jejunum with vascular pedicle identified in readiness for transfer to the neck

vessels prepared. Then the vascular pedicle of the jejunal flap is divided, and the graft transferred to the neck. A feeding gastrostomy is fashioned before the abdomen is closed. Microvascular anastomosis is usually completed before the graft is sewn into the pharyngeal defect as an interposition graft (Figure 15.10). Ensure that the graft is orientated correctly so that isoperistaltic movements are in the direction of swallowing. The carotid artery on the side of dissection is covered by the mesentery of the flap for protection in the case of fistula formation. Because the jejunal transfer is a buried flap a segment of mesentery can be mobilized on its blood supply and exteriorized (Figure 15.11) for ease of postoperative monitoring.

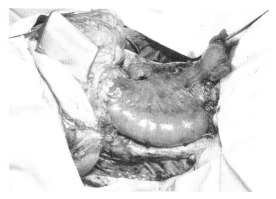

Figure 15.10 Jejunal free flap sutured in position after microvascular anastomosis. The upper end of the jejunal graft must be opened at the antimesenteric border to accommodate the larger lumen of the oropharynx. A separate portion of mesentery (inferiorly) will be exteriorized for monitoring flap viability (see Figure 15.11)

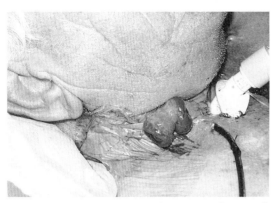

Figure 15.11 Postoperative view of a patient with a jejunal free flap, displaying a small exteriorized segment of mesentery for monitoring purposes

Table 15.8 Postoperative Green Lane Hospital enteric feeding protocol

Day 1	Glucose and electrolyte solution (Paedialyte) Start at 30 ml per hour and increase rate as patient tolerates. Nursing staff will manage this phase
Day 2	or when 100 ml/h glucose and electrolyte solution is tolerated Full strength feed; e.g. Isocal HN, or Osmolite HN. Rate: 50 ml/h
Day 3	Full strength feed Rate: 75 ml/h, if patient tolerates it
Day 4	Full strength feed. Rate: Increase rate as patient tolerates, to achieve acceptable caloric and fluid level.

If using feeds other than iso-osomolar feed, the regimen may be different. Some feeds may need to be diluted to half strength (i.e. elemental feeds)

Enteral feeding

The nutritional management of a patient having treatment for a pharyngeal tumour requires close liaison between medical and nursing staff, the dietitian, and speech therapist. Preoperatively the dietitian should assess the nutritional status of the patient according to weight and height, history of recent weight loss, and biochemical parameters (albumin, total protein, haemoglobin). In the nutritionally de-pleted patient (i.e. > 10% loss of body weight) or in patients having a jejunal free flap, we prefer total parenteral nutrition to be given for the first 7–10 postoperative days. Otherwise, enteral feeding may commence after the resumption of bowel sounds. Stomach tube feeding may be via a nasogastric, stoma-gastric, or direct percutaneous route but the principles remain the same. The aim is to ensure a caloric and protein intake that is adequate to maintain or gain weight, and a fluid intake to maintain hydration.

Iso-osmolar enteral feeds do not need dilution before introduction into the stomach. However, the volume of feeding is most important and should start at slow rates with incremental increases as tolerated by the patient. With an iso-osmolar solution, bloat-ing, vomiting, and diarrhoea reflect excessive vol-umes rather than problems with osmolarity. To regu-late volume, patients are best fed via continuous pump infusion but bolus (hourly) feeding is adequate. However, if the tube passes through into the duode-num and jejunum by peristalsis, bolus feeding is poorly tolerated. Tube position may be checked on an abdominal radiograph. The schedule employed in our institution is outlined in Table 15.8.

Oral intake is usually commenced between days 7 and 14. Patients who have had partial pharyngec-tomy with or without partial laryngectomy will have a tendency to aspirate, particularly if surgery has included the tongue base. After closure of the trache-ostomy site these patients should be started on fluids thickened with a food thickener before progressing to pureed food, with thickened then unthickened liquids, and finally to a soft diet with unthickened fluids. A patient who has undergone total laryngectomy (Figure 15.12) can instead start with liquids and rapidly progress to a soft diet.

During or following radiotherapy, severe mucositis may necessitate hospitalization for pain relief and enteral feeding. These patients can be commenced directly on full strength feed with incremental in-creases in volume rather than starting with an electro-lyte solution.

One should monitor the patient's nutritional status by regular weighing, and monitoring of serum albu-min and haemoglobin. Serum prealbumin and trans-ferrin have shorter half-lives and can give an earlier indication of changing status if necessary.

Effects and complications of treatment

There is no doubt that the consequences of uncon-trolled local and regional disease are dreadful and that radical therapy is justified in an attempt to achieve control. Nevertheless, the impact of such treatment is considerable.

Radiotherapy

The short-term effects of radiotherapy relate to local tissue reaction and systemic fatigue. During treat-ment the patients can lose a considerable amount of weight and deteriorate in their general condition. This is because of the radiation mucositis which leads to dysphagia and odynophagia. Many patients will have already lost weight as a result of their tumour. In Auckland, radiotherapy has resulted in an average loss per person of about 5% of body

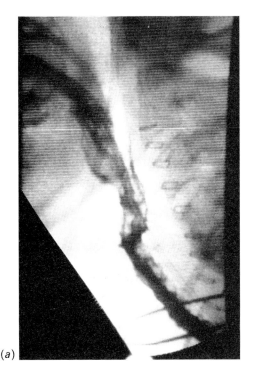

(a)

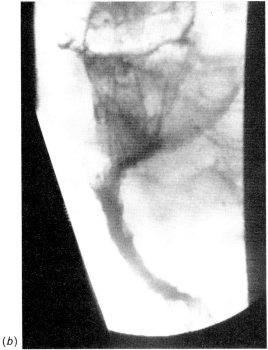

(b)

Figure 15.12 (a) and (b) Postoperative videofluoroscopic barium swallow of a patient with a jejunal microvascularized free flap repair after total laryngopharyngectomy. Note the lateralized position superiorly, due to opening of the antimesenteric border prior to suturing of the flap to the oropharyngeal mucosa

weight 3 months after treatment. This is superimposed on an average pre-treatment weight loss of 5%, and for some patients the total loss of body weight may be well in excess of 10–15% by the time radiotherapy has been completed. Some patients will therefore need hospitalization and tube feeding during treatment to prevent this. All require dietary advice and monitoring and early intervention if the treatment is to be tolerated.

If surgery has preceded radiotherapy then speech rehabilitation will be delayed by the radiotherapy, sometimes by many months. It is important to encourage the patient during this time. Sometimes an electric larynx needs to be supplied as a temporary measure to assist with communication.

Long-term, the problems from radiotherapy relate to fibrous tissue reaction, xerostomia and thyroid function. Fibrosis is not usually a problem unless there has been associated surgery. In that event stenosis of the pharyngeal repair and of the tracheal stoma may require revision surgery. Xerostomia is also more disabling if the patient has had surgery. If both submandibular glands and both parotid glands have been included in the radiotherapy fields then the patient is very miserable, usually unable to eat out socially, and constantly carrying a bottle of water for oral/pharyngeal lubrication.

Radiotherapy to the neck also renders early detection of nodal metastatic recurrence more difficult. Moreover, if there is nodal recurrence, it is less readily controlled with neck dissection, possibly because extranodal spread seems to be more prevalent than in the unirradiated neck.

Hypothyroidism is an important complication after radiotherapy. In patients who have had a hemithyroidectomy, more than 50% can be expected to become hypothyroid within a year; in patients in whom the thyroid remains intact, about 25% will become hypothyroid (Buisset *et al.*, 1991).

Surgery

The impact of surgery is very dramatic for the patient. The short-term effects relate to swallowing, breathing and talking. All patients require a feeding tube. Usually a nasogastric tube is used, but percutaneous, endoscopic gastrostomy (PEG) tubes are gaining popularity, especially in the USA. Our experience with PEG has been with long-term tube feeding, where it has been tolerated much better and with less morbidity than nasogastric tube feeding.

Resumption of oral intake is delayed if the pharyngeal repair fails and a pharyngocutaneous fistula develops. We have found that monitoring the wound amylase is a useful means of predicting which patients are likely to develop a fistula if oral feeding is started too soon (Fielder and Morton, 1989).

Once oral intake is resumed, those patients with

an intact laryngeal airway often aspirate at first. Techniques of assessment and management have been devised to deal with this problem, and most people are able to maintain a satisfactory nutrition, although many require some dietary modification. Liaison between speech therapist, dietitian and surgeon is important.

Late complications after surgery usually relate to pharyngeal stenosis, and local or regional recurrence.

A prospective study of our patients' quality of life after treatment has shown that they retain a surprisingly positive attitude and interest in life. The major problem has been that more than one-third cease eating out socially, as they are embarrassed or restricted too much by their residual swallowing disability, especially if they have had surgery plus radiotherapy. The effects of neck dissection are minimized if the accessory nerve can be preserved. Removal of the sternomastoid muscle leads to no great disability, but loss of trapezius function gives rise not only to disability but also to pain and discomfort in the shoulder.

Rehabilitation

Although swallowing is often impaired and the timing of pharyngeal constriction and function of the upper oesophageal sphincter are altered (Hannig *et al.*, 1991), most patients manage tolerably well and are able to maintain nutrition. The function of the base of the tongue becomes more important for pharyngeal emptying after total laryngectomy, and radiotherapy usually leads to a substantial, permanent loss of salivation. All this means that dry, and some solid food cannot be eaten and that patients have to modify their diet. This may lead to a degree of social reclusiveness, as they are often embarrassed by their difficulties with eating (see also above, Complications). This problem must be recognized, and attempts made to anticipate it and either to avoid it or overcome it. Some of these problems are compounded, rather than avoided, by preservation of some or all of the larynx, because of the added factor of aspiration and coughing during meals.

Schechter, Baker and Gilbert (1987) compared the functional results of pharyngeal reconstruction using gastric transposition, jejunal transfer, pectoralis musculocutaneous, and deltopectoral flaps. It took 6 months for all groups to achieve maximum rehabilitation. There was no significant difference in the ability to swallow, maintain weight, and to learn oesophageal speech between the two skin flap repairs. Jejunal free transfer produced significantly better scores for swallowing (see Figure 15.12) and ability to maintain weight compared to skin but scored lower for the acquisition of oesophageal speech. The gastric transposition group achieved higher scores than did the other reconstruction groups in all of the three functional categories.

Speaking is generally re-established after total laryngectomy by the use of tracheo-oesophageal puncture speech. This is covered in Chapter 11. Mendelsohn, Morris and Gallagher (1993) compared speech in patients after total laryngopharyngectomy with jejunal reconstruction and total laryngectomy alone. The laryngopharyngectomy group spoke at a lower frequency and produced intelligibility scores consistently lower than the laryngectomy group. Both groups were perceived as hoarse by naive listeners, but the pharyngolaryngectomy group also had a 'wet' quality, and shorter phonation times. The authors felt that autonomous jejunal contractions and excessive mucus from the grafts impaired fluency and control of pitch in the pharyngolaryngectomy group.

Surveillance/follow-up

Patients should be reviewed at regular intervals for evidence of local or regional recurrence, and for the development of a second primary tumour. Some recurrences cannot be treated curatively, but nodal metastases and small local recurrences can usually be treated.

Palliative care

In general, it is better to avoid treatment than to attempt to resect or irradiate and achieve only partial clearance or control. This is because the effects of the tumour will have only been very temporarily (if at all) alleviated, and the impact of the treatment will have added morbidity and discomfort. Patients, relatives and staff must be very clear what the objectives are when palliative treatment is given. Unrealistic expectations are to be avoided.

Pain can be managed usually without surgery or radiotherapy. Dyspnoea can be relieved by a tracheostomy, but many patients remain dependent on institutional care, and little is gained. Dysphagia can be managed by gastrostomy feeding. Loizou, Rampton and Bown (1992) reported the use of a modified celestin tube in the management of unresectable carcinoma of the cervical oesophagus in which they positioned the proximal end of the tube in the hypopharynx. This was remarkably well tolerated, and may well have application in palliation of some patients with postcricoid carcinoma.

References

AHLBOM, H. E. (1936) Simple achlorhydric anaemia, Plummer-Vinson syndrome and carcinoma of the mouth, pharynx and oesophagus in women. *British Medical Journal*, 2, 331–333

BARRA, S., BARON, A. E., FRANCESCHI, S., TALAMINI, R. and LA

VECCHIA, C. (1991) Cancer and non-cancer controls in studies on the effect of tobacco and alcohol consumption. *International Journal of Epidemiology*, **20**, 845–851

BATSAKIS, J. G. (1979) *Tumours of the Head and Neck*, 2nd edn. Baltimore: Williams & Wilkins

BIEL, M. A. and MAISEL, R. H. (1987) Free jejunal autograft reconstruction of the pharyngo-esophagus: review of a 10-year experience. *Otolaryngology – Head and Neck Surgery*, **97**, 369–375

BUISSET, E., LECLERC, I., LEFEBVRE, J., STERN, J., TON-VAN, J., GOSSELIN, P. *et al.* (1991) Hypothyroidism following combined treatment for hypopharyngeal and laryngeal carcinoma. *American Journal of Surgery*, **162**, 345–347

CHOI, S. Y. and KAHYO, H. (1991) Effect of cigarette smoking and alcohol consumption in the aetiology of cancer of the oral cavity, pharynx and larynx. *International Journal of Epidemiology*, **20**, 878–885

CHYOU, P. H., NOMURA, A. M., STEMMERMANN, G. N. and KATO, I. (1992) Prospective study of serum cholesterol and site-specific cancers. *Journal of Clinical Epidemiology*, **45**, 287–292

COLEMAN, J. J., SEARLES, J. M., HESTER, T. R., NAHAI, F., ZUBOWICZ, V., MCCONNEL, F. M. *et al.* (1987) Ten years experience with the free jejunal autograft. *American Journal of Surgery*, **154**, 394–398

EL BADAWI, S. A., GOEPFERT, H., FLETCHER, G. H., HERSON, J. and OSWALD, M. J. (1982) Squamous cell carcinoma of the pyriform sinus. *Laryngoscope*, **92**, 357–364

FIELDER, C. F. and MORTON, R. P. (1989) Wound amylase estimation and the prediction of pharyngo-cutaneous fistulae. *Clinical Otolaryngology*, **14**, 101–105

HAMMOND, E. C. (1964) Smoking in relation to mortality and morbidity. *Journal of the National Cancer Institute*, **32**, 1161–1188

HANNIG, C. E., WUTTGE-HANNIG, A. C., CLASEN, B., KELLER-MANN, S. L. and VOLKMER, C. K. (1991) Dysphagia of the treated laryngeal cancer – detection of functional and morphological changes by cineradiography. *Bildgebung*, **58**, 141–145

HARII, K., EBIHARA, S., ONO, I., SAITO, H., TERUI, S. and TAKATO, T. (1985) Pharyngoesophageal reconstruction using a fabricated forearm free flap. *Plastic and Reconstructive Surgery*, **75**, 463–474

HARRISON, D. F. N. (1970) Pathology of hypopharyngeal cancer in relation to surgical management. *Journal of Laryngology and Otology*, **84**, 349–367

HERITY, B., MORIARTY, M., BOURKE, G. J. and DALY, L. (1981) A case-control study of head and neck cancer in the Republic of Ireland. *British Journal of Cancer*, **43**, 177–182

HINDS, M. W., KOLONEL, L. N., LEE, J. and HIROHATA, T. (1980) Associations between cancer incidence and alcohol/cigarette consumption among five ethnic groups in Hawaii. *British Journal of Cancer*, **41**, 929–940

INOUE, T., SHIGEMATSU, Y. and SATO, T. (1973) Treatment of carcinoma of the hypopharynx. *Cancer*, **31**, 649–655

JACOBSSON, F. (1951) Carcinoma of the hypopharynx. A clinical study of 322 cases, treated at Radiumhemmet, 1931–1942. *Acta Radiologica*, **35**, 1–21

JOHNSON, C. R., SCHMIDT-ULLRICH, R. K. and WAZER, D. E. (1992) Concomitant boost technique using accelerated superfractionated radiation therapy for advanced squamous cell carcinoma of the head and neck. *Cancer*, **69**, 2749–2754

JONES, A. S. (1992) The management of early hypopharyngeal cancer: primary radiotherapy and salvage surgery. *Clinical Otolaryngology*, **17**, 545–549

JONES, A. S. and STELL, P. M. (1991) Squamous carcinoma of the posterior pharyngeal wall. *Clinical Otolaryngology*, **16**, 462–465

JUSSAWALLA, D. J. (1973) Cancer incidence patterns in the subcontinent of India. *Journal of the Royal Society of Medicine*, **66**, 308–312

KATO, I., NOMURA, A. M., STEMMERMANN, G. N. and CHYOU, P. H. (1992) Prospective study of the association of alcohol with cancer of the upper aerodigestive tract and other sites. *Cancer Causes Control*, **3**, 145–151

KEANE, W. M., ATKINS, J. P., WETMORE, R. and VIDAS, M. (1981) Epidemiology of head and neck cancer. *Laryngoscope*, **91**, 2037–2045

KELLER, A. Z. (1967) Cirrhosis of the liver, alcoholism and heavy smoking associated with cancer of the mouth and pharynx. *Cancer*, **20**, 1015–1022

KISSEN, B., KALEY, M. M., SU, W. H. and LERNER, R. (1973) Head and neck cancer in alcoholics. *Journal of the American Medical Association*, **224**, 1174–1175

KRAMER, S., GELBER, R. D., SNOW, J. B., MARCIAL, V. A., LOWRY, L. D., DAVIS, L. W. *et al.* (1987) Combined radiation therapy and surgery in the management of advanced head and neck cancer: final report of study 73–03 of the radiation therapy study group. *Head and Neck Surgery*, **10**, 19–30

LA VECCHIA, C., NEGRI, E., FRANCESCHI, S., D'AVANZO, B. and BOYLE, P. (1992) Tea consumption and cancer risk. *Nutrition and Cancer*, **17**, 27–31

LARSSON, L.-G., SANDSTROM, A. and WESTLING, P. (1975) Relationship of Plummer-Vinson disease to cancer of the upper alimentary tract in Sweden. *Cancer Research*, **35**, 3308–3316

LOIZOU, L. A., RAMPTON, D. and BOWN, S. G. (1992) Treatment of malignant strictures of the cervical esophagus by endoscopic intubation using modified endoprostheses. *Gastrointestinal Endoscopy*, **38**, 158–164

MCIVOR, N. P., MORTON, R. P. and DORMAN, E. B. (1991) Computed tomography and the clinically negative neck. *Head and Neck Surgery*, **13**, 74–75

MCIVOR, N. P., FREEMAN, J. L., SALEM, S. ELDEN, L., NOYEK, A. M. and BEDARD, Y. C. (1994) Ultrasonography and ultrasound-guided fine needle aspiration biopsy of head and neck lesions – a surgical perspective. *Laryngoscope*, **104**, 669–674

MARCIAL, V. A., PAJAK, T. F., CHANG, C., TUPCHONG, L. and STETZ, J. (1987) Hyperfractionated photon radiation therapy in the treatment of advanced squamous cell carcinoma of the oral cavity, pharynx, larynx and sinuses using radiation therapy as the only planned modality. *International Journal of Radiation Oncology, Biology and Physics*, **13**, 41–47

MARTINEZ, I. (1969) Factors associated with cancer of the oesophagus, mouth and pharynx in Puerto Rico. *Journal of the National Cancer Institute*, **42**, 1069–1094

MENDELSOHN, M., MORRIS, M. and GALLAGHER, R. (1993) A comparative study of speech after total laryngectomy and total laryngopharyngectomy. *Archives of Otolaryngology – Head and Neck Surgery*, **119**, 508–510

MENDENHALL, W. M., PARSONS, J. T., DEVINE, J. W., CASSISI, N. J., and MILLION R. R. (1987) Squamous cell carcinoma of the pyriform sinus treated with surgery and/or radiotherapy. *Head and Neck Surgery*, **10**, 88–92

MILLS, C. A. and PORTER M. M. (1950) Tobacco smoking habits and cancer of the mouth and respiratory system. *Cancer Research* **10**, 539–542

PETERS, L. J., GOEPFERT, H., ANG, K. K., BYERS, R. M., MARR, M.

H., GUILLAMONDEGUI, O. *et al.* (1993) Evaluation of the dose for postoperative radiation therapy of head and neck cancer: first report of a prospective randomized trial. *International Journal of Radiation Oncology, Biology and Physics*, **26**, 3–11

SCHECTER, G. L., BAKER, J. W. and GILBERT, D. A. (1987) Functional evaluation of pharyngoesophogeal reconstructive techniques. *Archives of Otolaryngology – Head and Neck Surgery*, **113**, 40–44

SCHMIDT, W. and POPHAM, R. E. (1981) The role of drinking and smoking in mortality from cancer and other causes in alcoholics. *Cancer*, **47**, 1031–1041

SCHOTTENFELD, D. (1979) Alcohol as a co-factor in the etiology of cancer. *Cancer*, **43**, 1962–1966

SPIRO, R. H., BAINS, M. S., SHAN, J. P. and STRONG, E. W. (1991) Gastric transposition for head and neck cancer: a critical update. *American Journal of Surgery*, **162**, 348–352

STELL, P. M. and SWIFT, A. C. (1987) Tumours of the hypopharynx. In: *Scott-Brown's Otolaryngology*, 5th edn., vol 5 *Laryngology*, edited by A. G. Kerr and P. M. Stell. London: Butterworths. pp. 250–263.

STELL, P. M., MISSOTTEN, F., SINGH, S. D., RAMADAN, M. F. and MORTON, R. P. (1983) Mortality after surgery for hypopharyngeal cancer. *British Journal of Surgery*, **70**, 713–718

STEMMERMANN, G. N., NOMURA, A. M., CHYOU, P. H., KATO, I. and KUROISHI, T. (1991) Cancer incidence in Hawaiian Japanese: migrants from Okinawa compared with those from other prefectures. *Japanese Journal of Cancer Research*, **82**, 1366–1370

TAKATO, T., HARII, K., EBIHARA, S., ONO, I., YOSHIZUMI, T. and NAKATSUKA, T. (1987) Oral and pharyngeal reconstruction using the free forearm flap. *Archives of Otolaryngology, Head and Neck Surgery*, **113**, 873–879

VAN DEN BREKEL, M. W., CASTELIJNS, J. A., STEL, H. V., LUTH, W. J., VALK, J., VAN DER WAAL, I. *et al.* (1991) – Occult metastatic neck disease: detection with US and US-guided fine needle aspiration cytology. *Radiology*, **180**, 457–461

VANDENBROUCK, C., ESCHWEGE, F., DE LA ROCHEFORDIERE, A., SICOT, H., MAMELLE, G., LE RIDANT, A. M. *et al.* (1987) Squamous cell carcinoma of the pyriform sinus: retrospective study of 351 cases treated at the Institut Gustave-Roussy. *Head and Neck Surgery*, **10**, 4–13

VIKRAM, B., MALAMUD, S., GOLD, J., NUSSBAUM, M., KIMMELMAN, C., LUCENTE, F. *et al.* (1991) Chemotherapy rapidly alternating with accelerated radiotherapy for advanced carcinomas of the hypopharynx and upper oesophagus: a feasibility study. *Head and Neck Surgery*, **13**, 415–419

WEBER, R. S., MARVEL, J., SMITH, P., HANKINS, P., WOLF, P. and GOEPFERT, H. (1993) Paratracheal lymph node dissection for carcinoma of the larynx, hypopharynx, and cervical esophagus. *Otolaryngology – Head and Neck Surgery*, **108**, 11–17

WEIR, J. M. and DUNN, J. E. (1970) Smoking and mortality: a prospective study. *Cancer*, **25**, 105–112

WHITAKER, E. L., MOSS, E., LEE, W. R. and CUNLIFFE, S. (1979) Oral and pharyngeal cancer in the North-West and West Yorkshire regions of England, and occupation. *British Journal of Industrial Medicine*, **36**, 292–298

WILLIAMS, R. R. and HORN, J. W. (1977) Association of cancer sites with tobacco and alcohol consumption and socioeconomic status of patients: interview from the third national cancer survey. *Journal of the National Cancer Institute*, **58**, 525–547

WYNDER, E. L., HULTBERG, G., JACOBSSOEN, F. and BROSS, I. J. (1957) Environmental factors in cancer of the alimentary tract. *Cancer*, **10**, 470–487

16

Benign diseases of the neck

A. G. D. Maran

Thyroglossal cysts

Terminology

Since it has not been established whether or not the tract connecting the thyroid gland to the foramen caecum persists as a solid tract, a hollow tube or a duct that becomes obliterated, terms such as 'thyroglossal duct cyst' or 'thyroglossal tract cyst' are best avoided and the general term 'thyroglossal cyst' should be used.

A sinus is an opening between an internal structure and an epithelial surface whereas a fistula is a connection between two epithelial surfaces. The term 'thyroglossal fistula' is often used but it is erroneous. Only one case of a congenital thyroglossal fistula has been described and its existence is rather tenuous. What most authors mean is a thyroglossal sinus and this is the preferred term. A fistula would suggest an opening between the base of the tongue and the skin surface of the neck and this clearly never occurs.

The discharge from a thyroglossal sinus is secreted mucus not saliva.

Embryology

The branchial arches and pharyngeal pouches develop at the beginning of the fourth week of embryonic life. Among other things the first arch forms the lingual swellings that make-up the bulk of the anterior two-thirds of the tongue; it is completed by the tuberculum impar which forms a median eminence behind the lingual swellings and eventually joins them. The posterior third of the tongue is formed by the merging of the ventral portions of the second and third branchial arches.

During the fourth week the thyroid anlage forms an outpouching from the floor of the pharynx between the tuberculum impar and the posterior third of the tongue. It enlarges caudally as a bilobed diverticulum following the descent of the heart and great vessels and grows into the loose parapharyngeal connective tissue. As it moves down it leaves a tract behind.

The hyoid bone develops later and joins from lateral to medial. It is possible, therefore, for the tract to be caught in this, resulting in the tract running through the bone. More commonly, however, the hyoid rotates to achieve its adult position and draws the thyroglossal tract posteriorly and cranially at the inferior edge of the body. Apart from this 'notch' behind the body or partly included in the body, the thyroglossal tract lies ventral to the body and the thyrohyoid membrane.

There is no natural internal opening of the tract. The tongue and foramen caecum form later than the descent of the thyroid and the blind tract. Sometimes found in association with the foramen caecum, is the lingual duct and represents the point of union between the paired anterior and posterior segments that form the tongue base.

The thyroglossal tract normally atrophies and disappears between the fifth and tenth weeks, but the caudal attachment may remain as the pyramidal lobe of the thyroid gland.

Pathogenesis

The prevalence of thyroglossal cysts depends on the author and the institution. While many authors claim it is the most common non-neoplastic neck mass and others that it represents 40% of all primary tumours in the neck, it is salutary to note that Sistrunk (1920), whose name is still attached to the operation for removal of the cyst, reported only 31 thyroglossal cysts in a series of 86 000 general paediatric patients.

The sex distribution is equal and the age range is from birth to 70 years with a mean age of 5.5 years. Of about half the published cases, 31.5% were under the age of 10, 20.4% were in the second decade, 13.5% in the third decade and 34.6% were older than 30 years. Ninety per cent lie in the midline and 10% are to one side of the midline; of those, 95% are on the left and 5% are on the right.

If this is a developmental abnormality and thus a congenital lesion, why should almost one in three not present until the patient is over the age of 30 years? The reason is not known but two possibilities are cited. The first suggests that recurrent throat inflammation may stimulate the epithelial remnants of the tract to undergo cystic degeneration. The second possibility is a retention phenomenon. A blocked thyroglossal duct may expand to form a cyst because of an accumulation of secretion. Most proponents of this theory, however, implicate the foramen caecum in the obstruction. The lingual duct has mucous and serous glands and the cyst may be a lingual cyst and not a true thyroglossal cyst. This might account for those cysts found in the tongue above the hyoid.

In the published series, where the position is analysed, 2.1% are intralingual, 24.1% suprahyoid, 60.9% thyrohyoid and 12.9% suprasternal. This means that about one in four is above the hyoid and three out of four are below (Figure 16.1).

A cyst may form on both sides of the hyoid resembling a dumb-bell lesion. The missing part of the dumb-bell may account for some recurrences after a Sistrunk operation. Sometimes multiple cysts are found. These are probably pseudocysts because they have no real lining and are only granulation tissue with extravasated mucus. They probably arise from continual mucus production in a blocked duct that gradually balloons out at its distal end to form a cyst that ruptures into the surrounding tissue.

Sinus openings are always secondary due to spontaneous or surgical drainage after infection. Sinus formation may also occur after a 'lumpectomy' operation leaving the hyoid and part of the tract if it is mucus secreting.

Thyroid tissue is present in the cyst wall in more than 60% of cases. Its presence is most probably due to the origin of the duct in relation to thyroid tissue, but benign thyroid metastases (compare endometriosis) have been postulated. It is from this tissue that thyroid carcinoma can arise.

The epithelial lining is variable; most commonly it is pseudostratified ciliated columnar but it may be squamous (Figure 16.2). Squamous carcinoma has also been reported in these cysts.

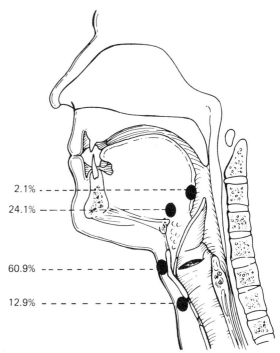

Figure 16.1 The site incidence of thyroglossal cysts

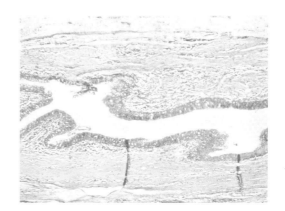

Figure 16.2 Photomicrograph showing a thyroglossal cyst lined by ciliated columnar epithelium

Clinical features

The patient will present with either a painless or an infected lump. One death has been reported due to respiratory obstruction from an intralingual cyst. If uninfected, the cyst may be soft, fluctuant and mobile, but very often it is so tense that it seems solid and, in this state, it can be wedged between the hyoid and the thyroid cartilage and thus appear fixed. It is, however, in the midline or just to the left and very few malignant lesions are at this site. Most cysts are prehyoid or infrahyoid and, since all are attached even by a tract to the hyoid, they move both on swallowing and protruding the tongue. Mobility depends on size (Figure 16.3).

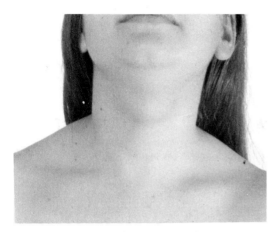

Figure 16.3 Thyroglossal cyst in a typical site

If infected, the lump will be painful, the patient will have odynophagia and the overlying skin will be red. Misguided attempts at abscess drainage here can cause problems when excision is attempted and the recurrence rate is measurably higher.

Sometimes a tract is seen or palpated from the cyst to the hyoid. Such a tract may also be found clinically if there is a sinus.

The differential diagnosis is from a dermoid cyst, an infected lymph node, lipoma, minor salivary gland tumour, sebaceous cyst, cartilaginous tumour of the thyroid, hypertrophic pyramidal lobe and choristoma.

If the cyst is intralingual, it might be a lingual thyroid and, if it is below the thyroid cartilage, it may be a thyroid adenoma. Finally, the possibility of a carcinoma in the thyroglossal remnant must be borne in mind.

It is almost impossible to differentiate a midline dermoid cyst from an uninfected thyroglossal cyst before operation. The content of a dermoid cyst is different. Instead of thick, viscous mucus, dermoid cysts contain cheesy semisolid material. The epithelial lining is keratinizing squamous epithelium with skin appendages in the wall. There is no evidence of a duct nor of inflammation.

Lipomas are more ill defined at the edges, but are tantalizingly fluctuant and so may cause diagnostic difficulty. They also move on swallowing.

Some of these alternative diagnoses may be clarified by needle biopsy.

Consideration should be given to ordering an ^{131}I scan in all suprahyoid and infrathyroid lumps. In 65–75% of patients with a lingual thyroid, there is no other thyroid tissue and it represents a complete failure of the gland to descend. It is three times more common in women because of the increased demands on the thyroid at puberty, pregnancy and the menopause. Although in former years there was not the same necessity to scan patients with lumps in the usual position between the thyroid and front of the hyoid the medico-legal position now dictates that all should have a thyroid scan.

Treatment

Wenglowski (1912) who performed much of the embryological study on neck cysts, first suggested that, not only the body of the hyoid, but a core of tissue between this and the foramen caecum be removed. Schlange (1893) was the first to remove the body of the hyoid, but Sistrunk (1920) still has his name applied to the present day operation. He adopted Wenglowski's suggestion and removed a core of tissue between the hyoid and the foramen caecum.

A horizontal incision is made at the inferior border of the mass and the skin carefully dissected off the mass. Sometimes there is a close connection between the mass and the skin and cyst rupture is a possibility. This makes further dissection difficult and there is then a risk of leaving part of the wall or pseudocysts behind.

The cyst is mobilized and the tract is often found in these cysts lying low in the neck, but in the higher ones there is little point in looking for a tract in and around the hyoid. Sometimes the tract is multiple and in sections its very thin wall is sometimes striking.

The body of the hyoid between the lesser horns is divided with shears or Mayo scissors. Medial to the lesser horns there is no danger of damaging the hypoglossal nerves. The genioglossus, mylohyoid and geniohyoid are attached to the body of the hyoid bone and a segment of these muscles is removed in continuity with the bony segment. There is no possibility of identifying a tract in this core of muscle, but failure to remove the core involves the risk of recurrence. The core is removed in a line drawn at 45° to the body of the hyoid aiming at the foramen caecum. There is no need, however, to open into the oral cavity.

The infected cyst

It is unwise to incise or excise an infected cyst. On the other hand, these may be very tense and painful and antibiotic penetration may be poor. The cyst should be aspirated with a wide bore needle to improve antibiotic penetration and allow resolution with a view to later removal.

Treatment of recurrence

If the hyoid body is not removed, the recurrence rate is 85%. Even if it is removed the reported recurrence rate varies from 2% to 8%. Recurrence is easily understood if the body of the hyoid is not removed, but it is not so easily explained if Sistrunk's procedure is performed. Possible causes of recurrence are:

1 Missing a dumb-bell cyst deep in the back of the hyoid pushing the thyrohyoid membrane back
2 Dealing with a cyst that has ruptured to form thin-walled pseudocysts
3 Rupturing a cyst and leaving part of the wall behind
4 Failing to realize that the tract may be multiple and taking too thin a core.

If Sistrunk's procedure has not been performed then revision surgery is simple and the body of the hyoid removed along with a core. If, however, Sistrunk's procedure has been carried out, further surgery is difficult and the removal of the recurrent cyst plus tract must be improvised.

Treatment of a sinus

A sinus is due to spontaneous or surgical drainage and is always secondary. Sistrunk's operation is performed, but an ellipse of skin is removed around the sinus.

If the sinus is high in the neck then the scar is a problem. If a healing scar is mobile then hypertrophy will possibly occur. The hyoid area moves constantly during swallowing and the patient should be warned of the scar problem. Dermabrasion, or breaking the line of the scar may be necessary.

Thyroglossal carcinoma

Two types of carcinoma have been described – one from the thyroid elements and one from the squamous elements.

The thyroid carcinomas are the more common and over 100 have been reported. Some have been diagnosed before operation for removal of thyroglossal cyst and some have been associated with coexisting thyroid gland cancer and only seven have had metastatic neck nodes. The age range is between 6 and 81 years with an average age of 39 years. The sex incidence is equal. The age and sex distribution is the same as for thyroid carcinoma. Eighty-five per cent are papillary adenocarcinomas and the remaining 15% are follicular adenocarcinomas, adenocarcinomas and squamous carcinomas.

With so few cases reported, no treatment plan has evolved and prognosis cannot be delineated. It does appear, however, that Sistrunk's operation plus suppressant doses of thyroxine offer a reasonable chance of a cure.

Branchial cysts, sinuses and fistulae

Terminology

It is now thought that branchial cysts, sinuses and fistulae are not all variants of the same thing originating from the branchial apparatus. The original papers linking them with the branchial apparatus did so more by acclamation than experimentation.

The cysts, also known as lateral cervical cysts, usually present in the lateral part of the neck deep to the sternomastoid at the junction of its upper third and lower two-thirds. A few cysts have a definite tract into the area of the posterior pillar of the tonsil but most have no evidence of a tract. There is doubt if these are of branchial origin.

Sinuses, or branchial pits, open along a line between the tragus and the sternoclavicular joint at the anterior border of the sternomastoid. These are almost certainly failure of completion of development of the branchial apparatus. As such, they are present at birth and reflect failure of development of the first, second, third and fourth arches. Sinuses may also occur with an internal opening only. These, however, may not always come to light but some may produce mucus, block off and become cysts with an identifiable tract.

On rare occasions, the estimated pit is demonstrated clinically and/or radiologically to have an internal opening at the posterior tonsillar pillar. Thus with two openings between epithelial surfaces there is a fistula. No case has been described with an external opening, an inclusion cyst in the tract and an internal opening.

Embryology

A 2-week embryo has on each side six branchial arches, five branchial clefts and five pharyngeal pouches. These arrangements are not parallel but tend to come together at the sixth arch. The first and second arches are important, the third and fourth less so, and the fifth and sixth vestigial.

The second pharyngeal pouch forms the palatine tonsils; the second arch grows downwards on its lateral side to meet the fifth arch thus enclosing the second, third and fourth clefts forming the cervical sinus of His. By the sixth week, the branchial apparatus has disappeared having formed the ear, tongue, hyoid, larynx, tonsils and parathyroids.

Theories of origin

The debate as to the origin of a branchial cyst reached a climax in the 1920s and 1930s. There are four theories of origin of branchial cysts, but because of the complicated development of the neck none has been proven by embryological investigation. Most of the theories have been an attempt to correlate clinical findings with known embryological facts and none can stand close scrutiny.

Branchial apparatus theory

These cysts may represent the remains of the pharyngeal pouches or branchial clefts or a fusion of these two elements. When branchial cysts have an internal opening, it is in the region of the tonsillar fossa indicating an origin from the second branchial pouch. Fistulae and sinuses from the second pouch would necessarily pass between the external and internal carotid arteries.

An origin from the third or fourth pouches is unlikely, as they would have to pass over the hypoglossal nerve to reach the skin and would be severed by the upward movement of that nerve during development.

A fourth arch tract would also have to pass below the subclavian artery on the right and the aortic arch on the left.

A third arch tract should have its internal opening in the pyriform fossa and a fourth arch tract below this. These have never been described, so that origin from these pouches can be discounted.

Origin from the first pouch is possible because high branchial cysts have been described lying under the parotid gland with an internal opening between the bony and cartilaginous meatus. If the branchial apparatus theory were to be upheld, many more cysts would be expected to have internal openings; it is a popular misconception that many branchial cysts have an internal opening. More cysts would also be expected to be present at birth, but this event has been described only once. The peak age incidence is in the third and fourth decades which is late for a congenital lesion (compare thyroglossal duct cysts).

Cervical sinus theory

This is an extension of the previous theory and considers that branchial cysts represent remains of the cervical sinus of His which is formed by the second arch growing down to meet the fifth. It is unlikely that this is true for those with an internal tract, since this is closed by fusion of its ectodermal lining from within towards the surface. This makes an internal opening difficult to achieve.

Thymopharyngeal duct theory

Cysts may be a remnant of the original connection between the thymus and third branchial pouch from which it originates. The originator of this theory presumed that the hyoid bone constituted the lower level of branchial derivatives. Not only is this false but a persistent thymic duct has never been described. Furthermore, no branchial cyst has ever been de-scribed deep to the thyroid gland nor have there been any examples of tracts between the pharynx and thymus.

Inclusion theory

King (1949) stated that there was insufficient evidence to show that cysts arose from the branchial apparatus and suggested that the cyst epithelium arose from lymph node epithelium. The following facts support this theory:

1 Most branchial cysts have lymphoid tissue in their wall and are found in the parotid and pharynx as well as in the lateral neck
2 The peak age incidence is later than expected for a congenital lesion
3 A branchial cyst in a neonate is almost unknown
4 Most branchial cysts have no internal opening or at best a tract with an ill-defined termination.

Pathogenesis

Cysts and sinuses are lined by stratified squamous epithelium but occasionally by non-ciliated columnar epithelium. The appearance of this latter epithelium probably represents a glandular metaplasia as a result of infection. This could account for the mucus production from sinuses but, if it were the sole cause of cyst formation the cysts would be expected to be filled with thick, viscous mucus like thyroglossal cysts. This is not the case, however, because the cysts contain straw-coloured fluid containing cholesterol crystals. It is the type of fluid that could only be derived from blood rather than from a mucous gland secretion. If mucus production from metaplastic epithelium was postulated as a cause of the cysts then it is unlikely that the wall would also contain lymphoid tissue, as more than 80% of cysts do. The lymphoid tissue often shows evidence of germinal centres which could only happen if the cyst formed inside a lymph node (Figure 16.4).

Squamous cysts within lymph nodes are also found in sites far removed from the branchial apparatus, such as the posterior triangle of the neck, the pharynx, the parapharyngeal space and even within the substance of the parotid gland.

Heterotopic salivary, thyroid and squamous epithelium within lymph nodes is well documented. Salivary tissue within lymph nodes in the parotid gland can undergo neoplastic change to form a monomorphic adenoma. Thyroid tissue may undergo carcinomatous change in the lateral neck and ectopic thyroid cancer is well recognized. Similarly, therefore, the squamous epithelium can undergo cystic change (as in branchial cysts) or neoplastic change as in branchogenic carcinoma.

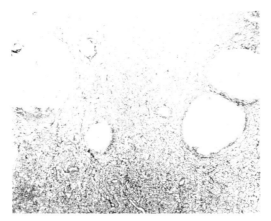

Figure 16.4 Photomicrograph of a branchial cyst showing lymphoid tissue with germinal centres in the wall and lining by squamous epithelium

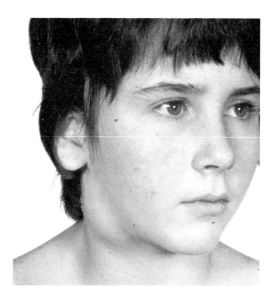

Figure 16.5 A branchial cyst in the typical position in the upper neck

Branchial sinuses and fistulae are present at birth as one would expect for a developmental defect of the branchial apparatus. The peak age incidence for branchial cysts is in the third decade, the range being 1–70 years.

Clinical features

Sixty per cent are in males and 40% in females. The peak age incidence is in the third decade for cysts; sinuses are often noted at birth and no cases are reported of sinuses appearing later in life unless by virtue of spontaneous or surgical drainage, always after infection. Sixty per cent are on the left and 40% on the right and a few are bilateral. Three-quarters are in the classical upper lateral neck position, the remainder being in the lower neck, the parotid, the pharynx and the posterior triangle (Figure 16.5).

The presenting features are:

continuous swelling	80%
intermittent swelling	20%
pain	30%
infection	15%
pressure symptoms	5%

Seventy per cent are cystic on palpation and 30% are firm, but this is probably just a measure of fluid content. Before the widespread use of fine needle aspiration biopsy, some patients had the long work-up for a metastatic node from no identifiable primary.

It is unknown why some cysts present suddenly as infected masses with overlying skin erythema. The infection might be blood borne, might reflect an internal opening and infection from the pharynx or it might be a chemical reaction within a squamous-lined cyst in a lymph node.

The differential diagnosis depends on the age of the patient.

In the patient under the age of 10 years, and especially the very young, the neck is relatively smaller than in the adult and division of the lateral neck into thirds is easier on paper than on the patient. In the newborn, a lymphangioma or dermoid cyst must be suspected; a lymphangioma is much softer than a branchial cyst and a dermoid cyst is very firm and tense. A lymphangioma does not have well-demarcated edges while dermoid and branchial cysts do. If the child is a little older, rhabdomyosarcoma is a possibility and, if it is tender, it might be lymphadenitis from the tonsil or even the teeth and pharyngeal spaces.

In the patient aged between 15 and 40 years, the most likely alternative diagnosis is adenitis from viral or bacterial causes, tuberculosis, lymphoma or a nerve sheath tumour.

In the patient over the age of 40 years, a metastatic node from a head and neck primary neoplasm is the diagnosis that must be excluded. Alternatives are lymphoma, tuberculosis, lipoma or nerve sheath tumour.

Diagnosis is by clinical examination and from fine needle aspiration biopsy if necessary. Radiology is not usually helpful but if the swelling pulsates then carotid angiography or CT scanning should be considered.

There is no differential diagnosis for branchial sinuses or fistula. To differentiate between a sinus and a fistula is important because all the tract must be removed to avoid recurrence. A sinogram will give this information (Figure 16.6).

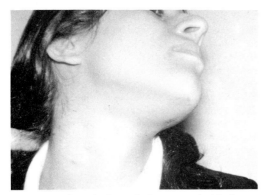

Figure 16.6 A branchial pit which connected with the oropharynx

Treatment of branchial cysts

These should be removed if they present as a mass both for diagnosis and cosmetic reasons. If left there is also the danger of infection.

A transverse incision is made in a neck crease and the sternomastoid retracted. When the cyst is mobilized, attempts are made to find a tract. This is not usually possible and very often surgeons who feel they 'ought' to find a tract, manufacture compressed areolar tissue and fascia into one going between the external and internal carotid arteries. If a true tract exists it traverses this path to the posterior pillar of the tonsil. Before the operation, careful examination of this area of the fauces under anaesthesia may reveal whether or not there is an internal sinus.

If the cyst presents as an infected mass it should be aspirated and treated with antibiotics. When the infection has settled excision is planned, but sometimes there is no mass to find when the time comes for incision. If this is the case, exploration of the neck should not be performed because it will be impossible to tell which of the many lymph nodes contains the cyst and which are reactive.

Treatment of branchial sinus and fistula

The mouth of the sinus is encompassed in an elliptical incision and the tract, which is often as thick as a medium-sized artery, is found just underneath the skin. It is dissected as high as possible and then another incision is made higher in the neck. Dissection is continued to the tonsillar area where the tract usually disappears.

If a periauricular pit is noted, the surgeon should be well versed in parotid surgery and also ear anatomy, because while the tract often goes up towards the temporal region, it may also go to the junction of the bony and cartilaginous external audi-tory meatus. The most troublesome route, however, is when the tract goes towards the facial nerve. In this instance, the surgeon should stop following the tract into the parotid and should formally identify and dissect the facial nerve.

Branchogenic carcinoma

In the 1940s, many cases of carcinoma in nodes in the neck were reported and the fashion was to ascribe the development of the squamous carcinoma to neoplastic growth of heterotopic squamous epithelium within lymph nodes: hence the name branchogenic carcinoma.

It became obvious that many of these cases were metastatic deposits in lymph nodes from primary tumours in the head and neck. This was the dawn of modern head and neck surgery and in order to discourage the haphazard treatment of metastatic neck nodes, it was decreed that before a branchial carcinoma could be claimed, four postulates had to be attained:

1 The carcinoma should be demonstrated as arising in the wall of a branchial cyst
2 The tumour should occur in a line running from a point just anterior to the tragus along the anterior border of the sternomastoid to the clavicle
3 The histology should be compatible with an origin from the tissue found in the branchial vestigia
4 No other primary should become evident in a 5-year follow up.

It is patently obvious why virtually no branchogenic carcinomas were reported over the next 20 years. The first postulate would be a matter of exquisite timing. The second is virtually meaningless. The third merely means squamous carcinoma, but was sufficiently vague as to be menacing, and the fourth is essential.

In spite of the above, several cases of branchogenic carcinoma have been reported in the last 20 years that undoubtedly are real. There is no doubt that heterotopic squamous epithelium can exist within lymph nodes. It would also be within the scope of normal biological developments for this squamous epithelium to undergo malignant change just as heterotopic tissue anywhere can.

While emphasizing that branchogenic carcinoma cannot be claimed until the possibility of an undiagnosed primary has been completely excluded, it is a real entity that is underdiagnosed. Perhaps many of the long-term survivors who orginally present with a metastatic neck node with a primary tumour that never comes to light, have this tumour.

Treatment is that of a node with no discoverable primary, i.e. is either radical neck dissection and postoperative radiotherapy or excision biopsy and postoperative radiotherapy.

Neurogenous tumours

Terminology

These tumours arise from the neural crest which differentiates into the Schwann cell and the sympathicoblast; this latter cell gives rise to paraganglionic cells from which arise carotid body tumours, glomus jugulare tumours, glomus vagale tumours and ganglionic cells from which arise benign and malignant gangliomas. The Schwann cell gives rise to the neurilemmoma (schwannoma) and the neurofibroma (Figure 16.7).

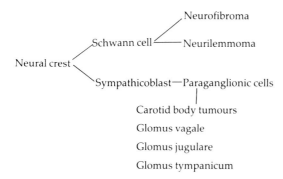

Figure 16.7 The tumour derivatives from the neural crest

The thin outer sheath of nerves is called the neurilemma and the inner sheath of Schwann is the neurolemma. Tumours arising from the inner nerve sheath are often called neurilemmomas which is incorrect, as is neuronoma. The preferred term is 'schwannoma' for tumours arising from nerve sheaths. A schwannoma shows well-developed cylindrical bands of Schwann's cells and delicate connective tissue fibres with a tendency towards pallisading of the nuclei about a central mass of cytoplasm (Verocay bodies). This form is known as Antoni type A tissue, whereas Antoni type B tissue is a loosely arranged stroma in which the fibres and cells form no distinctive pattern. The two types may also be mixed. It has no clinical significance, no surgical significance and no prognostic significance and is only mentioned because it forms part of the pathological catechism of these tumours.

Neurofibromas are often seen in association with von Recklinghausen's disease if they are multiple, but they need not be multiple and can exist as discrete entities. It is suggested that they arise from a disseminated neuroblastoma or aberrantly migrating neural crest cells. It is said that they are not as encapsulated as schwannomas and have an 8–10% chance of becoming malignant. Histologically they are characterized by a loose structure, abundant matrix, stout bundles of collagen fibres and spindle-shaped cells sometimes with waveform nuclei.

The difference between neurofibroma and schwannoma is histological, but it is not as clear cut as it might seem to the non-pathologist. A study by Horak, Szentirmay and Swgar (1983) has shown that these histological pictures can be mixed in the one tumour. From a prognostic viewpoint, these authors also show that the important difference is in the degree of cellularity rather than the classification.

Both of these tumours can show a plexiform pattern of growth. This applies especially to the cellular ones rather than to those showing the typical histological picture. The typical growth pattern is a lump that either arises from the sheath and grows outwards leaving the trunk of the nerve intact, but more often the growth involves the nerve trunk and fibres can be splayed around the tumour with apparently normal clinical function. In plexiform growths, the abnormal nerve tissue grows into adjacent tissue planes and is rather like a neural lymphangioma. It is difficult to remove and is liable to recur. These are known as plexiform neuromas.

Gangliomas or ganglioneuromas are very rare. They usually arise from a cervical sympathetic ganglion and are firm, smooth and well encapsulated. Microscopically they contain ganglion cells and neurites.

Postoperative neuromas are the result of uncontrolled growth of axons from the proximal stump of a nerve that has been cut. These are not true tumours, but represent attempts by the damaged nerve to repair itself; the axon cylinders become enmeshed in Schwann cells and scar tissue. If the process becomes hyperactive, the neuroma becomes clinically obvious and the patient experiences localized pain and tenderness.

Carotid body tumours were first termed 'chemodectomas'. This term has now lost favour because carotid body tumours appear to arise from paraganglionic cells rather than chemoreceptor cells. Paraganglionic cells are epithelioid in appearance, are derived from the neural crest and migrate in close association with autonomic ganglion cells. They are located chiefly along the aorta and great vessels with the largest accumulation in the adrenal medulla where they are chromaffin-positive producing catecholamines, adrenalin and noradrenalin and may give rise to phaeochromocytomas.

Formerly, tumours of the extra-adrenal chemoreceptor system were described as non-chromaffin paragangliomas, but in recent years catecholamines and secretory granules like those in the adrenal medulla have been found in the carotid body. Functioning tumours producing hypertension have been reported in the carotid body and the jugular body. Phaeochromocytomas have been described in association with carotid body tumours.

Paragangliomas have been reported in the following sites – aortic bodies, superior vagal ganglion (glomus jugulare), auricular branch of the vagus (glomus tympanicum), inferior vagal nodose ganglion (glomus vagale), superior laryngeal nerve (glomus laryngicum), mandible (alveolar body), ciliary ganglion (ciliary body), bifurcation of the pulmonary artery, pleura, femoral artery, retroperitoneal tissue, mesentery, coccyx and pineal body.

Pathogenesis

The growth pattern of nerve sheath tumours is either fusiform or plexiform as outlined in the previous section. Nerve paralysis on presentation is very rare, even though at surgery the nerve is found to be grossly distorted with the fibres widely stretched over the tumour. The histology has also been described and the fact highlighted, that features of neurofibroma and schwannoma can exist in the one tumour. These tumours both arise from the Schwann cell. On occasion, peripheral nerve tumours may be difficult to distinguish from other spindle cell mesenchymal lesions. The neural crest marker antigen, S100, is common to the supporting cells of the peripheral and central nervous system. Immunocytochemical staining using antibody to S100 is positive in the majority of tumours of Schwann cell derivation, although expression of the antigen is reduced in Antoni A or malignant areas. The use of antibody to neuron specific enolase may help to distinguish neurofibromas, although the method is less tissue specific.

They arise from any cranial or spinal nerve that has a sheath and this means any motor or sensory nerve other than the optic or olfactory. In the head and neck (apart from the acoustic nerve), the vagus is affected more commonly than any other nerve, but nerve sheath tumours have been described on the hypoglossal nerve, the facial, the spinal accessory, the sympathetic chain, the glossopharyngeal and branches of the cervical plexus.

While multiple neurofibromas can occur in association with von Recklinghausen's disease, little is known of the aetiology of other nerve tumours. In a long-term follow up of over 2000 patients who had been irradiated for tonsil and adenoid enlargement, Shore-Freedman *et al.* (1983) found 29 schwannomas, two neurofibromas and one ganglion neuroma. These tumours can, therefore, be radiation induced and they can continue to occur for at least 30 years after the radiation exposure. They are more common in women than in men. Most cases present in the 30–50-year age group. Malignant change in nerve sheath tumours in the head and neck is very rare. Das Gupta *et al.* (1969) described only one sarcomatous change in a series of 303 solitary nerve tumours. It is said that malignant change occurs in 10–15% of patients with multiple neurofibromatosis. The only thing that differentiates a neurogenous sarcoma from a fibrosarcoma is its origin from a nerve trunk. Malignant change is suggested by rapid growth, pain

and paraesthesia. They do not metastasize to regional lymph nodes but to the lungs.

The microscopic appearance of carotid body tumours does not relate to the future behaviour of the tumour. They are poorly encapsulated and extremely vascular, like haemangiomas, with an enveloping network of capillaries and areolar tissue arranged in concentric circles similar to an onion. They encroach upon and gradually surround the carotid bulb, invade it and extend along the carotid artery for long distances drawing blood from the vasa vasorum. The carotid system becomes progressively distorted and extended with the internal carotid artery being attenuated but never occluded. The adjacent cranial nerves are encased as may be muscles and even the base of the skull.

Glomus tumours of the vagus grow in the same manner and totally distort the anatomy at the skull base with bleeding tissue making dissection extremely difficult.

Less than 10% are frankly malignant with regional and distant metastases to lung and bone.

Due to the fact that chronic hypoxia at high altitudes leads to carotid body hyperplasia, there is a high incidence of carotid body tumours in Peru where the majority of the population live at altitudes of 2000–5000 metres. The average age of presentation ranges from 35 to 50 years, the youngest reported being 12 years old. The sex incidence is equal.

There is a striking family history of up to 10% and also a tendency to bilateral tumours, tumours of other similar cells and phaeochromocytomas. Twenty-five per cent are bilateral in those with a positive family history, compared with 3% in those with no family history.

Clinical features

Nerve sheath tumours of the vagus present as parapharyngeal space masses. They are nearly all fusiform and so do not expand out of the parapharyngeal space to cause a discrete lump at the angle of the jaw, but usually push the sternomastoid laterally. This gives an ill-defined neck mass deep to the muscle which may, however, have an anterior border but certainly no palpable superior border. Since the vagus lies deep in the parapharyngeal space tumours arising from it push the pharynx medially. Tumours of the deep lobe of the parotid push the tonsil and soft palate medially but vagal and carotid tumours push the posterior pillar and posterolateral oropharyngeal wall forward. They are painless masses that rarely cause nerve paralysis (Figures 16.8 and 16.9).

Tumours of the sympathetic trunk present in the same way, but tumours of the hypoglossal, accessory and cutaneous cervical nerves merely present as neck lumps in the appropriate area. Facial nerve tumours are invariably diagnosed as parotid tumours.

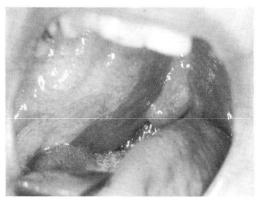

Figure 16.8 Palate pushed medially by a deep lobe parotid tumour

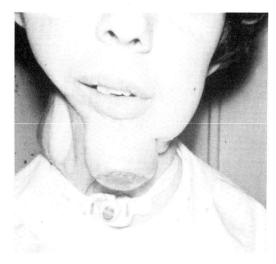

Figure 16.10 Huge postoperative neuroma of the mental nerve in a patient who had a commando operation

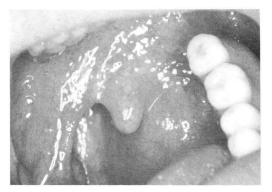

Figure 16.9 Posterior pillar pushed medially by schwannoma of the vagus

A postoperative neuroma is very tender and, on palpation, the patient experiences an electric shock type of sensation. There must be a previous history of neck surgery, such as a parotidectomy, or a radical neck dissection. The nerves most usually affected are the cutaneous branches of the cervical plexus, that is the great auricular, the lesser occipital and the anterior cutaneous nerve of the neck. They rarely form on a stump of the hypoglossal nerve after a XII–VII anastomosis (Figure 16.10).

Carotid body tumours present in the same space, but it is as usual for them to form a discrete neck mass as it is for them to present as a parapharyngeal mass pushing the pharyngeal wall medially. Noradrenalin-secreting tumours have been described which have properties similar to phaeochromocytomas. There is also an association with the neural crest lesions and the syndrome of multiple endocrine adenomatosis should be suspected. Cranial nerve paralysis is more common in carotid body tumours than in nerve sheath tumours.

Glomus vagale tumours may or may not present with vagal nerve paralysis but all present with a neck mass high under the sternomastoid.

On clinical examination, it is impossible to differentiate these tumours if they present, as they usually do, in the parapharyngeal space. Old clinical aids, such as moving masses side to side but not up and down, are fairly useless because any lesion attached to a structure that runs vertically in the neck like a vagus nerve, a carotid artery or the sternomastoid muscle will behave in such a fashion. Pharyngeal presentation will be the same for carotid or vagus masses, namely behind the posterior tonsillar pillar. Carotid body tumours are not pulsatile.

A CT scan will show if there is a mass in the parapharyngeal space and this will be very useful for smaller tumours that only give a suspicion of a lump clinically. A CT scan will not, however, always differentiate between a nerve sheath tumour and a carotid body tumour. Angiography is nearly always advisable if there is real suspicion of a carotid body tumour. This is not only diagnostic but gives an indication of the resectability of the tumour (Figure 16.11).

Fine needle aspiration biopsy is always worth carrying out but open biopsy should be avoided. Although much less frequent now, there is ample scope for surgical disaster by exploring these tumours unprepared for major vascular surgery. The disaster potential can be maximized by an approach through the mouth.

Treatment of nerve sheath tumours

There are three approaches to the parapharyngeal space:

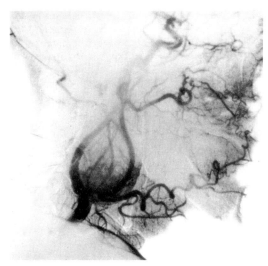

Figure 16.11 Carotid angiogram showing typical tumour blush of a chemodectoma

1 Transparotid
2 Transmandibular
3 Transcervical.

The transcervical route is best employed for these tumours. The sternomastoid muscle is retracted backwards, the tail of the submandibular gland swung forwards and the tail of the parotid gland lifted upwards. Adequate access to the skull base can be achieved by this route. The author's experience is that it has not been possible to remove nerve sheath tumours from this space, keeping the nerve intact. The first step is to make sure it is not a carotid body tumour or a glomus vagale. Once this is done, the nerve is dissected off the artery and excised with the tumour. The vocal cord paralysis is subsequently rehabilitated by a Teflon injection or a thyroplasty.

Treatment of carotid body tumours

Carotid body tumours should be removed if technically possible. If the tumour is not removed, then the patient is left with a progressively enlarging neck tumour of uncertain biological behaviour. The factor that limits resection is extension to the skull base. Unless there is an inch (2.5 cm) or so of carotid artery free of tumour at the skull base, it is impossible to attach a graft and resection should be abandoned. Usually it is possible to dissect these tumours from the carotid after freeing its whole length and rotating it. This is to allow access to the posterior aspect where a plane can often be entered. At all of these operations, however, there should exist the facility for immediate vascular grafting if required.

Radiation should not be used as a primary treatment. It should be reserved for poor risk patients, inoperable patients, malignant tumours and those who refuse surgery.

Lymphangiomas
Terminology

There are three types of lymphangioma:

1 Lymphangioma simplex
2 Cavernous lymphangioma
3 Cystic hygroma.

Embryology

The lymphatic system arises from five primitive sacs (two jugular sacs, two posterior sciatic sacs and a single retroperitoneal sac) developed from the venous system. Endothelial buds from these extend centrifugally to form the peripheral lymphatic system.

There are two theories of the origin of lymphangiomas: either they are sequestrations of lymphatic tissue derived from portions of the primitive sacs, which retain their rapid and proliferative growth potential and have no connection to the normal lymphatic system, or they arise from endothelial fibrillar membranes which sprout from the walls of the cyst, penetrate the surrounding tissue, canalize and produce more cysts.

Pathology

Lymphogenous conditions have been classified into three groups:

1 Lymphangioma simplex – composed of thin-walled capillary-sized lymphatic channels
2 Cavernous lymphangioma – composed of dilated lymphatic spaces often with a fibrous adventitia
3 Cystic hygroma – composed of cysts varying in size from a few millimetres to several centimetres in diameter.

All these can be regarded as one entity but site may play some part in the final version – the smaller lymphangiomas occur in the lips, tongue, cheek and where the tissue planes are tighter, whereas the cystic hygroma has more space to expand into the tissue planes of the neck. Simple lymphangiomas can occur anywhere in the mouth as pale soft fluctuant lesions and form one-third of all lymphangiomatous tumours. More common are cavernous lymphangiomas which form 40% of these lesions, mainly in the tongue. At the base of the tongue they must be differentiated from a lingual thyroid, a lingual carcinoma or an internal laryngocoele. They also occur on the lateral border of the tongue. Some cheek lesions reach an enormous size and are very difficult to eradicate since total excision produces an unacceptable cosmetic defect.

A cavernous lymphangioma of the floor of the mouth can be part of a cystic hygroma or a ranula. Macrocheilia usually affects only the upper lip.

A cystic hygroma consists of large multinodular cystic masses which may communicate or be isolated. The walls are thin and the contained fluid can be clearly seen. A hygroma occurs in the cervicofacial region spreading into the cheek, mouth, tongue, parotid and even the ear canal.

Histologically the cyst is lined by a single layer of flattened endothelium with fetal fat and cholesterol crystals. They are rare tumours forming 0.5% of large series of neck lumps. There is no sex or side predominance. Two out of three are noted at birth and nine out of 10 before the end of the second year.

Thirty-five per cent of lymphangiomas of all types occur in the cheek, tongue and floor of the mouth, 25% in the neck and 15% in the axilla.

Clinical features

Most of these tumours manifest themselves at birth or shortly afterwards. Lymphangiomas in the mouth can first appear in adult life, as can recurrences of cystic hygromas after surgery in infancy. Recurrences usually occur on the periphery of the facial area where the main mass originally presented, such as the ear, parotid or posterior triangle.

While size alone is the prominent first symptom and sign, if the cyst is big enough it can cause stridor (Figure 16.12). In very large cysts, lateral displacement of the trachea and even mediastinal widening may be seen on the radiograph.

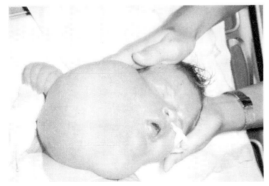

Figure 16.12 Cystic hygroma in a neonate

Sudden increase in size by spontaneous haemorrhage may be fatal. Brachial plexus compression with pain and hyperaesthesia may also occur.

The most common site is in the posterior triangle of the neck. Large masses can extend into the anterior triangle and across the midline. These anterior tumours may involve the floor of the mouth and the base of the tongue. Cystic hygromas often extend up into the cheek and parotid gland or down into the mediastinum or axilla.

If it is not the gross congenital swelling characteristically seen at birth, it can be discovered as a painless soft or semi-firm swelling in the neck. The tumour usually progressively enlarges, although some fluctuation in size is common. Depending on its mass and direction of growth, the lesion can encroach on the trachea, pharynx and oesophagus causing dyspnoea and dysphagia. A sudden increase in size of the tumour may be secondary to infection or haemorrhage and has caused death. Tumour swelling is usually related to upper respiratory tract infection and tumour pain, which is an unusual complaint, occurs only in the presence of infection. One case of facial nerve paralysis due to enlargement of the hygroma has been recorded.

The diagnosis is usually made on clinical grounds. CT scanning shows the extent and size of the lesion and also its relation to the important structures at the skull base.

Treatment

The treatment of lymphangiomas is surgical. Intraoral lymphangiomas should be removed from an external approach since they are almost certainly much more extensive than expected. Remnants will also be left in the tissue planes of the tongue. Lymphangiomas of the base of the tongue can often be dealt with by laser excision, repeated if necessary. Cryosurgery may also be helpful. Lymphangioma of the upper lip should be dealt with by a lip shave and vermilion advancement and excision of muscle and cyst to reach an acceptable size.

Recurrences usually appear within the first 9 months in about 10–15% of patients. The recurrence rate is higher with cavernous lymphangiomas than with cystic hygromas.

No patient with a cystic hygroma should have surgery unless he has had a chest radiograph to check for mediastinal extension. Since the child at birth looks like a monster to the mother, surgery should not be delayed. Total removal is impossible, but surgery is easiest at the first attempt, before there is infection and scarring, so as much as possible is removed. It is essential not to damage the child and so the carotid arteries, jugular vein, vagus nerve and facial nerve, if necessary, are dissected with great care. The first excision should be limited to the cervical area. After removal it will become apparent that there is a large amount of the tumour left in the parotid and cheek. Excision of this should be delayed as long as possible, taking into account the effect of an asymmetrical face on a child's psyche. The longer one waits, the bigger

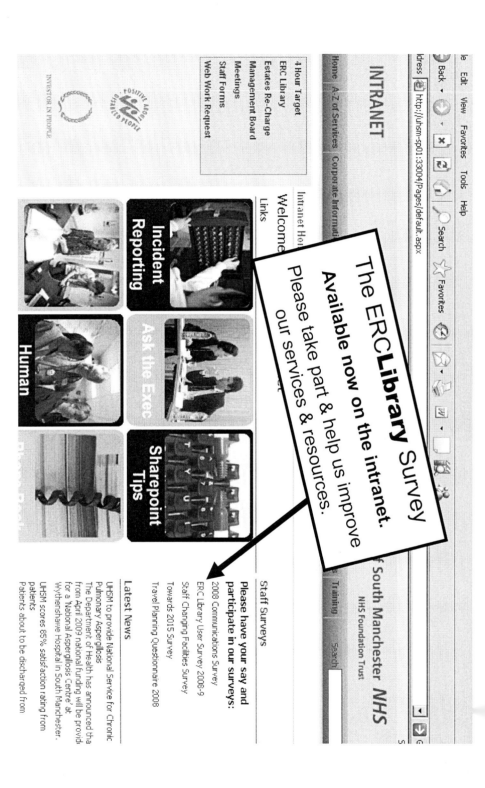

the facial nerve branches become and the safety of dissection increases. In the initial excision the nerves most likely to be damaged are the lower branch of the facial nerve, the spinal accessory and the vagus.

Radiotherapy should not be used because of the possible damaging effects on the growth of local structures and the potential induction of malignancy.

Injection of sclerosants has been suggested and tried, but the scarring is unpredictable because of the multiplicity of cysts and further surgery may be made very difficult.

Repeated aspirations should only be performed in the event of rapid increase in size causing pressure effects. The danger is infection and possibly haemorrhage into the cysts.

Broomhead (1964) claimed that in 15% of patients there is spontaneous regression but this view has not met with universal agreement.

After surgery, about one-third of patients will have nerve paralysis and more than half will have to undergo further surgery.

Dermoid cysts

Pathology

In the head and neck there are three varieties of dermoid cyst.

Epidermoid cyst

The epidermoid cyst has no adnexal structures, is lined by squamous epithelium and may contain cheesy keratinous material. This is the most common variety.

True dermoid cyst

The true dermoid cyst is lined by squamous epithelium and contains skin appendages such as hair, hair follicles, sebaceous glands and sweat glands. Dermoid cysts are either congenital or acquired.

The congenital type derives from ectodermal differentiations of multipotential cells pinched off at the time of closure of the anterior neuropore. It occurs, therefore, along the lines of fusion.

The acquired type is due to implantation of epidermis at the time of a puncture type of injury and is often solid with areas of cystic spaces containing sebaceous material.

Teratoid cyst

The teratoid cyst can be lined with squamous or respiratory epithelium and contains elements formed from ectoderm, endoderm and mesoderm – nails, teeth, brain, glands, etc. This is the rarest variety in the neck and is nearly always diagnosed in the first

year of life. Fewer than 10 examples of teratoid tumours of the neck have been described in adults.

Twenty per cent of all dermoid cysts are found in the neck, and 30% in the neck and face. Dermoid cysts form 28% of all midline cysts, and there is no sex predominance.

Clinical features

These cysts present as solid or cystic masses in the midline of the neck between the suprasternal notch and the submental region. They can also occur lateral to the submandibular gland. Painless swelling is the only symptom, but if the cyst is large, minor obstructive symptoms can occur.

About 20% of dermoid cysts occur in the mouth, either deep to the mylohyoid (sublingual) or superficial to it (submental). They present in the second and third decades but have probably been present since birth (Figure 16.13).

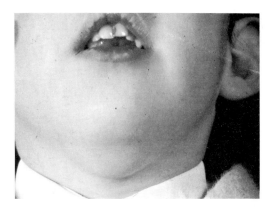

Figure 16.13 Dermoid cyst of the neck

Treatment

Complete excision is usually easy and should be carried out in all patients.

Infective neck masses

Tuberculosis

Pathology

The condition is not common in the USA or Europe, but it is still common in Asia or Africa. There are 32 000 new cases of tuberculosis in the USA each year and 5% of these develop cervical lymphadenitis.

Where the incidence of tuberculosis is low, primary infections are acquired later and so it is young adults who acquire tuberculous nodes. In the UK, the maximum age incidence is 5–9 years, but in 30% it occurs in patients over the age of 25 years many of whom are Asian immigrants.

The bacillus, which is usually the human variety, reaches the lymph nodes by direct drainage or by haematogenous spread. The incidence of coexisting pulmonary tuberculosis is less than 5%. In one series, almost half of the tonsils removed showed evidence of tuberculosis and it thus appeared that the tonsil was the source and that the cervical adenitis was precipitated by an attack of acute tonsillitis. Once the bacillus has entered the host, further exposure is not necessary to trigger off the adenopathy.

Clinical features

Most patients give a fairly long history and usually seek medical advice because the lumps have become painful. In Asia, the presentation is different: 20% have discharging sinuses, 10% a cold abscess and 10% are adherent to the skin; all these patients have a negative chest radiograph.

Ninety per cent are unilateral and 90% involve only one node group, the most common being the deep jugular chain followed by the nodes in the submandibular region and then those of the posterior triangle.

Diagnosis is by a positive tuberculin skin test and demonstration of acid and alkali fast bacteria in the biopsy. In the USA, patients should also have histoplasmin and coccidioidin skin tests. The differential diagnosis is between lymphoma and metastatic cancer. The absence of a primary tumour in a young adult and the length of history usually makes the latter diagnosis improbable.

Treatment

The treatment is an excisional biopsy followed by 9–12 months of antituberculous chemotherapy. If the glands are very large and matted, local removal is dangerous since the nodes are often attached to the internal jugular vein. A functional neck dissection should then be carried out preserving the sternomastoid, accessory nerve, and jugular vein if possible. In a child, it is usually wise to remove and examine histologically the tonsils before removing the lymph nodes.

If removal is not followed immediately by chemotherapy, a sinus forms with persistent drainage and, later, ugly scars.

Sarcoidosis

Sarcoidosis presenting as cervical adenitis with no other manifestation of the disease is extremely rare. The neck nodes are not often involved in this condi-

tion, even when it is generalized. It is almost impossible, therefore, to make a preoperative diagnosis and a biopsy is always needed. The histological characteristic is the absence of caseation. Diagnosis may be confirmed by the Kveim skin test.

AIDS

The head and neck manifestations of acquired immune deficiency syndrome (AIDS) include multiple cervical lymph nodes, multicentric simple parotid cysts, benign lymphoid hyperplasia, cutaneous, oral or pharyngeal lesions of Kaposi's sarcoma, hairy leukoplakia and aerodigestive lesions of *Candida*. Parotid enlargement is due to hyperplastic intraparotid lymph nodes which are also seen to be characteristically cystic on imaging.

Toxoplasmosis

Toxoplasmosis is a worldwide infection caused by *Toxoplasma gondii*, a protozoon transmitted by the ingestion of cysts excreted in the faeces of infected cats, or from eating undercooked beef or lamb. The manifestations of congenital infection are principally cerebral, including hydrocephalus or microcephaly. Many patients with acquired toxoplasmosis are asymptomatic. Acute symptoms include generalized aches and pains, fever, cough, malaise and a maculopapular rash. In the more chronic form there may simply be lymphadenopathy. The peripheral blood picture shows lymphocytosis with some atypical mononuclear cells similar to those seen with Epstein–Barr infection. Reactivation of latent toxoplasmosis may cause encephalitis in immunocompromised patients. Diagnosis is confirmed by the presence of serum antibodies, by lymph node biopsy or by examination of the cerebrospinal fluid. Where treatment is indicated, a combination of suphadimidine, pyrimethamine and folic acid is used and the blood count is monitored weekly.

Actinomycosis

This disease is now regarded as a bacterial infection and is caused by *Actinomycosis israelii*, an anaerobic organism which is a commensal in the healthy oral cavity. The organism may become pathogenic when the mucous membrane is injured. Infection usually affects the cervicofacial region and is nearly always associated with severe dental caries and periodontitis. Occasionally suppurative pneumonia and empyema may develop. A firm indurated mass with indefinite edges is found, usually lateral to the mandible. If untreated the mass spreads by direct invasion to adjacent tissue and becomes bony hard. Characteristically multiple sinuses develop which discharge pus and watery fluid containing sulphur grains. Treatment is by intravenous benzylpenicillin and may require to be continued for several weeks.

Cat-scratch disease

This is a slowly progressive chronic form of regional lymphadenopathy, associated with small pleomorphic Gram-negative bacilli within the walls of capillaries, and in lymph node macrophages, but the bacillus and its associated antibody are difficult to identify. The involved lymph nodes are acutely tender. Only one-third of patients are pyrexial but about 90% give a history of contact with cats, most commonly kittens. A primary papule or vesicle develops at the site of a scratch 1–2 weeks after contact with the cat. This subsides after a few weeks and may be helpful in diagnosis. Lymphadenopathy ensues 1–2 weeks later.

Brucellosis

This is primarily a disease of domesticated animals and causes contagious abortion or other reproductive problems in cattle (*Brucella abortus*), pigs (*B. suis*), goats (*B. melitensis*), dogs (*B. canis*), and sheep (*B. ovis*). Human spread occurs by direct contact of infected tissue with conjunctiva or broken skin, by ingestion of contaminated meat or dairy products and by inhalation of infectious aerosols. Pasteurization of milk and other measures have greatly reduced the incidence in the western countries, but stock producers, abattoir employees and veterinary surgeons remain at risk. The symptoms in humans are so variable that there is no characteristic clinical picture. The average incubation is 2–3 weeks and some infections are subclinical. In clinical cases most patients have drenching sweats, chills, fever and malaise. Although classically associated with undulating fever, the commonest pyrexia pattern is a slight elevation in the morning with an increase in the afternoon. About 20% of patients have cervical and inguinal lymphadenopathy and a similar percentage have splenomegaly. Relapses occur in 5% of patients but are uncommon in appropriately treated individuals. Complications include arthritis, meningitis, depression, genitourinary symptoms, abnormal liver function tests, pulmonary symptoms and blood dyscrasias. A definitive diagnosis is made by recovering the organism from blood, fluid or tissue specimens. Blood cultures should be processed using the Castaneda biphasic medium bottle. The diagnosis can also be made serologically.

Treatment is probably best effected by combination therapy as most single agents are associated with a 30% chance of relapse. The presently favoured World Health Organization recommendation is a combination of doxycycline 200 mg and rifampacin up to 900 mg daily for 6 weeks. Prevention is by reducing the incidence of brucellosis in animal populations, e.g. the vaccination of cattle with *B. abortus* strain 19 vaccine.

Infectious mononucleosis

The characteristic clinical triad is fever, sore throat and lymphadenopathy. About 5% of patients have a rash which is almost universal if ampicillin is inadvertently administered. Up to 50% have palatal petechiae or splenomegaly. More serious complications include autoimmune haemolytic anaemia, thrombocytopenia, splenic rupture, encephalitis and cranial nerve palsies. On rare occasions the degree of pharyngeal obstruction from swelling of the lymphoid tissue is such that tracheostomy is required to prevent acute upper airway obstruction.

The illness in the vast majority of patients subsides over 2–3 weeks. Elevation of hepatocellular enzymes is usually also self-limiting but alcohol is probably best avoided for a few months after the illness. Treatment is largely supportive. Contact sports or heavy lifting should be avoided during the first 2–3 weeks of the illness. Corticosteroids have a part to play in impending airway obstruction, in severe thrombocytopenia or haemolytic anaemia, and sometimes in the presence of other complications. The role of antiviral chemotherapy in the management of Epstein-Barr virus infections is likely to broaden as new agents are developed. Given the potential oncogenicity of Epstein-Barr virus, the risk of administration of inactivated Epstein-Barr virus as a vaccination has not yet been fully evaluated and immunization against Epstein-Barr virus has not been established.

Neck space infections

Neck space infections are very rare and there is confusion about how many neck spaces there are: estimates vary from 13 to 20. A fascial space is an area of loose connective tissue bounded by dense connective tissue called fascia. It is a matter of opinion how thick connective tissue must be before it is called fascia, and this is where the disagreement as to the number of spaces arises. Knowledge of the anatomy of the areas in which infection tended to collect was important in the pre-antibiotic days from the point of view of routes of spread, complications, and surgical drainage, but nowadays knowledge of three spaces (retropharyngeal, lateral pharyngeal and submandibular) will allow management of 90% of patients.

Anatomy

The spaces listed are described by Hollinshead (1954) and are shown in Table 16.1.

Table 16.1 Anatomy of neck spaces

Below the hyoid
  carotid sheath
  pretracheal space
  retrovisceral space
  visceral space
  prevertebral space
Above the hyoid
  submandibular space
  submaxillary space
  masticator space
  parotid space
Peripharyngeal area
  retropharyngeal space
  lateral pharyngeal (parapharyngeal) space
  submandibular space
Intrapharyngeal area
  paratonsillar space

Nowadays, abscesses usually only occur in the retropharyngeal, lateral pharyngeal (parapharyngeal) and submandibular spaces.

Retropharyngeal space

This space lies between the pharynx and the posterior layer of the deep fascia which bounds the prevertebral space. It separates the pharynx from the vertebral column and extends from the base of the skull to the posterior mediastinum as far as the bifurcation of the trachea. Anteriorly, it connects with the pretracheal space so that infections can spread by way of this latter space to the anterior mediastinum, though mediastinitis due to a retropharyngeal abscess is rare. In the infant this space contains one or two lymph nodes.

Lateral pharyngeal space

This is more commonly known as the parapharyngeal space; it lies lateral to the pharynx connecting with the retropharyngeal space posteriorly. Laterally, it is bounded by the lateral pterygoid muscles and the sheath of the parotid gland. It extends from the base of the skull to the level of the hyoid bone where it is limited by the sheath of the submandibular gland. This sheath is also connected to the sheaths of the stylohyoid muscle and the posterior belly of the digastric muscle.

The carotid sheath is bounded anterosuperiorly by the pterygomandibular raphe and the spaces around the floor of the mouth anteroinferiorly.

This space is prone to infection because of its close connection to the tongue, teeth, parotid, submandibular gland and tonsils.

Submandibular space

This is bounded above by the mucous membrane of the floor of the mouth and tongue and below by the deep fascia that extends from the hyoid to the mandible.

It is divided into two by the mylohyoid muscle and so the submandibular gland, which is wrapped around the mylohyoid muscle, extends into both parts of the space. The space superior to the mylohyoid muscle contains most of the sublingual gland. The space inferior to the muscle contains the submandibular gland. Anteriorly lies the submental space between the two anterior bellies of digastric.

Infections of this space are known as Ludwig's angina.

Clinical features and management

Retropharyngeal abscess

This abscess in infants is due to a lymphadenitis secondary to an upper respiratory tract infection. The child has a sore throat; examination shows a swelling behind an otherwise normal tonsil. The temperature is elevated to 38–39°C and the child is ill. The swelling may obstruct the posterior nares and push the soft palate down. Respiratory obstruction is an ever-present danger because the child's spine is short and the larynx is high. (In a 9-month-old infant, the epiglottis is at the level of the atlas.)

Radiographs of the neck show a large retropharyngeal swelling. Treatment is by incision and drainage in the tonsil position.

In an adult, a retropharyngeal abscess usually signifies a tuberculous infection of the cervical spine. It is of insidious onset with a low grade fever. Pus must be obtained to confirm the diagnosis which is also suggested on a radiograph of the cervical spine. Treatment is by antituberculous chemotherapy.

Parapharyngeal abscess

This is more common in adults than children. It is a complication of tonsillectomy or tonsillitis in about 60% of patients and a complication of infection or extraction of the lower third molar in a further 30% (Figure 16.14).

Infection of the petrous apex can rarely rupture directly into the space. Infection of the mastoid tip can also enter the space by way of the digastric sheath.

There is fever and marked trismus because of involvement of the medial pterygoid muscle. The tonsil is pushed medially but looks normal. The most

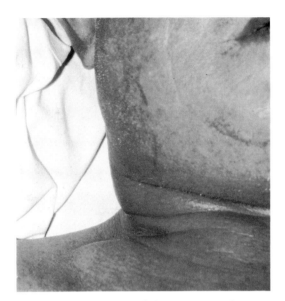

Figure 16.14 Parapharyngeal abscess occurring during a tonsillar infection

marked swelling is in the neck at the posterior part of the middle third of the sternomastoid. Each patient should be given at least 48 hours' treatment with an antibiotic, but by this time most patients have a swollen neck and incision and drainage will be required.

Ludwig's angina

This is a rapidly swelling cellulitis of the floor of the mouth and submandibular space secondary to soft tissue infection, tonsillar infection and infection of the lower premolar and molar teeth. Over 80% of patients have dental disease and, in these patients, the lower molars are set eccentrically with the roots closer to the inner than the outer side of the jaw, or the roots of the second and third molars may lie inferior to the mylohyoid line. Root abscesses of these teeth, therefore, drain into the submandibular space. This space may be affected with minimal discomfort from the tooth; pain comes from tension within the bone, but if this gives way and drains there is no dental pain. In cases of dental origin the most usual organisms are *Streptococcus viridans* and *Escherichia coli*.

When infection spreads to the sublingual space, the floor of the mouth becomes very swollen and appears as a roll of oedematous tissue rising to the level of the biting edge of the teeth. The tongue is elevated posterosuperiorly and respiratory obstruction is a danger. The patient is very ill with a temperature of over 38°C with pain, trismus and salivation.

Treatment is by antibiotics; incision and drainage should be postponed as long as possible.

Laryngocoele
Pathology

In the UK, the incidence of laryngocoele is approximately one per 2.5 million population per year. The sex incidence is 5:1 in favour of men and the peak age incidence is at 50–60 years. Only one case has been reported in a neonate, but it is possible that this was a laryngeal cyst; 82% were in Caucasians; 85% were unilateral and 15% bilateral. They can be external (30%), where the sac arises from the laryngeal ventricle and expands into the neck through the thyrohyoid membrane, or internal (20%) where it arises from the laryngeal ventricle and stays within the larynx presenting in the vallecula, or combined (50%). Laryngocoeles are lined by columnar ciliated epithelium, whereas simple laryngeal cysts are lined by squamous epithelium.

It has long been held that laryngocoeles are due to 'blowing' hobbies or jobs such as trumpet playing or glass blowing. A careful review of the published cases reveals at most four patients subject to these habits so this theory appears to be untrue. Of more importance is the coexistence of a carcinoma or papilloma of the larynx which acts as a valve allowing air under pressure into the ventricle. External laryngocoeles can be found in 16% of laryngectomy specimens for laryngeal carcinoma, as opposed to 2% in laryngectomy specimens for pyriform sinus cancer. The ventricle in these cases of laryngeal cancer was also significantly higher than that in patients with pharyngeal cancer due to increased air pressure consequent upon obstruction by the laryngeal carcinoma.

Lower animals have air sacs, e.g. the cheek pouch of monkeys, the fish pouch of pelicans, the tracheal sacs of emus, the syrinx of male quacking birds, etc. Lateral laryngeal sacs are well developed in certain anthropoid apes and are a means of enabling the animal to rebreathe while holding its breath for long periods.

Laryngocoeles in man, therefore, are almost certainly atavistic remnants corresponding to these lateral air sacs. On occasion they become manifest due to an increase in intralaryngeal air pressure due to blowing or coughing.

Clinical features

The most common presenting features are hoarseness and a swelling in the neck. The third most common symptom is stridor, which can come on very suddenly over a period of a few days or even hours in a patient who had previously only mild symptoms for months or years. Other presenting symptoms are dysphagia, sore throat, snoring, pain or cough. Ten per cent present with infected sacs (pyocoeles) and, because of the mixture of infection and air on the radiograph, a diagnosis of gas gangrene is sometimes made. On palpation, the swelling which is usually large and over the thyrohyoid membrane, can be emptied easily (Figure 16.15). A plain radiograph of the neck is diagnostic showing an air-filled sac. Nothing else except gas gangrene can produce this picture (Figure 16.16).

The most common presenting symptom of laryngocoeles is hoarseness with apparently normal vocal cords. To diagnose smaller laryngocoeles, therefore, every patient with hoarseness and normal vocal cords should have a plain anteroposterior neck radiograph with and without a Valsalva manoeuvre. Particularly

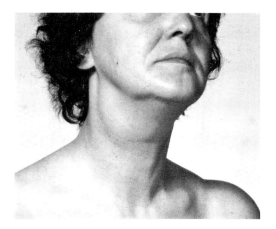

Figure 16.15 An inflated laryngocoele

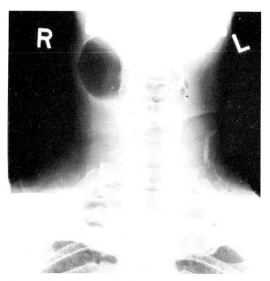

Figure 16.16 Radiograph showing a laryngocoele

if a unilateral laryngocoele is present, the patient should have a laryngoscopy to make sure there is no underlying carcinoma of the laryngeal ventricle. These tumours can act as valves allowing air into, but not out of, the saccule thus dilating it.

If an enlarged saccule does not penetrate the thyrohyoid membrane, it travels up behind the thyrohyoid membrane and the hyoid and bulges into the vallecula. This is an internal laryngocoele and, if the mouth of the sac is blocked, then it may be full of mucus and not radiolucent. These are often diagnosed during routine otolaryngological examination and may be quite symptomless. On occasion they can reach a reasonably large size and the patient complains of a feeling of a lump in the throat.

Treatment

Laryngocoeles discovered radiologically and that are contained within the larynx, require no treatment. The patients have the cause of the hoarseness explained to them and are kept under annual review. If surgery is attempted on these patients, the uninflated saccule is almost impossible to find and oversew.

Internal laryngocoeles may be uncapped to see if marsupialization and scarring will stop recurrence. If they recur then they should be excised with the approach used for the external laryngocoele.

An infected laryngocoele should be aspirated and treated with antibiotics. When the infection has subsided, formal excision should be carried out.

The best operation for a laryngocoele aims at excising the saccule at its neck. This is found by removing the upper half of one thyroid ala, or fracturing it downwards and replacing it. The method used depends on the state of ossification of the thyroid cartilage. Once access to the supraglottis is obtained, it is an easy matter to follow the neck of the laryngocoele down as far as possible. The neck is transected and closed in layers and oversewn. If the thyroid ala is not replaced then the thyroid perichondrium is sewn into the area.

Recurrence after this operation is extremely rare.

References

BROOMHEAD, I. W. (1964) Cystic hygroma of the neck. *British Journal of Plastic Surgery*, **17**, 285

DAS GUPTA, T. K., BRASFIELD, R. D., STRONG, E. W. and HAJDU, S. L. (1969) Benign solitary schwannomas (neurilemmomas). *Cancer*, **24**, 355

HOLLINSHEAD, W.H. (1954) *Anatomy for Surgeons*, vol. 1. London: Cassel

HORAK, E., SZENTIRMAY, Z. and SWGAR, J. (1983) Pathologic features of nerve sheath tumours with respect to prognostic signs. *Cancer*, **51**, 1159–1167

KING, E. S. J. (1949) The lateral lympho-epithelial cyst of the neck (branchial cyst). *Australian and New Zealand Journal of Surgery*, **19**, 109

SCHLANGE, H. (1893) Ueber die Fistula colli congenita. *Archives für klinische Chirurgie*, **46**, 390

SHORE-FREEDMAN, E., ABRAHAMS, C., RECANT, W. and SCHNEIDER, A. B. (1983) Neurilemmomas and salivary gland tumours of the head and neck following childhood irradiation. *Cancer*, **51**, 2159–2163

SISTRUNK, W. E. (1920) The surgical treatment of cysts of the thyroglossal tract. *Annals of Surgery*, **71**, 121–123

WENGLOWSKI, R. (1912) Veber die Halsfistein und Cysten. *Archives für klinische Chirurgie*, **65**, 172–176

Further reading

ALESSI, D. P. and DUDLEY, J. P. (1988) Atypical mycobacteria induced cervical adenitis: treatment by needle aspiration. *Archives of Otolaryngology – Head and Neck Surgery*, **114**, 664–666

AMIN, M. and MARAN, A. G. D. (1988) The aetiology of laryngocoele. *Clinical Otolaryngology*, **13**, 267–272

BENNHOFF, D. F. (1985) Actinomycosis: diagnostic and therapeutic considerations and a review of 32 cases. *Laryngoscope*, **94**, 1198–1217

CIVANTOS, F. J. and HOLINGER, L. D. (1992) Laryngoceles and saccular cysts in infants and children. *Archives of Otolaryngology – Head and Neck Surgery*, **118**, 296–300

COHEN, S. R. and THOMPSON, J. W. (1986) Lymphangiomas of the larynx in infants and children: a survey of pediatric lymphangioma. *Annals of Otolaryngology and Laryngology*, **127**, (Suppl.), 1–20

FLEMING, W. B. (1988) Infections in branchial cysts. *Australian and New Zealand Journal of Surgery*, **58**, 481–483

FRANKLIN, D. I., MOORE, G. F. and FISCH, U. (1989) Jugular foramen peripheral nerve sheath tumors. *Laryngoscope*, **99**, 1081–1087

FRIEDBERG, J. (1989) Pharyngeal cleft sinuses and cysts and other benign neck lesions. *Pediatric Clinics of North America*, **36**, 1451–1469

JACKSON, C. G., HARRIS, P. F. and GLASSCOCK, M. E. (1990) Diagnosis and management of paragangliomas of the skull base. *American Journal of Surgery*, **159**, 389–393

KATZ, A. D., PASSY, V. and KAPLAN, N. (1971) Neurogenous neoplasms of major nerves of the head and neck. *Archives of Surgery*, **103**, 51–56

KENNEDY, T. L. (1989) Cystic hygroma-lymphangioma: a rare and still unclear entity. *Laryngoscope*, **99** (suppl.), 1–10

LEVEQUE, H., SARACENO, A. A., TANG, C. K. and BLANCHARD, O. L. (1979) Dermoid cysts of the floor of the mouth and lateral neck. *Laryngoscope*, **89**, 296–305

MICHEAU, C., KLIJANIENKO, J., LUBOINSKI, B. and RUHARD, J. (1990) So called branchiogenic carcinoma is actually cystic metastases in the neck from a tonsillar primary. *Laryngoscope*, **100**, 878–883

MIKAELIAN, A. J., VARBEY, B., GROSSMAN, T. W. and BLATNIK, D. S. (1989) Blastomycosis of the head and neck. *Otolaryngology – Head and Neck Surgery*, **101**, 489–495

MITCHELL, O. B., IRWIN, C., BAILEY, O. M. and EVANS, J. N. G. (1987) Cysts of the infant larynx. *Journal of Laryngology and Otology*, **101**, 833–837

RADKOWSKI, D., ARNOLD, J. and HEALY, G. B. (1991) Thyroglossal duct remnants: pre-operative evaluation and management. *Archives of Otolaryngology – Head and Neck Surgery*, **117**, 1378–1381

RICCIARDELLI, E. J. and RICHARDSON, M. A. (1991) Cervicofacial cystic hygroma: patterns of recurrence and management of the difficult case. *Archives of Otolaryngology – Head and Neck Surgery*, **117**, 546–553

SHARP, J. F., KERR, A. K., CARDER, P. and SELLAR, R. J. (1989) Facial schwannoma without facial paralysis. *Journal of Laryngology and Otology*, **103**, 973–975

SHINKWIN, C., WHITFIELD, B. C. S. and ROBSON, A. K. (1991) Branchial cysts: congenital or acquired. *Annals of the Royal College of Surgeons of England*, **73**, 379–380

TUFFIN, J. R. and THEAKER, E. (1991) True lateral dermoid cyst of the neck. *International Journal of Oral and Maxillofacial Surgery*, **20**, 275–276

WILSON, J. A., MCLAREN, K. and MACINTYRE, M. A. (1988) Nerve sheath tumours of the head and neck. *Ear Nose and Throat Journal*, **67**, 103–110

YOUNG, E. J. (1983) Human brucellosis. *Review of Infectious Diseases*, **5**, 821–844

17

Metastatic neck disease

John Hibbert

The single most important factor in determining the survival of patients with a head and neck cancer at any site is the presence or absence of metastatic disease in the neck. It is therefore essential in treating patients with head and neck cancer to pay particular attention to the possibility of neck node metastases. Unfortunately medical opinion is divided on the best way of managing some of these problems. Thus controversy applies to topics such as the assessment of neck disease, the prophylactic treatment of metastatic nodes, the place of radical neck dissection as opposed to modified neck dissection and the place of radiotherapy.

Applied anatomy of the neck

A detailed knowledge of the surgical anatomy of the neck is essential for an understanding of the diagnosis and management of pathological processes occurring there. Surgical procedures in the neck are essentially exercises in applied anatomy and any surgeon operating in this region must have a complete knowledge of its anatomy.

Anatomical divisions of the neck

The divisions of the neck are illustrated in Figure 17.1 and it must be remembered that, although only shown in two dimensions these triangles are, in fact, three dimensional. The posterior triangle is bounded by the trapezius muscle, the middle third of the clavicle and by the posterior border of the sternomastoid muscle. The anterior triangle is bounded by the anterior border of the sternomastoid muscle, the

mandible and by the midline of the neck anteriorly. This apparently excludes the sternomastoid from the neck and what is more important excludes the structures deep to this muscle or makes it difficult to place them in a particular triangle. Since most of the important structures in the neck lie deep to the sternomastoid this is a ridiculous situation which has been handed down from anatomy text to anatomy text and has been transferred to surgical texts. By convention the structures deep to the sternomastoid are included within the anterior triangle as many of them emerge from the anterior border of the muscle. However, this anomalous situation would be easily

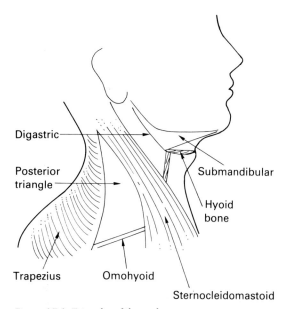

Figure 17.1 Triangles of the neck

avoided if the posterior limit of the anterior triangle was defined as the *posterior* border of the sternomastoid muscle so that the muscle and structures deep to it are included in the anterior triangle.

Further subdivisions of the two main triangles of the neck are usual. The posterior triangle is divided by the inferior belly of the omohyoid muscle into an occipital triangle and a supraclavicular triangle. The anterior triangle is divided into the submental, submandibular (or digastric), muscular and carotid triangles. In general each of the triangles of the neck contains connective tissue, blood vessels, nerves and lymph nodes. In addition certain triangles contain special organs or structures, e.g. the submandibular triangle contains the submandibular salivary gland, the anterior triangle contains the parotid gland above, the thyroid gland below and the larynx, pharynx and oesophagus in the midline.

Fascia and fascial spaces of the neck

The importance of the fascial spaces of the neck is that the localization and spread of neck space infections is dependent upon the fascial spaces. In addition, the fascia of the neck is important to surgeons because dissection is easier, better controlled and more bloodless if it proceeds along the fascial planes rather than through them. Removal of the fascia is an important part of a radical neck dissection mainly because it surrounds those tissues which need to be removed and also because dissection along the fascia protects important structures.

The superficial fascia of the neck is a single layer of fibrofatty tissue which lies superficial to the platysma muscle. The deep cervical fascia is much more extensive; it lies deep to the platysma muscle and occupies the spaces between muscles, blood vessels, lymph nodes and the viscera in the neck. In parts the deep cervical fascia is very thin forming little more than a thin sheet of areolar tissue, whereas in other situations it forms a dense fibrous layer surrounding various structures and allowing movement between structures. For descriptive purposes it is divided into three layers: the investing or external layer, the visceral or middle layer, and the internal layer. The investing part of the deep cervical fascia surrounds the whole of the neck and splits to surround the trapezius muscle posteriorly and the sternomastoid laterally. Above, its attachments are the superior nuchal line, the mastoid process and mandible. Below it is attached to the spine of the seventh cervical vertebra, the spine of the acromion, the clavicle and the manubrium. The investing layer also splits to provide a fascial sheath for the parotid and submandibular salivary glands and to form the carotid sheath which surrounds the internal and external carotid arteries, common carotid artery, internal jugular vein and the vagus nerve. Other cranial nerves are also surrounded by this fascia in the part of their course which is related to the carotid vessels and these are the glossopharyngeal, accessory and hypoglossal nerves (and the branch of the latter to the strap muscles, the ansa hypoglossi).

The middle layer of the deep cervical fascia surrounds the pharynx, larynx, oesophagus and trachea and allows these structures to move. The pretracheal fascia also surrounds the thyroid gland and usually the parathyroid glands are contained within this layer. The internal layer of the deep cervical fascia or prevertebral fascia surrounds the deep muscles of the neck, i.e. the erector spinae, the levator scapulae, the three scalene muscles, the longus capitis and longus colli. The prevertebral fascia has important relations with certain nerves in the neck. The cervical sympathetic trunk lies superficial to the prevertebral fascia deep and slightly medial to the carotid sheath. The branches of the cervical plexus lie deep to the fascia but pierce it as they become more superficial. The phrenic nerve lies deep to the prevertebral fascia as does the brachial plexus.

The lymphatic system of the head and neck

The lymph nodes of the head and neck consist of two main groups, an outlying group and a terminal group. The terminal group are the deep cervical nodes which lie along the internal jugular vein and which receive all the lymphatic drainage of the head and neck. The lymph may drain directly into the deep cervical group or may first pass through nodes of the outlying group. The deep cervical nodes are divided into upper and lower groups, and within these groups two more prominent either single nodes or groups of nodes can be identified. These are the jugulo-digastric nodes and the jugulo-omohyoid nodes. The jugulo-digastric nodes consist of one large and several smaller nodes situated in the triangle formed by the internal jugular vein, the facial vein and the posterior belly of the digastric muscle. They receive lymphatic vessels from the submandibular region, from the tonsil and from the tongue and floor of the mouth. The jugulo-omohyoid nodes are situated low in the neck close to the point where the omohyoid muscle crosses the internal jugular vein. This group of nodes receives lymphatic vessels from the anterior floor of mouth and from the tongue. The efferent vessels from the deep cervical nodes form into a jugular trunk which, on the right side ends at the junction of the internal jugular vein and subclavian vein or joins the right lymphatic duct, and on the left side usually joins the thoracic duct or may enter the junction of the internal jugular vein and subclavian vein separately (Figure 17.2).

The lymphatic drainage of the tissues of the head and neck is usually divided into superficial and deep,

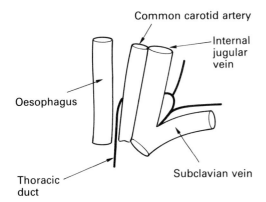

Figure 17.2 Termination of the thoracic duct

both systems draining either directly into the deep cervical nodes or first passing through outlying nodes.

The superficial system

The nodes which drain the superficial tissues of the head and neck consist of two circles of nodes, one in the head, the other in the neck. In the head these nodes are situated in groups, namely occipital, retroauricular, parotid and buccal (or facial); they drain the skin and underlying tissues of the scalp, eyelids and face. The superficial nodes in the neck consist of superficial cervical, submandibular, submental and anterior cervical. The superficial cervical nodes lie along the external jugular vein and the anterior cervical nodes along the anterior jugular veins.

The deep system

The deeper tissues of the head and neck drain either directly into the deep cervical group or indirectly after passing through a number of outlying nodes. The outlying nodes consist of the parotid, submandibular and submental groups already mentioned together with retropharyngeal, occasional lingual nodes (adjacent to the hyoglossus), infrahyoid, prelaryngeal, pretracheal nodes and paratracheal nodes.

In general the deeper tissues of the head and neck drain into the adjacent outlying nodes and deep cervical nodes. The nasopharynx and nasal cavities and sinuses drain into the upper deep cervical nodes having passed through retropharyngeal or submandibular lymph nodes. The oropharynx and tonsil drain into the upper deep cervical nodes either directly or via the retropharyngeal or submandibular nodes.

The oral cavity and tongue have a widely distributed system of drainage. The posterior parts of the tongue and oral cavity either drain directly into the upper deep cervical nodes or through the submandibular nodes. More anterior parts of the oral cavity and tongue also drain to these nodes but, in addition, lymph vessels pass to the submental nodes or directly to the jugulo-omohyoid nodes low in the neck. Since the tongue and floor of mouth are midline structures there is free communication between the two sides and contralateral drainage occurs. This is of course important when considering the spread of malignant disease.

The lymphatic drainage of the larynx is separated into lower and upper systems divided at the level of the true vocal cord. The supraglottis drains through vessels which accompany the superior laryngeal pedicle through the thyrohyoid membrane to reach the upper deep cervical nodes. The lower system drains directly into the deep cervical nodes through vessels which pass through or behind the cricothyroid membrane or drain into the prelaryngeal, pretracheal or paratracheal nodes before reaching the deep cervical nodes.

The lymphatic drainage of the pharynx is similar to the larynx and both may drain to each side of the neck, particularly areas which are close to the midline, e.g. epiglottis, posterior pharyngeal wall, postcricoid region. It should be noted that great variation occurs in the lymphatic drainage of the tissues of the head and neck and, in the case of malignant disease, this drainage may be greatly modified by surgery or radiotherapy to the area.

The patterns of spread of malignant disease to the neck

The spread of cancer to lymph nodes is dependent upon normal anatomical pathways but the pattern of spread may also depend upon distortion of drainage by disease and treatment such as radiotherapy and surgery (Larson, Lewis and Rapperport, 1965). In general the site of a metastasis in the neck is fairly predictable from the site of the primary tumour and Lindberg (1972) in a classical study of patients with head and neck cancer and palpable lymph nodes identified the most likely site of a metastasis related to the site of the primary tumour (Figure 17.3). It is usually accepted that these patterns of spread of obvious, palpable metastases are also applicable to subclinical microscopic metastases. The factors which affect the incidence of either palpable metastatic disease at presentation or microscopic disease are variable and depend both upon factors in the tumour and in the patient. These are difficult to identify with certainty but are very important in the management of disease. For example, if a particular tumour shows a very high incidence of occult metastases it is logical to consider treatment to these sites at the same time as treatment of the primary tumour. At the present time the treatment of patients with no palpable disease in the neck but who may have subclinical disease is the subject of much debate and is discussed

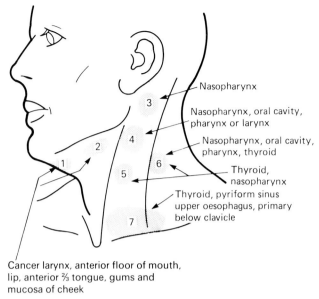

Nasopharynx

Nasopharynx, oral cavity,
pharynx or larynx

Nasopharynx, oral cavity,
pharynx, thyroid

Thyroid,
nasopharynx

Thyroid, pyriform sinus
upper oesophagus, primary
below clavicle

Cancer larynx, anterior floor of mouth,
lip, anterior ⅔ tongue, gums and
mucosa of cheek

Figure 17.3 The location of cervical lymph node groups most frequently affected by metastasis from named primary sites

below. The factors which affect the rate of metastasis are discussed below in terms of tumour and host factors. Certainly host factors are important, i.e. the patient's immunological response to the disease, but are much more difficult to identify and to quantify.

Site of the primary tumour

Tumours in certain sites show a very high incidence of both palpable metastases at presentation and occult metastases which appear subsequently, after successful treatment of the primary tumour. Thus nasopharyngeal, oropharyngeal, hypopharyngeal and oral cavity cancers have a very high incidence of palpable metastases on presentation. These same tumours show a high incidence of occult metastases of up to 40% in those patients whose necks are not treated at the time of treatment of the primary tumour. This information is obtainable partly from prophylactic neck dissection specimens in which occult disease is identified but also from the subsequent development of metastases in patients whose primary tumour has been successfully treated (Mendenhall, Million and Cassisi, 1980).

Size of the primary tumour

It is generally felt that the incidence of both palpable metastatic disease and occult metastatic disease is related to the size of the primary tumour (Spiro and Strong, 1971; Lindberg, 1972; Spiro *et al.*, 1974; Hibbert *et al.*, 1983). Similarly, studies have suggested that in those patients with no palpable metas-

tases on presentation the likelihood of metastases appearing at a later stage is increased in larger tumours (Biller, Davies and Ogura, 1971; Teichgracher and Clairmont, 1984).

Histological differentiation

The relationship between the histological differentiation of the primary tumour and its propensity to metastasize is not certain. Although it has been suggested that the poorer the differentiation the more likely the tumour is to metastasize (McGavran, Bauer and Ogura, 1961; Kirchner, Cornog and Holmes, 1974, Holm *et al.*, 1982), this is certainly not a particularly reliable relationship (Willen *et al.*, 1975). Of more importance is the characteristic of the interface between the edge of the tumour and the host; thus those tumours with an infiltrating margin are more likely to metastasize (McGavran, Bauer and Ogura, 1961). More recently the study of the infiltrative deep margin of the tumour in oral cancer has shown a close relationship between certain histopathological features and neck node metastasis and prognosis (Brync *et al.*, 1992).

Host factors

Although there can be little doubt that the immunological response of the host to the tumour is of vital importance in the spread and prognosis of head and neck cancer there is little in the way of definite evidence of this. Various attempts to assess the immunological response of patients with head and neck cancer have been made. Although there is correlation between immunological parameters and stage of disease and prognosis, these measures are relatively crude and not yet sufficiently well developed to allow predictions to be made (Katz, 1983; Mevio *et al.*, 1991).

Clinical staging of cervical metastases

Although the presence or absence of cervical metastases is the single most important factor in determining prognosis in head and neck cancer (Norris, 1963; Spiro *et al.*, 1974; Schuller *et al.*, 1980), the extent of the cervical metastases is also important. Thus staging of the metastasis is important both from the point of view of reporting disease but also in terms of management and prognosis in a particular patient. In an ideal staging system the prognosis should worsen as the stage of the disease increases. Because of differences in the importance of various factors the American Joint Committee (AJC) and the International Union against Cancer (UICC) until recently used a different nodal classification. Fortunately the most recent classifications suggested by the AJC and UICC are identical. These classifications apply to nodes from an unknown primary and from all primary tumours in the head and neck apart from the thyroid. The classification is shown in Table 17.1.

Table 17.1 TNM classification of regional nodes

Nx	Regional lymph nodes cannot be assessed
N0	No regional lymph node metastasis
N1	Metastasis in a single ipsilateral lymph node 3 cm or less in greatest dimension
N2	Metastasis in a single ipsilateral lymph node, more than 3 cm but not more than 6 cm in greatest dimension, or in multiple ipsilateral lymph nodes none more than 6 cm in greatest dimension, or in bilateral or contralateral lymph nodes, none more than 6 cm in greatest dimension
N2a	Metastasis in a single ipsilateral lymph node, more than 3 cm but not more than 6 cm in greatest dimension
N2b	Metastasis in multiple ipsilateral lymph nodes, none more than 6 cm in greatest dimension
N2c	Metastasis in bilateral or contralateral lymph nodes, none more than 6 cm in greatest dimension
N3	Metastasis in a lymph node more than 6 cm in greatest dimension

The present staging system has evolved from the previous systems where the UICC and AJC classifications differed significantly. The present system is based mainly upon the size of the node and attempts to relate the staging system to the prognosis of the patient. The nodal factors which affect prognosis are discussed in detail below. The present staging systems take no account of the position or level of the node in

the neck, although in the AJC classification, diagrammatic representation of the position of the node is encouraged. The importance of the position of the node in the neck is also discussed below.

Assessment of cervical lymph nodes

The assessment of cervical lymph nodes in a patient depends upon history, clinical examination and radiology. These are the limits of clinical staging for the TNM classification; examination of operative specimens by histopathology allows further staging and relation to prognosis.

History and clinical examination

The patient may be aware of a swelling in the neck, to which he may draw the clinician's attention. On the other hand one of the most important reasons for close follow up of patients who have had a head and neck malignancy is that cervical metastases may be detected by the clinician. Thus in follow-up examination careful inspection of both sides of the neck is essential. Each clinician will develop his own method of palpation but, in general, this should be from behind the patient, using both hands to palpate each side of the neck simultaneously and all regions of the neck should be examined. Thus a sequence of examination should be developed taking into account all regions. The present writer first examines the submandibular and submental triangles, then the neck anterior to the sternomastoid passing from above downwards, the supraclavicular fossa, then upwards into the posterior triangle and forwards across the sternomastoids to the nodes of the anterior triangle which are palpated a second time. If this sequence is adopted no area will be missed but, in addition the parotid region, the postauricular region, the pre- and post-vascular facial nodes and the thyroid gland should also be borne in mind in the relevant clinical situation.

Clinical examination still remains the most important method of assessing regional lymph nodes. Some nodes in the neck are more difficult to palpate than others. Thus retropharyngeal and parapharyngeal nodes are almost impossible to detect by palpation until they are very large and nodes in the supraclavicular fossa are often difficult to feel. Patients with short thick necks are more difficult to examine accurately.

Structures in the neck which may be mistaken for enlarged lymph nodes are the transverse process of the atlas, the carotid bifurcation and the submandibular salivary gland. In addition a lymph node may be enlarged because of infection or reactive hyperplasia rather than a metastatic deposit. Thus clinical examination of the neck has a variable reliability (Watkinson *et al.*, 1990). The false-positive rate of neck dissection is of the order of 20–30% (Beahrs and Barber, 1962; Ali, Tiwari and Snow, 1985) and the false-negative rate of the order of 30–40% (Beahrs and Barber, 1962; Cady and Catlin, 1989).

Radiology

Computerized tomography

CT scanning of the neck can certainly detect metastatic lymph nodes. As with clinical examination the sensitivity and specificity vary from series to series and depend upon the criteria used to define a node as metastatic or not. The three CT criteria which are used are size, peripheral enhancement (with i.v. contrast) and central necrosis (low attenuation area on CT). Different workers have used different size criteria, thus Friedman *et al.* (1984) used 1 cm as the maximum upper limit of a non-involved lymph node, whereas other workers have defined metastatic nodes as those larger than 1.5 cm on CT (Mancuso, Maceri and Rice, 1981; Stevens *et al.*, 1985). Probably the most reliable size criteria are that nodes up to 1.5 cm can be considered as non-metastatic in the submandibular and jugulo-digastric regions but up to 1 cm in other parts of the neck (Som, 1987). However, if central necrosis is present on CT or if there is a rim of enhancement around the periphery of the node, even small nodes are likely to be metastatic (Som, 1987). Uniform enhancement of a node is much more likely to indicate inflammatory rather than neoplastic disease.

In general, CT examination of the neck gives a similar sensitivity and specificity rate when compared with clinical examination (Feinmasser *et al.*, 1987), but when used in conjunction with clinical examination sensitivity and specificity may be improved (Friedman *et al.*, 1987). It is certainly not necessary to scan every patient but CT is of value in the assessment of necks which are difficult to palpate accurately (short, thick necks), in those where there is a high possibility of bilateral disease (midline primary tumours and extensive ipsilateral disease) and when invasion of the base of the skull and carotid artery are suspected. Routine scanning of the neck in a patient with head and neck cancer is probably not justifiable in terms of time and cost at the present time (Watkinson, 1993).

Magnetic resonance imaging

MRI is at present being evaluated in the assessment of cervical lymphadenopathy. Normal lymph nodes are rarely demonstrated but enlarged nodes and nodes with central necrosis are well demonstrated by MRI. At the present time CT is preferable to MRI for nodes smaller than 13 mm, but the two techniques are comparable for larger nodes except

that MRI differentiates nodes from surrounding tissues rather more clearly than CT (Dooms *et al.*, 1984).

Ultrasound

Metastatic lymph nodes in the neck can be demonstrated by ultrasound, but distinguishing between normal and metastatic nodes is difficult. Size has been used as one criterion (Hajek *et al.*, 1986) though malignant nodes may show a heterogeneous appearance with a mixed solid and cystic image. Ultrasound has been said to be more sensitive than clinical examination in the detection of cervical lymphadenopathy due to metastatic disease (Baatenburg de Jong *et al.*, 1988) and will demonstrate the relationship of metastatic nodes to the major vessels in the neck (Rothstein, Persky and Horii, 1988). Ultrasound can also be used in conjunction with fine needle aspiration cytology (Rothstein, Persky and Horii, 1988).

Radioisotopes

Scanning with radionuclides and using a gamma camera has been evaluated and metastatic nodes can be demonstrated with gallium (Teates, Preston and Boyd, 1980) and with cobalt-labelled bleomycin (Cummings *et al.*, 1981). These agents do not label normal lymph nodes and therefore have an advantage over CT and MRI scanning, but metastatic nodes are not demonstrated until they are at least 2 cm in size when, of course, they are nearly always palpable. Recently scanning with technetium-labelled DMSA (Watkinson *et al.*, 1991) has been shown to demonstrate metastatic lymph nodes. The use of labelled auto-antibodies to squamous carcinoma is, in theory, an ideal approach to the problem of demonstrating subclinical metastatic disease in the neck, but tumour specific auto-antibodies have yet to be found. Nevertheless, this technique offers possibilities for the future (Tranter, Fairweather and Bradwell, 1984; Soo *et al.*, 1987).

Finally positron emission tomography (PET scanning) has yet to be fully evaluated in the assessment of metastatic neck disease (Bailet *et al.*, 1992).

Fine needle aspiration cytology

On occasions fine needle aspiration cytology is helpful in demonstrating metastatic carcinoma in a lymph node (Friedman, Panahou and Fox, 1983; Baatenberg De Jong *et al.*, 1988). This technique is not valuable as a routine but may be helpful in the evaluation of a difficult clinical situation. For example in the assessment of a palpable node in the evaluation of a patient with an unknown primary tumour fine needle aspiration may be useful. In general negative aspiration cytology is not sufficiently reliable and should be ignored.

Treatment of metastatic neck disease

Although metastatic disease in the neck indicates a poorer prognosis than if disease is localized to the primary site, the patient is still distinctly curable if managed in the correct way and overall cure rates of up to 50% are still possible in patients with metastatic neck disease. Great controversies surround the correct management of a patient with metastatic neck disease and this is an important and very interesting subject. The issues which are most contentious are:

1 The management of the N0 neck, i.e. prophylactic or elective treatment to the neck (surgery or radiotherapy) in the absence of palpable nodes.
2 The management of metastatic neck disease in the absence of a primary lesion (unknown primary disease).
3 The place of radiotherapy in the treatment of metastatic neck disease either as primary or follow-up treatment.
4 The place of radical neck dissection or modified procedures preserving various structures such as the internal jugular vein, sternomastoid muscle and accessory nerve.
5 The value of treatment of bilateral disease in the neck.
6 The untreatable or inoperable disease in the neck such as that fixed to the carotid artery, prevertebral muscles, etc.

Participants in panel discussions or members of the audience in controversies in otolaryngology discussions may consider that the above issues are the burning questions of the present day. It is a sobering thought that all these issues were discussed in a symposium on head and neck cancer held in 1923 (Symposium, 1923) and frankly up to the present day we have accumulated virtually no well controlled scientific evidence which makes us any nearer solving these issues. The arguments surrounding these questions are just as vociferous as they were 70 years ago.

History of neck dissection

Although occasional attempts were made to remove metastatic lymph nodes in the neck in the nineteenth century the first description of radical neck dissection was by Crile in 1906. He described the classical radical neck dissection in which metastatic glands were removed together with the internal jugular vein, the sternomastoid muscle, the accessory nerve and the submandibular salivary gland. Following

Crile's description of this radical surgical procedure a number of surgeons advocated less radical operations, but these were condemned by Hayes-Martin who in 1951 published the results of 1450 radical neck dissections (Martin, Del Valle and Ehrlich, 1951). The next stage in the surgery of metastatic neck disease was a further promotion of modified procedures now called functional neck dissection (Bocca and Pignataro, 1967). Retrospective series have been published to support the claim that recurrence in the neck is no more common after a functional procedure than after the more radical operation (Molinari *et al.*, 1980; Bocca *et al.*, 1984). At the present time the argument continues and will be discussed in more detail below.

Management of metastatic neck disease

A number of different clinical situations arise in patients with metastatic neck disease and these are approached in different ways by different surgeons. In a patient with no obvious primary tumour but in whom a previous primary tumour has been treated, palpable lymphadenopathy in the neck is virtually always assumed to be metastatic. Reference has already been made to the false-positive rate in neck dissection but this approach is the safest in terms of cancer treatment. Occasionally needle biopsy or, more reliably, frozen section examination at the time of radical neck dissection is advisable if there is significant doubt. The differential diagnosis of a mass in the neck has been discussed in Chapter 16 but false-positive nodes arise in neck dissection mainly due to infective or reactive nodes or an enlarged submandibular salivary gland.

The treatment options for metastatic neck disease are radiotherapy, surgery (a variety of procedures) or a combination of the two. The place of these various treatments in different clinical situations is yet to be universally agreed. In addition what constitutes a hopeless situation, e.g. bilateral nodes, huge fixed nodes is not agreed nor its optional management.

Radiotherapy for metastatic neck disease

The role of radiotherapy in the treatment of metastatic neck disease remains uncertain. It has been used in a variety of situations: palpable metastatic disease, as an addition to surgery both preoperatively and postoperatively, prophylactically, i.e. in patients with no palpable disease but with a high risk of occult metastases, and palliatively.

There is no doubt that irradiation will cure a proportion of tumours in patients with palpable nodes in the neck. Most surgeons would claim that once disease is palpable in the neck the results of surgery are better than those of radiotherapy. This, however, has never been tested by a controlled trial.

It has been shown that cure of palpable nodes by radiotherapy is both dependent on the size of the nodes and the dose of radiation (Schneider, Fletcher and Barkley, 1975). In the above series cure rates of 90% were obtained for palpable nodes less than 3 cm in diameter when treated with at least 6500 cGy. Most head and neck specialists however would, except in special circumstances, treat patients with palpable metastatic disease in the neck by surgery. This includes both patients with a primary lesion and metastatic disease on presentation and those who develop a positive neck node after successful primary treatment. When the treatment of the primary tumour is radiotherapy, e.g. nasopharyngeal carcinoma, and metastatic nodes are present it is logical to treat both primary disease and neck disease by radiotherapy reserving surgery for persistent disease in the neck.

The use of radiotherapy as an adjunct to surgery in the treatment of metastatic neck disease has not been fully evaluated. There is, however, retrospective evidence that it is beneficial. Thus in one study, surgery followed by 5000–6000 cGy was shown to be superior either to surgery alone or to surgery and preoperative low dose radiotherapy (Vikram *et al.*, 1984). There are two prospective randomized trials which have evaluated this problem. In one trial (Strong, 1969) surgery was compared with surgery and preoperative radiotherapy (2000 cGy). The incidence of recurrence of disease in the neck was reduced by the addition of radiotherapy, particularly in patients with advanced nodal disease although the overall survival of patients was similar in both groups. The only other prospective study was in patients with oral and oropharyngeal carcinoma in which patients were treated with preoperative radiotherapy and surgery, surgery and postoperative radiotherapy and radiotherapy alone (Snow *et al.*, 1980). At 3 years there were no differences in survival in the three groups. The advantages of giving postoperative radiation have not been satisfactorily demonstrated. There is no firm evidence that it is beneficial though many believe that the addition of radiotherapy improves local control rates (Fletcher, 1979). It may not necessarily improve survival because a higher proportion of patients free of local disease will die of distant metastases or second primary tumours (De Santo *et al.*, 1982). This issue is unresolved and will remain unresolved until a properly conducted prospective trial is reported. Perhaps at the present time postoperative radiotherapy should be reserved for patients with advanced disease in the neck (extracapsular spread, large nodes, multiple nodes) when the prognosis is worse and this issue is discussed below (Snow *et al.*, 1982).

Perhaps the most widely accepted role of radiotherapy in metastatic neck disease is its use in situations where there are no palpable nodes but, nevertheless, a high likelihood of microscopic disease with nodes developing subsequently. Thus in patients with no palpable disease in the neck but a primary tumour in the oral cavity, oropharynx, nasopharynx, hypopharynx and supraglottic larynx, there is a high incidence of microscopic disease in the neck and a high risk of development of metastatic nodes if only the primary tumour is treated. Fletcher (1972) has shown that the risk of subsequent development of nodes can be reduced from about 25% to 5% by the use of prophylactic neck irradiation. This has also been confirmed in other series (Million, 1974; Mendenhall, Million and Cassisi, 1980). Although none of these series is prospective or randomized the evidence for the value of radiotherapy in this situation is fairly convincing. No one has yet demonstrated that this effect of radiotherapy actually improves survival figures.

Surgery for metastatic neck disease

The most widely accepted operation for palpable metastatic disease in the neck is the radical neck dissection originally described by Crile (1906). The purpose of this operation is to remove, as a single block, the lymph nodes of the lateral neck together with the superficial and deep layers of the deep cervical fascia. The limits of the operation are the mandible superiorly, the clavicle inferiorly, the trapezius muscle posteriorly and the strap muscles anteriorly. The dissection includes the lymph nodes of the submandibular triangle, the deep cervical lymph nodes, the posterior triangle nodes and the supraclavicular nodes. Certain lymph nodes are not removed in a radical neck dissection and these include superficial nodes in the preauricular, postauricular and occipital regions and nodes in the parotid gland, retropharyngeal, lateral pharyngeal, prelaryngeal and paratracheal nodes. In certain circumstances these nodes may be enlarged and will usually be removed in an in-continuity dissection of primary disease and radical neck dissection. A standard radical neck dissection also includes in the specimen the external and internal jugular veins, the sternomastoid and omohyoid muscles, the submandibular salivary gland, the tail of the parotid gland, the accessory nerve and sensory branches of the cervical plexus. The indications and contraindications of radical neck dissection are not easy to define because certain controversies exist in this area. Perhaps the following indications would be accepted by most:

1 Palpable neck disease in the presence of primary tumour in the upper aerodigestive tract where an in-continuity dissection with primary disease is probably the best chance of cure.
2 Palpable disease is present in the neck when the primary tumour has previously been controlled.

More controversial indications are:

1 In the presence of a large primary tumour which by its size, site and nature carries a high risk of

microscopic deposits though no cervical nodes are palpable. Such instances would be a large oral cavity tumour, hypopharyngeal tumour and transglottic laryngeal tumour. This is really the realm of 'prophylactic' or 'elective' neck dissection which is discussed below.

2 In patients with an extensive primary lesion which is being treated surgically, perhaps using a flap, it is illogical not to perform a radical neck dissection at the time of primary surgery.

3 When metastatic disease is present in the neck though no primary can be found, i.e. the 'unknown primary' also discussed below.

The contraindications for neck dissection are relative and include:

1 A patient who is unfit for major surgery because of a serious medical condition which is irreversible and renders anaesthesia and major surgery dangerous.

2 A patient whose primary tumour is untreatable.

3 A patient with extensive bilateral neck disease is generally incurable (perhaps with the exception of lesions of the supraglottic larynx) and extensive surgery offers little chance of cure and may increase the patient's discomfort. This is an area of controversy and the final decision must rest with the patient and the surgeon.

4 Patients with distant metastases.

The operation of radical neck dissection

This operation is classically an application of applied anatomy and in the performance of the operation as well as the answering of examination questions the detailed anatomy must be second nature to the surgeon. Although it is not the purpose of this text to discuss surgical procedures in detail this subject is so important that some description on anatomical lines is essential.

Many skin incisions have been used to perform a neck dissection (Figure 17.4). The most important considerations are the viability of the flaps and carotid artery protection though these are not so critical as in the past when surgery was often performed following a large dose of radiotherapy. At the present time this is much less of a problem because treatment has swung to primary surgery and radiotherapy is not so frequently used for advanced lesions and also the dose and delivery of radiotherapy are much better controlled. Other considerations when planning flaps are ease of access, particularly if bilateral operations are planned and cosmesis of the incisions (horizontal incisions tend to heal better than vertical incisions which may leave a scar contracture). The half-H or T on its side incision (horizontal T in Figure 17.4) provides good access, protects the carotid artery, and conforms to the main cutaneous blood vessels in the skin of the neck which tend to flow from above and

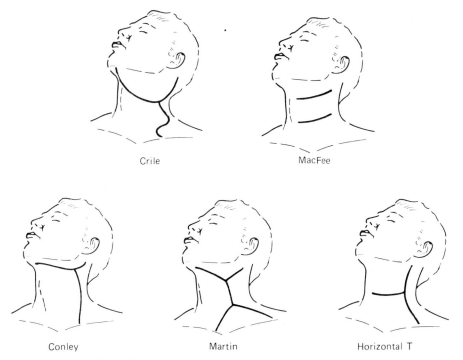

Figure 17.4 Incisions for radical neck dissection

below (facial and subclavian arteries) and the horizontal incision is in the anastomotic area between these two systems (Rogers and Freeland, 1976). Its disadvantage is that the vertical limb may heal with a scar contracture. The original Y incision of Crile (1906) is often used. Its main disadvantage is that the three-point junction may lie over the carotid artery. The double horizontal incision of MacFee (1960) is used if there are fears about the viability of neck skin, necrosis is unlikely with this incision though it does not strictly follow the arterial pattern described above. The main disadvantage is access which may be restricted particularly if a primary resection is being carried out at the same time.

The skin flaps are elevated to include the platysma muscle but the plane of dissection is superficial to the external jugular vein and anterior jugular veins. The plane of dissection is also superficial to the greater auricular nerve and other branches of the cervical plexus. In the submandibular region it may be reasonable (if there are no metastatic nodes in this area) to incise through the fascia over the submandibular salivary gland so that the plane of dissection is right down on the gland to protect the mandibular division of the VIIth nerve. The posterior part of the dissection is to the anterior border of the trapezius muscle and the accessory nerve may be encountered as the flaps are elevated as it runs rather superficially through the posterior triangle.

There are many ways to perform a radical neck dissection, an orderly sequence is necessary but may need to be modified if an in-continuity neck dissection with primary resection is being carried out. The first stage is division of the clavicular and sternal heads of the sternomastoid muscle and identification of the carotid sheath. The sheath is incised and the internal jugular vein ligated being sure that the vagus nerve which lies within the sheath between the common carotid artery and jugular vein is not divided. The thoracic duct may be seen on the left side of the neck. It may actually be identified having emerged from behind the carotid sheath to enter the lateral side of the internal jugular vein close to its junction with the subclavian vein. More usually the thoracic duct will be divided and a flow of lymph will be seen. The source of the lymph should be identified and oversewn. It is worth at this stage just carefully observing this area for a short time to be certain that a small flow of lymph is not overlooked.

The dissection next proceeds laterally and the fat and tissue overlying the scalene muscles and levator scapulae is incised and included in the specimen. In this part of the dissection the omohyoid muscle is divided and taken with the specimen as are the transverse cervical and external jugular veins. Some supraclavicular cutaneous nerves are also divided. The transverse cervical artery is usually divided and removed but not if a trapezius myocutaneous flap is contemplated. The phrenic nerve as it lies on the scalenus anterior deep to the prevertebral fascia and the trunks of the brachial plexus as they emerge between the scalenus anterior and scalenus medius are preserved. The cervical sympathetic trunk is much more medially placed behind the carotid sheath but superficial to the deep cervical fascia. In the supraclavicular fossa the subclavian vein may be visualized as it lies behind the clavicle. The dissection proceeds superiorly along the anterior border of the trapezius and the accessory nerve is divided as it enters the muscle.

The next stage is division of the superior part of the sternomastoid muscle close to the mastoid tip. Here it is usual to divide the tail of the parotid gland and remove it with the specimen. Others prefer to retract the parotid tail superiorly. The position of the facial nerve, particularly its mandibular division, should be borne in mind at this point. It can be damaged by dissection too superiorly and if the dissection needs to be taken very high then formal identification and preservation of the facial nerve is necessary by performing a superficial parotidectomy. Once the sternomastoid muscle has been divided the next landmark is the posterior belly of the digastric muscle which is crossed anteriorly by the posterior facial vein. Two arteries are related to the digastric muscle, one at its upper border, one at its lower. The posterior auricular artery is the more superior of the two and is usually not encountered. The occipital artery is divided as it crosses the carotid sheath at the inferior border of the digastric muscle. The digastric muscle is retracted superiorly and the internal jugular vein can be identified within the carotid sheath. The site of the internal jugular vein can easily be identified by palpating the transverse process of the atlas. The vein lies immediately anterior to this point. Lying superficially to the vein and running backwards is the accessory nerve. Anterior to the vein is the vagus nerve. After the jugular vein has been ligated the neck dissection specimen is freed from posterior to anterior by dissecting it off the prevertebral fascia immediately overlying the prevertebral muscles. Branches of the cervical plexus are divided and the phrenic nerve which lies deep to the prevertebal fascia is preserved.

The final part of the dissection involves dissection of the jugular vein out of the carotid sheath and superiorly the hypoglossal nerve must be preserved as it crosses the internal and external carotid arteries. Finally the submandibular triangle is dissected and in this region the lingual and hypoglossal nerves must be preserved. The facial vessels and the duct of the submandibular salivary gland are divided.

Complications of neck dissection

There are many possible complications of neck dissection and these can be classified into local and general. Up to 20% of patients will have a major complication following radical neck dissection and the mortality is about 1%.

General complications

Anaesthetic complications, postoperative atelectasis, and bronchopneumonia are the most important of these but urinary retention and deep vein thrombosis may occur.

Local complications

Haemorrhage

This may be peroperative or postoperative. Severe peroperative haemorrhage usually results from damage to the internal jugular vein at its upper or lower end before it has been ligated. Tearing of a tributary is usually the cause and if severe haemorrhage occurs pressure with a finger on the bleeding point, dissection of the vessel above and below the source of bleeding and then ligation of the vein is the solution. Damage to the carotid arterial system usually only occurs when the artery is invaded by tumour and attempts are being made to dissect the tumour off the vessel. This should be a situation which has been anticipated and is dealt with below.

Postoperative haemorrhage

This is usually of the reactionary type and avoided by meticulous attention to haemostasis at the end of the procedure. Secondary haemorrhage may occur as a result of a carotid artery rupture which is discussed below.

Wound infection

The four most important factors in the development of a wound infection after radical neck dissection are:

1 Contamination of the surgical field at the time of surgery.
2 Contamination of the surgical field because the operation involves an in-continuity radical neck dissection and primary excision (composite resection, pharyngeal and laryngeal resection).
3 Postoperative haematoma which becomes infected.
4 Flap necrosis and wound breakdown.

These factors vary in their importance and can be avoided most of the time by careful surgical technique. Prophylactic antibiotics are not necessary in a neck dissection alone but should always be used if the operation is part of a surgical procedure in which mucosal surfaces are opened to the neck (Becker and Parell, 1979; Raine, 1984).

Carotid artery rupture

Spontaneous rupture of the carotid artery is a result of necrosis of the arterial wall which is due to infection in and around the artery. A number of factors combine to produce this situation but it usually occurs in patients who have been treated by radiotherapy followed by surgery. It can occur after surgery alone but preoperative radiotherapy is certainly implicated in most series (Joseph and Shumrick, 1973; Shumrick, 1973). The situation which leads to rupture in most patients is following a major surgical procedure with excision of primary tumour and neck dissection in which a postoperative salivary fistula develops adjacent to the carotid artery. Removal of the adventitia of the artery during surgery devascularizes the vessel and predisposes to rupture (Kennedy, Krause and Loevy, 1977). Although carotid artery rupture may be totally unexpected usually it is predictable (i.e. in an irradiated patient who has developed a postoperative fistula with loss of neck skin). Surgical debridement and toilet with local and systemic antibiotics should be instituted. In many patients a warning or herald bleed occurs and when there is any significant bleeding the wound should be explored and the bleeding point located. If the bleeding is from the carotid artery this should be ligated. In a situation where a carotid bleed seems likely blood should be cross-matched and the patient should have a cuffed tracheostomy tube to protect the airway. When rupture occurs and emergency ligation of the artery is performed the complication rate is very high, e.g. a mortality of 38% and a hemiplegia rate of 50% was reported by Moore, Karlan and Sigler (1969). The complications are reduced if the ligation is elective when the blood pressure is normal, thus if local pressure can be applied to the bleeding vessel until volume replacement can be instituted, the complication rate may be reduced.

Chylous fistula

In dissections on the left side of the neck if the thoracic duct is seen it must be ligated. More usually a leak of fluid occurs when the lower end of the jugular vein is being dissected and the duct must be found and ligated. At the end of a neck dissection this area must be inspected for any fluid leak. The loss at this stage is not severe because the patient is starved but once postoperative feeding is instituted milky fluid pours out of the drain. Opinion is divided as to the correct management in this situation. The options are surgical exploration or conservative management. If the leak is mild, i.e. less than 100 ml a day, conservative management will almost always succeed. However, if the leak is major most surgeons will re-explore the wound, try to identify the source of the leak and oversew it. This is far from easy but probably an attempt should be made if the chylous fistula is producing large volumes such as 300 ml a day or more. Conservative management involves pressure dressings and parenteral feeding and may be successful without surgery when the leak is not severe. The problems of a chylous leak are the loss of protein and electrolytes. If conservative measures and exploration of the neck do not control the leak a lateral thoracotomy and a suture placed between the oesophagus and descending aorta in the inferior and posterior mediastinum will usually succeed.

Pneumothorax

If there is disease low in the neck the apical pleura may be damaged when the disease is being dissected free. This will usually be obvious because there will be an air leak at the time if the patient is being ventilated and the tear should be repaired.

Nerve injuries

In a standard radical neck dissection the nerves which are deliberately divided are:

1 Accessory nerve
2 Branches of the cervical plexus namely the lesser occipital, great auricular, transverse cutaneous nerve of the neck, supraclavicular nerves and probably some motor branches to the trapezius (see below)
3 The descendens hypoglossi.

A number of other nerves may be damaged by accident. These include:

1 The facial nerve or its mandibular division
2 The hypoglossal and lingual nerves
3 The vagus, sympathetic trunk, phrenic nerve or brachial plexus.

The effect of damage to these nerves is obvious but some discussion of division of the accessory nerve and its effects is worthwhile. Division of the accessory nerve during radical neck dissection gives rise to what Nahum, Mullall and Marmor (1961) call the shoulder syndrome: pain in the joint, limitation of abduction and drooping of the affected shoulder. It has been reported that this complication occurs in varying degrees, in 60% of patients after standard radical neck dissection (Leipzig, Suen and English, 1983). This has led to the introduction of accessory nerve saving procedures (Skolnik *et al.*, 1967) or operations in which the cervical nerve supply to the trapezius is preserved (Weitz, Weitz and McIlkinney, 1967; Jones and Stell, 1985). It must be said at the present time that the vast majority of head and neck surgeons when performing a radical neck dissection will almost always try to preserve the accessory nerve.

Cerebral oedema

A certain amount of cerebral oedema occurs after radical neck dissection, the intracranial pressure probably increasing about threefold (Jones, 1951). The dangers are much greater after bilateral neck dissection (McQuarrie, 1977) when the rise in pressure may be fivefold or more. These risks are still present but less so after staged neck dissection in which both internal jugular veins are ligated but at different operations. The vertebral venous system together with the occipital veins and superficial veins constitute the main venous drainage system when both jugular veins have been ligated. A patient with cerebral oedema will have a congested face and the blood pressure will rise and the pulse rate will fall. The patient should be nursed in a sitting position and given mannitol intravenously and dexamethasone. These patients often have pharyngeal and laryngeal oedema and any patient having bilateral neck dissection, whether simultaneous or staged, should have a tracheostomy.

Conservation or functional neck dissection

The sequelae and morbidity associated with radical neck dissection have stimulated the description of operations designed to preserve the more important structures in the neck. Thus operations have been described to preserve one or more of the following structures: accessory nerve, cervical plexus branches to the trapezius, sternomastoid muscle, internal jugular vein (or part of it). These operations are attractive from the functional point of view and have been proposed as alternatives to radical neck dissection for palpable unilateral disease, bilateral disease, and as elective neck dissections in patients classified as N0 but with a high risk of microscopic metastatic disease. The operation described by Bocca and his colleagues (Bocca and Pignataro, 1967; Bocca *et al.*, 1984) removes a specimen containing fascia and lymph nodes as a single block but preserves the internal jugular vein, the sternomastoid muscle and accessory nerve. As a surgical procedure this is an elegant operation, but although many reports have been cited to demonstrate that it is just as effective as radical neck dissection, all these reports are retrospective and not one prospective. It must also be remembered that these reports are based upon large series in which the participating surgeons were very experienced in this particular surgical procedure. It would be naive indeed to think that a surgeon performing the occasional 'Bocca operation' could achieve the same results.

A very similar operation to the one performed by Bocca has been described by Ballantyne at the MD Anderson Hospital, Houston, Texas and uses an anterior approach to clear the posterior triangle (Jesse, Ballantyne and Larson, 1978). Other operations in which the accessory nerve is preserved with or without the internal jugular vein are commonly performed and again retrospective studies have promoted the idea that these are safe procedures (Skolnik and Deutsch, 1983; Deutsch, Skolnik and Friedman, 1985). However, none of these operations has been tested by a randomized controlled trial and caution is needed. The main anxiety about these operations is that disease extending outside the capsule of a lymph node will be left behind in the neck. McKelvie (1974) showed that small lymph nodes with microscopic deposits of cancer in them could invade the adventitia of the internal jugular vein and Schuller, Platz and Krause (1978) showed that although metastatic disease was uncommon in the posterior triangle adjacent to the accessory nerve it was very common close to the accessory nerve in its more proximal part. Suprahyoid neck dissection is mentioned to dismiss it immediately. Removal of nodes above the level of the hyoid bone is totally inadequate in a disease in which metastases can occur low in the neck in the absence of palpable disease in the upper neck (Vandenbrouck *et al.*, 1980). Supra-omohyoid neck dissection is also another operation which can only be condemned. Basically it involves a dissection of the anterior triangle of the neck preserving the internal jugular vein, sternomastoid muscle and accessory nerve, but is not a logical treatment (Schuller, Platz and Krause, 1978).

With all these surgical options available to treat metastatic neck disease it is little wonder that there is divided opinion about what is appropriate. The present author is very anxious about operations which preserve the jugular vein in the presence of palpable disease and, unless bilateral neck dissections are being performed simultaneously, surely the possible disadvantages outweigh the advantages. However, accessory nerve preservation is often possible and unless there is disease high in the neck adjacent to the nerve an attempt should probably be made to preserve it. Thus the present author, in the presence of palpable disease or when the neck is being treated electively, i.e. no palpable disease but a high risk of microscopic deposits, performs a radical neck dissection with the object of preserving the accessory nerve. If there is disease in the vicinity of the nerve found at the time of the dissection the nerve is divided. When bilateral disease is present and yet the clinical situation suggests there is something to be gained by neck dissection, a radical neck dissection, with preservation of the XIth nerve, is performed on the side of the most extensive disease and an operation performed on the other side in which the internal jugular vein and XIth nerve are preserved. There seems little advantage in trying to save the sternomastoid muscle and the improved access obtained by dividing it makes the dissection easier and probably also more effective.

Elective neck dissection – treatment of N0 disease

It is well known and has been discussed earlier in this chapter that patients with carcinoma of the head and neck, particularly nasopharynx, oral cavity, pharynx, supraglottic larynx, who have no palpable disease in their necks nevertheless have a high incidence (20–40%) of subclinical disease. It is therefore thera-peutically tempting to treat the neck in these patients on the basis that this will avoid subsequent treatment which may not be as effective. On the other hand it will mean unnecessary treatment is given to 60%–80% of patients who do not have subclinical disease. The arguments for and against elective treatment of the neck have been put forward by Nahum, Bonbe and Davidson (1977).

Arguments for elective neck dissection:

1 The high incidence of occult metastatic disease
2 Neck dissection has low morbidity and mortality
3 If the neck has to be entered to remove the primary lesion, it is better to perform an in-continuity resection at the same time
4 It is impossible to provide the clinical follow up necessary to detect the earlier conversion of a neck from N0 to N1
5 Allowing neck metastases to develop increases the incidence of distant metastases
6 The cure rate for neck dissection is decreased if gland enlargement occurs or multiple nodes appear.

Arguments against elective neck dissection:

1 Cure rates are no lower if the surgeons waits for the neck to convert from N0 to N1.
2 Careful clinical follow up will allow detection of the earliest conversion from N0 to N1.
3 Radiation is as effective as neck dissection (this means in the elective situation, i.e. N0).
4 Elective neck dissection results in a large number of unnecessary surgical procedures and is associated with inevitable morbidity.
5 Elective neck dissection removes a barrier to the spread of disease and also has a detrimental immunological effect.

It is a sad reflection on head and neck surgeons that although radical neck dissection has been performed many times since early this century there is only one prospective trial to attempt to answer this critical issue. This trial (Vandenbrouck *et al.*, 1980) randomized patients with T1–3 N0 oral cavity cancer into two groups. One group was treated by interstitial implantation and an elective radical neck dissection within 2 months of implantation. The other group was treated by an implant and follow up, radical neck dissection being performed when nodes became palpable. There was no difference in survival at 5 years between the two groups. At the present time it would seem that elective neck dissection has no place unless the neck is being opened to provide access for surgical treatment of the primary tumour. Thus it would be ridiculous not to clear the neck of a patient with a large oral, oropharyngeal, hypopharyngeal and possibly transglottic laryngeal tumour which was being treated surgically. In other situations elective neck irradiation to both sides of the neck would seem to be a better option if elective treatment was felt to be necessary.

Bilateral neck disease

The presence of bilateral neck disease on presentation is a bad prognostic sign and 5-year survival figures of the order of 5% are usual for this group (Spiro *et al.*, 1974; Lederman, 1967). However, although the prognosis of patients with bilateral nodes is poor this may in part be due to the fact that these patients are not offered radical treatment in many series. In one series from the MD Anderson Hospital 3-year survival of patients with histologically proven bilateral neck disease was better than 50% (Ballantyne and Jackson, 1982). These patients were treated radically with radical neck dissection on one side, modified neck dissection on the other and often with postoperative radiotherapy.

Patients with fixed nodes

Because of the difficulty of assessing fixation of a neck mass this criterion has now been excluded from the nodal staging system of both the AJC and UICC. However, fixation does indicate a poor prognosis and should alert the surgeon to the possibility of both the difficulties of removing the mass entirely and increased likelihood of surgical complications. The incidence of true fixation of a neck mass is difficult to determine and varies from series to series partly depending on the variability of clinical assessment but also upon the population group studied. Thus figures vary from 23% in Stell's series (Stell *et al.*, 1984), 30% in Snow's (Snow *et al.*, 1982) and 50% in Hiranandani's (1971). The structure to which the gland is fixed is important. Fixation to the mandible, sternomastoid muscle or prevertebral muscles is less of a problem than fixation to the cervical spine, brachial plexus or carotid artery. Carotid artery fixation is said to occur in about 5% of neck dissections (Kennedy, Krause and Loevy, 1977). Cure of patients with fixed nodes is rare even with radical treatment with both radiotherapy and surgery. Thus survival figures of the order of 5% are usually quoted (Kennedy, Krause and Loevy, 1977; Stell and Green, 1976; Fee *et al.*, 1983; Stell *et al.*, 1984). Surgical management of these patients involves preoperative scanning with CT or MRI and angiography to assess not only the involved vessel but the rest of the carotid circulation. Resection of the carotid artery at neck dissection carries a high mortality (up to 12%) and a high risk of hemiplegia (33%) (Kornblut and Shumrick, 1971). Although numerous methods have been described to try to predict the safety of carotid artery ligation, the most reliable method is to measure the back pressure in the carotid artery at surgery. Unless the carotid stump pressure is greater than 70 mmHg resection alone carries a high morbidity and mortality, and vessel replacement should be performed.

Second radical neck dissection

It is usually felt that patients with bilateral metastatic disease in the neck have a poor prognosis but it has also been a belief that a reasonable proportion of patients developing nodes on the second side of the neck are potentially curable. Thus Lee and Krause (1975) reported a series of patients who underwent neck dissection for nodes on the second side following resection of the primary and neck dissection on the same side. Excluding patients with recurrent tumour at the primary site or the side of the first neck dissection there was a 44% 5-year survival which is similar to that for unilateral neck disease. Similarly Baffi, Razack and Sako (1980) reported a 38% 5-year survival in this group of patients. In a more recent study, Jackson and Stell (1990) showed that patients with a hypopharyngeal or oral cancer had about a 5% chance of developing nodes on the second side of the neck and this was mainly seen in patients with palpable nodes on one side at presentation and in patients with a poorly differentiated tumour. Overall the 5-year survival of this group was 35% with an operative mortality of about 2%.

Relationship of neck nodes to prognosis

Virtually all series investigating the prognosis of patients with head and neck cancer have demonstrated that patients with palpable nodes on presentation have a poorer prognosis. Thus palpable nodes on presentation reduce the survival by about one half. As well as the presence of nodes the staging of nodes is also important though not having such a profound effect. Spiro *et al.* (1974) showed that the size of the palpable nodes was significantly related to prognosis. Similarly Snow *et al.* (1982) showed nodal fixation to be a bad prognostic sign. Multiple nodes and the level of nodes in the neck have also been shown to be of significance (Kraus and Panje, 1982; Stell, Morton and Singh, 1983; Jones *et al.*, 1994), the prognosis worsening the lower in the neck the nodes are found. Although clinical factors (size, number, mobility and level) of metastatic nodes are important in determining prognosis it has been shown that histological factors are probably of greater importance and the presence of multiple positive nodes on histological examination and the presence of extracapsular spread are the most important factors (Snow *et al.*, 1982; Kalmins, Leonard and Sakok, 1977; Johnson *et al.*, 1981). The relation of histological factors to prognosis is important particularly when further treatment such as radiotherapy is being considered.

The unknown primary tumour

One of the practices which tends to provoke head and neck surgeons into criticism of their general surgical colleagues is open biopsy of neck nodes. Martin and Morfit (1944) for example criticized this practice and said, 'There can be no better example of ill-advised and needless surgery'. They were writing about the clinical situation where the patient presents with a lymph node in the neck as the primary complaint and the clinician involved goes straight to biopsy (either incisional or excisional) without investigating the patient for a primary tumour. In this situation if the biopsy proves to be a lymphoma nothing is lost but, if the node shows metastatic squamous carcinoma, the primary disease remains undiagnosed and many believe that the biopsy compromises the chances of cure. This latter point of course is important though the evidence for it is not very strong. The main paper quoted as evidence (McGuirt and McCabe, 1978) has many faults of design and a further paper (Razack, 1977) failed to demonstrate any difference in prognosis caused by biopsy. Nevertheless it is not good medicine to biopsy a neck node without a thorough search for a possible primary tumour. Thus when a patient presents with a palpable mass in the neck which is suggestive of metastatic cancer in a cervical node the patient should be investigated by history, clinical examination (general physical and detailed otolaryngological examination) and a chest radiograph. Detailed radiological examination should only be performed in the presence of a suggestive history or examination, e.g. dysphagia, dyspepsia, etc. Fine needle aspiration biopsy may be very helpful.

The next stage is full examination of the upper respiratory and alimentary tracts and biopsy of suspicious areas or if none is present biopsy of the nasopharynx at least. Some would remove the tonsil on the side of the lesion (Tytor and Olofsson, 1986). If all these investigations are negative, probably the correct course of action is to prepare the patient for neck dissection, perform a frozen section at the time of neck dissection and proceed as appropriate if the diagnosis is metastatic squamous carcinoma. Postoperative radiation should almost certainly be given to the neck and to the nasopharynx, oropharynx and hypopharynx. However, the alternative form of treatment is not to treat the patient by primary surgery but to irradiate the neck and likely sites of primary tumour (Fitzpatrick and Kotalik, 1974; Tytor and Olofsson, 1986). Jesse, Perez and Fletcher (1973) found little difference in survival between patients treated with radiotherapy, surgery or combined therapy. As in most controversial issues in medicine there are reasonable grounds for both sides of the argument. If the node is small then excisional biopsy and radiotherapy may be appropriate. If the node is much larger then perhaps primary neck dissection and postoperative radiotherapy is the correct course of action. Either way cure rates of the order of 25–40% are usual (Jones *et al.*, 1993).

Neck dissections for conditions other than squamous carcinoma

Non-squamous malignancy

For patients with a non-squamous primary tumour of the head and neck and metastases radical neck dissection with resection of the primary tumour is standard treatment. Similarly, neck dissection for recurrence of non-squamous malignancy in the neck nodes following successful treatment of the primary is valuable. Survival figures depend upon the site of the tumour and histology, thus patients with thyroid malignancy do best, those with anaplastic lesions and melanoma worst (Clarke and Jones, 1992). Malignant salivary gland lesions also carry a poor prognosis.

Non-malignant conditions

Occasionally radical neck dissection or a modification of it will be the treatment of choice for a benign condition. Thus extensive lymphangioma or haemlymphangioma are probably best dealt with by an approach similar to radical neck dissection. Also when a branchial fistula or branchial cyst has recurred following previous surgery identification of the residual disease in the presence of infection or sinus formation is virtually impossible and en bloc resection of the whole area by some form of modified radical neck dissection is probably the most likely operation to solve the problem.

References

ALI, S., TIWARI, R. M. and SNOW, G. B. (1985) False positive and false negative neck nodes. *Head and Neck Surgery*, **8**, 78–82

BAATENBERG DE JONG, R. J., RONGEN, R. J., DE JONG, P. C., LAMERIS, J. S. and KNEGT, P. (1988) Screening for lymph nodes in the neck with ultrasound. *Clinical Otolaryngology*, **13**, 5–9

BAFFI, R., RAZACK, M. S. and SAKO, K. (1980) Non simultaneous bilateral neck dissection. *Head and Neck Surgery*, **2**, 272–275

BAILET, J. W., ABEMAYOR, E., JABOUR, B. A., HAWKINS, R. A., HO, C. and WARD, P. A. (1992) Positron emission tomography: a new precise imaging modality for detection of primary head and neck tumours and assessment of cervical adenopathy. *Laryngoscope*, **102**, 281–288

BALLANTYNE, A. J. and JACKSON, G. L. (1982) Synchronous bilateral neck dissection. *American Journal of Surgery*, **144**, 452–455

BEAHRS, O. H. and BARBER, K. W. (1962) The value of radical dissection of structures of the neck in the management of carcinoma of the lip mouth and larynx. *Archives of Surgery*, **85**, 49–56

BECKER, G. D. and PARELL, G. J. (1979) Cefazolin prophylaxis in head and neck cancer surgery. *Annals of Otology, Rhinology and Laryngology*, **88**, 183–187

BILLER, H., DAVIES, W. and OGURA, H. H. (1971) Delayed

contralateral metastases with laryngeal and laryngopharyngeal cancers. *Laryngoscope*, **81**, 1499–1502

BRYNE, M., KOPPANG, H. S., LILLENG, R. and KJAERHEIM, A. (1992) Malignancy grading of the deep invasive margins of oral squamous cell carcinoma has high prognostic value. *Journal of Pathology*, **166**, 375–381

BOCCA, E. and PIGNATARO, O. (1967) A conservative technique in radical neck dissection. *Annals of Otology*, **76**, 975–987

BOCCA, E., PIGNATARO, O., OLDINI, C. and CAPPA, C. (1984) Functional neck dissection: an evaluation and review of 843 cases. *Laryngoscope*, **94**, 942

CADY, B. and CATLIN, D. (1989) Epidermoid carcinoma of the gum. A 20 year survey. *Cancer*, **23**, 551–569

CLARKE, R. W. and JONES, A. S. (1992) Neck dissection for non-squamous malignancy. *Clinical Otolaryngology*, **6**, 540–544

CRILE, G. (1906) Excision of cancer of the head and neck. *Journal of the American Medical Association*, **47**, 1780–1786

CUMMINGS, C. W., LARSON, S. M., DOBIE, R. A., WEYMULLER, E. A. JR., RUDD, T. G. and MERELLO, A. (1981) Assessment of cobalt 57 tagged bleomycin as a clinical aid in staging head and neck carcinoma. *Laryngoscope*, **91**, 529–537

DE SANTO, L. W., HOLT, J. J., BEAHRS, O. H. and O'FALLON, W. M. (1982) Neck dissection. Is it worthwhile? *Laryngoscope*, **92**, 502–509

DEUTSCH, E. C., SKOLNIK, E. M. and FRIEDMAN, M. (1985) The conservative neck dissection. *Laryngoscope*, **95**, 561–565

DOOMS, G. C., HRICAK, H., CROOKS, L. E. and HIGGINS, C. B. (1984) Magnetic resonance imaging of the lymph nodes: comparison with CT. *Radiology*, **153**, 719–728

FEE, W. E., GOFFINET, D. R., PARYANI, S., GOODE, R. L., LEVINE, P. A. and HOPP, M. L. (1983) Intra-operative iodine 125 implants: their use in large tumours in the neck attached to the carotid artery. *Archives of Otolaryngology*, **109**, 727–730

FEINMASSER, R., FREEMAN, J. L., NOYEK, A. M. and BIRT, B. D. (1987) Metastatic neck disease. A clinical radiographic/pathologic relative study. *Archives of Otolaryngology, Head and Neck Surgery*, **113**, 1307–1310

FITZPATRICK, P. J. and KOTALIK, J. F. (1974) Cervical metastases from an unknown primary tumour. *Radiology*, **110**, 659–661

FLETCHER, G. H. (1972) Elective irradiation of subclinical disease in cancers of the head and neck. *Cancer*, **29**, 1450–1454

FLETCHER, G. H. (1979) The role of irradiation in management of squamous cell carcinomas of the mouth and throat. *Head and Neck Surgery*, **1**, 441–457

FRIEDMAN, M., PANAHOU, A. M. and FOX, S. (1983) Needle aspiration cytology. *International Advances in Surgical Oncology*, **6**, 89–126

FRIEDMAN, M., SHELTON, V. K., MAFEE, M., BELLITZ, P., GRYBAUS-KAS, V. and SKOLNIK, E. (1987) Metastatic neck disease. Evaluation by computed tomography. *Archives of Otolaryngology, Head and Neck Surgery*, **113**, 1307–1310

HAJEK, P. C., SALOMONOWITZ, E., TURK, R., TSCHOLAKOFF, D., KUMPARI, W. and CZEMBIREK, H. (1986) Lymph node of the neck evaluation with ultrasound. *Radiology*, **158**, 739–742

HIBBERT, J., MARKS, N. J., WINTER, P. J. and SHAHEEN, O. H. (1983) Prognostic factors in oral squamous carcinoma and their relation to clinical staging. *Clinical Otolaryngology*, **8**, 197–203

HIRANANDANI, L. H. (1971) The management of cervical metastases in head and neck cancer. *Journal of Laryngology and Otology*, **85**, 1097–1126

HOLM, L. E., LUNDQUIST, P. G., SILFVESVARD, C. and SOBIN, A. (1982) Histological grading of malignancy in squamous cell carcinoma of the oral tongue. *Acta Otolaryngologica*, **94**, 185–192

JACKSON, S. R. and STELL, P. M. (1990) Second radical neck dissection. *Clinical Otolaryngology*, **16**, 52–58

JESSE, R. H., PEREZ, C. A. and FLETCHER, G. H. (1973) Cervical lymph node metastasis: unknown primary cancer. *Cancer*, **31**, 854–861

JESSE, R. H., BALLANTYNE, A. J. and LARSON, D. (1978) Radical or modified radical neck dissection: a therapeutic dilemma. *American Journal of Surgery*, **136**, 516–519

JOHNSON, J. T., BARNES, L., MYERS, E. N., SCHRAMM, V. L., BOROCHOVILZ, D. and SIGLER, B. A. (1981) The extracapsular spread of tumours in cervical node metastasis. *Archives of Otolaryngology*, **107**, 725–729

JONES, A. S., COOK, J. A., PHILLIPS, D. E. and ROLAND, N. (1993) Squamous cell carcinoma presenting as an enlarged cervical lymph node: the occult primary. *Cancer*, **72**, 1756–1761

JONES, A. S., ROLAND, N. J., FIELD, J. K. and PHILLIPS, D. E. (1994) The level of cervical lymph node metastases: their prognostic relevance and relationship with head and neck squamous carcinoma. *Clinical Otolaryngology*, **19**, 63–69

JONES, R. K. (1951) Increased intracranial pressure following radical neck surgery. *Archives of Surgery*, **63**, 599–605

JONES, T. A. and STELL, P. M. (1985) The preservation of shoulder function after radical dissection. *Clinical Otolaryngology*, **10**, 89–92

JOSEPH, D. and SHUMRICK, D. (1973) Risks of head and neck surgery in previously irradiated patients. *Archives of Otolaryngology*, **97**, 381–384

KALMINS, I. K., LEONARD, A. G. and SAKO, K. (1977) Correlation between prognosis and degree of lymph node involvement in carcinoma of the oral cavity. *American Journal of Surgery*, **134**, 450–454

KATZ, A. E. (1983) Immunobiologic staging of patients with carcinoma of the head and neck. *Laryngoscope*, **93**, 445–463

KENNEDY, J. T., KRAUSE, C. J. and LOEVY, S. (1977) The importance of tumour attachment to the carotid arery. *Archives of Otolaryngology*, **103**, 70–73

KIRCHNER, J. A., CORNOG, J. L. and HOLMES, R. E. (1974) Transglottic cancer its growth and spread within the larynx. *Archives of Otolaryngology*, **99**, 247–251

KORNBLUT, A. D. and SHUMRICK, D. A. (1971) Complications of head and neck surgery. *Archives of Otolaryngology*, **94**, 246–254

KRAUSE, E. M. and PANJE, W. R. (1982) Factors influencing survival in head and neck patients with giant cervical lymph node metastases. *Otolaryngology, Head and Neck Surgery*, **90**, 296–303

LARSON, D. L., LEWIS, S. R. and RAPPERPORT, A. S. (1965) Lymphatics of the mouth and neck. *American Journal of Surgery*, **110**, 625–630

LEDERMAN, M. (1967) Cancer of the pharynx. *Journal of Laryngology and Otology*, **81**, 151–172

LEE, J. G. and KRAUSE, C. J. (1975) Radical neck dissection: elective therapeutic and secondary. *Archives of Otolaryngology*, **101**, 656–659

LEIPZIG, B., SUEN, J. Y. and ENGLISH, J. L. (1983) Functional evaluation of the spinal accessory nerve after neck dissection. *American Journal of Surgery*, **146**, 528–530

LINDBERG, R. D. (1972) Distribution of cervical lymph node metastases from squamous cell carcinoma of the upper respiratory and digestive tract. *Cancer*, **29** 1446–1449

MACFEE, W. F. (1960) Transverse incisions for neck dissections. *Annals of Surgery*, **157**, 229–234

MCGAVRAN, M. H., BAUER, W. C. and OGURA, J. H. (1961) The incidence of cervical node metastases from epidermoid carcinoma of the larynx and their relationship to certain characteristics of the primary tumour. A study based on the clinical and pathological finding for 96 patients treated by primary en bloc laryngectomy and neck dissection. *Cancer*, **14**, 55–66

MCGUIRT, W. F. and MCCABE, B. F. (1978) Significance of node biopsy before definitive treatment of cervical metastatic carcinoma. *Laryngoscope*, **88**, 594–597

MCKELVIE, P. (1974) Metastatic routes in the neck. *Canadian Journal of Otolaryngology*, **3**, 473–479

MCQUARRIE, D. G. (1977) A physiologic approach to the problems of simultanous bilateral neck dissection. *American Journal of Surgery*, **134**, 455–460

MANCUSO, A. A., MACERI, D. and RICE, D. (1981) CT of cervical lymph nodes. *American Journal of Radiology*, **136**, 381–385

MARTIN, H. and MORFIT, H. (1944) Cervical lymph node metastasis as the first symptom of cancer. *Surgery, Gynecology and Obstetrics*, **78**, 133–137

MARTIN, H., DEL VALLE, B. and EHRLICH, H. (1951) Neck dissection. *Cancer*, **4**, 441–449

MENDENHALL, W. M., MILLION, R. R. and CASSISI, N. J. (1980) Elective neck irradiation in squamous cell carcinoma of the head and neck. *Head and Neck Surgery*, **3**, 15–20

MEVIO, E., BENAZO, M., GALIOTO, P., SPRIANO, P. and PIZZALA, R. (1991) Use of serum markers in the diagnosis and management of laryngeal cancer. *Clinical Otolaryngology*, **16**, 90–92

MILLION, R. R. (1974) Elective neck irradiation for T_xN_0 squamous cell carcinoma of the oral tongue and floor of the mouth. *Cancer*, **34**, 149–153

MOLINARI, R., CANTU, G., CHIESA, F. and GRANDI, C. (1980) Retrospective comparison of conservative and radical neck dissection of larynx cancer. *Annals of Otology*, **89**, 578–581

MOORE, O. S., KARLAN, M. and SIGLER, L. (1969) Factors influencing the safety of carotid ligation. *American Journal of Surgery*, **118**, 666–669

NAHUM, A. M. MULLALL, Y. W. and MARMOR, L. (1961) A syndrome resulting from radical neck dissection. *Archives of Otolaryngology*, **74**, 424–428

NAHUM, A. M., BONBE, R. C. and DAVIDSON, T. M. (1977) The case for elective prophylactic neck dissection. *Laryngoscope*, **87**, 588–599

NORRIS, C. M. (1963) Problems in classification and staging of cancer of the larynx. *Annals of Otology, Rhinology and Laryngology*, **72**, 83–96

RAINE, C. H. (1984) Chemoprophylaxis in major head and neck surgery. *Journal of the Royal Society of Medicine*, **77**, 1006

RAZACK, M. (1977) Influence of initial neck node biopsy on the incidence of recurrence in the neck and survival in patients who subsequently undergo curative resectional surgery. *Journal of Surgery and Oncology*, **9**, 347–352

ROGERS, J. H. and FREELAND, A. P. (1976) Arterial vasculature of cervical skin flaps. *Clinical Otolaryngology*, **1**, 325–331

ROTHSTEIN, S. G., PERSKY, M. S. and HORII, S. (1988) Evaluation of malignant invasion of the carotid artery by CT scan and ultrasound. *Laryngoscope*, **98**, 321–324

SCHNEIDER, J. J., FLETCHER, G. H. and BARKLEY, H. T. JR. (1975) Control by irradiation alone of non-fixed clinically positive lymph nodes from squamous cell carcinoma of the oral cavity, oropharynx, supraglottic larynx and hypopharynx. *American Journal of Radiology*, **123**, 42–47

SCHULLER. D. E., PLATZ, C. E. and KRAUSE, C. J. (1978) Spinal accessory lymph nodes. A prospective study of metastatic involvement. *Laryngoscope*, **88**, 439–449

SCHULLER, D. E., MCGIRT, W. F., MCCABE, B. F. and YOUNG, D. (1980) The prognostic significance of metastatic cervical lymph nodes. *Laryngoscope*, **90**, 557–570

SHUMRICK, D. (1973) Carotid artery rupture. *Laryngoscope*, **83**, 1051–1061

SKOLNIK, E. M., TENTAL, L. T., WINEIG, D. M. and TARDY, M. E. (1967) Preservation of the XI cranial nerve in neck dissection. *Laryngoscope*, **77**, 1304–1314

SKOLNIK, E. M. and DEUTSCH, E. C. (1983) Conservation neck dissection. *Journal of Laryngology and Otology*, Suppl. **8**, 105

SNOW, J. B., GELBER, R. D., KRAMER, S., DAVIS, L. W., MORCIAL, V. A. and LOWRY, L. D. (1980) Randomised pre-operative and post-operative radiation therapy for patients with carcinoma of the head and neck: preliminary report. *Laryngoscope*, **90**, 930–945

SNOW, G. B., ANNYAS, A. A., VAN SLOOTEN, E. A., BARTELINK, H. and HART, A. A. M. (1982) Prognostic factors of neck node metastasis. *Clinical Otolaryngology*, **7**, 185–192

SOM, P. M. (1987) Lymph nodes of the neck. *Radiology*, **165**, 593–600

SOO, K. C., WARD, M., ROBERTS, K. R., KEELING, F., CARTER, R. L., MCCREADY, V. R. *et al.* (1987) Radio-immunoscintigraphy of squamous carcinomas of the head and neck. *Head and Neck Surgery*, **9**, 349–352

SPIRO, R. H. and STRONG, E. (1971) Epidermoid carcinoma of the mobile tongue. *American Journal of Surgery*, **122**, 707–711

SPIRO, R. H., ALFONSO, A. E., FARR, H. W. and STRONG, E. W. (1974) Cervical node metastasis from epidermoid carcinoma of the oral cavity and oropharynx. *American Journal of Surgery*, **122**, 562–567

STELL, P. M. and GREEN, J. R. (1976) Management of metastases to the lymph glands of the neck. *Proceedings of the Royal Society of Medicine*, **69**, 411–412

STELL, P. M., MORTON, R. P. and SINGH, S. D. (1983) Cervical lymph node metastases, the significance of the level of the lymph node. *Clinical Oncology*, **9**, 101–107

STELL, P. M., DALBY, J. E., SINGH, S. D. and TAYLOR, W. (1984) The fixed cervical lymph node. *Cancer*, **53**, 336–341

STEVENS, M. H., HARNSBERGER, H. R., MANCUSO, A. A., DAVIS, R. K., JOHNSON, L. P. and PARKIN, J. L. (1985) Computed tomography of cervical lymph nodes. *Archives of Otolaryngology*, **111**, 735–739

STRONG, E. (1969) Pre-operative radiation and radical neck dissection. *Surgical Clinics of North America*, **49**, 271–279

SYMPOSIUM (1923) Head and neck cancer surgery. *Gynaecology and Obstetrics*, **36**, 159–177

TEATES, C. D., PRESTON, D. F. and BOYD, C. M. (1980) Gallium 67 citrate imaging in head and neck tumours. Report of the Co-operative Group. *Journal of Nuclear Medicine*, **21**, 622–627

TEICHGRACHER, J. and CLAIRMONT, A. (1984) The incidence of occult metastases from cancer of the oral tongue and floor of mouth: treatment rationale. *Head and Neck Surgery*, **7**, 15–21

TRANTER, R. M. D., FAIRWEATHER, D. S. and BRADWELL, A. R. (1984) The detection of squamous cell tumours of the head and neck using radiolabelled antibodies. *Journal of Laryngology and Otology*, **98**, 71–74

TYTOR, M. and OLOFSSON, J. (1986) Cervical lymph node metastases with occult primary. *Clinical Otolaryngology*, **11**, 463–467

VANDENBROUCK, C., SANCHO GARNIER, H., CHASSAGNE, D., SARAVENE, D., CACHIN, Y. and MICHEAU, C. (1980) Elective versus therapeutic radical neck dissection in epidermoid carcinoma of the oral cavity – results of a randomised clinical trial. *Cancer*, **46**, 386–390

VIKRAM, B., STRONG, E. W., SHAN, J. P. and SPIRO, R. (1984) Failure in the neck following multinodality treatment in advanced head and neck cancer. *Head and Neck Surgery*, **6**, 724–729

WATKINSON, J. C. (1993) Editorial. The clinically N_0 neck: investigation and treatment. *Clinical Otolaryngology*, **18**, 443–445

WATKINSON, J. C., JOHNSTON, D., JAMES, D., COADY, M., LAWS, D., ALLEN, S. *et al.* (1990) The reliability of palpation in the assessment of tumours. *Clinical Otolaryngology*, **5**, 405–410

WATKINSON, J. C., TODD, C. E. C., PASKIN, L., RANKIN, S., PALMER, T., SHAHEEN, O. H. *et al.* (1991) Metastatic carcinoma in the neck: a clinical radiological scintigraphic and pathological study. *Clinical Otolaryngology*, **16**, 187–192

WEITZ, J. W., WEITZ, S. L. and MCILHINNEY, A. J. (1983) A technique for preservation of spinal accessory nerve function in radical neck dissection. *Head and Neck Surgery*, **5**, 75–78

WILLEN, R., NATHENSEN, A., MOBERGER, G. and ANNEROTH, G. (1975) Squamous cell carcinoma of the gingiva. Histological classification and grading of malignancy. *Acta Otolaryngologica*, **79**, 146–154

18

The thyroid gland

O. H. Shaheen

Anatomy

The thyroid gland is composed of follicles, which are the secreting functional units of the gland, together with a rich vascular, lymphatic and neural network.

The gland comprises two large lobes situated on either side of the trachea, an isthmus which joins them and straddles the midline, and a pyramidal lobe which arises from the upper border of the isthmus, usually to the left of the midline.

The isthmus covers the second and third rings of the trachea to which it is loosely attached. The pyramidal lobe, which may take its origin from any part of the isthmus or indeed the adjacent medial part of a lobe, ascends for a variable distance lateral to the cricoid cartilage and thyroid ala. Although usually situated on the left, it may arise from the right side of the isthmus or close to the midline.

Each of the thyroid lobes has a pronounced conical upper pole, and a smaller less obvious rounded lower pole. Descriptions of the surfaces vary from one text to another, but for the surgeon it is simpler to refer to anterolateral and posteromedial surfaces and a posterior rounded margin where the two surfaces merge. Medially the lobes blend imperceptibly into the isthmus without there being any obvious indication as to where one becomes the other.

The gland is invested in a fascial capsule, sometimes referred to as the surgical capsule, which is in essence the pretracheal fascia. It is thin and closely applied to the external surface of the gland, although a plane of dissection exists between the two. The capsule is deficient on the posterior aspect of the isthmus and most of the posteromedial surface of each lobe, where the gland lies in intimate relationship to the trachea. Along the upper part of the posterior border of the thyroid lobe and the adjacent posteromedial surface the fascia is tough and thick,

and firmly attached to the trachea. This part of the fascia is called the ligament of Berry, and its importance is twofold. It binds the gland firmly to the trachea and must be freed when releasing a lobe surgically and secondly the recurrent nerve lies immediately behind the ligament of Berry just before it disappears into the larynx behind the cricothyroid joint.

Posteriorly, the surgical capsule extends backwards to blend with the prevertebral fascia, and laterally with the carotid sheath. Superiorly, it envelops the upper pole of the gland to extend upwards around the superior vascular pedicle for an indefinite distance. Along the upper border of the isthmus, the fascia attaches itself to the outer surface of the trachea and the cricoid. Inferiorly, the fascia passes into the mediastinum anterior to the trachea and contains a number of inferior thyroid veins.

Vascular supply

The principal arterial supply is from the superior and inferior thyroid arteries. The former originates from the external carotid artery, and loops downwards as a substantial trunk lying upon the inferior constrictor muscle of the pharynx and enters the upper pole of the gland, where it divides. The superior branch runs down along the medial surface of the upper pole and thence along the upper border of the isthmus to anastomose with its fellow of the opposite side. The inferior branch descends along the posterior border of the lobe to anastomose with the upper branch of the inferior thyroid artery.

The inferior thyroid artery originates from the thyrocervical trunk which is a branch of the subclavian artery. It approaches the thyroid gland deep to the common carotid artery and as it nears the gland, it divides into upper and lower branches which run respectively superiorly and inferiorly along the posterior border of the thyroid lobe. The former anastomoses with the inferior or descending branch of the superior thyroid artery; the latter runs downwards towards the inferior pole of the gland.

The inferior thyroid artery serves as an important surgical landmark for the recurrent laryngeal nerve and the parathyroid glands.

The nerve will either pass immediately superficial to the artery, deep to it, or between its two terminal branches. Finding the artery during thyroidectomy provides the surgeon with a reliable indication of the depth at which the nerve should be sought, after which the nerve should be exposed below the point where it approaches the artery.

The two terminal branches of the inferior thyroid artery furnish the blood supply of the superior and inferior parathyroid glands via subsidiary branches, and tracing these to their destination, is one method of locating the parathyroids. The thyroidea ima artery is a miniscule vessel which arises from the brachiocephalic (innominate) artery and ascends towards the lower border of the thyroid gland. It is of little importance.

Veins

There are three named groups which drain the thyroid gland, namely the superior, middle and inferior thyroid veins.

The superior thyroid vein accompanies the artery of the same name and ultimately joins the internal jugular vein. The middle thyroid vein originates from the anterolateral surface of the gland and passes laterally to join the internal jugular while the many inferior thyroid veins, which come away from the inferior border of the gland drain mainly into the left brachiocephalic (innominate) vein, but also into the internal jugular vein.

A small branch of the superior thyroid vein leaves the superior pedicle of the gland and passes upwards and medially towards the cricothyroid muscle. Its importance lies in its proximity to the external laryngeal nerve which innervates the cricothyroid muscle.

Lymphatics

The thyroid gland contains a rich interlacing network of lymphatics which ultimately merges into major lymphatic channels. These will leave the gland alongside the principal blood vessels to find their way to various clusters of lymph nodes. Thus upper, middle and lower deep cervical nodes receive lymph from the thyroid gland, together with pretracheal and paratracheal nodes, while the second echelon of nodes involved in thyroid disease comprises the supraclavicular and mediastinal nodes.

Nerves

The thyroid is innervated by the sympathetic nervous system, the fibres of which make their way to the gland alongside the principal arterial blood supply. The gland however, is related closely to the recurrent laryngeal nerves, and to a lesser extent to the external laryngeal nerves.

The recurrent nerve on the right side approaches the thyroid gland from a starting point behind the first part of the subclavian artery. It thus lies relatively laterally in the first part of its course, but veers medially as it ascends towards the gland; just below the level of the inferior thyroid artery, it comes to lie in its classical position in the tracheo-oesophageal groove (Figure 18.1). It crosses the inferior thyroid artery, either superficially, deeply, or between its terminal branches and beyond that part, lies immediately posterolateral to the ligament of Berry, before disappearing behind the cricothyroid joint. It is not uncommon for the nerve to divide into two or sometimes three terminal branches, the point of division being close to the level of or just below the inferior thyroid artery. It gives off small oesophageal and tracheal branches (to the trachealis muscle) as it ascends superiorly. As a very rare occurrence, it may be non-recurrent on the right side and then comes off the vagus nerve directly before passing medially

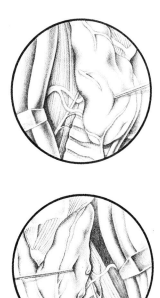

Figure 18.1 The right and left recurrent nerves. The right nerve inclines from lateral to medial in its ascent towards the larynx. The left nerve stays in the tracheo-oesophageal groove throughout its course

to reach the tracheo-oesphageal groove, thence to follow its usual course to the larynx (Figure 18.2).

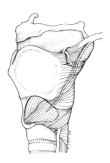 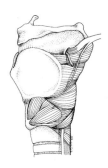

Figure 18.3 The external laryngeal nerve may not always be visible on the external surface of the inferior constrictor

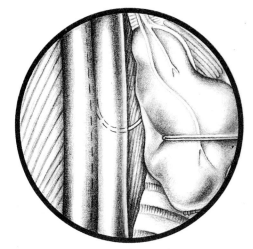

Figure 18.2 A non-recurrent laryngeal nerve comes directly off the right vagus

The left recurrent nerve lies in the tracheo-oesophageal groove throughout its length; like the nerve on the right, it is closely related to the inferior thyroid artery, and may also divide into two or more terminal branches.

Each nerve has a small visible blood vessel running lengthwise within its sheath (Rustad, 1956).

The external laryngeal nerve, which is a subdivision of the superior laryngeal nerve, passes anteroinferiorly upon the inferior constrictor muscle towards the cricothyroid muscle. As it approaches the muscle it lies in close proximity to the posteromedial aspect of the superior thyroid vascular pedicle. Occasionally it takes a somewhat more lateral course before veering medially behind the pedicle in the direction of the cricothyroid muscle; uncommonly it may get caught up in the fascial extension of the glandular surgical capsule surrounding the superior thyroid vessels. In some cases the nerve disappears out of sight into the inferior constrictor muscle before emerging again at its lower border to enter the cricothyroid muscle (Figures 18.3 and 18.4) (Durham and Harrison, 1964; Katz, 1973).

The parathyroid glands

There are two parathyroid glands on each side. They are inconstant in position, although the upper glands are less subject to variation in this respect. They are semilunar in shape and tend to have one rounded and one sharp edge. Measuring approximately 1–2 mm, they are ochre-coloured and invariably situated in a pad of fat, which generally lies outside the surgical capsule of the thyroid gland. Rarely they may be within the capsule, in which case locating them can

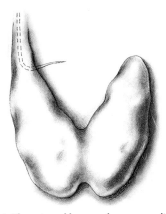

Figure 18.4 The external laryngeal nerve may lie in a lateral position behind the superior vascular pedicle of the thyroid gland

be very difficult. The upper parathyroid gland receives a branch from the upper division of the inferior thyroid artery, while the lower is supplied by the inferior terminal branch of the inferior thyroid artery.

The upper pair are generally situated at the level of the pharyngo-oesophageal junction, immediately behind and separate from the posterior border of the thyroid gland.

The inferior parathyroid glands are much more variable in position and are usually located a short distance from the lower pole of the thyroid. They tend to be more anteriorly and medially placed, and like the superior glands are found in a fat pad. They may be quite far removed from the thyroid gland and in unusual situations, such as the mediastinum.

Sometimes little nodular excrescences arising from the thyroid gland may be mistaken for a parathyroid gland, but whereas parathyroid glands can be rolled from side to side, surface thyroid projections are immovable (Shaheen, 1984).

Physiology of the thyroid gland

The functioning unit of the thyroid gland is the follicle, which is made up of a single layer of cells surrounding a lumen which contains a variable amount of colloid, depending on the state of cellular activity. The colloid is essentially a solution of proteins, the main constituent of which is thyroglobulin.

The thyroid epithelial cell possesses a basal plasma membrane abutting on a capillary, while the membrane adjacent to the lumen of the follicle exhibits microvilli which are responsible for the process of endocytosis of colloid (macropinocytosis), i.e. its active absorption back into the cell.

The thyroid has the property of selectively concentrating inorganic iodine, which is mainly dietary in origin but to a lesser extent the result of deiodination of existing thyroid hormones. Ninety per cent of the iodine absorbed by the thyroid gland is incorporated into thyroglobulin, which is essentially an iodinated glycoprotein.

Iodinated thyroglobulin is absorbed into and stored in the colloid filling the lumen of the thyroid follicles, but is actively absorbed back into the cell within droplets of colloid under the influence of thyroid stimulating hormone (TSH), by the process of macropinocytosis.

Within the cell cytoplasm, the droplets of colloid containing iodinated thyroglobulin fuse with lysosomes to form phagolysosomes, from which, by a process of hydrolysis, thyroglobulin releases iodo-amino acids into the cell cytoplasm, namely monoiodo- and diodotyrosine (MIT and DIT). Coupling reactions between DIT molecules lead to the formation of thyroxine (T4), while those between MIT and DIT form triiodothyronine (T3).

Only T3 and T4 are released into the circulation as hormones, while iodotyrosines are rapidly deiodinated within the cell to provide further iodide for hormone production. There may however, be some leakage of iodide and thyroglobulin into the blood stream when there is thyroid hyperplasia and thyroid cancer.

Thyroid hormones (T3 and T4) secreted into the blood stream, circulate in a bound form with globulin, prealbumin and albumin. Only about 1% of the total thyroid hormone content of the blood is in an unbound or free state and it is this fraction that is readily available for metabolic purposes. Since thyroxine binding proteins may be increased or decreased by certain physiological and pathological states, measurement of the total thyroxine content of the blood may not accurately reflect the metabolic state.

The thyroid-binding proteins which find their way into the extracellular fluid act as a buffer, regulating and stabilizing the end concentration of free or unbound hormones against rapid alterations in metabolism.

Peripherally, about one-quarter of the T4 concentration is deiodinated to form T3, this being over and above the concentration of T3 liberated by the thyroid gland. Whereas at one time it was thought that T4 was a precursor of T3 and that the latter was the active ingredient in peripheral metabolism, it is likely that both are significant in this respect.

The hypothalamic–pituitary–thyroid negative feedback system represents the major influence on hormone synthesis, constantly adapting the secretion of thyroid hormones to the peripheral needs of the body. An excess of free circulating T4 will diminish the secretion of TSH, whereas a reduction will have the opposite effect and may lead to hypertrophy of the thyroid gland.

Thyrotropin releasing hormone (TRH), which is produced by the hypothalamus and released into the pituitary portal circulation, stimulates the release of TSH and may influence its production. TSH, which is a glycoprotein, attaches itself to binding sites on the thyroid follicular cells and promotes the trapping of iodide, and the synthesis of both thyroglobulin and thyroxine. It also stimulates the release of T3 and T4 into the blood stream. In hypothyroidism, the low level of circulating thyroid hormones stimulates an increased production of TSH via the feedback system, and the level can be raised still further by injecting the patient with TRH. In hyperthyroidism, where the TSH level is low, an injection of TRH fails to increase TSH production to any significant degree. The use of TRH can thus be helpful in distinguishing between hyper- and hypothyroidism, and between primary pituitary failure and intrinsic disease of the thyroid gland (Beckers, 1993).

Calcitonin

Calcitonin is a peptide produced by the parafollicular or C cells of the thyroid gland. It reduces resorption of calcium from bone and lowers the serum calcium in opposition to parathormone. It is released in response to hypercalcaemia, gastrin, whisky and cholecystokynin-pancreozymin.

Thyroid antibodies

Autoantibodies are detected in the serum in several thyroid diseases. They are present significantly in hyperthyroidism and Hashimoto's autoimmune thyroiditis, and in some instances of multinodular goitre.

Some antibodies are more significant than others;

thyroid stimulating immunoglobulins to TSH receptors on thyroid cells are formed in hyperthyroidism, and are also referred to as LATS protector (LATS-P), and antibodies to thyroglobulin and cell microsomes are detectable in Hashimoto's disease. The titre of LATS-P in the blood represents a measure of the thyroid's potential to convert eventually from a hyperthyroid to a hypothyroid state under the influence of treatment.

Thyroid function tests

Total T4

This includes both free and protein bound T4 in the serum and may thus be affected by the level of thyroxine binding proteins in the circulation.

Thyroid hormone uptake test

This is also referred to as the T3 resin uptake test, and measures the competitive binding of radioactive T3 between serum thyroxine binding globulins and a resin. The radioactive T3 added to the system will bind preferentially to the resin if the thyroid binding sites on the thyroxine binding globulins are saturated with endogenous T3 and T4; in this instance the 'T3 uptake' on the resin will be high. It can be said therefore that the resin uptake of T3 is directly proportional to the fraction of free T4 in the serum, and inversely related to the thyroxine binding globulin binding sites. The uptake is thus high in hyperthyroidism and low in hypothyroidism. The test serves as an indirect measurement of the unbound fraction of T4 and is simpler to perform than other tests.

Free thyroxine index

Using a mathematical formula, an index of the free or unbound T4 in the serum can be arrived at from the total T4 and resin uptake test.

Serum TSH measurement

This is useful in the diagnosis of hypothyroidism, when levels of TSH are elevated at an early stage, and also for monitoring adjustments to treatment with oral thyroxine in hypothyroid patients.

The serum TSH is low in hyperthyroidism and also in hyperthyroid states due to an excess of T3. The response to injections of TRH in hyperthyroidism is minimal, the rise in TSH being barely perceptible.

Radioactive iodine uptake

Following the oral ingestion of radioactive iodine, I-131, the uptake by the gland is measured between 10 and 120 minutes after administration. Measuring the uptake at this stage, rather than at 24 hours, has the advantage that no appreciable discharge of radioactivity in the form of labelled hormone will have occurred.

In general, the rate with which the thyroid traps iodine reflects the rate of secretion of hormones into the circulation. Thus in hyperthyroidism both the proportion of the isotope taken up and the rate at which this occurs are increased.

The amount of radioactive iodine taken up is influenced by the amount of inorganic iodide in the serum, and if that is low, the uptake of I-131 by the thyroid will be increased, even though the amount of iodine entering the gland is normal. When stores of iodide are low the thyroid hypertrophies to maintain a normal output of hormone by trapping a greater proportion of the circulating iodide. This gives rise to the hyperplastic non-toxic goitre of iodine deficiency. A high radioactive iodine uptake in a patient with a simple goitre may then lead to a mistaken diagnosis of toxic goitre. Conversely, if the inorganic iodide stores are high, there is a decrease in the uptake of the isotope.

Before the radioactive iodine uptake test is performed, it would be as well to ascertain that the patient has not been taking foods containing iodine, or that there have not been any recent radiographic studies entailing the use of contrast agents.

The I-131 test should not be used in children or in pregnant women (Havard, 1975).

Thyroid suppression test

This is also known as the T3 suppression test, and is useful in differentiating hyperthyroidism from other causes of raised uptake such as iodine deficiency. It may also help to confirm the diagnosis of hyperthyroidism when the radioactive iodine uptake test is equivocal. Failure of suppression is characteristic of hyperthyroidism (Werner, Hamilton and Nemeth, 1952).

After an initial radioactive iodine uptake test, 120 μg of T3 are given daily for 5 days, after which the uptake is repeated. T3 is used in preference to T4 because of its more rapid effect and shorter half-life. In the euthyroid state the uptake is suppressed by this dose of exogenous hormone, while in hyperthyroidism no suppression occurs.

TRH stimulation test

This test measures the release of TSH in response to an injection of TRH. It serves to distinguish between diminished TSH production as a consequence of pituitary suppression from an autonomously operating hyperthyroid state and pituitary insufficiency. It is also useful in determining whether a dose of exogenous T4 is sufficient to suppress TSH production, as for instance after treatment of cancer of the thyroid gland.

TSH stimulation test

This test was introduced to distinguish between primary and secondary hypothyroidism. An injection of

TSH will cause an increase in uptake of radioisotope in patients with hypopituitarism, but not in patients with primary thyroid failure. This uptake is measured before and after an injection of bovine TSH, and the isotope of choice is technetium (Van Arsdel and Williams, 1956; Havard, 1975).

Imaging of the thyroid gland

Scanning

Automatic gamma cameras are used to obtain information on the size, shape and position of the gland and the distribution of the administered isotope within it.

Both Tc-99 and I-131 are used, the former more frequently than the latter. Technetium has the advantage of requiring a smaller dose, being less expensive, having a short half-life, and therefore allowing the scan to take place in 30 minutes. Iodine scans on the other hand are useful not only for morphological and topographical purposes, but also for assessing the function of the gland. They are indispensible for monitoring patients after total thyroidectomy for differentiated thyroid cancer, both in respect of identifying residual thyroid tissue which requires ablation, and the emergence of fresh deposits of disease (see section on scanning under neoplasms).

Both types of scan will distinguish between solitary and multiple nodules, and will confirm the presence of a retrosternal goitre. They will disclose the presence of a 'warm' nodule against a normally active background, and equally a 'hot' nodule against a suppressed or 'silent' background, indicating that the nodule has become autonomously hyperactive and has caused the remaining gland parenchyma to cease all activity (Figure 18.5).

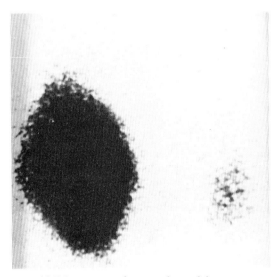

Figure 18.5 Isotope scan showing a hot nodule against a suppressed thyroid parenchyma

Ultrasound

The main benefit of ultrasound is the differentiation between solid and cystic lesions, but it also serves in the absence of istope scans to distinguish between a mononodular and a multinodular goitre.

When the precise position of a nodule is in doubt, ultrasound can be used to guide fine needle aspiration biopsy.

Radiology

Plain radiographs, CT scan, MRI

Plain films are sufficient to show features such as displacement and narrowing of the trachea such as occurs with retrosternal goitres (Figure 18.6).

Apart from revealing the extent of any thyroid enlargement, CT scans will reveal features such as compression of the trachea and oesophagus, and other distortions of anatomy.

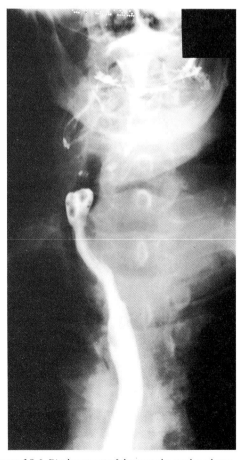

Figure 18.6 Displacement of the oesophagus by a large goitre

MRI is equally impressive in identifying the site and extent of disease in the thyroid gland, and its effect on adjacent structures (Figure 18.7).

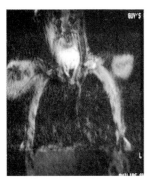

Figure 18.7 MRI of a large goitre causing displacement of the trachea

Fine needle aspiration biopsy

This is employed mainly in the work-up of patients with solitary thyroid nodules, or where a suspicion of cancer exists. It is useful in the identification of papillary, medullary, and poorly differentiated follicular carcinomas, but cannot distinguish between adenoma and carcinoma in a well-differentiated follicular lesion. It has, to a large extent, replaced open biopsy for the diagnosis of lymphoma (see neoplasms). Although useful in the diagnosis of Hashimoto's thyroiditis it is of little practical importance in other non-neoplastic thyroid diseases.

Diseases of the thyroid gland
Enlargement of the gland

Simple goitre

Simple goitre presents either as a diffuse symmetrical enlargement or as a multinodular goitre. The diffuse type may regress, persist unchanged, or develop into the multinodular variety. Simple non-toxic goitre is up to nine times more common in women than men.

There are a number of possible causes for a non-toxic goitre, but in each case the underlying basis of the enlargement is likely to be the same; namely glandular enlargement in response to oversecretion of TSH at a time when iodine reserves are deficient or not capable of being utilized. The resultant increase in thyroid mass is associated with an intensification of functional activity, so that hormone synthesis is maintained at a normal rate and the patient remains euthyroid.

In the case of diffuse goitre, the stimulus to increased TSH production may only be short-lived in which case the goitre will subside with the passage of time. If the stimulus is maintained or repeated cyclically, the symmetry of the goitre may eventually become disrupted and multinodularity occur (Marine, 1924).

One variant of the diffuse type is the physiological goitre seen in women at times of endocrine stress such as puberty, pregnancy, lactation and the menopause. Another is endemic goitre, which is seen in geographical areas of iodine shortage.

Goitre may be induced by the over-ingestion of vegetables of the brassica family, such as cabbages and turnips, the thiocyanate of which interferes with the proper utilization of iodine by the thyroid. Equally drugs may induce goitre, a common example today being carbimazole, which interferes with the organic binding of iodine. Other drugs causing goitre are lithium, para-aminosalicylic acid, phenylbutazone and excess of iodine.

There is some reason to suppose that goitres may run in families, possibly as a result of enzymic defects. One type of familial goitre, known to be inherited along mendelian laws, is associated with specific functional defects. In this type of dyshormonogeneic goitre there is deficient trapping of iodine and impaired organification of the element, a state which may be associated with congenital deafness and referred to as Pendred's syndrome. There may, in addition, be a defect of deiodinase activity, a relative failure to form thyroglobulin, and an inability of iodotyrosines to couple and form T_3 and T_4.

Diffuse non-toxic goitre

As the name implies, the enlargement is generalized, smooth and more or less symmetrical. Seen about nine times more commonly in women than men, the condition is usually associated with a euthyroid state, although in certain well-defined instances such as cretinism and endemic instances, the individual may be hypothyroid.

The histopathology of diffuse goitre depends on the duration and severity of the stimulus. At its most severe, there is hypertrophy and hyperplasia of follicular epithelium to the extent that the follicular lumen may be obliterated by papillary-like epithelial projections. The volume of colloid decreases, while at the same time, there may be an increase in vascularity. The histological picture differs from that seen in hyperthyroidism only in degree.

The goitre may be unsightly but rarely causes obstructive symptoms. Physiological goitre usually subsides once the cause is removed, but regression can be induced by the administration of small doses of T4.

Multinodular non-toxic goitre

This can be described as a non-symmetrical enlargement of the gland, characterized by structural and functional heterogeneity in the form of nodular change.

Multinodular goitre may be the sequel to an apparent diffuse goitre or may develop *ab initio*. As mentioned previously, the combination of intermittent TSH oversecretion in association with deficient iodine reserves, manifesting as bursts of cellular activity followed by involution, leads eventually to nodularity.

Alternatively, a variation in the sensitivity of thyroid follicles to the stimulus of TSH may account for the variegated appearance of this type of goitre. One study showed that as many as 50% of autopsies revealed previously undetected nodular change, suggesting that the process is much more prevalent than supposed (Mortensen, Woolner and Bennett, 1955).

Multinodular goitre may be sporadic or endemic, and is seen three to six times more commonly in women than men (Tunbridge *et al.*, 1977).

Pathologically, there is considerable variation in the size and shape of the nodules which are responsible for the increase in size of the gland. Some nodules would appear to be the result of the coalescence of colloid-filled follicles, while others present as solid follicular adenomas. Some present as cystic spaces in which haemorrhage may occur, while at the same time there may be calcification as well as areas of normal thyroid tissue in between. Malignant change in a multinodular goitre is allegedly rare, although reports now emerging would suggest that in some parts of the world this may not be the case (Al-Salah and Al-Kattan, 1994).

The changes described are consistent with the preservation of a normal level of hormone secretion, although with advancing years there may be a decline in activity, leading to hypothyroidism. The opposite may happen, when a nodule or parts of the gland become autonomously hyperthyroid, namely secondary hyperthyroidism or Plummer's disease.

Clinically, the goitre presents as a nodular swelling, usually more apparent on one side of the gland than the other. It will enlarge forwards, superiorly, laterally, medially and inferiorly. Enlargement of the goitre may cause tracheal displacement and compression, especially if there is downward extension into the mediastinum as a retrosternal goitre. In such a situation one side of the gland hypertrophies markedly and spreads downwards, although occasionally there is bilateral retrosternal extension. The part of the goitre lying in the mediastinum remains enveloped in the surgical capsule of the gland, and is devoid of venous attachments. It can thus be delivered from the mediastinum without fear of rupturing any veins. In most instances the recurrent nerve lies deep to the retrosternal extension, but at times the goitre will insinuate itself between the nerve and the trachea, so that the nerve comes to lie on the lateral aspect of the gland where it is vulnerable to damage (Figure 18.8).

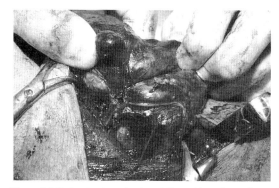

Figure 18.8 A retrosternal goitre delivered into the neck, with a recurrent laryngeal nerve lying plastered to the lateral surface of the goitre, out of its usual position

A retrosternal goitre may be the seat of 'hot' nodules which cause secondary hyperthyroidism, or it may represent the downward extension of a thyroid cancer.

Pressure from a retrosternal goitre is exerted principally on the trachea, causing displacement and eventually compression; it may, when very bulky, impede the venous return from the head and neck. The least common pressure symptom is dysphagia, since the oesophagus is posteriorly situated. Patients however, not infrequently complain of a sensation of a lump in the throat which may be misconstrued as dysphagia.

The patient with obstructive tracheal symptoms will have biphasic stridor, and difficulty in lying flat.

A technetium scan presents the typically mottled appearance of a multinodular goitre, together with an extension inferiorly. A plain radiograph of the chest will pick up the mass and the shift in the position of the trachea, as will a CT scan.

The clinical presentation of a multinodular goitre is such that in the majority of cases, it leaves little doubt about the diagnosis, and fine needle aspiration is unnecessary except in those rare instances when malignancy is suspected.

The two therapeutic avenues are suppression with exogenous T4 and surgery. The former may bring about a slow long-term reduction in size, but is often unsuccessful. Surgery on the other hand offers the prospect of an immediate and effective result, although if postoperative levels of TSH remain high there may be significant regrowth of residual thyroid tissue, unless this is suppressed by T4 therapy.

The indications for surgery are incipient or actual tracheal compression, retrosternal goitre, or massive enlargement of the gland, giving a cosmetic problem for the patient.

Surgery

This either takes the form of a total lobectomy on one side together with isthmusectomy, and a partial lobectomy on the other side; or alternatively entails removal of most of each thyroid lobe together with the isthmus, leaving the posterior part of each lobe behind. The operation of lobectomy is described in the section on neoplasms, while the description of the conventional operation of subtotal thyroidectomy follows below. The choice of operation depends on the configuration of the gland and the extent of the nodularity. If the nodules are exclusively unilateral a lobectomy would seem to be the appropriate procedure; whereas if the nodular change is more or less evenly distributed throughout the gland, a bilateral subtotal removal of glandular tissue is required.

Subtotal thyroidectomy

With the patient under general anaesthesia, intubated, and lying supine and the head fully extended, an incision is made horizontally above the suprasternal hollow to avoid subsequent thickening of the scar in its median third (Figure 18.9). One method is to outline the incision by pressing a piece of stretched linen or silk horizontally across the lower neck, and to mark the resultant impression with ink. The incision should not be so low that reaching the upper poles of the gland is going to be a struggle, but at the same time should not be so high as to be very conspicuous. Injection of the soft tissues with a large volume of 1:200 000 saline-adrenalin solution is optional, but considered by some to be helpful in reducing bleeding and separating the planes.

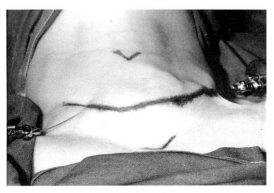

Figure 18.9 The incision for thyroidectomy

The incision is taken down through the subcutaneous tissue and platysma to the deep cervical fascia, and the flaps are raised superiorly and inferiorly (Figure 18.10).

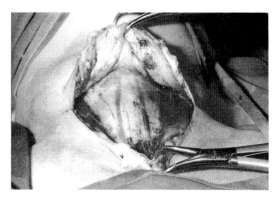

Figure 18.10 Superior and inferior flaps are elevated

The option now lies between a midline approach, or horizontal transection of the strap muscles. The latter is simpler, since it requires less retraction and is therefore more suitable for large goitres. The former is considered to be more physiological since the strap muscles and their nerve supply are not tampered with but, in practice, division of the straps rarely leaves any functional sequelae.

With the midline approach the deep cervical fascia is incised from the cricoid to the suprasternal notch, dealing with the anterior jugular veins and their tributaries if necessary. The two layers of the strap muscles are separated and retracted laterally to expose the thyroid lobe which is to be mobilized.

The surgical capsule of the gland is opened and dissection commenced between the gland surface and the capsule.

The common carotid artery is retracted and the inferior thyroid artery sought and isolated. This is the cardinal landmark for the recurrent laryngeal nerve, which is now sought in the space below the inferior thyroid artery (Figure 18.11). On the right side it approaches the tracheo-oesophageal groove with an inclination from lateral to medial, while on the left side, the nerve runs in a strictly vertical plane. Once the nerve has been located and its course up to the ligament of Berry has been fully exposed, attention is paid to the vessels, although the order with which these are secured is a matter of individual preference.

All the inferior thyroid veins are found and ligated. Dividing the inferior thyroid artery as opposed to simply ligating it has the advantage of facilitating the mobilization of the thyroid lobe. The superior vascular pedicle is cleared of its surrounding capsular extension and interrupted as close to the gland as possible to avoid the external laryngeal nerve.

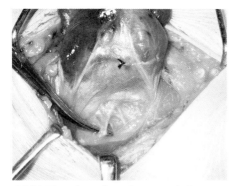

Figure 18.11 The inferior thyroid artery with the recurrent nerve below it

Mobilization of the lobe is continued until it is literally only attached to the trachea by the ligament of Berry. Two-thirds of the lobe are removed by a coronal transection taking care to ensure that the cut on the medial side of the lobe is away from the recurrent laryngeal nerve (Figure 18.12).

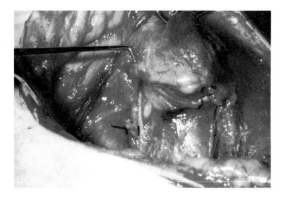

Figure 18.12 Mobilization of the thyroid lobe off the recurrent nerve

The lobe and isthmus are now lifted off the trachea, and the procedure repeated on the contralateral side. At the conclusion of the resection the raw surface of the posterior part of each thyroid lobe is either left exposed after haemostasis, the medial and lateral edges approximated and sutured, or the raw surfaces turned in onto the trachea to which they are sutured.

The wound is drained by a large bore suction drain, and the wound closed in layers, using clips for the skin. These should be removed by the third postoperative day.

Complications

The complication which is most feared is trauma to the recurrent laryngeal nerve, estimated to occur in between 1 and 10% of operations (Wade, 1955, 1960; Riddell, 1970).

The nerve may be cut, stretched or burnt, usually as a result of failure to recognize or dissect it out properly.

In unilateral paralysis the vocal cord is immobile in the paramedian position, a situation which leaves the patient with a weak, cracked, and breathy voice. A paralysis which has persisted for longer than 6 months is amenable to treatment by thyroplasty or Teflon injection.

Bilateral paralysis leads to severe airway obstruction, necessitating an urgent early tracheostomy in the majority of patients. Those patients who have a small chink between the vocal cords can sometimes breathe reasonably well at rest, but this is the exception rather than the rule. The treatment for bilateral palsy is laser cordectomy and arytenoidectomy on one side.

The external laryngeal nerve is traumatized more often than one supposes. Its close relationship to the superior vascular pedicle and an occasionally aberrant course predispose it to damage (Durham and Harrison, 1964). Diathermy of the small vein which passes from the superior thyroid vein to the lateral part of the cricothyroid muscle is a further cause of damage to this nerve.

Hypocalcaemia which is uncommon after subtotal thyroidectomy for multinodular goitre, may be the result of rough handling of the posterior aspect of the thyroid lobes, or interruption of the terminal branches of the main divisions of the inferior thyroid artery. Intravenous calcium gluconate (10%) administered slowly provides an immediate solution to the symptoms which vary from tingling in the extremities to frank tetany. Oral calcium (Sandocal) supplemented by 1-alphacalcidol should be instituted and the situation periodically reviewed.

Hypothyroidism, developing gradually over a period of months or years after operation, is a common though acceptable complication of subtotal thyroidectomy and is readily treated with T4 (Hedley *et al.*, 1972).

Metabolic diseases of the gland

Diffuse toxic goitre – Graves' disease

This disease is thought to be immunologically mediated by thyroid stimulating immunoglobulins which are part of the IgA class of antibodies. The probable mechanism is an interaction between thyroid stimulating immunoglobulins and specific sites on the membranes of follicular cells, possibly TSH receptor sites;

an override of the normal regulatory control of thyroid metabolism thus occurs.

Thyroid stimulating immunoglobulins are found in between 70 and 90% of patients with Graves' disease and are called LATS-P. The exophthalmos seen in hyperthyroidism may also be caused by thyroid stimulating immunoglobulins, since it is suspected that TSH receptors may be present in the retro-orbital fat cells, and may be subject to stimulation by the immunoglobulins. In infiltrative ophthalmopathy, the volume of the retro-orbital tissues is increased in response to an inflammatory reaction and its associated oedema. Graves' disease is seen in 3% of the population between the third and fourth decade of life and is seven to ten times more common in women than in men (Tunbridge *et al.*, 1977).

Hyperthyroidism is characterized by irritability, weight loss, increased appetite, emotional instability and heat intolerance. The patient sweats excessively, the skin is smooth, there is increased muscle tone and often a fine tremor. The pulse is rapid and bounding due to increased pulse pressure, even during sleep, and patients frequently complain of palpitations. Later still there may be cardiac arrhythmias such as atrial fibrillation.

There are specific eye signs to be looked for, namely lid lag, lid retraction, exophthalmos and ophthalmoplegia. In the worst cases there may be chemosis of the conjunctiva.

Lid lag can be demonstrated by asking the patient to follow a finger from above downwards, at which time the upper lid tends to lag behind the downward movement of the iris, exposing an area of sclera briefly. Lid retraction is defined as observance of an area of sclera between the upper lid and the iris with the patient looking ahead, while exophthalmos or proptosis is noted when the sclera is observed between the lower lid and the iris. Ophthalmoplegia is the most advanced stage of Graves' ophthalmopathy.

In Graves' disease, the thyroid is diffusely enlarged, to the extent that the pyramidal lobe may stand out above the rest of the gland, and by virtue of the increased vascularity, there may be a bruit heard over the gland on auscultation.

The clinical diagnosis can be confirmed in the laboratory by a number of tests. The serum T4 can be measured by immunoassay, but as the measurement is of the total thyroxine content, it cannot differentiate between hyperthyroidism and raised levels of thyroxine binding globulins.

The T3 resin uptake test is an indirect measure of the unoccupied thyroxine-binding sites on the proteins in the blood. In hyperthyroidism there are fewer unoccupied sites on the proteins, hence the resin uptake is increased. When there is an alteration in the concentration of thyroxine binding globulin, the serum T4 levels and the T3 resin uptake move in opposite directions. Thus in patients with an increase in thyroxine binding globulins, the serum T4 rises into the hyperthyroid range and, because of the increase in binding sites on the serum protein, the T3 resin uptake moves into the hypothyroid range. A mathematical combination of serum T4 and T3 resin uptake provides normal values in euthyroid patients with abnormal levels of thyroxine binding globulins. This combination is called the free thyroid index, and correlates closely with the level of free T4 in the serum.

The radioactive iodine uptake of the gland measured between 10 and 120 minutes after the administration of the isotope will be raised in Graves' disease, although it should be remembered that if the iodide stores in the body are low and the serum iodide level reduced, the uptake of I-131 will be increased, and could be wrongly attributed to increased activity of the gland. Conversely, if the inorganic stores of the body are increased as a result of over-ingestion, there is a decrease in the uptake of isotope.

The T3 suppression test is useful for differentiating thyrotoxicosis from other causes of raised uptake, such as iodine deficiency, and in studying the autonomy of thyroid nodules. It is helpful in the diagnosis of hyperthyroidism when the T3 resin uptake test is equivocal (Havard, 1974, 1975).

Pathology of Graves' disease

A diffuse toxic goitre is soft to firm in consistency, and under the influence of antithyroid medication becomes distinctly rubbery. The cut surface of the gland is red to brown, and glistening, and extremely vascular. Microscopically the follicles are lined by hyperplastic columnar epithelium with scant colloid filling the lumen of the follicles. The hyperplasia may be so intense that the epithelium bulges inwards in the form of papillary projections. There is frequently a lymphocytic infiltrate in keeping with the autoimmune nature of the condition.

Treatment

There are three effective methods of treatment available: antithyroid drugs, subtotal thyroidectomy, and radioactive iodine.

With antithyroid drugs the effect on the gland is reversible, while with the other two methods it is permanent. The choice of treatment will depend on a variety of factors – medical, logistical and social. None of the modalities mentioned has any influence on the underlying cause of the disease, but all are effective in controlling it. Exophthalmos, however, may not be affected by treatment, although it will occasionally subside under the influence of therapy. The medical factors influencing the choice of therapy include the duration and severity of the disorder, the age of the patient, the size and duration of the goitre, and the availability of surgical expertise.

Medical treatment

The thiouracils and imidazoles are the most frequently used drugs. Unlike potassium perchlorate which interferes with the trapping of iodide by the thyroid, they prevent the organic binding of iodine in the gland. Their main disadvantage is that treatment must be continued for at least 18 months, and that half the patients relapse after discontinuing treatment. These drugs are relatively free of side effects, and severe complications, such as agranulocytosis, occur in less than 0.5% of patients (Vanderlaan and Storrie, 1955).

As the drugs are absorbed and excreted rapidly they should be given in three divided doses spread out evenly over 24 hours. Carbimazole 10 mg eight-hourly is a satisfactory initial dose, reducing to 5 mg three times a day once control has been achieved.

The patient who is being scheduled for surgery should be euthyroid at the time of operation, and the aim should also be to shrink the gland with iodine, commencing 2 weeks before surgery.

Potassium iodide, 60 mg three times a day or Lugol's iodine, 5 drops t.d.s., should be commenced 14 days prior to operation, while tailing off conventional therapy.

As many of the clinical features of hyperthyroidism are due to sympathetic overactivity, treatment with beta-adrenergic antagonists such as propranolol complements the standard antithyroid regimen and serves as a useful adjunct in patients who are being prepared for surgery.

Radioactive iodine

This is the ideal treatment for the majority of patients since it carries virtually no risks. Given as a tasteless drink, it begins to exert its effect in 2–3 months and for several months thereafter. It is unwise to treat children with Graves' disease with this modality in view of possible carcinogenicity, and equally pregnant women should not be treated either, for fear of inducing carcinoma in the fetus' thyroid gland.

The minimum age for eligibility has dropped over the last three to four decades, so that is is now common practice to treat patients in their middle twenties. There is no increased risk of carcinoma or leukaemia and the only long-term effect is hypothyroidism (Harvard, 1974).

Surgical treatment

Subtotal thyroidectomy as described in a previous section is effective in the control of thyrotoxicosis.

The aim is to achieve a balance at operation between removing too much tissue and thus rendering the patient hypothyroid, and leaving too much behind so that the patient remains hyperthyroid. About 10% of patients remain hyperthyroid, while it is now accepted that as many as 40% of patients ultimately become myxoedematous. It is possible that the figure may be even higher than this (McNeil and Thomson, 1968; Hedley et al., 1972).

Subtotal thyroidectomy for Graves' disease

The steps are virtually the same as surgery for multinodular goitre, but the trend is to aim for a symmetrical removal of tissue so that the two remnants on either side are roughly the same in size. Opinions are divided on the precise volume of tissue to be left behind, and also the manner of estimating remnant size. The figure of 8 g of tissue continues to be mentioned, but unfortunately a standard figure cannot reasonably take into account variations in the severity of the disease or the autoimmune factor which is present in the majority of patients (Hedley et al., 1972; Pegg et al., 1973).

Complications

The complications mentioned in relation to subtotal thyroidectomy for multinodular goitre apply to the surgery of Graves' disease, but perhaps even more so, since the goitres are spongier and more vascular, and therefore somewhat more difficult to remove.

The incidence of residual hyperthyroidism is of the order of 10%, of long-term hypothyroidism 40% and tetany 10%. The incidence of recurrent nerve paralysis is between 1 and 10%, (Wade, 1955, 1960; Riddell, 1970; Hedley et al., 1972; Havard, 1974).

Thyroid crisis

This is an uncommon complication of surgery, and only likely to occur if the patient has not been properly prepared, i.e. when hyperthyroidism persists in spite of medical treatment. It may occur rarely in patients who have been adequately controlled medically, but who develop an active infection which upsets the body homeostasis.

The features are hyperthermia, tachycardia, intense irritability, profuse sweating, hypertension, extreme anxiety, prostration, and eventually hypotension and death. The precise mechanism is unclear, but is thought to be due to the synergistic effect of an adrenergic outburst together with an outpouring of thyroid hormone into the circulation.

The treatment consists of propranolol, potassium iodide and hydrocortisone (Havard, 1974).

Toxic nodular goitre – Plummer's disease

This is hyperthyroidism developing in an older person, usually a woman, with a nodular goitre. The onset is gradual and insidious, and the first sign may be a disturbance of the cardiac rhythm, such as atrial fibrillation. Eye signs are much less commonly seen than in primary hyperthyroidism (Graves' disease).

As with Graves' disease signs of toxicity are present, and the diagnosis is confirmed by the appropriate blood tests. Scanning with technetium reveals the typical patchy uptake of a nodular goitre, and an iodine scan will demonstrate areas of intense activity interspersed with areas of poor or non-existent function.

Contrary to some opinions, all three methods of treatment are effective in the management of toxic nodular goitre. It has been suggested that medical treatment and radioiodine may not be as effective as in primary hyperthyroidism, and that surgery is therefore the preferred treatment. There is no good evidence to support this supposition, and in the majority of patients the logical treatment is radioiodine. Medical treatment is not ideal for patients with large retrosternal extensions for fear of increasing the swelling under the influence of carbimazole and bringing on acute pressure symptoms. Retrosternal and large goitres remain the definitive indications for subtotal thyroidectomy.

Solitary hot or toxic nodule

While most solid solitary nodules are inactive or 'cold' there exists the possibility of a solitary follicular nodule becoming autonomously hyperactive, to the extent of suppressing TSH production from the anterior pituitary, and inhibiting hormone secretion from the rest of the gland.

Scanning with technetium or iodine will show a 'hot' nodule with little uptake in the remaining gland. A 'warm' nodule by contrast is a functioning adenoma, capable of trapping iodine, and appearing against a parenchyma which takes up isotope and continues to secrete hormone. The treatment of a hot nodule is either by excision or radioactive iodine and both are immediately curative. Up to 5% of warm nodules can become malignant and excision is therefore recommended. Hot nodules on the other hand virtually never become malignant.

Hypothyroidism

The symptoms and signs of hypothyroidism include apathy, lack of energy, inability to concentrate, and intolerance to cold. The skin is dry and there is loss of hair, especially noticeable in the lateral third of the eyebrows. There may be constipation and menstrual irregularity and weight gain; the voice may deepen, and the patient may complain of pins and needles in the fingers as a result of carpal tunnel compression. Ankle jerk reflexes are lost, and the ECG voltage may be reduced. Treatment is with T4, monitored by estimation of serum T4 and TSH levels.

Inflammatory conditions

Hashimoto's autoimmune thyroiditis

This is most commonly seen in middle-aged women, whose thyroid becomes asymmetrically enlarged, nodular, firm or rubbery. On section, the affected part of the gland stands out by contrast with the rest of the gland as being pale or even white. Microscopically there is a diffuse lymphocytic infiltrate followed later by variable obliteration of the follicles and fibrosis.

There is a high titre of circulating antibodies to thyroglobulin and thyroid cell microsomes, and reduced thyroid hormone secretion. Scanning shows a patchy uptake which may be confused with the changes seen in a multinodular goitre, but fine needle aspiration will readily differentiate the two conditions.

The correct treatment for this condition is to administer thyroxine.

Acute thyroiditis

Acute thyroiditis is sometimes associated with an upper respiratory or throat infection, but more often is due to an acute granulomatous infection secondary to tuberculosis, syphilis or actinomycosis. The disease is characterized by painful swelling and recurrent sinus formation (Figure 18.13). Recognition of the cause and treatment with the appropriate antibiotic is curative, although with actinomycosis there is a tendency to relapse.

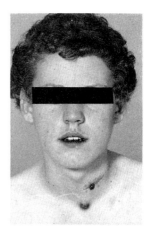

Figure 18.13 Actinomycosis of the thyroid with sinus formation

Subacute or de Quervain's thyroiditis

This usually follows an upper respiratory tract infection. The thyroid gland becomes diffusely swollen, painful and very tender. The ESR is raised, while the rest of the blood picture is unaffected and the patient's hormonal status remains unchanged. Treatment with hydrocortisone or prednisolone is effective, but in the absence of a rapid response, malignancy, either lymphoma or anaplastic carcinoma, should be suspected.

Thyroid neoplasms

Incidence of thyroid neoplasms

Malignant tumours of the thyroid gland represent less than 0.5% of all cancers in England and Wales (Yeung and Addison, 1983). In southern Sweden there are roughly two cases per 1 000 000 population per annum (Tennval, 1984), and in the USA the equivalent figure is slightly less than four (Third National Cancer Survey, 1971).

It is predominantly a disease of women, the female: male ratio being about 2.5:1.

Aetiology of thyroid neoplasms

Radiation

After reviewing all the available evidence, there is little doubt that radiation stands out as the most definite of all the possible aetiological factors.

The practice of irradiating the thymus was fashionable in the earlier part of the century, particularly in the USA, and for a time irradiation of the adenotonsillar lymphoid tissue also enjoyed a passing vogue in the years leading up to and including the Second World War.

After reviewing the histories of such patients, it was concluded that radiation to the head, neck, and thorax in small doses during childhood was liable to induce cancer of the thyroid gland in later life (Winship and Rosvoll, 1961).

Further evidence of the carcinogenic effect of radiation during childhood came from the survivors of the atomic bombs in Japan, 18% of whom developed cancers of the thyroid gland. Most patients were under the age of 10 years at the time of exposure, implying that susceptibility to the disease is most pronounced before puberty; furthermore most tumours were of the papillary type, the most common of the differentiated neoplasms (Sampson *et al.*, 1969).

Although the adolescent and adult gland is evidently less at risk, reports of cancers in adults who had previously been irradiated for Hodgkin's disease of the cervical lymph nodes 10–15 years before clearly indicate a continued susceptibility, albeit on a somewhat reduced scale (McDougall *et al.*, 1980). There is also some evidence to suggest that benign nodular disease may in some instances be linked to a history of previous radiation, possibly as much as 35 years previously (Favus *et al.*, 1976).

On the experimental level, Doniach (1953) demonstrated that rats fed on thiouracil and subsequently exposed to radiotherapy developed thyroid cancer. This led him to postulate that two factors were necessary for carcinogenesis, namely a high thyroid stimulating hormone (TSH) level, which one would normally expect in the prepubertal subject, and secondly ionizing radiation. The finding that most differentiated thyroid cancers regress if TSH is suppressed by the administration of thyroxine, supports this contention (Crile, 1966).

Hormonal causes

Experimental work on rats has shown that excessive production of TSH over prolonged periods, whether induced by the administration of thiouracil, by partial thyroidectomy, or by iodine-deficient diets, may induce benign and malignant tumours (Doniach and Williams, 1962). The addition of a specific carcinogen such as 2-acetylaminofluorene increases the incidence of cancer (Bielschowsky, 1944).

One should therefore expect a higher incidence of cancer in glands hypertrophied by high levels of TSH over prolonged periods of time, such as in areas where goitre is endemic (Wegelin, 1928). The evidence in support of this is, however, contradictory and the issue unlikely to be resolved by comparing the statistics of one country with those of another. In favour of the view that endemic goitre predisposes to carcinoma is the finding that the predominant pathological type in such areas is the follicular neoplasm, whereas for non-endemic goitre it is more often papillary.

Genetic factors

Familial medullary carcinoma, as opposed to the sporadic disease, is passed on as an autosomal dominant form of inheritance, with an increased predisposition to other tumours, mainly of neuroectodermal origin, such as phaeochromocytoma, epithelial neuroma, and parathyroid adenoma.

In the north-western coastal area of Norway, which is not particularly noted for endemic goitre and which until quite recently was isolated from the rest of the country, the incidence of differentiated thyroid cancer is high, a fact which has led to the suggestion that this may have resulted from inbreeding over a considerable period of time (Wade, 1975).

Autoimmune thyroiditis

Malignant lymphoma is a well-known sequel of Hashimoto's disease but the exact frequency of this change is difficult to assess.

Classification, pathology and natural history of thyroid neoplasms

Solitary non-functioning nodules of the thyroid gland are either cystic or solid, and the latter are either benign adenomas or cancers. Anything up to 20% of non-functioning solid nodules will prove to be cancers, although a more common figure is about 10% (Katz and Warren, 1976; Burrow *et al.*, 1978).

For a comprehensive review of the pathology of malignant tumours of the thyroid, the reader can do no better than refer to the paper by Woolner *et al.* (1961), which reviews a very large number of cases collected in a major centre. The two most common cancers, specifically of thyroid tissue origin, are papillary and follicular carcinoma. Because of their distinctive histological features and behaviour, they are sometimes grouped together and referred to collectively as differentiated tumours.

Medullary carcinoma arises from the parafollicular or C cells and is, therefore, not a true thyroid neoplasm, but because of its anatomical location and similarities in behaviour, it is included in discussions of thyroid neoplasms.

Papillary carcinoma

This tumour comprises about 60% of all malignant neoplasms in the larger American series, but figures a little less prominently in European reports. It is the type which most often follows previous irradiation. The histological appearance is one of papillary excrescences together with neoplastic follicles; in most cases encapsulation is absent.

Small papillary tumours not exceeding 1.5 cm in diameter and exhibiting marked desmoplasia and psammoma bodies are referred to as occult carcinomas. By contrast to their bulkier counterparts, they are usually detected by accident or their presence may be suspected when a metastatic node is discovered in the absence of palpable disease at the primary site.

Most papillary cancers present as discrete, hard, intrathyroid masses, but additional discrete deposits are found in other parts of the gland in as many as 40% of patients, most of these being microscopic. Whether these smaller deposits represent spread within the gland along lymphatic channels or entirely independent new tumours is impossible to say, but their presence has led some people to believe that papillary cancer is truly multifocal in origin.

The tumour generally grows slowly and is late to break through the capsule of the gland, although lymph node metastasis is not uncommon. The disease may occur at any age, but it is classically commoner in younger subjects, 42% being under the age of 40 (Woolner *et al.*, 1961).

The ratio of females to males for all papillary cancers in the same study was 2.4:1, but that in cases which had broken through the capsule of the gland was 1.5:1, and in inoperable cases 0.7:1. This suggests that the prognosis may be influenced by the sex of the individual, although other factors also need to be taken into account.

Once the tumour has become extrathyroid, it attaches itself to neighbouring structures and ultimately becomes invasive. Typically the tumour invades the strap muscles first and, although lacking a capsule, it may well provoke the formation of fibrous tissue at its leading edge, thus creating the impression of encapsulation.

Gross invasion of veins is virtually absent, but invasion of the trachea, larynx, oesophagus, and recurrent nerves takes place when the disease has extended beyond the confines of the gland.

Almost all papillary cancers exhibit a mixed papillary and follicular pattern, in varying proportions. At one end of the spectrum are tumours which are wholly papillary, while at the other end the proportion of papillary elements is overshadowed by a predominantly follicular pattern. Even those exhibiting a mainly follicular appearance lack a capsule and behave in a similar way to their papillary counterparts.

Nodal metastasis occurs in as many as 40% of patients (Woolner *et al.*, 1961). Deposits appear classically in the paratracheal nodes, but may present anywhere in the neck, so that lymphadenopathy in the carotid or supraclavicular triangles is common. Bilateral spread to the nodes is found in about 8% of patients.

Pulmonary metastasis is very uncommon at presentation, and only affects 4% of all patients, chiefly those in the older group and those with extrathyroid spread. It often presents as a diffuse, coarse, miliary infiltrate rather than a series of discrete rounded shadows.

Follicular carcinoma

Whereas the mean age for papillary cancer was 42 years in the series of Woolner *et al.* (1961), that for follicular carcinoma was 50. The sex ratio however, was similar at 2.6:1 in favour of females, and the total group comprised 18% of all malignant thyroid neoplasms.

Follicular carcinoma is typically encapsulated and, in those lesions with minimal invasive characteristics it may be mistaken for a follicular adenoma. The extent to which the capsule is invaded, and in particular the veins located within the capsule, provides an indication of the likelihood of metastasis. The term 'micro-angioinvasive' has been coined to describe those tumours with little evidence of venous invasion, and in which the potential for local invasiveness and distant metastasis is consequently low. Gross infiltration of capsular veins is a bad prognostic sign and generally portends distant dissemination of disease.

Besides this particular feature of follicular cancers, the pathologist may recognize a gradation from a well-differentiated to a poorly differentiated pattern, and this feature may also be used in forecasting the outcome. In some, dedifferentiation assumes an even more sinister quality so that the tumour ultimately becomes anaplastic.

Once follicular carcinoma becomes extrathyroid, the capacity for local invasion becomes more dramatic than in papillary cancer, although the tissues involved are essentially the same, namely the larynx, trachea, oesophagus and recurrent nerves. Curiously, the only structure which defies invasion in both types of neoplasm is the carotid artery. In the case of the larynx and trachea, cartilage is destroyed and intraluminal extension of disease causes airway obstruction and bleeding. Oesophageal invasion is uncommon and late, and usually manifests itself as an insinuation of the disease between trachea and oesophagus, followed by migration some distance up and down the muscle coat, and between muscle and mucosa. The tumour rarely penetrates the mucosa to enter the lumen of the oesophagus and is unlikely therefore to be recognized by preoperative endoscopy.

Nodal metastasis is uncommon in purely follicular cancers being found in about 4% of patients (Woolner *et al.*, 1961).

Metastases of angioinvasive tumours to bone and viscera are common, and the better differentiated of these may resemble normal thyroid tissue. In the lungs the radiological appearance is generally of multiple large rounded shadows and, in the bones, that of osteolytic lesions. The latter in fact may be extremely vascular, to the extent of resembling arteriovenous malformations.

In rare instances, the primary tumour may present as a hyperfunctioning nodule causing some degree of hyperthyroidism.

Medullary carcinoma

Medullary carcinoma, comprising between 5 and 10% of thyroid neoplasms, is a tumour of the para-follicular or C cells and, unlike differentiated thyroid neoplasms, is of neuroectodermal origin (Hazard, Hawk and Crile, 1959). It falls into one of two categories, namely the sporadic or the familial hereditary type of disease.

The former is generally seen between the third and seventh decade of life, with women again predominating over men. The latter, which is inherited as an autosomal dominant trait, may appear as early as the second decade, and affects both sexes equally.

Both types present as a single hard nodule, but in the familial group there is nearly always histological evidence of multicentricity. The tumour is solid and unencapsulated, and grows in sheets or nests surrounded by a hyaline fibrous stroma which stains strongly for amyloid.

The propensity for lymph node metastasis is exhibited by both familial and sporadic types, and as many as 75% of patients eventually develop lymphadenopathy. Like papillary cancer, medullary cancer may spread to any group of cervical lymph nodes, although the emphasis is frequently on the lower deep cervical, supraclavicular, and mediastinal nodes.

The natural tendency of the primary tumour is to enlarge and then to break through the capsule of the thyroid gland, first to attach to adjacent structures, and finally to invade them.

Medullary cancer is characterized by an elevation of the serum calcitonin, which tends to be relatively higher in the familial type of disease. Selective venous catheterization has been used in the past to determine the site of maximum calcitonin concentration in the gland, and is most useful for the detection of the site of any recurrent disease.

Infusion of calcium into the blood stream, or the ingestion of whisky, are potent stimuli for the release of calcitonin, a fact which is made use of in patients in whom occult tumours are suspected, or when screening the siblings of a person known to suffer from the disease. The greater the bulk of the disease, both at the primary site and at sites of metastasis, the higher the level of the serum calcitonin.

When the tumour is confined exclusively to the thyroid gland, eradication of the disease should in theory reduce the serum calcitonin level to normal (less than 0.1 mg/ml), but this is seldom achieved even when distant spread is absent.

There is good evidence to suggest that serotonin is secreted by some medullary cancers since flushing, headache, breathlessness, sweating and fainting are experienced by some patients, and both the serum 5-hydroxytryptamine (serotonin) and the urinary 5-hydroxyindoleacetic acid levels are raised. Prostaglandins and histaminase are also secreted, the concentration of the latter serving as a useful guide to the extent of metastatic disease.

The intractable and severe diarrhoea which is so typical of many patients with medullary carcinoma is almost invariably linked to the presence of gross metastatic disease, mainly in the liver, but its precise cause is not understood. Fifty per cent or more of the patients eventually suffer from this distressing symptom for which there is no specific treatment.

Blood-borne metastases are seen typically in the liver, but may also affect the lungs and the bones, at which site they may cause severe pain.

Other tumours are seen in about 10% of patients with familial medullary carcinoma, namely phaeochromocytoma, mucosal neuromas and parathyroid adenoma. Investigations should therefore include an estimate of the 24-hour urinary levels of vanylmandelic acid and the serum calcium.

Anaplastic carcinoma

The average age of patients in this group is about 60 years and once again women outnumber men. The tumour only accounts for about 5% of all thyroid neoplasms, and even this may be an overestimate, since many lymphomas were previously mistaken for anaplastic cancer.

Microscopically, the tumour is characterized by large cells with markedly irregular nuclei some of which may take on a bizzare giant appearance, while others assume a spindly look, hence the subdivision into giant-cell or spindle-cell anaplastic carcinoma.

Typically there is a history of a long-standing but asymptomatic goitre preceding the sudden and explosive onset of the disease. The clinical course is characterized by rapid growth with pain, early invasion of surrounding structures, and a swift decline. Patients rarely survive for longer than a year after the diagnosis is made.

Malignant lymphoma

Whereas anaplastic carcinoma is almost invariably fatal, the outlook in lymphoma is comparatively favourable.

The histology, which may bear some resemblance to anaplastic tumours, is usually distinctive, and there should rarely be any confusion between the two conditions.

The clinical course, however, may be almost as dramatic as anaplastic cancer, in that there is a sudden onset of swelling spreading to adjacent structures and causing acute respiratory embarrassment. Early treatment is essential for the prevention of complications, and this may then be followed by the appropriate investigations for staging the disease.

Follicular adenoma

This is a solitary encapsulated ovoid or rounded mass varying in consistency from soft to firm, depending on whether the growth has been the seat of haemorrhage, infarction, cyst formation, fibrosis, or calcification. The architecture of this neoplasm is one of multiple follicles of relatively uniform appearance with compression of the adjacent fibrous parenchyma. Care must be taken not to overlook a carcinoma, the key being the absence of venous or capsular invasion.

Adenomas may be non-functioning, or may exhibit some degree of activity, varying from slight to hyperactive. True 'toxic' adenomas are uncommon; usually a toxic nodule suppresses the remaining parenchyma of the gland.

Factors influencing prognosis in thyroid cancer

The two most important factors influencing prognosis in differentiated thyroid cancer are the age of the patient and the pathology of the tumour.

Most authors agree that survival is inversely related to age and that this effect is most evident from the age of 40 years onwards (Staunton and Skeet, 1979).

Opinions differ on the relation of the patient's sex to prognosis. It is generally accepted that men with differentiated thyroid cancer fare better than women, though Crile (1971) asserted that women under the age of 40 years unquestionably had a higher survival rate than men.

The histopathological criteria which govern the behaviour of a thyroid neoplasm are also considered to influence prognosis. Papillary carcinoma tends to be slow growing and, although lacking a capsule, provokes a fibrous reaction as the disease becomes extrathyroid. This may serve to lessen the tendency towards invasion, at least for a while. It would seem also that both occult tumours and papillary cancer induced by exposure to radiation in childhood carry a particularly favourable prognosis.

Follicular carcinoma exhibits a greater capacity for invasion, exemplified typically by its tendency to infiltrate the veins which lie in the tumour capsule. The degree of differentiation also has an important bearing on the final outcome, so that the expectations for a poorly differentiated follicular neoplasm must be lower than for a well-differentiated one.

In general, follicular tumours have a worse prognosis than purely papillary neoplasms, and papillary tumours with follicular elements are intermediate. Extrathyroid spread carries a worse prognosis than disease confined to the gland.

Nodal spread of papillary carcinoma apparently does not affect the prognosis adversely.

Symptoms and signs

Thyroid neoplasms whether benign or malignant present in the early or intrathyroid phase as solitary nodules, often of indeterminate consistency. They usually lie in one or other lobe, but occasionally arise in the isthmus of the gland. Even tumours which are eventually reported by the pathologist to be multicentric generally appear to be uninodular on clinical examination. For the vast majority of patients, the principal concern about which they seek advice is the presence of a swelling.

Attempts to draw conclusions about the nature of the swelling from its consistency are generally unrewarding, for by no means every cancer possesses the hardness of a squamous cancer, and in any case the interposition of numerous soft tissue layers between the palpating fingers and the neoplasms makes interpretation of the consistency difficult.

The distinction between benign and malignant in the later stages of the natural history of a thyroid swelling is usually much easier to make because adenomas do not become as overtly extrathyroid in the way that cancers do. Conversely large thyroid masses which blend imperceptibly into the adjacent anatomy so that their limits are indeterminate are rarely benign.

Fixation due to escape of the disease from the gland is therefore an important criterion of malignancy, and is evident by the failure of the mass to move up and down with swallowing.

Such is the diffuse extent of extrathyroid spread in some cases, that the carotid artery may be displaced quite far laterally, or even obscured by the overlying neoplasm so that distal pulsations may be reduced. The close relationship of the cervical sympathetic nerve to the posteromedial aspect of the carotid sheath explains the presence of a Horner's syndrome when spread is as extensive as this.

Displacement of the trachea to the contralateral side does not in itself signify the presence of malignancy, since any large goitre may do this, but compression and narrowing of the trachea leading to stridor and shortness of breath, especially when the patient lies down, should arouse suspicion of malignancy.

Haemoptysis, on the other hand, is a clear indication of an invasive process which has finally broken through into the tracheal lumen, and should leave the clinician in no doubt about the nature of the disease.

Dysphagia is a late phenomenon in the natural history of thyroid cancers, and usually signifies infiltration of the gullet, rather than simple displacement such as occurs when a very bulky goitre comes into contact with the oesophagus.

The laryngeal ala or the cricoid may be infiltrated, and the hypopharynx may be invaded when disease from the posterior aspect of the upper pole of the thyroid attaches itself to the pyriform sinus.

Hoarseness is common in such circumstances, and is later followed by dyspnoea and laryngeal stridor. Indirect laryngoscopy shows an oedematous mucous membrane encroaching on the laryngeal lumen.

Hoarseness, is, however, more likely to be due to paralysis of the vocal cord resulting from infiltration of the recurrent laryngeal nerves. It should be said that vocal cord mobility may be preserved for a long time in the face of obvious invasion of the recurrent nerve.

Lymphadenopathy is most apparent at those sites which are amenable to palpation, but the nodes which are most consistently involved, namely the paratracheal, are deep seated and are therefore rarely palpable.

As nodal disease enlarges, so the likelihood of fixation to the jugular vein and prevertebral fascia increases.

Retrosternal extension, a common feature of large follicular cancers, causes tracheal displacement and narrowing as well as engorgement of the neck and upper chest wall veins. At operation the retrosternal extension, unlike its benign counterpart, is often attached to adjacent structures in the mediastinum such as the pleura, trachea, recurrent nerves, oesophagus and prevertebral fascia.

The pathology of each thyroid nodule largely determines the pattern of symptoms in any given case. Follicular adenomas rarely give rise to any symptoms other than awareness of the presence of a swelling.

In papillary carcinoma, the primary tumour often fails to grow to any significant degree, and may be overshadowed by quite substantial lymphadenopathy.

Follicular and medullary cancers are similar in their behaviour since both diseases tend to be bulkier and to spread more readily. Hence the symptoms are related to the displacement and invasion of structures lying close to the thyroid gland.

Both lymphomas and anaplastic carcinomas are characterized by rapid growth, pain and respiratory obstruction.

Diagnosis

Thyroid scans

Patients undergoing scanning should not have received iodine compounds or thyroid supplements for 4–6 weeks before the procedure, as uptake of tracer is suppressed. The scan is carried out 20–30 minutes after an intravenous dose of technetium-99 or 24 hours after an oral dose of iodine-131 or iodine-123.

Just before the scan, the patient is given a glass of water to wash away any radionuclide which has found its way into the pharynx from the saliva. Anatomical landmarks, such as the suprasternal notch, are defined on the scan by means of a radioactive marker which is placed on the patient. This is important for the accurate localization of nodules and for identification of retrosternal extension.

Non-functioning solitary nodules, often referred to as 'cold' nodules, appear on the scan as localized areas of diminished or absent tracer uptake, but this does not indicate whether they are cystic and therefore unlikely to be malignant.

The converse of the 'cold' or non-functioning lesion is the 'hot' nodule, indicative of a biologically active circumscribed area of gland parenchyma. It is rare for such a nodule to be malignant but, exceptionally, malignant lesions may be 'hot' on technetium scanning and 'cold' on iodine scan.

There had been no specific radionuclide imagining technique for the demonstration of primary or metastatic medullary cell carcinoma until the development of the (Tc-99) dimercaptosuccinic acid (DMSA) and (I-131) meta-iodo-benzylguandine (MIBG). Both are specific for medullary carcinoma, but MIBG is considerably more expensive and therefore not often used (Clarke, Fogelman and Lazarus, 1986; Clarke *et al.*, 1988).

Ultrasound

This is a valuable complementary investigation to radionuclide imaging since it may distinguish between cystic and solid nodules. Although cancers could conceivably arise in cysts, or alternatively undergo cystic degeneration, such an eventuality is extremely rare and almost all cancers are solid.

The results of ultrasound scanning and the findings at operation are usually in agreement but disparities do occur, such as when a solid nodule has undergone cystic degeneration.

Radiology

Plain radiographs of the neck and the thoracic inlet will establish whether there is any displacement or compression of the trachea and will demonstrate the calcification which is sometimes present in papillary cancers.

Barium swallow complements the posteroanterior and lateral plain radiographs and will reveal the presence of oesophageal shift or narrowing.

CT and MRI are essential to the preoperative evaluation of patients with suspected thyroid carcinoma. They are especially valuable when assessing invasion of the trachea and oesophagus, and in determining the extent of nodal and mediastinal involvement.

A chest radiograph is carried out routinely to determine if there are pulmonary metastases, which appear as rounded shadows in follicular carcinoma and as a miliary infiltrate in papillary carcinoma.

Fine needle aspiration

Aspiration biopsy is a safe and easy preoperative investigation, but it requires the services of an experienced cytologist for the interpretation of the findings. Unlike larger needles such as the Vim-Silverman which extract a core of tissue, aspiration with a fine needle yields a liquid specimen which is smeared onto a slide and may be reported on in minutes.

With such a technique, it is possible to identify papillary and follicular cells as distinct entities, but the distinction between the follicular cells of an adenoma and a carcinoma is very difficult to make.

The simplicity of the technique and the fact that the percentage of false negatives may be as low as 2.2% recommends it as part of the routine work-up of patients with thyroid swellings (Lowhagen *et al.*, 1979).

Thyroglobulin estimation

This antibody is detectable in the blood of all patients with differentiated thyroid cancer and its level serves as a very sensitive marker of the extent of the disease. Patients who have been treated successfully lose all trace of thyroglobulin in their serum, and those who, after a period of quiescence, eventually develop a recurrence, once again demonstrate thyroglobulin in their blood.

The test is therefore useful for gauging the success or otherwise of treatment.

Calcitonin estimation

Calcitonin levels in the blood of patients with medullary carcinoma are abnormally high and, like thyroglobulin, the greater the bulk of the disease, the higher the level.

Unlike thyroglobulin, however, it does not often drop to the normal level of below 0.1 ng/ml in patients who have apparently been treated successfully.

Other investigations

Patients suffering from familial medullary carcinoma may also harbour other neoplasms, such as phaeochromocytoma and parathyroid adenoma.

To rule out the presence of such associated tumours, it is appropriate to estimate the level of vanillylmandelic acid in the blood together with that of the urinary catecholamines over 24 hours and, in addition, the serum calcium.

Patients suspected of metastases from primary follicular or mixed papillary-follicular carcinoma should undergo whole body radioiodine scans after ablation of the thyroid gland.

In the case of medullary carcinoma, scanning with technetium may be used, although Tc-99-DMSA, because of its specificity, is now increasingly the isotope of choice.

In its absence, general surveillance of metastatic medullary carcinoma may be carried out with technetium scans to show soft tissue deposits and bone scans to delineate osseous lesions.

Principles of treatment

With the exception of anaplastic carcinoma and lymphoma, the mainstay of treatment for all thyroid neoplasms is surgery. The contentious issue is whether the operation for differentiated lesions should be a partial or complete removal of the gland, bearing in mind that total thyroidectomy carries a higher morbidity.

The debate hinges on two points, namely whether the more radical of the two procedures improves the prognosis and whether its complication rate is as high as is claimed.

The morbidity of the operation should theoretically be easy enough to assess by reviewing the incidence of parathyroid gland insufficiency and that of recurrent nerve paralysis in the literature. But, as so often happens in large series, there is considerable variation in the clinical material and in the experience of those performing the surgery. If one group of patients has a significantly higher proportion of advanced cases, the morbidity in respect of the parathyroid glands and the recurrent nerves is bound to be higher.

Tollefsen, Shah and Huvos (1972), for example, quoted an incidence of 21% for hypocalcaemia after total thyroidectomy, whereas that in Mustard's (1970) hands was 12% and that reported by Bartolo, Kay and Talbot (1983) was nil.

Similarly the incidence of permanent recurrent nerve paralysis may be as high as 17% when secondary thyroidectomy is practised (Beahrs and Vandertoll, 1963) or as low as 4.8% after primary total thyroidectomy (Thompson and Harkness, 1970).

The point which is much more difficult to decide is whether total thyroidectomy achieves a higher cure rate than lobectomy in differentiated thyroid cancer. Arguments are marshalled in favour of each, but the truth of the matter is that comparisons between reported series are invalid because of too many variables.

In order to make matters simpler, the reasons for and against are discussed, and guidelines for the choice of one of the two options drawn up.

Papillary carcinoma

The protagonists of lobectomy argue that the incidence of recurrent disease in the contralateral remaining thyroid lobe is about 4%, in spite of the fact that as many as 40% of cases exhibit signs of multcentricity throughout the gland (Tollefsen and Decosse, 1963; Tollefsen, Shah and Huvos, 1972). It is further suggested that the recurrence rate might have been even lower if the patients had been maintained on thyroxine after operation by virtue of its suppressive effect on TSH (Crile, 1980).

On the other hand, the incidence of recurrence in the contralateral lobe after hemithyroidectomy may be considerably higher: 24% in one series (Rose *et al.*, 1963) and 17% in another (Hirabayashi and Lindsay, 1961). The large differences in recurrence rates can be explained on the basis of the age factor, since the prognosis of patients over the age of 40 years is much worse than that in younger subjects.

There are also some who speculate that some of the recurrences may have been sparked off by the administration of postoperative radioiodine, given with the intention of ablating remaining thyroid tissue after hemithyroidectomy. It has been postulated that this, rather than the inadequacy of the original operation, was responsible for recurrence of disease and that the tumour may also have been transformed from a well-differentiated to an anaplastic lesion in the process (Crile, 1971).

As regards the management of lymph node metastasis, most authors agree that removal of overtly diseased nodes by simple rather than radical dissection suffices in all but the most advanced cases. There is also general agreement that the presence of lymph node metastasis does not make the prognosis any worse.

With all these points in mind, how should one proceed when faced with a patient with a papillary carcinoma of the thyroid? Patients under the age of 40 years with intrathyroid disease, especially those with a previous history of exposure to radiation, may be managed by hemithyroidectomy with the local removal of any enlarged nodes. The risk of postoperative tetany is nil and that to the recurrent nerve is halved. However, it is vital that the patient is maintained permanently on an adequate dose of thyroxine. If Crile's (1971) comments on the inadvisability of postoperative radioiodine are accepted, a matter upon which not all are agreed, this treatment must clearly be withheld.

It would seem that the place for total thyroidectomy is in the management of the older patient, and in all patients who exhibit signs of extrathyroid escape of disease.

The case for ablating microscopic residues with radioiodine is much stronger in this group in view of the increased likelihood of recurrence if thyroid tissue is allowed to remain. The therapeutic value of such treatment lies both in the eradication of the soil in which microscopical tumour deposits reside and in the effect of the isotope on the tumour cells directly, many of which are derived from mixed papillary and follicular lesions and therefore likely to take up radioiodine.

For those patients with unequivocally papillary tumours which have escaped into the surrounding tissues, the alternative of postoperative external beam radiotherapy may be equally or more effective.

The management of neck nodes does not differ in the more advanced cases, although the need for radical neck dissection as opposed to 'berry picking' may be that much greater. It is mandatory to keep all patients on thyroxine and to monitor subsequent recurrence by regular scanning and serum thyroglobulin estimations.

Follicular carcinoma

Those who support the view that follicular carcinoma with minimal invasion of capsular veins is a relatively benign disease would go on to argue that a hemithyroidectomy is an adequate procedure for this neoplasm. Such an argument is based on the fact that the potential for spread is small and, consequently, the need for whole body scans to detect metastases after surgery is unnecessary.

However, one can never be certain that a follicular tumour, no matter how benign in appearance, will not metastsize, and since whole body scans for the detection of distant spread are unsuccessful when a significant bulk of normal thyroid tissue remains, the argument in favour of total thyroidectomy would appear to be stronger.

This, together with the fact that follicular carcinoma is seen in an older age group in whom the prognosis is considered to be generally worse, should steer the clinician in the direction of total removal rather than hemithyroidectomy.

Any residual thyroid tissue or distant deposits which are picked up by a postoperative whole body scan are managed by radioiodine therapy, and hormone therapy is withheld until such treatment is completed.

The propensity for lymph node metastasis in follicular cancer is low, but the principles of their management are the same as for papillary carcinoma.

Medullary carcinoma

The prognosis for this tumour is worse than for differentiated tumours. Whereas the presence of lymphadenopathy in papillary neoplasms does not appear to affect the outcome adversely, the same cannot be said of medullary carcinoma. Quite clearly the factors which influence survival are local escape of disease from the gland and malignant lymphadenopathy, both of which herald the appearance of distant spread.

Total thyroidectomy is the treatment of choice in all patients, be they sporadic or familial, and this includes members of a family who have raised calcitonin levels but who do not show signs of overt disease on clinical examination or on scanning.

Lymph node deposits are generally more diffusely spread than in differentiated thyroid cancer and the surgical clearance must, therefore, be more ambitious, to include the upper mediastinum as well as the cervical nodes.

The question as to whether or not external beam radiotherapy is useful in the control of local disease has not been addressed adequately so far, but there is no reason to suppose that it may not be helpful in the management of postoperative microscopic residues.

Anaplastic carcinoma

This disease advances with such rapidity that very few tumours are suitable for surgical excision. Those early cases which prove to be suitable for total thyroidectomy should receive postoperative radiotherapy to control local disease, even if distant metastases have already appeared.

Inoperable disease which threatens to cause respiratory obstruction should be managed by uncapping the trachea to avert imminent asphyxiation, followed by irradiation. The operation also yields a sample of tissue for histology.

Lymphoma

Resection of the isthmus for the purpose of averting or relieving respiratory embarrassment should be followed by immediate radiotherapy with the expectation of rapid recovery. During treatment the patient is fully investigated for the purpose of staging the disease and deciding whether chemotherapy will be required or not.

Surgery

The diagnosis of differentiated thyroid cancer is sometimes arrived at by accident following lobectomy for a supposedly benign solid nodule. After consideration of all the relevant factors, a decision must then be made as to whether the treatment thus far has been adequate or whether the contralateral thyroid lobe should also be removed.

Some surgeons, however, favour the operation of subtotal thyroidectomy as an alternative to total removal, the aim being to leave a sliver of normal thyroid tissue to protect the recurrent nerve and two parathyroid glands on the side of least disease.

It is not popular with others, however, because it leaves very little scope for the safe removal of the remaining thyroid tissue in the event of subsequent local recurrence at that site.

The operation generally referred to as lobectomy entails the removal of the diseased lobe, usually with some part of the thyroid isthmus, and is therefore in essence a hemithyroidectomy.

A description of this procedure follows and, as total thyroidectomy is simply a double hemithyroidectomy, it will not be described.

Lobectomy

The operation proceeds exactly as described for subtotal thyroidectomy. On one side the superior and inferior thyroid arteries are ligated and the recurrent laryngeal nerve is identified.

Once all the principal vascular channels have been secured, and the recurrent laryngeal nerve has been identified the surgeon can mobilize the thyroid lobe off the nerve. This is done by releasing the extension of the surgical capsule which passes back from the posterior border of the thyroid lobe to the prevertebral fascia, working from below upwards and dividing this fascial attachment in a plane just superficial to the nerve. The point of greatest adherence between the nerve and the thyroid gland is in the condensation of the surgical capsule which tethers the thyroid lobe to the trachea and to the prevertebral fascia, namely the ligamemt of Berry. This is the area where the nerve is at most risk since forward traction on the gland pulls the nerve anteriorly with it.

During the process of freeing the thyroid gland from its posterior attachments and from the nerve, every effort should be made to find the two parathyroid glands. The upper is generally found on the posterior border of the thyroid lobe, at the level of the pharyngo-oesophageal junction. It is nearly always placed within a pad of fat which is separate from the gland, and its feeding vessel is the upper branch of the inferior thyroid artery.

The lower is usually found a short distance from the lower pole of the thyroid and is more anteriorly and medially placed than the upper parathyroid, and therefore closer to the trachea. It too is within a pad of fat and is nourished by the inferior thyroid artery by way of its lower branch. Both parathyroid glands appear as flat, brown, pear-shaped structures, with one sharp edge, and are freely mobile when displaced. They are extremely vulnerable and must be handled very gently.

Once the thyroid lobe is freed from the side of the trachea, it is lifted forwards and medially to mobilize the isthmus of the gland, which is then transected just beyond the midline. After suturing the cut edge of the remaining isthmus with catgut the wound is drained and closed in layers.

Total thyroidectomy

This operation is simply a double thyroid lobectomy.

Postoperative management

After a total thyroidectomy the serum calcium is estimated daily to detect hypocalcaemia, but if signs of tetany appear, calcium gluconate is given by mouth or, if a rapid effect is required, by intravenous injection. At a later stage the degree of hypocalcaemia is reviewed and a decision taken as to the need for vitamin D3 supplements.

Patients who undergo lobectomy for cancer are prescribed thyroxine in a dosage between 0.1 and 0.3 mg daily, and the effectiveness of suppression of TSH output assessed later, by injecting TRH and estimating the level of TSH in the blood; those who are maximally suppressed by an effective dose of thyroxine will not show a rise of TSH.

By contrast, patients who have undergone total thyroidectomy and who are likely to receive radioiodine do not have replacement therapy for 3–6 weeks to allow their TSH levels to rise before ablating any residual thyroid tissue with radioiodine. It is usual to scan the patient immediately before the administration of the isotope to show the site and extent of the remaining thyroid tissue.

Once ablation with the isotope has been carried out, thyroxine is prescribed long term and is only discontinued for short periods before future diagnostic scans, at which time the serum thyroglobulin is also estimated. The need for repeat treatment with radioiodine is judged on the findings of each scan.

Complications

Recurrent nerve paralysis is an unlikely complication after lobectomy or total thyroidectomy when disease is purely within the thyroid gland. It is generally due to excessive traction, rough handling, coagulating vessels too close to the nerve, or catching the nerve in a ligature.

Paralysis is likely when disease has escaped from the gland and is involving the nerve or when a cancerous paratracheal node is stuck to the nerve. Attempts to peel neoplastic tissue off the nerve sheath are unrewarding; they contribute little to clearance of the disease, and are likely to paralyse a nerve which hitherto may have been functioning.

Under such circumstances a decision has to be made whether or not to dissect out the contralateral nerve, in view of the probability that the nerve on the diseased side is likely to be non-functional.

Unilateral nerve paralysis may require a vocal cord augmentation procedure, either by thyroplasty, the injection of Teflon or the insertion of cartilage strips in the paraglottic space (Shaheen, 1984). Bilateral nerve paralysis is managed by immediate tracheostomy, and later if desired by a partial cordectomy and arytenoidectomy using the carbon dioxide laser.

External laryngeal nerve palsy is also more likely to occur when disease is extrathyroid and, if present on its own, is expressed by the patient as a limitation in the register of the voice or an inability to sing. In conjunction with a unilateral recurrent nerve palsy, it manifests as a weak, breathy voice, and with a bilateral recurrent nerve palsy, as a severely compromised airway, although slightly less so than when a bilateral recurrent paralysis exists on its own.

Preservation of at least two parathyroid glands is necessary for the prevention of tetany, and care should be taken during a total thyroidectomy to identify as many of the glands as possible. Finding them is never easy, but attention to the finer points of surgical anatomy and the use of the operating microscope generally yield dividends. If no gland is found during the operation, the excised specimen should be inspected carefully and any parathyroid tissue which is considered to be free of disease is re-implanted into the patient. The value of such a manoeuvre is still the subject of debate, but nothing is lost by attempting it.

References

AL-SALAH, M. S. and AL-KATTAN, K. M.(1994) Incidence of carcinoma in multinodular goitre in Saudi Arabia. *Journal of the Royal College of surgeons of Edinburgh*, **39**, 106–108

BARTOLO, D. C. C., KAY, P. H. and TALBOT, C. H. (1983) Treatment of thyroid carcinoma in 107 cases. *Annals of the Royal College of Surgeons*, **65**, 301–303

BEAHRS, O. H. and VANDERTOLL, D. J. (1963) Complications of secondary thyroidectomy, *Surgery, Gynecology and Obstetrics*, **117**, 535–539

BECKERS, C., (1983) *Thyroid disease*. Paris: Pergamon Press. pp.. 1–21

BIELSCHOWSKY, F. (1944) Tumours of the thyroid produced by 2-acetylamino-fluorene and allyl-thiourea. *British Journal of Experimental Pathology*, **25** 90–95

BURROW, G. N., MIRJTABA, Q., LIVOLSI, V. and CORNOG, J. (1978) The incidence of carcinoma in solitary cold nodules'. *Yale Journal of Biological Medicine*, **51**, 13–17

CLARKE, S. E. M., FOGELMAN, I. and LAZARUS, C. R. (1986) (131I) MIBG uptake in medullary cell tumours – experience in diagnosis and treatment. *Nuclear Medicine Communications*, **7**, 297

CLARKE, S. E. M., LAZARUS, C. R., WRAIGHT, P., SAMPSON, C. and MAISEY, M. N. (1988) Pentavalent ^{99m}TcDMSA, ^{131}I MIBG and ^{99m}Tc MDP – an evaluation of three imaging techniques in patients with medullary carcinoma of the thyroid. *Journal of Nuclear Medicine*, **29**, 33–38

CRILE, G. (1966) Endocrine dependency of papillary cancer of the thyroid. *Journal of the American Medical Association*, **214**, 316–324

CRILE, G. (1971) Changing end results with papillary cancer of the thyroid. *Surgery, Gynecology and Obstetrics*, **132**, 460–468

CRILE, G. (1980) The treatment of papillary carcinoma of the thyroid occurring after irradiation. *Surgery, Gynecology and Obstetrics*, **150**, 850–852

DONIACH, I. (1953) Effect of radioactive iodine alone and in combination with methyl thiouracil upon tumour production in rat's thyroid gland. *British Journal of Cancer*, **7**, 181–202

DONIACH, I. and WILLIAMS, E. D. (1962) The development of thyroid and pituitary tumours in the rat two years after partial thyroidectomy. *British Journal of Cancer*, **16**, 222–231

DURHAM, C. F. and HARRISON, T. S. (1964) The surgical anatomy of the superior laryngeal nerve. *Surgery, Gynecology and Obstetrics*, **118**, 38–44

FAVUS, M. J., SCHNEIDER, A. B., STACHURA, M. E., ARNOLD, J. E., RYO, Y., PINSKY, S. M. *et al.* (1976) Thyroid cancer occurring as a late consequence of head and neck irradiation. *New England Journal of Medicine*, **294**, 1019–1025

HAVARD, C. W. H. (1974) The management of thyrotoxicosis. *British Journal of Hospital Medicine*, **11**, 893–908

HAVARD, C. W. H. (1975) The assessment of thyroid function. *British Journal of Hospital Medicine*, **14**, 239–250

HAZARD, J. B., HAWK, W. A. and CRILE, G. (1959) Medullary carcinoma of the thyroid. A clinicopathological study. *Journal of Clinical Endocrinology*, **19**, 152–161

HEDLEY, A. J., MICHIE, W., DUNCAN, T., HEMS, G. and CROOKS, J. (1972) The effect on remnant size in the outcome of subtotal thyroidectomy for thyrotoxicosis. *British Journal of Surgery*, **59**, 559–563

HIRABAYASHI, R. N. and LINDSAY, S. (1961) Carcinoma of the thyroid gland: a statistical study of 390 patients. *Journal of Clinical Endocrinology*, **21**, 1596–1610

KATZ, R. C. (1973) The identification of and protection of the laryngeal motor nerves during thyroid and laryngeal surgery: a new microsurgical technique. *Laryngoscope*, **83**, 59–78

KATZ, A. D. and WARREN, J. Z. (1976) The malignant cold nodule of the thyroid. *American Journal of Surgery*, **132**, 459–462

LOWHAGEN, T., GRANBERG, P. O., LUNDELL, G., SKINNARI, P., SUNDBLAD, R. and WILLENS, J. S. (1979) Aspiration biopsy cytology (ABC) in nodules of the thyroid gland suspected to be malignant. *Surgical Clinics of North America*, **59**, 3–18

MCDOUGALL, I. R., COLEMAN, C. N., BURKE, J. S., SAUNDERS, W. and KAPLAN, H. S. (1980) Thyroid carcinoma after high dose external radiotherapy for Hodgkin's disease. *Cancer*, **45**, 2056–2060

MCNEIL, A. D. and THOMSON, J. A. (1968) Long term follow-up of surgically treated thyrotoxic patients. *British Medical Journal*, **3**, 643–646

MARINE, D. (1924) Etiology and prevention of simple goitres. *Medicine*, **3**, 453–479

MORTENSEN, J. D., WOOLNER, L. B. and BENNETT, W. A. (1955) Gross and microscopical findings in clinically normal thyroid glands. *Journal of Endocrinology*, **15**, 1270–1280

MUSTARD, R. A. (1970) Treatment of papillary carcinoma of the thyroid with emphasis on conservative neck dissection. *American Journal of Surgery*, **120**, 697–703

PEGG, C. A. S., STEWART, D. J., BEWSHER, P. D. and MICHIE, W. (1973) The surgical management of thyrotoxicosis. *British Journal of Surgery*, **60**, 765–769

RIDDELL, V. (1970) Thyroidectomy: prevention of bilateral recurrent nerve palsy. *British Journal of Surgery*, **57**, 1–11

ROSE, R. G., KELSEY, M. P., RUSSELL, W. O., IBANEZ, M. I., WHITE, E. C. and CLARK, R. L. (1963) Follow up study of thyroid cancer treated by unilateral lobectomy. *American Journal of Surgery*, **106**, 494–500

RUSTAD, W. H. (1956) *The Recurrent Laryngeal Nerves in Thyroid Surgery*. Springfield, Illinois: Charles C. Thomas

SAMPSON, J. S., KEY, C. R., BUNCHER, C. R. and IJIMA, S. (1969) Thyroid carcinoma in Hiroshima and Nagasaki. Prevalence of thyroid carcinoma at autopsy. *Journal of the American Medical Association*, **209**, 65–70

SHAHEEN, O. H. (1984) *Problems in Head and Neck Surgery*. London: Balliere Tindall

STAUNTON, M. D. and SKEET, R. G. (1979) Thyroid cancer: prognosis in 469 patients. *British Journal of Surgery*, **66**, 643–647

TENNVAL, J. (1984) Carcinoma of the thyroid. Preoperative diagnosis and prognostic factors. *Doctoral dissertation*, Department of Oncology, University Hospital, Lund, Sweden

THIRD NATIONAL CANCER SURVEY, 1969, INCIDENCE (1971) *Preliminary Report*. Washington, DC: Department of Health, Education and Welfare, Publication No. (NIH) 72–128

THOMPSON, N. W. and HARKNESS, J. K. (1970) Complications of total thyroidectomy for carcinoma. *Surgery, Gynecology and Obstetrics*, **131**, 861–868

TOLLEFSEN, H. R. and DECOSSE, J. J. (1963) Papillary carcinoma of the thyroid: recurrence in the thyroid gland after initial surgical treatment. *American Journal of Surgery*, **106**, 728–734

TOLLEFSEN, H. R., SHAH, J. P. and HUVOS, A. G. (1972) Papillary carcinoma of the thyroid. Recurrence in the thyroid gland after initial surgical treatment. *American Journal of Surgery*, **124**, 468–472

TUNBRIDGE, W. M. G., EVERED, D. C., HALL, R., APPLETON, D., BREWIS, M. CLARK, F. *et al.* [1977] The spectrum of thyroid disease in a community. The Whickham survey. *Clinical Endocrinology*, **7**, 481–493

VAN ARSDEL P. D. and WILLIAMS, R. H. (1956) Simmond's disease; evaluation of certain laboratory tests used in diagnosis. *American Journal of Medicine,* 20, 4–14

VANDERLAAN, W. P. and STORRIE, V. M. (1955) Survey of factors controlling thyroid function with special reference to newer views on antithyroid substances. *Pharmacological Reviews,* 7, 301–334

WADE, J. S. H. (1955) Vulnerability of the recurrent laryngeal nerves at thyroidectomy. *British Journal of Surgery,* 43, 164–180

WADE, J. S. H. (1960) The morbidity of subtotal thyroidectomy. *British Journal of Surgery,* 48, 25–42

WADE, J. S. H. (1975) The aetiology and diagnosis of malignant tumours of the thyroid gland. *British Journal of Surgery,* 62, 760–764

WEGELIN, C. (1928) Malignant disease of the thyroid gland and its relationship to goitre in man and animals. *Cancer Review,* 3, 297–313

WERNER, S. C., HAMILTON, H. and NEMETH, M. (1952) Therapeutic effects from repeated diagnostic doses of I-131 in adult and juvenile hyperthyroidism. *Journal of Clinical Endocrinology,* 12, 1349–1355

WINSHIP, T. and ROSVOLL, R. V. (1961) Childhood thyroid carcinoma. *Cancer,* 14, 734–743

WOOLNER, L. B., BEAHRS, O. H., BLACK, M., MCCONAHEY, W. M. and KEATING, I. R. (1961) Classification and prognosis of thyroid carcinoma. A study of 885 cases observed in a thirty year period. *American Journal of Surgery,* 102, 354–387

YEUNG, C. K. and ADDISON, N. V. (1983) Presentation and prognosis of malignant tumours of the thyroid in the West Riding of Yorkshire. *Annals of the Royal College of Surgeons of England,* 65, 155–158

19

Non-neoplastic salivary gland disease

A. G. D. Maran

It is astonishing to consider how little is known of the pathological processes that affect any organ that is:

1 So near the surface
2 So accessible for clinical examination
3 So easily biopsied
4 So simple to obtain secretions from for analysis.

Pseudoparotomegaly

The parotid gland is in direct contact with the skin, the masseter muscle and the parapharyngeal space. It encloses the facial nerve and external carotid artery. It contains up to 20 lymph nodes within its parenchyma and has five to ten nodes on its surface.

Many conditions of these structures can mimic parotid gland enlargement.

Hypertrophy of the masseter

This is a condition which occurs almost exclusively in women. It is very distressing because it creates a square shape rather than an oval shape to the face (Figure 19.1). It usually affects younger women and so they are more sensitive to the change in facial appearance. Initially it presents as bilateral parotid enlargement, but the diagnosis becomes obvious when the patient is asked to clench the teeth; a bulging rippling masseter becomes obvious. It is an important diagnosis to make if only to stop unnecessary parotidectomies being performed. In the group of patients in whom it occurs, it must be distinguished from true parotomegaly that results from bulimia.

The reason for the muscular hypertrophy is not truly understood. It is too simplistic to blame all cases on bruxism, which is grinding of the molar teeth. Although some patients do this, it is unlikely that this can be held to be the cause unless the cusps of the molars show distinct signs of wear. It is sometimes seen in patients who have undergone long-term orthodontic treatment, perhaps as the result of the masseter setting the jaw in the new position. The most recent explanation is that it is due to kissing and that this is why it is predominantly a disease of females because the male has the stronger jaw.

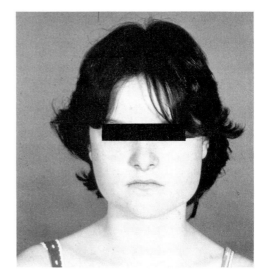

Figure 19.1 Twelve-year-old patient with hypertrophy of the masseter

Treatment is difficult but often very necessary because of the distress it causes to the patients who are so frequently young and female. There is little point in approaching the problem from an external route. This causes a facial scar, requires an unnecessary parotidectomy and puts the facial nerve at risk. It is unlikely that sufficient masseter could be removed without causing at least a temporary paralysis of the facial nerve and the disease certainly does not warrant this approach.

An intraoral approach is the recommended one. The jaw is splinted open and a cut is made along the ascending process of the mandible. The three heads of the masseter are identified and the inner two heads are removed. This leaves the outer head protecting the facial nerve. Care must be taken in this operation, however, not to penetrate the posterior limit of the masseter or else the main trunk of the facial nerve may be damaged. If bruxism exists, dental advice should be sought to prevent it. Even if this is treated however the muscle hypertrophy does not diminish.

Ageing

With the absorption of adipose tissue in the ageing process, the salivary glands become more obvious. It is usual that one can palpate the glands in the submandibular area in elderly patients. Patients are sometimes referred to otolaryngology/head and neck units with suspected metastatic disease of the submandibular nodes on the basis of absorption of fat from the submandibular area, leaving the glands obvious and palpable. Likewise the parotid glands become more prominent with age.

Dental causes

Dental infection can spread to the lymph nodes either within or surrounding the parotid gland and also to the lymph nodes in the submandibular area. Drainage of the lower incisor or canine teeth below the mylohyoid line can, on occasion, cause Ludwig's angina which involves the submandibular glands although the swelling is much more brawny. Tissue oedema within the infratemporal fossa and between the heads of the masseter muscle in turn may cause facial swelling (Figure 19.2).

Tumours in the parapharyngeal space

These are dealt with elsewhere in this volume. Chemodectomas, glomus vagale tumours, schwannomas of the vagus or sympathetic trunks and enlargement of lymph nodes with cyst, tuberculosis or metastatic

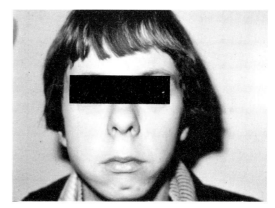

Figure 19.2 Facial swelling in the parotid region due to infection of an upper canine tooth

disease can fill this space and push the parotid gland outwards. This gives fullness in the parotid area that is not a true parotid swelling, but only a displacement. These tumours can also present between the tail of the parotid and the posterior border of the submandibular gland at the angle of the jaw and displace both structures.

Tumours of the infratemporal fossa

The infratemporal fossa is anterior to the parapharyngeal space and tumours in this area can mimic parotid swellings by escaping from the space through the mandibular notch or under the zygomatic arch. The author has had personal experience of this occurring with a haemangioma, a haemangiosarcoma, a leiomyosarcoma, a hydatid cyst, a liposarcoma and metastases to lymph nodes.

Mandibular tumours

Although tumours of the mandible are relatively rare, both osteosarcoma and chondrosarcoma of the ascending process of the mandible can mimic parotid gland enlargement as can tumours of the horizontal portion of the mandible in relation to the submandibular gland (Figure 19.3).

Mastoiditis

Mastoiditis in any form is now extremely rare in western and northern Europe, but there are parts of the world where it still occurs. A well pneumatized mastoid, if infected, can cause a subperiosteal abscess which, in turn, can drain into the sternomastoid muscle or the digastric muscle lifting the tail of the parotid gland and mimicking enlargement.

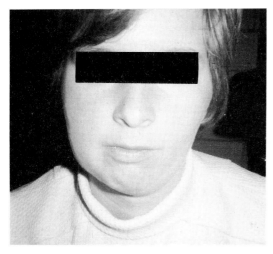

Figure 19.3 Thirty-two-year-old patient who had a parotidectomy for a chondrosarcoma of the mandible which was performed in error

Intraparotid lesions

1 Neuroma of the facial nerve
2 Aneurysms of the temporal artery
3 Lymph node enlargement in or around the parotid gland. This can occur from infections in adjacent areas such as the external auditory canal or ear lobe. Lymph nodes may also enlarge as a result of metastatic spread from skin cancers such as melanoma and squamous cell carcinoma
4 Parotid cysts.

These can be mimicked by cystic mixed cell tumours, Warthin's tumours, epithelial cysts in lymph nodes (branchial cysts) and hydatid cysts.

Parotitis

Pathogenesis

Parotitis is probably the most common infectious disease in childhood and is due to the mumps virus in this age group. What is less well known is that the incidence of viral parotitis in young adults is rising and is due to infection with one of the many strains of the echo- or coxsackieviruses. Bacterial parotitis used to be a common pre-mortem event prior to the advent of antibiotics. The cause of this was an ascending staphylococcal infection along the parotid duct in the dehydrated patient who lacked resistance to infection. Oral candidiasis is common but spread to the parotid gland via the duct is uncommon.

Parotitis can occur secondary to obstruction of the duct either by a stone, which is common in the submandibular gland, epithelial debris, which is common in the parotid gland, and stenosis of the parotid duct due to interdental problems. The patient usually recovers from the pain within a period of minutes or hours but, on occasion, infection can supervene and may even progress to parotid abscess formation (Figure 19.4).

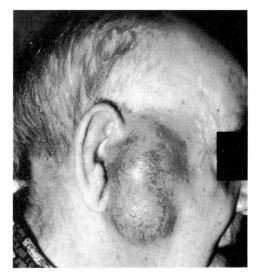

Figure 19.4 Parotid abscess secondary to bacterial parotitis

Infection of the parotid gland can be due to lymphadenitis. There are five to ten lymph nodes around the parotid gland and 15–20 within the parotid gland. These drain the skin of the side of the face, the scalp, the ear, the eye and the posterior part of the oral cavity. Lymphadenitis can thus be secondary to skin lesions and, in this regard, infected pierced ears are probably the commonest cause. Otitis externa frequently presents with preauricular pain and swelling due to lymph node enlargement. The relationship with dental infection of the molar teeth has already been mentioned and preauricular pits as a result of malformation of the branchial apparatus can result in recurrent infections which drain to the parotid lymph nodes. These nodes may resolve or they may proceed to abscess formation.

Chronic infection of the salivary glands can occur as the result of tuberculous infection. It is rare for tuberculosis to affect the stroma of the gland and, if the salivary glands do become affected by tuberculosis, then it is the surrounding lymph nodes that are infected. Sarcoid can similarly affect the area and rarely the parotid and submandibular glands can be affected by actinomycosis, leprosy or tularaemia.

The symptoms from parotitis prior to abscess formation come when saliva is produced. This happens when the patient attempts to eat and creates secretomotor stimulation of the salivary glands. If the ducts are oedematous or blocked with a stone or debris, then the flow of saliva is obstructed and the tense glands swell even more, causing severe pain. The parotid and the submandibular glands are covered with the investing fascia of the neck. Although this is not very obvious at surgery, it causes constriction of the salivary glands in the case of infection. It then becomes very difficult for the glands to expand causing severe pain.

Clinical features

Parotitis causes severe pain and elevation of temperature. It is made worse by eating and even if the patients are very hungry they do not eat because of the fear of pain. The pain and surrounding swelling cause spasm of the masseter, the temporalis and the pterygoid muscles; this causes trismus. The effect of trismus in a viral parotitis can be to create the environment in which a superadded opportunistic bacterial infection can occur due to poor oral hygiene. The area over and around the affected salivary gland is extremely tender. The diagnosis can be substantiated by asking the patient to sip a little lemon juice when there will be an acute worsening of the pain. This will not be the case, however, if the swelling is due to a lymph node.

Apart from the examination of the salivary glands, the oral cavity should be examined for the presence of dental infection and the molar teeth especially should be palpated, moved and tested with hot and cold stimuli. Some attempts should be made to see what material comes out of the salivary ducts with moderate pressure over the glands. Infection from pierced ears and otitis externa should be looked for.

It should also be borne in mind that the painful parotid gland may be a manifestation of Sjögren's syndrome, but this is not at all common.

Laboratory investigations

There will be an elevated white cell count with lymphocytes predominating if it is a viral infection, and neutrophils if it is a bacterial infection. The erythrocyte sedimentation rate will also be raised in keeping with the general condition of the patient but, if it is very elevated, then the possibility of Sjögren's syndrome arises.

Viral titres should be measured in every patient and, although the mumps titre is reliable, there are so many strains of the echo- and coxsackieviruses that to test for each strain is too expensive.

The important result is not a positive mumps titre but a negative one. This would strongly suggest that an infection was due to an echo- or coxsackievirus.

Bacteriology

Secretions from the ducts can be used to try to identify a viral infection and also can be plated for bacterial culture and sensitivity. Mycology should also be considered in every case.

If tuberculosis or sarcoidosis is suspected then the opinion of an ophthalmologist should be obtained to see if the patient has uveitis. This often accompanies parotitis in these two conditions and if present allows a diagnosis of Heerfordt's syndrome.

Radiology

Plain radiographs

Plain radiographs are useful in identifying the presence of stones. Occlusal films in the submandibular region show stones very well and are much better in this regard than lateral films. It is important to be able to assess whether or not the stone is in the oral cavity or in the gland.

Parotid stones are radiolucent and will not be seen on plain radiographs.

Sialography

The timing of a sialogram in parotitis is debatable. It would be universally agreed that a sialogram should not be performed during the acute phase. A week or two later, however, it might be therapeutic in washing out the duct system.

This examination is very useful because it will give some idea of duct blockage and will certainly give a diagnosis of sialectasis, if this is present. It may show duct distortion, although this is such a variable feature that it lacks any diagnostic specificity.

Scanning

Parotid gland scanning with technetium-99 has largely been abandoned because of so many false-positive and negative results.

Fine needle aspiration biopsy

Parotid gland histology is difficult and needle biopsy compounds the many problems. The diagnosis in parotitis is usually so obvious that fine needle aspiration is not required, but it may be carried out and if positive is helpful.

Conservative treatment

The patient will feel so ill that he probably should be confined to bed. In spite of trismus and pain, oral hygiene should be of a high standard and, although eating and drinking are very painful, the least painful nutrition is with high calorie milk drinks which do not carry any flavour. All patients will require the appropriate degree of analgesia and local heat applied to the affected gland is often comforting. Adrenalin should be applied to the appropriate salivary duct in the hope of reducing the oedema and causing some lessening of tension with drainage of saliva. It is doubtful if any antibiotic is truly effective, but the only antibiotic that is secreted in saliva is clindamycin and this can be used according to the circumstances. This does however carry the risk of severe enterocolitis as a side effect. If a diagnosis of tuberculosis is established then the appropriate chemotherapy can be begun with a high resolution rate.

Similarly, with leprosy, actinomycosis and tularaemia, a reasonable response to chemotherapy can be expected.

If the infection is due to lymphadenitis, then the primary source of infection should also be dealt with either surgically or with antibiotics.

Surgical treatment

The most successful situation for surgical intervention is where a stone blocks the submandibular duct with secondary sialadenitis. The stone can be removed perorally. This allows the abscess to drain and the condition to resolve with antibiotics. In the parotid gland abscess formation is often loculated and any serious attempt at drainage involves lifting a facial flap and carrying out multiple incisions over the gland. This is seldom warranted and local and antibiotic treatment is preferable.

Metabolic parotomegaly

The following conditions have traditionally been recorded as causes of parotomegaly – gout, Cushing's disease, myxoedema and diabetes mellitus. Investigators who have examined large series of patients with these endocrine disorders with special reference to their salivary glands, have not substantiated the original relationships and endocrine parotomegaly may be anecdotal.

The parotid gland is much more closely related to nutritional abnormalities. Since the Second World War, parotomegaly and enlargement of the submandibular glands have been noted in prisoners of war and other groups subject to starvation. This is probably a similar process to the one mentioned earlier in relation to ageing, namely the persistence of the substance of the salivary glands with the disappearance of surrounding adipose tissue. The histology of these glands does however show alveolar hypertrophy.

Obesity and the parotid

Wesley–Hadzija and Pigon (1972) reported that individuals fed on a carbohydrate diet in West Africa have increased salivary amylase activity irrespective of age and race and that amylase activity varied within 2 months of dietary modifications. There have also been several reports on parotid gland enlargement resulting from excessive ingestion of starch.

Hall and Schneyer (1977) showed that an increased functional activity of the parotid glands of rats resulted from feeding with a bulk diet which caused a compensatory enlargment of the parotid gland by an increase in acinar cell size.

The metabolism of fat within the parotid glands is ill understood. As well as the salivary glands maintaining their shape and form and the surrounding adipose tissue disappearing, fatty infiltration is very common in obese individuals. Furthermore, if these individuals lose a lot of weight then they are left with the original fat deposition in the salivary glands causing residual parotomegaly.

Bulimia

Although salivary gland enlargement is not noticed in anorexia nervosa, parotomegaly is a feature of bulimia where binge eating is followed by self-induced vomiting. The aetiology of parotomegaly in bulimia nervosa remains unknown. Du Plessis (1956) suggested that the cause is compensatory salivary gland hypertrophy due to the increase in work load while Stanstead, Koehn and Sessions (1955) attributed it to the associated malnutrition.

Riad *et al.* (1991) showed that the principal changes in the secretory patterns in bulimia are a reduction in salivary flow rate and an increase in salivary amylase levels. This mimics the pattern of stimulatory proteodyschylia and supports the presence of an abnormality of parotid sympathetic innervation in bulimic patients. Several of these patients have presented with parotomegaly and have not disclosed their binge eating. As a result some normal parotid glands have been removed. Histological examination of these glands, furthermore, has failed to reveal any abnormality or abnormal deposition of fat.

Drug-induced parotomegaly

In the laboratory, it has been shown that both isoprenaline and thiouracil make a rat's parotid gland swell. Nowadays, with the expert control of thyroid disease, it is very seldom that a patient with parotomegaly due to thyroid-related medication or isoprenaline is seen. The list made up by the Committee for the Safety of Medicines, however, shows over 40 drugs as affecting the salivary glands. Many of these reports are anecdotal and coincidental and there is little in the way of scientific evidence to show that drugs do cause parotomegaly. Although drug 'allergy' is mentioned in many reviews of parotomegaly, again there is no evidence for such an entity.

In clinical practice, the only drugs associated with parotomegaly or painful parotid glands with any frequency are dextropropoxyphene (Distalgesic) and high oestrogen oral contraceptive pills. The method of action of these latter drugs is to create epithelial shedding within the duct system, the creation of epithelial mud and the blockage of salivary ducts with the possible creation of stones in the submandibular area.

Radiotherapy and the parotid gland

Radiotherapy causes varying degrees of permanent damage to the salivary glands; the degree and permanence of the damage are primarily related to dose-time-volume factors. After radiotherapy to the head and neck most patients have a dry oral cavity with subsequent complications such as candidiasis.

Studies of the effects of irradiation on salivary gland parenchyma showed that the ductal cells are the least affected; damage to the acinar cells has been noted with a single dose of 100 cGy. Initial degenerative changes are followed by regeneration when the dosage is low; following high doses acinar regenerative activity is lost and duct proliferation becomes marked.

Irradiation also affects the extraglandular structures such as blood vessels and nerves and this may in turn have an effect on salivary gland function.

Parotomegaly and HIV infection

Bilateral parotid gland enlargement was first described as a sign of human immunodeficiency virus infection in adults in 1985 (Ryan, Joachim and Marmer, 1985). While some of these patients had malignant lymphoma or Kaposi's sarcoma, a number who just had multiple cyst formation were recognized as having early HIV infection. Nowadays, whenever multiple cysts in the parotid gland are found on CT or MRI then the clinician should be alert to the possibility of a diagnosis of AIDS.

The differential diagnosis includes sialosis, Sjögren's syndrome and lymphoma. However, when diffuse enlargement and multiple intrinsic cysts with or without associated focal mass lesions are found involving one or both parotid glands, HIV infection must be a prime consideration. If the diagnosis is established radiologically it can then be confirmed by ultrasound guided needle biopsy. This will probably prevent unnecessary further investigations and treatment.

Sialectasis
Pathogenesis

The cause of sialectasis is unknown. It is probably best regarded as a salivary gland analogue of bronchiectasis. There is a progressive necrosis and disintegration of the alveoli which ultimately coalesce forming cysts. The debris from these cysts passes along the duct and intermittently blocks areas of the duct causing hypertrophy, stenosis and duct dilatation. This is exactly what happens in bronchiectasis and, as with this disease, some patients have it from birth, and others develop it for no very good reason. In a few this debris is secondary to known obstructions, but occurrence in both the salivary glands and the lung is the exception rather than the rule. Congenital sialectasis has no adequate embryological explanation.

The parotid gland is a serous gland and is low in calcium. The epithelial debris, which could become calcified to form a stone, does not have the stimulus of the correct environment for calcification and remains as 'mud'. This is effective in blocking the duct system but not as effective as a stone would be. It is softer and does not impact so easily and is more easily removed with a build-up of saliva. Stones can form, however, in the parotid gland but they are of low density and are radiolucent.

The submandibular gland is a mixed seromucinous gland and is high in calcium. Epithelial debris here, therefore, calcifies easily and this is why stones are more common in the submandibular than in the parotid gland. The stones are of high density and are, therefore, radiopaque.

Although some texts list calculus disease as a separate entity, it is unlikely that stones can form *de novo*. They are probably all formed in a radiologically negative sialectatic gland.

The symptoms are produced when the ducts are blocked. If the main duct is blocked then the whole gland will swell up in response to the secretomotor stimulation of eating, or drinking. This is especially marked with citrus drinks or fruits which cause maximal salivary stimulation. The blockage may be in a more distal duct, in which case only a portion of the gland will swell up.

In most instances, the gland will clear itself. Sometimes the swelling stays for days but usually only for minutes or hours. If the swelling stays for some days, then it may become secondarily infected and abscess formation occur. The abscess may rupture or be drained, but more likely it will heal by fibrosis.

Clinical features
History

The patient typically complains of pain and swelling of the gland during a meal. The swelling is visible and can remain for minutes, hours or days. While the gland is swollen it is painful but, when the swelling goes down the gland is not painful. The patient does not feel unwell and does not have an elevation of temperature (Figure 19.5).

The condition can be particularly troublesome in children. This is the group of children that are diagnosed as having 'mumps' more than once. Fifty per cent of these cases resolve in time and only a few adult cases require surgical treatment.

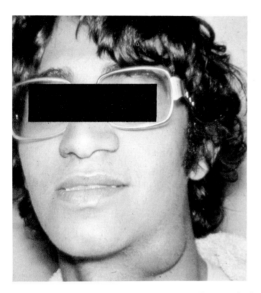

Figure 19.5 Swollen submandibular gland due to calculus obstruction secondary to sialectasis

Examination

On examination, a stone may be seen in the submandibular duct or palpated by bimanual palpation within the gland. The mouth of the duct may be oedematous and pouting.

The parotid duct may have the same appearance and it is useful to massage each parotid gland to see if there is any drainage of saliva from the duct.

Investigations

Laboratory investigations

There is little information to be gained from blood tests.

Radiology

The sialogram is diagnostic of this condition. A plain radiograph should be performed in all cases to see if a

radiopaque stone is visible and then one should proceed to a sialogram (Figure 19.6).

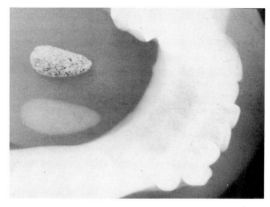

Figure 19.6 Radiograph of a stone in the submandibular duct together with the actual stone after removal

A sialogram may show six appearances:

1 It may be normal
2 It may be overfilled; an overfilled sialogram is often reported as sialectasis and one must be aware of this picture (Figure 19.7)
3 The radiologist may fail to cannulate the duct; most radiologists know that they should not persist with difficult cannulations for any period of time because the duct becomes oedematous

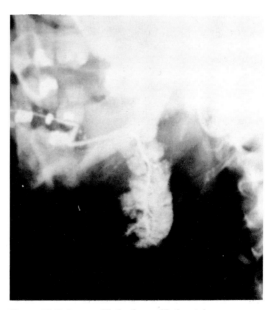

Figure 19.7 An overfilled submandibular sialogram

and it then becomes virtually impossible to cannulate; if cannulation in these cases is eventually successful then the radiologist's report will be of duct stenosis but it will be iatrogenic rather than real

4   The fourth possible picture is that of an obstructed duct; this will be obvious in the submandibular gland if a stone is seen on the plain film but, in the parotid gland, the dye may enter a little way along the duct and come to a halt, in which case it can be presumed that epithelial mud is blocking the main duct

5,6   There are two classical pictures of sialectasis: the first is cystic and the second is globular or saccular (Figures 19.8 and 19.9). Only one of these truly represents the pathology of the condition. Cystic sialectasis where the alveoli coalesce and form large spaces together with duct stenosis and dilatation, is the true picture of sialectasis. Thackray (1955) has shown that globular sialectasis represents no abnormality of the duct other than abnormal leakage where the lipiodol or radiopaque medium comes out of the alveoli

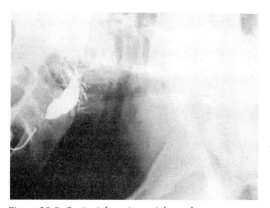

Figure 19.8 Cystic sialectasis on sialography

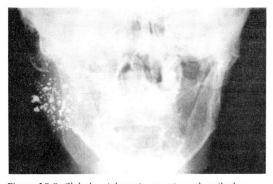

Figure 19.9 Globular sialectasis sometimes described as saccular

and lies in the stroma of the gland. Although popularly called saccular sialectasis, it is not related to the abnormality that was described akin to bronchiectasis.

As stated previously scans are unreliable. A sialogram together with a CT scan is of little value in this condition even though the films are attractive.

Treatment

No treatment

In many cases the sialogram is therapeutic. It washes out the duct and alveolar system and, thereafter, the patient may be advised to finish each meal with a citrus drink which will encourage the production of saliva, and then to massage the affected gland in order to wash out any epithelial debris and stop collections. This is successful in the vast majority of patients.

Peroral removal of a calculus

This can be carried out if a calculus is seen, usually in the submandibular gland. The duct is blocked proximally to stop the stone disappearing back into the gland during manipulation and the duct is marsupialized after the stone is removed.

Marsupialization of the duct

This must accompany any peroral removal of the stone and it can be undertaken in the parotid duct stenosis of dental origin. A cannula is placed into the duct and a 2.5–5 cm (1–2 inch) segment is opened and stitched carefully to the adjacent mucosa with 6–0 absorbable suture material.

Ligation of the duct

This is mentioned only to be dismissed as an illogical and inadequate present-day treatment.

Duct dilatation

The same applies to this method of treatment.

Tympanic neurectomy

This procedure was popular during the 1950s and 1960s. The aim of treatment is to divide Jacobson's nerve which crosses the promontory to form the tympanic plexus. It joins the jugular plexus and glossopharyngeal nerve to the greater superficial petrosal nerve and forms part of the reflex arc of salivary secretion. Some surgeons combine this with division of the chorda tympani nerve.

The procedure certainly works for up to 6 months

but, like all autonomic surgery, alternative pathways develop and symptoms eventually recur.

Removal of the submandibular gland

This is a straightforward procedure and carries little risk with it. If the gland shows evidence of sialectasis, or if there is a stone in the body of the gland, then the surgeon should have no hesitation in removing the submandibular gland as a whole. If there have been numerous attacks of sialadenitis, then the removal may be difficult, but care should be taken to avoid paralysing the mandibular branch of the facial nerve. Furthermore, one should make sure that the remnant of the submandibular duct in the oral cavity is clear of stones when the gland is removed, because it is quite possible to push stones from the gland into the duct remnant during manipulation. This is of little clinical significance, but the patient may be surprised to spit out a stone some days after the operation.

Total parotidectomy

Superficial parotidectomy is illogical for a disease which affects the whole parotid gland. By removing half of a sialectatic parotid gland, there is a high risk of fistula. In a superficial parotidectomy for tumour, a denervated normal deep lobe is left behind. This usually ceases to function and thus a fistula is rare. In sialectasis a cystic diseased deep lobe is left behind for which denervation does little. It continues to produce mucus and saliva and causes a salivary fistula.

Total parotidectomy is, therefore, the only logical operation for sialectasis and, in the gland which may be heavily fibrosed due to recurrent sialadenitis, the facial nerve is at more risk than it is in surgery for benign tumours.

Sjögren's syndrome

In 1888, Dr Mikulicz described the case of a 42-year-old East Prussian farmer with swelling of the submandibular, parotid and lacrimal glands (Mikulicz, 1937). He removed two-thirds of the submandibular gland and found it to be infiltrated with lymphocytes, and then removed the whole gland some months later with recovery of the patient. This was known as Mikulicz's disease and to it were added all the symptoms of other non-neoplastic salivary gland disease over the next 50 years. Mikulicz's syndrome included tuberculosis, sarcoid, actinomycosis, gout, etc. In 1925, Gougerot, a French dermatologist, introduced the concept of dryness when he described a series of patients with dry mouth, vulval dryness, skin dryness, etc. In 1933, Henrik Sjögren, a Stockholm ophthalmologist, described 33 women with the syndrome of xerostomia and keratoconjunctivitis sicca.

Twenty-three of these patients had rheumatoid arthritis. No mention was made of parotid gland disease. In 1952, Godwin at the Armed Forces Institute of Pathology in Washington, described the concept of enlargement of the parotid glands due to lymphocytic infiltration and related this to the future development of lymphoma. It was named benign lymphoepithelial lesion. In 1980, Strand and Talal described a further variety of this called aggressive lymphocytic behaviour.

The classification now is as follows:

1 Primary Sjögren's syndrome (sicca complex) – this consists only of xerostomia and xerophthalmia with no connective tissue component
2 Secondary Sjögren's syndrome – this consists of xerostomia, xerophthalmia and a connective tissue disease which, in nearly 50% of patients, is rheumatoid arthritis but may also be systemic lupus erythematosus, scleroderma and polymyositis
3 Benign lymphoepithelial lesion, otherwise known as myoepithelial sialoadenitis, which is localized to the parotid glands and some regard as a prelymphomatous condition
4 Aggressive lymphocytic behaviour which again is confined to the parotid glands and is almost a pseudolymphoma.

Epidemiology

Sjögren's syndrome is more common in the northern than the southern hemisphere and is more common in northern than in southern Europe. A proportion of older people have many of the symptoms of Sjögren's syndrome, but do not have the immunological profile. In a study of octogenarians, Whaley, Williamson and Chisholm (1972) showed that one in six had keratoconjunctivitis sicca. Three per cent of men and 20% of women had xerostomia, but only 2% had the immunological profile of the sicca syndrome. Eleven per cent of patients with rheumatoid arthritis had keratoconjunctivitis sicca, 1% had xerostomia but 100% had lymphocytic infiltration of the submaxillary glands when examined at autopsy. Thirty per cent of patients with rheumatoid arthritis will develop Sjögren's syndrome. It has a very wide range of autoantibodies and is the second most common autoimmune disease after rheumatoid arthritis.

Clinical features

Sjögren's syndrome is a multisystem disease affecting every system in the body but particularly the oral cavity, the eyes and the salivary apparatus.

The oral symptoms are those of a dry mouth with secondary candidiasis, stomatitis, glossitis and subsequent dental caries.

The eye symptoms are due to keratoconjunctivitis sicca; the patient has a foreign body sensation in the eye, burning, redness, itching, photosensitivity and an inability to tolerate contact lenses.

Only 40% feel salivary gland enlargement and only 20% show it clinically. It is nearly always in the parotid gland and those patients with parotomegaly from Sjögren's syndrome have a much higher chance of developing lymphoma. Two-thirds of the patients never have salivary gland enlargement.

Other associated systemic problems are primary biliary cirrhosis, chronic hepatitis, vasculitis, chronic graft versus host disease, cryoglobulinaemia, hyper-gammaglobulinaemic purpura and polyarteritis. Fifteen per cent will have thyroiditis and many will develop pancreatitis.

Achlorhydria, disorders of oesophageal motility and web formation may present to the otolaryngologist as may nasal crusting, epistaxis, serous otitis media, laryngitis sicca and a persistent cough with tenacious sputum, glazing of the oral mucosa and sticky secretions in the nasopharynx, etc.

General examination

The presence or absence of a connective tissue disorder should be established as should the presence of any of the above-mentioned abnormalities of other organs.

Investigations

Blood examination

The erythrocyte sedimentation rate is usually raised. A protein profile will show elevation of all the immunoglobulins especially IgG. Rheumatoid factor and antinuclear factor will probably be positive and there may well be a wide range of autoantibodies.

Specific immunological tests

These can only be carried out in a few places in the UK. When class 2 antigens such as HLA A1 and B8 and DR3 are examined, then almost three times as many patients with the sicca syndrome have these antigens when compared with patients with the secondary syndrome. Specific antigens for Sjögren's syndrome are called SSA and SSB. Again these are more common in patients with the sicca syndrome than in those with secondary Sjögren's syndrome with rheumatoid arthritis. The immediate clinical relevance of these immunological abnormalities is not known and it may be that they are *in vitro* epiphenomena.

Schirmer's test

This is carried out by putting special strips into the lower fornix (Figure 19.10). Wetting of less than 5

mm in 5 minutes represents a diagnosis of xerophthalmia. A diagnosis of keratoconjunctivitis sicca, however, cannot be made until the ophthalmologist examines the eye with Rose Bengal dye to see the filamentary keratitis.

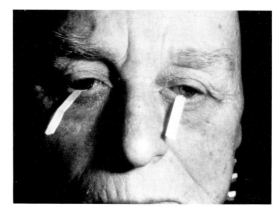

Figure 19.10 Schirmer's test is performed by placing special strips in the lower fornix and leaving them for 5 minutes

Salivary flow rate

This is measured using Carlsson–Crittenden cups (Figure 19.11); these are suction cups placed over the parotid duct. Maximum stimulation is created by asking the patient to suck a lemon. A flow of less than 0.5 ml in a minute represents xerostomia.

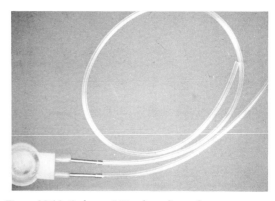

Figure 19.11 Carlsson–Crittenden salivary flow cup

Labial biopsy

This is performed by obtaining four globules of fat from the back of the lower lip. It can be performed under local anaesthetic and is the diagnostic test for Sjögren's syndrome. The pathologist must grade it according to the rules laid down.

Grade 1: slight lymphocytic infiltration
Grade 2: less than 50 lymphocytes per 4 mm^2

Grade 3: 50 lymphocytes per 4 mm^2
Grade 4: more than 50 lymphocytes per 4 mm^2.

The distribution of lymphocytes is important also because they cannot be diffuse, but must be periductal. In this test, false positives can be obtained in rheumatoid arthritis, scleroderma, subacute lupus erythematosus, sarcoid, amyloid and graft versus host disease.

Radiology

Sialography either shows a normal sialographic pattern or that of 'globular sialectasis'. This does not imply that the patients with Sjögren's syndrome have sialectasis. What it does imply is that there is an abnormality in the duct allowing leakage of lipiodol into the stroma of the gland.

Natural history

One in six patients with Sjögren's syndrome will go on to develop lymphoma. This will be a B-cell type non-Hodgkin's lymphoma. The immunological abnormality in Sjögren's syndrome is a loss of suppressor T-cell activity and an alteration in the T-suppressor-helper cell relationship. As well as a non-Hodgkin's lymphoma patients can develop Waldenström's macroglobulinaemia and immunoblastic sarcoma.

The present suggestion as to aetiology is that the cytomegalovirus infects salivary ducts and ducts elsewhere in the body. The ducts act as the antigen and B-lymphocyte proliferation occurs. As well as lymphoma, a peculiar type of anaplastic carcinoma can also develop in these patients. It has been reported predominantly but not solely in Eskimos.

Treatment

There is little of a specific nature that can be done to help these patients. Bouts of parotid gland swelling may be treated with steroids but the bouts are seldom so severe that they require other immunosuppressive drugs. Artificial tears and synthetic saliva provide limited comfort and bromhexine 40 mg/day sometimes helps a tenacious cough.

The most important feature of treatment, however, is to put these patients on a lymphoma follow up. Those who have parotid gland enlargement are at a higher risk of developing lymphoma and diagnostic parotidectomy should be considered.

Salivary gland cysts

Similar to vascular and lymphatic malformations, salivary gland cysts are benign swellings, and merit inclusion in this section.

Most cysts within the parotid or submandibular glands are secondary to sialectasis, or salivary tumours (pleomorphic adenoma, Warthin's tumour, cystic duct adenoma, mucoepidermoid tumour, adenocarcinoma). Cysts not related to other disease more commonly arise from minor salivary glands. In a series of 483 salivary gland cysts, 77% were minor salivary gland mucocoeles, and the remainder included parotid duct cysts (10.5%), lymphoepithelial cysts (6%), and ranulae (5%) (Seifert *et al.*, 1986).

Mucocoeles are spherical, painless swellings that contain mucus. There are two histological types – extravasation mucocoeles (80%), which probably follow repeated minor mucosal trauma, and retention mucocoeles (20%) due to duct obstruction by microliths, or inspissated secretions or to bends in the duct.

Extravasation mucocoeles (sometimes called a mucous granuloma) are commoner in younger adults, and show a predilection for certain sites (lower lip 80%, cheek and floor of mouth 15%, and palate, tongue and upper lips 5%). In contrast, retention mucocoeles present in older patients and do not have the marked predilection for certain sites. Treatment of either variety is simple excision.

A ranula is a specific type of salivary gland cyst which arises from the sublingual gland, and is discussed in Chapter 3.

Salivary fistulae

A salivary fistula usually originates from the parotid gland, although it sometimes arises from the submandibular gland. It can be internal or external, congenital or acquired. Internal fistulae drain into the mouth and are therefore often not noticed. Congenital fistulae are rare, and may arise from aberrant or accessory salivary tissue, or be associated with branchial cleft abnormalities.

A parotid fistula may be due to surgery, facial trauma, or sepsis within the gland parenchyma. A fistula which follows a partial parotidectomy (especially a lumpectomy) usually arises from the gland parenchyma, and generally drains through the suture line. This type of fistula will close spontaneously in most cases, and until this time, minor leakage will occur with meals. To help prevent such a fistula from developing, the parotid duct is often divided well forward, and ligated in some cases. Saliva may collect underneath the skin flap after surgery, and should be aspirated and a pressure dressing applied. Saliva has a high amylase content compared with fluid from a seroma.

In contrast to the above, a fistula which arises from the main duct system of the parotid leaks profusely, even at the thought of food, and invariably needs an operation to close it. This type of fistula is usually due to a deep facial wound, and the facial nerve may also be damaged. Such fistulae can be difficult to control, and three categories of treatment are described:

1 Reduction of saliva production; by drugs, irradiation, gland denervation, and duct ligation
2 Operations on the fistula; excision, diversion into the mouth, reconstruction of the damaged duct
3 Removal of the gland; partial or total conservative parotidectomy.

Reducing the output of saliva may promote closure of the fistula, and tympanic neurectomy provides a simple effective way of achieving this. Irradiation has been used, but the outcome is uncertain, and there is a risk of later carcinoma. A damaged main duct may be suitable for repair, and this may be demonstrated by a sialogram. However, the outcome of such surgery is uncertain, especially if the fistula has been present for some time, and in such cases parotidectomy may be necessary.

A salivary fistula from the submandibular gland is a much easier problem to deal with. If it does not close spontaneously the gland should be excised.

References

DU PLESSIS, D. J. (1956) Parotid enlargement in malnutrition. *South African Medical Journal*, 30, 700–710

GODWIN, J. T. (1952) Benign lymphoepithelial lesion of the parotid gland. *Cancer*, 5, 1089–1096

GOUGEROT, H. (1925) Progressive et atrophie des glands salivaires et muqueuses de la bouche de conjunctives. *Bulletin de la Société Françaises Dermatologie Syphilographie*, 32, 376–381

HALL, H. D. and SCHNEYER, C. A. (1977) Functional mediation of compensatory enlargement of the parotid gland. *Cell and Tissue Research*, 184, 249–254

MIKULICZ, J. (1937) Concerning peculiar symmetrical disease of lacrimal and salivary glands. *Medical Classics*, 2, 165–186

RIAD, M., BARTON, J. R., WILSON, J. A., FREEMAN, C. P. L. and MARAN A. G. D. (1991) Parotid salivary secretory pattern in bulimia nervosa. *Acta Otolaryngologica*, 111, 392–395

RYAN, J. R., JOACHIM, H. L. and MARMER, J. (1985) Acquired immune deficiency syndrome related lymphadenopathy presenting in the salivary gland lymph nodes. *Archives of Otolaryngology*, 111, 554–556

SEIFERT, G., MIEHLKE, A., HANBRICH, J. and CHILLA, R. (1986) Salivary gland cysts. In: *Diseases of the Salivary Glands*, translated by P. M. Stell. New York: Georg Thieme Verlag. pp. 91–100

SJÖGREN, H. (1933) Zur kenntnis der kerato-conjunctivitis sicca. *Acta Ophthalmologica*, Suppl. II, 1–151

STANSTEAD, H. R., KOEHN, C. and SESSIONS, S. M. (1955) Enlargement of the parotid gland in malnutrition. *American Journal of Clinical Nutrition*, 3, 198–200

STRAND, V. and TALAL, N. (1980) Advances in the diagnosis and concept of Sjögren's syndrome. *Bulletin of Rheumatic Diseases*, 30, 1046–1052

THACKRAY, A. C. (1955) Sialectasis. *Archives of Middlesex Hospital*, 5, 151–159

WESLEY-HADIJA, B. and PIGON, H. (1972) Effect of diet in West Africa on human salivary amylase activity. *Archives of Oral Biology*, 17, 1415–1420

WHALEY, K., WILLIAMSON, J. and CHISHOLM, D. (1972) Sjögren's syndrome. Sicca components. *Quarterly Journal of Medicine*, 42, 279–285

Further reading

BARTON, J. R., RIAD, M. A., GAZE, M. R., MARAN, A. G. D. and FERGUSON, A. (1990) Mucosal immunodeficiency in smokers and in patients with epithelial head and neck tumours. *Gut*, 31, 378–382

BECKERS, H. L. (1977) Masseteric muscle hypertrophy and its intraoral surgical correction. *Journal of Maxillo-facial Surgery*, 5, 28–35

BLATT, I. M. (1969) The parotid masseter hypertrophy-traumatic occlusion syndrome. *Laryngoscope*, 79, 624–630

BODNER, I., KUYATT, B. I., HAND, A. R. and BAUM, B. J. (1984) Rat parotid cell function in vitro following X-irradiation in vivo. *Radiation Research*, 97, 381–389

CHAPNIK, J. S., NOYEK, A. M., BERRIS, B., WORTZMAN, G., SIMOR, A. E. and HOUPT, J. B. (1990) Parotid gland enlargement in HIV infection. *Journal of Otolaryngology*, 19, 189–194

CHISHOLM, D. M. and MASON, D. (1968) Labial salivary gland biopsy in Sjögren's disease. *Journal of Clinical Pathology*, 21, 656–659

ENEROTH, C. M., HENDERIKSON, C. O. and JAKOBSSON, P. A. (1972) Effect of fractionated radiotherapy on salivary gland function. *Cancer*, 30, 1147–1151

LEVIN, P. A., FALKO, J. M., DIXON, K., GALLUP, E. M. and SAUNDERS, W. (1980) Benign parotid enlargement in bulimia. *Annals of Internal Medicine*, 93, 827–829

MARAN, A. G. D. (1986) Sjögren's syndrome. *Journal of Laryngology and Otology*, 100, 1299–1305

MAYNARD, J. D. (1965) Recurrent parotid enlargement. *British Journal of Surgery*, 52, 784–793

SCHWARTZ, A. W., THOMSON, M. G. and JOHNSON, C. L. (1966) Acute postoperative parotitis. *Plastic and Reconstructive Surgery*, 25, 51–58

SILVERMAN, M. and PERKINS, R. L. (1966) Bilateral parotid enlargement and starch ingestion. *Annals of Internal Medicine*, 64, 843–846

20

Benign salivary gland tumours

O. H. Shaheen

Historical perspective

Salivary gland surgery in the years leading up to the Second World War was viewed with diffidence, if not trepidation, for good reason.

A poor understanding of the natural history of salivary diseases in general, and tumours in particular, together with a fear of damaging the facial nerve stand out in retrospect as the main obstacles to progress. Despite being well-versed in the anatomy of the facial nerve there was little enthusiasm on the part of surgeons for confronting the nerve *in vivo*, a diffidence engendered in part by the difficult operating conditions of the time but also the fear of dissecting around the nerve. Safeguarding the physiological integrity of nerves by delicate handling was a concept familiar to neurosurgeons, whereas the saying that 'a nerve exposed is a nerve damaged' very much dominated the thinking in general surgical circles.

Operations on the submandibular gland were viewed with much less reluctance, and fears there were focused more on the danger of spread of infections through fascial spaces rather than the danger of damaging nerves such as the mandibular branch of the facial nerve.

The lack of a proper classification of salivary tumours and general ignorance of their natural history probably constituted the greater impediment to progress. For many years the belief existed that mixed tumours were a low-grade form of malignancy largely because of their propensity to recur after local enucleation. It was not appreciated that the degree of encapsulation of pleomorphic adenomas was variable and often incomplete, or that their surface was frequently bosselated; features which favoured recurrence if simple enucleation was practised.

Others ascribed the high recurrence rate of pleomorphic adenomas to a multifocal origin, little realizing

that the appearance of separate outlying foci was an artefact created by the plane of section passing not only through the main bulk of tumour but also through a number of surface excrescences. Serial sections ultimately established the continuity of the little foci to the parent tumour and redirected attention to the real cause of recurrence, namely inadequate surgical margins and spillage of tumour.

During the war years, the foundations of our present knowledge and expertise were laid through the efforts of a number of individuals working mainly in North America, France and England, with later contributions from these countries as well as Scandinavia.

McFarland (1942) attempted to correlate the histology of mixed tumours to their prognosis after surgery, while Foote and Frazell (1953) were largely responsible for placing the classification of salivary gland tumours on a sound basis and for providing a comprehensive account of their natural history.

The implantation of mixed tumours during the operation of enucleation, long suspected as a cause of recurrence, was eventually demonstrated in a most convincing manner by Patey and Thackray (1957–8) and the belief that they were multifocal in origin was finally put to rest.

Bailey (1941) was the first in Britain to practise formal dissection of the facial nerve in operations for benign parotid gland tumours, while Redon (1945) in France was advocating total parotidectomy with conservation of the facial nerve at much the same time. The former considered the parotid gland to be essentially a bilobed structure separated by an anatomical plane containing the facial nerve, a concept which we now know to be fallacious, but which in no way detracts from Bailey's valuable contribution to parotid gland surgery. Redon on the other hand believed that all mixed tumours were multifocal in origin and consequently advocated removal of both superficial and deep parts of the parotid gland after freeing the facial nerve.

Although this belief was finally and irrevocably refuted, Redon's contribution should not be minimized since it broadened the technical repertoire of parotid gland surgeons and demonstrated that the facial nerve is much more robust than had hitherto been considered.

Surgical anatomy

The parotid gland

A horizontal section through the parotid gland offers a better perspective of the normal disposition of salivary gland tissue than might be otherwise gained by lateral inspection. Such a section would clearly demonstrate that most of the gland actually lies in the retromandibular sulcus rather than on the external aspect of the masseter muscle and would thus explain why the majority of tumours are to be found in that segment (Figure 20.1). Since the facial nerve bisects this area unequally into a major portion lateral to the facial nerve and a much smaller part medial to it, it is not surprising that most tumours are to be found superficial to the nerve.

The gland is incompletely invested by a continuation of the deep cervical fascia, which posteriorly surrounds the sternomastoid muscle and anteriorly overlies the masseter. The surface component of the parotid fascia is exceedingly tough but as it extends medially over the anteromedial and posteromedial aspects of the gland it thins out progressively (Figure 20.1). Where the gland lies close to the styloid process the fascia blends with a tough band of fibrous tissue which joins the styloid to the posterior aspect of the angle of the mandible, thus forming the stylomandibular ligament (Figure 20.2).

The toughness of the fascia on the external surface of the gland inevitably means that benign tumours are slow to project outwards to any great extent, and hence it takes years for them to present as large unsightly bulges. The facial nerve is often displaced by the tumour either inwards, where there is little resistance from the deep component of the parotid fascia, or upwards or downwards, depending on the relationship of the nerve to the tumour.

The facial nerve emerges from the fallopian canal and runs anteriorly, inferiorly and laterally to enter the posteromedial surface of the gland. The segment of the nerve which lies in the interval between the stylomastoid foramen and the parotid is extremely short, but is the ideal location for finding the facial nerve before the parotidectomy properly commences. It is best found by searching in the tympanomastoid sulcus, which is formed by the edge of the bony external meatus on the one hand and the anterior face of the mastoid process on the other. The nerve emerges from the stylomastoid foramen some 3–4 mm deep to the outer edge of the bony external canal (Conley, 1978) (Figure 20.3).

The second most reliable landmark for finding the nerve is the posterior belly of the digastric muscle which lies just inferior to the nerve. The styloid process is a useful confirmatory landmark but to depend on it for finding the nerve is to court trouble

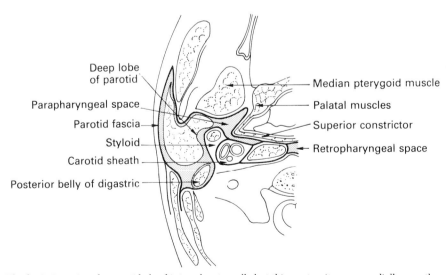

Figure 20.1 The fascia investing the parotid gland is tough externally but thins out as it passes medially over the anteromedial and posteromedial surfaces of the gland

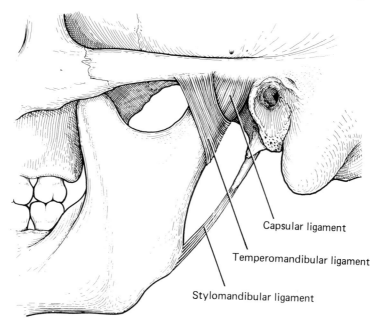

Figure 20.2 The stylomandibular ligament

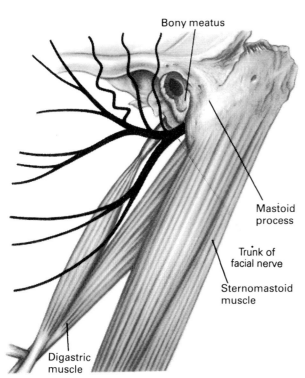

Figure 20.3 The facial nerve in the tympanomastoid sulcus above the digastric muscle

since it lies medial and anterior to the nerve's point of emergence from the mastoid. The posterior auricular artery frequently bleeds during the process of looking for the facial nerve since it lies below and just lateral to the nerve.

The cartilaginous pointer described by Conley (1978) is an artificially created landmark formed by posterior traction on the external auditory canal. The backward pull on the cartilage causes the meatus to assume the shape of a horn, the curved extremity of which allegedly points to the position of the facial nerve. Of all the landmarks mentioned, this is probably the least reliable since it very much depends on the configuration of the cartilaginous meatus.

The facial nerve divides into upper and lower divisions about 1 cm beyond its point of entry into the parotid gland; these divisions diverge sharply.

The upper division proceeds upwards, forwards and very much outwards towards the zygomatic arch and gives off temporal, upper zygomatic, lower zygomatic and buccal branches. This division is almost invariably stouter than the lower and can therefore withstand more handling. In elderly or obese individuals its branches are often tortuous both mediolaterally and anteroposteriorly, a feature which makes them liable to damage if efforts to keep the tissues constantly on the stretch are neglected while the nerve is being dissected. As with the lower division the pattern of branching is variable both in terms of the number of branches and their point of origin (Figure 20.4). The lower zygomatic branch, however, is constant in one respect, in that it almost

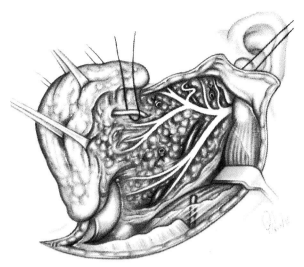

Figure 20.4 The division of the facial nerve into two main segments and the arborization of the branches

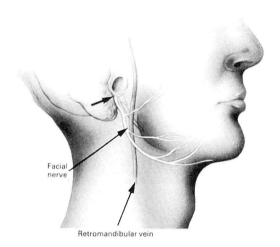

Figure 20.5 The position of the mandibular branch of the facial nerve in relation to the retromandibular vein

invariably lies just superior to the parotid duct, a point to be remembered when attempting to deal with duct stenoses or stones.

The lower division passes downwards and forwards but lacks the outward inclination of the upper division and by comparison therefore lies deeper. It gives off buccal branches, a mandibular and a cervical branch, and it thins progressively as it becomes more peripheral. Occasionally a buccal branch may arise from the bifurcation itself.

The thinness of the branches of the lower division, and the mandibular branch in particular, makes paralysis of the depressor anguli oris a common complication of parotidectomy. The very fine interlacing nerve fibres between one branch and another could well explain why the facial nerve will withstand more than a modest degree of handling at operation and yet still recover. These communicating fibres are often absent between the lower buccal and mandibular branches, hence the propensity to paralysis of the muscles supplied by the latter.

The mandibular branch invariably emerges from the tail of the parotid gland immediately anterior to the retromandibular vein and then passes downwards and forwards on the outer aspect of the deep cervical fascia to enter the submandibular triangle. The proximity of the mandibular branch of the facial nerve to the retromandibular vein at its point of emergence from the tail of the parotid gland provides an alternative method of locating the nerve if the usual method is for any reason not possible. By working backwards along the nerve, the two divisions, the other branches, and the main trunk can be found in turn (Figure 20.5).

The retromandibular vein lies in the deep lobe of the gland immediately medial to the facial nerve and

its branches, although very occasionally it may be superficial to it. It gives off small tributaries which pass outwards between the nerve branches and which may be a source of troublesome bleeding when dissecting out the nerve. Deep to the vein lies the continuation of the external carotid artery which gives off in turn transverse facial, internal maxillary and superficial temporal branches as it proceeds superiorly within the deep lobe of the gland. These branches with their venous counterparts must be ligated when the deep lobe of the gland is removed.

Deep to the parotid gland lies the parapharyngeal space which, if followed upwards above and behind the medial pterygoid muscle, merges with the infratemporal fossa.

The parapharyngeal space is roughly pyramidal in shape, the apex lying superiorly at the point where the medial pterygoid muscle is inserted into the inner aspect of the lateral pterygoid plate and where the superior constrictor muscle is attached to the posterior edge of the medial pterygoid plate. It is bounded medially by the lateral wall of the pharynx, and laterally by the medial or undersurface of the medial pterygoid muscle, while further posteriorly the lateral boundary is the deep part of the parotid gland.

Anteriorly, the parapharyngeal space narrows into the cul-de-sac formed by the pterygomandibular raphe and the posterior part of the buccinator muscle, while posteriorly the space is open and bounded by the prevertebral fascia.

The parapharyngeal space is occupied posteriorly by the internal carotid artery, internal jugular vein and the upper part of the last four cranial nerves and superior cervical ganglion of the sympathetic chain.

It is crossed from lateral to medial and from above downwards by the styloid process and its muscles, and by the pharyngeal branch of the vagus and the superior laryngeal nerve.

The submandibular gland

The gland lies in the triangle of that name, covering the mylohyoid and hyoglossus muscles, and overlapping the inferior margins of the triangle, namely the anterior and posterior bellies of the digastric and their common tendon. The gland itself is overlapped by the horizontal ramus of the mandible which forms the upper margin of the triangle. Inferiorly the gland approaches the greater wing of the hyoid which serves as a useful landmark when marking the incision for the operation to remove the gland (Figure 20.6).

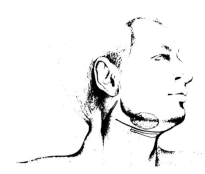

Figure 20.6 The incision for the removal of the submandibular gland should be sited just above the greater wing of the hyoid bone

Although ovoid in appearance when viewed from a lateral direction, the gland is in fact U-shaped in sagittal section, possessing a large outer component which lies outside the mylohyoid muscle, and a smaller inner component giving origin to the duct on the inner aspect of this muscle. The portion of the gland joining these two parts curves round the posterior free edge of the mylohyoid. In operations to remove the gland, retraction of the mylohyoid forwards will facilitate exposure of the deep part of the gland and the duct.

The gland is invested in a loose fine surgical capsule which is derived from the overlying deep cervical fascia. If dissection of the gland is limited to a plane within this capsule any important structure lying outside it will not come to any harm. The deep cervical fascia provides a further external protection since the mandibular branch of the facial nerve and

its subsidiary branches lie plastered to its outer aspect and never make contact with the gland or its capsule.

However, it must be appreciated that the most inferior of the branches of the mandibular nerve lies close to the lower border of the submandibular gland and could be damaged when gaining entry to the plane of dissection at the beginning of the operation (Figure 20.7).

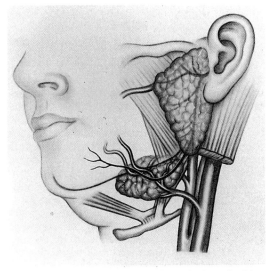

Figure 20.7 The branches of the mandibular branch of the facial nerve may be very low down in the submandibular triangle

The hypoglossal nerve with its venae comitantes lies on the hyoglossus but is separated from the deep aspect of the gland by a potential space. Escape of disease from the deep aspect of the gland would be the only likely circumstance to put the nerve at risk when removing benign tumours.

The lingual nerve arches gently downwards just above the deep part of the submandibular gland to which it is attached by a ganglionic connection, alongside which is a small blood vessel. The nerve subsequently passes below the duct then round its outer aspect in the form of a broad loop before heading for the mucosa of the tongue. It is at risk when the deep part of the gland is being mobilized.

The sublingual gland

Also ovoid in shape and about 2 cm in size the sublingual gland lies below the submandibular duct between the genioglossus on the one hand, and the mandible and mylohyoid on the other. About half of its ducts drain into Wharton's duct and the remainder directly onto the sublingual papilla.

Incidence of salivary gland tumours

Although the geographical incidence varies somewhat, salivary tumours are in general uncommon. In a population of 2.8 million living in an area comprising Liverpool, Merseyside, North Wales and the Isle of Man, the incidence of neoplasms of all types was of the order of 1.1 per 100 000 persons. This can be compared with a slightly higher incidence of 1.5 per 100 000 Caucasians in the USA, rising to 1.6 for non-white men and 2.5 for non-white North American women. The highest incidence would appear to be among the Eskimos in whom the majority of tumours are of the malignant kind (Evans and Cruickshank, 1970).

Salivary gland tumours represent about 3% of all neoplasms. Approximately 80% are located in the parotid gland, 10% in the submandibular gland, the remainder being distributed between the sublingual gland and the countless minor salivary glands (Snow, 1979). This last group comprises the innumerable tiny submucosal serous and mucinous glands to be found in the oral cavity, nose, sinuses, postnasal space, oropharynx, larynx and trachea.

Benign tumours are more common than malignant, although the ratio will vary from one site to the next. In the parotid gland for instance, 80% of tumours are benign whereas in the submandibular gland this drops to 60% and in the oral cavity malignant tumours may well outnumber the benign.

Among the white population of Europe and the USA the sex distribution is about equal but among non-whites in North America and Africa, women outnumber men and if the parotid gland is considered in isolation, there is a preponderance of tumours in women (Evans and Cruickshank, 1970).

Benign tumours of the major salivary glands may occur in children but are exceedingly rare. Although fractionally more common in adolescence they are, nevertheless, still infrequent and the vast majority of patients present in the age range 30–70 years, the average being about 45.

Aetiology

Little is known about the aetiology of salivary gland tumours and much of what has been written is speculative.

The inoculation of new-born mice with polyoma virus is reported to provoke the formation of salivary gland neoplasms although there is nothing to suggest that this is the mechanism in humans. Hydrocarbons implanted into the salivary glands of rats and guinea-pigs are also known to result in tumour formation.

The evidence that low dose radiation may induce tumours in humans is much more convincing and is derived from studies of people exposed to the effects of the atomic bomb at Hiroshima. In this group of individuals the incidence of tumours at all sites is significantly greater than that expected in persons who have never been previously exposed to radiation (Ju, 1968; Takeichi, Hirose and Yamamoto, 1976).

Surgical pathology

Approximately 80% of all salivary gland tumours arise in the parotid gland, the remainder being distributed between the submandibular, sublingual and minor salivary glands. Eighty per cent of tumours in the parotid gland are benign, whereas in the submandibular gland the figure drops to 60% and at other sites to something just under 50%.

Of the benign tumours which occur in the parotid gland about 80% are pleomorphic adenomas and the remainder include monomorphic adenomas, Warthin's tumours (otherwise known as cystadenomas or papillary cystadenoma lymphomatosum), oxyphil adenomas or oncocytomas, and vascular and lymphatic swellings.

In the submandibular gland and at other sites the only benign tumour to occur with any degree of frequency is the pleomorphic adenoma or mixed tumour.

Benign tumours in the parotid gland seem to occur most commonly in the lower posterior part of the gland, namely in that portion which fills the retromandibular sulcus. They may present less commonly in the preauricular region or even further forwards over the masseter, or alternatively in the deep lobe and parapharyngeal space. Tumours at these sites seem to have a slightly greater tendency to become malignant and should therefore always be viewed with a modicum of suspicion.

There is no obvious site of election in the submandibular gland for mixed tumours, and more often than not, at operation, the tumour is found to be larger than previously suspected and virtually replacing the entire gland. Benign tumours are rare in the sublingual gland, but not all that uncommon in the hard and soft palates where they are nearly always pleomorphic adenomas. At sites other than the parotid gland the distinction between benign and malignant is not always easy to make on clinical grounds, and a relatively common alternative which may be confused with mixed tumours is adenoid cystic carcinoma.

There is a group of tumours in which both clinical and histological characteristics are difficult to reconcile with the picture of malignancy and yet whose progression ultimately proves to be overtly nefarious. Included in this group are the acinic cell tumours and some mucoepidermoid tumours.

Vascular and lymphatic malformations

Although not strictly speaking tumours in the accepted sense of the word, vascular and lymphatic malformations are very much benign surgical swellings and merit inclusion in this section.

The vascular type differs from the lymphatic in certain specific respects. Such tumours tend to be more obviously confined to an anatomical compartment by comparison with lymphangiomas and although lacking a proper capsule, their limits are relatively easy to define. The larger the vascular spaces within the swelling the greater the tendency for there to be significant feeding vessels originating from recognizable local arteries.

Haemangiomas are to be found in the parotid gland, and may make their appearance at birth. The congenital variety present as large bilateral bluish spongy swellings which tend to swell when the infant cries, coughs, or is placed horizontally. They are often associated with haemangiomas elsewhere, notably on the lips and in the subglottic compartment of the larynx. There is some evidence that this type of haemangioma will atrophy as the infant grows, the age of 2 years usually being considered the turning point (Williams, 1975). Other parotid haemangiomas may appear later, in which case atrophy cannot be expected and surgery is required.

Vascular malformations are also seen in the submandibular and sublingual glands and may then present beneath the oral mucosa.

Lymphatic malformations are by contrast no respectors of anatomical compartments. They are diffuse, occupy large tracts of tissue and cross from one plane to another. They lack a precise boundary, infiltrate muscles, glands, and completely engulf nerves and vessels.

Lymphangiomas of the parotid gland for example surround the facial nerve, infiltrate the temporalis muscle and fascia, and spread downwards into the sternomastoid, and forwards and downwards into the submandibular gland. Those which are primarily related to the submandibular gland invade the mylohyoid, the muscles of the tongue, and even the intraoral mucous membrane.

Lymphangiomas are difficult to remove because of their indeterminate boundaries, their far-flung and deep-seated extensions, and their tendency to surround vital structures. It is always advisable to dissect out important nerves beyond the periphery of the malformation and then to follow them into the swelling itself.

Sometimes these malformations appear to be a mixture of vascular and lymphatic tissue and often bleed excessively during their removal (Figure 20.8).

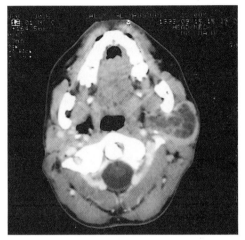

Figure 20.8 CT scan of haemangiolymphangioma of the parotid gland

Pleomorphic adenoma

This is the commonest of all benign tumours and is characterized by slow growth and a clinically benign course. It is essentially an epithelial tumour of complex morphology, possessing epithelial and myoepithelial elements arranged in a variety of patterns and surrounded by a mucopolysaccharide stroma. Its capsule is the result of fibrosis of the surrounding salivary parenchyma which is compressed by the tumour, and is referred to as a false capsule (Figure 20.9). Since the capsule is formed in response to expansion by the neoplasm, it is frequently incomplete, and

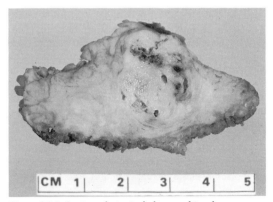

Figure 20.9 Section of a typical pleomorphic adenoma surrounded by its false capsule

tumour may be seen projecting through the dehiscences as small bosselations which contact the surrounding gland tissue (Eneroth, 1964).

The projections are sometimes seen in histological sections as small outlying foci of tumour, seemingly separated from the parent tumour by normal glandular tissue, and it is this appearance which prompted the belief at one time that mixed tumours were multifocal in origin. This view was eventually rejected when serial sections demonstrated continuity of the excrescences with the main body of the tumour (Figure 20.10). Mixed tumours are often soft in consistency, almost with a myxomatous appearance, and may be subject to cystic or haemorrhagic degeneration, features which make them susceptible to rupture when handled too enthusiastically.

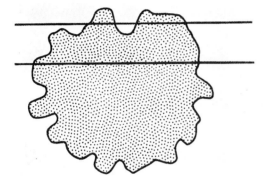

Figure 20.10 Serial sections of pleomorphic adenomas demonstrate the continuity of the surface bosses with the main body of the tumour

The lack of a complete capsule and their softness are compelling reasons for removing them with as wide a margin as possible, and this is generally possible at all the sites from which these tumours arise. The operation of enucleation, which has now been largely abandoned in favour of parotidectomy, resulted in an unacceptably high rate of recurrence, often as high as 40% over a 25 or 30-year period, but one should mention that some mixed tumours of the parotid cannot be removed adequately with a satisfactory surrounding margin. Very large tumours replacing the parotid parenchyma, or those sitting on the facial nerve or external auditory canal are just such instances and the operation to remove them can only be described as a compromise between a parotidectomy and an enucleation. Pleomorphic adenomas which arise from the deep lobe of the gland grow primarily in a medial direction across the parapharyngeal space towards the pharynx, which is eventually displaced inwards by the tumour. If their site of origin within the parotid gland is substantial,

they may lie in intimate contact with the undersurface of the facial nerve and cause the superficial lobe of the gland to bulge outwards as a conspicuous swelling (Figure 20.11).

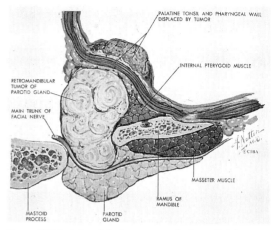

Figure 20.11 A deep lobe tumour may be immediately beneath the facial nerve

In order to negotiate a passage into the parapharyngeal space, the tumours have to pass through the hiatus bounded on the one hand by the posterior edge of the ascending ramus of the mandible, and on the other by the tough condensation of fascia called the stylomandibular ligament which takes origin from the styloid process and inserts into the angle of the mandible (see Figure 20.2). Growth is unrestricted across the parapharyngeal space, but as the tumour enlarges, it displaces the medial pterygoid muscle upwards and outwards and the soft palate, tonsil and anterior faucial pillar are pushed forwards and inwards.

Not all so-called deep lobe tumours of the parotid gland arise from the deep lobe. A significant number arise from detached islands of salivary tissue which lie in the parapharyngeal space and come to fill the space with little external displacement of the parotid gland (Figure 20.12). This distinction between a truly intraparotid gland origin and one in the parapharyngeal space can usually be made on CT scanning (Figure 20.13).

Provided removal is complete, pleomorphic adenomas arising from the deep lobe of the parotid gland or the parapharyngeal space do not commonly recur after surgery in spite of the fact that the operation to remove them is little better than a grand enucleation. The reason for this could well be their tendency to acquire a thicker and more complete capsule than is usually the case at other sites. Recurrence, when it occurs, is due to rupture of the swelling, nearly always because the dissection and removal are carried out within a confined space.

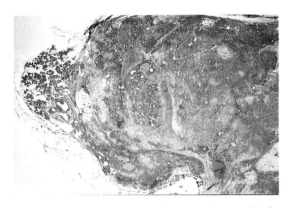

Figure 20.12 Pleomorphic adenoma arising from an island of salivary tissue within the parapharyngeal space

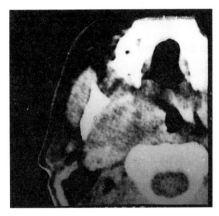

Figure 20.13 Pleomorphic adenoma arising from within the parapharyngeal space, separate from the deep lobe of the parotid gland

The concept of removal with a margin is eminently practicable when mixed tumours arise in the sub-mandibular gland since it takes many years for the neoplasm to break through the capsule of the gland. It is also feasible when the site of origin is the hard or soft palate, although a surgically created fistula may be necessary to ensure adequate removal.

A recurrent mixed tumour is to be feared, since it presents not as a discrete mass but a multiplicity of nodules (Figure 20.14a and b). In the case of the parotid gland it is common to find nodules in the previous scar, subcutaneous tissue, parotid parenchyma both superficial and deep, the sheath of the facial nerve and the perichondrium of the external meatus. Further surgical attempts are often fruitless given the widespread nature of the condition, and may well cause damage to the facial nerve.

Pleomorphic adenomas may, after several years' growth, become overtly malignant. It is estimated that the incidence of malignancy is approximately 6%, although the most important factor which determines this tendency is the length of time the tumour has been present.

Warthin's tumour

This is primarily a tumour of men, although not exclusively so, and seen generally in middle and old age. Curiously it is nearly always found in heavily built or obese individuals with short fat necks and prominent jowls. It is occasionally bilateral and often more than one tumour is found in any given gland.

Ovoid in shape, the tumour is rather like a lymph node and is characteristically situated in the tail of the parotid gland (Figure 20.15).

Histologically it is made up of areas of lymphoid tissue intermingling with cystic spaces lined by a tall tubular or papillary epithelium. The presence of lymphoid tissue within the tumour makes it susceptible to inflammation, often secondary to upper respiratory infections, with enlargement of the tumour, pain and tenderness. The clinical features therefore include fluctuation in size and intermittent pain. Rarely, the inflammatory reaction is so severe as to cause the swelling to enlarge massively and to ulcerate, even to the extent that a malignancy may be suspected.

Removal with a margin such as one would practise for a mixed tumour will generally suffice. When cut across the fresh specimen is often found to contain a viscous chocolate-like fluid. Recurrence after surgery is very rare.

Oxyphil adenoma (oncocytoma)

This is a rare tumour composed of large pleomorphic eosinophilic cells replete with mitochondria not unlike the oncocytes seen in ageing normal salivary glands. It nearly always arises from the outer part of the parotid gland, but there are reports of it developing in the submandibular gland and oral cavity. It may exceptionally become malignant.

Benign lymphoepithelial lesion

This is considered by some to be a solid variant of Warthin's tumour, and by others not to be a tumour at all. As its name implies it is composed of lymphoid and epithelial components which form a well-defined tumour-like mass indistinguishable from any other benign tumour. It may surround nerve fibres and thus appear malignant, but a frozen section usually settles the issue.

It too has a malignant counterpart which is rare.

Symptoms

Patients with benign salivary gland tumours generally complain of little more than the presence of a swelling, whose growth is so slow as to be barely perceptible from one year to the next. A sudden increase in size strongly suggests malignant transformation, although infection of a Warthin's tumour may result in rapid enlargement. Similarly pain must be regarded as unusual in benign tumours unless infection or haemorrhage have occurred in a cyst.

Pressure from a benign tumour never causes facial paralysis even when the nerve is engulfed by the growth as in benign lymphoepithelial hyperplasia. Facial palsy signifies either malignancy, tuberculosis, or sarcoidosis. Enlargement of the subparotid nodes is a frequent accidental finding during operations for the removal of benign tumours and is invariably due to non-specific reactive hyperplasia.

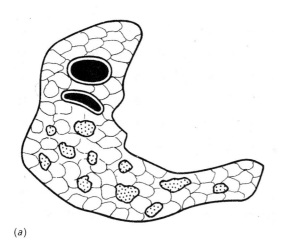

(*a*)

Examination

The precise anatomical site of the lesion must be defined during the clinical examination to establish whether or not a swelling is likely to have arisen from a salivary gland. Swellings in the retromandibular sulcus, the immediate preauricular region, and over the masseter are, in most cases, of parotid gland origin. Lumps in the submandibular triangle either arise in the salivary gland or turn out to be enlarged lymph nodes. Non-ulcerative swellings of the oral cavity, especially on the hard and soft palates, but also in the floor of the mouth or palatofaucial region, are likely to be benign salivary gland tumours. In the last case the tumour is likely to have arisen from the deep lobe of the parotid gland or parapharyngeal space, and to have filled the space before displacing the palatofaucial region inwards. Exceptionally the tumour may arise from the fauces and grow backwards and laterally into the parapharyngeal space.

Vascular or lymphatic swellings are softer and spongier than most benign tumours and may present with a blue or purplish tinge, while exceptionally, the larger variety may produce a vascular hum audible on auscultation.

In the parotid gland pleomorphic adenomas present as round, firm, reasonably well-demarcated tumours, with a tendency to nodularity as they grow. Their site of election is between the ascending ramus of the mandible anteriorly, and the mastoid process and sternomastoid posteriorly, usually in the tail of the gland (Figure 20.16). Occasionally they arise in the immediate preauricular region, where they tend to be small, and very occasionally they occur still further forwards.

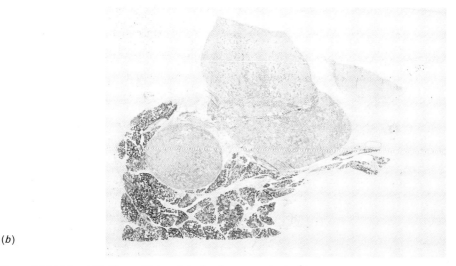

(*b*)

Figure 20.14 (*a*) and (*b*) The multiple nodularity of a recurrent mixed tumour

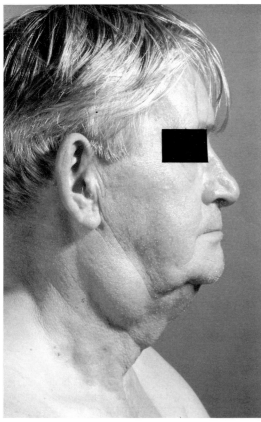

Figure 20.15 The ovoid shape and low position of a typical Warthin's tumour

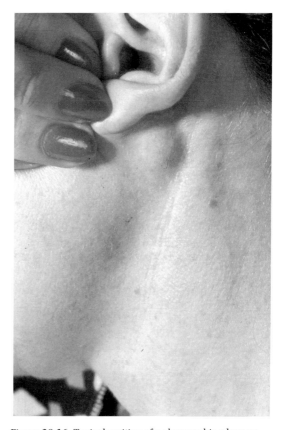

Figure 20.16 Typical position of a pleomorphic adenoma in the lower half of the parotid gland

Recurrent mixed tumours present as multiple nodules, or as a nodular thickening, although what is generally palpable represents only a fraction of the full extent of the disease, much of which is microscopic.

Warthin's tumours by contrast lie almost invariably in the lower pole of the gland, are ovoid in shape, and vary in consistency between soft and firm, depending on whether or not they have been exposed to previous inflammation. They may well be bilateral.

It is often difficult to distinguish between a tumour arising within the submandibular gland or an enlarged node close to the gland or on its outer surface. Bimanual palpation is essential to differentiate between the two, since a node lying on the outer surface of the salivary gland is unlikely to be palpated by a finger in the mouth, whereas a tumour of the gland itself is more readily compressible bimanually. Pleomorphic adenomas of the submandibular gland are usually large, quite hard, and nodular, but may be confused with a slowly growing malignancy such as an adenoid cystic carcinoma.

Tumours of the hard or soft palate are often fusiform, firm to hard in consistency and nodular. Again the distinction between mixed tumour and adenoid cystic carcinoma may be difficult to make. Apart from the obvious difference in growth rate, the latter tumour is often discoloured by telangiectases or bleeding into the tumour.

For parapharyngeal masses presenting in the palato-faucial region, the presence or absence of an associated external swelling visible and palpable in the parotid gland region is a point of considerable importance.

Swelling detectable both in the pharynx and parotid gland region indicates an origin from within the deep lobe of the parotid gland, and a very bulky tumour which has displaced the superficial lobe of the gland outwards and grown across the parapharyngeal space to push the palate and fauces inwards. Such a swelling may well be visible externally, but the technique of bimanual palpation will elicit the characteristic sign of ballotement between the examining fingers, typical of masses occupying such a wide area. The absence of both a visible swelling in the parotid gland and ballotement suggests an origin exclusively in the parapharyngeal space.

Investigations

There are only three useful investigations for benign salivary gland tumours: CT scanning, MR scanning and fine needle aspiration. Sialography may sometimes show up a tumour as a punched out area against a background of contrast-filled ducts and acini, but the time and trouble expended, and uncertainty of outcome, have virtually relegated this investigation to the past.

Equally, isotope imaging of the salivary gland with technetium, while once enjoying a brief vogue, has been superceded by CT scanning which is quick, painless and precise, and which can, if necessary, be combined with sialography to optimize definition (Figure 20.17). Given the resources, MRI is now recognized as the investigation of choice for benign salivary gland tumours, and may even on occasions display the relationship of the tumour to the facial nerve (Figure 20.18).

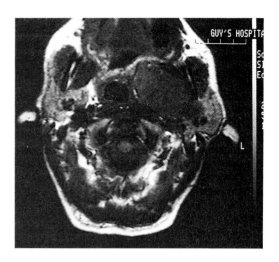

Figure 20.18 MRI of pleomorphic adenoma taking origin from within the deep lobe of the parotid and crossing the parapharyngeal space. The outer aspect of the tumour must be very close to the facial nerve

Whereas open biopsy or large needle biopsy carries the danger of implanting seedlings into the biopsy track, fine needle aspiration appears not to have this disadvantage.

Surgical treatment
Partial parotidectomy

This is the operation most often performed for benign tumours since most tumours of the parotid gland lie superficial to the facial nerve.

The patient is placed in the supine position with the neck extended and the head turned away from the surgeon. Tilting the table in a head-up position facilitates the surgery by reducing the venous pressure. The towels should be so arranged that the corner of the eye and mouth are accessible for inspection.

The incision begins in the preauricular crease and descends to the point where the lobule joins the skin of the face, at which point it inclines backwards at first, then downwards and forwards into a cervical skin crease well below the mandible (Figure 20.19). A skin flap is elevated to uncover the area which the parotid gland occupies. The posterior extremity of the gland is separated from the external auditory canal, the mastoid process and sternomastoid muscle so that sufficient room is created to find the surgical landmarks for the facial nerve. Using the tympano-

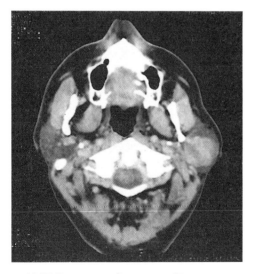

Figure 20.17 Benign parotid tumour on CT

Fine needle aspiration has now finally come to stay. There is little doubt it has much to offer in the hands of a person practised in the interpretation of small samples of tissue. However, evaluation of the findings may be difficult if the aspirate has been contaminated with blood, or even misleading if sampling of the swelling has been haphazard. Under these circumstances, a negative diagnosis for malignancy should never be considered as final.

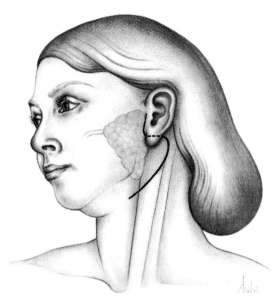

Figure 20.19 The incision used for superficial parotidectomy

mastoid sulcus as the starting point, the nerve is found and followed into the parotid gland.

That part of the parotid gland which lies superficial to the facial nerve is then peeled off the nerve together with the enclosed tumour (see Figure 20.4). The wound is then drained and the incision closed in layers. Tumours of the deep lobe of the parotid gland and parapharyngeal space are generally removed either by total conservative parotidectomy, a submandibular approach or a transmandibular technique (Shaheen, 1986).

Operations for deep lobe parotid gland and parapharyngeal space tumours

Tumours lying deep to the facial nerve and confined to the deep lobe of the parotid gland are removed by total conservative parotidectomy, the details of which are described below. Tumours arising from within the deep lobe and invading the parapharyngeal space are also removed by this technique. Such large tumours are quite difficult to disengage from the deep-seated and enclosed space in which they lie, and great care has to be taken to avoid their rupture while freeing and delivering them.

Tumours taking their origin from the parapharyngeal space exclusively, as judged radiologically, may be resected without removing the parotid gland. The options are either a submandibular approach, not favoured by the author, or a transmandibular/oral/pharyngeal approach which provides excellent access to the parapharyngeal space (see below).

Total conservative parotidectomy

This is the approach for tumours occupying the deep lobe of the parotid gland, but is also employed when tumours extend into or arise from the parapharyngeal space. It is based on the principle that the tumour will be delivered through a gap between the branches of the facial nerve, or will be scooped out inferiorly from under the facial nerve.

A superficial parotidectomy as described above is performed, but with the superficial lobe pedicled inferiorly rather than anteriorly. Alternatively the lobe may be removed altogether, and the deep lobe and tumour removed as a separate specimen. The branches and main trunk of the facial nerve are dissected off the underlying deep lobe, and the attachments of the deep lobe to adjacent structures freed by blunt or sharp dissection.

Those vessels which traverse the deep lobe of the parotid gland, namely the retromandibular vein, external carotid, internal maxillary and superficial temporal arteries, are ligated at their points of entrance and exit from the parotid gland. Thereafter, the deep lobe together with the contained tumour is mobilized as one unit, taking care not to rupture the neoplasm (Figure 20.20). This is not easy, since the mass may fill the parapharyngeal space, and the areas through which it may be delivered are usually confined.

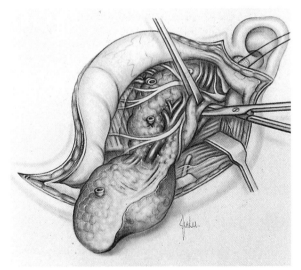

Figure 20.20 Mobilization of the deep lobe of the parotid from beneath the facial nerve

Smaller tumours may be lifted out between the divisions or branches of the facial nerve, but larger growths have to be delivered from below and beneath the facial nerve. To assist the process of delivery of the tumour, the stylomandibular ligament should be divided, and possibly also the styloid process.

At the conclusion of the operation there is a large

dead space deep to the facial nerve, which lies limply across it. Suction drainage should be avoided in case the nerve is sucked into the openings or tip of the drainage tube.

Submandibular approach to the parapharyngeal space

This approach is applicable to deep lobe or parapharyngeal tumours. A horizontal incision is made just above the level of the hyoid bone extending from the midline to a point just behind the anterior edge of the sternomastoid muscle.

The submandibular gland is excised and the tumour approached as it lies beneath the medial pterygoid muscle, bounded laterally by the deep lobe of the parotid gland.

Separation from adjacent tissue should not prove difficult, except possibly superiorly and laterally. The superior part of the tumour cannot be seen, and dissection must of necessity be blind, and defining the lateral margin of the tumour if it arises from within the deep lobe may also be problematical. If access to the upper part of the neoplasm is restricted, dividing the horizontal ramus of the mandible immediately anterior to the ascending ramus will improve matters. This, however, entails peeling off the mandibular periosteum and overlying masseter muscle from below, with the concomitant risk of damaging the mandibular branch of the facial nerve.

The line of division through the bone is best inclined downwards and forwards in order to ensure subsequent stability of the bone fragments, and the ascending ramus is everted laterally and upwards to facilitate access to the upper part of the tumour (Figure 20.21).

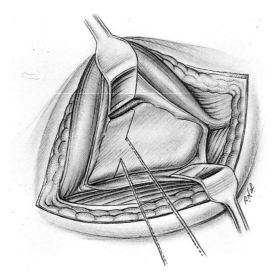

Figure 20.21 Division of the horizontal ramus of the mandible for access to the parapharyngeal space

At the conclusion of the operation the bone fragments are realigned and either plated or wired together and the wound is drained with suction.

Midline transmandibular oropharyngeal approach to parapharyngeal salivary gland tumours

This is the best approach for large tumours occupying the parapharyngeal space but not arising from the deep lobe of the parotid gland. The patient is positioned as for excision of the submandibular gland. The lower lip is divided by a staggered incision, either curved or a V lying on its side. At the point of the chin, the incision inclines downwards and laterally, preferably in a skin crease, just above the level of the hyoid bone (Figure 20.22). The submandibular gland is removed and the mandible divided in the midline. As the mandible is retracted laterally the reflection of the mucous membrane on the inner aspect of the mandible is divided together with the attachment of the mylohyoid to the bone, thus assisting retraction of the mandible laterally. The proximal course of the lingual nerve should be exposed by this manoeuvre.

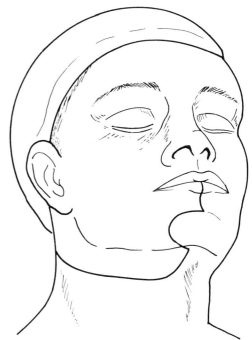

Figure 20.22 Incision for the midline transmandibular oropharyngeal approach to the parapharyngeal space

The incision of the mucous membrane is carried backwards and upwards onto the anterior faucial pillar, ending on the soft palate. The incision is deepened to open the parapharyngeal space and the tumour exposed and mobilized (Figure 20.23).

After removing the tumour, the oral soft tissues

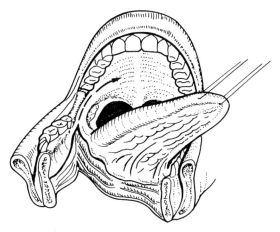

Figure 20.23 The soft tissue incision in the palatofaucial region to open the parapharyngeal space

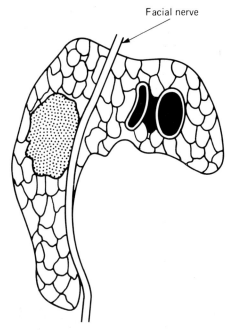

Facial nerve

Figure 20.24 Tumours may sit on the facial nerve preventing removal other than by enucleation

are closed in layers and the mandible plated or wired. The wound is closed with drainage using a suction tube.

Recurrent pleomorphic adenoma

Recurrence of this tumour occurs when it is enucleated without a margin of healthy tissue, or when it is breached accidentally during the course of an operation to remove it, or deliberately, as with a biopsy. Spillage of tumour is apt to occur when the tumour is particularly large and tense, or soft, or when it is awkwardly situated. Examples of the latter are large tumours impacted between the mandible and the mastoid, deep-seated growths, or tumours sitting intimately on the facial nerve (Figure 20.24).

As previously mentioned, recurrence presents as multiple nodules scattered not only within the parotid gland parenchyma but also in the overlying tissues (see Figure 20.14).

If the initial operation which led to the recurrence was simply an enucleation, salvage surgery in the form of a superficial or even total conservative parotidectomy is generally feasible. If however, the first operation was a parotidectomy with exposure of the nerve, any subsequent attempt to excise the residual disease without compromising the facial nerve is difficult to say the least. Under such circumstances, it may be possible to find the nerve in the mastoid, but even then the process of following it through a mass of fibrous tissue and neoplastic nodules which are so typical of recurrent mixed tumour is complicated and hazardous. More often than not the nerve and its branches disappear from view into the surrounding fibrous tissue so that further dissection is technically impossible without damaging the nerve. Given this

sort of scenario and the fact that neoplastic nodules are commonly embedded within the sheath of the facial nerve, the surgeon might be forgiven for opting for a radical parotidectomy.

There is however an alternative strategy which offers the possibility of preventing recurrence in high risk cases and of dealing with it once it has become established.

It has been common knowledge for many years that postoperative radiotherapy following a limited operation such as enucleation will reduce the recurrence rate of mixed tumours to that expected after parotidectomy, namely about 3–4% (Rafla, 1970). The rationale for this is that the operation serves to remove the bulk of the disease, leaving scattered microscopic residues which are more readily amenable to sterilization by radiotherapy, notwithstanding the known relative radioresistance of mixed tumours. The application of this philosophy to the management of those patients undergoing adequate surgery by present day standards, but who are deemed to be at risk, should minimize the risk of recurrence still further. Such cases would include patients with tumours sitting on the facial nerve, those stuck to the external auditory meatus, or those which have ruptured during removal.

In practice, the irradiation of such patients has proved to be satisfactory and has eliminated recurrences altogether.

The same approach can be adopted for patients who have an established recurrence. Here the approach is to remove all macroscopic disease by total conservative parotidectomy if this procedure is feasible and to follow this with radiotherapy.

In those patients where the integrity of every branch of the facial nerve is impossible to safeguard, the surgeon cuts his losses by resorting to a total parotidectomy, with every attempt being made to preserve as much of the nerve as possible. Deficits are restored by immediate nerve grafting, and surgery is followed some weeks later by radiotherapy.

Generally between 4000 and 5000 cGy are given by a lateral field and preferably by linear accelerator. The results of treating established recurrences by this method have been equally rewarding, recurrence having been abolished.

This naturally raises the ethical question of whether it is proper to irradiate patients with benign disease. There are indeed isolated reports of patients developing cancers of the parotid gland after radiotherapy but many of these date back to the era when low dosage therapy was used in the management of lymphoid tissue hypertrophy in childhood (Watkin and Hobsley, 1986a and b). Most radiotherapists with whom one discusses the matter are sceptical about the likelihood of a properly administered course of irradiation eventually causing cancer of the parotid gland, although it is conceivable that adjacent areas such as the postnasal space might be at risk.

The pros and cons of the issue will doubtless continue to be debated but, in the final analysis, the decision whether to use radiotherapy or not has to be a personal one.

Removal of the submandibular gland

The position of the patient is the same as for parotidectomy. A horizontal skin incision is made just above the hyoid bone preferably in a skin crease (see Figure 20.6). The incision is deepened through subcutaneous fat, platysma, and deep cervical fascia until the surgical capsule at the lower limit of the gland is reached. This is then opened along the lower border of the gland and a large superior flap elevated in the plane between the surgical capsule and the gland.

The facial vessels are ligated both at the inferolateral corner of the gland and at its upper border.

The gland is mobilized until it is pedicled on its deep part, whereupon the mylohyoid muscle is retracted forwards to permit separation of the gland from the lingual nerve (Figure 20.25). Finally the duct is severed and the wound closed in layers with drainage.

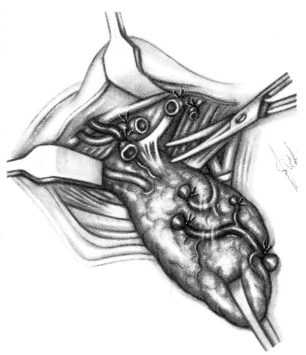

Figure 20.25 Retraction of the mylohyoid muscle forwards to allow separation of the submandibular gland from the lingual nerve

Removal of the sublingual gland

This may be done intraorally after injecting an adequate volume of a vasoconstrictor solution immediately beneath the mucous membrane to lessen bleeding.

An incision medial to the line of Wharton's duct provides access to the gland, but care has to be taken to avoid injuring the lingual nerve which winds round the duct. With the submandibular duct and lingual nerve retracted medially out of the way, the gland and tumour may be removed.

Removal of a pleomorphic adenoma from the hard palate

The patient should be placed in the supine position with a sandbag beneath the shoulders and the head fully extended. The table should be in the Trendelenburg position so that, with a Boyle-Davis gag separating the jaws, a clear view of the operation site is obtainable. Illumination with a headlight and adequate suction are imperative.

The incision through the mucous membrane and down to the bone of the hard palate is best made with the cutting diathermy to lessen the bleeding, and should be sited a short distance away from the tumour to ensure an adequate surrounding margin of normal tissue.

Enucleation of the tumour by dissection from the underlying bone is not safe unless the bone is then drilled away virtually through its whole thickness. The safest approach is to fenestrate the palate so that the tumour is cut out en-bloc. In either case provision should be made for the wearing of a protective denture, with or without an obturator, depending on the size of the defect.

Complications of surgery
Parotidectomy

Haematoma

This is fairly common in view of the dead space resulting from the removal of a substantial segment of glandular tissue. A large suction drain sited away from the facial nerve together with adequate pressure from a suitable dressing will minimize this complication.

Facial weakness

This is generally temporary if it occurs after an uneventful operation. It usually affects the mandibular and frontal branches of the facial nerve and is more prone to occur in the elderly, in those with slender as opposed to stout facial nerves, and when there has been an unusual degree of trauma in the vicinity of the nerve. Pressure or traction on the nerve, constant suction on its surface, excessive dryness of its sheath, and heat from the coagulating diathermy are all factors contributing to facial weakness.

Anaesthesia

Anaesthesia of the lower half of the pinna and preauricular skin results from division of the great auricular nerve and is therefore an inevitable sequel of parotidectomy. The area of numbness gradually diminishes in size and ultimately becomes confined to the lobule of the pinna. Sensation in the surrounding skin rarely returns to complete normality and in some patients a degree of increased sensitivity can assume distressing proportions and is attributable to the presence of an amputation neuroma of the greater auricular nerve. Excision of the neuroma and alcohol injection into the cut end of the nerve will resolve the problem by substituting complete anaesthesia for hyperaesthesia.

Fistula formation

This is very uncommon and probably results from an overproduction of saliva in the remaining glandular tissue. A pressure bandage and continuous suction suffice to dry up the wound and permit normal healing.

Gustatory swelling

This condition is thought to be due to misrouting of parasympathetic secretomotor fibres into cutaneous nerves during the healing phase following parotidectomy. The precise origin of these fibres is uncertain, having been thought to have come via the otic ganglion and to have accompanied the auriculotemporal nerve to their final destination in the parotid gland. There is some reason to suppose that this is not the only source of secretomotor fibres and that some may come via the facial nerve itself.

Most patients develop some degree of Frey's syndrome, but in many the condition is so mild as to be barely noticeable. The complaint is of sweating in the preauricular and subparotid regions at meal times, although many patients imagine at first that it is an escape of liquid through a small opening in the surgical scar. It may on occasions be so bad as to be a severe social embarrassment.

Contrary to reports in the literature, tympanic neurectomy has not been successful in controlling the condition and the effectiveness of other techniques such as the interposition of fascial grafts between skin and the underlying parotid bed is also doubtful.

More recently pilocarpine cream 1% and aluminium hydrochloride solution have been applied with some success (Shaheen, 1984).

Trismus

Some degree of trismus may occur for a short while following parotidectomy.

Approaches to the parapharyngeal space

The transparotid approach is characterized by a greater postoperative incidence of neuropraxia, which tends to persist longer than usual. If trauma to the nerve is particularly severe, involuntary contractions and mass movement of the face may be permanent sequelae. The likelihood of temporary trismus of the jaw is greater than with superficial parotidectomy.

The submandibular approach is complicated by trismus postoperatively and permanent mental anaesthesia if the jaw has been divided.

The main by-product of the transmandibular/oral approach is long-standing trismus, but damage to the inferior dental and lingual nerves may also occur.

Submandibular gland excision

Paralysis of the depressor anguli oris

This is due to damage to the marginal mandibular branch of the facial nerve and is best avoided by gaining access to the correct plane of dissection, well away from the nerve, from the very outset.

Attempts to dissect out the mandibular branch are likely to do more harm than good, and if the nerve is badly traumatized the likelihood of recovery is remote.

Damage to the hypoglossal and lingual nerves

Both these complications are uncommon and generally speaking cannot be rectified (Shaheen, 1984).

References

BAILEY, H. (1941) The treatment of tumours of the parotid gland. *British Journal of Surgery*, **28**, 337–346

CONLEY, J. J. (1978) Search for and identification of the facial nerve. *Laryngoscope*, **88**, 172–175

ENEROTH, C. M. (1964) Histological and clinical aspects of parotid tumours. *Acta Otolaryngologica Supplementum*, **191**, 1–99

EVANS, R. W. and CRUICKSHANK, A. H. (1970) *Epithelial Tumours of the Salivary Glands*. Philadelphia: W. B. Saunders. p. 11

FOOTE, F. W. and FRAZELL, E. I. (1953) Tumours of the major salivary glands. *Cancer*, **15**, 1065–1133

JU, D. M. C. (1968) Salivary gland tumours occurring after radiation of the head and neck area. *American Journal of Surgery*, **116**, 518–523

MCFARLAND, J. (1942) The histopathological prognosis of salivary gland mixed tumors. *American Journal of Medical Science*, **203**, 502–519

PATEY, D. H. and THACKRAY, A. C. (1957–1958) The treatment of parotid tumours in the light of pathological study of parotidectomy material. *British Journal of Surgery*, **28**, 477–487

RAFLA, S. (1970) *Mucous and Salivary Gland Tumours*. Springfield, Illinios: Charles C. Thomas. p. 104

REDON, H. (1945) Technique de la parotidectomie totale avec conservation du nerf facial. *Journal de Chirurgie (Paris)*, **61**, 14–20

SHAHEEN, O. H. (1984) *Problems in Head and Neck Surgery*. London: Bailliere Tindall. pp. 22–49

SHAHEEN, O. H. (1986) Partial and complete parotidectomy – removal of the submandibular gland. In: *Operative Surgery*, edited by J. Ballantyne. London: Butterworths. pp. 409–431

SNOW, G. B. (1979) Tumours of the parotid gland. *Clinical Otolaryngology*, **4**, 457–468

TAKEICHI, N., HIROSE, F. and YAMAMOTO, H. (1976) Salivary gland tumours in atomic bomb survivors, Hiroshima, Japan. *Cancer*, **38**, 2462–2468

WATKIN, G. and HOBSLEY, M. (1986a) The influence of local surgery and radiotherapy on the natural history of pleomorphic adenomas. *British Journal of Surgery*, **73**, 74–76

WATKIN, G. and HOBSLEY, M. (1986b) Should radiotherapy be used routinely in the management of benign parotid tumours? *British Journal of Surgery*, **73**, 601–603

WILLIAMS, H. B. (1975) Hemangiomas of the parotid gland in children. *Plastic and Reconstructive Surgery*, **56**, 29–34

21

Malignant salivary gland tumours

Michael Gleeson

Fewer than 3% of all neoplasms originate in salivary glands (OPCS Cancer Statistics, 1983) and at least 75% of these tumours are benign. In England and Wales (1985), the registration rate of malignant salivary gland tumours developing in major glands was 1.2 per 100 000 population. By comparison, rates of 142.7 for trachea, bronchus and lung, 86.9 for breast and 6.9 for larynx were recorded (OPSC Cancer Statistics, 1985). By all standards, therefore, malignant salivary gland tumours are uncommon. From a clinical standpoint, it is unfortunate that the vast majority of malignant salivary gland tumours have no features that distinguish them from benign tumours at presentation; the diagnosis being made at or after an operation designed to control benign disease and, therefore, often not as radical as it might have been. Furthermore, despite the benign nature of the most frequently encountered salivary gland tumour, pleomorphic adenoma, even this can pose considerable management problems as it recurs locally if inadequately resected, ruptured or biopsied. More importantly, it also has the potential to undergo carcinomatous change. Furthermore, the malignant character of some salivary gland tumours has only recently been appreciated as their natural history must be measured in decades rather than years. The slow growth pattern of these tumours does not lessen their malignant nature. Despite treatment they can recur and be manifest as metastatic disease many years later and thus exert a considerable morbidity and mortality.

Normal structure and pathological classification

Normal salivary tissue has a complex structure consisting of secretory cells, which may be either serous or mucous, arranged in acini and drained by a duct system. The major glands – the parotid, submandibular and sublingual – are composed of collections of acini of differing character which secrete into a complex duct system. Around the acini lie myoepithelial cells which display features common to both epithelial and smooth muscle cells. Their probable action is to propel the contents of the acini along the duct system. While the parotid gland is predominantly serous, the submandibular and sublingual glands produce mucoid secretions. There are numerous collections of salivary acini scattered throughout the oral and oropharyngeal mucosa. These are referred to as the minor glands (Figure 21.1).

The histopathology of salivary gland neoplasms poses many problems to the pathologist. Like most other tumours they are rarely homogeneous in structure, many present a variety of patterns and some are so uncommon that few pathologists have the opportunity to acquire expertise in their diagnosis.

A widely recognized system of classification was established by Thackray and Sobin (1972) which divided these lesions into four subgroups: epithelial, non-epithelial, unclassified tumours, and a group of conditions that may give rise to diffuse or discrete salivary gland enlargement. Epithelial tumours predominate in all series. This classification has recently been reviewed and changed (Seifert and Sobin, 1991), so that a clearer distinction can be drawn between tumours of similar pathological type but widely differing prognosis. There are now six groups of tumours and one other group devoted to tumour-like disorders (Table 21.1).

Distribution

Salivary gland tumours are more common in the parotid gland than in any of the other glands. The

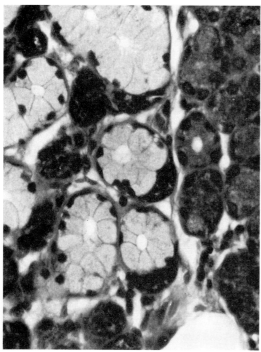

(a)

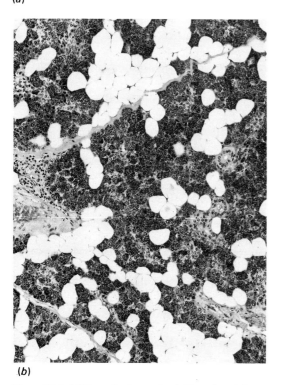

(b)

Figure 21.1 (*a*) Normal salivary gland. The pale staining cells are mucous cells and the darker cells serous secreting cells. (*b*) Normal parotid gland. Both serous and mucous cells can be seen. The presence of fat is a common finding

Table 21.1 Histopathological classification of salivary gland tumours

I   Adenomas
Pleomorphic adenoma
Myoepithelioma (myoepithelial adenoma)
Basal cell adenoma
Warthin's tumour (adenolymphoma)
Oncocytoma (oncocytic adenoma)
Canalicular adenoma
Sebaceous adenoma
Ductal papilloma
    Inverted ductal papilloma
    Intraductal papilloma
    Sialadenoma papilliferum
Cystadenoma
    Papillary cystadenoma
    Mucinous cystadenoma

II   Carcinomas
Acinic cell carcinoma
Mucoepidermoid carcinoma
Adenoid cystic carcinoma
Polymorphous low-grade (terminal duct)
    adenocarcinoma
Epithelial-myoepithelial carcinoma
Basal cell adenocarcinoma
Sebaceous carcinoma
Papillary cystadenocarcinoma
Mucinous adenocarcinoma
Oncocytic carcinoma
Salivary duct carcinoma
Adenocarcinoma
Malignant myoepithelioma (myoepithelial carcinoma)
Carcinoma in pleomorphic adenoma (malignant mixed
    tumour)
Squamous cell carcinoma
Small cell carcinoma
Undifferentiated carcinoma
Other carcinomas

III   Non-epithelial tumours

IV   Malignant lymphomas

V   Secondary tumours

VI   Unclassified tumours

VII   Tumour-like disorders
Sialadenosis
Oncocytosis
Necrotizing sialometaplasia (salivary gland infarction)
Benign lymphoepithelial lesion
Salivary gland cysts
Chronic submandibular sialadenitis (Küttner tumour)
Cystic lymphoid hyperplasia in AIDS

frequency of malignant tumours varies according to the site, being relatively lower in the parotid than elsewhere (Table 21.2). Malignancy is far more frequent, in relative terms, in the submandibular, sublingual and minor glands. Even within the minor gland group there is much variation in the proportion of

Table 21.2 Frequency (%) of all primary epithelial salivary gland tumours and malignancy (%) analysed by site

Site	Absolute no.	Frequency (%)	Malignant (%)
Parotid	1756	72.9	14.7
Submandibular	257	10.7	37.0
Sublingual	7	0.3	85.7
Minor glands (oropharyngeal)	336	14.0	46.4
Unknown	54	2.2	0.0
Total	2410		

(Eveson, J. W. and Cawson, R. A., 1985. British Salivary Gland Tumour Panel data)

frankly malignant tumours, the lip being the least common site, while those tumours arising in the sublingual glands, albeit rare, are usually malignant (Table 21.3). The most common sites for tumours of the minor glands are the palate, lip and buccal mucosa.

Table 21.3 Distribution of salivary gland tumours in minor glands and malignancy (%)

Site	Absolute no.	% of total	Malignant (%)
Palate	183	54.3	47.0
Lip	71	21.1	26.7
Buccal mucosa	38	11.3	50.0
Tongue	12	3.6	92.0
Pharynx	12	3.6	50.0
Tonsil	6	1.8	50.0
Retromolar	5	1.5	50.0
Alveolar ridge	5	1.5	100.0
Tuberosity	3	0.9	100.0
Ethmoid	1	0.3	100.0
Total	336		

(Eveson, J. W. and Cawson, R. A., 1985. British Salivary Gland Tumour Panel data)

Benign tumours (the mono- and pleomorphic adenomas) outnumber malignant tumours at all sites except in the sublingual glands. The available data show that the relative incidence of the more common varieties of malignant neoplasm differs widely between the major and minor glands (Table 21.4). Thus mucoepidermoid carcinomas and adenoid cystic carcinomas are the most common malignant neoplasms overall.

Malignant salivary gland tumours are more frequent in women than men and have a peak age incidence in the seventh decade. Adenomas and non-epithelial tumours present at a much younger age and, indeed, many have been reported in infancy. Even discounting congenital anomalies, the salivary gland tumours arising in infancy have a different distribution from those of adult life (Table 21.5). Pleomorphic adenoma still predominates but, in infants, the mucoepidermoid tumour is the most common malignancy (Byers, Piorkowski and Luna, 1984).

Epidemiology

The reported, worldwide, incidence of salivary gland tumours from countries with reliable registries is variable, for example 2.5 per million in Norway, 7.5 per million in Sweden and 15 per million in Caucasians living in the USA (Dorn and Cutler, 1959; Soder, 1973). The developing nations appear to experience a similar incidence (Davies, Dodge and Burkitt, 1964; Loke, 1967).

The peak incidence of salivary neoplasms is in the sixth and seventh decades for both men and women. In the major series, salivary gland tumours have been found to be slightly more common in women than men. This tendency, while present throughout life, becomes most marked in the eighth and ninth decades when there is a female predominance in the population and ratios of 1.6:1 and 1.9:1 are recorded respectively.

Predisposing and associated factors

Several possible predisposing factors have been postulated including race, diet, occupation, Epstein-Barr virus, etc. (Lanier *et al.*, 1976; Lennox *et al.*, 1978; Saemundsen *et al.*, 1982; Spitz *et al.*, 1984). Previous radiation alone has been shown convincingly to have a significant influence. In a study of survivors of the Hiroshima atomic bomb, Takeichi, Hirose and Yamamoto (1976) found that the incidence of benign and malignant salivary gland tumours was 2.6 times higher than that of a comparable non-exposed population, while that of malignant tumours was 10 times greater. This risk of salivary gland malignancy was higher in those closest to the hypocentre of the explosion and in those returning early to the city. As with similarly induced thyroid neoplasms there would appear to be a latent period of 15–25 years after exposure before development of the tumour. In a later study of the same population it was established that this increased susceptibility was shared by both the parotid and submandibular glands (Takeichi *et al.*, 1983). Patients given low dosage radiotherapy to

Table 21.4 Frequency (%) of primary epithelial salivary gland tumours by site

Tumour type	Parotid	Submandibular	Sublingual	Minor
Benign				
Pleomorphic adenoma	63.3	59.5	0.0	42.9
Adenolymphoma	14.0	0.8	0.0	0.0
Oxyphil adenoma	0.9	0.4	0.0	0.0
Other monomorphics	7.1	1.9	14.2	11.0
Malignant				
Mucoepidermoid carcinoma	1.5	1.6	0.0	8.9
Acinic cell tumour	2.5	0.4	0.0	1.8
Adenoid cystic carcinoma	2.0	16.8	28.6	13.1
Adenocarcinoma	2.6	5.0	14.2	12.2
Epidermoid carcinoma	1.1	1.9	0.0	1.2
Undifferentiated carcinoma	1.8	3.9	14.2	2.1
Carcinoma ex pleomorphic adenoma	3.2	7.8	28.6	7.1
Total no. cases	1756	257	7	336

(Eveson, J. W. and Cawson, R. A., 1985. British Salivary Gland Tumour Panel data)

Table 21.5 Distribution of juvenile salivary gland tumours by site and type

Tumour type	Site					
	Parotid (%)	Submandibular (%)	Sublingual (%)	Intraoral (%)	Lip (%)	Unknown (%)
Pleomorphic	26 (55)	14 (29.8)	0	4 (8.5)	0	3 (6.4)
Warthin's	1 (100)					
Monomorphic	1 (100)					
Mucoepidermoid	3 (50)	2 (33)		1 (17)		
Acinic cell	1 (100)					
Adenoid cystic	1 (100)					
Adenocarcinoma				1 (50)	1 (50)	
Undifferentiated	1 (33)				2 (67)	
Unclassified	1 (100)					
Others	9 (90)	1 (10)				
Total number	44 (61)	17 (24)		6 (8)	3 (3.5)	3 (3.5)

(British Salivary Gland Tumour Panel data, 1986)

the tonsil and nasopharyngeal area for benign conditions have also shown identical trends (Shore-Freedman *et al.*, 1983).

Some authors have found that patients with salivary gland tumours are more likely to develop a second primary tumour at any site. A link with hormone-dependent tumours has been suggested as the breast is structurally similar to salivary gland tissue. Women are more likely to develop a later breast tumour, but in men skin cancer is the only growth with a significantly increased incidence, despite early claims suggesting an association with prostatic carcinoma (Prior and Waterhouse, 1977; Abbey *et al.*, 1984; Spitz *et al.*, 1985).

Histopathology and natural history of the common tumour types

Carcinomas

Mucoepidermoid carcinoma

Mucoepidermoid carcinoma is the most common salivary gland neoplasm to arise in childhood but only the second most common salivary gland malignancy overall (see Table 21.5). The parotid and minor glands are the most frequently affected sites and, of the latter group, the palatal glands predominate.

Mucoepidermoid carcinomas grow slowly and recur locally. Lymph node metastases arise in up to

30% of patients and are present *ab initio* in 15%. Metastases to the lungs, bones and brain develop in approximately 15%. It has been claimed that recurrence and survival rates are strongly influenced by the histological grading of the tumour and its size at presentation. Low grade tumours are said to be compatible with an 80% 15-year determinate cure rate, while a comparable figure for high grade tumours is reported to be only 33% (Spiro *et al.*, 1978). However, even cytologically benign tumours can be unexpectedly invasive. Cytophotometric assessment of DNA content can aid the distinction between potentially aggressive and clinically benign mucoepidermoid carcinomas. Those carcinomas with a diploid profile have been reported to have a more favourable outcome (Hamper *et al.*, 1989).

Mucoepidermoid carcinoma is composed of two distinct cell types: epidermoid cells and mucous cells, both of which may show varying degrees of differentiation (Figure 21.2). Mucus is secreted into the stroma of the tumour often giving rise to a partially cystic structure. This neoplasm has been graded according to its cellular content (Batsakis and Luna, 1990). Tumours are designated high grade if 90% or more of their area is made up of tumour cells and less than 10% of intracystic spaces. Low grade tumours display a reversal of this ratio (Evans, 1984). Increased mi-totic activity is not necessarily seen even in high grade tumours – a feature partially responsible for the unpredictable nature of this particular neoplasm.

Low grade tumours should be managed by local resection and prolonged follow up. High grade lesions require more radical resection with adjunctive radiotherapy. Local recurrence is likely to appear within 12 months of the primary procedure.

Acinic cell carcinoma

Acinic cell carcinoma accounts for 2.5% of all salivary gland tumours and predominantly affects the parotid gland. A very small proportion may be bilateral. Like adenoid cystic carcinoma this tumour is very slow growing, a feature that belies its malignant potential. Local recurrence or the development of metastases after a prolonged disease-free interval are common. This tumour exerts a mortality many years after other salivary neoplasms would have been considered cured. Determinate survival rates of 85%, 65% and 50% for 5, 10 and 15 years respectively, have been reported (Batsakis *et al.*, 1979; Perzin and LiVolsi, 1979; Hickman, Cawson and Duffy, 1984).

Microscopically, a solid pattern is usually seen with varying degrees of organization into an acinar arrangement. Microcystic, or rarely papillary-cystic, follicular and poorly differentiated patterns are also recognized, but are rare (Figure 21.3), tumours are

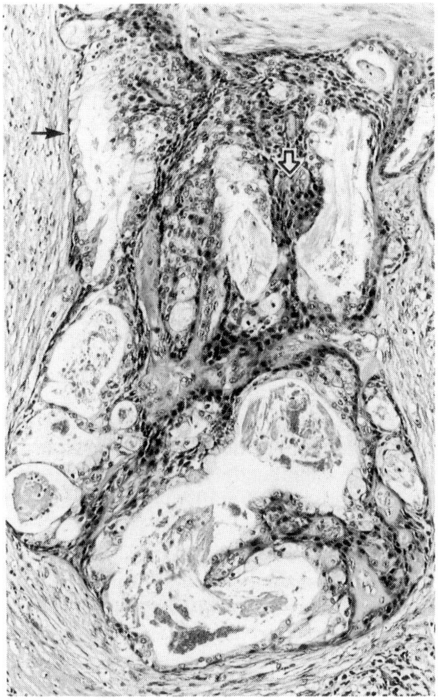

Figure 21.2 Mucoepidermoid tumour. Mucus secreting cells with basally located nuclei (solid arrow) are intermixed with epidermoid cells (open arrow)

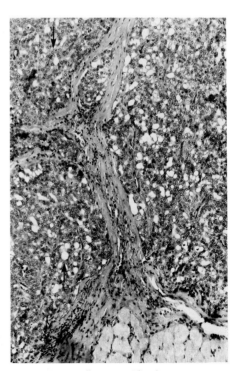

Figure 21.3 Acinic cell tumour. The classic arrangement of the cells into acini is well illustrated (arrow)

often not homogeneous and some are multifocal. The constituent cells contain zymogen granules, thus bearing a close resemblance to the serous salivary gland cell. No histological features or grading scheme appear to correlate with poor prognosis and what data are available concerning the value of cytophotometric DNA analysis would appear to be conflicting (Hamper *et al.*, 1990; El-Naggar, Batsakis and Luna, 1990).

The management of this carcinoma is excision of the gland with conservation of all uninvolved nerves. Since nodal disease is uncommon and develops in no more than 10%, elective neck dissection is not indicated.

Adenoid cystic carcinoma

Adenoid cystic carcinoma is the most common malignant salivary gland neoplasm. As with the other tumours, its distribution varies between sites. It is far more common in the submandibular, sublingual and minor glands, where it constitutes 16%, 28% and 13% of all neoplasms in these glands respectively. However, in the parotid gland only 2% of tumours are of this type (see Table 21.4).

Adenoid cystic carcinoma grows slowly and insidiously with a characteristic propensity for perineural infiltration and spread along the haversian systems and neural canals of bones. Widespread infiltration by this route is often achieved with little, if any, apparent bone erosion. This pattern is reflected in the local recurrence and cumulative mortality rates for this tumour, namely 5-year survival – 62%; 10-year survival – 39%; 15-year survival – 26%; and 20-year survival – 21% (Spiro, Huvos and Strong, 1974). Nodal involvement is normally the result of direct spread of tumour rather than lymphatic spread. Metastases develop late in the disease and are usually pulmonary (Shannon Allen and Marsh, 1976). Local recurrence is common and appears in at least 50% of patients, but even multiple local recurrences or distant metastases are compatible with prolonged survival (Conley and Dingman, 1974). Indeed, while 33% of patients die within one year of the recognition of their metastatic disease, 20% of those with pulmonary secondaries survive with this increased tumour load for longer than 5 years.

Clinically, adenoid cystic carcinoma usually presents as a mass or a submucosal swelling which can be either painless or painful. It is usually non-ulcerated unless it is traumatized. Facial palsy develops in up to 20% of parotid gland tumours and palpable lymph node involvement or direct invasion of adjacent tissues is found in 15%.

Four histological patterns can be recognized, namely cribriform, basaloid or solid, cylindromatous, and tubular (Batsakis and Regezi, 1979; Batsakis, Luna and El-Naggar, 1990) (Figure 21.4). The type and grade of tumour appear to affect survival. The more solid types are reported to have the worst prognosis, display greater cellular atypia and, thus, are of higher grade than the tubular and cribriform varieties. These latter types are usually better differentiated, of lower grade and are reported to impart a superior survival rate (Perzin, Gullane and Clairmont, 1978; Szanto *et al.*, 1984, Seifert *et al.*, 1986).

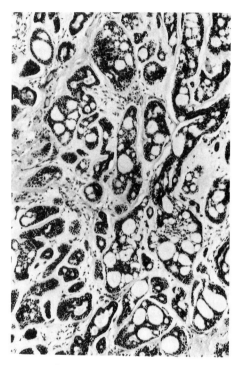

Figure 21.4 Adenoid cystic carcinoma. This illustrates the cribriform variety with its multiple cystic spaces resembling a 'Swiss cheese' pattern

The management of this tumour is by the widest possible excision followed by radiotherapy to improve local control. For a parotid gland tumour this implies total parotidectomy. The facial nerve is conserved only if there is no evidence of invasion by tumour. Subtotal petrosectomy has been advocated for patients with clinical evidence of facial nerve invasion. It is essential to appreciate that this tumour spreads perineurally both peripherally and centrally. Great care must therefore be given to excision of the neural spread in both directions. Part of the mandible, maxillary tuberosity and the contents of the infratemporal fossa must also be resected in some of these patients. Radical neck dissection is only indicated for those patients with obvious nodal disease or those in whom a large soft tissue cuff must be removed. The treatment plan must take full account of the patient's age, their general health and attitude to their illness, the realistic extent of microscopic disease and the likely benefit that the patient might derive from mutilating surgery.

Submandibular disease is best managed by a monobloc resection of the gland encompassing the lingual, hypoglossal and marginal mandibular nerves, together with a suprahyoid nodal clearance. Palatal tumours require wide local resection to include the floor of the maxillary sinus at least. Perhaps it is because this is a relatively simple surgical procedure that disease at this site enjoys slightly better survival rates (Eneroth, Hjertman and Moberger, 1968).

Recurrent tumour is best dealt with by surgery followed by radiotherapy if possible. Advanced and incurable disease is sometimes palliated by radiotherapy which, in a few, makes salvage surgery feasible (Simpson, Thawley and Matsuba, 1984; Matsuba *et al.*, 1984).

Adenocarcinoma

This is an uncommon tumour which, by virtue of the overall higher incidence of parotid growths, is most frequently found at that site. However, it constitutes only 2.5-4% of all parotid neoplasms and forms a much larger proportion of the tumours in other glands – 5% of submandibular tumours and 12–14% of sublingual and minor gland neoplasms (see Table 21.4).

Clinically, 80% of adenocarcinomas present as masses, half of which are fixed; 85% have been present for less than 5 years, but only 35% for less than 12 months. About 20% are painful but, of those arising in the parotid gland, only 5% produce a facial palsy. Nearly 20% of patients have nodal disease at presentation and a further 10% develop it later. Failure to control disease is usually manifest as local or regional recurrence, but distant metastasis, usually to the lungs, is also common.

Several histological patterns of adenocarcinoma are now recognized, non-mucin producing types being the most common. Mucinous, papillary, trabecular, clear cell and sebaceous variants are also seen and are more frequent in the minor glands. As a group they display a wide structural range, but have in common neoplastic duct or tubule formation and, by definition, lack any evidence of pre-existing pleomorphic adenoma (Figure 21.5). The grade of the neoplasm as judged by mitotic rate, cellular pleomorphism and stromal invasion correlates better than the clinical stage and outcome. Most of the high grade tumours are the non-mucin producing type, while the rarer variants are usually of a lower grade. The high grade neoplasms tend to present with locally advanced disease, often with nodal involvement, and are reported to have a significantly poorer prognosis (Spiro, Huvos and Strong, 1982).

A subset of adenocarcinoma, the polymorphous low-grade adenocarcinoma, has been recognized in recent years (Batsakis *et al.*, 1983). This tumour

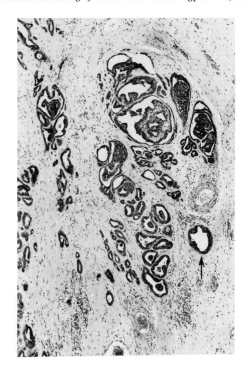

Figure 21.5 Adenocarcinoma. The neoplastic cells are arranged into tubular structures which are infiltrating a fibrous stroma

affects the minor salivary glands, particularly those of the palate, and usually presents as a firm painless swelling which is sometimes ulcerated. Its histological appearance is varied, often with aggressive features such as perineural and perivascular invasion. These appearances are misleading as the tumour rarely metastasizes but, if not adequately excised, local recurrence needs to be dealt with (Evans and Batsakis, 1984; Mitchell, Eveson and Ord, 1989).

The clinical management of this tumour is determined by the histological grade and the circumstances of the patient. It would be inappropriate to manage an elderly patient with a high grade tumour with anything other than palliation, whereas an identical tumour in a younger patient ought to be treated aggressively. Surgical treatment should be planned to provide a generous cuff of healthy tissue around the tumour.

Rare epithelial neoplasms

Of these only the undifferentiated carcinoma and squamous cell carcinoma are sufficiently frequent to deserve mention.

Undifferentiated carcinoma usually presents in middle age and constitutes 1.8% of all epithelial tumours. These neoplasms can be subdivided into small cell and large cell types, the small cell variety being twice as common as the large cell type (Nagao *et al.*, 1982). Some of the lesions included in this group could be very poorly differentiated adenocarcinomas or epidermoid carcinomas. The acinar arrangement of very poorly differentiated adenocarcinoma can be demonstrated by immunocytochemistry, thus facilitating a distinction between the groups (Heyderman *et al.*, 1985). Such distinction is essentially academic as this disease is very aggressive and requires radical surgery combined with postoperative radiotherapy to achieve a 5-year survival rate of 20–30%.

Squamous cell carcinoma of the salivary glands is very unusual but represents 1.1% of all salivary epithelial neoplasms. It tends to be restricted to the elderly. From a clinical standpoint, it is essential to establish that such a lesion does not represent a metastasis from a distant or regional site.

Carcinoma in pleomorphic adenoma

Rapid growth of a pleomorphic adenoma, the development of facial palsy, or the onset of pain, all suggest malignant change. Carcinoma in pleomorphic adenoma is a rare entity and is in fact a collective term for three or more main tumour types. Almost all are adenocarcinomas or undifferentiated carcinomas which are clearly seen to arise close to, or within, a pleomorphic adenoma (Figure 21.6). The majority of these carcinomas have been found to develop in recurrences (Seifert *et al.*, 1986). This subtype is termed 'carcinoma ex pleomorphic adenoma'. It is an aggressive disease with reported 5-year survival rates of 50%, and all patients died in whom the carcinoma extended more than 8 mm beyond the residual benign tumour, its capsule or invaded bone (Tortoledo, Luna and Batsakis, 1984). Perhaps this is a pessimistic assessment of this disease

as many more may have been missed due to the limitations of processing large pleomorphic tumours. Radical local resection and radiotherapy offer the best chance of control.

Rare variants of carcinoma in pleomorphic adenoma

The other subtypes of carcinoma in pleomorphic adenoma are exceptionally rare. A highly malignant, biphasic neoplasm composed of both epithelial and mesenchymal elements – a carcinosarcoma – is occasionally found (Bleiweiss *et al.*, 1992). Another type of tumour is completely indistinguishable from a benign pleomorphic adenoma but is found to metastasize to the lungs and bones (Batsakis, 1982; Wenig *et al.*, 1992). By definition, the diagnosis of this neoplasm is made at a time when therapeutic options are very limited. Indeed, experience with this tumour is anecdotal.

Lymphomas

Lymphomas comprise 40% of non-epithelial tumours and constitute the majority of the malignant lesions in this category. Non-Hodgkin's lymphomas predominate, grade 1 tumours being more common than grade 2. Three-quarters of these lymphomas are found in the parotid gland, and it is therefore possible that they arise in lymph nodes normally present within the gland. However, for staging purposes they are categorized as an extranodal site. Most lymphomas arise between the fifth and seventh decades of life and some are found in association with a benign lymphoepithelial lesion. There is increasing evidence to suggest that there is malignant transformation of the lymphocytic infiltrate in salivary glands of

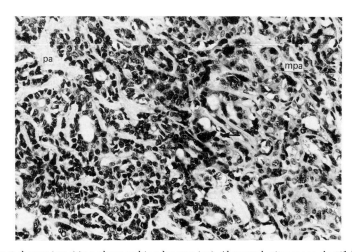

Figure 21.6 Malignant change (mpa) in a pleomorphic adenoma (pa). Abnormal mitoses are plentiful (arrowed)

patients with Sjögren's syndrome and that this usually presents as an extrasalivary lymphoma (Falzon and Isaacson, 1991).

Clinically, these lesions are firm and rapidly enlarging, and most give little more than a 6-month history. Pain and facial palsy are not prominent features, but the development of regional lymph node involvement is to be expected in those with delayed presentation.

In some instances, diagnostic suspicion may be so high as to justify open biopsy of a regionally involved node (Watkin, MacLellan and Hobsley, 1984), however, in view of the comparative rarity of these lesions this practice cannot be recommended for the inexperienced surgeon. The clinical stage and histological type of the lymphoma dictate the treatment regimen. Median survival for patients with this disease is 4 years. However, unlike other salivary gland tumours, advanced clinical stage does not appear to influence prognosis (Gleeson, Bennett and Cawson, 1986).

Management of malignant salivary gland tumours

Very few salivary gland tumours have specific features which are pathognomonic. In other words, unless very advanced, a large number are clinically indistinguishable from benign tumours. Open biopsy is almost totally contraindicated in these lesions, the exception being neoplasms of the minor glands. Tumour spilt by biopsy will seed the area and result in the development of multiple recurrences within the biopsy scar. The precise histological diagnosis can only be made from tissue obtained at the operation. Despite this, a strong suspicion of malignancy can be aroused by the clinical history, examination and preoperative investigations.

Most salivary gland neoplasms arise as painless masses which grow slowly. Rapid growth or acceleration of growth in a pre-existing lesion is a strong indication of malignancy, as is pain. It is almost impossible to distinguish by palpation alone whether a salivary gland mass is benign, malignant or inflammatory. Very few salivary gland tumours, including those that arise in the minor glands, present as ulcers from the outset. Facial, lingual and hypoglossal nerve palsies or evidence of infratemporal fossa infiltration (trismus) denote malignancy, but are uncommon. Similarly, enlarged regional lymph nodes or distant metastases, although indicative of malignancy, are a most uncommon presentation.

A staging system has been devised for malignant tumours arising within the major glands. Significant features for staging purposes are tumour size, local extension or fixation, neural involvement, nodal disease and distant metastases. The criteria for both the

TNM and clinical staging systems are shown in Table 21.6 (Levitt *et al.*, 1981; American Joint Committee on Cancer, 1988).

The preoperative and intraoperative diagnosis of these lesions relies upon the interpretation of CT and

Table 21.6 TNM classification system for malignant salivary tumours in major glands

Primary tumour (T)

TX	Primary tumour cannot be assessed
T0	No evidence of primary tumour
T1	Tumour 2 cm or less in greatest dimension
T2	Tumour > 2 cm but not more than 4.0 cm in greatest dimension
T3	Tumour > 4 cm but not more than 6.0 cm in greatest dimension
T4	Tumour > 6 cm in greatest dimension

All categories subdivided into:
  (*a*) no local extension
  (*b*) evidence of local extension
Local extension is defined as *clinical* evidence of invasion of either skin, soft tissue, bone or nerve.

Regional lymph nodes (N)

NX	Regional lymph nodes cannot be assessed
N0	No regional lymph node metastases
N1	Metastases in a single ipsilateral lymph node, 3 cm or less in greatest dimension
N2	Metastases in a single ipsilateral lymph node > 3 cm but not more than 6 cm in greatest dimension, or in multiple ipsilateral lymph nodes none more than 6 cm in greatest dimension, or in bilateral or contralateral lymph nodes none more than 6 cm in greatest dimension
	N2a Metastasis in single ipsilateral lymph node > 3 cm but not more than 6 cm in greatest dimension
	N2b Metastasis in multiple ipsilateral lymph nodes, none more than 6 cm in greatest dimension
	N2c Metastasis in bilateral or contralateral lymph nodes, none more than 6 cm in greatest dimension
N3	Metastasis in a lymph node > 6 cm in greatest dimension

Distant metastases (M)

MX	Presence of distant metastases cannot be assessed
M0	No distant metastases
M1	Distant metastases

Stage grouping

Stage I	T1a	N0	M0
	T2a	N0	M0
Stage II	T1b	N0	M0
	T2b	N0	M0
	T3a	N0	M0
Stage III	T3b	N0	M0
	T4a	N0	M0
	T < 4b	N1	M0
Stage IV	T4b	Any N	M0
	Any T	N2, N3	M0
	Any T	Any N	M1

MR images, aspiration cytology and frozen section histopathology, all considered in the context of the clinical findings.

Radiological evaluation of malignant salivary gland disease

CT and MR imaging have rendered other methods of demonstrating malignant salivary gland disease obsolete, for example contrast sialography and isotope studies (McGahan, Walter and Bernstein, 1984). The precise relation of the tumour to major structures – the external and internal carotid arteries, facial nerve and retromandibular vein – can be identified in parotid disease. Careful scrutiny of the integrity of the fibrofatty planes that demarcate the major glands from their surrounding structures gives valuable information about the tumour margin and any regional extension. Obliteration of this plane and obvious infiltration of the surrounding muscles indicate malignancy (Figure 21.7). The general consistency of the mass is also significant. Non-homogeneous tumours are more likely to be malignant than those displaying a homogeneous structure. Coronal sections of the facial canal may show expansion secondary to tumour infiltration in those patients with a facial palsy (Figure 21.8). However, tumour spread will always be far more proximal than the image indicates.

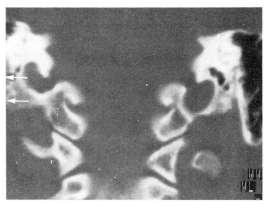

Figure 21.8 Coronal reconstruction of a CT scan from a patient with an adenoid cystic carcinoma of the parotid gland. Tumour has infiltrated the facial nerve and expanded the fallopian canal (arrows)

There is little doubt that MR images are superior to those derived by CT (Schaefer *et al.*, 1985). Tumour margins are seen with better clarity and the consistency of the lesions is more accurately depicted (Figure 21.9). Perhaps its most significant advantages

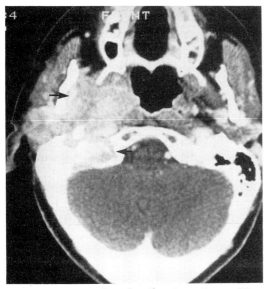

Figure 21.7 CT scan of an adenoid cystic carcinoma of the parotid (long arrow) which has obliterated the normal fatty tissue planes and is eroding the base of the skull (short arrow)

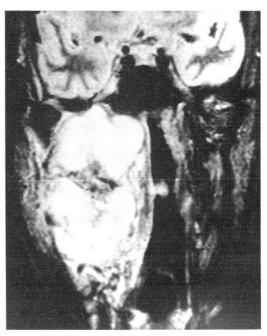

Figure 21.9 Coronal STIR (short tau inversion recovery) sequence MR scan of a deep lobe parotid pleomorphic adenoma. Part of the tumour has undergone malignant change which is represented by an area of decreased signal in its centre

are the lack of artefact from dental restorations, which often degrade CT images of this region, and sensitivity to small volumes of disease (Chaudhuri *et al.*, 1992a, b).

The choice between CT and MR will ultimately be determined by such factors as cost, availability, degree of suspicion of malignancy and site of the tumour. As stated previously, it is impossible to predict the malignant nature of every salivary gland mass and, without doubt, not every salivary gland mass needs to be scanned. However, CT or MR imaging is mandatory if any other investigation suggests malignancy.

The role of biopsy in the management of suspected salivary gland malignancy

Open biopsy of lesions in the major glands is totally contraindicated. Seeding of the area with neoplastic cells at the time of biopsy is inevitable, leading to local recurrence. Open biopsy as a prelude to treatment is only justified when the tumour arises in a minor gland, for example the palate. In these sites the overlying and adjacent mucosa should be removed as part of the definitive resection and therefore the extent and outcome of the procedure remains uninfluenced. This is not feasible in a major gland where the overlying skin is normally preserved and only has to be excised if it is infiltrated by tumour or if previous biopsy has been performed.

The concern about tumour spillage at the time of diagnostic biopsy has been overcome by fine needle aspiration biopsy. Seeding of salivary gland tumours by this technique has not been documented. The technique has two distinct limitations. First, the sample may miss a critical area in the tumour, for example a focus of malignant change within a pleomorphic adenoma. Second, accurate interpretation of smears requires considerable experience and skill on the part of the cytologist. At best a diagnostic accuracy of 85% can be achieved, but only by a few cytologists (Eneroth, Franzen and Zajicek, 1967; Sismanis *et al.*, 1981), and this degree of cytological expertise is rare. Notwithstanding this criticism, the distinction between benign and malignant disease can be made in over 90% of patients and this has immense clinical value. It is prudent therefore to consider such information in conjunction with that obtained by perioperative frozen section biopsy.

However, even frozen section analysis of salivary gland tumour tissue is difficult. Accurate histopathological diagnosis of neoplastic salivary gland tissue is not often achieved and false-negative (malignant called benign) rates of 5–12% are commonplace (Hillel and Fee, 1983; Wheelis and Yarrington, 1984). In providing a sample for frozen section it is essential that the pathologist receives a representative sample and that this includes part of the tumour capsule and adjacent normal glandular tissue.

It is evident that, in the majority of patients, histological diagnosis will prove impossible before surgery and that in a minority the definitive diagnosis will change from benign to malignant on examination of paraffin sections. The surgeon should be aware of this possibility and not compromise his surgical technique when the clinical findings conflict with the frozen section or cytological diagnosis.

Surgical management of malignant salivary gland disease

The high incidence of local recurrence following simple excision encouraged a more aggressive approach to the management of neoplastic salivary gland disease. Radical surgery, the removal of the entire gland, and more recently supraradical surgery, that is resection *en bloc* of the gland with its surrounding tissues and lymphatic drainage field, have been advocated for some tumours regardless of their stage (Conley and Dingman, 1974). There is little to suggest that these larger operations improve survival unless there is preoperative evidence of neural infiltration or lymph node metastases.

Parotid gland

The operative details of parotidectomy are described in Chapter 20. The fundamental principles of surgery for malignant parotid disease are adequate resection of tumour together with the branches or main trunk of the facial nerve when these are either directly involved or potentially so. Frozen section confirmation of tumour clearance in the ends of the resected facial nerve is a prerequisite before any attempt at reconstruction. There should be no hesitation to combine parotidectomy with removal of the mandibular ramus, infiltrated masticatory muscles and maxillary tuberosity in order to obtain a monobloc clearance. In some cases it will be necessary to perform a subtotal petrosectomy or mastoidectomy for tumour removal or to facilitate facial nerve repair.

If the facial nerve must be resected as many of its peripheral branches as possible should be identified at the outset, particularly those supplying the sphincters of the eye and mouth. The main trunk can be prepared at a site free from disease within the temporal bone. Bifurcated or multiple cable grafts can then be interposed to restore continuity. Suitable graft material may be obtained from the greater auricular nerve, sural nerve or cervical plexus. Meticulous attention to the accurate approximation and stabilization of the nerve and graft is essential for a good functional result (Fisch, 1974).

Neck dissection is definitely indicated if there is palpable neck disease, strong evidence of lymph node involvement on CT examination, or to facilitate myocutaneous flap repair of the defect. A strong case can be made for prophylactic neck dissection in specific tumour types which have a relatively poor prognosis, for example adenocarcinoma, squamous and undifferentiated carcinomas (Spiro, Wang and Montgomery, 1992). Albeit uncommon, it should be remembered that it is most unlikely that a patient can be salvaged if he or she subsequently develops neck disease. The definitive operation must include excision of the scar and overlying skin or mucosa if the patient has previously undergone open biopsy or incomplete removal of the tumour.

Submandibular gland

It is unusual for a submandibular salivary gland neoplasm to present as a mass associated with a palsy of the hypoglossal nerve, lingual nerve or mandibular branch of the facial nerve. More commonly suspicion is aroused by the consistency of the growth which tends to be hard and craggy when malignant. It is also unusual for a tumour to present as duct obstruction with a history of recurrent pain and swelling at meal times. In these patients a radiograph of the floor of the mouth will fail to reveal a calculus and therefore help to distinguish between a tumour and chronic sialadenitis.

The principles concerning preoperative biopsy hold as well for the submandibular gland as they do for the parotid. If fine needle aspiration and frozen section diagnosis indicate malignancy, the resection should include all nerves in close proximity to the tumour together with all suprahyoid lymph nodes.

The technique of removal of the submandibular gland is described in Chapter 20.

Minor salivary gland tumours

Approximately 85% of these lesions arise in either the palate, lip or buccal mucosa. At these sites the differential diagnosis is from a retention cyst or squamous cell carcinoma. The clinical distinction of a cyst by palpation is usually easy.

Resection with an adequate cuff of soft tissue can be achieved in most cases. The commonest site for one of these tumours is the hard palate which may be treated by partial maxillectomy. Since the overlying mucosa is removed in continuity with the tumour, it is permissible to biopsy lesions of the minor glands.

Great care must be taken in the assessment of tumours arising in the tonsillar and lateral oropharyngeal region. The clinically unwary may mistake a deep lobe parotid gland tumour for one arising in a minor gland. Deep lobe tumours must be removed by an external approach and previous biopsy increases the complications.

The role of radiotherapy

Radiotherapy should only be used as an adjunct to surgery in the treatment of malignant salivary gland tumours. The sole exception to this rule is that of early stage lymphomas which can be cured by radiation alone. There is a good case for reserving radiotherapy for specific types of tumour. It is certainly indicated for any tumour that shows locally aggressive features, for example perineural invasion, extensive soft tissue infiltration, lymph node spread and extranodal extension. It should also be given to those in whom the presence of residual disease is suspected after surgery, those whose disease lies close to a preserved facial nerve and in all who have undergone surgery for recurrent disease. It is claimed that with this management policy local recurrence rates are diminished. It is hard to prove these claims in diseases which are uncommon and run a very prolonged course. However, this treatment policy has become established for most tumour types (Jackson, Luna and Byers, 1983; Simpson, Thawley and Matsuba, 1984; Spiro, Wang and Montgomery, 1992). Until such data become available patients should not be denied possible benefit, a local dose of 6000 cGy being the accepted norm. However, radiotherapy should be withheld from some patients, for example those with low grade and early stage tumours that have been adequately excised. The side effects of radiotherapy, xerostomia and eustachian tube dysfunction, may then outweigh its potential benefits. Similarly, careful consideration should be given before irradiating benign tumours in young patients in whom the possibility of inducing a subsequent neoplasm is high.

Radiotherapy also has a role in the palliation of inoperable tumours. Pain can be alleviated to an extent and tumour progress retarded. Complete regression of tumour has been reported with fast neutron therapy but, to date, the experience with this modality has not been uniform (Catterall, Blake and Rampling, 1984).

The role of chemotherapy

Whether chemotherapy has a part to play in the management of these tumours has yet to be determined. Complete and partial responses to the administration of both single and multiple agents have been reported and either type of regimen would seem to be equally effective. Cisplatin, 5-fluorouracil and doxorubicin have all been claimed to be useful. No study to date has been able to determine whether chemotherapy prolongs survival time, but it is clear that in a large proportion of inoperable cases regression of disease and pain can be achieved, albeit temporarily (Suen and Johns, 1982).

Prognosis of salivary gland malignancy

Survival times vary widely according to many factors, namely histological type of salivary gland tumour, grade and stage of disease, age and sex of the patient, method of diagnosis and type of treatment administered. Of these, it is suggested that the stage of disease at presentation correlates the best with the ultimate outcome, as perhaps would be expected. Unfortunately, the data from which survival figures have been calculated are based on clinical material collected over decades. During this time considerable advances in diagnosis, operative technique and radiotherapy have been made, all of which influence the validity and accuracy of any conclusions. As a guide to the natural behaviour of the epithelial tumours irrespective of their treatment, grade and stage, the figures in Table 21.7 are the compilation of all reliable

Table 21.7 Prognosis of specific types of salivary gland tumours

Tumour type	No. cases	5-year survival (%)	10-year survival (%)
Acinic cell tumour	101	82	67.6
Mucoepidermoid tumour	749	70.7	50
Adenoid cystic carcinoma	1065	62.4	38.9
Malignant mixed tumour	383	55.7	31

(From Hickman, Cawson and Duffy, 1984)

series collected between 1964 and 1982 based on 2298 malignant salivary gland tumours. From this it can be seen that the malignant mixed tumour is the least favourable with a collective 5-year survival rate similar to that of carcinoma of the breast, while the acinic cell tumour has the best prognosis (Hickman, Cawson and Duffy, 1984).

References

ABBEY, L. M., SCHWAB, B. H., LANDAU, G. C. and PERKINS, E. R. (1984) Incidence of second primary breast cancer among patients with a first primary salivary gland tumour. *Cancer*, 54, 1439–1442

AMERICAN JOINT COMMITTEE ON CANCER (1988). *Manual for Staging of Cancer*, 3rd edn, edited by O. H. Beahrs, D. E. Henson, R. V. Hutter, and M. H. Myers. Philadelphia: J. B. Lippincott Company

BATSAKIS, J. G. (1982) Malignant mixed tumour. *Annals of Otology, Rhinology and Laryngology*, 91, 342–343

BATSAKIS, J. G. and LUNA, M. A. (1990) Histopathologic grading of salivary gland neoplasms. 1. Mucoepidermoid carcinomas. *Annals of Otology, Rhinology and Laryngology*, 99, 835–838

BATSAKIS, J. G. and REGEZI, J. A. (1979) The pathology of head and neck tumours: salivary glands, part 4. *Head and Neck Surgery*, 1, 340–349

BATSAKIS, J. G., LUNA, M. A. and EL-NAGGAR, A. (1990) Histopathologic grading of salivary gland neoplasms: III. Adenoid cystic carcinoma. *Annals of Otology, Rhinology and Laryngology*, 99, 1007–1009

BATSAKIS, J. G., CHIN, E. K., WEIMERT, T. A., WORK, W. P. and KRAUSE, C. J. (1979) Acinic cell carcinoma: a clinico-pathologic study of thirty-five cases. *Journal of Laryngology and Otology*, 93, 325–340

BATSAKIS, J. G., PINKSTON, G. R., LUNA, M. A., BYERS, R. M., SCIUBBA, J. J. and TILLERY, G. W. (1983) Adenocarcinoma of the oral cavity: a clinicopathologic study of terminal duct carcinomas. *Journal of Laryngology and Otology*, 97, 825–835

BLEIWEISS, J. W., ZIMMERMAN, M. C., ARNSTEIN, D. P., WOLLMAN, J. S. and MICKEL, R. A. (1992) Carcinosarcoma of the submandibular salivary gland. *Cancer*, 69, 2031–2035

BYERS, R. M., PIORKOWSKI, R. and LUNA, M. A. (1984) Malignant parotid tumours in patients under 20 years of age. *Archives of Otolaryngology*, 110, 232–235

CATTERALL, M., BLAKE, P. R. and RAMPLING, R. P. (1984) Fast neutron treatment as an alternative to radical surgery for malignant tumours of the facial area. *British Medical Journal*, 289, 1653–1655

CHAUDHURI, R., BINGHAM, J. B., CROSSMAN, J. E. and GLEESON, M. J. (1992a) Magnetic resonance imaging of the parotid gland using the STIR sequence. *Clinical Otolaryngology*, 17, 211–217

CHAUDHURI, R., GLEESON, M. J., KELLY, P. and BINGHAM, J. B. (1992b) MR evaluation of the parotid gland using STIR and gadolinium-enhanced imaging. *European Radiology*, 2, 357–364

CONLEY, J. and DINGMAN, D. L. (1974) Adenoid cystic carcinoma in the head and neck (cylindroma). *Archives of Otolaryngology*, 100, 81–90

DAVIES, J. N. P., DODGE, O. G. and BURKITT, D. P. (1964) Salivary gland tumours in Uganda. *Cancer*, 17, 1310–1322

DORN, M. F. and CUTLER, S. J. (1959) Morbidity from cancer in United States. *Public Health Monograph, No. 56*. Washington, DC: US Government Printing Office

EL-NAGGAR, A. K., BATSAKIS, J. G. and LUNA, M. A. (1990) DNA flow cytometry of acinic cell carcinomas of major salivary glands. *Journal of Laryngology and Otology*, 104, 410–416

ENEROTH, C. M., FRANZEN, S. and ZAJICEK, J. (1967) Cytologic diagnosis on aspirate from 1000 salivary gland tumours. *Acta Otolaryngologica Supplementum* 244, 168–171

ENEROTH, C. M., HJERTMAN, L. and MOBERGER, G. (1968) Adenoid cystic carcinoma of the palate. *Acta Otolaryngologica*, 66, 248–260

EVANS, H. L. (1984) Mucoepidermoid carcinoma of salivary glands: a study of 69 cases with special attention to histologic grading. *American Journal of Clinical Pathology*, 81, 696–701

EVANS, H. L. and BATSAKIS, J. G. (1984) Polymorphous low-grade adenocarcinomas of minor salivary glands: a study of 14 cases of a distinctive neoplasm. *Cancer*, 53, 935–942

EVESON, J. W. and CAWSON, R. A. (1985) Salivary gland tumours. A review of 2410 cases with particular reference to histological types, sites, age and sex distribution. *Journal of Pathology*, 146, 51–58

FALZON, M. and ISAACSON, P. G. (1991) The natural history of benign lymphoepithelial lesion of the salivary gland in which there is a monoclonal population of B cells. A report of two cases. *American Journal of Surgical Pathology*, **15**, 59–65

FISCH, U. (1974) Facial nerve grafting. *Otolaryngologic Clinics of North America*, **7**, 517–529

GLEESON, M. J., BENNETT, M. H. and CAWSON, R. A,. (1986) Lymphomas of salivary glands. *Cancer*, **58**, 699–704

HAMPER, K., SCHMITZ-WÄTJEN, W., MAUSCH, H.-E., CASELITZ, J. and SEIFERT, G. (1989) Multiple expression of tissue markers in mucoepidermoid carcinomas and acinic carcinomas of the salivary glands. *Virchows Archives [A]*, **414**, 407–413

HAMPER, K., MAUSCH, H.-E., CASELITZ, J., ARPS, H., BERGER, J. and ASKENSTEN, U. (1990) Acinic carcinoma of the salivary glands: the prognostic relevance of DNA cytophotometry in a retrospective study of long duration (1965–1987). *Oral Surgery, Oral Medicine and Oral Pathology*, **69**, 68–75

HEYDERMAN, E., LARKING, S. E., ALSOP, J. E., GLEESON, M. J., EVESON, J. W. and CAWSON, R. A. (1985) Epithelial markers in salivary gland tumours. *Journal of Pathology*, **146**, 265a

HICKMAN, R. E., CAWSON, R. A. and DUFFY, S. W. (1984) The prognosis of specific types of salivary gland tumours. *Cancer*, **54**, 1620–1624

HILLEL, A. D. and FEE, W. E. (1983) Evaluation of frozen section in parotid gland surgery. *Archives of Otolaryngology*, **109**, 230–232

JACKSON, G. L., LUNA, M. A. and BYERS, R. M. (1983) Results of surgery alone and surgery combined with post-operative radiotherapy in the treatment of cancer of the parotid gland. *American Journal of Surgery*, **146**, 497–500

LANIER, A. P., BENDER, T. R., BLOT, W. J., FRAUMENI, J. F. and HURLBURT, W. B. (1976) Cancer incidence in Alaska natives. *International Journal of Cancer*, **18**, 409–412

LENNOX, B., CLARKE, J. A., DRAKE, F. and EWEN, S. W. B. (1978) Incidence of salivary gland tumours in Scotland: accuracy of national records. *British Medical Journal*, **1**, 687–689

LEVITT, S. H., MCHUGH, R. B., GOMEZ-MARIN, O., HYAMS, V. J., SOULE, E. H., STRONG, E. W. *et al.* (1981) Clinical staging system for cancer of the salivary gland: a retrospective study. *Cancer*, **47**, 2712–2724

LOKE, Y. W. (1967) Salivary gland tumour in Malaya. *British Journal of Cancer*, **21**, 665–674

MCGAHAN, J. P., WALTER, J. P. and BERNSTEIN, L. (1984) Evaluation of the parotid gland. *Radiology*, **152**, 453–458

MATSUBA, H. M., THAWLEY, S. E., SIMPSON, J. R., LEVINE, L. A. and MAUNEY, M. (1984) Adenoid cystic carcinoma of major and minor salivary gland origin. *Laryngoscope*, **94**, 1316–1318 1316–1318

MITCHELL, D. A., EVESON, J. W. and ORD, R. A. (1989) Polymorphous low-grade adenocarcinoma of minor salivary glands: a report of three cases. *British Journal of Oral and Maxillofacial Surgery*, **27**, 494–500

NAGAO, K., MATSUZAKI, O., SAIGA, H., SUGANO, I., SHIGEMATSU, H., KANEKO, T. *et al.* (1982) Histopathologic studies of undifferentiated carcinoma of the parotid gland. *Cancer*, **50**, 1572–1579

OPCS CANCER STATISTICS (1983) *Survival series MBI No. 3. 1983.* London: HMSO

OPCS CANCER STATISTICS (1985) *Registration Series MB1 No 18.* London: HMSO

PERZIN, K. H., GULLANE, P. and CLAIRMONT, A. C. (1978) Adenoid cystic carcinomas arising in salivary glands. A correlation of histological features and clinical course. *Cancer*, **42**, 265–282

PERZIN, K. H., and LIVOLSI, V. A. (1979) Acinic cell carcinomas arising in salivary glands. *Cancer*, **44**, 1434–1457

PRIOR, P. and WATERHOUSE, J. A. H. (1977) Second primary cancers in patients with tumours of the salivary glands. *British Journal of Cancer*, **36**, 362–368

SAEMUNDSEN, A. K., ALBECK, H., HANSEN, J. P. H., NIELSEN, N. A., ANVRET, M., HANLE, W. *et al.* (1982) Epstein-Barr virus in nasopharyngeal and salivary gland carcinomas of Greenland Eskimos. *British Journal of Cancer*, **46**, 721–728

SCHAEFER, S. D., MARAVILLA, K. R., CLOSE, L. G., BURNS, D. K., MERKEL, M. A. and SUSS, R. A. (1985) Evaluation of NMR versus CT for parotid masses: a preliminary report. *Laryngoscope*, **95**, 945–950

SEIFERT, G. and SOBIN, L. H. (1991) Histological classification of salivary gland tumours. *World Health Organization, International Histological Classification of Tumours*. Berlin: Springer-Verlag

SEIFERT, G., MIEHLKE, A., HAUBRICH, J. and CHILLA, R. (1986) In: Adenoid cystic carcinoma. *Diseases of the Salivary Glands*. Stuttgart, New York: George Thieme Verlag: pp. 239–248

SHANNON ALLEN, M. and MARSH, W. L. (1976) Lymph node involvement by direct extension in adenoid cystic carcinoma. *Cancer*, **38**, 2017–2021

SHORE-FREEDMAN, E., ABRAHAMS, C., RECANT, W. and SCHNEIDER, A. (1983) Neurolemmomas and salivary gland tumors of the head and neck following childhood irradiation. *Cancer*, **51**, 2159–2163

SIMPSON, J. R., THAWLEY, S. E. and MATSUBA, H. M. (1984) Adenoid cystic salivary carcinoma: treatment with irradiation and surgery. *Radiology*, **151**, 509–512

SISMANIS, A., MERRIAM, J. M., KLINE, T. S., DAVIS, R. K., SHAPSAY, S. M. and STRONG, M. S. (1981) Diagnosis of salivary gland tumors by fine needle aspiration biopsy. *Head and Neck Surgery*, **3**, 482–489

SODER, P. O. (1973) The incidence of malignant tumours in the mouth-pharynx region in Sweden 1958–1967. *Swedish Dental Journal*, **66**, 419–428

SPIRO, R. H., HUVOS, A. G. and STRONG, E. W. (1974) Adenoid cystic carcinoma of salivary origin. A clinicopathological study of 242 cases. *American Journal of Surgery*, **128**, 512–520

SPIRO, R. H., HUVOS, A. G. and STRONG, E. W. (1982) Adenocarcinoma of salivary origin. Clinicopathologic study of 204 patients. *American Journal of Surgery*, **144**, 423–431

SPIRO, R. H., HUVOS, A. G., BERK, R. and STRONG, E. W. (1978) Mucoepidermoid carcinoma of salivary gland origin. A clinicopathologic study of 367 cases. *American Journal of Surgery*, **136**, 461–468

SPIRO, I. J., WANG, C. C. and MONTGOMERY, W. W. (1992) Carcinoma of the parotid gland. Analysis of treatment results and patterns of failure after combined surgery and radiation therapy. *Cancer*, **71**, 2699–2705

SPITZ, M., TILLEY, B., BATSAKIS, J., GIBEAU, J. and NEWELL, G. (1984) Risk factors for major salivary gland carcinoma. *Cancer*, **54**, 1854–1859

SPITZ, M. R., NEWELL, G. R., GIBEAU, J. M., BYERS, R. M. and BATSAKIS, J. G. (1985) Multiple primary cancer risk in patients with major salivary gland carcinoma. *Annals of Otology, Rhinology and Laryngology*, **94**, 129–132

SUEN, J. Y. and JOHNS, M. E. (1982) Chemotherapy for salivary gland cancer. *Laryngoscope*, **92**, 235–239

SZANTO, P. A., LUNA, M. A., TORTOLEDO, M. E. and WHITE, R. A.

(1984) Histologic grading of adenoid cystic carcinoma of the salivary glands. *Cancer*, **54**, 1062–1069

TAKEICHI, N., HIROSE, F. and YAMAMOTO, H. (1976) Salivary gland tumours in atomic bomb survivors, Hiroshima, Japan. *Cancer*, **38**, 2462–2468

TAKEICHI, N., HIROSE, F., YAMAMOTO, H., EZAKI, H. and FU-JIKURA, T. (1983) Salivary gland tumours in atomic bomb survivors, Hiroshima, Japan. *Cancer*, **52**, 377–385

THACKRAY, A. C. and SOBIN, L. H. (1972) Histological typing of salivary gland tumours. *International Histological Classification of Tumours No. 7*, Geneva: WHO. pp. 16–27

TORTOLEDO, M. E., LUNA, M. A. and BATSAKIS, J. G. (1984) Carcinomas ex pleomorphic adenoma and malignant mixed tumours. *Archives of Otolaryngology*, **110**, 172–176

WATKIN, G. T., MACLELLAN, K. A. and HOBSLEY, M. (1984) Lymphomas presenting as lumps in the parotid region. *British Journal of Surgery*, **71**, 701–702

WENIG, B. M., HITCHCOCK, C. L., ELLIS, G. L. and GNEPP, D. R. (1992) Metastasising mixed tumor of salivary glands. A clinicopathologic and flow cytometric study. *American Journal of Surgical Pathology*, **16**, 845–858

WHEELIS, R. F. and YARRINGTON, C. T. (1984) Tumours of the salivary glands. Comparison of frozen-section diagnosis with the final pathologic diagnosis. *Archives of Otolaryngology*, **110**, 76–77

22

Tumours of the infratemporal fossa and parapharyngeal space

O. H. Shaheen

The division of the space lying below the skull base and lateral to the pharynx into two entities, namely the infratemporal fossa and parapharyngeal space, appealing though it may be to traditionalists, is of dubious practical significance. The surgical literature has tended to treat these two spaces separately, while on occasions blurring the distinction between the two, and has failed to acknowledge sufficiently that they are often the seat of one and the same disease.

Ostensibly separated by the medial pterygoid muscle, the two spaces intercommunicate freely behind this muscle, and it is difficult therefore to understand why they should be looked upon as separate compartments. Nevertheless, for the sake of clarity and to appreciate what has been written before, the shape, size, boundaries, and relationship of the two spaces to each other need to be clearly visualized in the mind of the surgeon, while accepting the concept that the one space is merely an extension of the other.

As stated above, the dividing line between the infratemporal fossa and parapharyngeal space is essentially the medial pterygoid muscle; the former lies above it and the latter below it, and the hiatus which exists behind the posterior free edge of the muscle is where the two spaces merge freely with each other. In essence therefore, the two compartments are separated by the medial pterygoid in their anterior halves, but posteriorly there is nothing between them (Figure 22.1).

Anatomy

The infratemporal fossa

This compartment lies below the base of the skull deep to the ascending ramus of the mandible. Shaped rather like an inverted pyramid, it possesses a roof, anterior, lateral and medial walls, a posterior edge,

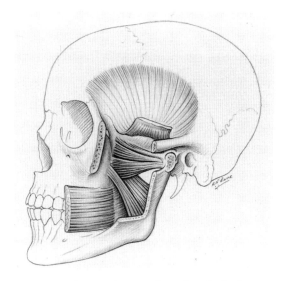

Figure 22.1 The medial pterygoid muscle is the dividing line between the infratemporal fossa and parapharyngeal space

and an apex inferiorly. It is filled with muscles, nerves and blood vessels and it communicates with adjacent anatomical spaces by fissures and openings.

The roof is formed by the infratemporal surface of the greater wing of the sphenoid bone and further back by a small part of the squamous temporal bone. The gap between the lateral edge of the bony roof and the upper limit of the lateral boundary accommodates the temporalis muscle and communicates superiorly with the temporal fossa (Figure 22.2).

Inferiorly, the fossa is limited by the upper surface of the medial pterygoid and the attachment of this

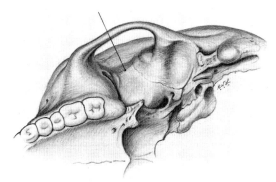

Figure 22.2 The roof of the infratemporal fossa is formed mainly by the greater wing of the sphenoid

muscle to the inner aspect of the lower part of the ascending ramus of the mandible. Behind the muscle, lies the hiatus which communicates below with the parapharyngeal space.

The lateral pterygoid plate represents the anterior half of the medial wall of the infratemporal fossa, with the tensor palati and superior constrictor forming the posterior half of the medial wall.

On the lateral side, the inner aspect of the zygomatic arch, the masseter and temporalis muscles, the ascending ramus of the mandible, the uppermost part of the deep lobe of the parotid gland and the styloid apparatus constitute the external boundary.

The anterior wall of the fossa is the rounded posterolateral wall of the maxillary antrum, and the posterior margin the innermost part of the tympanic plate.

The infratemporal fossa communicates with the pterygopalatine fossa through the pterygomaxillary fissure, which occupies the junction of anterior and medial walls (Figure 22.3).

The inferior orbital fissure similarly forms a connection with the orbit at the junction of the roof and anterior walls (Figure 22.4). The gap between the anterior edge of the ascending ramus of the mandible and the posterolateral wall of the maxilla represents a potential channel of communication between the infratemporal fossa and the oral cavity.

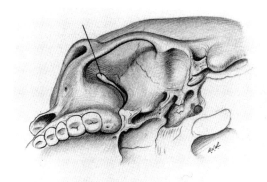

Figure 22.4 The inferior orbital fissure

The muscles which fill the infratemporal fossa are the medial and lateral pterygoids and the temporalis. The maxillary artery crosses the fossa, giving off its five named branches on the way to the infraorbital and pterygomaxillary fissures. The fossa abounds with thin walled veins, some of which are grouped together within and overlying the pterygoid muscles as the pterygoid venous plexus. The mandibular division of the Vth cranial nerve, its anterior and posterior subdivisions and their branches traverse the length of the fossa, mainly in a downward and lateral direction, between the pterygoid muscles (Figure 22.5).

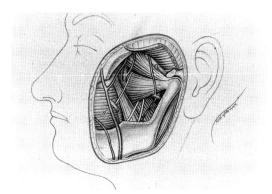

Figure 22.5 The muscles and the nerves of the infratemporal fossa

The parapharyngeal space

This space has had a number of names in the past including the pterygomaxillary space, lateral pharyn-

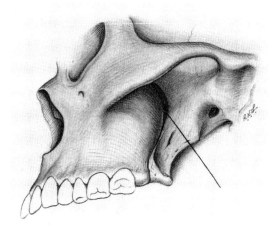

Figure 22.3 The pterygomaxillary fissure

geal space, and pharyngomaxillary space, but the present term which has come to stay evokes the clearest image of its location. It is distinct from the retropharyngeal space, which lies between the posterior aspect of the pharynx, and the prevertebral fascia and underlying prevertebral muscles.

The roof of the parapharyngeal space is the sharp angle formed by the insertion of the medial pterygoid muscle into the inner aspect of the lateral pterygoid plate on the one hand, and by the superior constrictor muscle on the other (Figure 22.6). The medial boundary is the lateral wall of the pharynx, while the lateral limit superiorly is formed by the medial or undersurface of the medial pterygoid muscle, and further posteriorly by the deep lobe of the parotid gland and styloid apparatus. Shaped rather like a boat the parapharyngeal space narrows anteriorly where the superior constrictor is attached to the pterygomandibular raphe, whereas it is somewhat broader posteriorly where the carotid sheath separates it from the prevertebral muscles, and where it merges medially with the retropharyngeal space.

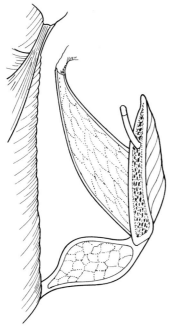

Figure 22.6 The roof of the parapharyngeal space is the junction between the medial pterygoid muscle and superior constrictor

Superiorly, the anterior half of the parapharyngeal space is separated from the infratemporal fossa by the medial pterygoid muscle, while the posterior half is continuous with it. Inferiorly, the parapharyngeal space descends into the neck medial to the carotid sheath.

Unlike the infratemporal fossa, which is filled with named arteries, veins, and nerves, the parapharyngeal space is relatively devoid of such structures. Its lower extremity which descends into the neck is traversed by the superior laryngeal nerve and further down the pharyngeal branch of the vagus nerve.

The parapharyngeal space contains loose fibroalveolar tissue and small islands of salivary gland tissue, derived presumably from the deep lobe of the parotid gland. There are no lymph nodes within it, by contrast with the adjacent retropharyngeal space which harbours a small number of longitudinally arranged nodes.

Pathology of tumours arising from or invading the infratemporal fossa and parapharyngeal space

Primary tumours of the infratemporal fossa are uncommon, whereas those arising from within the parapharyngeal space are somewhat more frequent. In each instance, tumours may enlarge to fill the compartment in which they arose, and then spill over to occupy the adjacent compartment.

Invasion of either, or both spaces by disease arising in adjacent structures is not infrequent.

Primary tumours arising in the infratemporal fossa include extracranial meningiomas, fibrosarcomas, chondrosarcomas, histiocytosis X, lymphomas and angiomas (Conley, 1964; Arena and Hilal, 1976; Shaheen, 1982). Primary tumours arising within the parapharyngeal space are mainly pleomorphic adenomas originating from detached islands of salivary gland tissue (Work and Gates, 1969; Som, Biller and Lawson, 1981).

Invasion of both spaces from adjacent structures and anatomical areas is not uncommon. Typical examples of benign swellings are angiofibromas, ameloblastomas of the upper and lower jaws, and pleomorphic adenomas arising within the deep lobe of the parotid gland and escaping into the parapharyngeal space. Angiofibromas make their way into the infratemporal fossa via the pterygopalatine fossa first, and then through the pterygomaxillary fissure, while ameloblastomas extend directly into the infratemporal fossa. The passage of mixed tumours arising from within the deep lobe of the parotid gland into the parapharyngeal space occurs through the tunnel bounded by the posterior edge of the ascending ramus of the mandible and the styloid process and stylomandibular ligament.

Other examples of obliteration of the parapharyngeal space by benign swellings are carotid body and glomus vagale tumours, neurilemmomas and neurofibromas. As they grow upwards, they ultimately come to fill the infratemporal fossa. Glomus jugulare tumours will extend downwards and expand the carotid sheath, but rarely invade the parapharyngeal space. Superiorly, however, they will extend along the skull base in the direction of the carotid foramen and will thus lie in the infratemporal fossa.

Chordomas will displace the prevertebral muscles forwards into both spaces and eventually come to fill the infratemporal fossa. Cancers of the nasopharynx, maxillary antrum, and oral cavity all invade the infratemporal fossa. In the last instance spread may occur either through the hiatus between the maxilla and ascending ramus of the mandible, or along the inferior dental canal of the mandible.

Specific common tumours of the infratemporal fossa and parapharyngeal space

Angiofibroma

It is now accepted that angiofibromas arise in or close to the sphenopalatine foramen, and either grow into the nasopharynx or outwards into the pterygo-palatine fossa or both. As they escape laterally through the pterygomaxillary fissure, they push the posterolateral wall of the antrum anteriorly, produc-ing the classical radiological feature of bowing of the posterior antral wall (Figure 22.7). Eventually, they come to fill the infratemporal fossa and further expan-sion is by way of the inferior orbital fissure into the orbit, or into the space between the maxilla and ascend-ing ramus of the mandible. Erosion of the undersur-face of the sphenoid bone also takes place and the swelling becomes intimately attached to the dura.

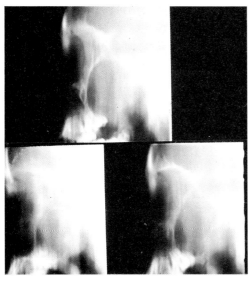

Figure 22.7 Bowing of the posterior antral wall

Chordoma

This tumour is derived from the primitive notochord and presents as a swelling in the prevertebral region behind the nasopharynx. It pushes the posterior wall of the nasopharynx forwards so that, on clinical examination, a smooth non-ulcerating swelling is noted in the posterior wall and roof of the nasopha-rynx. Expansion laterally and anterolaterally forces the prevertebral fascia forward with escape of disease eventually into the infratemporal fossa. As the disease grows it picks off the last four cranial nerves and this may be how it first presents. The tumour itself is soft in consistency, almost gelatinous, and for that reason it is virtually impossible to ensure its complete re-moval. When operating on chordomas much of the tumour finds its way into the sucker because of its almost liquid consistency.

Meningioma

This tumour may arise rarely as a primary extracra-nial tumour of the infratemporal fossa, taking its origin from the dural sheath which surrounds the trunk of the mandibular division of the trigeminal nerve as it makes its exit from the foramen ovale. It presents as a hard or firm nodular swelling which fills the infratemporal fossa, extends into nooks and crannies which represent points of escape from the fossa, and eventually extends downwards into the parapharyngeal space.

Escape of an intracranial meningioma through the base of the skull is by comparison a likelier event, rare though it may be in itself. With large intracranial meningiomas, escape may occur through more than one orifice, depending on the site of origin of the tumour within the skull. Posterior fossa neoplasms may grow through the foramen magnum and anter-ior condylar and jugular foraminae, while middle fossa tumours may come through the foramen lacerum and ovale. Once outside the skull, such tumours display an alarming propensity to spread inferiorly, first into the infratemporal fossa and then the parapharyngeal space which is obliterated from above downwards as far as the carotid triangle of the neck. Structures which lie in the way are either displaced, become attached, or completely encircled by the downward growth of the tumour. It is usual to find that the last four cranial nerves and internal carotid artery are either fused to the growth or encom-passed by it to the point that their preservation is impossible (Figure 22.8).

Ameloblastomas

The majority of these tumours are benign and rarely grow to the extent of filling the infratemporal fossa or parapharyngeal space. Those arising from the maxilla may expand posteriorly into the infratemporal fossa without involving or invading the structures therein. The mandibular ameloblastoma more often than not arises from the horizontal ramus of the mandible and is likely therefore to bulge into the parapharyngeal

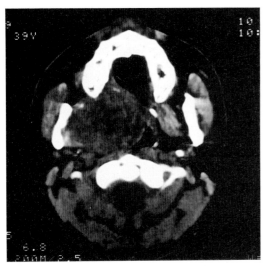

Figure 22.8 Extracranial meningioma filling the infratemporal fossa and parapharyngeal space

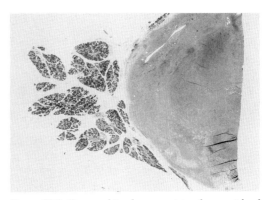

Figure 22.9 Pleomorphic adenoma arising from an island of salivary tissue in the parapharyngeal space

space rather than the infratemporal fossa but, if spread into the ascending ramus has occurred, the infratemporal fossa may become involved secondarily. Apart from the possible risk of rupture during surgical excision the mere fact of spread into either space should not be considered alarming since ameloblastomas which have broken through the cortex of the bone from which they arose are contained by the tough inner periosteum. Their rare malignant counterparts are however destructive, and involvement of the infratemporal fossa or parapharyngeal space is characterized by adherence to structures initially, and infiltration subsequently. The extent of spread is such that attempts to encompass the escape of disease into these spaces are usually unsuccessful.

Pleomorphic adenomas

These are by far the most common tumours to involve the parapharyngeal space primarily and the infratemporal fossa secondarily. They may arise from detached islands of normal salivary gland tissue which lie in the parapharyngeal space medial to the deep lobe of the parotid gland (Figure 22.9). As they fill the space they displace the medial pterygoid muscle upwards and laterally, the parotid gland outwards and the palatofaucial region of the oropharynx medially. They do not become attached to these structures, but in the case of the medial pterygoid, its muscular bundles become stretched out over the expanding tumour.

Only in the event of these tumours being biopsied, which sadly continues to occur, will they become adherent to the overlying soft tissues through which the biopsy has been taken.

Pleomorphic adenomas may also arise from within the deep lobe of the parotid gland and grow into the parapharyngeal space, eventually filling it and displacing the pharynx inwards (Figure 22.10). Their route of escape from the deep lobe of the parotid gland into the parapharyngeal space is invariably through the so-called stylomandibular tunnel, a hiatus bounded on one side by the posterior edge of the ascending ramus of the mandible and on the other by the stylomandibular ligament and styloid process. The dimensions of this space are relatively small, so that the tumour is constricted as it passes through it, hence the overall appearance of a dumb-bell with enlarged inner and outer components and a narrow waist lying in the stylomandibular tunnel. It should be emphasized that the term dumb-bell tumour applies to the situation just described, as opposed to a pleomorphic adenoma which involves both superficial and deep lobes and which displays an area of constriction as it passes between the divisions of the facial nerve or, above or below the main trunk of the nerve.

Enlargement of deep lobe or primary parapharyngeal pleomorphic adenomas is eventually limited by the confined space which they come to occupy. Once the parapharyngeal space is filled, expansion continues into the infratemporal fossa as high up as the base of the skull with the tumour coming to rest on the eustachian tube. However, the consistency of pleomorphic adenomas is rarely tough enough to cause bone erosion in the manner of angiofibromas.

Malignant tumours of the parotid gland

The deep lobe of the parotid gland is sometimes the seat of malignancy, usually adenoidcystic carcinoma. Growth occurs medially and laterally, and structures blocking the path of the growing tumour are infiltrated. Extension medially quickly involves the medial

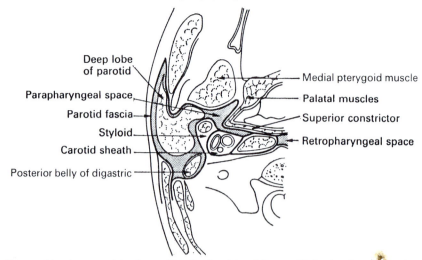

Figure 22.10 Pleomorphic adenoma arising from within the deep lobe of the parotid gland and traversing the parapharyngeal space

pterygoid muscle, while upward extension into the infratemporal fossa involves the base of the skull and eustachian tube.

Lateral growth into the superficial lobe of the parotid gland picks off the facial and auriculotemporal nerves, and eventually the posterior fibres of the masseter. Erosion of bone is uncommon, but occurs when the tumour is no longer free to expand through soft tissues.

Neurogenic tumours

Neurogenic tumours are divided into three categories, namely neurilemmomas, otherwise referred to more accurately as schwannomas, and neurofibromas and ganglion neuromas.

The schwannoma is the most common of the neurogenic tumours in the head and neck, and possesses a rare malignant counterpart which infiltrates adjacent tissues and metastasizes. The tumour takes it origin from the Schwann cells which surround motor and sensory nerve axons. These tumours grow longitudinally along the length of the nerve, assuming a fusiform appearance but without compromising the morphological or functional integrity of the nerve. They can therefore be separated surgically from their nerve of origin, leaving it more or less intact. In practice, however, the process of separation is likely to result in a disturbance of function, although this does not preclude an eventual return to normality.

These tumours are firm to hard in consistency and on section are often studded with areas of cystic degeneration, haemorrhage or lipid deposition.

Neurofibromas have a double origin from the Schwann cells and perineurium and are inextricably intertwined with the nerve from which they arise. They cannot therefore be separated from the nerve, which has to be sectioned above and below the tumour. Macroscopically, they resemble schwannomas in appearance, and the distinction can only be made microscopically.

Ganglion neuromas, which are exceedingly rare, arise as the name implies from ganglia and, in the head and neck, the likeliest site of origin is the superior cervical ganglion of the sympathetic trunk, which lies posteromedial to the internal carotid artery just below the base of the skull.

The nerves which give rise to schwannomas and neurofibromas are chiefly the vagus and its branches, the hypoglossal nerve, and branches of the cervical plexus. Tumours of the first two nerves, namely the vagus and hypoglossal, will encroach significantly on the posterior half of the parapharyngeal space. If the site of origin is high up, they may splay out the internal carotid artery and internal jugular vein, causing the former to be displaced anteromedially further into the parapharyngeal space and the latter outwards. Ganglion neuromas will displace the internal carotid forwards and also annexe the posterior part of the parapharyngeal space. Surgical resection of the tumour is not problematical when dealing with benign variants of these tumours, but the greatest single problem is one of access.

Chemodectomas

Carotid body tumours, glomus vagale and glomus jugulare tumours all arise from chemoreceptor bodies, which are situated at the carotid bifurcation, along the trunk of the vagus, on its ganglion nodosum, and on the jugular bulb. They are more common in women and those living at high altitudes, and are not uncommonly bilateral. Occasionally they secrete catecholamines, and rarely present as a malignancy which metastasizes regionally and distantly.

Carotid body tumours

These arise beneath the adventitia in the carotid bifurcation and grow upwards between the internal and external carotid arteries, displacing the adventitia of each vessel superiorly, splaying the one vessel anteromedially and the other laterally.

They may ultimately reach the base of the skull, and in so doing, come to occupy the parapharyngeal space and the infratemporal fossa.

Nerves in close proximity to the tumour such as the vagus, the pharyngeal branch of the vagus, the superior laryngeal nerve, and the hypoglossal, become fused to the capsule of the advancing tumour and cannot be easily saved at operation.

Carotid body tumours are characterized by a rich blood supply and a surface vasculature of small blood vessels which bleed readily on touch, thus rendering their excision a slow and laborious process. They are often firmly embedded in the wall of the carotid bifurcation, to the extent that a tear in the vessel wall often results as the tumour is being prised away from the bifurcation.

Glomus vagale tumours

These are almost indistinguishable in appearance from carotid body tumours, but certain features are characteristic. They lie somewhat more posteriorly and tend to push the internal carotid artery forwards, and the internal jugular vein laterally, rather than splaying out the two carotid arteries as does a carotid body tumour. They do not arise from the carotid bifurcation, and their surface vasculature is much less evident, so that excision is much more straightforward. Rarely, however is it possible to save the vagus nerve when resecting these tumours.

Glomus jugulare tumours

The glomus jugulare tumours, unlike the aforementioned neoplasm, lack a distinct capsule. Much of their impact is on the petrous bone, but they grow downwards in and around the internal jugular vein to a limited extent, and also forwards beneath the base of the skull towards the carotid foramen, in parallel with intraosseous spread towards the bony carotid canal. They may thus come to occupy the posterior and uppermost part of the infratemporal fossa (Figure 22.11).

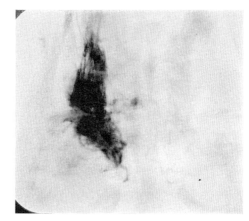

Figure 22.11 Downward extension of a glomus jugulare tumour within and around the internal jugular vein

Invasion of the infratemporal fossa and parapharyngeal space by squamous carcinoma

The nasopharynx, maxillary antrum and oral cavity are all related to the infratemporal fossa and parapharyngeal space and therefore squamous carcinoma arising at these sites may invade both spaces.

Escape of cancer from the fossa of Rosenmüller into the infratemporal fossa probably occurs more often than one suspects, even in the absence of overt involvement of the mandibular division of the Vth cranial nerve. Extensive invasion results in trismus, as much from infiltration of the lateral and medial pterygoids as invasion of the nerve itself.

In the past, such invasion was presumed on the basis of clinical signs, but modern scanning facilities can demonstrate this at an earlier stage.

Similarly, erosion of the posterior antral wall by squamous carcinoma arising from within the antrum allows tumour to enter the infratemporal fossa, and by infiltrating the pterygoids, to cause trismus. Tumour will track proximally along the posterior superior dental nerves towards the pterygomaxillary fissure and pterygopalatine fossa, and then along the maxillary nerve into the foramen rotundum (Figure 22.12). Extended maxillectomy offers a means of maximizing the excision of all bulk disease, leaving microscopical residues to be destroyed by radiotherapy.

The route by which oral cancer escapes posteriorly depends on its precise location. Tumours of the floor of mouth will generally escape along the pathway of the lingual nerve into the infratemporal fossa, in much the same way as carcinoma of the alveolus follows the inferior dental nerve into the infratemporal fossa. Buccal and retromolar trigone tumours, once past the pterygomandibular raphe, will choose the closest avenue to spread backwards into either

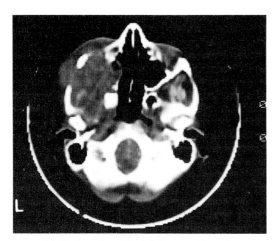

Figure 22.12 Invasion of the infratemporal fossa by carcinoma of the antrum

the infratemporal fossa or parapharyngeal space. Tonsillar tumours on the other hand by virtue of a more posteriorly placed position will invade the parapharyngeal space rather than the infratemporal fossa. The net result is similar in all instances in terms of symptoms and signs which are related to infiltration of the medial pterygoid muscle and involvement of branches of the mandibular division of the Vth nerve and the glossopharyngeal nerve.

Rare tumours affecting the infratemporal fossa

During the course of a busy career, the head and neck surgeon will encounter a small number of exceptionally rare tumours which affect the infratemporal fossa. These will vary in degree of malignancy, and may be amenable to resection. At the lower end of the spectrum of malignancy are osteoblastomas arising from the greater wing of the sphenoid, histiocytosis X, and desmoid tumours, previously referred to as fibrosarcomas. Quite often the symptoms produced by these growths are minimal, and the condition only comes to light because of the presence of a swelling.

More aggressive are chondrosarcomas arising from the skull base or the pterygoid plates and infiltrating and destroying soft tissues and bone, with symptoms and signs to match.

Tumours of lymphatic origin and lymph node metastases

Although traversed by lymphatic channels, there are no lymph nodes in the infratemporal fossa, and those related to the parapharyngeal space are found at its outer and inner extremities. The node of Rouviere and retropharyngeal nodes actually lie in the retropharyngeal space, with which both spaces communicate, and are situated on the prevertebral fascia lateral to the midline. The upper deep cervical nodes lie

lateral to the internal jugular vein and are therefore at the very edge of the parapharyngeal space.

Metastatic carcinoma in the upper deep cervical nodes may on occasions grow to such a size as to occupy the parapharyngeal space. Similarly cancer in a lymph node with no known primary, may present as a parapharyngeal mass.

The node of Rouviere is at times the seat of metastatic disease from carcinoma of the nasopharynx, and will extend laterally into both spaces. Such metastatic disease may present as a posterior or posterolateral swelling of the naso- and oropharynx, with little sign of any primary mucosal disease, and thus be mistaken for a neurogenic tumour.

Disease in the lymph aggregates within the parotid gland does not invade the parapharyngeal space, since the 15 or so follicles or 'nodes' mostly lie in the superficial lobe of the gland.

Lymphoma of the nodes bordering the parapharyngeal space and infratemporal fossa will invade both spaces and present as a large mass, but curiously lymphoma may also arise at sites which are known not to contain lymphoid tissue, such as the infratemporal fossa, and presents with the classical signs of an infratemporal fossa tumour.

Clinical aspects
Infratemporal fossa

Benign primary tumours cannot be seen or felt while still confined within the boundaries of the fossa. It is not until expansion has occurred via the various channels of escape that they make their presence known.

Pain or discomfort is minimal in such patients, and little more than a dull ache. Clinically a bulge in the temple above the zygomatic arch indicates upward extension into the temporal fossa deep to the temporalis muscle (Figure 22.13). Occasionally a small bulge may be noticeable in the small lateral hiatus of the infratemporal fossa represented by the coronoid notch (Figure 22.14). The lateral wall of the nasopharynx may be pushed inwards, indicating displacement of the superior constrictor muscle and pharyngobasilar fascia behind the medial pterygoid plate. Similarly there may be proptosis as a result of orbital invasion through the inferior orbital fissure.

Escape of benign primary tumours of the infratemporal fossa to the oral cavity is rarely detected by inspection, since the oral mucous membrane in the area is inelastic and resists forward extension of the tumour. However the tumour may be palpable in the gap between the ascending ramus of the mandible and the maxilla.

Pressure of a hard mass in the infratemporal fossa is likely to cause either collapse or dysfunction of the eustachian tube with consequent secretory otitis media.

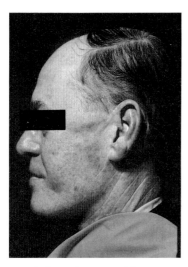

Figure 22.13 A bulge in the temporal fossa is typical of a large space-occupying lesion of the infratemporal fossa

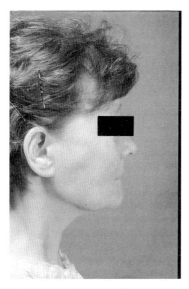

Figure 22.14 A bulge in the coronoid notch suggests a mass in the infratemporal fossa

Malignant primary or secondary swellings of the infratemporal fossa are characterized by pain, often very severe, anaesthesia in the distribution of the mandibular division of the Vth nerve, and trismus, in addition to swelling as outlined above.

Parapharyngeal space

Benign swellings are painless and detected either by the patient or during the course of a routine examina-tion. In patients where the swelling has reached large proportions, there may in addition be the typical signs of an infratemporal fossa tumour.

Swelling is noted in two specific areas, namely the oropharynx and the neck, including at times the parotid gland region. Pleomorphic adenomas arising in the parapharyngeal space cause a bulge of the homolateral soft palate, tonsil and faucial pillars. They rarely cause much external swelling of the parotid gland. To palpation they feel firm and rub-bery, and the classical sign of ballotement elicited by bimanual palpation, with one finger on the palato-fauces and a hand on the parotid area, is often indeterminate (Figure 22.15).

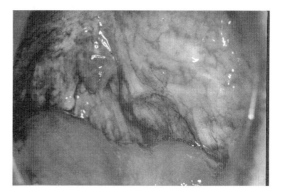

Figure 22.15 Pleomorphic adenoma presenting as a swelling in the palatofaucial region

Tumours arising from within the deep lobe of the parotid and crossing the parapharyngeal space will cause swelling of the palatofaucial region and obvious swelling of the parotid gland. Here the sign of ballote-ment is positive (Figure 22.16).

Large tumours of either kind will ultimately come to exert pressure on the eustachian tube with result-ing serous otitis.

Benign tumours of nerve origin and chemodecto-mas present as painless swellings in the carotid trian-gle of the neck, extending upwards deep to the mandi-ble and parotid gland, causing the parotid gland to bulge outwards. Like pleomorphic adenomas, they often present in the oral cavity as a bulge, which can be mistaken for a tumour of salivary gland origin. The inexperienced have fallen into the trap of assum-ing the oral swelling to be a quinsy, with unfortunate consequences, but the absence of trismus effectively rules out an inflammatory condition.

Uncommonly, a carotid body tumour will present with a nerve palsy, either vagal or hypoglossal, and this should not be taken to signify malignant transfor-mation. The cause is not clear since there is rarely any doubt about the benign nature of the swelling, but could be related to stretching or distortion of the nerve in question by the tumour. Some carotid body tumours are associated with headache, or a tendency

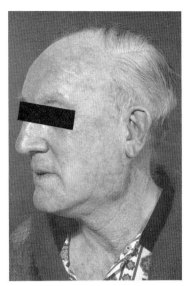

Figure 22.16 Pleomorphic adenoma arising from within the deep lobe of the parotid gland and invading the parapharyngeal space will cause an external bulge in the parotid area

to syncope, calling into question the possibility that they may be secreting catecholamines. When examining a seemingly unilateral carotid body tumour, the possibility of a small contralateral growth or other chemodectomas should not be forgotten.

Malignant swellings in or bordering the parapharyngeal space are associated with pain, trismus, and loss of nerve function.

Investigations

Radiology

The refinements in modern radiological techniques have been of considerable benefit to the clinician, particularly when dealing with potentially complex problems such as those involving the infratemporal fossa and parapharyngeal space. A good example is the accurate definition of extrapharyngeal extensions of angiofibromas which show up with remarkable clarity, and which allows the clinician to select the appropriate surgical strategy. Before the advent of computerized methods, such extensions were overlooked, and resulted in operations being unnecessarily difficult and dangerous. MRI and CT scanning permit the precise assessment of size, shape, and consistency of a lesion, the definition of its margins, and its relationship to surrounding structures. Perhaps most important of all is the opportunity to decide on what is technically removable or not. The statement that MRI is better for soft tissues and CT for bone is broadly true, but in the absence of one or

the other, the information gained from either method is adequate for the majority of cases. Ideally both should be used as they complement each other, and often one method will fill in details which are absent in the other.

CT scanning, digital subtraction angiography and carotid angiography are of considerable use in the overall assessment of angiofibromas, and have removed the need for biopsy, which is invariably attended by severe haemorrhage.

So far as pleomorphic adenomas are concerned, CT and MRI will display the extent to which such neoplasms fill the parapharyngeal space and infratemporal fossa and establish whether the tumour is intrinsically of deep lobe origin or arising independently of the parotid gland. If the latter, there will actually be a narrow space between the tumour and parotid gland, thus introducing the possibility of removing it without dissection of the facial nerve. CT with enhancement will diagnose the majority of carotid body and glomus vagale tumours. Either digital subtraction angiography and arteriography are useful to confirm the diagnosis, demonstrate the full extent of the tumour and its proximity to the base of the skull, and outline the carotid system and its relationship to the neoplasm. A tumour splaying the external and internal carotid arteries mediolaterally is likely to arise from the carotid body, whereas a tumour pushing the internal carotid artery forwards is probably a glomus vagale tumour.

The sophistication of modern angiology using Doppler techniques allows the clinician to determine the risks of sacrificing the internal carotid artery in any given patient. The ultrasonic investigation assesses the adequacy of circulation across the circle of Willis, while compressing one internal carotid, and provides the surgeon with the confidence to ablate the vessel if previously assured of good cross-flow. It has to a large extent superseded ophthalmodynamometry, and progressive clamping of the common carotid artery under local anaesthesia (Padayachee *et al.*, 1986).

An alternative to external compression, is to monitor the effects of inflating a balloon placed in the internal carotid artery in an awake patient, by observing clinical responses and changes in the EEG. The availability of detachable balloons offers the surgeon the means of occluding that part of the internal carotid artery lying distal to a large vascular tumour, and dividing the vessel just below the level of the balloon. This has simplified the task of securing a transected carotid artery just below the skull base, a procedure which is technically difficult to achieve by suturing, given the difficult access.

When a glomus jugular tumour is suspected, plain radiography is a quick and inexpensive way of comparing the size of the jugular foramen on each side. The diagnosis is usually made by CT with enhancement, and for greater detail by digital subtraction angiography and arteriography. Jugular venograms are rarely performed now, and their only value is to determine whether the internal jugular vein is blocked and if so, at what level.

Tissue diagnosis

In dealing with many of the conditions discussed, open biopsy is either unnecessary because the diagnosis is obvious, discouraged because of the relative inaccessibility of the lesion, or overtly dangerous as with angiofibromas and chemodectomas.

There are occasions when quite clearly a tissue sample is deemed useful before operation, and the trend now is to perform fine needle aspiration. This does not always yield a precise diagnosis, but may provide some indication as to the nature of the disease, or equally exclude preconceived diagnoses.

Treatment

With the exception of lymphomas which may be treated primarily by radiotherapy and/or chemotherapy, all the other tumours mentioned are treated preferentially by surgery.

A number of surgical approaches has been devised for access to the infratemporal fossa and the parapharyngeal space and in some instances a given procedure will double for both spaces.

The infratemporal fossa can be approached through temporal, palatal, maxillary, and oral routes (Shaheen 1982), and techniques for exploring the petrous apex, skull base, clivus, parasellar, and parapharyngeal regions via the infratemporal fossa have been devised (Fisch and Pillsbury, 1979).

Experience has shown that no procedure is versatile enough to cope with every contingency, and that the best means of access to the infratemporal fossa can only be determined by judging the position, extent, and type of disease. The configuration of the fossa is such that complete eradication of extensive malignant disease is rarely possible, and therefore only patients thought to have disease with limited involvement of the fossa should be considered for operation. Unfortunately, there are occasions when despite careful preoperative assessment the disease is subsequently found at operation to be more extensive than previously anticipated. This possibility should always be borne in mind, especially in cases of high grade tumour, and prompt the surgeon to adopt a somewhat more cautious policy. No such inhibitions should restrain the surgeon when it comes to dealing with benign tumours, or even low grade malignancies, provided the surgical strategy is carefully thought out.

The parapharyngeal space can be approached by transparotid, submandibular, and midline trans-mandibular oropharyngeal approaches, each method having its advantages and disadvantages.

The lateral transparotid approach is suitable for deep lobe tumours which invade the parapharyngeal space. It is direct, but hampered by the need to dissect out the trunk and every branch of the facial nerve, in order to lift the nerve away from the underlying deep lobe and tumour. It is therefore associated with a high incidence of temporary facial palsy.

The submandibular route is appropriate for smaller parapharyngeal space tumours which are independent of the parotid gland, but access to the higher reaches of the parapharyngeal space and infratemporal fossa is difficult through this approach.

The transmandibular route is excellent for both the parapharyngeal space and infratemporal fossa but entails a lip-splitting incision, which is not always acceptable, and inflicts a significant degree of trismus on the patients for many months after the operation.

Transparotid approach

Total conservative parotidectomy

This operation is suitable for patients with pleomorphic adenomas arising from within the deep lobe of the parotid gland and invading the parapharyngeal space.

A superficial parotidectomy is performed at the end of which the superficial lobe is left pedicled inferiorly instead of anteriorly. The pedicle ideally should lie between the cervical and mandibular branches of the facial nerve. Alternatively, the superficial lobe can be excised completely and the deep lobe removed as a separate specimen. The branches and the main trunk of the facial nerve are dissected off the underlying deep lobe, using small scissors to divide the fascial attachments of the nerve to the underlying gland. This manoeuvre is helped by lifting and supporting the nerve and its branches with a nerve hook (Figure 22.17).

The deep lobe is separated from the posterior border of the ascending ramus of the mandible and from the temporomandibular joint as well as the digastric muscle and the bony external auditory meatus. Its deep aspect is gently separated from the styloid process to which it may have some fibrous attachments.

The posterior facial or retromandibular vein is divided at the point where it emerges from the deep lobe of the gland, and the superficial temporal vein is secured superiorly and just below the zygomatic arch. Similarly, the external carotid artery is divided at its point of entry into the deep lobe of the gland, just above the stylohyoid muscle and the superficial temporal artery is interrupted at its point of emergence from the gland.

The internal maxillary and transverse facial branches of the external carotid artery are divided in the interval between the deep lobe of the gland and the ascending ramus of the mandible.

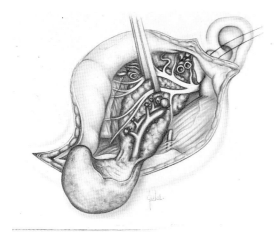

Figure 22.17 Elevation of the facial nerve from the underlying deep lobe of the parotid gland before mobilization and removal of the deep lobe

Mobilization of the tumour, which lies medial to the deep lobe of the gland, is commenced using blunt dissection, but leaving the lateral extremity of the tumour attached to the gland. Care is taken not to breach its substance, for although most deep lobe pleomorphic adenomas are firm and reasonably well-encapsulated, a softer variant which is prone to rupture is not uncommonly encountered.

To improve access to the deep part of the tumour the stylomandibular ligament needs to be divided and the styloid process possibly also fractured and removed.

Once the tumour is reasonably free from its surroundings, it is extricated in a lateral and downward direction from beneath the facial nerve, together with the deep lobe of the parotid gland, which has already been freed from its attachments during the earlier stages of the operation.

Any remaining bleeding points are secured, taking care not to damage the exposed facial nerve and its branches which may overlie points of bleeding in the depths of the wound.

Temporary weakness of the muscles of the face may commonly occur following this operation as the result of stretching of the nerve. If the tumour is spilled during the course of surgery, the wound should be washed thoroughly with distilled water to avoid a subsequent multinodular recurrence.

Conservative lateral approach

This is a more ambitious extension of a total conservative parotidectomy and is suitable for removing well-circumscribed benign tumours from the infratemporal fossa in patients reluctant to submit to a lip-splitting incision.

The access provided by this route is somewhat restricted but the author has used it for extracranial meningiomas, deep lobe tumours and recurrent pleomorphic adenomas of the parotid gland, and fibrosarcomas.

A superficial parotidectomy is performed through an extended parotidectomy incision (Figure 22.18), and the branches of the facial nerve traced as far distally as possible (Figure 22.19). The branches are also freed from underlying structures such as the temporalis fascia, zygomatic arch, and masseter muscle. The temporalis fascia is separated from the upper border of the zygomatic arch, and the arch divided anteriorly at the zygomaticomalar suture and posteriorly at its root. The zygomatic arch, together with attached masseter muscle, is allowed to drop beneath the overlying branches of the facial nerve to expose the ascending ramus of the mandible or, alternatively, the zygomatic arch is removed with the intention of replacing it at the end of the procedure (Figure 22.20).

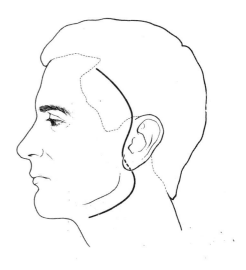

Figure 22.18 Extended parotidectomy incision

The ascending ramus of the mandible is sectioned in a trifurcate manner (Figure 22.21) above the level of the lingula, and the coronoid segment with attached temporalis muscle is reflected superiorly, if necessary threading it under a branch or two of the facial nerve to obtain adequate exposure. Alternatively the coronoid process can be removed altogether.

The lower fragment of the ascending ramus of the mandible is retracted inferiorly and the infratemporal fossa entered (Figure 22.22). Encapsulated masses can be freed without undue difficulty and delivery facilitated by having an assistant insert a finger into

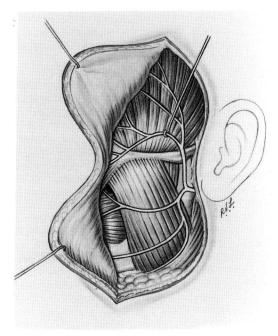

Figure 22.19 The branches of the facial nerve are dissected as far distally as possible

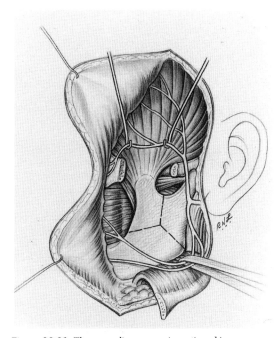

Figure 22.21 The ascending ramus is sectioned in a trifurcate manner

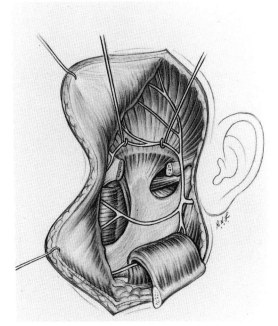

Figure 22.20 Detachment and downward displacement of the zygomatic arch and masseter muscle

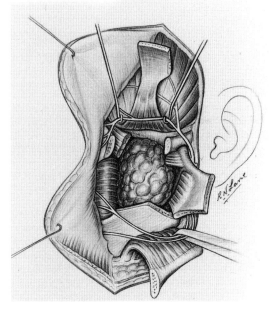

Figure 22.22 Retraction of the bony fragments exposes the infratemporal fossa

the nasopharynx and push the lateral nasopharyngeal wall outwards. More extensive masses may require division or resection of the medial and lateral pterygoid muscles, for better exposure of the deeper and upper aspects of the tumour.

Once the tumour has been removed the mandible and zygomatic arch are rewired and the wound closed with drainage.

Great care must be taken not to stretch the branches of the facial nerve unduly, for neuropraxia is not uncommon after this operation. The inferior dental bundle and lingual nerve may be damaged in spite of attempts to preserve them, but more likely will be sacrificed with the removal of the tumour mass. Postoperatively there will be some trismus.

Radical lateral approach

This is suitable in patients with cancer of the parotid gland invading the infratemporal fossa or carcinoma of the external ear and middle ear cleft invading the parotid gland and extending deeply into the fossa.

A resection of the parotid gland including the facial nerve, ascending ramus of the mandible, and zygomatic arch exposes the contents of the infratemporal fossa, the base of the skull, and the lateral aspect of the skull. A formal resection of the external auditory meatus and middle ear, either by osteotomies in the classical manner or by drilling, can be incorporated into the overall procedure.

The internal carotid artery can be traced upwards to the base of the skull and the carotid canal uncapped if necessary, using rongeurs and the drill. The cartilaginous eustachian tube is identified and may be dissected out of its groove in cases of middle-ear carcinoma, and the bony tube drilled away. The temporal lobe dura can be widely exposed and the petrous temporal bone drilled out.

Clearly it is desirable to establish operability at an early stage when embarking on a procedure of this kind, and in surgery for middle-ear carcinoma, for instance, exposure of the dura early on in the operation will allow the surgeon to make a decision whether to proceed with exenteration of the infratemporal fossa or not.

Obliteration of the large dead space and cover for the internal carotid artery is achieved by transposition of muscle, or when skin has been resected, by a suitable myocutaneous flap.

Anterior transantral approach

This approach was designed for the removal of benign well circumscribed masses, angiofibromas being a good example.

A Weber-Ferguson or facial degloving incision is used to expose the anterior surface of the maxilla. In the case of the Weber-Ferguson incision a cheek flap is reflected laterally and the infraorbital nerve transected with a cuff of soft tissue around it. If a degloving approach is used, the soft tissues of the face and lower nose are elevated superiorly to expose the maxilla.

The pyriform aperture of the nose is identified and the nasal mucosa elevated away from it by blunt dissection. The anterior, lateral, posterior, and medial antral walls are drilled out or removed with rongeurs, leaving the orbital floor and superior alveolus intact. The lateral nasal wall, incorporating mucosa and the inferior and middle turbinates, is removed (Figure 22.23).

That part of the angiofibroma which extends behind the antrum into the infratemporal fossa is identified and mobilized by blunt dissection. Mobilization pro-

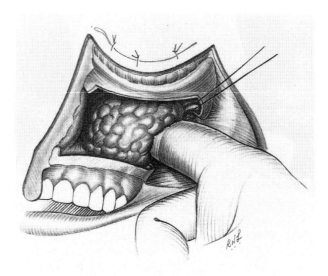

Figure 22.23 Removal of anterior, medial, posterior and lateral antral walls, leaving the orbital floor and superior alveolus, provides access to the infratemporal fossa

ceeds from lateral to medial, the tumour being displaced into the dead space provided by the antrum, and in the process exposing the internal maxillary artery as it approaches the tumour. The artery is divided and mobilization of the tumour continued towards the nasopharynx. Removal of the vertical plate of the palatine bone which constitutes the posterior part of the bony lateral nasal wall is essential if the neck of the 'dumb-bell' which occupies the enlarged sphenopalatine foramen is to be released (Figure 22.24). Separation of the nasopharyngeal component of the tumour from the skull base is effected, and the tumour finally excised with its mucosal covering. The dead space is filled with ribbon gauze impregnated with bismuth-iodoform-paraffin paste and the wound is closed in layers. Major haemorrhage has not been a problem so far with this type of approach. The only complications have been infraorbital anaesthesia, which younger subjects seem not to notice, and a mild degree of temporary ectropion of the lower eyelid.

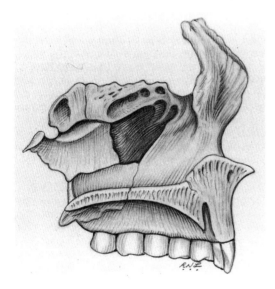

Figure 22.24 The sphenopalatine foramen is the site of origin of angiofibromas and the waist of dumb-bell tumours. (The arrow points to the foramen)

Superior approach

This approach allows satisfactory access to the upper lateral part of the infratemporal fossa but, as exposure is relatively restricted, its usefulness for most tumours in this area is limited. It might be considered as a useful approach for the removal of osteoblastomas of the skull base, low-grade malignancies, or simply as a safe avenue for biopsy. Because the dissection is carried out beneath the temporalis muscle, the facial nerve is not placed at risk in this procedure.

The incision, which is shown in Figure 22.25, is taken down to bone and the pinna reflected downwards and forwards after dividing the external auditory meatus. The temporalis muscle is detached from the side of the skull with the periosteal elevator and the muscle pushed downwards and forwards.

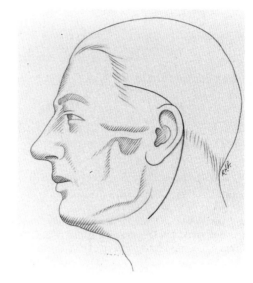

Figure 22.25 The incision for the superior approach to the infratemporal fossa

The temporalis fascia is separated from the upper border and inner aspect of the zygomatic arch, working from behind forwards. To increase exposure, the arch may be fractured at its most anterior and posterior limits, and the lateral margin of the wound retracted outwards by a retractor placed deep to the temporalis muscle and zygomatic arch (Figure 22.26). To gain further exposure of the skull base, the infratemporal crest is drilled away until the dura is exposed and the bone work extended medially along the greater wing of the sphenoid.

The approach may also be incorporated within the framework of an operation directed at the middle ear and mastoid.

Inferior approach

This approach is appropriate to both the parapharyngeal space and infratemporal fossa. It does however suffer the disadvantage that access to the most superior part of the infratemporal fossa is restricted given the distance between the submandibular triangle and the base of the skull.

A horizontal incision is made just above the level

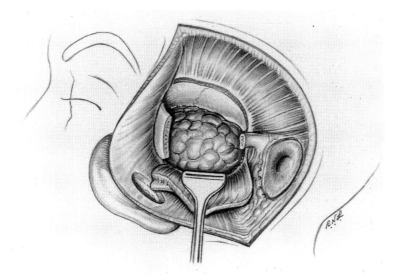

Figure 22.26 The zygomatic arch may be outfractured to increase exposure to the infratemporal fossa

of the hyoid bone, extending from the midline to a point which overlaps the sternomastoid muscle and the submandibular gland is excised (Figure 22.27). With the submandibular gland out of the way, the approach to a tumour lying in the parapharyngeal space is commenced. It has to be stressed that much of the procedure is carried out blind because, apart from the lower part of the neoplasm which is visible, the upper part is largely hidden from view. A plane of separation is established by blunt dissection between the tumour on the one hand and the inner aspect of the medial pterygoid muscle and the deep lobe of the parotid gland on the other. If the tumour lies in the infratemporal fossa, the insertion of the medial pterygoid into the mandible is divided to facilitate access. Dissection continues around the rest of the neoplasm in all directions. Medially and anteromedially, where it abuts against the superior constrictor muscle, separation is easy to perform unless a prior biopsy through the oropharynx has been performed, in which case the neoplasm is generally firmly stuck to the pharyngeal wall.

Separation superiorly may also be difficult if the tumour is large and reaches the base of the skull. Dissection at this level is restricted and not helped by the fact that it is performed entirely by blind blunt dissection.

Access to the upper part of the neoplasm may be helped by dividing the horizontal ramus of the mandible immediately anterior to the ascending ramus (Figure 22.28). This entails freeing enough of the masseter muscle and mandibular periosteum off the bone, proceeding from below upwards. The osteotomy may be accomplished either with an oscillating or Gigli saw, and the fracture line directed downwards and forwards to stabilize the bony fragments when subsequently realigned.

The inferior dental artery will bleed and this will have to be stopped, either by coagulation or by the insertion of bone wax into the inferior dental canal.

Once the mandible is divided the ascending ramus may be everted upwards and laterally, to facilitate access to the upper part of the tumour. After removal of the swelling, the mandibular fragments are wired together or alternatively plated, and the wound is drained with a suction drain and closed in layers.

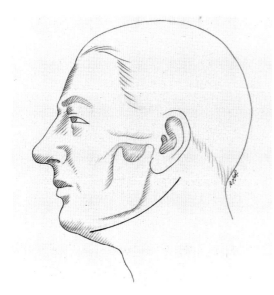

Figure 22.27 The incision for the inferior approach

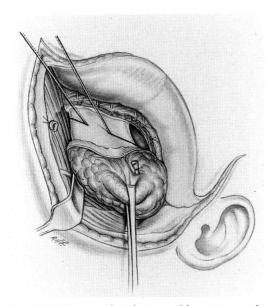

Figure 22.28 Access to the infratemporal fossa is improved by dividing the horizontal ramus of the mandible

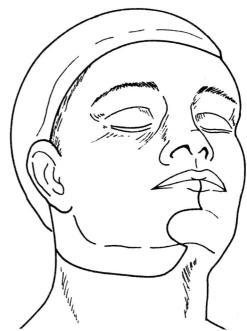

Figure 22.29 The incision for the midline transmandibular oropharyngeal approach

Damage to the mandibular branch of the VIIth nerve may occur, either during removal of the submandibular gland or subsequently if traction on the upper flap is excessive. Division of the mandible results in permanent mental anaesthesia and if realignment and fixation of the bone fragments is imperfect, instability may occur.

Midline transmandibular oropharyngeal approach

This is entirely suitable for both the parapharyngeal space and infratemporal fossa, and is the preferred operation for very large primary parapharyngeal pleomorphic adenomas.

A staggered incision through the lower lip is carried out and may take the form of a 'V' on its side or alternatively a vertical line drawn to the upper part of the protuberance of the chin, with a curve thereafter which surrounds and hugs the contour of the chin to its lower extremity (Figure 22.29).

At the point of the chin, the incision inclines downwards and laterally, preferably in a skin crease, just above the level of the hyoid bone. It ends at the anterior border of the sternomastoid or just beyond.

The submandibular part of the incision is deepened through the platysma and deep cervical fascia, again at a level just above the hyoid bone, and the submandibular gland is removed.

The removal of the gland has the advantage of releasing the lingual nerve from its attachment to the deep part of the salivary gland, so that when the

intraoral part of the operation takes place there may be some chance of preserving the lingual nerve, as it crosses the floor of the mouth from lateral to medial.

At the site where the mandible is to be divided a metal plate is laid on the chin and drill holes made through this for subsequent plating. The midline of the mandible is then split in a staggered manner to enhance subsequent stability, and the mucous membrane of the mouth entered.

The mucosal incision at the midline is then carried backwards and laterally, just inside the horizontal ramus of the mandible, and deepened to include division of the mylohyoid muscle close to its insertion into the inner aspect of the horizontal ramus of the mandible.

This will assist eversion of the horizontal ramus of the mandible and help to identify the course of the lingual nerve from lateral to medial (Figure 22.30).

The incision in the mucous membrane is continued backwards, onto the anterior faucial pillar ending on the soft palate; it is deepened to include division of the superior constrictor muscle, and the parapharyngeal space is opened. The osteoplastic flap containing the mandible is retracted as far out as possible to allow the surgeon full access to the parapharyngeal space, and after dividing the medial pterygoid muscle the tumour is separated from the adjacent structures by blunt dissection and excised.

The dehiscent muscles and mucous membrane are repaired and the mandible plated. The parapharyngeal space is drained with a large bore suction drain.

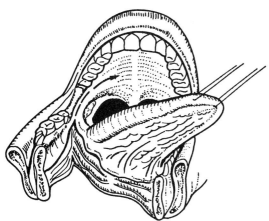

Figure 22.30 Division of the insertion of the mylohyoid into the mandible allows eversion of the bone, and broadens the access to the parapharyngeal space

Lingual anaesthesia may commonly be caused by damage to the lingual nerve, and the patient may also experience temporary trismus for a period of weeks after the operation.

Extended anterolateral approach

This operation was devised for dealing with carcinoma of the antrum extending posteriorly into the infratemporal fossa, and it may be combined with exenteration of the orbital contents. It may also be modified for selected operations for mouth cancer, such as retromolar, faucial and tonsillar lesions where invasion of the fossa is judged to have taken place.

The incisions are as depicted in Figure 22.31. The lower incision, which splits both lip and mandible, is extended backwards into the submandibular triangle and the contents of the submandibular triangle mobilized. The mucosa of the floor of the mouth and mylohyoid muscle are incised as close to the inner aspect of the horizontal ramus of the mandible as possible, and the medial pterygoid muscle identified and divided at its point of insertion into the lower inner aspect of the ascending ramus.

The upper incision resembles that of the classical Weber-Ferguson, but is made to surround the eye and is carried upwards in the midline of the forehead, curving slightly outwards as it proceeds backwards. To ensure that the orbicularis oculis muscle is not denervated at the outer canthus of the eye, the muscle is transected obliquely in the medial third of both upper and lower lids.

The cheek, lid, and forehead flap is lifted off the bone at the maxilla, malar bone, zygomatic arch and side of the skull deep to the periosteum. In order to free this enormous flap, the superior attachment of the temporalis fascia must be divided. The branches of the facial nerve are all contained within the substance of the flap and are therefore not at risk.

The oral mucosa is divided along the upper gingivo-buccal sulcus, at the posterior end of which the incision is curved downwards, just medial to the pterygomandibular raphe, to join up with the floor of the mouth incision.

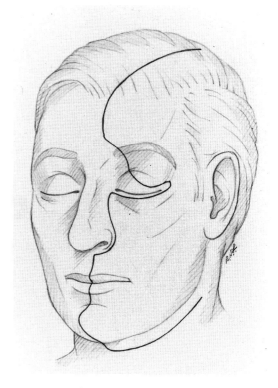

Figure 22.31 The incisions for the extended anterolateral approach

The zygomatic arch is divided at its anterior and posterior ends, and the temporalis muscle detached from the coronoid process of the mandible. The lateral pterygoid muscle is divided close to its point of insertion into the condyle of the mandible, the inferior dental nerve divided, and the mandible rotated almost 90° from the sagittal axis (Figure 22.32).

The infratemporal fossa is now fully exposed and its contents are ready for removal in conjunction with a maxillectomy, which in turn may include resection of the malar bone and orbital exenteration. Alternatively the infratemporal fossa dissection may be incorporated within the framework of an operation for the removal of a mouth cancer.

Once all soft tissue has been cleared, the bone of the greater wing of the sphenoid can be removed if judged to be involved and the pterygoid plate complex divided at its base and also removed. Once this block of bone is out of the way, the infratemporal fossa can be properly inspected and if necessary the maxillary

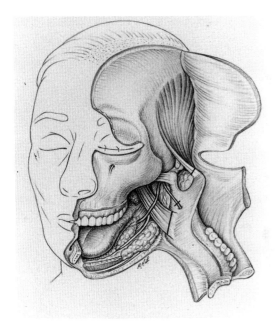

Figure 22.32 The enhanced exposure achieved by lateral eversion of the mandible

nerve removed flush with the foramen rotundum. The fibro-fatty contents of the fossa are also exenterated and any suspicious residua diathermized.

At the conclusion of the operation the divided mandible is rewired or plated, the soft tissues approximated in two layers, and the lower wound drained. Complications have included mental, lingual, and infraorbital anaesthesia, and limited soft tissue necrosis. Trismus is not uncommon and slow to improve.

Combined treatment

Postoperative radiotherapy in the management of malignant tumours of the head and neck is increasingly accepted as an integral and necessary part of treatment. It is, if anything, even more desirable in treating neoplasms of the infratemporal fossa and parapharyngeal space since the risk of leaving small or microscopic residues at surgery is likely to be higher than at other sites.

It is particularly effective in dealing with low grade malignancies such as desmoid tumours which would almost certainly recur without it and, subject to staging, is the preferred primary treatment for lymphoma.

There is good reason to believe that when pleomorphic adenomas have ruptured during operation spilling their contents, postoperative radiotherapy offers the surest means of averting subsequent recurrence (Rafla, 1970). The same applies to pleomorphic adenomas which have been previously biopsied, or when surgical excision is deemed to be incomplete. There is some debate however about the wisdom of such a policy given the possibility of inducing malignancy at a later date (Watkin and Hobsley, 1986 a, b).

References

ARENA, S. and HILAL, E. Y. (1976) Neurilemmomas of the infratemporal space. *Archives of Otolaryngology*, **102**, 180–184

CONLEY, J. J. (1964) Tumours of the infratemporal fossa. *Archives of Otolaryngology*, **79**, 498–504

FISCH, U. and PILLSBURY, H. C. (1979) Infratemporal fossa approach to lesions in the temporal bone and base of skull. *Archives of Otolaryngology*, **105**, 99–107

PADAYACHEE, T. S., KIRKHAM, F. J., LEWIS, R. R., GILLARD, J., HUTCHINSON, M. C. and GOSLING, R. G. (1986) Transcranial measurement of blood velocities in the basal cerebral arteries: a method of assessing the circle of Willis. *Ultrasound in Medicine and Biology*, **12**, 5–14

RAFLA, S. (1970) *Mucous and Salivary Gland Tumours.* Springfield, Illinois: Charles C. Thomas. p. 104

SHAHEEN, O. H. (1982) Swellings of the infratemporal fossa. *Journal of Laryngology and Otology*, **96**, 817–836

SOM, P. M., BILLER, H. F. and LAWSON, W. (1981) Tumours of the parapharyngeal space. Preoperative evaluation, diagnosis and surgical approaches. *Annals of Otology, Rhinology and Laryngology*, **90** (suppl. 80/4), 3–15

WATKIN, G. and HOBSLEY, M. (1986a) The influence of local surgery and radiotherapy on the natural history of pleomorphic adenomas. *British Journal of Surgery*, **73**, 74–76

WATKIN, G. and HOBSLEY, M. (1986b) Should radiotherapy be used routinely in the management of benign parotid tumours. *British Journal of Surgery*, **73**, 601–603

WORK, W. P. and GATES, G. A. (1969) Tumours of the parotid gland and parapharyngeal space. *Otolaryngologic Clinics of North America*, **2**, 497–514

23

Cysts, granulomas and tumours of the jaws, nose and sinuses

A. D. Cheesman and P. Jani

Cysts of the jaws

A cyst is a pathological cavity filled with fluid or semi-fluid which has not been created by pus (Kramer, 1974). Cysts of the jaws are more common than in any other bone and the majority, but not all, are lined by epithelium. Although the pathogenesis of several of these cysts is still not clearly understood they can be divided into three main groups according to the suspected origin of the epithelium lining the cyst:

Odontogenic cysts: the epithelial lining is derived from the epithelial remnants of the tooth-forming organ. These cysts can be further subdivided into developmental or inflammatory according to their aetiology.

Non-odontogenic cysts: the lining is derived from sources other than the tooth-forming organ. This group includes those cysts which were previously referred to as fissural cysts, and were thought to arise from epithelium trapped in the lines of fusion of the embryonic frontonasal and maxillary processes. However, this postulated pathogenesis is no longer accepted and fissural cysts are not included in the World Health Organization's classification (1992).

Non-epithelial cysts: these include the unusual solitary bone cyst and the aneurysmal bone cyst.

The classification is given in Table 23.1 and is based on that recommended by the World Health Organization.

The residual epithelial tissue which persists following completion of tooth development can be from three sources, each is responsible for a particular cyst (Figure 23.1):

Table 23.1 Classification of cysts of the jaws

Epithelial
1 Developmental
  a Odontogenic
     Gingival cyst of infants
     Gingival cyst of adults
     Lateral periodontal cyst
     Botryoid odontogenic cyst
     Glandular odontogenic cyst
     Dentigerous (follicular) cyst
     Eruption cyst
     Odontogenic keratocyst
  b Non-odontogenic
     Nasopalatine duct cyst
     Nasolabial (nasoalveolar) cyst
     Midpalatal cyst of infants
     So-called fissural cysts
       median palatine
       median alveolar
       median mandibular cysts
       globulomaxillary cyst
2 Inflammatory
    Radicular cyst
     Apical
     Lateral
     Residual
Non-epithelial
Solitary bone cyst (traumatic, simple or haemorrhagic)
Aneurysmal bone cyst

(Modified from Histological typing of odontogenic tumours, WHO publication, 1992).

1 The epithelial cells remaining following dissolution of the dental lamina are called *the cell rests of Serres.* They give rise to the odontogenic keratocyst

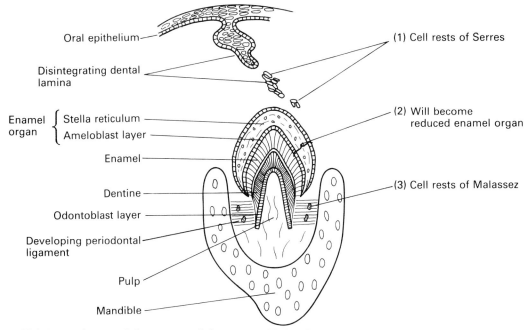

Figure 23.1 Potential source of odontogenic epithelium responsible for odontogenic cysts and tumours: (1) cell rests of Serres; (2) reduced enamel organ; (3) cell rests of Malassez

and probably to the developmental lateral periodontal cyst and the adult gingival cyst
2 *The reduced enamel organ* is derived from the post-functional enamel organ after completion of tooth crown development and this tissue gives rise to the dentigerous cyst and the rare paradental cyst
3 *The cell rests of Malassez* arise following fragmentation of Hertwig's root sheath which is responsible for the formation of the root. All radicular cysts originate from these cell rests.

Odontogenic cysts of the jaws

Gingival cysts of infants (Bohn's nodule)

Gingival cysts of infants are small keratinized cysts frequently seen on the alveolar ridge of infants. They arise from epithelial remnants of the dental lamina and are called Epstein pearls. The epithelial remnants of the dental lamina (glands of Serres) have a proliferative tendency and develop multiple microcysts with keratin formation from the fetal age of 10 weeks (Moskow and Bloom, 1983). In a study of 32 human fetuses, Moreillon and Schroeder (1982) demonstrated development of keratinized microcysts from the dental lamina, which increased in number from the twelfth to the twentieth week with a maximum of 190 cysts per fetus. It is postulated that these microcysts develop into the gingival cysts of infants.

Clinical features

The cysts are white or cream coloured nodules, approximately 2–3 mm in diameter and are found along the crest of the alveolar ridges. Monteleone and McLellan (1964) found the cysts in 85% of infants and they were more common on the maxillary dental ridge than the mandibular ridge. The highest incidence is at birth and the cysts are rarely seen after 3 months.

Histology

The cysts are usually round or ovoid in histological sections and are lined by a thin layer of parakeratinizing stratified squamous cells. The basal cell layer is flat, unlike that of the keratocyst where it is undulating. The cyst cavity is filled with concentric layers of keratin often containing flattened nuclei (Moskow and Bloom, 1983).

Treatment

The majority of gingival cysts are small, though cysts up to 1 cm in size have been described (Garlick *et al.*, 1989). Spontaneous resolution is usual by the age of 3 months making treatment unnecessary. Most of these cysts undergo involution and the keratin is digested by macrophages. Some rupture through the surface epithelium, become marsupialized and the cyst lining fuses with the oral epithelium (Shear, 1992). They are extremely rare over the age of 3 months (Saunders, 1972).

Gingival cyst of adults

Gingival cysts of adults arise in the soft tissue of the gingiva and present as a gingival swelling usually without any bony involvement. However, large cysts may produce erosion of the adjacent alveolar ridge and mimic the lateral periodontal cyst. As a consequence until recently most published series have combined gingival cysts of adults and lateral periodontal cysts making it difficult to obtain any meaningful data. Further confusion is caused by the fact that many other cysts in the lateral periodontal position, such as keratocysts and radicular inflammatory cysts adjacent to an accessory root canal, are misdiagnosed as true gingival cysts.

Many theories of origin have been proposed but most authorities now accept that the gingival cyst of adults arises from the reduced enamel epithelium (Shear, 1992).

Clinical features

Shear (1992) reported that 14 of 2616 jaw cysts in his series were gingival cysts of the adult, an incidence of 0.5%. Buchner and Hansen (1979) noted an incidence of 0.15% over an 11-year period.

The usual history is of a slowly enlarging, well circumscribed painless swelling arising in the gingiva or the interdental papillae. It is normally less than 1 cm in diameter and invariably on the buccal surface of the alveolar ridge. The soft fluctuant swelling has a smooth surface, and is usually pink or bluish in colour. Occasionally, when filled with blood, secondary to trauma, the cyst may be bright red.

It is more common in the mandible (73% in the series of Buchner and Hansen, 1979), the most frequent site being adjacent to a lower premolar or canine tooth. It is seen at any age but the majority occur in the fifth and sixth decades. Twenty nine of the 40 patients with true gingival cysts reported by Reeve and Levy (1968), Buchner and Hansen (1979) and Nxumalo and Shear (1992) were seen in patients between the ages of 40 and 59 years. Wysocki *et al.* (1980) reported a mean age of 50.7 years. In most cases there is no bony involvement, however, in large cysts there may be erosion of the cortical bone which appears on radiographs as a faint circumscribed radiolucency.

Histology

Histology is variable. Most cysts are lined by epithelium consisting of cuboidal cells, one to three layers thick, which closely resembles the reduced enamel epithelium. In others the lining may be of a rather thicker stratified squamous nature without rete pegs. Occasionally localized epithelial thickenings or plaques may be present with a whorled configuration.

Treatment

Excision biopsy under local anaesthesia is the preferred treatment.

Lateral periodontal cyst

The lateral periodontal cyst has been defined in the WHO classification as 'a cyst occurring on the lateral aspect or between the roots of vital teeth and arising from odontogenic epithelial remnants, but not as a result of inflammatory stimuli'. This cyst must be distinguished from collateral odontogenic keratocysts, gingival cysts of adults as well as from cysts of inflammatory origin on the lateral aspect of the root. As with the gingival cysts of adults, several reported series have pooled data relating to lateral periodontal cysts, with that of gingival cysts of adults, lateral inflammatory periodontal cysts and collateral keratocysts. Accurate clinical data are therefore sparse.

Clinical features

Lateral periodontal cysts accounted for 0.7% of 2616 jaw cysts reported by Shear (1992) over a 17-year period. Over three-quarters of these cysts are found in the mandible, the majority being adjacent to canine or premolar teeth (Cohen *et al.*, 1984). Fantasia (1979) reported a series of 12 patients with mandibular cysts which all fulfilled the diagnostic criteria of lateral periodontal cysts and all were adjacent to premolar or canine teeth. Shear's series (1992) of 18 cysts is unusual in that the majority of lesions (56%) were found in the maxilla. Rasmusson, Magnusson and Borrman (1991) reported that 88% of 32 cysts in their series were in the mandible.

These cysts can present between the second and eighth decades. When 15 of the cysts reported by Shear are pooled with those of Cohen *et al.* (1984) and Rasmusson, Magnusson and Borrman (1991) the peak incidence is in the sixth decade and 82% were in the 40–69-year age group.

Approximately two-thirds of the lesions are found in men. Seventy-six (61%) of the 124 patients pooled from the recently reported series by Wysocki *et al.* (1980), Cohen *et al.* (1984), Shear (1992) and Rasmusson, Magnusson and Borrman (1991) were in men.

These cysts are usually asymptomatic and are discovered by chance during routine dental radiography. However, they may present as a gingival swelling on the buccal aspect of the alveolar ridge and therefore need to be differentiated from other cysts in this area. Lateral periodontal cysts are classically less than 1 cm in diameter but cysts as large as 3 cm have been reported. If untreated the estimated growth rate is 0.7 cm per year (Rasmusson, Magnusson and Borrman, 1991). They may occasionally be painful (Cohen *et al.*, 1984; Shear, 1992) and tender on palpation (Eliasson, Isacsson and Kondell, 1989). It is important to note that the associated canine and premolar teeth are vital and therefore must not be extracted when the cyst is excised.

Characteristically the radiographic appearance is that of a round or oval, well circumscribed radiolucency less than 1 cm in diameter, with a sclerotic margin. The cysts lie between the apex of the root and the cervical margin of the crown. Resorption of the root by the enlarging cyst has not been reported.

Pathogenesis

It is now widely accepted that the lateral periodontal cyst is developmental and has an odontogenic origin. The lining of the cyst is a thin non-keratinizing epithelium which resembles the reduced enamel epithelium. Sheafer, Hine and Levy (1983) suggest that these cysts are a variant of the dentigerous cyst which develops on the lateral aspect of the tooth. Following eruption, the dentigerous cyst comes to lie on the lateral aspect of the tooth and becomes a lateral periodontal cyst. It has been proposed that the lateral periodontal cyst originates from the reduced enamel epithelium and this hypothesis has gained further support following histochemical studies by Hormia *et al.* (1987) who showed cytokeratin 18 expression in dentigerous cysts only and not in the other odontogenic cysts. Heikinheimo *et al.* (1989) reported strong expression of cytokeratin 18 in a botryoid variety of a lateral periodontal cyst suggesting a common origin for the dentigerous and lateral periodontal cyst. It is therefore likely that the lateral periodontal cyst is a variant of the dentigerous cyst which has developed in a lateral position and arises from the reduced enamel epithelium.

Histology

The lateral periodontal cyst is lined by a thin non-keratinizing squamous or cuboidal epithelium, one to five cell layers thick. Two-thirds of the specimens contain glycogen rich clear cells (Wysocki *et al.*, 1980; Altini and Shear, 1992). Another interesting feature is the presence of epithelial thickenings (plaques) which may protrude into the cyst cavity. Half of the cases described are multicystic containing two or more cystic spaces. The botryoid variety (described later) typically has several cystic spaces and is usually substantially larger.

If the cyst lining consists of distinctly keratinizing stratified squamous epithelium then a diagnosis of a keratocyst should be made rather than lateral periodontal cyst. Rasmusson, Magnusson and Borrman (1991) demonstrated that epithelial cells reacted positively for NADH2, NADPH2, diaphorase, glutamate dehydrogenase and lactate dehydrogenase. This differs from keratocysts which show increased acid phosphatase activity (Magnusson, 1978).

Treatment

Lateral periodontal cysts which appear unilocular on dental radiographs should be treated by enucleation, preserving the adjacent teeth if possible. Occasionally cysts which appear unilocular on radiographs are multilocular on histological examination. These have a greater tendency to recur (Greer and Johnson, 1988) and therefore should be followed up.

Botryoid odontogenic cyst

This is now recognized to be a variant of the lateral periodontal cyst. It was first reported by Weathers and Waldron (1973) who described two examples of multilocular cystic lesions where the gross specimen resembled a cluster of grapes (Greek, botryoid). A further three examples have been reported by Kaugars (1986), 10 by Greer and Johnson (1988), one by Heikinheimo *et al.* (1989) and four by Shear (1992).

Botryoid cysts are larger than lateral periodontal cysts and multilocular on radiographic and histological examination. The mean age at presentation is the fifth decade. Heikinheimo *et al.* (1989) demonstrated the presence of cytokeratin 18 in the lining. This is of interest as this polypeptide had previously been shown to be present only in dentigerous cysts.

Kaugars (1986), Greer and Johnson (1988), Heikinheimo *et al.* (1989) and Phelan *et al.* (1988) have all documented the tendency for this cyst to recur.

Treatment

Botryoid odontogenic cysts should be excised as recurrence following enucleation is common.

Glandular odontogenic cyst (sialo-odontogenic cyst)

This cyst has only recently been described and as yet there is no consensus regarding its name. Both the above names are used in the WHO classification (1992). The glandular odontogenic cyst has some features in common with both the lateral periodontal cyst and the botryoid odontogenic cyst. It was first reported in 1987 by Padayachee and Van Wyk who coined the term 'sialo-odontogenic cyst'. Sadeghi *et al.* (1991) used the term mucoepidermoid odontogenic cyst because of the presence of both glandular and squamous epithelial elements. Typically this cyst is an intraosseous, multilocular cyst which may recur if not adequately excised. The multicystic spaces are lined by non-keratinized squamous epithelium with occasional epithelial thickenings (plaques). The lining also has a prominent glandular component with mucous and ciliated epithelial cells. Mucinous material is commonly found within the cyst space.

Gardner *et al.* (1988), reporting a further eight cases, confirmed the cyst's propensity to grow to a large size and to recur. Patron, Colmenero and Larrauri (1991) reported a further three cases and pooled their data with that of Padayachee and Van Wyk and Gardner *et al.* In the 13 cases summarized the age range was 19 to 85 years, the majority occurred in the mandible (10 out of 13) and nine were in men. The radiographic features were not diagnostic and showed a large well defined uni-or multilocular radiolucency.

Treatment

Information from the small number of cases reported suggests that this lesion should be resected rather then enucleated to reduce the risk of recurrence.

Dentigerous cyst

The dentigerous cyst, also known as the follicular cyst is defined as a cyst which envelops the whole or part of the crown of an unerupted tooth, and is attached to its neck (amelocemental junction). This definition should be strictly adhered to as other cysts may present in a dentigerous relationship radiographically; e.g. keratocysts of the envelopmental variety (Main, 1970), follicular keratocyst (Altini and Cohen, 1982) and a unilocular ameloblastoma involving an adjacent unerupted tooth.

Clinical features

The dentigerous cyst is a common odontogenic cyst. Shear (1992) reported that 433 of 2616 jaw cysts seen over a 32-year period were dentigerous cysts. They occur at any age but have the highest incidence in the third and fourth decades. They are much more common in men than women (Killey, Kay and Seward, 1977) and five times more likely to occur in the white population than the black (Mourshed, 1964; Shear, 1992). Brown *et al.* (1982) showed that the white population in South Africa has a significantly greater incidence of unerupted or impacted teeth than the black population and this is the likely reason for the increased incidence of the dentigerous cyst in the white population.

The cysts are twice as common in the mandible as the maxilla and most frequently involve teeth which are impacted or erupt late. The majority are associated with mandibular third molars and then in decreasing frequency the maxillary canine, mandibular premolar and maxillary third molar (Shear, 1992). Rarely, they may be associated with supernumerary teeth (Lustmann and Bodner, 1988) and complex or compound odontomes (Kaugars, Miller and Abbey, 1989).

The majority are discovered on routine dental radiographs, taken because of missing teeth or retained deciduous predecessors. Otherwise they escape detection until they have enlarged sufficiently to produce expansion of the jaw. Pain is not a feature unless the cyst becomes infected.

Radiographs show a well defined radiolucency associated with the crown of an unerupted tooth (Figure 23.2). The tooth may be displaced a considerable distance by the enlarging cyst. The cavity is unilocular but an erroneous multilocular effect may be produced by occasional bony trabeculations.

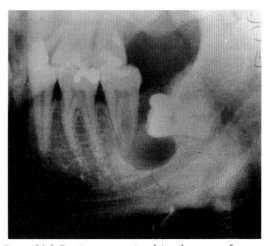

Figure 23.2 Dentigerous cyst involving the crown of a third molar

Radiographically the cyst may be related to the crown of the unerupted tooth in three ways (Figure 23.3):

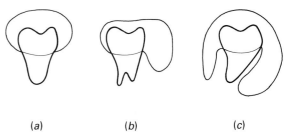

(a)   (b)   (c)

Figure 23.3 Morphological types of dentigerous cyst. (*a*) Central, (*b*) lateral, (*c*) circumferential

1 Central type: cyst completely surrounds the crown of the tooth. This is the commonest type
2 Lateral type: cyst projects laterally from the side of the tooth and does not completely envelop the

crown. This is most commonly seen in a horizontally impacted mandibular molar

3 Circumferential cyst: when the entire tooth appears enveloped by the cyst.

Dentigerous cysts have a greater tendency than other jaw cysts to resorb the roots of the adjacent teeth (Struthers and Shear, 1976). Expansion of the cyst and resorption of the adjacent root may be facilitated by the secretion of cytokines by the fibroblasts in the cyst wall (prostaglandins E2, E3, PGF2, interleukin 1) which in turn induce osteoclastic activity (Harris *et al.*, 1973; Matejka *et al.*, 1985; Meghji, Harvey and Harris, 1989).

Pathogenesis

There is little doubt that dentigerous cysts develop around the crowns of unerupted teeth. However, the frequency of dentigerous cysts is only of the order of 1.5 per 100 unerupted teeth (Mourshed, 1964; Toller, 1967). Furthermore, the difference in incidence in race and sex suggests that there may be a genetic role in determining whether a cyst develops.

The cyst develops by the accumulation of fluid between the reduced enamel epithelium and the enamel, or between the layers of the reduced enamel epithelium. Main (1970) suggested that compression of the follicle by the erupting tooth obstructs venous outflow, thereby increasing the venous pressure and inducing transudate formation. The transudate so formed is thought to separate the reduced enamel epithelium from the crown of the tooth leading to cyst formation.

The expansion of the cyst is facilitated by:

1 Increased osmotic pressure in the cyst fluid caused by the release of glycosaminoglycans by the cyst wall (Smith, Smith and Browne, 1984, 1986, 1988a,b)

2 Increased osteolytic activity induced by the release of cytokines from the cyst wall fibroblasts.

Histology

The cysts are lined by a layer of non-keratinized stratified squamous epithelium, two to five cells thick. It resembles the reduced enamel epithelium from which it is derived. Mucous metaplasia is common and increases with the age of the patient (Browne, 1972). The lining is supported by fibrous connective tissue free from inflammatory cell infiltrate. The contents consist of a protein rich yellow fluid with cholesterol crystals.

Hormia *et al.* (1987) showed increased cytokeratin 18 expression in two of their dentigerous cysts but this polypeptide was not present in any of the other odontogenic cysts.

Treatment

In a growing child dentigerous cysts require early intervention as these cysts grow rapidly in children and because the involved tooth should be given the chance to erupt.

Every effort should be made to preserve the space of the missing tooth in the dental arch and to this end orthodontic treatment may be required.

The best results are obtained with marsupialization as enucleation may lead to damage to the involved tooth. In the adult the tooth is unlikely to erupt and therefore enucleation together with removal of the associated tooth is the preferred option.

Eruption cyst

The eruption cyst is in fact a dentigerous cyst occurring in the soft tissues and results when a tooth is impeded during its eruption within the soft tissues.

Clinical features

It is an uncommon cyst and is seen throughout childhood. Both deciduous and permanent teeth can be involved and the majority of cysts are anterior to the first molar. They present as bluish, smooth swellings over the erupting tooth. The swelling is soft and fluctuant and usually painless. It often bursts spontaneously.

Treatment

The treatment of choice is marsupialization. The dome of the cyst is incised to expose the crown, allowing it to erupt.

Odontogenic keratocyst (primordial cyst)

The odontogenic keratocyst is a relatively uncommon cyst which has aroused considerable interest as it can grow to a large size and has a tendency to recur following surgical treatment. It arises from the remnants of the dental lamina. The term 'odontogenic keratocyst' was first introduced by Philipsen (1956). The term 'keratocyst' was used to include all cysts with a significant degree of keratinization. Shear (1960) recognized this lesion as a distinct entity and coined the term 'primordial cyst'. However, the term 'odontogenic keratocyst' is firmly established in the literature (WHO Classification, 1992).

Robinson (1945) used the term 'primordial cyst' to describe a cyst which arises from the breakdown of the enamel organ before mineralization has taken place; i.e. the cyst develops in place of the tooth. There is no evidence of such a pathogenesis and this cyst is therefore not recognized.

Clinical features

Shear (1992) reviewed 19 published series and quoted the frequency as 1.5–21.8% of all jaw cysts. In his own series he noted that 11.2% of the 2616 jaw cysts registered were odontogenic keratocysts. The cyst is much more common in the white population and rare in the black population, especially in black women. Odontogenic keratocysts have a bimodal age distribution with the first peak in the second and third decades and the second peak in the fifth and sixth decades (Woolgar, Rippen and Browne, 1987a). The clinical and histological features of these two groups are identical and therefore they are unlikely to represent variants of the keratocyst (Rachanis, Altini and Shear, 1979). Patients with multiple keratocysts which are part of the naevoid basal cell syndrome present earlier (mean age is 26.2 years), with a single peak in the second and third decades (Woolgar, Rippen and Browne, 1987b). Odontogenic keratocysts are twice as common in men as women.

Approximately three-quarters of keratocysts arise in the mandible (Ahlfors, Larsson and Sjoren, 1984) and the majority of these are found at the angle. They may extend into the ramus or forwards into the body of the mandible. They can, however, occur anywhere in the maxilla and mandible.

The majority of the cysts are symptomless and are found on routine radiological examination. However, they may give rise to pain, swelling and discharge in the presence of infection. Where the cyst is large, the mandible is weakened and a pathological fracture may result. In large cysts, teeth may be displaced and, rarely, in maxillary cysts there may be displacement or destruction of the orbital floor causing proptosis and diplopia (Lund, 1985). The cysts tend to grow in an anteroposterior direction within the medulla of the bone causing bony expansion only in the later stages.

Some patients have multiple keratocysts which may be part of the naevoid basal cell syndrome. Multiple odontogenic keratocysts have also been reported with Noonan's syndrome.

Naevoid basal cell syndrome

The naevoid basal cell syndrome was first recognized by Blinkley and Johnson (1951) and established as a syndrome by Gorlin and Goltz in 1960. The inheritance is autosomal dominant with marked penetrance and variable expressivity.

The main features are:

1 Multiple odontogenic keratocysts which develop throughout the lifetime of the patient (Figure 23.4)
2 Multiple naevoid basal cell carcinomas which may arise anywhere in the body and are not confined to sun-exposed areas. They first appear around puberty
3 Skeletal abnormalities, especially bifid ribs and vertebral anomalies, are frequently seen
4 Abnormal facies with frontal and temporal bossing, hypertelorism, mild mandibular prognathism and a broad nasal bridge.

An important clinical feature of keratocysts is their tendency to recur after surgical treatment. The recurrence rate has variously been reported from 10% to 60% (Stoelinga and Bronkhorst, 1988). It is likely that the recurrence rate is falling with better recognition of the problem and improved management. The likely reasons for recurrence are:

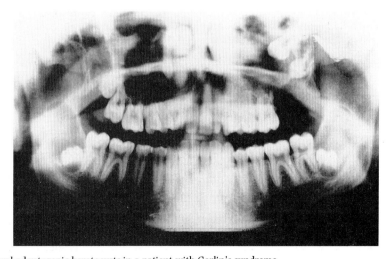

Figure 23.4 Bilateral odontogenic keratocysts in a patient with Gorlin's syndrome

1 Incomplete removal of cyst lining. This is especially so if the cyst margins are scalloped or an attempt is made to retain adjacent teeth. Forssell, Forssell and Kahnberg (1988) showed that the recurrence rate was approximately 50% in those cysts which were removed piecemeal, and extremely rare when the lining was removed in one piece.

2 Some recurrences are likely to be new cyst formation rather than true recurrence.

3 There may be microscopic satellite cysts present around the main lesion which may give rise to new cysts. These are commonly seen in the naevoid basal cell carcinoma syndrome (Woolgar, Rippen and Browne, 1987c).

Radiological features

Radiographically the cysts appear as unilocular or multilocular radiolucencies with well defined sclerotic margins. They tend to be small and ovoid in the maxilla. In the mandible they extend into the body and ramus with little or no bony expansion (Figure 23.5). However, in children expansion is more common and may be considerable.

They may appear in the periapical region of vital teeth and therefore can be confused with radicular cysts (Wright, Wysocki and Larder, 1983). There is often a dentigerous relationship and a misdiagnosis of a dentigerous cyst can be made. Occasionally they occur in the lateral periodontal area and are referred to as collateral keratocysts; in this region they must not be confused with the true lateral periodontal cyst.

Odontogenic keratocysts may displace unerupted teeth and produce resorption of adjacent roots (Partridge and Towers, 1987).

Histology

Odontogenic keratocysts are now widely believed to arise from remnants of the dental lamina (Shear, 1992). Some cysts however are located entirely in the ramus of the mandible and have no relationship with the dental lamina. Stoelinga and Peters (1973) have suggested that such cysts arise from basal cell ingrowths from the basal cell layer of the overlying oral mucosa.

The cyst wall is usually folded and composed of keratinized stratified squamous cell epithelium approximately five to eight cells thick. Parakeratosis predominates but there may be areas of orthokeratosis. The surface cells desquamate and fill the cyst cavity. The fibrous capsule is thin and devoid of inflammatory cells. There may be satellite cysts around the main lesion which are microscopic in size and more commonly associated with the naevoid basal cell carcinoma syndrome.

The cyst contains thick cheesy material and was referred to as a cholesteatoma in the earlier literature. A fine needle aspirate containing keratinizing squames and a protein content of less than 4 g/dl gives a reliable preoperative diagnosis of a keratocyst (Kramer and Toller, 1973). Other authors have confirmed this finding and have reported a virtual 100% preoperative diagnosis by fine needle aspiration cytology and protein estimation (Smith, Smith and Browne, 1986).

Kuusela, Ylipaavalniemi and Thesleff (1986) demonstrated an antigen which is found in the fluid of keratocysts but not in other cysts. They called it keratocyst antigen (KCA) and suggested it may be useful for preoperative diagnosis.

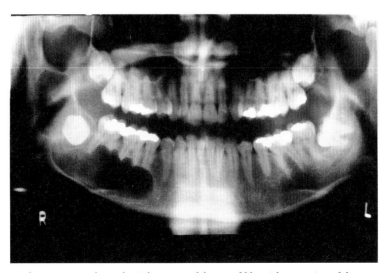

Figure 23.5 Odontogenic keratocyst involving the right ramus of the mandible, with resorption of the roots of adjacent teeth

Treatment

At present there is significant controversy about the optimum treatment of odontogenic keratocysts. Meiselman (1994) advocated a conservative approach and recommended careful enucleation of the cyst in one piece; this manoeuvre ensures that satellite cysts within the fibrous wall are also removed. In addition, any portion of the soft tissue of the oral cavity which is adherent to the cyst wall should also be excised (Brannon, 1977). If there is any doubt about the adequacy of the enucleation then an ostectomy should be carried out. Meiselman (1994) suggested that recurrent cysts are amenable to repeated conservative intervention. He stated that radical excision should be reserved for those cases which have breached the lower border of the mandible, those which involve the condyle and those which have undergone ameloblastic change or transformed to a carcinoma.

Williams and Connor (1994), on the other hand, prefer a more aggressive approach. They stated that enucleation alone is not adequate in view of the recurrent potential of keratocysts. Once the diagnosis has been established by an incisional biopsy, they recommended enucleation followed by mechanical curettage using methylene blue as a marking agent. This is then followed by a 3 minute application of Carnoy's solution (absolute alcohol, chloroform, glacial acetic acid and ferrous chloride). They believed that mechanical and chemical curettage is necessary to eradicate the satellite cysts. Recurrent cysts should be treated by resection of the involved bone.

Malignant potential

Odontogenic keratocysts are considered benign cysts with a propensity for local aggressive growth and recurrence after excision. Atypia of the cyst lining is uncommon. Brannon (1977) noted two cases of epithelial atypia out of 312 specimens. Rud and Pindborg (1969) found atypical cells in three out of 21 cysts. Frank malignant transformation is extremely rare and only nine cases have been reported in the literature. Seven of these were at the angle of the mandible, one in a patient with the naevoid basal cell carcinoma syndrome and one in a recurrent keratocyst.

Non-odontogenic cysts

In these cysts the epithelial lining is derived from sources other than the tooth-forming organ. This group of cysts includes lesions previously classified as 'fissural cysts' which were presumed to arise from epithelium entrapped along the lines of closure of embryonic processes during facial development. However doubt has been cast on this concept and the exact origin of these lesions is still unclear.

Recently, the existence of median palatine and median alveolar cysts as separate entities has also been questioned and these cysts have been excluded from the WHO classification (1992). They were misnamed as 'fissural cysts' but are now recognized to be anatomical variations of the nasopalatine duct cyst; median palatine cyst being a posterior extension and the median alveolar cyst being an anterior extension of the nasopalatine duct cyst.

Nasopalatine duct (incisive canal) cyst

The nasopalatine duct cyst is a distinct entity and is the commonest of all non-odontogenic developmental cysts. It arises from the epithelial remnants of the nasopalatine duct which connects the oral and nasal cavities in the embryo.

Clinical features

Shear (1992) reported that 11% of the 2616 jaw cysts in his series were nasopalatine duct cysts. However, he also included those previously diagnosed as median palatine cysts and cysts of the palatine papillae. Killey, Kay and Seward (1977) found only two nasopalatine duct cysts during examination of 2394 dry skulls. Nasopalatine duct cysts most commonly present in the third, fourth and fifth decades and approximately three-quarters are found in men (Swanson, Kaugars and Gunsolley, 1991).

The cyst may be asymptomatic and is discovered during routine radiography, alternatively it can present as a slowly enlarging swelling in the anterior part of the palate just behind the incisors. It may also present in the midline of the upper labial sulcus. If large, a protuberance may be seen in the floor of the nose. Secondary infection may lead to pain and discharge. The discharge may be mucoid with a salty taste or purulent with a foul taste.

On radiographs nasopalatine duct cysts are well defined ovoid or heart-shaped radiolucencies with sclerotic margins (Figure 23.6). They are usually symmetrical about the midline but may be displaced to one side. The cyst must be distinguished from a normal incisive fossa. Killy, Kay and Seward (1977) examined 2394 dry skulls have suggested that a radiolucency of less than 6 mm may be regarded as normal. Chamda and Shear (1980) reported that a radiolucency of up to 10 mm in the negroid population may be normal. The nasopalatine duct cyst must be distinguished from radicular cysts by confirming the vitality of adjacent teeth. Displacement of adjacent roots is common together with some degree of resorption.

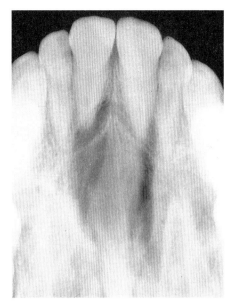

Figure 23.6 Nasopalatine cyst. (Courtesy of M. Hosseini)

Histology

The nasopalatine duct cyst may be lined by a variety of different epithelia. Stratified squamous, pseudo-stratified ciliated columnar, cuboidal or any combination of the above may be seen. Goblet cells may be present. A valuable diagnostic feature of nasopalatine duct cysts is the presence of a neurovascular bundle in the fibrous capsule. Mucous glands may be seen in the capsule.

Treatment

The standard treatment is enucleation using a palatal flap under a local or general anaesthetic.

Nasolabial cyst (nasoalveolar cyst)

The nasolabial cyst is a rare soft tissue lesion which arises in the upper lip just below the alar margin of the nose. Although it arises in soft tissue it is traditionally grouped with jaw cysts as it was previously regarded as 'fissural' in origin. The previously held view that it is a fissural cyst has now been discounted. Many authors support Bruggemann's (1920) theory that it arises from the epithelial remnants of the nasolacrimal apparatus.

Clinical features

The age distribution ranges from 12 to 75 years with a peak incidence in the fifth decade (Kuriloff, 1987). Over 75% of the cysts occur in women. An uncomplicated swelling is often the presenting feature. Rarely patients may complain of pain and nasal obstruction and occasionally of a poorly fitting upper denture. As the cyst enlarges it fills out the nasolabial fold, distorting the nostril and producing a protuberance in the floor of the nose. It can be palpated as a fluctuant swelling intraorally within the labial sulcus.

The enlarging cyst causes bone resorption of the labial surface of the maxilla and this scalloped concavity appears as a radiolucency above the roots of the incisor teeth.

Histology

The cyst is lined by non-ciliated pseudostratified columnar epithelium with some goblet cells. Patches of squamous metaplasia are seen. The cyst wall consists of loose connective tissue with occasional mucous glands.

Treatment

The cyst lies supraperiostially, high in the labial sulcus. It is therefore best removed via a labial sulcus approach together with the periosteum.

Midpalatal cysts of infants (Epstein pearls)

Although not of odontogenic origin, midpalatal cysts share many features of the gingival cysts of infants. They arise from epithelial inclusions at the line of fusion between the embryonic palatal folds and the nasal process.

They are twice as frequent as gingival cysts (Cataldo and Berkman, 1968) and are found along the midpalatal raphe. The clinical behaviour, histological appearances and the lack of need for treatment is similar to the gingival cyst of infants.

Fissural cysts (median palatine, median alveolar, median mandibular, globulomaxillary cysts)

Previously fissural cysts were thought to have developed from epithelium entrapped during embryonic fusion of the frontonasal and maxillary processes. However, embryological studies have shown that the surface bulges referred to as frontonasal and maxillary processes are not in fact prolongations with free ends but mere elevations and ridges which correspond to centres of growth in the underlying mesenchyme (Shear, 1992). Other than at the medial palatal raphe, there is no ectodermal to ectodermal contact which requires epithelial dissolution prior to fusion. Therefore the concept of fissural cyst has had to be reconsidered and has been discarded.

Median palatine and median alveolar cysts are now recognized to be varieties of the nasopalatine duct cyst; median palatine cyst being a posterior extension and the median alveolar cyst being an anterior extension of the nasopalatine duct cyst. Cysts do occur in the middle of the mandible but these are no longer referred to as median mandibular cysts of fissural origin. Those reported in the literature almost certainly have an odontogenic origin (Gardner, 1988).

Globulomaxillary cysts which have also traditionally been classified as fissural cysts are now not recognized to be an entity. Christ (1970), Wysocki (1981) and Shear (1992) have reviewed previously reported globulomaxillary cysts and found these to be a collection of odontogenic cysts, giant cell granulomas, myxomas and hamartomous bone cysts.

Radicular inflammatory cysts

Radicular cysts derive their epithelium from odontogenic remnants in the periodontal ligament (cell rests of Malassez) and are a result of chronic inflammation. The inflammation is usually a result of pulp death and therefore the cysts are commonly found at the apices of teeth (apical cysts). They may also be found at the lateral aspect of the root adjacent to an accessory root canal (lateral cysts). Radicular cysts may persist following extraction of the offending tooth when they are called residual cysts (Figure 23.7). The cyst associated with the cervical margin of the tooth and which arises due to inflammation in the gingival crevice is called an inflammatory collateral cyst.

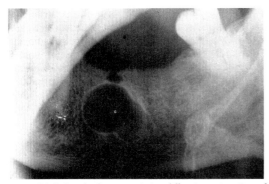

Figure 23.7 Residual cyst persisting following extraction of carious teeth

Clinical features

Radicular cysts are the commonest cystic lesion in the jaw and account for over half of all jaw cysts (68%, Killey, Kay and Seward, 1977). The peak frequency is in the fourth decade and there is a gradual decrease over subsequent decades. Approximately 60% are found in the maxilla especially associated with anterior teeth. The majority are detected on routine radiographs of non-vital teeth. They may present as slowly enlarging swellings; egg shell cracking may be elicited when the cortical bone is grossly thinned. Occasionally a sinus may be present discharging into the oral cavity. Radicular cysts are rare in deciduous teeth.

Radiographs

The cysts are round or ovoid radiolucencies with a sclerotic margin which extends from the lamina dura of the tooth (Figure 23.8).

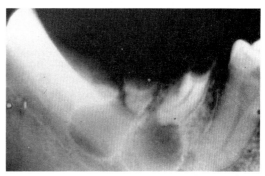

Figure 23.8 Two apical cysts associated with retained roots

Histology

Radicular cysts arise from the cell rests of Malassez within a chronic periapical granuloma. Approximately 1% of periapical granulomas progress to cyst formation. The mechanics involved in cyst formation are controversial but persistence of a chronic inflammatory stimulus is essential.

Cysts are lined by non-keratinized stratified squamous cell epithelium supported by a chronically inflamed capsule. Metaplasia into ciliated respiratory epithelium is rarely seen. Cholesterol crystals may be seen within the fibrous capsule. The cyst contents vary from a straw-coloured fluid to a cheesy brownish paste.

Treatment

Treatment involves removing the inflammatory source by root canal filling, apicectomy or extraction of the offending tooth and enucleation of the cyst.

Non-epithelial cysts

Solitary bone cyst

Solitary bone cysts are non-epithelialized bone cysts seen most commonly in the long bones of children, but occasionally they present in the jaws, almost exclusively in the mandible. They are rare and account for less than 1% of all jaw cysts. Solitary bone cysts occur mainly in childhood and adolescence. Howe (1965) reported that 78% of patients presented in the second decade. Kaugars and Cale (1987) reported 161 patients with solitary bone cysts of the jaws of which 95% were in the mandible. The majority of the cysts in the mandible are found in the body and symphysis, although some lesions have been reported in the ramus (Hosseini, 1979) and the mandibular condyle (Telfer *et al.*, 1990).

Clinical features

Most solitary bone cysts are diagnosed by chance following dental radiographs. In 25% of patients there is expansion of the mandible usually in a buccal or labial direction. Pain is infrequent and very occasionally patients complain of labial paraesthesia. Multiple cysts have been reported in 11% of patients (Kaugars and Cale, 1987).

Radiographs

The cyst appears as an irregular radiolucent area with slight cortication (Figure 23.9). Scalloping is a prominent feature particularly between teeth. Root resorption may be present.

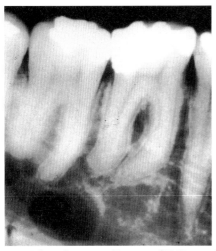

Figure 23.9 Solitary bone cyst. (Courtesy of M. Hosseini)

Pathogenesis

The pathogenesis of solitary bone cysts is not known. It has been suggested that trauma is the initiating factor which leads to a blood clot which fails to resolve and forms a cavity. However, in the majority of patients there is no history of related trauma (Kaugars and Cale, 1987). Hosseini (1979) suggested that there is a failure of differentiation in osteogenic cells, but there is no evidence to support this hypoth-

esis. At operation the cyst cavity is frequently empty, but may be filled with blood or serosanguineous fluid.

Treatment

Although the natural history of the cyst is to resolve spontaneously, surgery is required to confirm the diagnosis. The cyst cavity is opened to confirm its nature then tightly packed before closing.

Aneurysmal bone cyst

The aneurysmal bone cyst is a non-neoplastic lesion of bone of unknown pathogenesis and has been reported in most bones of the skeleton. It was first reported by Jaffe and Lichtenstein (1942) who proposed the term 'aneurysmal bone cyst'; Bernier and Bhaskar (1958) described the first case in the craniofacial skeleton. These cysts are most frequently seen in the long bones and vertebral spine and are rare in the jaws. Struthers and Shear (1984) found 42 cases in the literature. Aneurysmal bone cysts constituted 0.5% of the 2616 jaw cysts reported by Shear (1992) and 1.9% of all aneurysmal bone cysts of the skeleton.

The cysts occur predominantly in children and adolescents with the peak incidence in the second decade. There is a female preponderance. Approximately 60% are found in the mandible (Struthers and Shear, 1984), especially at the angle. Case reports of unusual locations include the floor of the orbit and the zygomatic arch (Shear, 1992).

The lesion presents as a firm localized swelling which is painful in about half the patients. Malocclusion may arise as result of displacement of teeth. The cyst erodes the cortical bone but is limited by the formation of new periosteal bone and therefore extension into soft tissues is rare. Egg shell cracking may be felt on palpation. At operation the periosteum is usually intact and the covering bone is thin. When the overlying bone is removed the cavity wells up with blood, and bleeding can be profuse.

Radiographs

The radiographic features are not diagnostic. The cyst produces a radiolucent ovoid expansion which is usually unilocular but may occasionally be multilocular. The multiple septation and trabeculations produce a 'soap bubble'-like appearance.

Pathogenesis

Trauma has been implicated in the past but there is little evidence to support this. Aneurysmal bone cysts may be found with other benign bone lesions such as non-ossifying fibroma, giant cell granuloma, fibrous dysplasia and myxofibroma (Biesecker *et al.*, 1970).

These authors postulated that a primary lesion of bone initiates an osseous arteriovenous malformation which leads, via its haemodynamic forces, to a secondary bone lesion which is termed an aneurysmal bone cyst.

Other reported series confirm the finding of associated bone lesions (El-Deeb, Sedano and Waite, 1980; Struthers and Shear, 1984). Struthers and Shear (1984) examined primary lesions of bone such as giant cell granulomas, fibrous dysplasia and ossifying fibromas and found microcysts at the periphery. They suggested that enlargement of these microcysts leads to aneurysmal bone cysts.

Histology

The inner architecture of the involved bone is destroyed. The predominant histological feature is multiple blood-filled spaces lined by flat spindle cells, not by endothelial cells. The solid areas of the lesion consist of sheets of vascular tissue containing large numbers of multinucleate giant cell, and fibroblasts with haemosiderin, giving the appearance of a giant cell granuloma. Other solid parts of the cyst may have histological features suggestive of fibrous dysplasia or ossifying fibroma.

Treatment

The treatment of aneurysmal bone cysts must be determined by the nature of the associated bony lesion. Following curettage recurrence is common. El-Deeb, Sedano and Waite (1980) reported a 26% recurrence rate. Cysts which recur or continue to expand should be resected.

Odontogenic tumours of the jaws

Over the years a number of authors have attempted to classify odontogenic tumours (Pindborg and Clausen, 1958). The task is difficult, partly due to the complexity of the tissues involved and partly because of the rarity of these lesions, this latter fact making it difficult to accumulate large series for clinicopathological study. The WHO has recently published a classification of odontogenic tumours (Table 23.2). The authors however acknowledged that some of the lesions included are certainly not neoplasms but hamartomas. They also acknowledged that some of the lesions given separate designations may in fact be a single lesion in different stages of evolution. Those lesions considered to be hamartomas will not be discussed further in this chapter.

Table 23.2 Odontogenic tumours of the jaws

Benign odontogenic neoplasms
Epithelial lesions
Ameloblastoma
Squamous odontogenic tumour
Calcifying epithelial odontogenic tumour (Pindborg)
Clear cell odontogenic tumour
Epithelial and mesenchymal lesions
Ameloblastic fibroma
Ameloblastic fibrodentinoma
Ameloblastic fibro-odontoma
Odontoameloblastoma
Adenomatoid odontogenic tumour
Calcifying odontogenic cyst
Complex odontoma
Compound odontoma

Malignant odontogenic tumours
Carcinomas
Malignant ameloblastoma
Primary intraosseous carcinoma
Malignant change in odontogenic cysts
Sarcomas
Ameloblastic fibrosarcoma
Ameloblastic fibrodentinosarcoma
Ameloblastic fibro-odontosarcoma

(Modified from Histological typing of odonotogenic tumours; WHO publications 1992)

Benign tumours

Ameloblastoma

The ameloblastoma is a benign but locally invasive neoplasm. The first detailed description of this tumour was given by Falkson in 1879 and the term ameloblastoma was introduced by Churchill (cited by Baden, 1965). The exact origin of the neoplastic epithelium is unclear although the strong resemblance to ameloblasts supports an odontogenic origin. The possible sources of epithelium are residues of the dental lamina, the enamel organ, the root sheath of Hertwig or the epithelial lining of other odontogenic cysts. The predominant opinion is that it is derived from the remnants of the dental lamina. Two variants, unicystic ameloblastoma and peripheral ameloblastoma (extraosseous ameloblastoma), have been described but these have a sufficiently different clinical behaviour to merit a separate mention later in the chapter.

Clinical features

Ameloblastomas are the most common odontogenic tumours but only account for approximately 1% of all oral tumours. In a review of 706 odontogenic tumours Regezi, Kerr and Courtney (1978) found that 11% were ameloblastomas. They are usually diagnosed in the fourth and fifth decades although cases have been reported in the newborn and the elderly. The mean age of presentation is 38.9 years

(Small and Waldron, 1955). The distribution between the sexes is equal.

About 80% of the tumours occur in the mandible of which three-quarters are in the molar region and the ascending ramus, 20% in the premolar region and 10% in the incisor region. Of the 24 maxillary tumours reported by Tsaknis and Nelson (1980), 80% were in the posterior part of the upper jaw.

Ameloblastomas are slow growing and usually asymptomatic in the early stages. Most are discovered on routine radiographs. As the lesion enlarges it causes bony expansion which can lead to facial deformity. The expansion is bony hard, but in advanced cases egg shell cracking may be apparent due to thinning of the cortical plate. Perforation of the cortex and extension into the soft tissues is an advanced feature. In the maxilla, expansion is uncommon as the lesion can expand into the maxillary sinus and into the pterygomaxillary space (Tsaknis and Nelson, 1980). Other clinical manifestations include loose teeth, ill fitting dentures, malocclusion, ulceration, discharge and nasal obstruction (Mehlisch, Dahlin and Masson, 1972).

On radiographs ameloblastomas most commonly appear as multilocular radiolucencies with well defined borders and distinct compartmentalization (Figure 23.10). There may be erosion of adjacent roots. The tumour may become associated with an unerupted tooth, especially the third molar, when it is indistinguishable from a dentigerous cyst. The unilocular ameloblastoma is a distinct variant and has a different clinical behaviour.

Histology

There is considerable variation in the histopathology of ameloblastoma and many patterns are described. Several of these varieties often coexist. It is important to appreciate that there appears to be no difference in clinical behaviour between the various histological types:

1 *Follicular:* this is the commonest histological pattern and consists of discrete islands of epithelium each resembling the enamel organ of the developing tooth germ
2 *Plexiform:* the tumour epithelium is arranged in strands and bounded by a layer of cuboidal cells resembling a stellate reticulum. Cyst formation may be present
3 *Acanthomatous:* this term is used when squamous metaplasia takes place and there is keratin production. This pattern is often found coexisting with the follicular type
4 *Basal cell:* the epithelium bears a strong resemblance to basal cell carcinoma and the cuboidal cells are arranged in sheets
5 *Granular:* in this variety the stellate reticulum-like cells undergo transformation into large, granular, eosinophilic cells. The granules represent lysosomal aggregates.

Behaviour and treatment

A typical intraosseous ameloblastoma is locally invasive with islands of tumour infiltrating cancellous marrow spaces without causing bone resorption. As a consequence simple curettage is not sufficient and recurrence rates of 55% (Gardner and Corio, 1983) to 90% (Sehdev, Havos and Strong, 1974) have been reported with enucleation. Rare reports of pulmonary metastases have been documented but these have been attributed to aspiration of tumour cells.

The recommended treatment is radical resection of the affected part of the jaw.

Unicystic ameloblastoma

This type usually affects a younger age group and presents in the second and third decades. It predominantly occurs in the region of the third molar (Robinson and Martinez, 1975). Radiographically, the cyst is a well defined unilocular radiolucency, which may be associated with unerupted teeth. Clinically and radiographically they are indistinguishable from dentigerous cysts or keratocysts and are only diagnosed after histological examination. This lesion may represent an ameloblastomous change in a pre-existing odontogenic cyst.

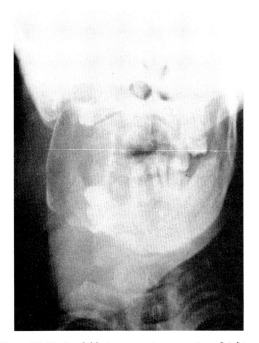

Figure 23.10 Ameloblastoma causing expansion of right ramus of mandible

The histological appearance is of a cyst with intraluminal growths of ameloblastoma. The lining consists of a basal layer of columnar cells covered by a loose layer of stellate epithelial cells.

Treatment

The recurrence rate is low. Eversole, Leider and Strub (1984) reported a recurrence rate of 18% following curettage. These lesions should therefore be enucleated and long-term follow up is required. Recurrences may be treated by repeated conservative treatment.

Extraosseous ameloblastoma

Rarely, ameloblastomas have been reported in the gingiva or alveolar soft tissue without any bone involvement (Moskow and Baden, 1982). They resemble an epulis. The common sites are the lingual gingiva of the mandible and the soft tissue tuberosity of the maxilla. Microscopically they have an acanthomatous pattern. The recurrence rate following local excision is less than 20%.

Squamous odontogenic tumour

The squamous odontogenic tumour was first described by Pullon, Shafer and Elzay in 1975. It is a rare lesion which presents with few symptoms except for local tenderness and tooth mobility. It probably arises from the remnants of the dental lamina or cell rests of Malassez.

The lesion usually presents in the third decade, but can be found from the second to the seventh decades (Cataldo, Less and Giunta, 1983). There is no sex predilection and both the jaws are equally affected.

The radiographic features are a well circumscribed radiolucency with a sclerotic margin associated with the roots of teeth. On histological examination, islands of well differentiated squamous epithelial cells are seen surrounded by a mature connective tissue stroma. The epithelial islands have a peripheral layer of cells resembling ameloblasts. In addition there may be microscopic cystic degeneration or calcification.

Recurrence after enucleation may occur but is rare and the choice of treatment is local curettage.

Calcifying epithelial odontogenic tumour

The calcifying epithelial odontogenic tumour is a rare neoplasm first recognized as a distinct entity by Pindborg in 1958. It is thought to arise from the elements of the enamel organ but the pathogenesis has not been firmly established.

Clinical features

The lesion accounts for less than 1% of all odontogenic tumours (Regezi, Kerr and Courtney, 1978).

It can present at any age between 8 and 90 years, but the majority occur in the fourth decade and there is an equal sex distribution (Franklin and Pindborg, 1976). Over two-thirds affect the mandible and of these most are found in the molar region. A calcifying epithelial odontogenic tumour arising in the maxillary antrum causing nasal obstruction has been described (Baunsgaard, Lontoff and Sorensen, 1983). The majority of lesions are intraosseous, although extraosseous tumours have been reported (Wertheimer, Zielinski and Wesley, 1977).

The tumour presents as a slowly growing painless mass and is usually discovered incidentally on dental radiographs. Symptoms of pain, nasal obstruction, epistaxis and proptosis have been reported.

The radiographic appearance is of an irregular radiolucent area containing radiopaque masses of various sizes which tend to be located close to the crown of an unerupted tooth.

Histology

Histologically the tumour shows considerable variation. There are strands of epithelial cells with well defined borders within a fibrous stroma. A characteristic feature is the presence of homogeneous amyloid-like material between sheets of cells which may be calcified.

Treatment

Since the recurrence rate is low, the preferred treatment is local curettage.

Clear cell odontogenic tumour

This is an extremely rare tumour which presents as an intraosseous mass in the maxilla or the mandible. Representative clinical data are not available as very few cases have been reported. Those which have been, occurred mostly in women over 50 years of age. The tumour is thought to arise from residues of the dental lamina.

Radiographs show a unilocular radiolucency with a poorly defined margin. Strands of epithelial cells, with clear cytoplasm, rich in glycogen are seen on histological examination.

Clear cell odontogenic tumours are aggressive tumours being locally invasive. The recurrence rate is high following enucleation and therefore it is recommended that they are resected with a margin of normal bone.

Ameloblastic fibroma

This rare tumour contains both epithelial and connective tissue elements. The mesenchymal component is also neoplastic unlike the ameloblastoma where only the epithelium is neoplastic. Ameloblastic fibromas usually occur in the younger age group and are uncommon over the age of 20 years. They present as slowly enlarging, painless masses most frequently in the premolar and the molar area. The lesion may interfere with the eruption of adjacent teeth. Over 80% occur in the mandible, the majority of which are in the molar region (Slootweg, 1981).

Radiographs show a well defined radiolucency with sclerotic margins. Approximately 70% are multilocular and are usually associated with unerupted teeth.

Histology

The histological features are proliferating strands of epithelium within a highly cellular fibroblastic tissue. The appearances are similar to the ameloblastoma, but there is a proliferative mesenchymal component.

Treatment

Unlike ameloblastomas recurrence is very rare and the treatment recommended is local curettage only.

Ameloblastic fibrodentinoma and ameloblastic fibro-odontoma

These lesions have been defined in the WHO classification (1992) as lesions similar to ameloblastic fibroma but also showing evidence of mineralization; there is dentine formation in ameloblastic fibrodentinoma and dentine and enamel formation in ameloblastic fibro-odontoma. It is unclear if these lesions are distinct from ameloblastic fibromas or just single lesions at various stages of development.

They occur mostly in children under the age of 10 years. There is no tendency to recur and are best treated by enucleation.

Odontoameloblastoma

The odontoameloblastoma is a very rare tumour which is locally aggressive. Clinically it behaves like an ameloblastoma but also shows evidence of dentine and enamel formation (LaBriola, Steiner and Bernstein, 1980). It is very difficult to distinguish an odontoameloblastoma from a developing complex odontoma which also show the same basic tissue elements.

Recurrence rates following enucleation are high and radical resection is therefore recommended.

Adenomatoid odontogenic tumour

Philipsen and Birn (1969) first proposed the term adenomatoid odontogenic tumour, distinguishing the lesion from the ameloblastoma. Since then about 500 cases have been reported in the literature (Philipsen *et al.*, 1991) and the lesion is now recognized as a distinct entity in the WHO classification (1992).

It is a rare tumour and its origin is still a source of dispute. However, most authors agree that it has an odontogenic origin as it occurs exclusively in the tooth-bearing areas and is closely associated with unerupted teeth. Some authorities still believe that it is a hamartoma rather than a neoplasm (Courtney and Kerr, 1975). Adenomatoid odontogenic tumours account for 3.3 to 6.6% of all odontogenic tumours (Bhaskar, 1968; Ajagbe *et al.*, 1985). The majority are found in the maxilla, especially in the canine region. They are usually asymptomatic and the only clinical finding is a bony swelling. Very rarely extra-osseous lesions may be found, mostly in the gingiva, clinically presenting as an epulis (Philipsen *et al.*, 1991).

The radiographic features include a well defined radiolucency with occasional calcification within the cavity. They are almost always associated with unerupted teeth.

Histology

Histological examination shows a well encapsulated lesion which is partly solid and partly cystic. Occasionally it may be entirely cystic. The epithelium is arranged in sheets and whorls of spindle cells. Rings of columnar cells give rise to a duct-like appearance, hence the name 'adenomatoid'. There is little supporting stroma. Calcification is sometimes seen and may be extensive, and very rarely enamel matrix may be present within the tumour.

Treatment

The adenomatoid odontogenic tumour is readily enucleated and does not recur.

Calcifying odontogenic cyst

The calcifying odontogenic cyst is classified in the WHO publication (1992) as a tumour and is defined as 'a locally invasive neoplasm characterized by the development of intraepithelial structures, probably of an amyloid like nature which may become calcified and which may be liberated as the cells break down'. Praetorius *et al.* (1981) recognized the calcifying odontogenic cyst as consisting of two entities, a cyst and a neoplasm. However Shear (1992) still referred to this lesion as a developmental cyst of odontogenic origin.

Clinical features

Buchner (1991) has reviewed the literature and found only 215 cases. Shear (1992) reported that 1% of his 2616 jaw cysts were calcifying odontogenic cysts. The age at presentation ranged from 5 to 82 years with a mean age of 30.3 years. The highest incidence is in the second decade. There is an equal sex distribution, and a racial predilection is not apparent.

Calcifying odontogenic cysts occur equally between the mandible and maxillae and the majority (65%) are in the incisor and canine regions. In the mandible the cyst may cross the midline but this is unusual in the maxilla. Extraosseous or peripheral cysts have been documented (Buchner *et al.*, 1991) and these are located mainly in the gingiva. Gorlin *et al.* (1964) reported one case arising in the parotid gland.

Most of the cysts are symptomless and are discovered on routine radiography. They may present as hard swellings of the maxilla or mandible. Pain is rare, occurring in association with secondary infection. Displacement of the teeth has been described and occasionally the lesion may perforate the cortical plate and extend into the soft tissues.

The radiological features are characteristic, the cysts appearing as unilocular radiolucencies with well defined margins. In approximately half a variable amount of calcified material is seen within the radiolucency. The calcifying odontogenic cyst may be associated with a complex odontome or an unerupted tooth. Root resorption of the adjacent teeth is a frequent finding.

Histology

The calcifying odontogenic cyst is often cystic but may be solid. The cyst cavity is lined by epithelium which shows a well defined basal layer of columnar, ameloblast-like cells. A characteristic feature is the presence of smooth, keratinizing epithelial cells referred to as 'ghost cells'. Irregular masses of dentine-like material are frequently found in the fibrous tissue. Five cases of malignant transformation have been reported.

Treatment

Uncomplicated cases of calcifying odontogenic cysts should be treated by enucleation. If the lesion is associated with another odontogenic tumour such as an ameloblastoma or ameloblastic fibroma then radical resection is recommended.

Malignant odontogenic tumours

Most of the carcinomas found in the mandible and maxilla have invaded bone from lesions of the oral cavity. Some may be metastatic deposits of primary lesions elsewhere in the body. Primary endosteal carcinoma of the jaws is exceedingly rare and arises from odontogenic epithelial residues in the jaws and are therefore called odontogenic carcinomas.

Odontogenic carcinomas have various origins:

1 They may develop by malignant transformation of an ameloblastoma and are called 'malignant ameloblastomas'
2 Some may develop directly from the epithelial remnants of odontogenic epithelium left after completion of tooth development. These are called 'primary intraosseous carcinoma'
3 They may result from malignant transformation of odontogenic cysts.

Subdivision into the above three categories is of academic interest only as these three groups behave similarly from a clinicopathological point of view.

Malignant ameloblastoma

Malignant ameloblastoma has been defined in the WHO classification as 'a neoplasm in which the pattern of an ameloblastoma and cytological features of malignancy are shown by the primary growth in the jaws and/or by any metastatic growth'. Tumours meeting these criteria may arise as a result of malignant change in a pre-existing ameloblastoma, or possibly as a primary malignant ameloblastoma not preceded by an ordinary ameloblastoma.

Previously these malignancies were subclassified into malignant ameloblastoma and ameloblastic carcinoma according to the degree of differentiation (Elzay, 1982). These terms are still used currently in the literature (Fertilo *et al.*, 1982; Dorner, Sear and Smith, 1988; Nagai *et al.*, 1991), but are not recognized in the WHO classification (1992) and the two groups should be treated as one.

The ordinary ameloblastoma that endangers life through direct invasion of vital structures (such as the cranium) should not be called malignant ameloblastoma. Care should also be taken to distinguish intraosseous salivary gland tumours (e.g. intraosseous mucoepidermoid tumour) from malignant ameloblastomas.

Nagai *et al.* (1991) reviewed 46 cases of malignant ameloblastomas. Most were found in the mandible (80%). The mean age at presentation was 40 years and there was a slight predilection for men. Metastases have been reported in lungs, lymph nodes, spleen, kidney and the lower ribs.

Treatment

The recommended treatment is radical excision of the primary tumour together with neck dissection if there is evidence of neck node involvement. Radiotherapy has been used for distant metastases. The malignant ameloblastoma is a rare tumour and therefore information about long-term survival and response to chemotherapy is not available.

Primary intraosseous carcinoma

The primary intraosseous carcinoma arises within the jaw and has no connection with the oral mucosa. It is therefore presumed to develop from odontogenic epithelial remnants. The histological appearance may be indistinguishable from an oral squamous cell carcinoma.

To *et al.* (1991) summarized 21 cases of primary intraosseous carcinoma reported in the literature and provide a detailed analysis. The mean age at presentation was 50 years. Three times as many men were affected as women. Sixteen cases were found in the posterior part of the mandible, the maxilla being involved in only three patients. The tumour may be an incidental finding on radiographs or it may present with swelling, pain, discharge, paraesthesia of the lip and tongue or a pathological fracture. Radiographs show a radiolucency with poorly defined margins. In the three new cases reported by To *et al.* (1991) preoperative radiographs did not contribute diagnostically. Neck node and lung metastases have been reported.

Histology

In some cases the histological appearance is indistinguishable from a squamous cell carcinoma of the oral mucosa. In others, the tumour has a distinct odontogenic pattern with squamous metaplasia and keratin formation similar to that seen in the acanthomatous variety of the ameloblastoma. It may therefore be difficult to decide whether a tumour should be classified as a malignant ameloblastoma or a primary intraosseous carcinoma.

Treatment

Radical resection with or without radiotherapy is the optimal treatment. Shear (1960) estimated the 5-year survival at 40%. To *et al.* (1991) reported a 46% 5-year survival in their series.

Malignant change in odontogenic cysts

Several reports have described lesions which clinically and radiographically were diagnosed as odontogenic cysts such as radicular, residual, dentigerous and keratocysts but, on histological examination, were found to be carcinomas (Van der Waal, Rauhamaa and Van der Kwast, 1985; Maxymiw and Wood, 1991; Dabbs *et al.*, 1994). Such lesions could have resulted from malignant transformation of the benign cysts although cystic degeneration of an existing carcinoma cannot be excluded.

Ameloblastic fibrosarcoma

The ameloblastic fibrosarcoma is defined as a neoplasm similar in structure to an ameloblastic fibroma but in which the mesenchymal component shows features of a sarcoma. The lesion is called an ameloblastic fibrodentinosarcoma when dentine is present and ameloblastic fibro-odontosarcoma when both enamel and dentine are present. These lesions are rare and there is a paucity of clinical data in the literature.

The average age at presentation is 31 years (Leider, Nelson and Trodahl, 1972) and the sex distribution is equal. Over two-thirds are found in the posterior part of the mandible. Ameloblastic fibrosarcomas may present with pain, swelling, paraesthesia of the lip, bleeding and ulceration. Radiographs show a poorly defined multilocular radiolucency with gross thinning of the cortex. Root resorption is common. Metastases to neck nodes have been reported (Howell and Burkes, 1977). There are several documented cases of ameloblastic fibrosarcomas arising from an ameloblastic fibroma or an ameloblastic fibro-odontoma (Howell and Burkes, 1977; Adekeye, Edwards and Goubran, 1978).

Treatment

From the limited information available it is clear that radical surgery should be the primary mode of treatment. Radiotherapy has not been helpful (Howell and Burkes, 1977).

Non-healing granulomas

The non-healing granulomas and tumours of the nose and sinuses both present with nasal obstruction and epistaxis. A tumour-like mass is seen on nasal inspection and the diagnosis is usually made by biopsy.

Many chronic inflammatory conditions of the nose are characterized by the formation of granulation tissue infiltrated by chronic inflammatory cells. Most of these granulomas are the result of a specific infectious organism and are termed 'specific granulomas'. In others, the aetiology is less clear and they are termed 'non-specific granulomas' or more familiarly to the otolaryngologist as the 'midline non-healing granulomas.'

Generally, the correct diagnosis can be established by either histological or microbiological examination. Table 23.3 lists some of the more common types of nasal granulomas. The specific granulomas are discussed in Chapter 8 of Volume 4 of this book.

Non-specific granulomas, more frequently called non-healing midline granulomas of the nose, have for many years been the cause of considerable confusion to both clinicians and pathologists. There have been many apparently different clinical entities described with detailed but non-specific histological appearances. Fortunately, over the last decade both clinical and pathological studies have clarified the

Table 23.3 Nasal granuloma

Specific	Syphilis
	Tuberculosis
	Lupus vulgaris
	Leprosy
	Sarcoidosis
	Rhinosporidiosis
	Mucormycosis
	Aspergillosis
	Histoplasmosis
	Blastomycosis
	Sporotrichosis
	Leishmaniasis
Non-specific	Wegener's granulomatosis
	Lethal midline granuloma (midfacial lymphoma)

situation and most clinicians recognize two main groups: Wegener's granulomatosis and the lethal midline granuloma (nasal lymphoma). Both groups have an appropriate therapeutic regimen and, provided the correct diagnosis is made early, the prognosis has been dramatically improved.

Wegener's granulomatosis

Wegener's granulomatosis is a systemic vasculitis of probable autoimmune aetiology. It may present to the otolaryngologist at various sites in the head and neck, but primarily it involves the upper and lower respiratory tracts and the kidneys. Other parts of the body are less commonly involved. It is distinguished histologically from polyarteritis nodosa by the typical formation of granulomas.

Wegener's description of rhinogenic granulomatosis in 1939 was a classical paper in which he described both the clinical and pathological features of the condition. The essential histological features are: necrotizing granulomas of the upper and lower respiratory tracts; focal necrotizing glomerulonephritis of the kidneys; and systemic vasculitis.

Clinical features

The original concept of the condition was of a fulminating disease leading to early death from renal failure. The patient often presents with a persistent 'cold', complicated by a blood-stained nasal discharge. Nasal examination at this stage reveals thickening of the mucosa with some ulceration and crust formation. The appearances are similar to atrophic rhinitis, but the patient is obviously unwell. Biopsy of the nasal granulations may be reported as non-specific chronic granulation by an inexperienced patholo-

gist, but careful examination of multiple biopsies will generally demonstrate the diagnostic epithelioid necrotizing granulomas, fibrinoid necrosis and focal vasculitis. However, the rapid clinical deterioration with evidence of systemic involvement of both the lungs and kidneys confirms the diagnosis. The chest radiograph shows localized areas of infarction which may proceed to cavity formation (Figure 23.11). Urinalysis will often show red cells and casts, and tests of renal function will demonstrate a decreased creatinine clearance. The erythrocyte sedimentation rate is raised. Untreated, the patient rapidly progresses to renal failure and death within 6 months.

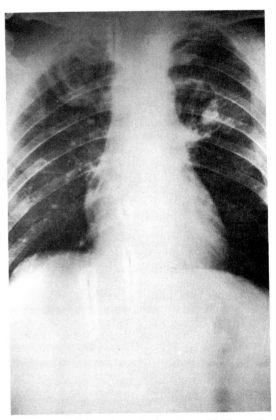

Figure 23.11 Chest radiograph of a patient with Wegener's granulomatosis showing bilateral apical cavities

However, it is now recognized that there is a more limited form of Wegener's granulomatosis with a relatively benign natural history (Friedman, 1995). One or other of the main sites is primarily involved with little obvious involvement of the other sites. Careful investigation will generally confirm the diagnosis by demonstrating decreased renal or pulmonary function. This modified presentation, when primarily involving the nose, is the usual source of confusion to the otolaryngologist. The patient complains of nasal obstruction, crusting and occasional epistaxis, and the initial diagnosis is atrophic rhinitis. Sinus radiographs will show a thickened lining membrane, and culture of the nasal secretions often grows *Staphylococcus aureus*. In such cases the true diagnosis will only be obvious on investigation and it is important to obtain an erythrocyte sedimentation rate, urinalysis, creatinine clearance and chest radiograph. The nasal biopsy is important and should be referred to an experienced head and neck pathologist for an opinion. The need for a confirmatory renal biopsy in such patients is best discussed with the renal physician, for early diagnosis and treatment will prevent the development of the crucial renal failure.

Other sites in the head and neck, occasionally involved either by direct spread or as separate entities, are the middle ear, eyes and orbit, the palate, oral cavity and larynx. Systemically the skin, joints and central nervous system may be involved.

Autoantibody estimation (ANCA titres)

Over the last 5 years the discovery of autoantibodies to neutrophil cytoplasmic antigens (ANCA) in patients with Wegener's granulomatosis has been of considerable importance both in diagnostic and therapeutic terms, as well as supporting an autoimmune aetiology.

In microscopic polyarteritis nodosa, similar autoantibodies are found; however their antigenic target is mainly perinuclear and the antibodies are termed perinuclear (P-ANCA). In Wegener's granulomatosis the autoantibodies generally have a cytoplasmic target (C-ANCA), although these may also be found with the P-ANCA antibodies in microscopic polyateritis nodosa (Lockwood *et al.*, 1987).

Equally important, the titre of C-ANCA correlates well with the disease activity and allows monitoring of therapy, although in cost terms the ESR gives similar information more cheaply. Raised C-ANCA titres are said to be diagnostic and while this is true for the acute phase it is not always the case in subacute disease when the degree of tissue damage is not very great. Unfortunately this is not uncommon in patients with early disease presenting in the head and neck and a negative ANCA test certainly does not exclude the condition.

Treatment

The essential aim is to control the renal involvement as the usual cause of death is renal failure. High doses of steroids (40–60 mg prednisolone/day) often result in a rapid clinical improvement, but long-term control or cure depends on the use of the cytotoxic drugs, azathioprine or cyclophosphamide. Cyclophosphamide, a widely used alkylating agent, is the drug of choice in North America (used in doses of 2 mg/kg per day.) Its main side effects are well documented, but the occurrence of haemorrhagic cystitis may be confusing in Wegener's granulomatosis. With the long-term use of steroids necessary in Wegener's granulomatosis, sterility, particularly in men, is a problem. In the UK the drug of choice has been the antimetabolite azathioprine (3 mg/kg per day). This drug is also used widely as an immunosuppressant in transplant surgery. Its main side effects on the liver and bone marrow are dose related and, with the control of the condition, the dosage can usually be decreased. The variation of the dosage requires considerable experience, and is best monitored by the clinical improvement and by the fall in the erythrocyte sedimentation rate (Figure 23.12) and ANCA titre. In particularly severe cases, both drugs can be used concurrently with benefit. Long-term use of cytotoxic agents beyond the period of active disease is probably necessary to prevent relapse.

A relapse often presents with minor changes in the patient's well-being and can be detected from either an increase in the ESR or ANCA titres. With relapses it is important to exclude concurrent sinus infection in an immunosuppressed patient with disordered nasal anatomy and physiology. Opportunistic fungal infections are not uncommon. After a prolonged period of inactive disease some patients are able to stop all medication, but continued close supervision is necessary. Management of the nasal cavities during the active phase requires regular irrigations and the use of glucose-in-glycerine nose drops to reduce crusting. Sinus drainage surgery is necessary if there is an associated sinus infection. Correction of the common saddle deformity of the nose is best left until control of the disease is well established.

Angiocentric lymphoma (non-healing midline granuloma)

The terminology of this condition has been confusing. The current recommended term is angiocentric lymphoma (Cleary and Batsakis, 1994; Friedman, 1995).

Clinically, the condition can readily be differentiated from Wegener's granulomatosis – the slowly progressive destruction of the nose and midfacial region by an apparent chronic inflammatory response is much greater than seen in the latter. There is remarkably little systemic disturbance and no evidence of pulmonary or renal involvement, death eventually following intercurrent infection or cachexia.

Originally described by McBride in 1897, the condition has been of interest and confusion to both clinicians and pathologists over the years with a variety of causes being suggested. More recently the consensus of opinion has been that the condition is probably a malignant lymphoma (Kassel, Echevarria and Guzzo, 1969), the variable clinical picture being the result of different degrees of immunological control in individual patients. Harrison (1974) on clinical

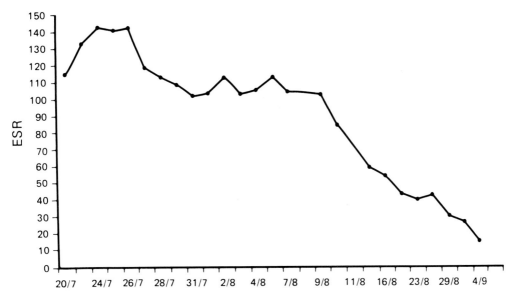

Figure 23.12 Fall in erythrocyte sedimentation rate following treatment of Wegener's granulomatosis with azathioprine and prednisolone

grounds, used radiotherapy with success and, in 1977, Michaels and Gregory found common histological features suggestive of lymphoma in a group of patients with this disorder. The features of widespread necrosis with atypical cells was termed 'necrosis with atypical cellular exudate' (NACE) by them and was considered to be consistent with a histiocytic lymphoma. Furthermore, four of their cases had similar lymph node metastases confirming their view that this was a malignant lymphoma. More recently Ishii *et al.* (1982), using immunofluorescent techniques, demonstrated that the cell-surface markers of the malignant cells in lethal midline granuloma had the same cell-surface phenotype as is usually found in human peripheral T cells. Consequently, they concluded that lethal midline granuloma was a nasal T-cell lymphoma. T-cell lymphomas tend to develop in such extralymphatic sites as the skin and nasal mucosa. They also found the histological appearances to be consistent with T-cell lymphoma. With the increased use of immunocytochemistry in histological diagnosis most cases of midline granuloma are now identified as T-cell lymphomas (Ramsay, Michaels and Harrison, 1988). Epstein-Barr virus is thought to play a role in the oncogenesis as it is found in most high grade midface lymphomas (Medeiros *et al.*, 1992).

Treatment

The condition responds well to local radiotherapy, consistent with the diagnosis of lymphoma (Figure 23.13). Initially low non-curative doses appeared satisfactory for control, but with experience, relapses became common and now full lymphoma curative doses of at least 50 Gy are used to the midfacial region and regional lymph nodes. The use of steroids and cytotoxics has been completely without success, supporting the different aetiology of Wegener's granulomatosis, and the malignant nasal lymphoma. This latter group contains the polymorphic reticuloses. Whether there is a third small group of 'idiopathic' midline granulomas of non-lymphoma origin is becoming increasingly uncertain and, with full experienced pathological investigation, this possibility will probably disappear completely.

Nasal tumours

A wide variety of tumours of different histological type is found in the nasal cavities and paranasal sinuses. The more common types are listed in Table 23.4. Benign tumours are not uncommon, but malignant tumours are rare constituting less than 1% of all malignancies (3% of head and neck tumours). The presenting symptomatology of all tumours is similar and with advanced imaging using both CT and MRI a presumptive diagnosis can often be made. However, careful histological examination with immunocytochemistry is necessary to decide the nature of any particular tumour.

Benign tumours

Papilloma

Squamous papillomas of the skin of the nasal vestibule and anterior septum are quite common. Usually they are treated in the outpatient department by

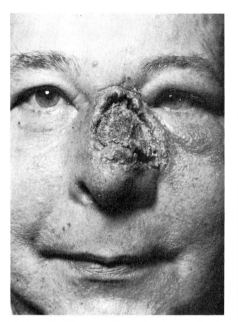 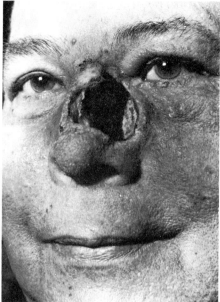

Figure 23.13 Case of midline granuloma showing results of surgical debridement following radiotherapy

cautery or cryosurgery. However, if they recur they should be excised for histological examination, as the early case of squamous carcinoma of this area is

Table 23.4 Tumours of the nose and paranasal sinuses

Benign	Malignant
Epithelial	
Adenoma	Squamous cell carcinoma
Papilloma	Adenocarcinoma
	Anaplastic carcinoma
	Transitional cell carcinoma
	Malignant melanoma
	Salivary gland tumours
	Adenoid cystic carcinoma
	Mucoepidermoid
	Malignant pleomorphic
	Aesthesioneuroblastoma
Non-epithelial	
Fibroma	Fibrosarcoma
Haemangioma	Angiosarcoma
Nasal glioma	Haemangiopericytoma
Neurilemmoma	Meningioma
Chondroma	Chondrosarcoma
Osteoma	Osteogenic sarcoma
	Lymphosarcoma
	Rhabdomyosarcoma
	Plasmacytoma
	Chordoma
Odontogenic tumours	
Fibro-osseous tumours	

readily curable whereas the missed case is often incurable. More persistent papillomas may benefit from the use of the argon laser.

Transitional cell papilloma or inverted papilloma was originally described by Ringertz (1938), and its potential for malignancy was discussed by Osborn (1970) and Hyams (1971). The diagnosis is made histologically, the deep invaginations of the epithelium into the stroma being the typical features (Figure 23.14). They are usually found unilaterally, and there is a male predominance of 5:1. They may be present at any age, but are found most commonly in

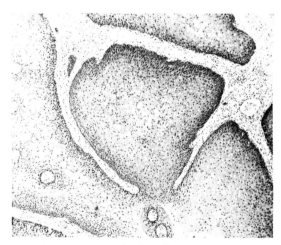

Figure 23.14 Transitional cell papilloma (× 65)

the fifth decade. Treatment is by surgical removal (radiotherapy is not indicated, even for recurrences). Local intranasal removal tends to be followed by recurrence, probably due to the difficulty in seeing the extent of the involved mucosa in the complex anatomy of the lateral nasal wall. CT imaging in both coronal and axial planes as for sinus disease will often clearly delineate the suspect areas and the experienced endoscopic sinus surgeon is becoming increasingly successful in the removal of these tumours. In those patients where repeated or rapid recurrence occurs, removal by a medial maxillectomy is indicated and this is increasingly being achieved by a midfacial degloving approach with excellent cosmesis. The important feature of these tumours is their tendency to undergo malignant change, in about 2–5% of patients. It must also be remembered that the papilloma may be present simultaneously with carcinoma in about 5–10% of patients, consequently careful follow up and examination of all material removed surgically is important.

Haemangioma

Haemangiomas may be found anywhere in the nasal cavities, but commonly are found on the anterior part of the nasal septum, where they are called the 'bleeding polypus of the septum'. They are probably not true tumours but vascular malformations (Osborn, 1959). Recurrence is common unless the base of the haemangioma is excised from the septum.

Fibroma

Simple fibromas are occasionally seen as single firm polyps in the nose, but do not tend to grow very large.

Neurofibroma

Neurofibromas involving any of the nerves inside the nose may grow to quite a large size and a lateral rhinotomy approach is often necessary to allow complete excision. Careful histological examination is essential as some of these tumours have a degree of low grade malignancy.

Osteomas and other osseous tumours

Harrison (1984) reviewed this group of tumours and emphasized the need to correlate the clinical features with both radiological and histopathological findings in order to understand the natural history of each tumour and plan its management. The benign osteomas are the commonest tumours in this group and are often found as an incidental finding in the frontal sinus on radiographs. The majority are asymptomatic and do not progress rapidly. However, they tend to occur at an earlier age in the Arabic races and often grow to quite large sizes in this ethnic group. Surgical excision is indicated when osteomas are sympto-

matic and demonstrate an increase in size. Complete removal is essential and the base attachment must be included. As the base is often in contact with the underlying dura a craniofacial type of approach is occasionally indicated.

Fibrous dysplasia, originally described by von Rechlinghausen in 1891, is now divided into two types – the multiple polyostotic lesions of Albright's syndrome and the monostotic lesions more familiar to the otolaryngologist involving the bones of the skull. The management of the monostotic foci consists of limited surgery to reduce the cosmetic defect. Radiotherapy may cause malignant change and is contraindicated.

Tumours and cysts of dental origin

The ameloblastoma and dental cysts are discussed at the beginning of this chapter.

Malignant tumours

Cancer of the nasal cavities or paranasal sinuses is a highly lethal condition and particularly unpleasant by its obvious nature both to the patient and the family. The results in the past have been unsatisfactory with a 30% overall 5-year survival. Frazell and Lewis (1963) commented that the unsatisfactory results could be attributed to a number of factors:

1 The disease was invariably advanced on presentation
2 The complex anatomy of the region and close relationship to the orbit and skull base
3 The reluctance of surgeon and radiotherapist to treat aggressively for fear of increasing the natural mutilation of the disease.

The increasing use of craniofacial resections for these tumours over the last two decades has done much to overcome Frazell and Lewis's comments and we are now able to offer these patients a reasonable prognosis with excellent cosmesis and functional rehabilitation.

The rarity of these tumours, which constitute less than 1% of all malignancies (3% of head and neck tumours), means that many primary physicians will not see a single patient with this disease in the whole of their professional careers. Their consequent relative unawareness of the condition and the similarity of the symptoms with the more common inflammatory conditions of the upper respiratory tract result in a failure to think of the true diagnosis before the tumour extends beyond the bony margins of the sinus. The average delay between the first noticeable symptom and diagnosis is 6 months. Unfortunately, this situation is unlikely to improve in the UK due to the scarcity of primary physicians with extra training in otolaryngology.

The best hope for early diagnosis lies in the greater use of CT imaging for the assessment of chronic rhinosinusitis where the radiological picture will suggest the correct diagnosis. Already we are seeing the earlier referral of those patients whose symptoms take them to other specialties such as neurology and ophthalmology, where CT and MR imaging are essential parts of the diagnostic assessment.

There is an increasing tendency to refer these patients to major centres, and this generally results in better management. The surgeon and radiotherapist being more experienced are more able to provide the very individual treatment regimen that is so often necessary with these tumours. The use of CT and MR imaging enables the precise delineation of the tumour extent, and careful planning of both the radiotherapy and subsequent surgical resection.

Aetiology

The upper jaw is one of the few sites in the head and neck where a definite aetiology has been established for some tumour types (Lund, 1991).

Adenocarcinoma of the nasal cavity and sinuses is known to be common among woodworkers (Acheson *et al.*, 1968). Esme Hadfield in her Hunterian Lecture (1970) showed the incidence of adenocarcinoma to be 10 times greater in High Wycombe compared with the rest of Buckinghamshire, and Acheson *et al.* (1982) showed the skilled furniture makers particularly the machinists, had a cumulative risk of at least 1 in 120 during their industrial lifetime (similar to carcinoma of the bronchus). The occupational risk was recognized by the Government and, in 1969, in the UK, adenocarcinoma of the nasal sinuses in woodworkers in the furniture industry became a prescribed disease under the 1959 National Insurance (Prescribed Diseases) Regulations: Reference D6, and it is the duty of the doctor to inform patients of their rights. Currently the patient needs to refer to leaflet BI 95 of the Benefits Agency. The particular type of wood machined also appears to be significant, African mahogany being the most dangerous. It is interesting to note that this wood is often used in fires by the Bantu tribesmen of South Africa who have the highest incidence of upper jaw cancer in the world, although in these patients, squamous cell carcinoma is the more common type.

Experimentally in rats there is a close relationship between exposure to a combination of formaldehyde vapour and wood-dust and the development of squamous metaplasia and, in one rat, squamous carcinoma (Holmstrom and Wihelmsson, 1988). Although this combination of irritants is common in industrial practice there is, as yet, no clinical demonstration of a correlation with squamous cell carcinoma in humans.

Barton (1977) discussed the role of nickel as a carcinogen in squamous cell carcinoma in nickel workers. In Norway, the modification of the industrial process and a screening programme among the workers has resulted in a decline in incidence. In the UK squamous cell carcinoma of the paranasal sinuses in nickel workers is also a prescribed disease, Reference C22.

Pathology

A large variety of different tumour types has been described in the upper jaw, and Table 23.4 lists the more common types. The most common histological type is squamous cell carcinoma, representing about 80% of all cases.

The primary site is not always easy to determine with several different sinuses commonly involved by the time the patient presents. The majority (60%) of tumours appear to be of antral origin, 30% arise in the nasal cavities, and the remaining 10% arise from the ethmoids. Primary frontal and sphenoid tumours are very rare.

Palpable cervical lymphadenopathy is present in about 15% of patients on presentation. This small figure is because the lymphatic drainage of the paranasal sinuses is to the retropharyngeal nodes and thence to the lower deep cervical chain. Consequently, the early involved nodes are not easily palpated in any area of the neck.

Presentation

The presentation of each particular patient depends on the primary site and the direction and extent of spread. Nasal cavity tumours present with the nasal symptoms of obstruction and epistaxis. Ethmoidal tumours also present with nasal symptoms, but also may have early orbital symptoms such as proptosis and epiphora, with diplopia being a late symptom. Frontal sinus tumours tend to present solely with orbital symptoms. Sphenoid sinus tumours generally present late to neurologists with neurological symptoms.

It is instructive to look at the potential presentation of antral tumours. Tumours within the antral cavity are unlikely to present early unless fortuitously they involve the infraorbital nerve giving a change in facial sensation, or alternatively bleed giving rise to epistaxis. Any epistaxis in an elderly patient who is not hypertensive requires radiological investigation, but the sinus radiographs are best deferred for 7–14 days to allow resolution of any inflammation associated with nasal packing or better still CT scans should be obtained. When the tumour breaches the antral walls, definite signs and symptoms become more obvious, their exact nature depending on the particular wall eroded.

Invasion of the nasal cavity leads to nasal obstruction and epistaxis and the tumour is often clearly seen. Less commonly, the tumour causes ethmoidal polyposis and apparently normal nasal polyps are seen; hence it is essential to examine histologically all material removed from the nose. Inferior spread to involve the palate and alveolus may result in presentation to the dentist with either an ill-fitting denture or loose tooth. Frank ulceration of the palate is a late symptom. Anterolateral spread into the soft tissues of the face may result in epiphora by involving the lacrimal sac. Facial swelling, disordered sensation and pain are more common. Anterior spread is more likely to result in palpable cervical lymphadenopathy. Posterior spread into the infratemporal fossa and skull base may cause less obvious symptomatology, loss of trigeminal function and trismus occurring from involvement of the pterygoid muscles. Spread into the nasopharynx may result in deafness as a result of eustachian tube dysfunction. Superior spread into the orbit causes early proptosis by increasing the volume of the orbital contents, direct involvement of the nerves and muscles occurring late.

Investigation

The objectives of investigation are to obtain a histological diagnosis and to determine the extent of the tumour. A biopsy may be readily obtained from tumour presenting in the nasal or oral cavities. If the tumour is within the antrum, a biopsy is best obtained by an intranasal antrostomy which will also provide drainage during radiotherapy. Biopsy by a Caldwell-Luc approach was previously recommended because it allowed better visualization of the tumour within the sinus and also palpation of the antral walls. This is more appropriately done by CT scanning, and there is always a potential danger of removing the bony barrier between tumour and the facial soft tissues, even if subsequently radiotherapy 'sterilizes' the area. In making the biopsy, good representative samples must be taken, and with any overlying necrotic tissue removed.

Modern imaging gives excellent delineation of tumour extent (Figure 23.15). Plain sinus radiographs have no value and the minimum requirement is CT scanning in two planes, axial and true coronal in the submentovertical position. High resolution scans with bone windows demonstrate bone erosion or often bone displacement with expansile tumours. The use of contrast gives useful information regarding soft tissue spread but does not readily distinguish between secondary inflamed mucosa and tumour. This distinction requires MRI scanning with gadolinium enhancement and subtraction scans give even more information. Images produced automatically in three planes are another virtue of MRI. Although modern imaging has an enormous potential in diagnosis, it is important to remember that the results are only as good as the staff operating the equipment and with these rare tumours it is essential for the rhinologist to explain his requirements to the radiologist and he will gain considerable advantage if he can be present at the time of the scan.

Angiography other than for vascular tumours has little to offer.

Nasendoscopy may be valuable in early tumours, but with the tumours usually encountered the associated bleeding and mucocoele formation make the procedure difficult, and the information obtained is generally inferior to radiology.

Classification

The classification of tumours is considered an essential feature of cancer management. It enables the individual clinician to plan an appropriate method of treatment based on experience, and also allows comparison between different treatment regimens. Unfortunately, the complex anatomy and late presentation with extensive disease involving more than one site has made classification difficult, different systems have been suggested and there has been a failure to agree on a standard UICC (International Union Against Cancer) classification. The first practical classification was proposed by Sebileau (1906) and he divided the upper jaw into three regions: suprastructure, mesostructure and infrastructure. Lederman (1970) adapted Sebileau's classification of the TNM system, but unfortunately it has not found wide acceptance (Figure 23.16). Harrison (1978) has discussed in detail the problems with the various classifications. The main objection to all systems is the doubt that individual cases can be accurately recorded as to site and extension. With the advent of CT and MRI scanning, this objection has been largely overcome and it is to be hoped that a universally acceptable classification will be found. At the present time the only accepted classification is the American Joint Committee on Cancer (AJCC) system for the maxillary antrum (Figure 23.17).

Treatment

There is no widespread agreement on treatment regimens for upper jaw cancer. This is due to several factors:

1 The relative rarity of the tumours, which means few clinicians develop a wide experience
2 The lack of a standard system of classification prevents meaningful comparisons between different centres
3 The wide variation in tumour extent on presentation
4 The differing response depending on histological type.

The condition is naturally mutilating and death tends to be delayed and unpleasant; consequently most patients require some form of active treatment, if only for palliation. No single modality of treatment

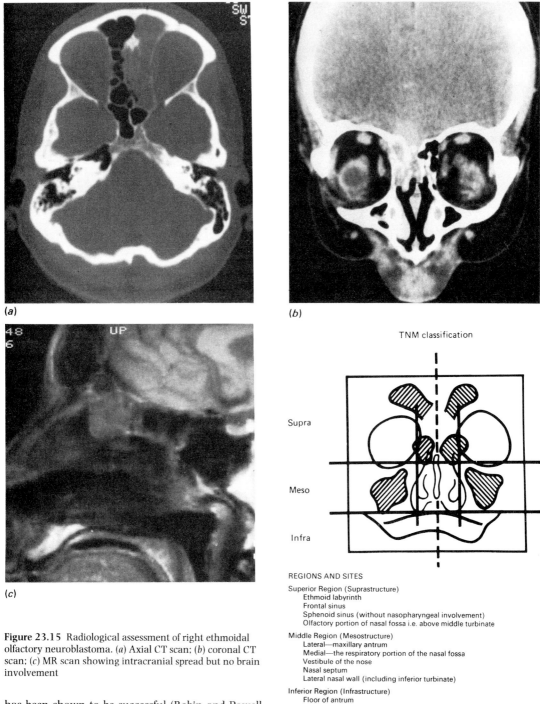

(a)

(b)

(c)

Figure 23.15 Radiological assessment of right ethmoidal olfactory neuroblastoma. (*a*) Axial CT scan; (*b*) coronal CT scan; (*c*) MR scan showing intracranial spread but no brain involvement

TNM classification

Supra

Meso

Infra

REGIONS AND SITES

Superior Region (Suprastructure)
  Ethmoid labyrinth
  Frontal sinus
  Sphenoid sinus (without nasopharyngeal involvement)
  Olfactory portion of nasal fossa i.e. above middle turbinate

Middle Region (Mesostructure)
  Lateral—maxillary antrum
  Medial—the respiratory portion of the nasal fossa
  Vestibule of the nose
  Nasal septum
  Lateral nasal wall (including inferior turbinate)

Inferior Region (Infrastructure)
  Floor of antrum
  Floor of nose
  Tumours involving simultaneously
  Hard palate and antrum
  Hard palate and floor of nose
  Dental tumours

has been shown to be successful (Robin and Powell, 1981) and in most centres a combination of radiotherapy and surgery is used. Both systemic and intra-arterial chemotherapy have been used, but results have been disappointing, and there is also some suggestion that such regimens encourage systemic

Figure 23.16 Proposed TNM classification for tumours of the upper jaw (Lederman, 1970)

PARANASAL SINUSES (ICD-O 160.9)

Data Form for Cancer Staging

Patient identification
Name _____
Address _____
Hospital or clinic number _____
Age _____ Sex _____ Race _____

Institutional identification
Hospital or clinic _____
Address _____

Oncology Record

Anatomic site of cancer _____
Chronology of classification*   [ ] Clinical-diagnostic (cTNM)
                                [ ] Surgical-evaluative (sTNM)
Date of classification _____

Histologic type† _____ Grade (G) _____
[ ] Postsurgical resection–pathologic (pTNM)
[ ] Retreatment (rTNM)   [ ] Autopsy (aTNM)

Definitions: TNM Classification

Primary Tumor (T)

[ ] TX Minimum requirements to assess the primary tumor cannot be met.
[ ] T0 No evidence of primary tumor
[ ] Tis Carcinoma *in situ*
[ ] T1 Tumor confined to the antral mucosa of the infrastructure with no bone erosion or destruction
[ ] T2 Tumor confined to the suprastructure mucosa without bone destruction, or to the infrastructure with destruction of medial or inferior bony walls only
[ ] T3 More extensive tumor invading skin of cheek, orbit, anterior ethmoid sinuses, or pterygoid muscle
[ ] T4 Massive tumor with invasion of cribriform plate, posterior ethmoids, sphenoid, nasopharynx, pterygoid plates, or base of skull

Nodal Involvement (N)

[ ] NX Minimum requirements to assess the regional nodes cannot be met.
[ ] N0 No clinically positive nodes
[ ] N1 Single clinically positive homolateral node 3 cm or less in diameter
[ ] N2 Single clinically positive homolateral node more than 3 cm but not more than 6 cm in diameter or multiple clinically positive homolateral nodes, none more than 6 cm in diameter
  [ ] N2a Single clinically positive homolateral node more than 3 cm but not more than 6 cm in diameter
  [ ] N2b Multiple clinically positive homolateral nodes, none more than 6 cm in diameter
[ ] N3 Massive homolateral node(s), bilateral nodes, or contralateral node(s)
  [ ] N3a Clinically positive homolateral node(s), one more than 6 cm in diameter
  [ ] N3b Bilateral clinically positive nodes (in this situation, each side of the neck should be staged separately, i e , N3b right, N2a left, N1)
  [ ] N3c Contralateral clinically positive node(s) only

Distant Metastasis (M)

[ ] MX Minimum requirements to assess the presence of distant metastasis cannot be met
[ ] M0 No (known) distant metastasis
[ ] M1 Distant metastasis present
        Specify _____

*Use a separate form each time a case is staged
†See reverse side for additional information

Site-Specific Information

Status before treatment anywhere is noted here.

Location of Tumor

[ ] Antrum
[ ] Infrastructure
[ ] Suprastructure
[ ] Both
[ ] Nasal Cavity
[ ] Septum
[ ] Roof
[ ] Lateral wall
[ ] Floor
[ ] Ethmoid
[ ] Anterior
[ ] Posterior
[ ] Sphenoid
[ ] Frontal

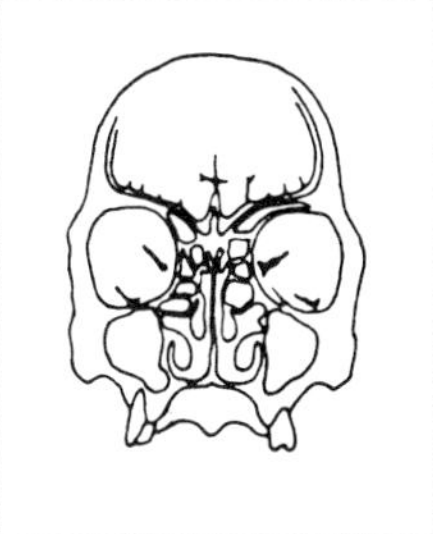

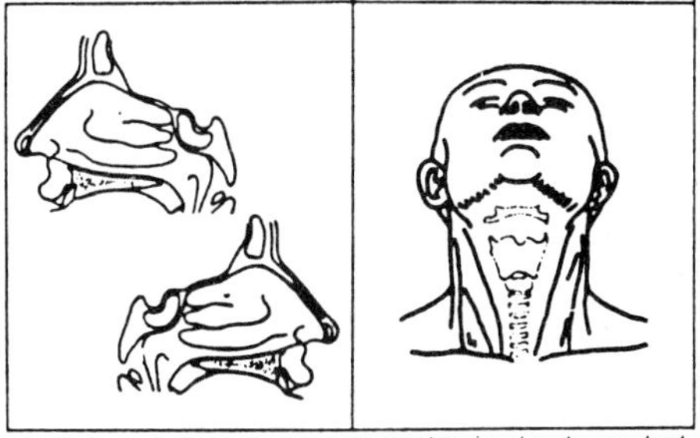

Indicate on diagram primary tumor and regional nodes involved.

Characteristics of Tumor

[ ] Radiographic destruction of bone
[ ] Invasion of adjacent areas
  [ ] Skin   [ ] Orbit
  [ ] Palate   [ ] Base of skull
  [ ] Nasopharynx   [ ] Pterygoid muscles
  [ ] Cribriform plate [ ] Pterygoid bone

Examination by _____ M D
Date _____

Figure 23.17 AJCC classification for paranasal sinuses (by courtesy of the American Joint Committee on Cancer)

metastases. There have been sporadic reports from Japan of good results following topical chemotherapy, but this treatment generally has not found favour in the West. However, a carefully controlled study in Rotterdam (Kneght *et al.*, 1985) of subtotal resection followed by twice weekly applications of topical 5-fluorouracil cream and repeated debridement of the resulting dead tissue continued for a period of 4 weeks has demonstrated excellent results particularly for adenocarcinoma and warrants further consideration.

General principles of management

In the absence of definite treatment schedules it is best to consider each patient individually and plan a treatment protocol based on general principles.

Patient factors

The consultation and subsequent investigation of the patient will establish the primary aim of treatment. There is a choice between treatment for cure and palliative treatment. In considering palliative treatment it is necessary to note the patient's symptoms and how they impinge upon his life, the extent of the disease and whether distant metastases are present, the patient's general medical condition and, most importantly the informed opinion of the patient and the relatives. In coming to a conclusion one must remember the relatively long natural history and propensity to facial mutilation of the disease and many experienced surgeons will advocate local debulking surgery with adjunctive radiotherapy as palliative treatment to improve the patient's quality of life.

Modality of treatment

Although most centres recommend a combination of radiotherapy and surgery there is still dispute as to whether the irradiation should be used before or after surgery. Preoperative radiotherapy has traditionally been advocated; it is more appropriate in radiobiological terms and the criticism that it interferes with healing should not be true with modern radiotherapeutic regimens (given with the intention of proceeding to subsequent surgery and not for primary cure). Those clinicians who favour postoperative irradiation cite the value of preliminary tumour debulking and accurate identification of tumour spread. Postoperative radiotherapy may be more valuable in slow growing tumours such as adenoid cystic carcinoma and chondrosarcoma.

Contraindications

These are very relative and reflect more on the experience and expertise of the treatment centre. The patient's wishes and poor health are probably the main factors. Local invasion of the anterior fossa and skull base are not contraindications with modern skull base surgery, but distant intracranial or systemic metastases mean a poor prognosis. Involvement of the facial skin is not a contraindication to treatment, and in practice many such patients do well. The involved area is best excised and repaired with a rotation flap of skin from either the forehead or cervical region, and occasionally microvascular free flaps have a part to play.

The authors' encouraging experience with craniofacial surgery has led them to advocate radical surgery for even early disease with the objective of obtaining an en-bloc clearance of the tumour. Adjunctive radiotherapy is also necessary.

Careful imaging demonstrates tumour extent and then a transnasal debulking of the tumour is performed before primary radiotherapy with curative doses of 60–65 Gy over 6 weeks. Approximately 6 weeks after the completion of radiotherapy the patient undergoes planned craniofacial resection to encompass completely any residual tumour. This regimen is recommended for even early stage disease and the results of such an approach have seen considerable improvements in local control but systemic metastases remain a problem.

Rehabilitation

High quality prosthetic rehabilitation is essential and requires the help of a maxillofacial laboratory. With a palatal resection the defect must be sealed with an obturator fitted with teeth to restore both speech and normal deglutition. Orbital resections leave an obvious cosmetic deformity and the Branemark system of titanium implants has revolutionized the fitting of facial prostheses, and radiotherapy is not a contraindication to their use.

Surgery of upper jaw tumours

A variety of operations has been described depending on the extent of the bone removed.

Partial maxillectomy

This entails partial removal of the upper jaw skeleton. Two variants are used regularly:

1 Medial maxillectomy involves the clearance of the lateral wall of the nose including the ethmoid sinuses
2 Palatal resection along with the adjacent alveolus is used for tumours of the oral cavity that involve the hard palate.

A further variant called palatal fenestration was originally described for placing radium implants into the cavity of the antrum. It has also been advocated as it allows good visualization of the cavity post-treatment but is rarely used these days.

Total maxillectomy

This entails the total removal of the upper jaw, preferably as a bony box containing the tumour.

Extended maxillectomy

An extended maxillectomy is required when the tumour extends beyond the upper jaw. If this involves the skull base the term craniofacial resection is used.

To facilitate the various bone resections it is necessary to use an appropriate soft tissue approach.

Three different soft tissue approaches are used.

LATERAL RHINOTOMY

This approach is usually attributed to Moure (1902) but was originally described by Michaux in 1854 and gives excellent exposure of both the nasal cavities and medial maxilla with a cosmetically acceptable incision in the lateral nasal crease.

WEBER-FERGUSSON

Again this approach is incorrectly attributed to both Fergusson and Weber although it was originally described by Gensoul in 1833.

MIDFACIAL DEGLOVING

This approach is used as a more cosmetic alternative to both the Moure's lateral rhinotomy and Weber-Fergusson approaches. Originally proposed by Rouge it has recently been rediscovered (Casson, Bonnano and Converse, 1974).

The basic technique of each operation is well described in the standard textbooks of operative surgery, but many points require special emphasis to ensure good tumour clearance and rapid rehabilitation. The selection of the operation depends on the preoperative assessment, but generally if the palate or zygoma is involved a total maxillectomy is indicated; in most other tumours a lateral rhinotomy or midfacial degloving approach will usually give good access for medial maxillectomy and requires little rehabilitation. Extensive tumours require some form of craniofacial approach.

Anaesthesia

Skilled anaesthesia is essential; topical anaesthesia of the nasal mucosa with Moffet's solution and hypotensive general anaesthesia are of considerable benefit to the surgeon. If the cranial cavity is opened, brain shrinkage is essential and is achieved by either mannitol infusion or by hyperventilation to lower the end-tidal Pco_2 to about 24 mmHg which induces decreased cerebral blood flow and brain shrinkage. The authors prefer the latter method as it gives better control of the situation. If the anterior fossa is opened, anticonvulsant drugs (phenytoin 100 mg twice daily) are given prophylactically and continued for 3 months. The placing of the endotracheal tube through the mouth may interfere with the fitting of a prosthesis after maxillectomy and a nasal tube through the uninvolved nostril is preferable. Some surgeons advocate preliminary tracheostomy.

Maxillectomy (Figure 23.18)

SOFT TISSUE APPROACH

The maxilla is best exposed by the Weber-Fergusson incision. The transverse limb should be placed close to the lid margin to prevent postoperative oedema of the lower lid. In the medial canthal region where the potential for skin loss as a result of radiotherapy is greatest, it is helpful to curve the incision forward over

the nasal bones for additional support postoperatively. A midline upper lip incision, if closed in three layers, is cosmetically more acceptable than a stepped incision. The mucosal incision along the midline of the hard palate turns laterally at the junction with the soft palate passing behind the maxillary tuberosity and then round the alveolus anteriorly. The facial skin flap is raised and all the soft tissue incisions are gently dissected free of the bone to allow the subsequent osteotomies.

OSTEOTOMIES

The maxilla is freed from the skull by osteotomies through the frontal process of the maxilla, through the body of the zygoma, through the midline of the palate, and the pterygoid plates need to be freed posteriorly. The palatal osteotomy is placed in the floor of the nasal cavity and may be made either with a fissure burr or gigli saw. The pterygoid plates are best separated from the maxilla with a curved osteotome, and subsequently dissected free from the muscles. The final two osteotomies are made with a fissure burr medially through the ethmoid cells and frontal process of the maxilla after dividing the lacrimal sac; laterally the osteotomy is made through the body of the zygoma, except for those laterally placed tumours where the zygoma needs to be included in the resection then the osteotomy is made in the lateral orbital wall below Whitnall's tubercle and through the zygomatic arch.

The remaining bony attachments are the posterior ethmoid cells and posterior antral roof, and these break readily on mobilizing the maxilla. The remaining soft tissue attachments are freed with Mayo scissors, and the maxilla removed. Bleeding from the internal maxillary artery is controlled initially by packing and then by application of a Ligaclip.

COMPLETION OF RESECTION

Following removal of the maxilla, further tissue must be removed to ensure complete tumour clearance and promote drainage from the remaining sinuses. The ethmoid cells should be exenterated totally, and both the sphenoid and frontal sinuses opened widely. If there is obvious involvement of the orbital periosteum, orbital exenteration is generally indicated. The support of the globe is complex and virtually all the medial and inferior orbital walls can be removed without the eye sinking. However, the lateral removal of Whitnall's tubercle results in lack of support for the eye which is best corrected by transposing the temporalis muscle medially. Orbital exenteration is achieved by an extraperiosteal dissection and transection of the muscle cone at the apex with Mayo scissors. Bleeding from the ophthalmic artery stops with local pressure. Following orbital exenteration, the eyelids are preserved but the lid margins and tarsal plates are excised to give a smooth skin lined cavity which accepts an onlay prosthesis satisfactorily (Figure 23.19).

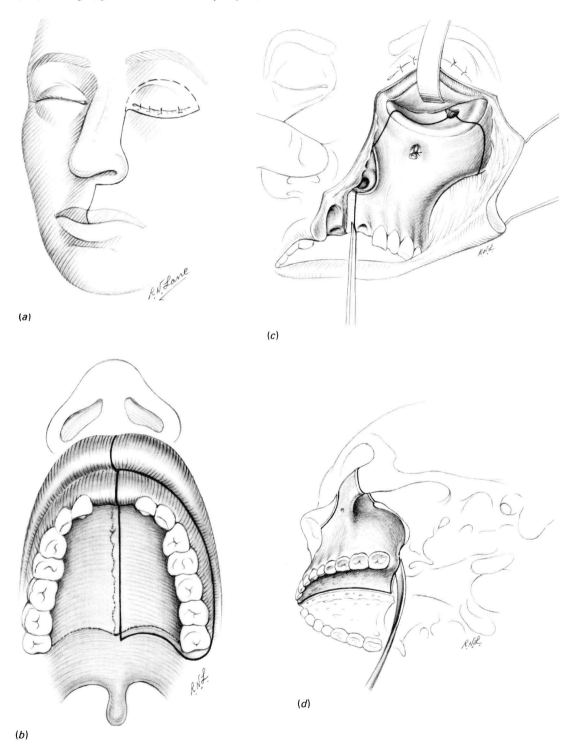

Figure 23.18 Classic maxillectomy: (*a*) Weber–Fergusson incision; (*b*) palatal incision; (*c*) following elevation of the facial flap, the maxilla is freed with osteotomies through the zygoma, palate and frontal process of the maxilla; (*d*) freeing the pterygoid plates. (From *Operative Surgery: Nose and Throat*, 4th edn, 1986, edited by J. Ballantyne and D. F. N. Harrison, with permission of the authors)

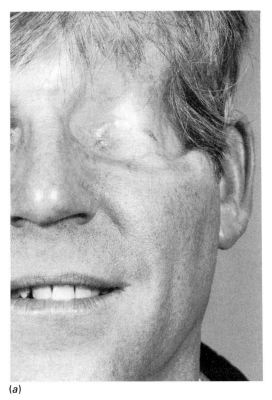

(a)

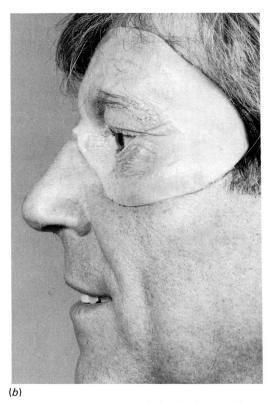

(b)

Figure 23.19 Orbital exenteration: (*a*) the lid margins and tarsal plates are excised leaving a smooth skin-lined cavity; (*b*) removal of the lateral wall of the orbit allows the on-lay prosthesis to be fitted more posteriorly with the medial canthus in its correct position

Postoperative spread into the pterygoid muscles is best managed by an alternative craniofacial procedure as further dissection after maxillectomy is complicated by venous bleeding from the pterygoid plexus.

REHABILITATION

Careful rehabilitation ensures minimal cosmetic and functional defect following maxillectomy. Healing of the bony cavity is fairly rapid, but it is advantageous to apply a split-skin graft to the back of the facial skin flap. After resuturing the facial incision, the cavity should be immediately fitted with an obturator. An initial cover plate should have been constructed preoperatively to fit the palate. This is then built up with gutta percha to fill the cavity and to restore the normal facial contours. The main problem with this type of prosthesis is its weight, and help in retention is necessary. Retention is aided medially by creating a ledge on the floor of the nasal cavity by resecting the inferior part of the septum, and laterally a mucosal ledge can be made by suturing the anterior margin of the soft palate to the lateral labial mucosa over a short distance. If the prosthesis still tends to fall into the mouth, it can be secured by a circumzygomatic wire.

The primary prosthesis is generally changed after 14 days, and the progressively more sophisticated prostheses can be made over the next 4–8 weeks. The final prosthesis should be no more problem than a bulky upper denture (Figure 23.20).

Medial maxillectomy using the lateral rhinotomy approach (Figure 23.21)

This approach gives good access to the nasal cavities, the ethmoids, and nasopharynx and sphenoid, and also to the pterygopalatine fossa. For more extensive tumours, an en-bloc resection can be achieved by combining this operation with an anterior craniofacial approach. The incision is cosmetically very acceptable as it passes along the lateral border of the nose to the upper edge of the alar margin, preservation of the lower alar rim, if still giving adequate access, improves cosmesis. The upper end should start just above the level of the medial canthus. The upper lateral cartilage is freed from the nasal bones at the pyriform opening and the soft tissue flap is elevated from the frontal wall of the maxilla and nasal bones. The orbital periosteum is elevated as for an external ethmoidectomy, and the lower part of

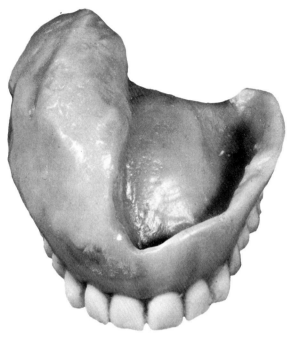

Figure 23.20 Permanent prosthesis with teeth used after total maxillectomy

the lacrimal sac is exposed by nibbling away the anterior lacrimal crest. The orbital contents can then be completely freed medially by dividing the sac low down, and also by freeing the insertion of the inferior oblique tendon and trochlea by sharp dissection from the orbital rim. Access to the anterior nasal cavities can be increased by removing the nasal bones with little cosmetic defect. However, it is more usual to include the lateral nasal wall and ethmoid complex in the resection. The bone is freed by osteotomies cut with a fissure burr. The first is through the anterior wall of the maxilla just medial to the inferior orbital foramen curving medially into the nasal cavity. Further osteotomies are made along the lower border of the lateral nasal wall in the inferior meatus, and across the floor of the orbit towards the foramen of the anterior ethmoidal artery. Finally an upper osteotomy is continued forward through the frontal process of the maxilla and nasal bone then down to the pyriform aperture. This frees the whole block of the lateral nasal wall and ethmoid complex, apart from their posterior attachments just in front of the optic and sphenopalatine foramina. In this region the bone is very thin and easily fractured by elevating the block medially. Virtually all the mucosa of the nose can be included as a cuff with the main specimen, the posterior and antral mucosal attachments being freed by scissors. The view obtained following the removal of this main block of tissue is excellent and the resection is extended into the sphenoid and frontal sinuses or alternatively into the pterygopalatine fossa. At the completion of the procedure, the operative cavity is packed with a Whitehead's varnish pack for 7–10 days.

Other surgical procedures

Palatal fenestration

This operation was originally designed for the implantation of radium into the maxillary antrum, and was claimed to allow good postoperative visualization of the cavity. However, with the alveolus left intact the view is very limited and with modern prostheses the operation has no advantage over the classical maxillectomy.

Midfacial degloving approach

This combines a bilateral sublabial approach to the anterior wall of the maxilla with a midline mobilization of the cartilaginous nose using rhinoplasty techniques to elevate the facial skin off the middle third of the face (Casson, Bonnano and Converse, 1974). This gives excellent exposure to the nasal cavities, postnasal space, antra and pterygopalatine fossae. In selected cases good exposure of the ethmoids is obtained but for ethmoid malignancy the lateral rhinotomy incision gives better exposure. This approach, when combined with either a Le Fort 1 osteotomy or maxillotomy, gives a very wide approach to the clivus and skull base and is of immense value for those extensive tumours which involve this region (Archer, Young and Uttley, 1987; James and Crockard, 1991).

Anterior craniofacial resections (Figure 23.22)

Involvement of the cribriform plate region has long been known as one of the major reasons for failure to control ethmoidal neoplasms; some surgeons even saw it as a contraindication to surgery. Smith, Klopp and Williams (1954) described a surgical approach to this region which was subsequently developed by Ketcham *et al.* (1973) and Clifford (1977). The present authors' team has been using a modified craniofacial technique for 15 years (Cheesman, Lund and Howard, 1986) but with experience it has become clear that the originally described procedure was not appropriate in all patients. In particular it tended to give a poor clearance for tumours in the region of the frontonasal duct and lacrimal sac. Similarly, it was found that more extensive involvement of the anterior fossa was better managed by more conventional combined procedures with the neurosurgeons.

More recently a more logical approach to tumours of this region has been published describing three different approaches (Cheesman and Reddy, 1995).

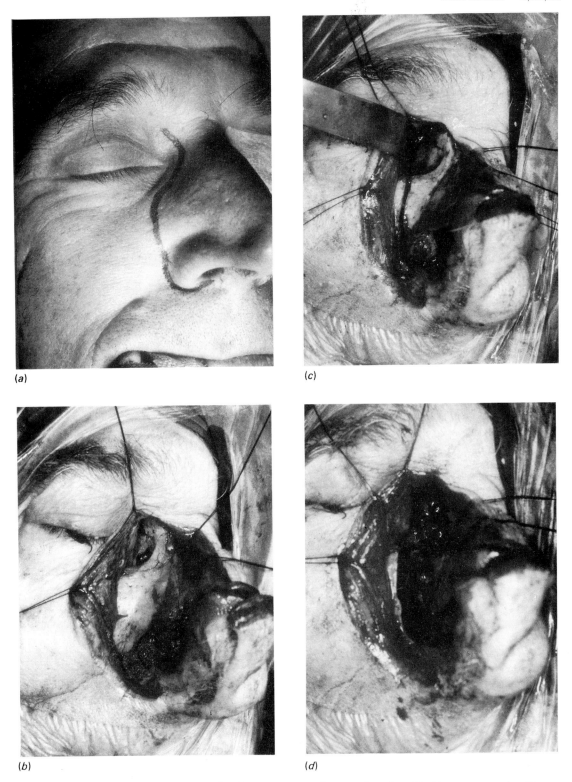

(a)

(b)

(c)

(d)

Figure 23.21 Lateral rhinotomy: (*a*) incision; (*b*) soft tissue exposure of anterior face of maxilla; (*c*) osteotomy made with fissure burr to free lateral wall of nose; (*d*) large single cavity at the end of the resection

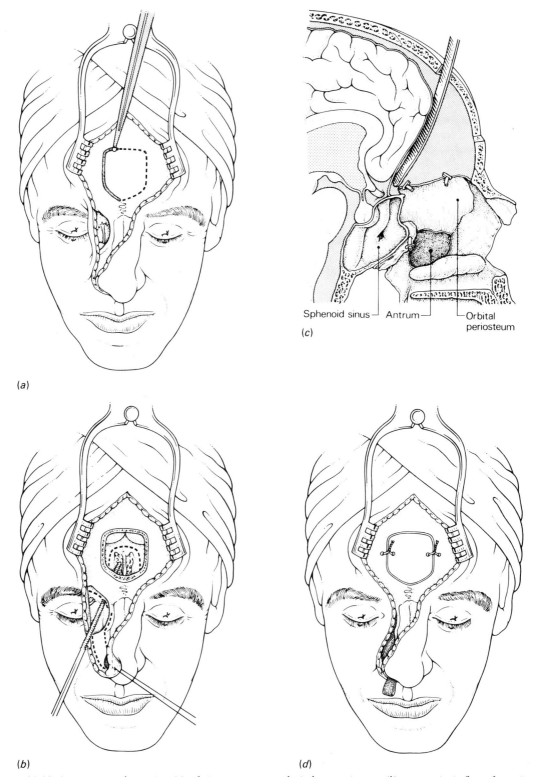

(a)

(b)

(c)

Sphenoid sinus ⎿ Antrum ⎿   ⎿ Orbital
                                   periosteum

(d)

Figure 23.22 Anterior cranial resection: (*a*) soft tissue exposure and window craniotomy; (*b*) osteotomies in floor of anterior fossa and medial wall of orbit; (*c*) sagittal section showing extent of resection; (*d*) the cavity is packed with Whitehead's varnish and the bone flap replaced. (From *Operative Surgery: Nose and Throat*, 4th edn, 1986, edited by J. C. Ballantyne and D. F. N. Harrison, with permission of the authors)

Type 1 craniofacial (transorbital) resection

This procedure is essentially an extended medial max-illectomy using a lateral rhinotomy incision. The operation entails a careful exploration of the anterior nasal cavities using the operating microscope and frozen section histological control. The wide exposure allows resection and repair of both the ethmoid roof and orbital periosteum if indicated. A similar approach has been described by Draf (1989).

Type 2 craniofacial (window craniotomy) resection

This procedure is essentially the original operation described in 1986 (Cheesman, Lund and Howard). A lateral rhinotomy approach is used for anterior access and extended superiorly in a frown line to expose the frontal bone. A small midline 'window' craniotomy is made giving access to the floor of the anterior cranial fossa. After shrinkage of the brain with controlled hyperventilation to reduce the end-tidal Pco_2 to 22 mmHg, the dura is elevated from the roof of the ethmoids and cribriform plate and the area is encompassed with a cranial osteotomy. This osteotomy, in conjunction with those of the lateral rhinotomy, allows the en-bloc resection of both ethmoid complexes. Involved dura can be excised and repaired with fascia lata. Involved brain can be excised, but cure is unlikely for disease at this late stage, although palliation is excellent. The window bone flap is replaced and fixed with mini-plates and the soft tissue is closed with remarkably little cosmetic defect. The combined approach not only gives excellent visualization of the ethmoid region, but readily allows extensions of the resection into the sphenoid, the orbit, the pterygopalatine fossae and the skull base centrally.

Type 3 craniofacial resection

This operation is performed in conjunction with a neurosurgeon and combines a transfacial approach with a neurosurgical approach such as a frontolateral craniotomy, to allow the resection of extensive tumours. The role of the neurosurgeon in such procedures remains subject to discussion. The growth of skullbase surgery as a subspecialty has exposed many otolaryngologists to neurosurgical techniques and has obviated the need for the immediate assistance of a neurosurgeon, but a neurosurgical opinion should be sought during the preoperative work up. He may be able to offer significant help and will be forewarned in the event of a neurosurgical complication.

A recent review of the first 10 years' experience shows a gratifying improvement in overall cure rates (Cheesman and Reddy, 1995). The series is now well over 230 patients and in the first 10 years 145 were treated with at least a 5-year follow up. The overall crude 5-year survival is 63%, for squamous cell carcinoma 45%, adenocarcinoma 50% and olfactory neuroblastoma 82%.

Lateral craniofacial resections

The routine use of CT scanning shows that many antral tumours extend posteriorly to involve the infratemporal fossa. In the past, attempts to clear the infratemporal fossa anteriorly have not been very successful mainly due to venous bleeding from the pterygoid plexus. A middle fossa extradural approach to the foramen rotundum allows the roof of the infratemporal fossa to be freed and an en-bloc resection of the medial infratemporal fossa is possible as part of a classical maxillectomy. The combination of this approach with an anterior fossa resection allows the en-bloc removal of the orbit for extensive tumours involving this region.

Orbital exenteration

Attempts to preserve the orbital contents and reduce mutilation have, in the past, often resulted in orbital recurrence, requiring a second operation and decreased cure rate. Ketcham *et al.* (1973) clearly showed that orbital exenteration for involvement of the orbital periosteum doubled the cure rate from 32% to 62%, even in more advanced tumours. Consequently, it was the authors' initial practice to remove the orbital contents if the orbital periosteum was involved with tumour. Histological examination however showed that the tumour rarely penetrated the orbital periosteum to involve the orbital fat. Currently, the authors' team practises resection of the orbital periosteum and, in the absence of involvement of the underlying orbital fat on frozen section, preserves the orbital contents. This has been achieved with little disturbance of ocular function and there has been no significant deterioration in overall cure. Medial defects in the orbital periosteum are repaired with split-skin grafts, but inferior resections must be repaired with fascia to prevent prolapse of the globe.

Special problems

Malignant melanoma

Malignant melanoma of the nasal mucosa is very rare, about 1% of all malignant melanomas. Usually they have a pigmented appearance, but an amelanotic tumour is not uncommon, and is often diagnosed as anaplastic carcinoma unless the intracytoplasmic pigment is sought. Melanomas respond poorly to radiotherapy; chemotherapy is equally unsuccessful, and may aggravate the situation by altering the patient's immune status. Consequently, wide surgical excision is used, but the success of the operation probably depends more on the patient's immune competence. Virtually the whole of the nasal mucosa can be removed by a lateral rhinotomy approach and experience indicates that there is nothing to be gained by a full craniofacial resection. Lymph node metastases in the neck are usually isolated and can be removed individually, there being no evidence to support the use of a radical neck dissection. Local recurrences can often be controlled for many years with no active treatment and symptomatic debulking can be achieved using the laser or cryoprobe. Death from melanomatosis often follows some mild immunological challenge such as influenza.

Aesthesioneuroblastoma (olfactory neuroblastoma)

This malignant tumour is derived from the neuroectoderm. It may present to the rhinologist as a nasal tumour or alternatively to the neurosurgeon as an anterior fossa mass. Many of these tumours produce vasoactive hormones, and urinary assays of the metabolites, dopamine and 3-methoxy-4-hydroxymandelic acid, have been used to monitor recurrence. The realization that this tumour is distributed on both sides of the cribriform plate and requires a craniofacial resection has resulted in an improved prognosis. For an early tumour, craniofacial resection offers the chance of complete cure, although at this time adjunctive curative radiotherapy is still recommended.

Adenoid cystic carcinoma

These tumours have a propensity to spread along the perineural spaces, and recurrences often occur at distant sites along the course of nerves supplying the primary area, many years after apparently successful local cure. They are not radiocurable, but do respond to radiotherapy. A combination of surgery and radiotherapy is indicated for these patients, surgery being used first to remove the bulk of the tumour and to indicate the likely areas of perineural spread. In the young patient, long-term cure is sought by attempting to include the involved nerves as centrally as possible. In terms of an antral lesion, this entails a lateral craniofacial approach dividing the maxillary nerve at the foramen rotundum before it enters the wall of the cavernous sinus. If tumour is found within the nerve at this level, it is best controlled with radioactive implants, and iodine-125 seeds with their long half-life, are a promising source for this type of tumour (Russell *et al.*, 1993; Glaser *et al.*, 1995).

Adenocarcinoma

The adenocarcinoma or wood-workers' cancer generally involves the ethmoid sinuses. It is a relatively slow-growing tumour and rarely metastasizes. It is said to be less radiosensitive than the squamous cell carcinoma and long-term cure rates are poor (less than 20% over 5 years). The initial results of craniofacial resections for these tumours in the ethmoid are encouraging and the current policy is to debulk the tumour intranasally initially. This is followed by a full course of radiotherapy and then 6 weeks later by

a planned craniofacial resection of the ethmoids, usually a type 1 approach. The results of Kneght *et al.* (1985) with topical chemotherapy however must be considered as an alternative method of treatment which does not prevent the subsequent use of a more radical procedure.

Tumours of the nasal cavity

These tumours are more common in men and, although 5% are bilateral, there is a predominant involvement of the right side of the nose, possibly related to the trauma of nose picking. The lateral wall is most commonly involved, 50% on the turbinates and, with decreasing frequency, the septum, vestibule, posterior choana and floor. Squamous cell carcinoma is the commonest histological type. As a group they do better than paranasal sinus tumours with a 50% 5-year survival. For most sites either radiotherapy or surgery is used, but tumours of the vestibule and septum are best treated surgically. Tumours in these sites look innocuous, but there is a real danger of spread along the tissue planes of the cartilaginous part of the nose and also into the upper lip. Local radical excision with careful histological control of the specimen is essential and, if the tumour is found near excision margins, postoperative radiotherapy should be given. If the tumour is restricted to one side of a cartilage plane local resection is possible, but if it breaches the cartilage boundary, cartilaginous rhinectomy is necessary. Prosthesis rehabilitation should be used initially until tumour recurrence can be excluded. Delayed nasal reconstruction is possible, but many patients prefer a prosthesis which can be cosmetically very acceptable.

References

ACHESON, E. D., COWDELL, R. H., HADFIELD, E. H. and MACBETH, R. G. (1968) Nasal cancer in woodworkers in the furniture industry. *British Medical Journal*, **2**, 587

ACHESON, E. D., WINTER, P. D., HADFIELD, E. and MACBETH, R. G. (1982) Is nasal adenocarcinoma in the Buckinghamshire furniture industry declining? *Nature*, **299**, 263–265

ADEKEYE, E. O., EDWARDS, M. B. and GOUBRAN, G. F. (1978) Ameloblastic fibrosarcoma. *Oral Surgery, Oral Medicine, Oral Pathology*, **46**, 254–259

AHLFORS, E., LARSSON, A. and SJOREN, S. (1984) The odontogenic keratocyst: a benign cystic tumour? *Journal of Oral and Maxillofacial Surgery*, **42**, 10–19

AJAGBE, H. A., DARAMOLA, J. D., JUNAID, T. A. and AJAGBE, A. O. (1985) Adenomatoid odontogenic tumour in a black African population: report of thirteen cases. *Journal of Oral and Maxillofacial Surgery*, **43**, 683–687

ALTINI, M., and COHEN, M. (1982) The follicular primordial cyst (odontogenic keratocyst). *International Journal of Oral Surgery*, **11**, 175–182

ALTINI, M. and SHEAR, M. (1992) The lateral periodontal cyst: an update. *Journal of Oral Pathology and Medicine*, **21**, 245–250

ARCHER, D. J., YOUNG, S. and UTTLEY, D. (1987) Basilar aneurysms: a new transclival approach via maxillotomy. *Journal of Neurosurgery*, **67**, 54–58

BADEN, E. (1965) Terminology of the ameloblastoma: history and current usage. *Journal of Oral Surgery*, **23**, 40–49

BARTON, R. T. (1977) Nickel carcinogenesis of the respiratory tract. *Journal of Otolaryngology*, **6**, 412–422

BAUNSGAARD, P., LONTOFF, E. and SORENSEN, M. (1983) Calcifying epithelial odontogenic tumour (Pindborg tumour): an unusual case. *Laryngoscope*, **93**, 635–638

BERNIER, J. L. and BHASKAR, S. N. (1958) Aneurysmal bone cysts of the mandible. *Oral Surgery, Oral Medicine, Oral Pathology*, **11**, 1018–1028

BHASKAR, S. N. (1968) Oral pathology in dental office: survey of 20 575 biopsy specimens. *Journal of the American Dental Association*, **76**, 761–766

BIESECKER, J. L., MARCOVE, R. C., HUVOS, A. G. and MIKE, V. (1970) Aneurysmal bone cysts. A clinicopathological study of 66 cases. *Cancer*, **26**, 615–625

BLINKLEY, G. W. and JOHNSON, H. H. (1951) Epithelioma adenoides cysticum: basal cell nevi, agenesis of the corpus callosum and dental cysts. *American Medical Association Archives of Dermatology and Syphilology*, **63**, 73–84

BRANNON, R. B. (1977) The odontogenic keratocyst. A clinico-pathological study of 312 cases. Part 2. Histological features. *Oral Surgery, Oral Medicine, Oral Pathology*, **43**, 233–255

BROWN, L. H., BERKMAN, S., COHEN, D., KAPLAN, A. L. and ROSENBERG, M. (1982) A radiological study of the frequency and distribution of impacted teeth. *Journal of the Dental Association of South Africa*, **37**, 627–630

BROWNE, R. M. (1972) Metaplasia and degeneration in odontogenic cysts in man. *Journal of Oral Pathology*, **1**, 145–158

BRUGGEMANN, A. (1920) Zysten als Folge von Entwicklungsstorungen im Naseneingang. *Archives of Laryngology and Rhinology*, **33**, 101–105

BUCHNER, A. (1991) The central (intraosseous) calcifying odontogenic cyst: an analysis of 215 cases. *Journal of Oral and Maxillofacial Surgery*, **49**, 330–339

BUCHNER, A. and HANSEN, L. S. (1979) The histomorphological spectrum of the gingival cyst in the adult. *Oral Surgery, Oral Medicine, Oral Pathology*, **48**, 532–539

BUCHNER, A., MERRELL, P. W., HANSEN, L. S. and LEIDER, A. S. (1991) Peripheral (extraosseous) calcifying odontogenic cyst. A review of forty five cases. *Oral Surgery, Oral Medicine, Oral Pathology*, **72**, 65–70

CASSON, P. R., BONNANO, P. C. and CONVERSE J. M. (1974) The midface degloving procedure. *Plastic and Reconstructive Surgery*, **53**, 102–103

CATALDO, E. and BERKMAN, M. D. (1968) Cysts of the oral mucosa in newborns. *American Journal of Diseases of Childhood*, **116**, 44–48

CATALDO, E., LESS, W. C. and GUINTA, J. L. (1983) Squamous odontogenic tumour: a lesion of the periodontium. *Journal of Periodontology*, **54**, 731–735

CHAMDA, R. A. and SHEAR, M. (1980) Dimensions of incisive fossae on dry skulls and radiographs. *International Journal of Oral Surgery*, **9**, 452–457

CHEESMAN, A. D. and REDDY, K. (1995) Craniofacial resection. A 10-year experience. *Proceedings of the 15th European Rhinologic Congress*

CHEESMAN, A. D., LUND, V. J. and HOWARD, D. J. (1986) Craniofacial resection for tumours of the nasal cavity and paranasal sinuses. *Head and Neck Surgery*, **8**, 429–435

CHRIST, T. F. (1970) The globulomaxillary cyst – an embryologic misconception. *Oral Surgery, Oral Medicine, Oral Pathology*, **30**, 515–526

CLEARY, K. R. and BATSAKIS, J. G. (1994) Sinonasal lymphomas – pathology consultation. *Annals of Otology, Rhinology and Laryngology*, **103**, 911–915

CLIFFORD, P. (1977) Transcranial approach for cancer of the antro-ethmoidal area. *Clinical Otolaryngology*, **2**, 115–130

COHEN, D. A., NEVILLE, B. W., DAMM, D. D. and WHITE, D. K. (1984) The lateral periodontal cyst. *Journal of Periodontology*, **55**, 230–234

COURTNEY, R. M. and KERR, D. A. (1975) Adenomatoid odontogenic tumour. A comprehensive study of twenty new cases. *Oral Surgery, Oral Medicine, Oral Pathology*, **39**, 424–435

DABBS, D. J., SCHWEITZER, R. J., SCHWEITZER, L. E. and MANTZ, F. (1994) Squamous cell carcinoma arising in recurrent odontogenic keratocyst: case report and literature review. *Head and Neck*, **16**, 375–378

DORNER, L., SEAR, A. J. and SMITH, G. T. (1988) A case of ameloblastic carcinoma with pulmonary metastases. *British Journal of Oral and Maxillofacial Surgery*, **26**, 503–510

DRAF, W. (1989) Surgery of space-occupying lesions of the anterior skull base. In: *Surgery of the Skull Base*, edited by M. Samii and D. Draf. Berlin: Springer–Verlag

EL-DEEB, M., SEDANO, H. O. and WAITE, D. E. (1980) Aneurysmal bone cyst of the jaws. Report of a case associated with fibrous dysplasia and review of the literature. *International Journal of Oral Surgery*, **9**, 301–311

ELIASSON, S., ISACSSON, G. and KONDELL, P. A. (1989) Lateral periodontal cysts. Clinical, radiographic and histopathological findings. *International Journal of Oral and Maxillofacial Surgery*, **18**, 191–193

ELZAY, R. P. (1982) Primary intraosseous carcinoma of the jaws: review and update of odontogenic carcinomas. *Oral Surgery, Oral Medicine, Oral Pathology*, **54**, 299–303

EVERSOLE, L. R., LEIDER, A. S. and STRUB, D. (1984) Radiographic characteristics of cystogenic ameloblastoma. *Oral Surgery*, **57**, 572–577

FANTASIA, J. E. (1979) Lateral periodontal cyst. An analysis of 46 cases. *Oral Surgery, Oral Medicine, Oral Pathology*, **48**, 237–243

FERTILO, A., RECHER, G., CALZAVARA, M. and BONINO, M. (1982) Malignant ameloblastoma of the mandible. *American Journal of Otolaryngology*, **3**, 57–60

FORSSELL, K., FORSSELL, H. and KAHNBERG, K. E. (1988) Recurrence of keratocysts. A long-term follow-up study. *International Journal of Maxillofacial and Oral Surgery*, **17**, 25–28

FRANKLIN, C. D. and PINDBORG, J. J. (1976) The calcifying epithelial odontogenic tumour: a review and analysis of 113 cases. *Oral Surgery*, **42**, 753–765

FRAZELL, E. L. and LEWIS, J. S. (1963) Cancer of the nasal cavity and accessory sinuses. *Cancer*, **16**, 1293–1313

FRIEDMAN, I. (1995) Ulcerative/necrotizing diseases of the nose and paranasal sinuses. *Current Diagnostic Pathology*, **2**, 236–255

GARDNER, D. G. (1988) An evaluation of reported cases of median mandibular cysts. *Oral Surgery, Oral Medicine, Oral Pathology*, **65**, 208–213

GARDNER, D. G. and CORIO, R. L. (1983) The relationship of plexiform unicystic ameloblastoma to conventional ameloblastoma. *Oral Surgery*, **56**, 54–60

GARDNER, D. G., KESSLER, H. P., MORENCY, R. and SCHAFFNER, D. L. (1988) The glandular odontogenic cyst: an apparent entity. *Journal of Oral Pathology*, **17**, 359–366

GARLICK, J. A., CALDERON, S., METZKER, A., ROTEM, A. and ABRAMOVICI, A. (1989) Simultaneous occurrence of a congenital lateral upper lip sinus and congenital gingival cyst: a case report and discussion of pathogenesis. *Oral Surgery, Oral Medicine, Oral Pathology*, **68**, 317–323

GENSOUL, P. J. (1833) *Lettre Chirurgicale sur quelques maladies graves du sinus maxillaire et de l'os maxillaire inferieur.* Paris: Bailliere

GLASER, M. G., LESLIE, M. D., COLES, I. and CHEESMAN, A. D. (1995) Iodine seeds in the treatment of slowly proliferating tumours in the head and neck region. *Clinical Oncology*, **7**, 105–108

GORLIN, R. J. and GOLTZ, R. W. (1960) Multiple nevoid basal cell epithelioma, jaw cysts and bifid rib: a syndrome. *New England Journal of Medicine*, **262**, 908–912

GORLIN, R. J., PINDBORG, J. J., REDMAN, R. S., WILLIAMSON, J. J. and HANSEN, L. S. (1964) The calcifying odontogenic cyst. A new entity and possible analogue of the cutaneous calcifying epithelioma of Malherbe. *Cancer*, **17**, 723–729

GREER, R. O. and JOHNSON, M. (1988) Botryoid odontogenic cyst: clinicopathological analysis of ten cases with three recurrences. *Journal of Oral and Maxillofacial Surgery*, **46**, 574–579

HADFIELD, E. H. (1970) A study of adenocarcinoma of the paranasal sinuses in woodworkers in the furniture industry. *Annals of the Royal College of Surgeons of England*, **46**, 301–319

HARRIS, M., JENKINS, M. V., BENNETT, A. and WILLS, M. R. (1973) Prostaglandin production and bone resorption by dental cysts. *Nature*, **245**, 213–215

HARRISON, D. F. N. (1974) Non-healing granulomata of the upper respiratory tract. *British Medical Journal*, **4**, 205–209

HARRISON, D. F. N. (1978) Critical look at the classification of maxillary sinus carcinomata. *Annals of Otology, Rhinology and Laryngology*, **88**, 1–7

HARRISON, D. F. N. (1984) Osseous and fibro-osseous conditions affecting the craniofacial bones. *Annals of Otology, Rhinology and Laryngology*, **93**, 199–203

HEIKINHEIMO, K., HAPPONEN, R. P., FORSELL, K., KUUSILEHTO, A. and VIRTANEN, I. (1989) A botryoid odontogenic cyst with multiple recurrences. *International Journal of Oral and Maxillofacial Surgery*, **18**, 10–13

HOLMSTROM, M. and WIHELMSSON, B (1988) Respiratory systems and pathophysiological effects of occupational exposure to wood dust and formaldehyde. *Scandinavian Journal of Work and Environmental Health*, **14**, 306–311

HORMIA, M., YLIPAAVALNIEMI, P., NAGLE, R. B. and VIRTANEN, I. (1987) Expression of cytokeratins in odontogenic jaw cysts: monoclonal antibodies reveal distinct variation between different cyst types. *Journal of Oral Pathology*, **16**, 338–346

HOSSEINI, M. (1979) Two atypical solitary bone cysts. *British Journal of Oral Surgery*, **16**, 262–269

HOWE, G. L. (1965) 'Haemorrhagic cysts' of the mandible. *British Journal of Oral Surgery*, **3**, 55–75

HOWELL, R. M. and BURKES, E. J. (1977) Malignant transformation of ameloblastic fibro-odontoma to ameloblastic fibrosarcoma. *Oral Surgery, Oral Medicine, Oral Pathology*, **43**, 391–401

HYAMS, V. J. (1971) Papillomas of the nasal cavity and paranasal sinuses. A clinicopathological study of 315 cases. *Annals of Otology, Rhinology and Laryngology*, **80**, 192–206

ISHII, Y., YAMANAKA, N., OGAWA, K., YOSHIDA, Y., TAKAMI, T., MATSUURA, A. *et al.* (1982) Nasal T-cell lymphoma as a type of so-called 'Lethal Midline Granuloma'. *Cancer*, **50**, 2336–2344

JAFFE, H. L. and LICHTENSTEIN, L. (1942) Solitary unicameral bone cyst with emphasis on the roetgen picture, the pathological appearance and the pathogenesis. *Archives of Surgery*, **44**, 1004–1025

JAMES, D. and CROCKARD, H. A. (1991) Surgical access to the base of skull and upper cervical spine by extended maxillotomy. *Neurosurgery*, **29**, 411–416

KASSEL, S. H., ECHEVARRIA, R. A. and GUZZO, F. P. (1969) Midline malignant reticuloses (so-called lethal midline granuloma). *Cancer*, **23**, 920–935

KAUGARS, G. E. (1986) Botryoid odontogenic cyst. *Oral Surgery, Oral Medicine, Oral Pathology*, **62**, 555–559

KAUGARS, G. E. and CALE, A. E. (1987) Traumatic bone cyst. *Oral Surgery, Oral Medicine, Oral Pathology*, **63**, 318–324

KAUGARS, G. E., MILLER, M. E. and ABBEY, L. M. (1989) Odontomas. *Oral Surgery, Oral Medicine, Oral Pathology*, **67**, 172–176

KETCHAM, A. S., CHRETIEN, P. B., VAN BUREN, J. M., HOYE, R. C., BEAZLEY, T. M. *et al.* (1973) The ethmoid sinuses: A reevaluation of surgical resection. *American Journal of Surgery*, **126**, 469–476

KILLEY, H. C., KAY, L. W. and SEWARD, G. R. (1977) *Benign Cystic Lesions of the Jaws, their Diagnosis and Treatment*, 3rd edn. Edinburgh: Churchill Livingstone

KNEGHT, P. P., DE JONG, P. C., VAN ANDEL, J. G., DE BOER, M. G., EYKENBOOM, W. and VAN DER SCHANS, E. (1985) Carcinoma of the paranasal sinuses. *Cancer*, **56**, 57–62

KRAMER, I. R. H. (1974) Changing views on oral disease. *Proceedings of the Royal Society of Medicine*, **67**, 271–276

KRAMER, I. R. H. and TOLLER, P. A. (1973) The use of exfoliative cytology and protein estimations in preoperative diagnosis of odontogenic keratocysts. *International Journal of Oral Surgery*, **2**, 143–151

KURILOFF, D. B. (1987) The nasolabial cyst – nasal hamartoma. *Otolaryngology – Head and Neck Surgery*, **96**, 268–272

KUUSELA, P., YLIPAAVALNIEMI, P. and THESLEFF, I. (1986) The relationship between the keratocyst antigen (KCA) and keratin. *Journal of Oral Pathology*, **15**, 287–291

LABRIOLA, J., STEINER, M. and BERNSTEIN, M. L. (1980) Odontoameloblastoma. *Journal of Oral Surgery*, **38**, 139–143

LEDERMAN, M. (1970) Tumors of the upper jaw: natural history and treatment. *Journal of Laryngology and Otology*, **84**, 369–401

LEIDER, A. S., NELSON, J. F. and TRODAHL, J. N. (1972) Ameloblastic fibrosarcoma of the jaws. *Oral Surgery*, **33**, 559–569

LOCKWOOD, C. M., JONES, S., MOSS, D. W., BAKES, D., WHITAKER, K. B. and SAVAGE, C. O. S. (1987) Association of alkaline phosphatase with an autoantigen recognised by circulating anti-neutrophil antibodies in systemic vascultis. *Lancet*, i, 716–720

LUND, V. J. (1985) Odontogenic keratocyst of the maxilla: a case report. *British Journal of Oral and Maxillofacial Surgery*, **23**, 210–215

LUND, V. J. (1991) Malignancy of the nose and sinuses, epidemiological and aetiological considerations. *Rhinology*, **29**, 57–68

LUSTMANN, J. and BODNER, L. (1988) Dentigerous cysts associated with supernumerary teeth. *International Journal of Oral and Maxillofacial Surgery*, **17**, 100–102

MCBRIDE, P. (1897) Case of rapid destruction of the nose and face. *Journal of Laryngology and Otology*, 12, 64–66

MAGNUSSON, B. C. (1978) Odontogenic keratocysts: a clinical and histological study with special reference to enzyme histochemistry. *Journal of Oral Pathology*, 7, 8–18

MAIN, D. M. G. (1970) Epithelial jaw cysts: a clinicopathological reappraisal. *British Journal of Oral Surgery*, 8, 114–125

MATEJKA, M., PORTEDER, H., ULRICH, W., WATZEK, G. and SINZINGER, H. (1985) Prostaglandin synthesis in dental cysts. *British Journal of Oral and Maxillofacial Surgery*, 23, 190–194

MAXYMIW, W. G. and WOOD, R. E. (1991) Carcinoma arising in a dentigerous cyst: a case report and review of the literature. *Journal of Oral and Maxillofacial Surgery*, 49, 639–643

MEDEIROS, L. J., JAFFE, E. S., CHEN, Y. Y. and WEISS, L. M. (1992) Angiocentric immunoproliferative lesions. Localization of EBV virus genome. *American Journal of Surgical Pathology*, 16, 439–447

MEGHJI, S., HARVEY, W. and HARRIS, M. (1989) Interleukin-1 like activity in cystic lesions of the jaw. *British Journal of Oral and Maxillofacial Surgery*, 27, 1–11

MEHLISCH, D. R., DAHLIN, D. C. and MASSON, J. K. (1972) Ameloblastoma: a clinicopathological report. *Journal of Oral Surgery*, 30, 9–22

MEISELMAN, F. (1994) Surgical management of the odontogenic keratocyst: conservative approach. *Journal of Oral and Maxillofacial Surgery*, 52, 960–963

MICHAELS, L. and GREGORY, M. M. (1977) Pathology of 'non-healing (midline)' granuloma. *Journal of Clinical Pathology*, 30, 317–327

MICHAUX (1854) Resections de la machoire superieure. *Bulletin de l'Academie Royale de Medecine de Belgique*, iii, 1–118

MONTELEONE, L. and MCLELLAN, M. S. (1964) Epstein's pearls (Bohn's nodules) of the palate. *Journal of Oral Surgery*, 22, 301–304

MOREILLON, M. C. and SCHROEDER, H. E. (1982) Numerical frequency of epithelial abnormalities, particularly microkeratocysts, in the developing human oral mucosa. *Oral Surgery, Oral Medicine, Oral Pathology*, 53, 44–55

MOSKOW, B. S. and BADEN, E. (1982) The peripheral ameloblastoma of the gingiva: case report and literature review. *Journal of Periodontology*, 53, 736–742

MOSKOW, B. S. and BLOOM, A. (1983) Embryogenesis of the gingival cyst. *Journal of Clinical Periodontology*, 10, 119–130

MOURE, E. J. (1902) Traitement des tumeurs malignes primitives de l'ethmoide. *Revue Hebdomadaire de Laryngologie, d'Otologie et de Rhinologie*, 47, 402–412

MOURSHED, F. (1964) A roentgenographic study of dentigerous cysts. Analysis of 180 cases. *Oral Surgery, Oral Medicine, Oral Pathology*, 18, 466–473

NAGAI, N., TAKESHITA, N., NAGATSUKA H., INOUE, M., NISHIJIMA, K., NOJIMA, T. *et al.* (1991) Ameloblastic carcinoma: case report and review. *Journal of Oral Pathology and Medicine*, 20, 460–463

NXUMALO, T. N. and SHEAR, M. (1992) The gingival cyst of adults. *Journal of Oral Pathology and Medicine*, 21, 309–313

OSBORN, D. A. (1959) Haemangiomas of the nose. *Journal of Laryngology and Otology*, 73, 174–179

OSBORN, D. A. (1970) Nature and behaviour of transitional tumours in the upper respiratory tract. *Cancer*, 25, 50–60

PADAYACHEE, A. and VAN WYK, C. W. (1987) Two cystic lesions with features of both the botryoid odontogenic cyst and the central mucoepidermoid tumour: sialo-odontogenic cyst? *Journal of Oral Pathology*, 16, 499–504

PARTRIDGE, M. and TOWERS, J. F. (1987) The primordial cyst (odontogenic keratocyst): its tumour like characteristics and behaviour. *British Journal of Oral and Maxillofacial Surgery*, 25, 271–279

PATRON, M., COLMONERO, C. and LARRAURI, J. (1991) Glandular odontogenic cyst: clinicopathological analysis of three cases. *Oral Surgery, Oral Medicine, Oral Pathology*, 72, 71–74

PHELAN, J. A., KRITCHMAN, D., FUSCO-RAMER, M., FREEDMAN, P. D. and LUMERMAN, H. (1988) Recurrent botryoid odontogenic cyst (lateral periodontal cyst). *Oral Surgery, Oral Medicine, Oral Pathology*, 66, 345–348

PHILIPSEN, H. P. (1956) cited by Shear (1992)

PHILIPSEN, H. P. and BIRN, H. (1969) The adematoid odontogenic tumour. *Acta Pathologica Microbiologica Scandinavica*, 75, 375–398

PHILIPSEN, H. P., REICHART, P. A., ZHANG, K. H. and YU, Q. X. (1991) Adenomatoid odontogenic tumour: biologic profile based on 499 cases. *Journal of Oral Pathology and Medicine*, 20, 149–158

PINDBORG, J. J. and CLAUSEN, F. (1958) Classification of odontogenic tumours; suggestion. *Acta Odontologica Scandinavica*, 16, 293–295

PINDBORG, J. J. (1958) A calcifying epithelial odontogenic tumour. *Cancer*, 11, 838–843

PRAETORIUS, F., HJORTING-HANSEN, E., GORLIN, R. J. and VICKERS, R. A. (1981) Calcifying odontogenic cyst. Range, variations and neoplastic potential. *Acta Odontologica Scandinavica*, 39, 227–240

PULLON, P. A., SHAFER, W. G. and ELZAY, R. P. (1975) Squamous odontogenic tumour: report of six cases of a previously undescribed lesion. *Oral Surgery*, 40, 616–630

RACHANIS, C. C., ALTINI, M. and SHEAR, M. (1979) A clinicopathological comparision of primordial cyst (keratocysts) in two different age groups. *Journal of Dental Research*, 58D, 2324 (abstract)

RAMSAY, A. D., MICHAELS, L. and HARRISON, D. F. N. (1988) Lethal midline granuloma – a T-cell lymphoma. *Journal of Pathology*, 154, 56A

RASMUSSON, L. G., MAGNUSSON, B. C. and BORRMAN, H. (1991) The lateral periodontal cyst. A histopathological and radiographic study of 32 cases. *British Journal of Oral and Maxillofacial Surgery*, 29, 54–57

REEVE, C. M. and LEVY, B. P. (1968) Gingival cysts: a review of the literature and a report of four cases. *Periodontics*, 6, 115–117

REGEZI, J. A., KERR, D. A. and COURTNEY, R. M. (1978) Odontogenic tumours: analysis of 706 cases. *Journal of Oral Surgery*, 36, 771–783

RINGERTZ, N. (1938) Pathology of malignant tumours arising in the nasal and paranasal cavities and maxilla. *Acta OtoLaryngologica Supplementum*, 27, 33–41

ROBIN, P. E. and POWELL, D. J. (1981) Treatment of carcinoma of the nasal cavity and paranasal sinuses. *Clinical Otolaryngology*, 6, 401–413

ROBINSON, H. B. G. (1945) Classification of cysts of the jaws. *American Journal of Orthodontics and Oral Surgery*, 31, 370–375

ROBINSON, L. and MARTINEZ, M. G. (1975) Unicystic ameloblastoma. *Cancer*, 40, 2278–2285

RUD, J. and PINDBORG, J. J. (1969) Odontogenic keratocysts: a follow-up study of 21 cases. *Journal of Oral Surgery*, 27, 323–330

RUSSELL, J. D., BLEACH, N. R., GLASER, M. G. and CHEESMAN, A. D. (1993) Brachytherapy for recurrent nasopharyngeal and naso-ethmoidal tumours. *Journal of Laryngology and Otology*, **107**, 115–120

SADEGHI, E. M., WELDON, L. L., KWON, P. H. and SAMPSON, E. (1991) Mucoepidermoid odontogenic cyst. *International Journal of Oral and Maxillofacial Surgery*, **20**, 142–143

SAUNDERS, I. D. F. (1972) Bohn's nodules – a case report. *British Dental Journal*, **132**, 457–458

SEBILEAU, P. (1906) Les formes clinques du cancer du sinus maxillaire. *Annales des Maladies d'Oreille, du Larynx, Nes et Pharynx*, **32**, 430–450

SEHDEV, M. K., HAVOS, A. G. and STRONG, E. W. (1974) Ameloblastoma of maxilla and mandible. *Cancer*, **33**, 324–333

SHEAFER, W. G., HINE, M. K. and LEVY, B. M. (1983) *A Textbook of Oral Pathology*, 4th edn. Philadelphia: Saunders

SHEAR, M. (1960) Primordial cysts. *Journal of the Dental Association of South Africa*, **15**, 211–217

SHEAR, M. (1992) *Cysts of the Oral Regions*, 3rd edn. Bristol: Wright

SLOOTWEG, P. J. (1981) An analysis of the inter-relationship of the mixed odontogenic tumours – ameloblastic fibroma, ameloblastic fibro-odontoma and the odontomas. *Oral Surgery*, **51**, 266–276

SMALL, I. A. and WALDRON, C. A. (1955) Ameloblastomas of the jaws. *Oral Surgery*, **8**, 281–297

SMITH, G., SMITH, A. J. and BROWNE, R. M. (1984) Glycosaminoglycans in fluid aspirates from odontogenic cysts. *Journal of Oral Pathology*, **13**, 614–621

SMITH, G., SMITH, A. J. and BROWNE, R. M. (1986) Analysis of odontogenic cyst fluid aspirates. *IRCS Medical Science*, **14**, 304–306

SMITH, G., SMITH, A. J. and BROWNE, R. M. (1988a) Histochemical studies on glycosaminoglycans of odontogenic cysts. *Journal of Oral Pathology*, **17**, 55–59

SMITH, G., SMITH, A. J. and BROWNE, R. M. (1988b) Quantification and analysis of the glycosaminoglycans in human odontogenic cyst linings. *Archives of Oral Biology*, **33**, 623–626

SMITH, R. R., KLOPP, C. T. and WILLIAMS, J. M. (1954) Surgical treatment of cancer of the frontal sinus and adjacent areas. *Cancer*, **7**, 991–994

STOELINGA, P. J. W. and BRONKHORST, F. B. (1988) The incidence, multiple presentation and recurrence of aggressive cysts of the jaws. *Journal of Cranio-Maxillo-Facial Surgery*, **16**, 184–195

STOELINGA, P. J. W. and PETERS, J. H. (1973) A note on the origin of keratocysts of the jaws. *International Journal of Oral Surgery*, **2**, 37–44

STRUTHERS, P. J. and SHEAR, M. (1976) Root resorption produced by ameloblastomas and cysts of the jaws. *International Journal of Oral Surgery*, **5**, 128–132

STRUTHERS, P. J. and SHEAR, M. (1984) Aneurysmal bone cysts of the jaws. 1: Clinicopathological features. *International Journal of Oral Surgery*, **13**, 92–100

SWANSON, K. S., KAUGARS, G. E. and GUNSOLLEY, J. C. (1991) Nasopalatine duct cyst: an analysis of 334 cases. *Journal of Oral and Maxillofacial Surgery*, **49**, 268–271

TELFER, M. R., JONES, G. M., PELL, G. and EVESON, J. W. (1990) Primary bone cyst of the mandibular condyle. *British Journal of Oral and Maxillofacial Surgery*, **28**, 340–343

TO, E. H. W., BROWN, J. S., AVERY, B. S. and WARD-BOOTH, R. P. (1991) Primary intraosseous carcinoma of the jaws. Three new cases and a review of the literature. *British Journal of Oral and Maxillofacial Surgery*, **29**, 19–25

TOLLER, P. A. (1967) Origin and growth of cysts of the jaws. *Annals of the Royal College of Surgeons of England*, **40**, 306–336

TSAKNIS, P. J. and NELSON, J. F. (1980) The maxillary ameloblastoma: an analysis of 24 cases. *Journal of Oral Surgery*, **38**, 336–342

VAN DER WAAL, I., RAUHAMAA, R. and VAN DER KWAST W. A. M. (1985) Squamous cell carcinoma arising in the lining of odontogenic cysts. *International Journal of Oral Surgery*, **14**, 140–152

VON RECHLINGHAUSEN, F. (1891) *Die fibrose oder deformirende ostitis die osteomalacie carcinose in ihren gegenseitigen beziehungen*. Berlin: Reimer

WEATHERS, D. R. and WALDRON, C. A. (1973) Unusual multilocular cysts of the jaws (botryoid odontogenic cysts). *Oral Surgery, Oral Medicine, Oral Pathology*, **36**, 235–241

WEGENER, F. (1939) Uber eine eigenartige rhinogene Granulomatose mit besonderer Beteiligung des Arteriensystems und der Nieren. *Beitrage zur Pathologischen Anatomie und zur Allgemeinen Pathologie*, **102**, 36–68

WERTHEIMER, F. W., ZIELINSKI, R. J. and WESLEY, R. K. (1977) Extraosseous calcifying odontogenic epithelial tumour (Pindborg tumour). *International Journal of Oral Surgery*, **6**, 266–269

WILLIAMS, T. P. and CONNOR, F. A. (1994) Surgical management of the odontogenic keratocyst: aggressive approach. *Journal of Oral and Maxillofacial Surgery*, **52**, 964–966

WOOLGAR, J. A., RIPPEN, J. W. and BROWNE, R. M. (1987a) The odontogenic keratocyst and its occurence in the nevoid basal cell carcinoma syndrome. *Oral Surgery, Oral Medicine, Oral Pathology*, **64**, 727–730

WOOLGAR, J. A., RIPPEN, J. W. and BROWNE, R. M. (1987b) A comparative study of the clinical and histological features of recurrent and non-recurrent odontogenic keratocysts. *Journal of Oral Pathology*, **16**, 124–128

WOOLGAR, J. A., RIPPEN, J. W. and BROWNE, R. M. (1987c) A comparative histological study of odontogenic keratocysts in basal cell naevus syndrome and control patients. *Journal of Oral Pathology*, **16**, 75–80

WORLD HEALTH ORGANIZATION (1992) *Histological typing of Odontogenic Tumours*, edited by I. R. H. Kramer, J. J. Pindborg and M. Shear. Berlin: Springer-Verlag

WRIGHT, B. A., WYSOCKI, G. P. and LARDER, T. C. (1983) Odontogenic keratocysts presenting as periapical disease. *Oral Surgery, Oral Medicine, Oral Pathology*, **56**, 425–429

WYSOCKI, G. P. (1981) The differential diagnosis of globulomaxillary radiolucences. *Oral Surgery, Oral Medicine, Oral Pathology*, **51**, 281–286

WYSOCKI, G. P., BRANNON, R. B., GARDNER, D. G. and SAPP, P. (1980) Histogenesis of the lateral periodontal cyst and the gingival cyst of the adult. *Oral Surgery, Oral Medicine, Oral Pathology*, **50**, 327–334

Further reading

BALLANTYNE, J. C. and HARRISON, D. F. N. (eds) (1986) *Operative Surgery. Nose and Throat.*, 4th edn. London: Butterworths

BATSAKIS, J. G. (ed.) (1969) *Tumours of the Head and Neck: Clinical and Pathological Considerations*, 2nd edn. Baltimore: Williams and Wilkins

HARRISON, D. F. N. and LUND, V. J. (1993) *Tumours of Upper Jaw*. Edinburgh: Churchill Livingstone

MCGREGOR, I. A. and HOWARD, D. J. (eds) (1992) *Head and Neck Surgery, Part 2*, 4th edn. London: Butterworth-Heinemann

SUEN, J. Y. and MYERS, E. N. (eds) (1981) *Cancer of the Head and Neck*. New York: Churchill Livingstone

24

The oesophagus in otolaryngology

Janet Ann Wilson

It is well known that patients with obstructive or functional disorders of the intrathoracic oesophagus or gastro-oesophageal junction can present with symptoms referred to the neck. It is, therefore, encumbent upon the otolaryngologist to be aware of these more distal diagnostic possibilities and to have a working knowledge of their diagnosis and management.

Current concepts of oesophageal physiology

Upper oesophageal sphincter function

Several studies, mostly carried out in North America, now strongly point to the posterior third of the tongue as the major driving force for bolus propulsion (McConnel, Cerenko and Mendelsohn, 1988). An integral part of this concept is that there is a retrolingual bolus loading chamber which accumulates the bolus in the oropharynx preparatory to the voluntary initiation of the swallow 'reflex' (Buchholz, Bosma and Donner, 1985). Clearly many of the complex interrelated functions of swallowing do operate as a reflex. We are not aware of having to suspend respiration, or to initiate apposition of the vocal cords which is a very early event in each swallow cycle. Nonetheless, the swallow reflex is not a standardized preset pattern but is subject to peripheral feedback from factors such as bolus volume, or consistency (Wilson et al., 1989a).

The use of synchronous manometry and radiology (manofluorometry) has also highlighted important details of upper oesophageal function during each swallow. Upper oesophageal sphincter activity during swallowing can be divided into five phases: relaxation; opening; distension by the bolus; collapse; and closure (Jacob et al., 1989). Upper oesophageal sphinc-

ter relaxation occurs during laryngeal elevation and precedes opening by around 0.1 s. Opening is now defined as an active process, distinct from bolus distension and effected by the upwards and forwards pull of the suprahyoid musculature and shortening of the thyrohyoid membrane. Distension is sometimes accompanied by a slight rise in upper oesophageal sphincter relaxation pressure. Active closure is achieved by the arrival of the pharyngeal stripping wave, which pursues rather than propels the tail of the bolus. The extent of upper oesophageal sphincter opening is a function of bolus volume. As the bolus volume increases, the sphincter not only opens more widely as one might expect but also opens more rapidly. The magnitude of laryngeal elevation is also related to the volume swallowed (Kahrilas et al., 1986). Synchronized manometric electromyographic videolaryngoscopy recordings confirm that swallow-induced vocal cord adduction precedes movement of the hyoid bone, base of tongue movement, and even submental EMG activity (Shaker et al., 1990).

Oesophageal motility

The oesophagus is a 21 cm muscular tube whose proximal centimetre, like the upper oesophageal sphincter, consists of striated muscle. The middle third is mixed with an increasing proportion of smooth muscle and the distal half is entirely smooth muscle. The bundles of the outer longitudinal muscle arise laterally from the cricoid cartilage and fuse approximately 3 cm below its posterior lamina. There is thus a posterior triangle (Laimer's triangle) that is devoid of longitudinal muscle. In the smooth muscle, the enteric neurons of the myenteric plexus between the longitudinal and circular muscle layers relay between the vagus and the smooth muscle. Their function in the striated muscle is obscure. The submucosal (Meissner's) plexus is exceedingly sparse in the human oesophagus (Christensen, 1987). Primary oesophageal peristalsis is initiated by the swallow reflex and proceeds at 2–4 cm/s.

The smooth muscle portion of the oesophagus is capable of secondary peristalsis in the absence of extrinsic innervation. A second swallow occurring while a peristaltic contraction is in progress will completely inhibit the contraction induced by the first swallow (Vanek and Diamant, 1987). Peristalsis in the striated muscle part of the oesophagus results from sequential activation of excitatory vagal motor units. The vagus also controls primary peristalsis in the smooth muscle of the oesophagus, e.g. diversion of a bolus by a cervical oesophagostome in an experimental animal does not eliminate primary distal peristalsis. The vagal control is, however, more complex and can induce either excitatory or inhibitory responses in the oesophageal musculature depending on the stimulus. Excitatory neurons of the myenteric plexus induce contraction of longitudinal and circular muscle layers by muscarinic cholinergic receptors, while inhibitory neurons principally operate on the circular muscle layer via a non-adrenergic, noncholinergic neurotransmitter.

Lower oesophageal sphincter barrier function

Recent detailed anatomical studies indicate that the maximal thickness of the circular lower oesophageal sphincter muscle is at the greater curvature of the stomach. The ring is split into two portions, one which forms transverse muscle clasps around the oesophagus and the other, long loops to the stomach. The resting tone of the lower oesophageal sphincter is around 10–30 mmHg relative to intragastric pressure. The barrier pressure tends to be lower after meals and to be elevated at night. Lower oesophageal sphincter tonic contraction appears to be an intrinsic muscular property rather than under extrinsic neural control. Sphincter tone may be maintained by a continuous release of intracellular calcium, perhaps mediated by inositol phosphate whose concentration is higher in the lower oesophageal sphincter than in the adjacent circular muscle. Swallowing induces inhibition of lower oesophageal sphincter tone (receptive relaxation) by a mechanism similar to the inhibition of circular oesophageal smooth muscle following swallows. In addition to intrinsic tonic activity, lower oesophageal sphincter pressure at any instant reflects the balance between excitatory and inhibitory vagal fibres.

The lower oesophageal sphincter is also subject to frequent, abrupt spontaneous relaxations which appear to be related to the majority of episodes of gastrooesophageal reflux both in healthy volunteers and in patients with gastro-oesophageal reflux disease (Mittal and McCallum, 1988). Transient lower oesophageal sphincter relaxations are usually of longer duration than swallow-induced relaxations by up to 30 seconds and in healthy volunteers only 35% are reflux-associated. The factors which determine the occurrence of gastro-oesophageal reflux during these relaxations are incompletely understood. Occasionally reflux is prevented by a swallow manoeuvre which intervenes between the onset of relaxation and the onset of the consequent reflux.

Clinical features of oesophageal disease
Dysphagia

It has long been known that the level at which a subject experiences dysphagia is not a reliable guide to the level of obstruction, except in so far as the obstruction is always perceived to be *above* the level of the relevant lesion. This is probably because of referred neural sensation, a mechanism which may be of relevance in the generation of other symptoms such as globus sensation or the laryngeal manifestations of gastro-oesophageal reflux. Dysphagia is a confusing and potentially misleading symptom. The derivation of the word (dys – difficulty; phagia – eating) suggests a difficulty in eating; the term is commonly used to refer to a difficulty in swallowing, but by far the most useful concept for differential diagnosis is that dysphagia should indicate food sticking. Patients are perhaps more likely to construe a difficulty in swallowing as a difficulty in food transfer prior to the initiation of the swallow reflex. Similarly, patients may also perceive regurgitation of food or aspiration as difficulty in swallowing while diagnostically they should really be regarded as separate entities. A further confusing factor is the coexistence of globus sensation with dysphagia. In fact around 20% of patients with true globus pharyngis and no structural or functional cause to account for their symptom will also complain on direct questioning of some difficulty in swallowing food. The food does not stick but they are aware that the swallow feels different. This is not true dysphagia in the motor sense.

It is often said that patients with neurological dysphagia have greater dysphagia for liquids than for solids. It should be borne in mind, however, that many subjects with achalasia of the lower oesophageal sphincter also complain of dysphagia which is greatest for cold liquids (and, interestingly alleviated by carbonated drinks). Patients with intermittent dysphagia must be questioned directly about the environment in which their symptom occurs. Certain subjects with functional dysphagia will experience most of their symptoms when in certain environments, usually when eating in company, particularly in restaurants. This is probably due to a combination of factors including less attention being paid to the process of eating, simultaneous eating and talking, and probably the effect of increased levels of stress. Thus in

North America recurrent bolus obstruction in otherwise healthy meat eaters has come to be known as 'steakhouse' spasm (DiPalma and Brady, 1987). In trying to determine the significance of the dysphagia symptom, the patient must also be asked whether or not any weight has been lost (subjects are frequently unable to define the amount precisely), and whether or not the diet taken comprises normal foodstuffs, has selected exclusions, or consists of only soft foods, or liquids.

Heartburn

Around 10% of individuals in western societies experience daily heartburn, while over one-third of the population have intermittent symptoms. Heartburn is a retrosternal burning sensation which tends to radiate towards the mouth and may be associated with a sour taste in the mouth. The importance of the underlying gastro-oesophageal reflux disease as a cause of dysphagia is discussed below. The term dyspepsia is less clearly defined and is typically associated with eating, including epigastric discomfort, nausea or bloating in various combinations. It must be remembered, however, that one of the commoner causes of epigastric pain is, in fact, gastro-oesophageal reflux disease. Gastro-oesophageal reflux disease may also be 'silent' or give rise to a variety of atypical symptoms (see below).

Chest pain

There is a wide variety of oesophageal causes for non-cardiac chest pain. These include gastro-oesophageal reflux, oesophageal motility disorders, hiatus hernia and altered visceral sensation. It can be extremely difficult to differentiate cardiac from non-cardiac chest pain. Gastro-oesophageal reflux can be triggered by exercise and thus mimic angina. Investigation of 50 consecutive patients with non-cardiac chest pain indicated an oesophageal disorder in 60%, most commonly gastro-oesophageal reflux and diffuse oesophageal spasm. These abnormalities, however, require more detailed investigation than simple radiology and upper gastrointestinal endoscopy. Thus if no major abnormality is detected at endoscopy, oesophageal transit studies, oesophageal manometry and ambulatory pH monitoring are indicated (Caestecker *et al.*, 1985).

Globus sensation

Globus sensation is also extremely common, having been experienced at some time in 45% of the population (Thompson and Heaton, 1982). While globus sensation is typically defined as a feeling of something in the throat, many subjects in fact are aware of a lump located in the suprasternal notch, i.e. in the region of the cervical oesophagus rather than the oropharynx. The female sex, stable or increasing weight, non-smoking and anxious diathesis of the typical subject are of immense diagnostic help to the clinician. Older male patients or those whose degree of difficulty in swallowing is harder to elucidate may require at least a radiological investigation and perhaps direct examination of the laryngopharynx.

Symptoms of gastro-oesophageal reflux

An aetiological association with gastro-oesophgeal reflux has been proposed for a wide range of laryngeal diseases including subglottic stenosis, laryngospasm, carcinoma, contact ulcer, posterior laryngitis and non-specific dysphonia. The substantiating investigations have, however, been somewhat haphazard and the mechanism by which gastro-oesophageal reflux might induce these conditions is unknown. The role of direct contact of acid with laryngopharyngeal structures has not yet been assessed adequately nor has the occurrence of oesophagopharyngeal reflux in healthy individuals. All that can be said at the present state of knowledge is that reflux should be borne in mind in patients who present with pharyngeal burning, unexplained chronic cough, laryngitis disproportionate to other aetiological factors and indeed in certain patients with asthma who may suffer a vagally mediated reflex bronchospasm (Wilson, 1992).

Investigations
Radiology

The first radiological evaluation of swallowing took place within a year of Roentgen's discovery of X-rays (Cannon and Moser, 1898). Single image radiology techniques of the 1920s gave way to cineradiography which had been perfected by the late 1940s. This in turn was superseded in the 1980s by the technique of videorecording which offers up to 50 frames per second but with a considerably lower radiation exposure than cineradiography (Curtis, Ekberg and Montesi, 1991). The wide availability of high quality fibreoptic endoscopes and manometric investigations of oesophageal disorders has led many radiologists interested in swallowing to concentrate on the pharyngo-oesophageal phase where the videofluoroscopic method described by Logemann (1986) remains the standard. The technique involves not only liquid barium swallows but also swallows of varying consistencies, e.g. quarter 'cookie'. Videorecording techniques allow radiological evaluation of the rapid sequence of oropharyngeal events including palatal closure, glottic closure, bolus transport through the pharynx, upper oesophageal sphincter relaxation and forward traction of the relaxed upper oesophageal sphincter by the anterior movement of the hyoid (Dodds, Stewart and Logemann, 1990).

Effective radiological evaluation of the tubular oesophagus requires a combination of four techniques (Ott *et al.*, 1986). The 'full column' study requires rapid filling of the oesophagus with barium in the prone patient (Figure 24.1). Oesophageal motility is best assessed in this position by multiple single swallows of barium. The method shows hiatus hernia, lower oesophageal mucosal rings and peptic strictures. The tubular oesophagus is seen to terminate as a bell-shaped structure called the oesophageal vestibule. The junction between the tubular oesophagus and the vestibule is known as the 'A level'. A portion of the oesophageal vestibule is intra-abdominal under normal resting conditions. The squamocolumnar mucosal transition is often called the 'E level'. This lies at the lower margin of the vestibule in the normal individual. The lower oesophageal mucosal ring (Schatzki's ring) is a thin, annular structure at the inferior margin of the oesophageal vestibule and is an important cause of episodic dysphagia for solids. The diameter of the ring reflects the severity of the dysphagia which may be intermittent with rings 13–20 mm in diameter but is almost always present with rings less than 13 mm diameter. Radiological demonstration of the ring requires distension of the oesophagogastric region beyond the diameter of the ring, which is best achieved by the full column technique. Two further techniques – mucosal relief and double contrast – must be used to detect smaller oesophageal neoplasms, oesophagitis and varices. Double contrast films are obtained by coating the oesophagus with a dense barium suspension and distending the organ with gas. The final technique is fluoroscopic observation and motion recording which may supplement the other techniques where an oesophageal motility disorder is suspected. The observation of single swallows of barium in the recumbent patient compares favourably with oesophageal manometry. Individuals with reflux, dysphagia, heartburn or an abnormal pharyngo-oesophageal swallow can also be given a solid substance, e.g. bread dipped in barium, designed as a 'stress test' to provoke dysfunction (Curtis, Ekberg and Montesi, 1991).

The principal value of CT scanning in oesophageal disease (Figure 24.2) is in the staging of oesophageal tumours. It appears, however, that the accuracy of the technique is greater for tumours of the gastro-oesophageal junction than of the thoracic oesophagus where adverse prognostic signs such as local invasion, aortic contact, tracheobronchial tree compression and lymph node involvement may be underestimated in one to two-thirds of patients (Consigliere *et al.*, 1992). Endoscopic ultrasonography (endosonography) has been shown to be superior to CT in evaluating oesophageal carcinoma (Tio *et al.*,

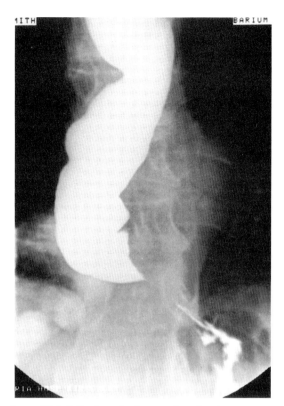

Figure 24.1 Full column barium swallow showing achalasia of the lower oesophageal sphincter

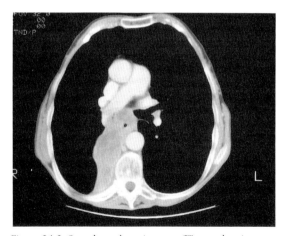

Figure 24.2 Oesophageal carcinoma – CT scan showing gross narrowing of the oesophageal lumen and posterior mediastinal lymphadenopathy

1989; Tytgat and Tio, 1990). The oesophagus is examined by one of two methods: in the water filled balloon method, the ultrasonic transducers are surrounded by a balloon filled with water. Alternatively, a transducer may be placed in direct contact with the oesophageal mucosa. The latter technique shows up the structures outside the oesophagus but the oesophageal wall itself is less well defined. Using the balloon method, the oesophageal wall has five echo layers, corresponding to the histological layers. While endosonography appears superior to CT in evaluation of the depth of tumour infiltration (89%, compared with 59% for CT scanning), CT scanning is more accurate in the detection of liver metastases.

Endoscopy

Within the past 15 years, oesophagoscopy has become the primary diagnostic method for many oesophageal disorders, while therapeutic endoscopy is increasingly the primary modality for numerous diseases. Rigid oesophagoscopy is useful for foreign body extraction, examination of the cervical oesophagus and dilatation of pliable strictures but, for most other indications, flexible oesophagoscopy provides improved visualization with lower morbidity (Bacon and Hendrix, 1992). While rigid oesophagoscopy is contraindicated in patients who are unfit for general anaesthesia, who have a precarious cervical spine or extremely tight fibrous strictures, there are few contraindications to flexible oesophagoscopy. In the diagnosis of carcinoma the more generous biopsies obtained through the rigid oesophagoscope are of greater diagnostic value. However, if six to 10 specimens are taken with a flexible oesophagoscope then the diagnostic accuracy of the two methods is similar. Newer endoscopic diagnostic modalities include chromoscopy which is the staining of the gastrointestinal mucosa by the application of dyes such as Lugol's iodine, toluidine blue and methylene blue. Lugol's solution stains normal squamous epithelium brown due to a reaction with cell glycogen. Injured, abnormal or metaplastic cells have less abundant glycogen and, therefore, stain less deeply. Ectopic mucosa, ulcer, cancer and severe dysplasia remain unstained after the application of Lugol's solution. The method is clinically valuable to detect early oesophageal cancer. Toluidine blue can also be used to stain dysplastic or neoplastic epithelium because the dye accumulates in nuclear DNA which is more abundant in pathological epithelial cells. Methylene blue can be used to delineate normal squamous epithelium from the intestinal metaplasia of Barrett's oesophagus.

Other novel endoscopic developments include the non-invasive endoscopic measurement of variceal pressure. The most reliable method is direct fine needle puncture of varices (Staritz, Poralla and Buschenfeld, 1985). In the past 10 years endoscopic neodymium-yttrium aluminium garnet (Nd-YAG) laser therapy has become an accepted palliation for oesophageal cancer with relief of dysphagia in up to 70% of patients. The endoscopic insertion of oesopha-

geal stents in patients who have failed palliative therapy or who have an oesophagorespiratory fistula may benefit 20% of patients with advanced oesophageal cancer. The stent should be 5–6 cm longer than the endoscopically assessed tumour length. Such stents may also be passed under radiographic control. Both rigid and flexible fibreoptic endoscopes have been used to perform sclerotherapy of oesophageal varices with agents such as ethanolamine or alcohol. In general the technique is more effective than balloon tamponade or treatment with vasopressin alone, and the long-term mortality from variceal haemorrhage may be reduced by 25%. Other novel endoscopic developments include the use of a cuffed foam prosthesis which self-inflates within the oesophagus, thus forming a tight seal to close an oesophagorespiratory fistula. Endoscopically placed endoluminal iridium irradiation can be combined with Nd-YAG laser therapy in the treatment of carcinomas.

Radionuclide transit

Radionuclide transit with technetium-99 sulphur colloid has been shown to be a useful non-invasive screening test for oesophageal motility disorders (Russell *et al.*, 1981). The subject is studied in the supine position under a low energy gamma camera, the colloid is swallowed in a single swallow with a further 'dry' swallow 30 seconds later. The swallowing sequences are recorded at 0.4 s intervals for 50 s (Figure 24.3). The method allows measurement of the oesophageal retention time of the bolus and the dynamics of bolus progression. There is some evidence to suggest that if the radionuclide transit time is normal then there is no requirement for manometry. Transit times in normal subjects are highly reproducible (Blackwell *et al.*, 1983) and there is at least an 84% concordance with conventional oesophageal manometry. Radionuclide oesophageal transit is more sensitive than video-radiology but it must be remembered that radionuclide studies are unable to differentiate clearly functional from organic obstruction (Llamas-Elvira *et al.*, 1986).

pH monitoring

The patient who presents with a classical history of gastro-oesophageal reflux disease, i.e. heartburn that comes on post-prandially or posturally with associated regurgitation of food or acid, and who responds symptomatically to a trial of antacids, probably requires no special investigations. If the symptoms are atypical or do not respond to a trial of medical treatment then more precise diagnostic assessment is necessary. This is particularly relevant to otolaryngological practice where atypical symptoms are the rule rather than the exception. Prolonged ambulatory pH

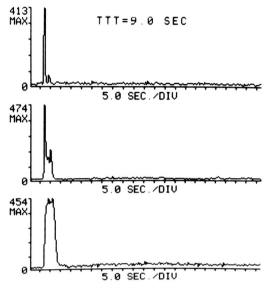 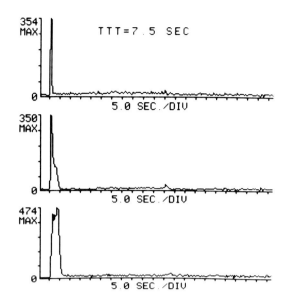

Figure 24.3 Radionuclide oesophageal transit study

monitoring remains the gold standard for the diagnosis of gastro-oesophageal reflux disease. A pH sensitive probe is placed 5 cm above the proximal margin of the manometrically determined lower oesophageal sphincter and linked to a digital microprocessor. During the 24-hour period the subject notes any symptoms present, activities such as eating and sleeping or cigarettes smoked. Some investigators preclude the ingestion of low pH foods during the test. Downloading of the microprocessor data onto the relevant PC-based software package generates a graphical printout of distal oesophageal acid exposure time throughout the test period and a calculation of various oesophageal pH parameters. The two most discriminant parameters of pH monitoring appear to be total oesophageal acid exposure time (under pH 4) and the number of reflux episodes longer than 5 minutes' duration (Schlesinger *et al.*, 1985). It is vital to select the appropriate control data for the accurate interpretation of pH monitoring. It is known that more reflux occurs, particularly during the daytime, when a patient is freely ambulatory in his own home environment compared with inpatient studies. Also the data from pH monitoring are not normally distributed and a 95th centile cut-off is, therefore, preferred to the use of an upper limit of mean + 2 standard deviation total acid exposure time. It has recently been appreciated that it is important to correlate reflux episodes recorded during the test with the patient's subjective symptoms. The use of such an 'index' should limit the number of false-negative results (Caestecker, 1989). It is important to remember that there is not, however, a direct relationship between mucosal acid sensitivity, symptomatic gastro-

oesophageal reflux and abnormal oesophageal acid exposure time. Although related these should be regarded as separate aspects of reflux disease. In other words, some patients have symptomatic reflux or a positive acid perfusion (Bernstein) test despite having normal oesophageal acid exposure and pH monitoring. A possible explanation is that these patients have an 'irritable' oesophagus which can respond to different stimuli by producing the same pattern of symptoms (Howard *et al.*, 1991). Heartburn, for example, may also occur during belching even when it is not associated with reflux, presumably as a result of acute gaseous distension of the oesophagus.

In the investigation of so-called atypical or cervical symptoms of gastro-oesophageal reflux, there is a clear logic in performing pharyngo-oesophageal rather than distal oesophageal pH monitoring. Two reports of pharyngeal pH monitoring in a total of 33 healthy volunteers (Wiener *et al.*, 1989; Wilson, Pryde and Maher, 1993) indicated that oesophago-pharyngeal reflux does not occur in the asymptomatic individual. Genuine oesophagopharyngeal reflux appears fairly uncommon in the small number of subjects studied to date (Wiener *et al.*, 1989). There may be some false negatives using current technology, however, as a small amount of acid refluxed into the capacious hypopharynx may not register contact with a fine pH probe.

Manometry

Accurate measurements of oesophageal pressures were made possible by the development of low compliance perfusion systems (Arndorfer, 1977). To some extent these have been superseded by the recording of oesophageal pressure by miniature intraluminal strain gauges. These are frequently used in conjunction with a solid state computer recorder rather than the conventional chart recorder (Wilson *et al.*, 1989a, 1990b). A non-perfused system has particular advantages in the pharynx, first because the irrigation of the hypopharynx with water can cause pharyngeal irritation and secondly because intraluminal strain gauges have a very much more rapid frequency response than perfused catheter sideholes, and are thus able to capture the rapid high pressure transients. Solid state recording in conjunction with a microprocessor has also opened the way for ambulatory pressure studies, frequently in conjunction with prolonged ambulatory pH monitoring (Figure 24.4). In the tubular oesophagus and lower oesophageal sphincter, manometry has a diagnostic potential for the definition of oesophageal motility disorders.

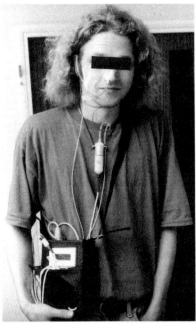

Figure 24.4 Patient undergoing ambulatory outpatient pH monitoring and manometry, with a portable microprocessor

Active measurement of lower oesophageal sphincter tonic pressure is not simple. The lower oesophageal sphincter has radial asymmetry and exhibits a respiratory pressure fluctuation which must be allowed for in pressure measurement. Also the presence of a hiatus hernia can confuse the investigator. Techniques of rapid pullthrough at 1 cm/s or station pullthrough of the catheter at 0.5 or 1 cm stations

with 20 seconds at each station are said to yield similar results. The recording of distal oesophageal peristalsis is usually performed by the assessment of a series of 5 ml water swallows with a suitable interval between each swallow to allow motor recovery. The normal pattern of such peristalsis has now been well defined (Richter *et al.*, 1987). Double peaked waves are frequently seen in normal subjects after both wet and dry swallows and non-peristaltic contractions may occur after up to 18% of dry swallows. Recent work has demonstrated decreased amplitude of contractions in the distal oesophagus of patients with gastro-oesophageal reflux. Such a disorder may in fact precede oesophagitis in such patients. Contraction amplitudes in excess of 180 mmHg are greater than two standard deviations above the normal and are found in fewer than 3% of the normal population, but occur in 48% of patients with a possible oesophageal cause of non-cardiac chest pain. The manometric pattern associated with specific disorders is discussed below. The concordance between manometric and radiographic analysis of swallows is over 90%. However, in difficult cases the tests give complementary information because radiology assesses bolus movement rather than the quantitative pressure data generated by manometry (Hewson *et al.*, 1990). Interrupted peristaltic waves have somewhat surprisingly been shown radiologically to clear nearly all of the bolus from the oesophagus, while to and fro movement of the barium in the mid-oesophagus corresponds to simultaneous manometric contractions.

The upper oesophageal sphincter demonstrates even greater radial and axial asymmetry than the lower oesophageal sphincter (Figure 24.5). It has also recently been discovered that the pharynx does not operate like the tubular oesophagus but, at least in its distal portion, close to the upper oesophageal sphincter, also has marked radial asymmetry with the greatest pressures exerted in the posterior plane (Wilson *et al.*, 1992b). When using a solid state recorder a sample speed of at least 32 Hz is necessary to capture the rapid pharyngeal transients. Any pharyngo-oesophageal pressure measurement is influenced by the diameter of the recording catheter because of the stretch tension response of muscle fibres. This response is, however, greatest in the striated muscle of the upper oesophagus and pharynx where the catheter diameter exerts an enormous influence on recorded pressure. It can be seen that, as with pH monitoring, the definition of abnormal manometric findings in an individual patient requires that the recording laboratory must establish its own normal data for the parameter in question and that direct comparison of absolute values among different centres is difficult. As in the lower oesophageal sphincter it is not known what constitutes the most significant parameter of upper oesophageal sphincter barrier function. The greatest pressures are in the anteroposterior plane, and reflect to some extent the mass of

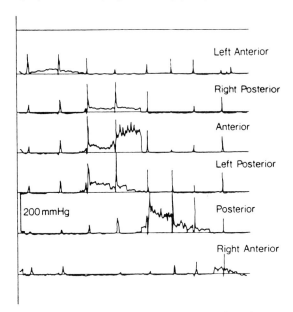

Figure 24.5 Station pull-through of upper oesophageal sphincter showing radial and axial asymmetry

the superimposed laryngeal structures. Whether this constitutes the primary barrier or whether the lateral pressures should also be included in the calculation of upper oesophageal sphincter tonic pressure has not been resolved. A more sophisticated way to analyse barrier function is the performance of a vector volume analysis by the computer recorder. While this technology is useful to study sphincter alteration, e.g. after surgical procedures, its diagnostic capacity remains limited. Indeed the use of upper or pharyngo-oesophageal manometry in isolation has a fairly restricted place in the diagnosis of pharyngo-oesophageal motility disorders.

Ambulatory pressure measurements have become possible due to the development of microprocessor technology such as is used in pH-monitoring and also in the creation of automated pressure analysis – it has been estimated that manual analysis of a 24 hour ambulatory pressure recording would take the observer up to 2 weeks! Development of ambulatory technology has opened the possibility for the generation of a symptom correlation, as with pH-monitoring, between patients' oesophageal symptoms and demonstrated manometric abnormalities. The technique has also highlighted enormous differences between the manometric pattern of 'free range' eating and the ordered peristaltic wave associated with single water swallows in the laboratory. Thus many subjects are now asked to undertake bread swallows and to attempt to reproduce their normal eating pattern during stationary manometry in the laboratory. This type of test has suggested that some patients experience dysphagia associated with aperistal-

sis as a response to the increased frequency of the swallowing (Howard, Pryde and Heading, 1989). The value of 24-hour ambulatory pressure monitoring has proved somewhat disappointing (Janssens, Vantrappen and Ghillebert, 1986). The technique has, however, supported the concept of the irritable oesophagus by defining certain patients in whom either reflux or an oesophageal motor disorder can provoke non-cardiac chest pain.

Evolving technology

Over the past 5 years, an increasing number of centres have developed techniques to combine manometric and radiological techniques. The methods have considerably advanced the understanding of the physiology of swallowing, although their importance in the investigation of patients with dysphagia, compared with a separate performance of manometry and radiology remains to be established. One of the main stimuli to its development was the difficulty in manometric interpretation due to the movement of the pharyngo-oesophageal segment relative to the pressure catheter during swallowing. It is the detailed analysis of manofluorographic tracings that has led to the conclusion that the bolus precedes the pharyngeal stripping wave for example.

Most workers now use a solid state manometric catheter to register pharyngeal pressure. Three recordings are generated – the independent pressure and radiographic tracings which are both marked simultaneously with a resettable video timer so that equivalent time points can be identified and related, and a manofluorograph which is the simultaneous presentation of both tracings (McConnel, Cerenko and Mendelsohn, 1988). Early analysis of manofluorometric tracings suggested that the tongue driving pressure and the negative pressure developed in the pharyngo-oesophageal segment appeared considerably more important than the pharyngeal clearing wave in successful bolus propulsion. The separate manometric and radiographic traces are required because sometimes the resolution of the combined trace is less clear, due to it being displayed on computer rather than a video monitor screen. Use of a computer in this way does, however, allow 'frame grabbing' of individual images which may then be subjected to digital measurement analysis by the computer, e.g. allowing precise estimation of the hyoid excursion (Kahrilas *et al.*, 1989). Radiopaque markers may be placed on anatomical landmarks, e.g. over the cervical spine, at the angle of the mandible and used as a reference point for such measurements. As the principal driving force is applied to the bolus the tongue base 'plunger' and the movement of the laryngopharynx upwards, embracing the bolus as it is pushed downwards, allows patients with paralysis of the pharyngeal constrictors to have an almost normal swallow. In such individuals there may be a residium of bolus aspirated after the completion of a swallow due to inefficiency of the pharyngeal clearing wave in 'mopping up' the tail of the bolus (Cerenko, McConnel and Jackson, 1989).

Further advances in computer and video technology have allowed the merging of more than two images. For example it is possible to combine a video signal of laryngeal events obtained through a transnasal fibreoptic laryngoscope with the other modalities (Shaker *et al.*, 1990). Most of the recording remains on videotape rather than on computer hard disc because of the memory requirement of stored images. As automated analysis programs are already available for the analysis of swallow pressures, it is possible to envisage that at some point in the future the computer may be able to analyse both captured images and recorded pressures to generate a very sophisticated analysis of swallowing abnormality.

A further recent development is the application of electromyography (EMG) to the pharyngo-oesophageal segment. While it is easy to perform new physiological studies of the suprahyoid musculature such as geniohyoid and mylohyoid with either transcutaneous or bipolar needle electrode recordings, recording transmucosal EMG signals from the pharyngeal constrictors is considerably more difficult. One of the difficulties is that the mucosa moves relative to the muscles with loss of the signal. This has led to the development of bipolar suction electrodes for surface EMG of the pharyngeal constrictors and upper oesophagus (Tanaka, Palmer and Siebens, 1986). The method has advantages over traditional hooked wire and needle electrodes as the thinness of the pharyngeal constrictors lends itself more readily to surface than to needle recording. Also because the mucosa and submucosa are thin and there is a high nerve to muscle fibre ratio, i.e. very few muscle fibres per motor unit, analysis of individual potentials by surface recording is at least theoretically possible. The wires may be passed transnasally, allowing the subject to swallow comfortably. The technique can obviously be adapted to the submucosal muscles of the oral cavity or larynx. Needle or hooked wire electrodes are, however, essential for access to deep muscles. Both hooked wires and suction electrodes are stable on movement whereas needle electrodes can become displaced during the laryngopharyngeal deglutition movement. A further disadvantage of the needle electrode is the associated discomfort. The analysis of individual electrical potentials is, however, optimal with a bipolar needle electrode and the topic is well reviewed by Palmer, Tanaka and Siebens (1989). EMG studies of the cricopharyngeus and inferior constrictor muscles appear to reveal only minimal activity in the inferior constrictor at rest, whereas the cricopharyngeus proper has a conspicuous resting tone (Elidan *et al.*, 1990). Palmer's group has been able to demonstrate EMG abnormalities in patients with neurological dysfunction due to lower motor neuron disorders such as

cranial nerve injury, poliomyelitis or unilateral bulbar palsy. Although time consuming and technically difficult, the methods offer the potential to classify more precisely the specific abnormalities in disorders such as motor neuron disease where there may be a combination of upper and lower motor neuron lesions.

The use of endosonography to delineate structural abnormalities of the tubular oesophagus has already been mentioned. In the oropharynx, ultrasound can also be of benefit in the recording of tongue movement with the obvious advantage of eliminating radiation exposure. In addition the technique offers a means of assessing tongue activity (Stone and Shawker, 1986) which is critical in normal swallowing and difficult to quantify. Real time mechanical sector ultrasound imaging of the oral cavity is now being used also to analyse speech production. The probe must be placed submentally as ultrasound does not penetrate bone. As the oral cavity is filled by air, the upper surface of the tongue and soft tissue anatomy of the floor of the mouth are clearly visible. Images may be recorded on videotape for frame by frame or slow motion analysis. Any delay in the initiation of the swallow reflex can be quantified and the images can be integrated with manometric recordings (Sonies and Baum, 1989).

Motility disorders
Upper oesophageal sphincter

Hundreds of patients have been subjected to cricopharyngeal myotomy because of a putative diagnosis of 'upper oesophageal sphincter spasm.' Sometimes this diagnosis is based on radiological criteria, sometimes on a clinical history or recurrent bolus obstruction and sometimes even on clinical grounds alone. It is only in recent years, however, that the comparative rarity of true upper oesophageal sphincter spasm (increased resting tone) or achalasia (failure of relaxation) has been recognized. Two independent studies of the functional significance of cricopharyngeal impressions (Figure 24.6) have failed to demonstrate either upper oesophageal sphincter hypertonicity or failure of relaxation in the majority of subjects (Dantas *et al.*, 1990; Wilson *et al.*, 1992a). Indeed, upper oesophageal sphincter achalasia appears to be extraordinarily rare. This is perhaps not surprising as the recording of complete manometric relaxation in this area requires only that the anterior wall of the sphincter is pulled forward sufficiently to lose its contact with a fine bore recording device. Upper oesophageal sphincter resting hypertonicity was present in around one-third of patients with cricopharyngeal impressions in one series (Wilson *et al.*, 1992a). A detailed manofluorometric analysis carried out on six patients with an isolated cricopharyngeal bar (Dantas *et al.*, 1990) confirmed normal axial upper oesophageal sphincter pressure and relaxation and normal bolus flow across the sphincter. The

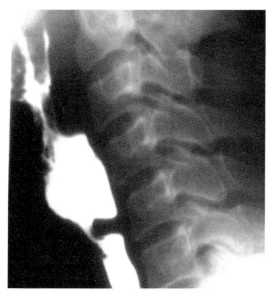

Figure 24.6 Persistent cricopharyngeal impression

duration of upper oesophageal sphincter opening was also normal but there was a reduced maximum dimension of opening during the trans-sphincteric flow of barium. There appears, therefore, to be a restrictive defect of upper oesophageal sphincter opening in these patients rather than a true motility disorder. Whether or not this restrictive opening may be one of the abnormalities which leads in later life to the development of a pharyngeal pouch remains speculative.

Hypofunction of the upper oesophageal sphincter (chalasia) remains a poorly defined entity as there is nearly always some residual manometric high pressure due to the anterior mass of the larynx. If techniques of cricopharyngeal EMG were more widely available then the disorder might be diagnosed more frequently. It does appear that certain elderly individuals and some patients with multiple neurological problems do have very poor upper oesophageal sphincter tone and are at risk from intraoesophageal air entry with each inspiration and also, conversely with oesophagopharyngeal reflux during recumbency.

Oesophageal body

Several manometric syndromes associated with hyperactivity of the oesophageal musculature have been defined. These cannot be identified precisely from the history, although if structural oesophageal or cardiac disease has been excluded approximately 30% of patients with non-cardiac chest pain will have a primary oesophageal motility disorder, the most common being nutcracker oesophagus. Diffuse oesophageal spasm and achalasia tend to present with dysphagia rather than chest pain.

The term nutcracker oesophagus refers to a manometric abnormality with an average distal oesophageal peristaltic pressure greater than two standard deviations above normal (> 180 mmHg) in a symptomatic patient. The aetiology is unknown, although psychological profiles are similar to those of the irritable bowel syndrome and globus sensation with higher scores on somatization, anxiety and depression. All patients have otherwise normal peristalsis and barium studies are usually normal. Some success may be achieved by treatment with calcium channel antagonists such as nifedipine or diltiazem. Bougienage and surgical myotomy are reserved for the rare non-responders.

Diffuse oesophageal spasm on the other hand is associated with radiological abnormalities and has, therefore, been recognized for over a century. The aetiology is unknown and the radiographic findings are variable. While proximal peristalsis is usually normal tertiary activity in the distal oesophagus produces the 'rosary bead' appearance on barium swallow. The disorder can be diagnosed accurately only by manometry. Current criteria require the presence of simultaneous contractions in more than 10% of wet swallows, intermixed with some normal peristalsis. Simultaneous contractions may, however, be seen in other motility disorders such as diabetes, scleroderma, amyloid and alcoholic neuropathies. Many patients with early or vigorous achalasia demonstrate high amplitude contractions, all of which are simultaneous. Repetitive or multipeaked waves are seen with variable frequency, depending on the definition used. Probably only wave forms with three or more peaks should be considered abnormal. These are present in about 30% of patients with diffuse oesophageal spasm. The patient should be reassured that there is no sinister cause for the dysphagia. Nitrates decrease radiographic abnormalities and reduce chest pain but the most popular agents remain the calcium channel antagonists, which decrease the amplitude of contractions in the oesophageal body and also reduce lower oesophageal sphincter pressure. Oesophageal dilatation with pneumatic dilators is of benefit in some patients. Because of the rarity of the disease, there are only three series reported of more than 15 patients and only one with 5-year follow up (Leonardi, Shea and Crosier, 1977). In general, the prognosis should be excellent, although transition to achalasia has been documented and may occur in 3–5% of patients (Katz, 1992). Oesophageal surgeons are not, however, in agreement as to whether the myotomy should involve the division of the lower oesophageal sphincter musculature (necessitating an associated fundoplication) or whether it should be confined to the distal two-thirds of the oesophagus.

The oesophagus can be involved in many other disorders affecting the central nervous system, vagus nerve, intraneural nerve plexus or oesophageal muscle (Weinstock and Clouse, 1987). Over half the patients with scleroderma have oesophageal involvement, generally occurring in association with Raynaud's phenomenon. The abnormalities occur only in the smooth muscle oesophagus and include low amplitude peristalsis, aperistalsis and reduced lower oesophageal sphincter pressure. The disease occurs in the third and fourth decades, is more common in women and is generally prolonged and progressive. It is not clear whether the observed smooth muscle atrophy is secondary to neurogenic damage. More common disorders such as diabetes mellitus may also interfere with oesophageal motility. The commonest cause of non-specific motility disorder is, however, gastro-oesophageal reflux which is associated not only with reduction in lower oesophageal sphincter tone but also with poor propagation of peristaltic waves in the distal oesophagus. It remains unclear whether this disorder precedes the reflux or results from it.

Lower oesophageal sphincter

Achalasia of the cardia is associated with degeneration of the ganglion cells in the myenteric plexus between the circular and longitudinal smooth muscle layers of the oesophagus. The dorsal motor nucleus and the nucleus ambiguus of the vagus are also affected. The vagus nerves show degeneration of axonal and Schwann cells. There are two types of achalasia, the classical type where the oesophageal body shows simultaneous non-propulsive low amplitude contractions and the so-called 'vigorous variant' where the simultaneous contractions are high amplitude, repetitive and of prolonged duration. This is thought to represent the early or 'compensated phase' of achalasia. The aetiology is unknown. Only a few cases occur in families and the similarity to the South American Chagas' disease (infection with *Trypanosoma cruzi*) suggests a possible infection of the myenteric plexus with a neurotropic virus. Physiological studies have confirmed denervation of the smooth muscle, e.g. exaggerated contractions are seen in the oesophageal body and lower oesophageal sphincter when achalasic patients are given a parenteral acetylcholine analogue. It is postulated that the lower oesophageal sphincter hypertonicity results from a combination of loss of ganglion cells, particularly of inhibitory neurons, and of a reduction in vagal inhibitory stimulation to lower oesophageal sphincter musculature.

The disease shows an equal sex incidence, affecting one to two subjects per 200 000 population per annum. The onset is usually in the third to fifth decades, although up to 5% have symptoms before adolescence. The average patient has a 2-year history before presentation. Patients may report specific manoeuvres which improve oesophageal emptying such as raising the arms above the head, or standing very erect in an attempt to increase intraoesophageal pressure. The regurgitation of undigested foods may be confused with functional eating disorders such as bulimia. Some patients find that the dysphagia is alleviated by ingestion of carbonated drinks, although these can in fact also alleviate bolus obstruction caused by a benign oesophageal stricture (Karanjia and Rees, 1993).

A chest radiograph is normal in the early stages but a para-aortic tubular mass or mediastinal widening with an air fluid level may be visible at a later stage (Figure 24.7). Also classical is the absence of the gastric fundal gas shadow. At barium swallow examination, the dilated oesophagus tapers symmetrically to a 'bird's beak' or 'rat tail' appearance. Endoscopy is essential to exclude a submucosal infiltrating carcinoma of the distal oesophagus which can be associated with 'pseudo achalasia' (Carter and Brewer, 1975). Typical endoscopic findings include dilatation of the oesophageal body and a closed lower oesophageal sphincter which does not open during the procedure. Under gentle pressure, however, the endoscope passes into the stomach. At manometry, no true peristaltic propagation is seen but transient intraoesophageal pressure rises may be recorded simultaneously in different sensors – the common cavity phenomenon due to the detection of pressure changes in a closed chamber. The lower oesophageal sphincter may show increased resting tone but more important is the demonstration of incomplete lower oesophageal sphincter relaxation.

The treatment of achalasia is either by forceful

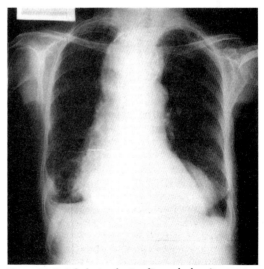

Figure 24.7 Achalasia: chest radiograph showing gross mediastinal widening

dilatation or myotomy. Medical therapy with such agents as aminophylline or nifedipine may give temporary relief. Forceful dilatation can be achieved with mechanical, hydrostatic or pneumatic dilators. The most popular of these is now pneumatic dilatation with an air filled balloon, e.g. Browne McHardy and Hurst–Tucker mercury pneumatic dilators. The bag is placed across the lower oesophageal sphincter and inflated under fluoroscopic control to obliterate the constriction. This may require a pressure of up to 600 mmHg. An alternative method is to use a series of bags of increasing diameter such as the Sippy dilating bag. Two to four dilations are usually necessary. The early complications include pain, oesophageal perforation, bleeding and aspiration, with an associated mortality of 0.3%.

The results of oesophagomyotomy are also excellent and the procedure may be advocated as first line treatment when there is severe oesophagitis or another abnormality requiring surgery. It may also be indicated in instances where dilatation is likely to be unsuccessful, e.g. when the dysphagia is very long-standing or when the patient is an infant or young child. Although Heller's original description involved division of both anterior and posterior lower oesophageal sphincter musculature, the results of anterior oesophagomyotomy appear equally satisfactory. The procedure may be carried out through a transthoracic approach if there is a requirement to deal with an associated abnormality such as an epiphrenic diverticulum. The transabdominal approach is favoured in the more frail subject but is associated with a higher instance of complicating postoperative gastro-oesophageal reflux and, therefore, requires an associated anti-reflux procedure to be carried out, such as an incomplete fundic wrap. The mortality is 0.2% with a mucosal perforation in about 10% of patients.

Gastro-oesophageal reflux
Pathophysiology

Over the past few years, the perception of a hypotonic lower oesophageal sphincter as the cause of gastro-oesophageal reflux has become more specific and the importance of transient lower oesophageal sphincter relaxations is now appreciated. Only a minority of reflux episodes occur because of an absence of sphincter pressure (Holloway and Dent, 1990). In patients with severe oesophagitis, however, up to one-third of reflux episodes may occur in the absence of lower oesophageal sphincter relaxation. Although the lower oesophageal sphincter relaxes reflexly with every normal swallow, it is in fact quite rare for reflux to occur during swallow-induced relaxation, because the duration of the relaxation is very brief and any reflux is further limited by the oncoming peristaltic wave. About 60% of reflux episodes occur during

spontaneous, transient lower oesophageal sphincter relaxations which last up to 30 seconds, appear to be neurally mediated and can be provoked by gastric distension. There is inconsistent evidence that these transient relaxations are associated with increased submental electromyographic activity and they, therefore, represent the response to an incomplete swallow (Mittal and McCallum, 1988), otherwise the basis for defective basal lower oesophageal sphincter pressure is poorly understood. It may be that the lower oesophageal sphincter pressure is occasionally normal but interspersed with periods of defective pressure, suggesting a defect of sphincter control rather than an intrinsic abnormality of the lower oesophageal sphincter smooth muscle. Reflux can, however, occur during episodes of increased intra-abdominal pressure or spontaneously in association with reduced lower oesophageal sphincter tonic pressure (Dodds *et al.*, 1982). The relationship between hiatus hernia and reflux remains controversial. Only 50–60% of patients with a hiatus hernia have endoscopic oesophagitis, whereas up to 94% of patients with oesophagitis have a hiatus hernia. It seems most likely that the hernia impairs lower oesophageal sphincter function particularly during straining when the crural diaphragm plays a role in the anti-reflux barrier (Mittal, 1990). It has been postulated that the pressure gradients caused by the smooth muscle of the oesophagus and stomach are counteracted by the lower oesophageal sphincter smooth muscle while the pressure gradients caused by the skeletal muscles (raised intra-abdominal pressure) are counteracted by the crural diaphragm.

Although gastro-oesophageal reflux is an almost universal occurrence even in asymptomatic healthy subjects, the comparative rarity of severe reflux oesophagitis as a result of the incompetence of the anti-reflux barrier highlights the importance of 'tissue resistance'. This resistance is based on the intraluminal mucous layer which acts as an alkaline microenvironment close to the epithelial surface, defended by its stratified squamous structure and tight, high electrical resistance characteristics. It has been stated that the presence of spontaneous gastro-oesophageal reflux in a well-sedated patient during endoscopy is pathological but there is no proof of this assertion. Particularly in patients being examined with rigid oesophagoscopes under general anaesthesia, it is possible for the significance of 'free reflux' to be over-interpreted. It was proposed in 1970 that the changes in the squamous epithelium itself rather than the inflammatory cell infiltrates were the key to the diagnosis of gastro-oesophageal reflux disease. However, it appears that some epithelial changes such as basal cell hyperplasia also occur in healthy individuals (Geisinger and Wu, 1985).

A variety of endoscopic grading systems of reflux oesophagitis has been developed. The most commonly used remains the Savary-Miller classification, and its variants (Miller, 1992). The original description is as follows:

Grade I: linear, non-confluent erosions
Grade II: longitudinal, confluent, non-circumferential erosions
Grade III: longitudinal, confluent, circumferential erosions that bleed easily
Grade IVa: one or several oesophageal ulcerations in the mucosal transition zone which can be accompanied by stricture or metaplasia
Grade IVb: with the presence of a stricture but without erosion or ulceration.

The treatment of gastro-oesophageal reflux disease is traditionally on lifestyle measures such as weight reduction, elevation of the head of the bed, reduction in fat intake and elimination of eating meals late in the evening. Reduction in smoking and alcohol intake is also beneficial and simple antacids or antacid-alginate combinations are a useful supplement to these measures. If they fail to control the symptoms then a dose of an H_2-antagonist, somewhat greater than that required to control duodenal ulceration, may be used (e.g. ranitidine 300 mg b.d. or cimetidine 800 mg b.d.), although these drugs relieve symptoms in most patients, both are somewhat disappointing in their ability to heal endoscopic oesophagitis.

The proton pump inhibitor, omeprazole, has a higher symptomatic response and a much higher incidence of endoscopic healing (over 80%) than H_2-antagonists. The synthetic gastrointestinal prokinetic drug, cisapride, which enhances the release of acetylcholine from the myenteric plexis has been shown to increase lower oesophageal sphincter pressure, and to increase the contractability of the middle and distal thirds of the oesophagus with a reduction in oesophageal transit time (Eriksen *et al.*, 1990) and in gastro-oesophageal reflux. It may, therefore, be considered a first line drug where dysphagia predominates. The indications for the surgical treatment of gastro-oesophageal reflux disease may be summarized as follows:

1 Failure of medical therapy
2 Development of complications such as stricture or Barrett's oesophagus
3 Reflux induced oesophageal dysmotility
4 Reflux in childhood
5 Postoperative gastro-oesophageal reflux.

Although the most commonly performed operation is the fundoplication, this has the major disadvantage of creating a 'super-competent' sphincter. The complete wrap described by Nissen can be modified in a loose complete wrap, or in a partial wrap. Incomplete wraps leave varying segments of the anterior wall of the oesophagus unsupported. The Angel Chik prosthesis effectively controls gastro-oesophageal reflux but is now appreciated to have significant complications, including gas-bloat and dysphagia in up to 50% of patients. The principle of Hill's posterior gastropexy is the plication of the lower oesophagus and maintenance of the intra-abdominal length of the oesophagus by fixation of this repair to the median crural ligament of the diaphragm. The most favoured thoracic operation is the Belsey mark IV which is a successful procedure but technically difficult.

Barrett's oesophagus

When Barrett first described his eponymous oesophageal abnormality in 1950, he misinterpreted his observations as those of a congenitally short oesophagus. He subsequently altered his view and suggested that the condition should be described as a lower oesophagus lined by a columnar epithelium (Hennessy, 1992). Areas of ectopic, probably embryonic epithelium are not infrequently seen in the proximal oesophagus. These do not constitute Barrett's oesophagus which is characterized by distal columnar epithelium associated with marked inflammation. Patients have repeatedly been shown to have greater oesophageal acid exposure times and poorer oesophageal acid clearance than controls. Similarly patients with achalasia who have undergone Heller's myotomy also have an increased incidence of Barrett's oesophagus. Bile reflux has also been implicated and the condition is associated with a low pressure short lower oesophageal sphincter with an inadequate intra-abdominal segment, under 1 cm.

Unequivocal evidence is provided by the finding of intestinal metaplasia which develops as a function of age and is almost invariably present in those patients who develop adenocarcinoma. The mucosa appears tubular with gastric folds and is a deeper red than the stomach and in marked contrast to the pale squamous mucosa of the healthy tubular oesophagus. Symptoms include heartburn, regurgitation and, if stricture is present, dysphagia. A Barrett ulcer may give rise to deep seated pain which radiates through to the back or life-threatening haemorrhage. The incidence of Barrett's type epithelium in the general population is not known. The autopsy prevalence has suggested one in 100 cases, similar to the incidence at routine endoscopy. There are two peak ages, 0–15 years and 40–80 years. Even more important than the association of the condition with oesophageal ulceration and stricture is the risk of oesophageal carcinoma which is in excess of 40 times that of the general population. A cumulative lifetime risk is, however, less than 1% (Hennessy, 1992). It has been suggested that high grade dysplasia correlates strongly with Barrett's carcinoma but the role of endoscopic tumour surveillance remains controversial. It has been estimated that in order to demonstrate a reduction in mortality from this surveillance, at least 2000 patients would need to be followed up for a minimum of 10 years.

Medical treatment includes the use of an H_2-receptor antagonist and conventional alginates. Cisapride may improve distal oesophageal acid clearance and in patients resistant to H_2-receptor antagonists, omeprazole may be indicated. Antireflux surgery is, however, a more effective method of abolishing reflux and, in addition to relieving symptoms and healing an ulcer, may also promote stricture resolution. There is, however, no evidence that such surgery reduces the risk of adenocarcinoma. High grade dysplasia may be an indication for an oesophageal resection particularly in a young fit patient who is also known to be a smoker and drinker. The risk of a fatal outcome from resection (5–8%) has, however, also to be borne in mind. Resection, if undertaken should at least include the Barrett segment with an anastomosis to healthy squamous epithelium.

Reported otolaryngological manifestations of gastro-oesophageal reflux

A wide variety of otolaryngological symptoms have occasionally been reported in association with gastro-oesophageal reflux (Hallewell and Cole, 1970; Bain *et al.*, 1983; Koufman, 1991). The commonest among these are probably chronic cough, pharyngeal burning, repeated swallowing and aerophagy, halitosis, and a choking sensation. The association with less frequently reported symptoms such as apnoeic episodes, otitis media and subglottic stenosis remains much more tenuous. The putative association between gastro-oesophageal reflux and oesophageal webs or Zenker's diverticula remains unproven in the context of an adequate, controlled study. Early reports of a relationship between posterior pharyngeal diverticula and hiatus hernia were based on illustrative case histories and the authors themselves emphasized the need for further investigation of this theory (Smiley, Caves and Porter, 1970). A more recent retrospective review of the radiological findings in 104 patients with a diagnosis of Zenker's diverticulum indicated a 39% incidence of concomitant hiatus hernia, compared with a 16% incidence of hiatus hernia in the control patients who had had a barium swallow as part of their head and neck malignancy workup (Gage-White, 1988). The 58 control patients were, however, not age matched with the group with Zenker's diverticulum and the study suffers from the usual problems of this type of retrospective analysis. As Dr Gage–White pointed out, moreover, the absence of a hernia in the majority of her patients indicates that hiatus hernia or reflux disease is far from being the sole aetiological factor in pharyngeal pouch. A review of 28 patients with a variety of head and neck symptoms possibly attributable to gastro-oesophageal reflux were investigated prospectively by various modalities including oesophageal scinti-graphy. The battery of tests showed gastro-oesophageal reflux in only three patients (Kuriloff *et al.*, 1989). Although the authors quoted a prevalence of gastro-oesophageal reflux in the population of up to 30%, it should not be surprising that much smaller numbers of patients present with atypical symptoms.

Up to 10% of patients with gastro-oesophageal reflux disease appear to have pulmonary symptoms secondary to reflux and it is now recognized that gastro-oesophageal reflux may be an important cause of intrinsic asthma and other respiratory conditions in both children and adults (Barish, Wu and Castell, 1985). A variety of mechanisms may explain the association between reflux and bronchospasm (Boyle *et al.*, 1985). These include overt micro-aspiration of liquid gastric contents associated with chemical pneumonitis; micro-aspiration with resultant stimulation of upper airway receptors; and stimulation of oesophageal mucosal receptors. Bronchospasm in turn may trigger reflux by increasing transdiaphragmatic pressure. Furthermore, specific bronchodilator therapy may cause relaxation of the lower oesophageal sphincter and thus promote reflux. A study of 100 patients with abnormal gastro-oesophageal reflux on ambulatory oesophageal pH monitoring, of whom 48 were suspected to be aspirators clinically, showed documented episodes of aspiration, i.e. drop in oesophageal pH, followed by acid taste and onset of cough or wheezing in only eight patients (Pellegrini *et al.*, 1979). Aspiration does not, therefore, appear to be the mechanism by which reflux is associated with asthma in about 50–60% of patients. It is likely that acid in the inflamed oesophagus of asthmatic patients, therefore, acts on exposed receptors and increases bronchial reactivity via a vagally-mediated reflex (Goldman and Bennett, 1988).

In infants, some cases of laryngospasm appear attributable to gastro-oesophageal reflux (Henry and Mellis, 1982; Orenstein, Orenstein and Whittington, 1983). Respiratory arrest due to acid aspiration has been proposed as a cause of sudden infant death syndrome but is exceptional in adults although isolated cases have been reported (Bortolotti, 1989). Patients have also been reported with refractory subglottic stenosis attributable to silent laryngeal penetration of gastric acid, which is known to produce experimental subglottic lesions in animals (Little *et al.*, 1985). There has also been recent interest in the suggestion that in the small proportion of patients with laryngeal carcinoma who are non-smokers, the disease may be reflux related. Morrison (1988) reported a series of six non-smokers with carcinoma of the larynx and symptoms and radiographic evidence of gastro-oesophageal reflux. A further series of 138 patients with carcinoma of the larynx included 14% of lifetime non-smokers, all of whom were reported to have moderate severe symptomatic reflux, while more than half had hiatus hernia or peptic ulceration (Ward and Hanson, 1988). No detailed investigations were performed, however, and the patients were not unselected new otolaryngological referrals – many had been under long-term follow up for lesions such as leukoplakia and granulomas when their cancers developed. More recently, Price, Jansen and Johns (1990) have found pathological evidence of Barrett's oesophagus in one-third of 24 patients undergoing laryngopharyngo-oesophagectomy for advanced hypopharyngeal carcinoma.

Reflux and laryngitis

In the early 1960s, vocal abuse was considered to be the primary cause of contact ulcer of the larynx, a rare disease which occurs predominantly in men and appears to be rare in European otolaryngological practice (Brodnitz, 1961). Brodnitz also observed an occasional association between contact ulceration and gastric or duodenal ulceration. Thereafter, Cherry and Margulies (1968) reported three patients with refractory contact ulcer, symptomatic gastro-oesophageal reflux and positive acid barium meal examinations. In a companion paper (Delahunty and Cherry, 1968), the effects of 20 minutes of daily experimental application of gastric juice to the vocal cords of two dogs per month were shown to produce granulation tissue and epithelial breakdown. The authors subsequently reported a series of 12 patients, largely men, with burning pharyngitis, throat clearing and occasional globus sensation (Cherry *et al.*, 1970). Only three had radiological evidence of hiatus hernia or oesophagopharyngeal reflux but the majority had a positive acid barium meal examination. Delahunty later described a syndrome of intractable posterior laryngitis which he attributed to nocturnal oesophagopharyngeal reflux on the basis of strongly positive acid barium swallow studies (Delahunty, 1972). Subsequent reports have indicated that posterior vocal cord granuloma can respond to anti-reflux surgery (Goldberg, Noyek and Pritzker, 1978). It has even been suggested that contact ulcer should be renamed 'peptic granuloma' because of its aetiology and histological appearance (Miko, 1989). Some believe that the aetiology requires a combination of gastro-oesophageal reflux and harsh throat clearing, which itself may result from oesophagopharyngeal reflux (Ward *et al.*, 1980). This combination was found in many patients of one North American series of 58 males with contact ulceration (Ohman *et al.*, 1983). One of the problems, however, in analysing contact ulceration is its relative rarity. Furthermore, the various aspects of oesophageal dysfunction which have been demonstrated do not explain the predominance of unilateral lesions. The male preponderance is usually explained on the basis of 'clashing' arytenoid opposition, although there may have been a small increase in the prevalence of contact ulceration among women in recent years, perhaps due to the taking up by women of high vocal demand employment (Watterson, Hansen-Magorian and McFarlane, 1990).

The reported incidence of gastro-oesophageal reflux in patients with more non-specific inflammation in the posterior third of the larynx depends very much on patient selection, and also on the degree of rigour with which the patients are investigated. In one series, all but two of 44 patients with posterior laryngitis had proven gastric hypersecretion on the basis of clinical examination by a gastroenterologist (Kambic and Radsel, 1984). Ward's group accrued 86 patients over 7 years with an 80% radiological incidence of hiatus hernia, although Ward stressed the response to therapy as the real evidence for the implication of gastro-oesophageal reflux (Ward and Berci, 1982). The therapeutic trial is, however, uncontrolled and incorporates not only traditional anti-reflux manoeuvres but also a variety of other measures such as smoking cessation, broad-spectrum antibiotic therapy and even a short course of steroids. The most systematic study of posterior laryngitis, specifically white plaques in the interarytenoid area, showed that a majority of patients with gastro-oesophageal reflux alone or in association with intrinsic asthma had evidence of such lesions at laryngoscopy (Larrain *et al.*, 1981). Other causes may have been responsible for some of the white plaques in asthmatics, however, such as reaction to inhaled pulmonary therapy, second to candidiasis and of course cigarette smoking.

It is clear that so far no single laryngeal abnormality has been linked unequivocally with reflux but the association has enduring appeal. More recent studies have examined the importance of reflux in association with chronic hoarseness rather than with a specific laryngeal lesion. Wiener *et al.* (1987) pioneered the use of dual probe ambulatory pH monitoring where one of the antimony pH electrodes is sited 5 cm above the lower oesophageal sphincter with another 2 cm above the upper oesophageal sphincter. No normal subject was found with a documented episode of pharyngeal reflux. Pharyngeal reflux was also uncommon in the patient group (who had hoarseness, laryngeal cancer or respiratory symptoms), although 26 of the 33 patients had abnormal pH monitoring, only three had episodes of pharyngeal reflux (Wiener *et al.*, 1989). A comparison of the results of distal oesophageal pH monitoring with posterior laryngeal and distal oesophageal biopsy in 97 voice clinic attenders who had symptoms or signs perhaps due to 'acid laryngitis' (heartburn, burning pharyngeal discomfort, nocturnal choking or interarytenoid pachydermia) showed that 14% had gastro-oesophageal reflux alone, 25% had laryngitis alone and 17% had both laryngitis and gastro-oesophageal reflux (Wilson *et al.*, 1989c). The most recent study (Jacob *et al.*, 1991) has shown a significant increase in proximal oesophageal acid exposure in patients with laryngeal symptoms compared with patients who have gastro-oesophageal reflux disease alone, although hypopharyngeal contamination was unfortunately not evaluated. Also only 10 of the 25 patients with cervical symptoms in this study had detectable laryngoscopic abnormalities.

It is clear from the above that the precise abnormalities with which gastro-oesophageal reflux may be associated in the larynx remain unknown. As the mechanism, either local direct, or distant, indirect, is not known, the optimum method for assessing gastro-oesophageal reflux in this context likewise remains to be established. What is certain, however, is that an uncontrolled trial of antacid therapy in pharyngeal disorders which are notorious for having a strong functional component is not an adequate method of addressing the question. The role of the upper oesophageal sphincter in the generation of acid laryngitis is also not known. There is no evidence that the upper oesophageal sphincter undergoes any protective augmentation during experimental upper oesophageal acid exposure or spontaneous episodes of gastro-oesophageal reflux (Kahrilas *et al.*, 1987; Vakil *et al.*, 1989; Wilson *et al.*, 1990a). It appears that the reflux responsible for laryngitis may occur predominantly in an upright position (Wiener *et al.*, 1987) in which case the transient upper oesophageal sphincter relaxations which accompany belching may be of some relevance (Kahrilas *et al.*, 1986).

Oesophageal cancer

Demography

In the past decade, cancer of the oesophagus has become the sixth most common cancer in the world, notably in the developing countries where it occupies fourth place. Environmental factors are believed to account for the remarkable international and re-gional variations in incidence (Figure 24.8). The highest mortality rates occur in the Asian oesophageal cancer belt. This stretches from European Russia and Turkey to Eastern China. Very high rates are also found in certain black communities of southern Africa, including the Transkei and Zimbabwe. The tumour is, however, rare in North and West Africa (Higginson, Muir and Munoz, 1992). In North America, the rate in Blacks is three to four times higher than that in Whites and the only major time trend is the dramatic increase in squamous carcinoma observed in the last two decades in North American Blacks. In Europe, the highest incidence is in France. The age-specific incidence rates increase rapidly with age, and there is a clear male predominance in the West. As with laryngeal cancer, certain areas of France have a very high sex ratio which can approach 20 to 1. This is in contrast to the high risk Asian belt where some areas show even a female excess and to the situation in Scotland where women also have a remarkably high incidence. The large difference in incidence within short distances supports a major role for exogenous aetiological factors. Between Jurjev Town at the head of the Caspian Sea and the towns in Georgia, 500 hundred miles away, the incidence of cancer of the oesophagus drops 70 fold for men and 230 fold for women (Cook-Mozaffari, 1989).

Predisposing factors

The small number of oesophageal cancers associated with tylosis are due to a single autosomal dominant gene. Tylosis is a condition in which there is marked thickening of the skin of the palms and soles, and

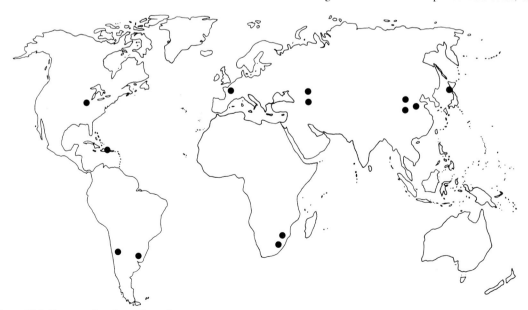

Figure 24.8 Demography of oesophageal cancer

frequently, hyperhidrosis. It is type A which occurs between the ages of 5 and 15 years that is associated with cancer of the oesophagus. Type B which occurs in infancy does not share the association. Much more important is the role of environmental agents, notably alcohol and tobacco. Studies in North America indicate a fivefold increase in risk for those taking 3 or 4 units of alcohol daily and who smoke more than 20 cigarettes per day compared with non-smokers and non-drinkers. The Epidemiological Centre in Britanny has also shown a clearly multiplicative effect of the two factors with the relative risk of over 130 for those who smoke more than 20 g of tobacco and drink more than 120 g of ethanol a day. Several studies also indicate that the effect of alcohol with a little tobacco smoking is greater than the effect of smoking accompanied by a little alcohol intake (Cook–Mozaffari, 1989). Spirits carry a greater risk than wine or beers and the data from Brittany and Normandy suggest an association with home distillation. In contrast, in those regions of the Middle East with a high incidence and where alcohol is not consumed for religious reasons, there may be an association with opium intake.

The exceptionally high incidence in certain populations such as the women of North Eastern Iran, among whom the consumption of alcohol and tobacco is negligible, stimulated interest in other possible aetiological factors and dietary deficiency of vitamin A, riboflavin and vitamin C has been implicated. These vitamins are believed to maintain the integrity of the oesophageal mucosa. Postcricoid carcinoma has been associated with Paterson Brown–Kelly syndrome in Northern European countries. In addition, there appears to be an increased risk associated with low socioeconomic status. This may relate to the dietary deficiencies of animal protein and fat, fruit and vegetables. It has long been known that strictures of the oesophagus following corrosive damage can lead to the subsequent development of malignant tumours. Lesser degrees of oesophageal trauma may also be relevant, e.g. the consumption of hot liquids such as mate in Brazil and abrasive seeds in bread in the high incidence areas in Iran. Endoscopic surveys in Iran and China also show that chronic oesophagitis is more prevalent in areas where oesophageal cancer is endemic. The prevalence of oesophageal cancer in patients with achalasia is approximately 3–7%. The average interval between the onset of symptoms of achalasia and the detection of malignancy is 17 years, and oesophageal cancer appears to occur at an earlier age in the achalasics than in the general population (Yakshe and Fleischer, 1992). There is also accumulating evidence to support an aetiological role for human papilloma virus which may induce cytopathic changes the progression of which to dysplasia then sets the scene for the development of carcinoma *in situ*.

Pathology

Various macroscopic appearances of *squamous cell carcinoma* are recognized. Fungating lesions appear as lobulated or polypoid intraluminal masses while ulcerating lesions are of variable depth with irregular, raised margins and necrotic bases. These tumours are deeply invasive and frequently extend into adjacent mediastinal tissues. Early tumours may appear as flat, erythematous patches or focally eroded pale plaques. Histologically squamous cell carcinoma is classified as at other sites, i.e. as well, moderately, or poorly differentiated and as keratinizing or non-keratinizing. The histological distinction between early and advanced lesions depends on the depth of invasion. Advanced lesions involve the muscularis mucosa. Well-differentiated carcinoma has epithelial stratification, intercellular bridges and keratinization. The degree of differentiation does not, however, affect prognosis (Earlam and Cunha–Melo, 1980). Poorly differentiated carcinoma by definition is characterized by near absence of the morphological features indicative of squamous origin. Extensive longitudinal spread is common and satellite tumours may appear in the mucosa some distance from the main tumour. Proximal extension is more common and up to 13% of patients exhibit a bronchial or tracheal fistula.

The true incidence of *adenocarcinoma* of the oesophagus is only 1%. It may arise from residual islands of columnar epithelium or in the submucous glands. The glands may also give rise to adenoid cystic carcinoma of the oesophagus. Five-year survival is reported to be under 3% (Turnbull and Goodner, 1968). The overwhelming majority of adenocarcinomas arise on Barrett's epithelium although rarely ectopic gastric mucosa near the oesophageal inlet may give rise to an adenocarcinoma. There have been frequent reports of *oat cell* tumours occurring in the oesophagus. Some comprise primary bronchial tumours with oesophageal extension and some are probably undifferentiated squamous tumours. New secretory granules have been identified (Rosen, Moon and Kim, 1975) and ACTH secretion has been reported. The rare *adenosquamous carcinomas* have both squamous and glandular features, most commonly in the lower third of the oesophagus. One of the most plausible explanations is the so-called collision theory whereby an adenocarcinoma from the oesphageal junction area meets and fuses with a distal squamous lesion. *Carcinosarcomas* present as polypoid masses in the mid and lower oesophagus and are very rare. The tumour is largely composed of spindle cells with a less prominent squamous epithelial element.

Diagnosis

The diagnosis of oesophageal carcinoma is usually made by barium study or endoscopy. The advantages of using CT scanning in pre-therapy staging are increasingly apparent, however, many tumours are beyond curative treatment at presentation. Early oesophageal cancer is defined as cancer limited to the mucosa or submucosa without lymph node metastases. Such early lesions are asymptomatic and require diagnosis by population screening. Endoscopic ultrasound may be more reliable than CT in predicting wall penetration and lymph node involvement (Gayet *et al.*, 1990).

Oesophageal cell specimens may be obtained easily using a variety of blind and endoscopic techniques including lavage, brushing, balloon sampling and fine needle aspiration. Since the development of fibreoptic endoscopy, lavage has been largely superseded by endoscopic brushings. Balloon abrasive cytology is an effective tool for detecting early squamous cancer in high risk populations and was developed in China 30 years ago. Endoscopic fine needle aspiration is still under evaluation, although it has a particular potential for malignant submucosal neoplasms. The normal oesophageal mucosa has infrequent mitotic figures which occur only in the basal zone and keratohylin granules are rare or absent. The presence of keratin formation suggests chronic mucosal irritation or an underlying premalignant or malignant lesion. The cytological appearance of invasive squamous cell carcinoma is variable and depends on the degree of differentiation of the tumour. Well differentiated cancers are characterized by large pleomorphic cells with abundant eosinophilic cytoplasm and large irregular nuclei. Bizarre forms with giant nuclei, spindle or tadpole cells are common. Poorly differentiated carcinomas are characterized by large or small cells with scanty basophilic cytoplasm and irregular markedly enlarged nuclei. There is considerable variation in cell size and shape and cells may occur singly or as small irregular aggregates – syncytia. Cytologically the distinction between poorly differentiated adenocarcinoma and other poorly differentiated malignant neoplasms may be difficult (Teot and Geisinger, 1992).

Endoscopic evaluation is essential to obtain histological or cytological confirmation of the diagnosis. Early lesions may only show subtle changes from normal and local areas of elevation, depression or colour change may be the only indication of malignancy. Lugol's solution can be used to delineate abnormal areas and vital staining has been attempted with toluidine blue. A mixture of 1% toluidine blue is applied to the mucosa and rinsed off 7–10 minutes later with 1% acetic acid. Determination of the distal extent of a lesion may be difficult at endoscopy if the tumour cannot be negotiated with the endoscope. In this situation, a preliminary careful dilatation may be necessary. Sometimes it is possible to pass a fine bore bronchoscope through the obstruction.

Staging

CT scanning has an important role in identifying lateral spread of the tumour to involve other mediastinal structures and also to identify nodal involvement. Conversely it can also provide information on a clear space between the oesophagus and the aorta confirming that the tumour is operable. Endoscopic ultrasound has made a significant contribution as outlined above, and may be comparable to CT in the assessment of spread. Sensitivity of invasion predicted by CT is high, approximately 98%, while the accuracy of nodal staging on endosonography is around 89% (Murata *et al.*, 1987). A mediastinoscopy and node biopsy may also have an important role in surgical planning and to define whether any resection is likely to be palliative or curative. The primary aim of palliative resection is a wide proximal and distal clearance to avoid anastomotic recurrence. Treatment is unlikely to be curative if there is local involvement of nodes or extension beyond the oesophageal wall, although such a palliative resection may still be feasible. More distant metastasis to liver or bone is rarely identifiable at presentation.

Radical treatment

As indicated above, occasionally resection of oesophageal tumours is undertaken with palliative intent. Less heroic palliative measures are discussed below. To be a candidate for resection, distant metastases should be absent, respiratory and cardiac function adequate, and there should be no evidence of fixation to the larynx or trachea, recurrent laryngeal nerve paralysis or oesophagobronchial fistula. If at operation, complete removal is impossible, a palliative resection may then be undertaken. Unfortunately there are insufficient data from adequate prospective controlled trials to form a scientific judgement of which patients should undergo radical radiotherapy as opposed to surgical resection.

Many patients are severely malnourished and would benefit from a high calorie, high protein diet preoperatively. Tumours of the lower third of the oesophagus are usually removed en bloc with the greater part of the stomach, part of the pancreas, and the spleen. Infradiaphragmatic lesions are best treated by total rather than partial gastrectomy (McKeown, 1979). Although the classical approach for these procedures is a left thoraco-abdominal incision, this may result in diaphragmatic herniation postoperatively. The use of an abdominal incision with the thorocotomy incision and preservation of an intact diaphragm results in better postoperative respiratory function.

Tumours of the middle third of the oesophagus are usually dealt with by mobilizing the stomach through a midline epigastric incision and performing an oesophago-gastric anastomosis. Patient survival is critically dependent on the security of the anastomosis as leakage is a disaster with a very high mortality (Hennessy and Cuschieri, 1992). McKeown's total three stage oesophagectomy (McKeown, 1976) with mobilization of the stomach to the cervical region allows greater proximal clearance of high intrathoracic tumours, although the overall mortality if high risk cases are included can approach 15%. Blunt dissection of the oesophagus without thorocotomy was described by Gray Turner in 1933 and was used by Le Quesne and Ranger (1966) for pharyngolaryngo-oesophagectomy. Recent developments with endoscopic surgery, however, are likely to replace blunt transhiatal oesophagectomy in the near future. The gastric mobilization and Kocherization of the duodenum and the cervical dissection are performed in the standard manner but the oesophageal dissection is carried out endoscopically, followed by a hand sewn anastomosis.

The single most important factor predicting the response to radical radiotherapy is the size of the primary oesophageal tumour (Arnott, 1989). An excellent response can be expected in growths less than 5 cm in diameter but only around one-third of those given radical treatment will have tumours within this range. Women appear to show a higher response rate at least with tumours up to 8 cm in length. Overall the one-year survival following radical radiotherapy is only 39% and it is thus difficult to justify protracted treatment techniques. It, therefore, seems appropriate to recommend limited treatment volumes and doses of 5000–5500 cGy given in 20 daily fractions over 4 weeks. A good 5-year survival is around 9% which is not dissimilar to that obtained following surgery. Multimodality therapy is, therefore, worthy of consideration. Unfortunately the majority of trials to date have been phase II trials without randomization, although phase III trials are now underway. Ten different chemotherapeutic agents have been used either singly or in combination. There are theoretical advantages to administering chemotherapy preoperatively, including the limitation of drug resistance. Improved resection rates have also been reported following chemotherapy, e.g. with cisplatin and 5-fluorouracil (Carey *et al.*, 1986). When a combination of irradiation and chemotherapy is used, however, despite improved resectability rates, there appears to be an increase in perioperative mortality primarily due to pulmonary toxicity (Leichman, Steiger and Seydel, 1984).

Palliative treatment

In modern oesophageal practice, dilators without guide wire systems are considered obsolete. The preferred system is the endoscopic placement of a guide wire over which a series of olive shaped dilators is passed (Figure 24.9). Those available include the

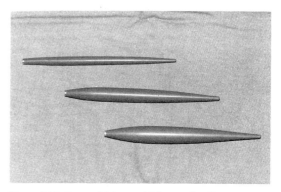

Figure 24.9 Keymed Advanced Dilators: the olives are introduced over a guide wire

Eder-Puestow, Celestin, Savary and the KeyMed advanced dilator. The Eder-Puestow system has a spring tipped guide wire which is passed under endoscopic control. The endoscope is then withdrawn leaving the guide wire *in situ*. The system requires repeated passage of a coiled carrier spring with metal olive shapes for increasing size. The Celestin system requires the passage of only two dilators and is, therefore, quicker, smoother and more acceptable to the patient. There are several types of pneumatic dilators with balloons designed to have a very low compliance, i.e. to rupture if excess pressure is exerted. Rubber dilators weighted with mercury, e.g. the rounded tip or Hurst dilator and the tapered tip or Maloney dilator are principally used in home selfbouginage by patients. Permanent in-dwelling tubes for the relief of malignant dysphagia have been used for almost 100 years. Most tubes currently used have a diameter of around 12 mm and all have a flange proximally to abut against the proximal margin of the tumour. The Mousseau-Barbin and Celestin tubes were designed for insertion after laparotomy and gastrotomy. It is now possible, however, to carry out an Eder-Puestow dilatation and to introduce the tube over a flexible guide wire from above, e.g. preliminary dilatation followed by the use of a Nottingham introducer and an Atkinson or Celestin tube (Atkinson and Ferguson, 1977). The complications include perforation, tube migration and blockage. An average hospital stay is around 5–7 days with a mean survival of between 6 and 11 months, according to different series.

Superior palliation has been reported following laser therapy with the neodymium-YAG laser (Carter and Smith, 1986). The possibility of superior palliation, however, may not outweigh the repeated treatment required in patients with a limited life span and of course the capital cost of the equipment. The issue can only be addressed by a randomized prospective trial. Intracavitary irradiation using after loading plastic tubes with iridium can be used in isolation or in combination with external beam irradiation or laser therapy. Other leak-proof radioactive materials such as caesium-137 may also be used and an 8 mm external diameter applicator is introduced under fluoroscopic control over a previously inserted guide wire. The caesium sources are then transferred along an inert tube and locked within the external tube. The treatment length is 13 cm and the procedure may be done under sedation and local anaesthetic. The whole oesophagus may be treated in two applications (Pagliero, 1989). Having positioned the applicator, it is maintained in position by an attachment to a face mask strapped to the patient's head. The patient is transferred for attachment to the Selectron machine. A dose of 1500 cGy may be achieved in around 1 hour giving a treated volume 2 cm in diameter and 13 cm in length. There is considerably less morbidity than is associated with external beam radiation. A more effective response may be possible by the use of a sensitizing chemotherapeutic agent such as 5-fluorouracil or methotrexate. Use of laser recanalization followed by after loading therapy is reported to give complete relief from dysphagia in 77% of patients and with a very low restenosis rate (Bader *et al.*, 1986).

Traumatic lesions of the oesophagus

Rupture

Spontaneous rupture of the oesophagus was first documented by Hermann Boerhaave in 1724 (McFarlane and Munro, 1990) in his description of the autopsy of a gluttonous Admiral who collapsed having taken a self-prescribed emetic. At postmortem, Boerhaave found a distended stomach and fluid smelling of roast duck in both pleural cavities. Spontaneous rupture has been reported to follow abdominal straining, not infrequently in association with oesophageal lesions such as Barrett's ulceration. At the other end of the spectrum, a small superficial tear in the oesophageal mucosa, known as a Mallory-Weiss laceration occurs with vomiting (often alcohol induced). A clinical triad of full blown spontaneous rupture is of vomiting, often after a heavy meal in an adult male, low thoracic pain and cervical emphysema. The pain may, however, present largely in the abdomen and haematemesis is not uncommon. The condition is often misdiagnosed initially, because of its rarity. Furthermore, the chest radiograph is usually abnormal but not specifically diagnostic. The commonest site of a spontaneous rupture is in the left distal oesophagus.

Instrumental perforation

The incidence of oesophageal perforation following routine diagnostic fibreoptic upper gastrointestinal endoscopy is only 0.018–0.03%. The risk of perforation, however, increases greatly when therapeutic manoeuvres are introduced, e.g. a perforation rate of 0.61% has been described following dilatation with metal olive dilators (Silvis *et al.*, 1976; Dawson and Cockel, 1981). The instance of perforation following rigid oesophageal examination is overall higher than that of routine fibreoptic endoscopy. It must be borne in mind, however, that the majority of fibreoptic endoscopy in the UK is carried out for non-oesophageal disorders while rigid examinations, by definition relate to an oesophageal disease and reported series are thus not directly comparable. When rigid endoscopy is employed with dilatation, the perforation rates vary from 0.2% to 0.9% (Anderson, 1990). A substantial perforation may be diagnosed at the time of endoscopy. If not, then the presence of subcutaneous surgical emphysema is pathognomonic, but not universal. Almost all patients complain of pain, initially well localized to the site of the perforation. The vast majority of patients will have confirmatory findings on plain radiography such as prevertebral gas in the case of a cervical oesophageal perforation or mediastinal emphysema where the intrathoracic portion of the oesophagus has been perforated (Hishikawa, Tanaka and Miura, 1986). An uncommon diagnostic 'V' sign is a triangular lucency seen through the heart perhaps due to emphysema in the lower pulmonary ligament and diaphragmatic pleura. A confirmatory barium swallow is more likely to be positive in a thoracic perforation than a cervical perforation. Only 60% of the latter may be demonstrable on barium swallow.

The optimum management is undecided. There is no doubt that early diagnosis and management improves outcome but while the traditional management was aggressively surgical (Grillo and Wilkins, 1975), over the past 10 years, certain centres have advocated non-operative management. In the cervical oesophagus, where the overall mortality from perforation of the oesophagus is considerably lower than in the thorax, the early institution of broad-spectrum antibiotic therapy and withholding of oral feeding can result in radiological closure within 5–7 days. For cervical perforations presenting later than 24 hours, and with established infection, then in addition to conservative treatment, drainage of the neck and occasionally the mediastinum may be required. Attempting to suture the margins of an inflamed perforation will be futile. Any resulting fistula will probably close spontaneously providing there is no distal obstruction.

Conservative management for thoracic oesophageal perforations has become increasingly popular since the report by Wesdorp *et al.* (1984) of the successful non-operative management of all but five of 54 consecutive fibreoptic instrumental perforations of the oesophagus. Thirty five of the 54 perforations occurred during intubation of malignant strictures, with a mortality of 8.6%. There were no deaths in the non-malignant group. The results were attributed to early diagnosis (most within 2 hours) and active conservative management, i.e. no oral intake, broad-spectrum antibiotic therapy, intravenous feeding and continuous naso-oesophageal suction for 5–7 days via a special tube with multiple side holes above and below the site of the perforation. Although the fatalities occurred in the malignant group, it is in precisely this group that early aggressive surgical management for a perforation may seem the least appropriate, and indeed may prove technically impossible if the tumour is extensive.

Conversely in circumstances where there is a distal oesophageal stricture whose dilatation has resulted in the perforation, spontaneous closure is less likely because of the distal obstruction, and in any case the patient may require definitive surgical treatment for the stricture. In such patients primary surgical intervention remains the treatment of choice. For oesophageal perforations detected within 24 hours, ideally in less than 12 hours, it may be possible to carry out a primary repair of a perforation. This is less likely where the perforation is diagnosed after 24 hours where the mortality is higher because of mediastinal contamination. The necrosis of oesophageal muscle around the site of the perforation leads many authors to advocate buttressing the repair with a variety of tissues including pericardium, stomach, diaphragm or jejunum while others, however, recommend resection of the oesophagus (DeMeester, 1986). There is no established place for conservative management of late oesophageal perforations but surgically or endoscopically placed Celestin tubes may be used in association with an appropriate drainage while the more traditional approach of surgical drainage and diversion to defunction the necrotic segment still has its proponents (Murphy and Roufail, 1991).

Foreign bodies

An estimated 1500 to 2750 individuals die annually in the USA following the ingestion of foreign objects. The normal oesophagus has four anatomical sites of narrowing which are preferential locations for the impaction of such objects: the cricopharyngeus muscle; the aortic arch; the left main bronchus; and the lower oesophageal sphincter. It is large and angulated objects such as coins and safety pins which are most commonly trapped in the proximal oesophagus (Taylor, 1987), although overall the cervical oesophagus is the commonest site of foreign body impaction. Pathological narrowing of the oesophagus due to peptic stricture or a distal oesophageal ring is also an important cause of foreign body impaction, which is surprisingly rare in oesophageal cancer. Eighty per cent of foreign bodies are seen in children who frequently swallow coins among other objects. A review of 57 children investigated because of possible coin

ingestion showed that in 22, the coin was in the stomach, and these were allowed to pass spontaneously (Lancet, 1989). Interestingly of the 30 with a coin lodged in the oesophagus, nine were entirely asymptomatic. The rest had the anticipated symptoms of dysphagia, drooling, pain, vomiting, cough or stridor. Children are noted to ingest more foreign bodies during the school holidays (Chaikhouni, Kratz and Crawford, 1985).

Adults who deliberately ingest foreign bodies are usually suffering from mental impairment or psychiatric illness. Prisoners, however, often ingest foreign objects to derive potential secondary gain from hospitalization. Most obstructions in adults are, however, due to swallowed food. Food bolus impaction is different from impaction of a foreign body in that it is usually in association with oesophageal disease, it is more frequently in the distal oesophagus and it generally occurs in older subjects and often in association with denture wearing. In addition to the typical symptoms outlined above, patients may complain of increased salivation and a persistent foreign body sensation. Factors resulting in delayed diagnosis include mild initial symptoms, radiolucency of the object and absence of a history of ingestion leading the diagnosis to be unsuspected. It should be remembered that dental plates are not radiopaque (Von Haacke and Wilson, 1986).

Oesophageal pain is more likely to be referred proximally than distally and, therefore, discomfort in the xiphisternal area is more reliable than is a sensation in the suprasternal notch. Cervical foreign bodies are, however, fairly accurately located by the patient. Foreign bodies which are lateralized in the suprahyoid region can usually be visualized in the oropharynx. Objects lodged in the cricopharyngeal area are usually felt somewhat lateral to the trachea but certainly above the clavicles. A lateral view for a foreign body should always be taken. Not only may this reveal some foreign bodies which might otherwise be missed but on occasion a child may have ingested two foreign bodies, one smaller than the other which is tucked out of sight on the anteroposterior neck/chest radiograph. Objects such as wood, aluminium, glass, plastics, meat and, as indicated, dental plates may not be visible without the use of contrast solutions. One helpful sign on the lateral cervical soft tissue film is the presence of a prevertebral gas shadow above an impacted foreign body in the upper oesophagus. (This is not infrequently overlooked by accident and emergency department staff who presumably are more intent on seeking out evidence of the foreign body itself.) Where the history is clear, it is probably not wise to carry out a barium swallow because endoscopy will be complicated by the obscuring presence of the barium.

Flexible fibreoptic endoscopy has been used in the removal of foreign bodies since the early 1970s. However, protection of the upper airway from the inadvertent aspiration of saliva or retained oesophageal gastric contents may require intubation, general anaesthesia and rigid endoscopy. The endoscopist should always be competent in emergency airway management. Flexible endoscopy does, however, offer the advantage of allowing examination of the stomach and duodenum in the event of no foreign body being found in the oesophagus. Pharmacological agents such as glucagon have been used successfully in promoting the passage of meat boluses since first described by Ferrucci and Long (1977). The method is thought to work by reducing lower oesophageal sphincter pressure (Smith, 1986). The technique works in around 40% of patients presumably because it does not affect the diameter of strictures or rings. A 1–2 mg intravenous bolus may cause nausea, vomiting or hyperglycaemia but is usually well tolerated. Historical attempts to digest meat boluses enzymatically with proteolytic agents such as papain have now fallen from favour because of two potentially life-threatening complications of enzymes – transmural digestion (Holsinger, Fuson and Sealy, 1968) of the oesophagus and haemorrhagic pulmonary oedema if the compound is aspirated. An alternative conservative measure is to use agents which release gas into the oesophagus thus raising intraluminal pressure, distending the oesophagus against a closed cricopharyngeal muscle and thus interiorly forcing the bolus into the stomach. The gas forming agents include simple carbonated drinks, a cocktail of tartaric acid and sodium bicarbonate and carbex effervescent granules (sodium bicarbonate, activated dymethicone and citric acid). A period of observation of a coin impacted in the *distal* oesophagus of a child of up to 12 hours is acceptable due to the relatively high incidence of spontaneous coin passage. Coins which reach the stomach generally transit uneventfully and do not require extraction unless they fail to appear within 7–10 days. In children, whether or not a flexible endoscope is used, poor cooperation usually necessitates the use of general anaesthesia.

Battery ingestion

Almost every household now contains several items operated by miniature batteries. Even 10 years ago, up to 1000 battery ingestions were estimated to occur annually in the USA. Of these around 400 are reported annually to the National Button Battery Ingestion Hotline at the National Capital Poison Center, Georgetown University (Smith and Peura, 1992). The majority involve button-type batteries in children under 5 years of age. The disc batteries are encountered in watches, clocks, calculators, games, toys and, most commonly, in hearing aids. A battery lodged in the oesophagus poses a severe hazard from caustic damage. A typical button battery is an anode and cathode separated by an electrolyte soaked fabric, usually a 45% solution of potassium hydroxide (Lito-

vitz, 1983). Tissue destruction can occur rapidly and can culminate in an oesophageal perforation after several hours. It is the leakage of caustic alkaline which results in tissue liquefaction. Other mechanisms of injury are direct pressure from the battery itself and low voltage electrical burns. Following prompt radiographic confirmation of the battery's presence which may show a double density shadow produced by a bilaminar disc battery, the child should be prepared for endoscopic removal. The removal is difficult because of the associated inflammation and the fact that the object tends to slip out of the teeth of the grasping forceps. Where batteries are reported to have been manipulated into the stomach, there is usually little damage to the lower gastrointestinal tract, although one case of intestinal perforation has been reported when a battery lodged in a Meckel's diverticulum (Willis and Ho, 1982). If the battery cannot be retrieved or manipulated into the stomach then open removal may be necessary. Following removal of a battery from the oesophagus, follow-up radiology should be arranged at intervals to exclude the late development of a stricture.

Chemical injury

The hazards of ingestion of caustic alkalis were observed by Chevalier Jackson, developer of the first distal lighted oesophagoscope, whose lobbying resulted in legislation to control their sale. Nonetheless, caustic oesophageal injuries are still not uncommon, most often following the ingestion of liquid cleaners (and button batteries as mentioned above). Occasionally seen in children (Anderson, Rouse and Randolph, 1990), the vast majority of ingestions are in the 20–40-year-old range and are suicide attempts. The mortality has markedly reduced following improvement in the management not only of the acute phase of the ingestion but also of the chronic stricture which ensues. Acidic material causes a coagulation rather than a liquefaction necrosis and, therefore, the damage caused by acids is more limited and less likely to penetrate the muscular layer. Alkaline oesophageal injury is associated with oedema of the submucosa, inflammation of the submucosa with thrombosis, sloughing of the superficial layers, necrosis of the muscular layer, fibrosis of the deep layer and finally delayed re-epithelialization (Browne and Thompson, 1991). The superficial necrotic tissue sloughs at about one week while the re-epithelialization phase does not take place until after almost one month. The clinical picture is widely varying and its severity is not related directly to the extent of the oesophageal injury. Patients may present with fairly acute airway obstruction from glottic and laryngeal oedema and this finding is highly correlated with significant oesophageal injury. Other symptoms and signs include pain, odynophagia, mucosal ulceration, tongue oedema, salivation, chest, back or abdominal pain, vomiting or haematemesis. Any patient with oral mucosal burns should be carefully monitored for signs of impending airway obstruction which may necessitate tracheostomy because of the obvious difficulties in intubation. Marked dyspnoea and pulmonary signs may suggest aspiration or mediastinitis.

Most investigators now advocate early endoscopy to assess the extent of the oesophageal burn as soon as possible after ingestion. First degree burns are manifest by variable amounts of erythema while second degree burns involve whitish exudate and varying degrees of ulceration. Third degree burns are transmural with oedema and necrosis which frequently obliterate the lumen. The areas of anatomical narrowing discussed above are the sites of predilection for oesophageal burns. There is a possibility of tracheo-oesophageal fistula formation at the upper oesophageal and mid-oesophageal narrowings. Where possible, therefore, any patient with a third degree anterior burn in these areas should undergo tracheoscopy. The procedure should be performed by an experienced endoscopist and if any difficulties are encountered, the burned area should not be negotiated. If at all possible, however, careful full length endoscopy and caustic injury may reveal more significant life-threatening burns distal to the first circumferential burn.

First degree burns require observation for dysphagia and infection. The treatment for second degree burns remains controversial. The range of measures available include supportive therapy, steroids, antibiotics, antacids, oesophagectomy for necrosis and oesophageal stenting. One controlled prospective study, however, showed no benefit from the use of steroids in 60 paediatric patients (median age 2 years) studied over an 18-year period (Anderson, Rouse and Randolph, 1990). The use of steroids has been noted to reduce the incidence of stricture from around 80% to 70% (Browne and Thompson, 1991). Steroids should, however, be avoided in a deep third degree burn because there is an increased incidence of oesophageal perforation. The prevention of stricture may be promoted by the use of agents which reduce cross-bonding in new collagen, e.g. N-acetylcysteine (Liu and Richardson, 1985) or penicillamine (Thompson, 1987). Some workers also advocate the insertion of a nasogastric tube as a means of reducing the incidence of stricture. This should remain in place for 3 weeks. More severe burns may be managed for a similar period with a silastic stent inserted by a gastrotomy. Once radiological evidence of stricture formation has occurred, regular dilatation should be instituted at once. If this fails to control dysphagia then oesophageal replacement, where possible, by a blunt rather than a thorocotomy approach is advocated. Many patients can be taught to pass mercury filled bougies for use at home. Dilatation should not, however, be attempted in very long, narrow, or tortu-

ous strictures which have an increased risk of perforation. Colon is the preferred method of bypass (De-Meester *et al.*, 1988) because of often associated gastric involvement. The operative mortality is around 5–9%. Because of the risk of carcinoma developing in a caustic stricture, there is a theoretical advantage in performing prophylactic excision of the damaged segment, although the actual risk is probably less than 5% with an interval from the injury of 24–46 years.

Benign obstructive lesions of the oesophagus

Tumours

Although rare, the leiomyoma is the commonest benign tumour in the oesophagus. It usually occurs in middle age, twice as frequently in men and largely in the lower and middle thirds of the oesophagus. About 50% of patients are asymptomatic. The usual presentation is of retrosternal pain, dysphagia and occasionally bleeding. Barium swallow examination shows the characteristic smooth filling defect. Multiple tumours should be distinguished from diffuse leiomyotosis which occurs in adolescents. At diagnosis, the leiomyoma should be removed even if asymptomatic as malignancy cannot otherwise be excluded and the condition is progressive.

Oesophageal cysts are rare, being three times less common than leiomyomas. Small retention cysts are clinically insignificant but enterogenous cysts may become symptomatic. These duplication cysts run parallel to the main lumen and may communicate with it at one or both ends. Bronchial glands and cartilage are sometimes present and compression of a main bronchus is possible. Oesophageal polyps may have very long pedicles – isolated reports describe regurgitation into the mouth or even aspiration into the larynx. Most can be removed endoscopically with electrocoagulation of the pedicle.

Diverticula

By far the commonest diverticula affecting the oesophagus are pharyngo-oesophageal or Zenker's diverticula (see Chapter 10). True oesophageal diverticula are usually classified as mid-oesophageal or epiphrenic. There is no real basis for the long-held belief that mid-oesophageal diverticula are traction diverticula (Bancewicz, 1992). As the thoracic oesophagus is, however, a simple tube, there is no alternative explanation of why asymmetrical pulsion out-pouchings should arise from this structure. Most patients with pulsion diverticula have an associated motility disorder such as vigorous achalasia or diffuse oesophageal spasm. Similar abnormalities are found in patients with epiphrenic diverticula (although when analysing the results of investigation in patients with established diverticula, as with pharyngo-oesophageal diverticula, the mechanical effect of the pouch itself must be considered).

Small asymptomatic diverticula found incidentally on investigation of other symptoms require no treatment. Gastro-oesophageal reflux is often found in association and should be treated where documented. Multiple diverticula may disappear following the treatment of oesophagitis. Where necessary, surgical excision should include myotomy down to the cardia to correct any obstruction of the distal oesophagus, and the surgical correction of gastro-oesophageal reflux where present. If possible, the approach should be through the left chest which gives the widest range of therapeutic options. A nasogastric tube should be avoided and oral intake restricted for 5–7 days.

Webs

These are encountered predominantly in midde-aged women. Cervical dysphagia occurring in combination with anaemia and an upper oesophageal web (Figure 24.10) has long been associated with the names of

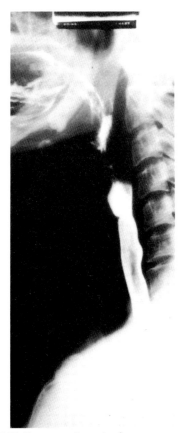

Figure 24.10 Upper oesophageal web

Brown-Kelly (1919), Paterson (1919) and Vinson (1922). These early workers recognized that the association of the various components of this syndrome was not a simple one. Both Paterson and Brown-Kelly considered that the female preponderance was not a reflection of neurosis in view of the established higher incidence of postcricoid carcinoma in female patients. Brown-Kelly also distinguished the syndrome from hysteria by the absence of globus sensation and of intermittent symptoms and proposed that the cervical dysphagia found in association with oesophageal webs is due to cricopharyngeal spasm secondary to an innervation imbalance. Vinson on the other hand failed to demonstrate very convincing radiological findings and took this to imply a hysterical condition which could be distinguished from globus hystericus by the obstruction to the passage of food. The most consistent finding, in other words, is of cervical dysphagia. The importance of the web in the story is unclear. Wynder and Fryer (1958) found iron deficiency anaemia related to geographical, nutritional and menstrual factors in a study of 150 patients (133 female) with Paterson Brown-Kelly syndrome, of whom 47% were anaemic and 77% had a past history of dysphagia. Jacobs (1962) found iron deficiency anaemia in 31% of patients with postcricoid carcinoma and described pernicious anaemia in a smaller number. A subsequent study of 50 patients (only three with upper oesophageal webs) showed almost half to be deficient in vitamin B_{12}. It was proposed that iron deficiency was secondary to the atrophic gastritis of pernicious anaemia (Jacobs and Kilpatrick, 1964). In the same year, however, Elwood *et al.* (1964) performed a unique epidemiological study of over 4000 subjects in Wales to find the incidence of cervical dysphagia in the general population. A definite history of dysphagia localized between the hyoid bone and the suprasternal notch was obtained in 1% of men and 5% of women. Only 15% of those with dysphagia had evidence of upper oesophageal webs. There was little evidence that women with dysphagia either alone or in association with a web had iron deficiency. It was thus concluded that previous studies of hospital-based inpatient populations may have over-estimated the haematological associations and that postcricoid dysphagia could best be regarded as a single symptom, in some cases associated with a web or stricture. The absence of iron deficiency is in keeping with the demographic pattern of the syndrome which is hardly recognized in Africa despite a high incidence of severe iron deficiency.

It can be concluded, therefore, that the presence of an upper oesophageal web in a patient with cervical dysphagia may be an incidental finding. Alternatively, it may, in a smaller proportion of patients, represent an integral part of an iron deficiency mucosal change (i.e. Paterson Brown-Kelly syndrome). Microscopically a cervical oesophageal web is a fold of normal oesophagus with some underlying loose connective tissue. Occasionally webs occur as part of a syndrome of multiple oesophageal webs in patients with dermatological disorders such as epidermolysis bullosa and benign mucous membrane pemphigoid. In addition, the mid-oesophagus may be involved in patients who have had bone marrow transplantation with chronic graft versus host disease.

The diagnosis is essentially a radiological one. The web is seen as a thin projection from the anterior surface of the oesophagus in the postcricoid area at barium swallow examination. The differential diagnosis includes a ventral venous plexus and ectopic gastric mucosa at the oesophageal inlet. The web is usually ruptured during diagnostic endoscopy and is, therefore, not well characterized during this examination. Patients with cervical webs should undergo estimation of iron and iron stores in addition to measurement of the haemoglobin as the web may precede the development of anaemia. Tests for pernicious anaemia should only be carried out if the mean corpuscular volume is elevated.

Lower oesophageal rings (Schatzki's rings) are seen in up to 14% of routine barium examinations. Symptomatic rings are much less common and are a cause of dysphagia in patients over the age of 40 years. The intermittent dysphagia tends to be provoked by hurried eating and is a cause of patients presenting with bolus obstruction. Endoscopically most patients have a normal distal oesophagus and gastro-oesophageal reflux probably plays no role in pathogenesis. Symptomatic muscular rings are extremely rare and are usually located 2 cm proximal to the squamocolumnar junction. Radiologically the appearance of the ring may alter as peristalsis progresses down the tubular oesophagus. In countries such as Sweden where Paterson Brown–Kelly syndrome was once common, the incidence of postcricoid carcinoma in women has slowly changed so that this cancer has a similar pattern to other head and neck cancers, i.e. a male preponderance, but the possibility of an associated carcinoma in the upper aerodigestive tract should always be borne in mind and a careful examination carried out on such patients.

Globus pharyngis

Globus sensation, a feeling of something in the throat, from the Latin *globus*, a ball, was observed by Hippocrates and constituted the graphic 'suffocation of the Mother' which was known to Shakespeare and was one of the definitive symptoms of hysteria in the seventeenth century. Mild forms of globus sensation occur in 35% of men and 53% of women in the general population (Thompson and Heaton, 1982). Globus now accounts for around 4% of otolaryngo-

logical referrals. A wide variety of organic explanations has been proposed to account for these more severe or persistent forms of the sensation. During the 1950s interest centred on hypertrophy of the lingual tonsils and anterior cervical osteophytes. Although a substantial minority of globus patients appeared in one study to have enlarged lingual tonsils (Kiviranta, 1957), an uncontrolled trial of lingual tonsillectomy in 23 globus patients produced symptom relief in only four (Miyake and Matsuzaki, 1970). Granular pharyngitis and sinusitis have also been proposed as causative factors but these common conditions appear frequently in the absence of marked globus sensation and are likely to represent a chance association of common conditions. There have been several reports of globus sensation and cervical dysphagia due to osteophytes but the high incidence of cervical spondylosis in the general population makes a causative association hard to establish. Overclosure of the bite was reported as a cause of globus sensation by Campbell (1962) and led to a placebo-controlled trial of occlusive adjustment in a selected group of globus patients, all but one of whom also had symptoms referrable to the temporomandibular joint. The use of splints improved symptoms in six of 13 patients (Kirveskari and Puhakka, 1985). A placebo response was, however, noted in three of nine patients treated by mock adjustment.

The most popular organic aetiological theory of recent years has been that globus sensation is an atypical manifestation of gastro-oesophageal reflux. Henry (1958) noticed oesophagitis in 50% of globus sensation patients undergoing endoscopy and thereafter several radiological studies supported an association between the symptom and oesophageal reflux. Clearly many patients have reflux without globus sensation and it was proposed that the link between reflux disease and globus sensation might be referred sensation or an increase in pharyngo-oesophageal tone due to the habit of dry swallowing caused by the sensation (Malcomson, 1966, 1968). Breuninger (1974) also noted a compulsive throat clearing in globus sensation, with secondary voice changes and suggested that dysphonia could develop into the principal symptoms in those patients who were heavy voice users. The reflux theory enjoyed a wave of popularity for almost 10 years until Mair *et al.* (1974) showed that the sex of the patient rather than the degree of radiological abnormality was an important predictor of therapeutic response. Moloy and Charter (1982) also noted that over 20% of globus sensation patients were resistant to a variety of treatments and that while the response to anti-reflux therapy was sex related, it was again independent of the presence of gastro-oesophageal reflux and of the effects of therapy on the associated dyspepsia. A report of pH-monitoring in globus sensation (Batch, 1988) concluded that it was reflux related in 60% of patients although there was a 69% incidence of normal oesophageal biopsy in those undergoing endoscopy. A subsequent study of 87 patients with globus sensation reported that analysis of consecutive globus sensation patients using prolonged ambulatory pH-monitoring demonstrates abnormally elevated oesophageal acid exposure time in fewer than one-third of patients (Wilson *et al.*, 1989b). The reflux theory does not in any case explain the location or the sex incidence of globus sensation. In addition, the only published placebo-controlled trial of globus sensation therapy (Kibblewhite and Morrison, 1990) failed to show an improvement in symptoms. Physical abnormalities such as reflux or postnasal drip may initiate or exacerbate a globus sensation but do not explain the occurrence of this pharyngeal sensation in only a minority of sufferers from these common symptoms.

It appears unlikely that there will be a unified organic aetiological theory for globus sensation. Somewhat like tinnitus or headache, it is a sensation which may arise by a variety of pathways in susceptible individuals. Globus sensation is clearly a sensory symptom but many patients experience a mild alteration in the motor function of swallowing. The first manometric investigation of globus sensation was carried out by Calderelli, Andrews and Derbyshire (1970) who studied 10 patients with a water-filled catheter. Chronic upper sphincter pressures were not significantly different from those of six control subjects. In contrast, Watson and Sullivan (1974) used a similar perfused system to study nine globus sensation patients and 22 controls. Levels of upper oesophageal sphincter tonic pressure recorded in the globus sensation group were significantly higher than those of controls and indeed seemed so high as to compromise upper oesophageal sphincter blood flow. In addition, the controls were heterogeneous including patients with gastro-oesophageal reflux, achalasia and unexplained chest epigastric pain. It is not surprising, therefore, that the results were not replicated in a subsequent study (Flores *et al.*, 1981) although upper oesophageal sphincter tonic pressure does appear to be augmented by stress (Cook, Dent and Collins, 1989). It was later shown using a more appropriate non-perfused pressure measurement system that globus sensation patients have elevated upper oesophageal sphincter after contraction pressures during water swallows compared with healthy controls (Wilson *et al.*, 1989b). This is perhaps more likely to represent a secondary response to the presence of a globus sensation rather than a primary motor disorder. Interestingly, normal women also have elevated after contraction pressures compared with normal male controls. Schatzki (1964) has proposed that repeated dry swallowing in tense individuals with heightened bodily awareness might be an important cause of globus sensation in some patients. This idea was expanded by Gray (1983) who described 'inferior constrictor strain swallows' in globus

sensation. Like Schatzki, Gray believed that a strain swallow caused by increased awareness of contact between the epiglottis and the lingual tonsils could provoke a vicious cycle of dry saliva swallows with increased frequency of swallowing, reduction in inter-swallow interval, aerophagy and failure of upper oesophageal sphincter relaxation. Ardran (1982) also proposed a vicious cycle mechanism in globus sensation but related this cycle to reflux and felt that it was the reduction in peristaltic amplitude secondary to gastro-oesophageal reflux which induced an increase in swallow frequency. Resultant deglutitive inhibition was thought further to impair acid clearance.

The ancients explained the propensity of women to certain psychological conditions by attributing them to a uterine origin – hence 'hysteria' from the Greek *hystera*, a womb. The uterus (mother) was thought to migrate and produce symptoms in women. The semantic ambiguity and pejorative overtones which have since surrounded the term 'hysteria' have limited its usefulness and threatened its viability (Lloyd, 1986). Hysteria was the principal condition studied in the development of psychoanalytic theory by Freud who considered that hysterical symptoms arose from the conversion of repressed ideas. Glaser and Engel (1977) related globus sensation to the close association of feeding and crying in infancy which they believed provided the basis for a sensation of a lump in the throat during inhibited crying. There is now a growing body of evidence that at least a substantial minority of female globus sensation patients is psychologically distressed. Small studies have suggested that these were neurotic (Wilson, Deary and Maran, 1988), depressed (Brown *et al.*, 1986) or suffering from panic attacks (Liebowitz, 1987). Larger series have indicated that female (not male) globus sensation patients show increased introversion, free floating anxiety, somatic concern and depression (Deary *et al.*, 1989; Deary, Smart and Wilson, 1991). Depression seems to be a feature of some male globus sensation patients. The associated personality traits, like the sensation itself, appear to be remarkably persistent over time but there has been no long-term study of the outcome of the mood disorders (Wilson, Deary and Maran, 1991). As recently as 1985, globus sensation was found to be the fourth discriminating symptom of conversion disorder, after vomiting, aphonia and painful extremities (Othmer and Desousa, 1985) and the classical attitude to globus sensation is maintained by the National Library of Medicine which still classifies globus sensation as a conversion disorder.

As with the physical abnormalities in globus sensation, psychological findings do not of themselves explain the symptom. Why should not, after all, the globus sensation patient have some other 'somatoform disorder'? In globus sensation, the personality predisposition might underlie a syndrome that is partly throat based, partly psychological distress. It is possible to postulate that the psychological abnormalities predisposed to globus sensation, e.g. that introverts are more sensitive to bodily sensations and introversion is associated with globus sensation. It is also possible, however, to postulate that the physical and psychological aspects of globus sensation are two sides of a psychosomatic coin which might best be viewed as an anxiety disorder variant. Increasing research is pointing to the importance of anxiety and panic disorder to be at least as important if not more important than depression in globus sensation.

To the experienced clinician, globus sensation patients rarely present any diagnostic difficulty. These are not the elderly male smokers with weight loss who are suspected of having pyriform fossa cancer, these are nearly all healthy looking individuals although by no means all women. The history is of a primary sensory problem, no actual sticking of food and there is often a typical pattern. The symptoms are worse in the evening when perhaps there is more time to focus on them. The patient will frequently admit to repeated throat clearing and dry swallowing. Absence of classical features or presence of atypical ones such as weight loss should indicate a need for investigation. By no means every patient needs any further investigation other than a careful otolaryngological examination however. Furthermore embarking on an apparent search for a physical cause of the sensation may lead to a disappointed patient who feels that something has been missed by the relevant tests. Any clinician who deals regularly with globus sensation patients should be willing to ask about the possible associated lifestyle factors such as precipitating life events which are not infrequent and indeed sometimes quite conspicuous. Also unless symptoms of panic disorder, e.g. in supermarkets, are specifically sought, they will never be volunteered spontaneously in an otolaryngological clinic by a patient who cannot be aware of their possible relevance.

In other words, the resource which a globus sensation patient should consume in greatest abundance is clinic time spent in consultation rather than on radiological or endoscopic services. If there is a strong history of heartburn, it is probably well worth a trial of antacids. In this situation a very powerful antacid such as omeprazole can be useful as it will give a fairly clear cut response/no response answer within a few weeks. Two messages must be got over to the patient. The first is that the more they clear and dry swallow, the worse and more persistent the sensation will be. An analogy may be drawn with scratching an itchy patch. Secondly it must be accepted by the patient that the throat is a naturally 'lumpy' area which is naturally closed at rest. It is, therefore, in fact not abnormal for it to feel lumpy and closed-off. An analogy may be drawn here with tinnitus. Something, whether exogenous or endogenous, has unlocked the patient's throat sensory awareness and this door will not be readily closed. Globus sensation patients have to learn to accept some element of throat awareness on a persisting basis. If they continue to believe that they might manage eventually to cough up their sensation if it is given one last push, then they will simply degenerate into a downward spiral and become more and more despondent. If facilities permit, it can be quite helpful to arrange for patients to meet each other in a small group whether for relaxation or social purposes. There is so little in the popular literature about globus sensation that patients, unlike their physicians, are frequently rather surprised to find there are so many other local sufferers.

References

ANDERSON, J. R. (1990) The changing face of the management of instrumental perforation. *Gullet*, **1**, 10–15

ANDERSON, K. D., ROUSE, T. M. and RANDOLPH, J. G. (1990) A controlled trial of corticosteroids in children with corrosive injury of the esophagus. *New England Journal of Medicine*, **323**, 637–640

ARDRAN, G. M. (1982) Feeling of a lump in the throat: thoughts of a radiologist. *Journal of the Royal Society of Medicine*, **75**, 242–244

ARNDORFER, R. C. (1977) Improved infusion system for intraluminal esophageal manometry. *Gastroenterology*, **73**, 23–27

ARNOTT, S. J. (1989) Radiotherapy and cytotoxic chemotherapy In: *Management of Oesophageal Carcinoma*, edited by R. L. Hurt. London: Springer Verlag. pp. 223–241

ATKINSON, M. and FERGUSON, R. (1977) Fibreoptic endoscopic palliative intubation of inoperable oesophagogastric neoplasms. *British Medical Journal*, **1**, 266–267

BACON, C. K. and HENDRIX, R. A. (1992) Open tube versus flexible esophagoscopy in adult head and neck endoscopy. *Annals of Otology, Rhinology and Laryngology*, **101**, 147–154

BADER, M., DITTLER, H. J., ULTSCH, B., RIES, G. and SIEWERT, J. R. (1986) Palliative treatment of malignant stenoses of the upper gastrointestinal tract using a combination of laser and afterloading therapy. *Endoscopy*, **18** (suppl. 1), 27–31

BAIN, W. M., HARRINGTON, J. W., THOMAS, L. E. and SCHAEFFER, S. D. (1983) Head and neck manifestations of gastroesophageal reflux. *Laryngoscope*, **93**, 175–179

BANCEWICZ, J. (1992) Oesophageal diverticula. In: *Surgery of the Oesophagus*, edited by T. P. J. Hennessy and A. Cuschieri. Oxford: Butterworth Heinemann. pp. 215–227

BARISH, C. F., WU, W. C. and CASTELL, D. O. (1985) Respiratory complications of gastroesophageal reflux. *Archives of Internal Medicine*, **145**, 1882–1888

BATCH, A. J. G. (1988) Globus pharyngeus. I and II. *Journal of Laryngology and Otology*, **102**, 152–158; 227–230

BLACKWELL, J. N., HANNAN, W. J., ADAM, R. D. and HEADING, R. C. (1983) Radionuclide transit studies in the detection of oesophageal dysmotility. *Gut*, **24**, 421–426

BORTOLOTTI, M. (1989) Laryngospasm and reflex central apnoea caused by aspiration of refluxed gastric content in adults. *Gut*, **30**, 233–238

BOYLE, J. T., TUCHMAN, D. N., ALTSCHULER, S. M., NIXON, T. E., PACK, A. I. and COHEN, S. (1985) Mechanisms for the association of gastroesophageal reflux and bronchospasm. *American Review of Respiratory Diseases*, **131** (suppl.), S16–S20

BREUNINGER, H. (1974) Zur Differentialdiagnose: chronische pharyngitis, globusgefuhl, hyperkinetische dysphonie. *Laryngologie Rhinologie Otologie*, **53**, 6–13

BRODNITZ, F. S. (1961) Contact ulcer of the larynx. *Archives of Otolaryngology*, **74**, 70–80

BROWN-KELLY, A. (1919) Spasm at the entrance to the oesophagus. *Journal of Laryngology, Rhinology and Otology*, **24**, 285–289

BROWN, S. R., SCHWARTZ, J. M., SUMMERGRAD, P. and JENIKE, M. A. (1986) Globus hystericus syndrome responsive to antidepressants. *American Journal of Psychiatry*, **143**, 917–918

BROWNE, J. D. and THOMPSON, J. N. (1991) Caustic injuries of the esophagus. In: *The Esophagus*, edited by D. O. Castell. Boston: Little, Brown and Company. pp. 669–685

BUCHHOLZ, D. W., BOSMA, J. F. and DONNER, M. W. (1985) Adaptation, compensation and decompensation of the pharyngeal swallow. *Gastrointestinal Radiology*, **10**, 235–239

CAESTECKER, J. S. de (1989) Twenty-four-hour oesophageal pH monitoring: advances and controversies. *Netherlands Journal of Medicine*, **34**, S20–S39

CAESTECKER, J. S. de, BLACKWELL, J. N., BROWN, J. and HEADING, R. C. (1985) The oesophagus as a cause of recurrent chest pain: which patients should be investigated and which tests should be used? *Lancet*, ii, 1143–1146

CALDARELLI, D. D., ANDREWS, A. H. and DERBYSHIRE, A. J. (1970) Esophageal motility studies in globus sensation. *Annals of Otology, Rhinology and Laryngology*, **79**, 1098–1100

CAMPBELL, J. (1962) Facial paraesthesia accompanying facial pain. *British Dental Journal*, **112**, 108–113

CANNON, W. B. and MOSER, S. (1898) The movements of food in the esophagus. *American Journal of Physiology*, **1**, 435–444

CAREY, R. W., HILGENBERG, A. D., WILKINS, E. N., CHOI, C. N., MATHISEN, D. J. and GRILLO, H. (1986) Pre-operative chemotherapy (5FU-DDP) as initial component in multimodality treatment program for esophageal cancer. *Journal of Clinical Oncology*, **4**, 697

CARTER, R. and SMITH, J. (1986) Oesophageal carcinoma: a comparative study of laser recanalization versus intubation in the palliation of gastro-oesophageal carcinoma. *Laser Medicine and Science*, **1**, 245–252

CERENKO, D., MCCONNEL, F. M. S. and JACKSON, R. T. (1989) Quantitative assessment of pharyngeal bolus driving forces. *Otolaryngology Head and Neck Surgery*, **100**, 57–63

CHAIKHOUNI, A., KRATZ, J. M. and CRAWFORD, P. A. (1985) Foreign bodies in the esophagus. *American Journal of Surgery*, **51**, 173–179

CHERRY, J. and MARGULIES, S. I. (1968) Contact ulcer of the larynx. *Laryngoscope*, **78**, 1937–1940

CHERRY, J., SIEGEL, C. I., MARGULIES, S. I. and DONNER, M. (1970) Pharyngeal localization of symptoms of gastroesophageal reflux. *Annals of Otology, Rhinology and Laryngology*, **79**, 912–914

CHRISTENSEN, J. (1987) Motor functions of the pharynx and esophagus. In: *Physiology of the Gastrointestinal Tract*, edited by L. R. Johnson, New York: Raven Press. pp. 595–612

CONSIGLIERE, D., CHUA, C. L., HUI, F., YU, C. S. and LOW, C. H.

(1992) Computed tomography for oesophageal carcinoma: its value to the surgeon. *Journal of the Royal College of Surgeons of Edinburgh*, **37**, 113–117

COOK, I. J., DENT, J. and COLLINS, S. M. (1989) Upper esophageal sphincter tone and reactivity in patients with a history of globus sensation. *Digestive Diseases and Science*, **34**, 672–676

COOK-MOZAFFARI, P. (1989) Epidemiology and predisposing factors. In: *Management of Oesophageal Carcinoma*, edited by R. L. Hurt. London: Springer Verlag. pp. 31–38

CURTIS, D. J., EKBERG, O. and MONTESI, A. (1991) Swallowing: a radiological perspective. *Gastroenterology International*, **4**, 47–54

DANTAS, R. O., COOK, I. J., DODDS, W. J., KERN, M. K., LANG, I. M. and BRASSEUR, J. G. (1990) Biomechanics of cricopharyngeal bars. *Gastroenterology*, **99**, 1269–1274

DAWSON, J. and COCKEL, R. (1981) Oesophageal perforation at fibreoptic endoscopy. *British Medical Journal*, **283**, 583

DEARY, I. J., SMART, A. and WILSON, J. A. (1991) Depression and hassles in globus pharyngis. *British Journal of Psychiatry*, **161**, 115–117

DEARY, I. J., WILSON, J. A., MITCHELL, L. and MARSHALL, T. (1989) Covert psychiatric disturbance in patients with globus pharyngis. *British Journal of Medical Psychology*, **62**, 381–389

DELAHUNTY, J. E. (1972) Acid laryngitis. *Journal of Laryngology and Otology*, **86**, 335–342

DELAHUNTY, J. E. and CHERRY, J. (1968) Experimentally produced vocal cord granulomas. *Laryngoscope*, **78**, 1941–1947

DEMEESTER, T. R. (1986) Perforation of the oesophagus. *Annals of Thoracic Surgery*, **42**, 285–298

DEMEESTER, T. R., JOHANSSON, K. E., FRANZE, I., EYPASCH, E., LU, C.-T., MCGILL, J. E. *et al.* (1988) Indications, surgical technique and long term functional results of colon interposition or bypass. *Annals of Surgery*, **208**, 460–474

DIPALMA, J. A. and BRADY, C. E. (1987) Steakhouse spasm. *Journal of Clinical Gastroenterology*, **9**, 274–278

DODDS, W. J., DENT, J., HOGAN, W. J., HELM, J. F., HAUSER, R., PATEL, G. K. *et al.* (1982) Mechanisms of gastroesophageal reflux in patients with reflux esophagitis. *New England Journal of Medicine*, **307**, 1154–1552

DODDS, W. J., STEWART, E. T. and LOGEMANN, J. A. (1990) Physiology and radiology of the normal oral and pharyngeal phases of swallowing. *American Journal of Roentgenology*, **154**, 953–963

EARLAM, R. and CUNHA-MELO, J. R., (1980) Oesophageal squamous cell carcinoma: a critical review of surgery. *British Journal of Surgery*, **67**, 381–391

ELIDAN, J., SHOCHINA, M., GONEN, B. and GAY, I. (1990) Electromyography of the inferior constrictor and cricopharyngeal muscles. *Annals of Otology, Rhinology Laryngology*, **99**, 466–469

ELWOOD, P. C., JACOBS, A., PITMAN, R. G. and ENTWHISTLE, C. C. (1964) Epidemiology of the Paterson–Kelly syndrome. *Lancet*, ii, 716–720

ERIKSEN, C. A., SUTTON, D., KENNEDY, N. and CUSCHIERI, A. (1990) Effect of cisapride on oesophageal transit: results of a prospectively randomised clinical trial. *Gullet*, **1**, 31–35

FERRUCCI, J. T. and LONG, J. A. (1977) Radiologic treatment of esophageal food impaction using intravenous glucagon. *Radiology*, **125**, 25–28

FLOKES, T. C., CROSS, F. S. and JONES, R. D. (1981) Abnormal esophageal manometry in globus hystericus. *Annals of Otology, Rhinology and Laryngology*, **90**, 383–386

GAGE-WHITE, L. (1988) Incidence of Zenker's diverticulum with hiatus hernia. *Laryngoscope*, **98**, 527–530

GAYET, B., PALAZZO, L., VILGRAIN, V. *et al.* (1990) Prospective study comparing endoscopic ultrasonography and computer tomography in 56 resected esophageal carcinomas. In: *Diseases of the Esophagus: Malignant Diseases*, edited by M. K. Ferguson, A. C. T. Little and D. B. Skinner. New York: Futura Publishing. **14**, 117–123

GEISINGER, K. R. and WU, W. C. (1985) Endoscopy and biopsy. In: *Gastroesophageal Reflux Disease. Pathogenesis Diagnosis Therapy*, edited by D. O. Castell, W. C. Wu and D. J. Ott. Mount Kisco, NY: Futura Publishing. pp. 149–166

GLASER, J. P. and ENGEL, G. L. (1977) Psychodynamics, psychophysiology and gastrointestinal symptomatology. *Clinical Gastroenterology*, **6**, 507–531

GOLDBERG, M., NOYEK, A. M. and PRITZER, K. P. H. (1978) Laryngeal granuloma secondary to gastro-esophageal reflux., *Journal of Otolaryngology*, **71**, 196–202

GOLDMAN, J. and BENNETT, J. R. (1988) Gastro-oesophageal reflux and respiratory disorders in adults. *Lancet*, **ii**, 493–495

GRAY, L. P. (1983) The relationship of the inferior constrictor swallow and globus hystericus or the hypopharyngeal syndrome. *Journal of Laryngology and Otology*, **97**, 607–618

GRILLO, H. C. and WILKINS, E. W. (1975) Esophageal repair following late diagnosis of intrathoracic perforation. *Annals of Thoracic Surgery*, **20**, 387–399

HALLEWELL, J. D. and COLE, T. B. (1970) Isolated head and neck symptoms due to hiatus hernia. *Archives of Otolaryngology*, **92**, 499–501

HENNESSY, T. P. J. (1992) Barrett's esophagus. *Journal of the Royal College of Surgeons of Edinburgh*, **37**, 69–73

HENNESSY, T. P. J. and CUSCHIERI, A. (eds) (1992) Tumours of the oesophagus. In: *Surgery of the Oesophagus*, 2nd edn. Oxford: Butterworth–Heinemann. pp. 275–327

HENRY, G. A. (1958) An objective approach to the complaint, lump in the throat. *Laryngoscope*, **68**, 1257–1266

HENRY, R. L. and MELLIS, C. M. (1982) Resolution of inspiratory stridor after fundoplication: Case report. *Australian Paediatric Journal*, **18**, 126–127

HEWSON, E. G., OTT, D. J., DALTON, C. B., CHEN, Y. M., WU, W. C. and RICHTER, J. E. (1990) Manometry and radiology. Complementary studies in the assessment of esophageal motility disorders. *Gastroenterology*, **98**, 626–632

HIGGINSON, J., MUIR, C. S. and MUNOZ, N. (1992) Human cancer: epidemiology and environmental causes. *Cambridge Monographs on Cancer Research*. pp. 263–272

HISHIKAWA, Y., TANAKA, M. and MUIRA, T. (1986) Esophageal fistula associated with intracavitary irradiation for esophageal carcinoma. *Radiology*, **159**, 549–551

HOLLOWAY, R. H. and DENT, J. (1990) Pathophysiology of gastroesphageal reflux: lower esophageal sphincter dysfunction in gastroesophageal reflux disease. *Gastroenterology Clinics of North America*, **19**, 517–535

HOLSINGER, J. W., FUSON, R. L. and SEALY, W. C. (1968) Esophageal perforation following meat impaction and papain ingestion. *Journal of the American Medical Association*, **204**, 734–735

HOWARD, P. J., PRYDE, A. and HEADING, R. C. (1989) Oesophageal manometry during eating in the investigation of patients with chest pain and dysphagia. *Gut*, **30**, 1179–1186

HOWARD, P. J., MAHER, L., PRYDE, A. and HEADING, R. C. (1991) Symptomatic gastro-oesophageal reflux, abnormal oesophageal acid exposure and mucosal acid sensitivity are three separate, though related aspects of gastro-oesophageal reflux disease. *Gut*, **32**, 128–132

JACOB, P., KAHRILAS, P. J. LOGEMANN, J. A., SHAH, V. and HA, T. (1989) Upper esophageal sphincter opening and modulation during swallowing. *Gastroenterology*, **97**, 1469–1478

JACOBS, A. (1962) Post cricoid carcinoma in patients with pernicious aneamia. *British Medical Journal*, **2**, 91–92

JACOBS, A. and KILPATRICK, G. S. (1964) The Paterson-Kelly Syndrome. *British Medical Journal*, **2**, 79–82.

JANSSENS, J., VANTRAPPEN, G. and GHILLEBERT, G. (1986) 24-hour recording of esophageal pressure and pH in patients with non cardiac chest pain. *Gastroenterology*, **90**, 1978–1984

KAHRILAS, P. J., DODDS, W. J., DENT, J. WYMAN, J. B., HOGAN, W. J. and ARNDORFER, R. C. (1986) Upper esophageal sphincter function during belching. *Gastroenterology*, **91**, 133–140

KAHRILAS, P. J., DODDS, W. J., DENT, J., HAEBERLE, B., HOGAN, W. J. and ARNDORFER, R. C. (1987) Effect of sleep, spontaneous gastroesophageal reflux and a meal on upper esophageal sphincter pressure in normal human volunteers. *Gastroenterology*, **92**, 466–471

KAHRILAS, P. J., DODDS, W. J., DENT, J., LOGEMANN, J. A. and SHAKER, R. (1989) Upper esophageal sphincter function during deglutition. *Gastroenterology*, **95**, 52–62

KAMBIC, V. and RADSEL, Z. (1984) Acid posterior laryngitis; aetiology, histology, diagnosis and treatment. *Journal of Laryngology and Otology*, **98**, 1237–1240

KARANJIA, N. D. and REES, M. (1993) The use of Coca-Cola in the management of bolus obstruction in benign oesophageal stricture. *Annals of the Royal College of Surgeons of England*, **75**, 94–95

KATZ, P. O. (1992) Disorders of increased contractility. In: *The Esophagus*, edited by D. O. Castell. Boston: Little, Brown and Company. pp. 261–275

KIBBLEWHITE, D. J. and MORRISON, M. D. (1990) A double-blind controlled study of the efficacy of cimetidine in the treatment of the cervical symptoms of gastroesophageal reflux. *Journal of Otolaryngology*, **19**, 103–109

KIRVESKARI, P. and PUHAKKA, H. (1985) Effect of occlusal adjustment on globus symptom. *Journal of Prosthetic Dentistry*, **54**, 832–835

KIVIRANTA, U.K. (1957) 'Globus hystericus' and tonsils. *Practica Otorhinolaryngologica*, **19**, 1–24

KOUFMAN, J. A. (1991) The otolaryngologic manifestations of gastroesophageal reflux disease. In: *Ambulatory Esophageal pH Monitoring*, edited by J. E. Richter. New York: Igaku-Shoin. pp. 129–149

KURILOFF, D. B. CHODOSH, P., GOLDFARB, R. and ONGSENG, F. (1989) Detection of gastroesophageal reflux in the head and neck: the role of scintigraphy. *Annals of Otology, Rhinology and Laryngology*, **98**, 74–80

LANCET (1989) Swallowed coins (editorial). **ii**, 659–660

LARRAIN, A., LIRA, E., OTERO, M. and POPE C. E. (1981) Posterior laryngitis: a useful marker of esophageal reflux (abstract). *Gastroenterology*, **80**, 1204

LE QUESNE, L. and RANGER, D. (1966) Pharyngolaryngectomy with immediate pharyngogastric anastomosis. *British Journal of Surgery*, **53**, 105–109

LEICHMAN, L. STEIGER, Z. and SEYDEL, L. (1984) Combined prospective chemotherapy and radiation for cancer of esophagus. *Seminars in Oncology*, **11**, 75

LEONARDI, H. K., SHEA, J. A. and CROZIER, R. E. (1977) Diffuse spasm of the oesophagus: clinical, manometric and surgical considerations. *Journal of Thoracic and Cardiovascular Surgery*, **74**, 736–743

LIEBOWITZ, M. R. (1987) Globus hystericus and panic attacks (letter). *American Journal of Psychiatry*, **144**, 390–391

LITOVITZ, T. L. (1983) The Button battery ingestion: a review of 56 cases. *Journal of the American Medical Association*, **249**, 2495–2500

LITTLE, F. B., KOUFMAN, J. A., KOHUT, R. I. and MARSHALL, R. B. (1985) Effect of gastric acid on the pathogenesis of subglottic stenosis. *Annals of Otology, Rhinology and Laryngology*, **94**, 516–519

LIU, A. J. and RICHARDSON, M. A. (1985) Effect of N-acetylcysteine on experimentally induced esophageal lye injury. *Annals of Otology, Rhinology and Laryngology*, **94**, 477–482

LLAMAS-ELVIRA, J. M., MARTINEZ-PARADES, M., SOPENA-MONFORTE, R., GARRIGUES, V., CANOTEROL, C. and VELASCO-LAJO, T. (1986) Value of radionuclide oesophageal transit in studies of functional dysphagia. *British Journal of Radiology*, **59**, 1073–1078

LLOYD, G. G. (1986) Hysteria: a case for conservation? (editorial). *British Medical Journal*, **293**, 1255–1256

LOGEMANN, J. A. (1986) *Manual for the Videofluorographic Study of Swallowing*. San Diego: College-Hill Press.

MCCONNEL, F. M. S., CERENKO, D. and MENDELSOHN, M. S. (1988) Manofluorographic analysis of swallowing. *Otolaryngologic Clinics of North America*, **21**, 625–635

MCFARLANE, G. A. and MUNRO, A. (1990) The changing face of the management of ruptured oesophagus: Boerhaave's syndrome. *Gullet*, **1**, 16–23

MCKEOWN, K. C. (1976) Total three-stage oesophagectomy for cancer of the oesophagus. *British Journal of Surgery*, **63**, 259–262

MCKEOWN K. C., (1979) Carcinoma of the oesophagus. *Journal of the Royal College of Surgeons of Edinburgh*, **24**, 253–274

MAIR, I. W. S., SCHRODER, K. E., MODALSLI, B. and MAURER, H. J. (1974) Aetiological aspects of the globus symptom. *Journal of Laryngology and Otology*, **88**, 1033–1040

MALCOMSON, K. G. (1966) Radiological findings in globus hystericus. *British Journal of Radiology*, **39**, 583–586

MALCOMSON, K. G. (1968) Globus hystericus vel pharyngis. *Journal of Laryngology and Otology*, **82**, 219–230

MIKO, T. L. (1989) Peptic (contact ulcer) granuloma of the larynx. *Journal of Clinical Pathology*, **42**, 800–804

MILLER, L. S. (1992) Endoscopy of the esophagus. In: *The Esophagus* edited by D. O. Castell. Boston: Little, Brown and Company. pp. 89–141

MITTAL, R. K. (1990) Current concepts of the antireflux barrier. *Gastroenterology Clinics of North America*, **19**, 501–516

MITTAL, R. K. and MCCALLUM, R. W. (1988) Characteristics and frequency of transient relaxations of the lower esophageal sphincter in patients with reflux esophagitis. *Gastroenterology*, **95**, 593–599

MIKAYE, H. and MATSUZAKI, H. (1970) Studies on abnormal feeling in the throat. *Practica Otorhinolaryngologica*, **32**, 364–372

MOLOY, P. J. and CHARTER, R. (1982) The globus symptom. *Archives of Otolaryngology*, **108**, 740–744

MORRISON, M. D. (1988) Is chronic gastroesophageal reflux a causative factor in glottic carcinoma? *Otolaryngology, Head and Neck Surgery*, **99**, 370–373

MURATA, Y., MUROI, M., YOSHIDA, M., IDE, H. and HANYU, F.

(1987) Endoscopic ultrasonography in the diagnosis of oesophageal carcinoma. *Surgical Endoscopy*, **1**, 11–16

MURPHY, D. W. and ROUFAIL, W. M. (1991) Rupture and perforation. In: *The Esophagus*, edited by D. O. Castell. Boston: Little, Brown and Company, pp. 747–757

OHMAN, L. OLOFSON, J., TIBBLING, L. and ERICSON, G. (1983) Esophageal dysfunction in patients with contact ulcer of the larynx. *Annals of Otology, Rhinology and Laryngology*, **92**, 228–230

ORENSTEIN, S. R., OREINSTEIN, D. M. and WHITTINGTON, P. F. (1983) Gastroesophageal reflux causing stridor. *Chest*, **84**, 301–302

OTHMER, E. and DESOUSA, C. (1985) A screening test for somatisation disorder (hysteria). *American Journal of Psychiatry*, **142**, 1146–1149

OTT, D. J., GELFAND, D. W., WU, W. C. and CHEN, Y. M. (1986) Radiological evaluation of dysphagia. *Journal of the American Medical Association*, **256**, 2718–2721

PAGLIERO, K. M. (1989) Brachytherapy (intercavitary irradiation) In: *Management of Oesophageal Carcinoma*, edited by R. L. Hurt. London: Springer Verlag. pp. 243–246

PALMER, J. B., TANAKA, E. and SIEBENS, A. (1989) Electromyography of the pharyngeal musculature: technical considerations. *Archives of Physical Medicine and Rehabilitation*, **70**, 283–287

PATTERSON, D. R. (1919) A clinical type of dysphagia. *Journal of Laryngology and Otology*, **24**, 289–291

PELLEGRINI, C. A., DEMEESTER, T. R., JOHNSON, L. F. and SKINNER, D. B. (1979) Gastroesophageal reflux and pulmonary aspiration. *Surgery*, **86**, 110–119

PRICE, J. C., JANSEN, C. J. and JOHNS, M. E. (1990) Esophageal reflux and secondary malignant neoplasia at laryngoesophagectomy. *Archives of Otolaryngology – Head and Neck Surgery*, **116**, 163–164

RICHTER, J. E., WU, W. C., JOHNS, D. N., BLACKWELL, J. N., NELSON, J. L., CASTELL, J. A. *et al.* (1987) Esophageal manometry in 95 healthy adult volunteers: variability of pressures with age and frequency of 'abnormal' contractions. *Digestive Diseases and Sciences*, **32**, 583–592

ROSEN, Y., MOON, S. and KIM, B. (1975) Small cell epidermoid carcinoma of the esophagus. An oat-cell like carcinoma. *Cancer*, **36**, 1042–1049

RUSSELL, C. O. H., HILL, L. D., HOLMES, E. R., HULL, D. A., GANNON, R. and POPE, C. E. (1981) Radionuclide transit: a sensitive test for esophageal dysfunction. *Gastroenterology*, **80**, 887–892

SCHATZKI, R. (1964) Globus hystericus. *New England Journal of Medicine*, **270**, 670

SCHLESINGER, P. K., DONAHUE, P. E., SCHMID, B. and LAYDEN, T. J. (1985) Limitations of 24-hour intraesophageal, pH monitoring in the hospital setting. *Gastroenterology*, **89**, 797–804

SHAKER, R., DODDS, W. J., DANTAS, R. O., HOGAN, W. J. and ARNDORFER, R. C. (1990) Coordination of deglutitive glottic closure with oropharyngeal swallowing. *Gastroenterology*, **98**, 1478–1484

SILVIS, S. E., NEBEL, O., ROGERS, A., SUGAWA, C. and MANDELSTAM, P. (1976) Endoscopic complications. Results of the 1974 American Society for Gastrointestinal Endoscopy Survey. *Journal of the American Medical Association*, **235**, 928–930

SMILEY, T. B., CAVES, P. K. and PORTER, D. C. (1970) Relationship between posterior pharyngeal pouch and hiatus hernia. *Thorax* **25**, 725–731

SMITH, J. C. (1986) Use of glucagon and gas-forming agents

in acute esophageal food impaction. *Radiology*, **159**, 567–568

SMITH, M. T. and PEURA, D. A. (1992) Foreign bodies. In: *The Esophagus*, edited by D O Castell. Boston: Little, Brown and Company. pp. 383–400

SONIES, B. C. and BAUM, B. J. (1989) Evaluation of swallowing pathophysiology. *Otolaryngological Clinics of North America*, **21**, 637–648

STARITZ, M., PORALLA, T. and BUSCHENFELDE, K. H. M. (1985) Intraoesphageal variceal pressure assessed by endoscopic fine needle puncture under basal conditions, Valsalva's manoeuvre and after glyceryltrinitrate application. *Gut*, **26**, 525–530

STONE, M. and SHAWKER, T. H. (1986) An ultrasound examination of tongue movement during swallowing. *Dysphagia*, **1**, 78–83

TANAKA, E., PALMER, J. and SIEBENS, A. (1986) Bipolar suction electrodes for pharyngeal electromyography. *Dysphagia*, **1**, 39–40

TAYLOR, R. B. (1987) Esophageal foreign bodies. *Emergency Medical Clinics of North America*, **5**, 301–311

TEOT, L. A. and GEISINGER, K. R. (1992) Diagnostic esophageal cytology and its histologic basis. In: *The Esophagus*, edited by D. O. Castell. Boston: Little, Brown and Company. pp. 187–216

THOMPSON, D. G. and HEATON, K. W. (1982) Heartburn and globus in apparently healthy people. *Canadian Medical Association Journal*, **126**, 46–68

THOMPSON, J. N. (1987) Corrosive esophageal injuries. *Laryngoscope*, **97**, 1191–1202

TIO, T. L., COHEN, J., COENE, P. P., UDDING, J., HARTOG JAGER, F. C. A. den and TYTGAT, G. N. J. (1989) Endosonography and computed tomography of esophageal carcinoma. *Gastroenterology*, **96**, 1478–1486

TURNBULL, A. D. M. and GOODNER, J. T. (1968) Primary adenocarcinoma of the esophagus. *Cancer*, **22**, 915–918

TYTGAT, G. N. J. and TIO, T. L. (1990) Techniques for staging oesophageal cancer. *Gullet*, **1**, 4–9

VAKIL, N. B., KAHRILAS, P. J., DODDS, W. J. and VANAGUNAS, A. (1989) Absence of an upper esophageal sphincter response to acid reflux. *American Journal of Gastroenterology*, **84**, 606–610

VANEK, A. W. and DIAMANT, N. E. (1987) Responses of the human esophagus to paired swallows. *Gastroenterology*, **92**, 643–650

VINSON, P. P. (1922) Hysterical dysphagia. *Minnesota Medicine*, **5**, 107–108

VON HAACKE, N. P. and WILSON, J. A. (1986) Missing denture as a cause of recurrent laryngeal nerve palsy. *British Medical Journal*, **292**, 664

WARD, P. H. and BERCI, G. (1982) Observations on the pathogenesis of chronic non-specific pharyngitis and laryngitis. *Laryngoscope*, **92**, 1377–1382

WARD, P. H. and HANSON, D. G. (1988) Reflux as an etiological factor of carcinoma of the laryngopharynx. *Laryngoscope*, **98**, 1195–1199

WARD, P. H., ZWITMAN, D., HANSON, D. and BERCI, G. (1980) Contact ulcers and granulomas of the larynx: new insights into their etiology as a basis for more rational treatment. *Otolaryngology, Head and Neck Surgery*, **88**, 262–269

WATSON, W. C. and SULLIVAN, J. N. (1974) Hypertonicity of the cricopharyngeal sphincter: a cause of globus sensation. *Lancet*, **ii**, 1417–1419

WATTERSON, T., HANSEN–MAGORIAN, H. J. and MCFARLANE, S.

c. (1990) A demographic description of laryngeal contact ulcer patients. *Journal of Voice*, **4**, 71–75

WEINSTOCK, L. B. and CLOUSE, R. E. (1987) Esophageal physiology: normal and abnormal motor function. *American Journal of Gastroenterology*, **82**, 399–405

WESDORP, I. C. E., BARTELSMAN, J. F. W. M., HUIBREGTSE, K., DEN HARTOG JAGER, F. C. A. and TYTGAT, G. N. (1984) Treatment of instrumental oesophageal perforation. *Gut*, **25**, 398–404

WIENER, G. J., KOUFMAN, J. A., WU, W. C., COOPER, J. B., RICHTER, J. E. and CASTELL, D. O. (1987) The pharyngoesophageal dual ambulatory pH probe for evaluation of atypical manifestations of gastroesophageal reflux (GER) (abstract). *Gastroenterology*, **92**, 1694

WIENER, G. J., KOUFMAN, J. A., WU, W. C., COOPER, J. B., RICHTER, J. E. and CASTELL, D. O. (1989) Chronic hoarseness secondary to gastroesophageal reflux disease: documentation with 24-H ambulatory pH monitoring. *American Journal of Gastroenterology*, **84**, 1503–1508

WILLIS, G. A. and HO, W. C. (1982) Perforation of Meckel's diverticulum by an alkaline hearing aid battery. *Canadian Medical Association Journal*, **126**, 497–498

WILSON, J. A. (1992) Reflux and the larynx. *Gullet*, **2**, 11–18

WILSON, J. A., DEARY, I. J. and MARAN, A. G. D. (1988) Is globus hystericus? *British Journal of Psychiatry*, **153**, 335–339

WILSON, J. A., DEARY, I. J. and MARAN, A. G. D. (1991) The persistence of symptoms in patients with globus pharyngis. *Clinical Otolaryngology*, **16**, 202–205

WILSON, J. A., PRYDE, A. and MAHER, L. (1993) Pharyngooesophageal pH-metry in healthy volunteers (abstract). *Clinical Otolaryngology*, **18**, 89–90

WILSON, J. A., PRYDE, A., MACINTYRE, C. C. A. and HEADING, R. c. (1989a) Normal pharyngoesophageal motility: a study of 50 healthy subjects. *Digestive Diseases and Sciences*, **34**, 1590–1599

WILSON, J. A., PRYDE, A., PIRIS, J., ALLAN, P. L., MACINTYRE, C. C. A., MARAN, A. G. D. et al. (1989b) Pharyngoesophageal dysmotility in globus sensation. *Archives of Otolaryngology – Head and Neck Surgery*, **115**, 1086–1090

WILSON, J. A., WHITE, A., HAACKE, N. P., MARAN, A. G. D., HEADING, R. C., PRYDE, A. et al. (1989c) Gastroesophageal reflux and posterior laryngitis. *Annals of Otology, Rhinology and Laryngology*, **98**, 405–410

WILSON, J. A., PRYDE, A., MACINTYRE, C. C. A. and HEADING, R. c. (1990a) The effect of esophageal acid exposure on upper esophageal sphincter pressure. *Journal of Gastrointestinal Motility*, **2**, 117–120

WILSON, J. A., PRYDE, A., MACINTYRE, C. C. A., MARAN, A. G. D. and HEADING, R. C. (1990b) The effects of age, sex and smoking on normal pharyngoesophageal motility. *American Journal of Gastroenterology*, **85**, 686–691

WILSON, J. A., PRYDE, A., ALLAN, P. L. and MARAN, A. G. D. (1992a) Cricopharyngeal dysfunction. *Otolaryngology, Head and Neck Surgery*, **106**, 163–168

WILSON, J. A., PRYDE, A., MAHER, L., MACINTYRE, C. C. A., BINGHUA, S. and HEADING, R. C. (1992b) The influence of biological and recording variables on pharyngeal pressure measurement. *Gullet*, **2**, 116–120

WYNDER, E. L. and FRYER, J. H. (1958) Etiologic considerations of Plummer-Vinson (Paterson–Kelly) syndrome. *Annals of Internal Medicine*, **49**, 1106–1128

YAKSHE, P. N. and FLEISCHER, D. E. (1992) Neoplasms of the esophagus. In: *The Esophagus*, edited by D. O. Castell. Boston: Little, Brown and Company. pp. 278–298

25

Facial plastic surgery

Michael P. Stearns

Facial plastic surgery has become an important sub-specialty of otolaryngology, the more so as the specialty has developed and surgeons have become conscious of patient demands for aesthetic surgery, whether this be an end in itself, or in conjunction with tumour excision, or an attempt to improve function.

General principles of facial plastic surgery

The skin of the face and neck has a rich blood supply derived mainly from the external carotid artery and thyrocervical trunk. Because of a generally abundant collateral supply to this part of the body there is the possibility of using a number of different skin flaps for tissue repair. These may be either random flaps or axial flaps and a number of variations on these will be discussed later in the chapter.

The direction of incisions in the skin of the face and neck should always be made after due consideration of the aesthetics of the subsequent scar. Clearly it is preferable to disguise a scar and make it as inconspicuous as possible. This can be achieved by camouflaging the scar by hiding it within a hair-bearing area such as the scalp, and by ensuring that it does not cross anatomical boundaries and contours, e.g. from the lateral aspect of the nose onto the cheek. Incisions should be made so that they blend into a natural crease line, such as the nasolabial groove.

All incisions should be made wherever possible in relaxed skin tension lines. These were described by Borges and Alexander in 1962 and are similar to Langer's lines of natural tissue tension (Langer, 1861). Langer, when mapping out these contours,

used cadavers rather than living subjects and although relaxed skin tension lines generally run in the same direction as Langer's lines, this is not always the case. When skin incisions are made in the direction of relaxed skin tension lines, the scar will heal with the minimum of tissue tension and should be therefore as fine as possible (Figure 25.1). If incisions are made across the relaxed skin tension lines they will tend to heal with maximum tension

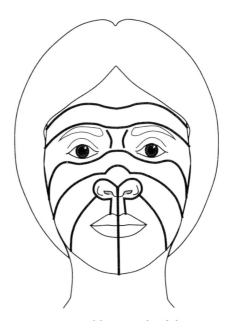

Figure 25.1 Direction of the main relaxed skin tension lines in the face

and will be spread and possibly hypertrophic. Clearly the direction of incisions, particularly when flaps are being raised, should be along the lines of supplying blood vessels rather than across them.

Tissue handling

The soft tissues of the face and neck should be handled with great care and delicacy, particularly around wound edges. Incision lines, if handled roughly with tissue forceps, may be traumatized so that unsightly marks are left along them, and small areas of the wound edge may become ischaemic. The use of skin hooks is to be recommended wherever possible because these are less traumatic to the skin than tissue holding forceps. If forceps are used they are best applied to the deeper tissues rather than the skin edges themselves.

Suturing

Wound closure in the head and neck may be performed using a variety of suture materials and suture methods. Generally speaking the use of monofilament, non-reactive materials such as nylon or steel wire, including clips, will reduce the likelihood of suture marks along a wound edge. Multifilament materials act as wicks, along which infection may pass; the resulting inflammatory reaction may produce an obvious suture mark. The use of absorbable materials such as catgut may also cause a tissue reaction especially if used as a cutaneous suture. This is particularly true for the more slowly absorbed catgut, such as chromic catgut, and less so for the newer, rapidly absorbed catguts. The extremely slowly absorbing materials such as polyglycolic acid may cause an excessive tissue reaction with fibrosis and are best avoided in the face even as a subcutaneous suture because of the possibility of producing an unsightly scar.

Sutures in the face may generally be removed at around 5 days. Skin closure may be augmented with the use of tissue glue such as Tisseal where this is available but, of course, this will not allow accurate skin apposition.

Skin replacement

Defects in the skin may be replaced with free skin grafts and also with local and distant flaps.

Free grafts

The free grafts which can be used are split skin grafts, full thickness grafts (Wolfe grafts), composite grafts and free grafts with microvascular anastomosis.

Split skin grafts

Split skin grafts consist of epidermis and a varying thickness of dermis. They are between 0.01 inch (0.25 mm) and 0.025 inch (0.64 mm) thick. They may be harvested using a blade such as a Humby knife or by the use of an electric dermatome. The graft may be harvested in large sheets from an area which is inconspicuous such as the thigh or buttock. The donor site generally heals in 10 days or so, and once healed, can be used as the donor site for further grafts if necessary. Split skin grafts may be applied to the skin defect either immediately or they may be stored on a backing of paraffin gauze and refrigerated. The graft may then be applied after a period of a few days. The advantage of applying a split skin graft as a delayed procedure is that one can wait until there is a completely dry field before applying it. This will improve the prospect of a successful graft.

Split skin grafts should be applied to the recipient site under moderate pressure, using either a pressure dressing, or using quilting sutures to tack the graft in place.

Split skin grafts have several advantages. They may be used to cover large areas, their success rate is extremely high, particularly if there is a delay in applying the graft, and the operating time needed is relatively short.

The disadvantages of these grafts are that they produce a large amount of fibrosis and scarring, which may be a major disadvantage, both functionally and cosmetically. The colour match is poor when used in the skin of the neck and face. Because the graft is thin the normal contours of the area are not followed, and a hollow area may be left, e.g. in repairing the defect after elevating a forehead flap. The consequence of these disadvantages is, that in practice, split skin grafts are now used infrequently in surgery of the skin of the face and neck.

Full thickness grafts (Wolfe grafts)

These grafts consist of full thickness epidermis and dermis denuded of all the underlying fat. These grafts can be harvested from areas where there is available soft tissue, with a similar colour match to the skin of the face or neck. Because the donor site has to be sutured and leaves a linear scar, the graft should be harvested from an inconspicuous area. Typically, in grafts for the face and neck, they are harvested from the postauricular area and supraclavicular fossa, these sites offering a good colour match for cervicofacial skin. The disadvantages of Wolfe grafts are that the take rate is not as good as in the split skin graft, because there is a thicker segment of skin to be revascularized. Furthermore, only small grafts can be harvested because of the constraints of providing wound closure at the donor site. Full thickness grafts heal with less fibrosis and scarring than split skin grafts. They are especially suitable for the repair of small skin defects around the face, e.g. after removal of epithelial tumours up to 2 cm diameter. Full thickness grafts should be applied to the recipient site with a pressure dressing, which is normally sutured into place.

Composite grafts

Composite grafts are grafts containing skin and cartilage. Their main use is for the repair of defects on the nose, particularly in repairing alar margin defects. These grafts are normally harvested from the pinna by excising a segment of pinna as a wedge and the cut edges subsequently being apposed as a linear suture line. The composite graft, thus obtained, consists of two layers of skin with an intervening layer of cartilage. This may then be used as a free graft to close defects of the alar margin of the nose. Two layer grafts may also be used, commonly on the dorsum of the nose to replace defects of skin and bone or cartilage. The success rate of these grafts is related to their size. Stucker, Bryarly and Shockley (1986) suggested that the graft should be less then 1.5 cm in its greatest diameter. Great care must be taken to ensure adequate haemostasis before applying the graft.

Composite grafts harvested from the nasal septum, with its mucosal layer, may be used in the repair of defects of the conjunctiva and tarsal plate of the eyelid.

Free-flaps with microvascular anastomosis

These flaps may be harvested with skin alone or with bone and/or muscle. The material is harvested so that it has a feeding artery and draining vein readily available. These vessels may then be anastomosed to appropriate vessels in the local area of the recipient site. There are several advantages to this type of free graft: extensive areas of tissue may be covered; muscles may be transferred and their motor nerves may be grafted onto local nerves in the recipient area, e.g. in reanimation of the paralysed face. Microvascular anastomosis may be used in the transfer of bone as a vital graft, e.g. in the reconstruction of the mandible.

The main disadvantage of this type of graft is the length of time needed to anastomose the vessels. This type of graft is not appropriate for smaller defects of the face and neck, but is, of course, eminently suitable for any of the more major head and neck oncological procedures.

Skin flaps

The three types of skin flap available are random flaps, axial flaps and myocutaneous flaps.

Random flaps are dependent for their blood supply on unnamed, small vessels, usually capillaries. In general, these flaps should be of the ratio of 1 : 1, length to width. In the face and neck because of the excellent blood supply in this area, random flaps may be 2 : 1, twice as long as they are broad. Such flaps can be moved with safety.

Axial flaps are those which have a named blood vessel, or branch of a named vessel, running along their length. This means, therefore, that there is no constraint on the proportions of the flap. It may be as long as the length of the supplying artery. An example of an axial flap commonly used in head and neck surgery is the deltopectoral flap, in which branches of the internal thoracic artery run through the flap. The forehead flap is another example and has the superficial temporal artery running along its course (Figure 25.2).

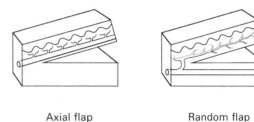

Axial flap   Random flap

Figure 25.2 The large vessel contained in the axial flap, whereas the random flap contains only capillaries

Axial flaps are the safest flaps to use out of all the possibilities for skin cover, because they have an extremely reliable blood supply. Providing that they are handled carefully, and care is taken not to damage the arterial supply, these flaps will have the most predictable behaviour of all skin flaps. The disadvantages of axial flaps are that frequently their use will imply a two-stage procedure where the graft will have to be separated from its pedicle at a later stage. Often the donor site will require secondary skin grafting, with a split skin graft for example. As these flaps may come from quite distant sites, the colour and texture of the skin may not be as good as skin from more adjacent sites. However, this is not true of all axial flaps. Some may be used as local flaps (i.e. the nasolabial flap, with its branches of the facial artery) for repairing small defects around the nose.

Myocutaneous flaps consist of skin and underlying muscle, the skin deriving its blood supply from the muscle. Use of these flaps may be made in a number of situations in head and neck surgery. They are generally used as island flaps with an island of skin on the muscle pedicle.

Random flaps

Random flaps are frequently used in the head and neck because the face has such an excellent blood supply. They are extremely predictable flaps with good colour match and texture because they are taken from local skin. The design of all these flaps is based on the transfer of tissue from an area where there is a relative excess of skin to one where there is a relative paucity of skin, e.g. a recipient site. The types of random flap available are advancement, rotation and transposition flaps.

Advancement flaps

These are of two types, the rectangular advancement flap and the V–Y advancement flap. The rectangular flap has limited use in the face because of the limited elasticity of the skin. The flap is constructed as a rectangle adjacent to a skin defect. The skin is then stretched to fill the defect. Bilateral advancement flaps may effectively be used to fill larger defects. The horizontal margins of the flap should be placed in relaxed skin tension lines. The distal edge of the flap may be curved slightly or even serrated, to form a W-plasty, to camouflage the end of the flap. Advancement flaps are ideally suited for filling defects in the forehead (Figure 25.3).

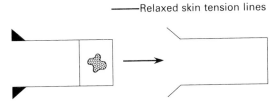

Figure 25.3 Single advancement flap. Above the diagram is shown the direction of the relaxed skin tension lines

V–Y advancement flaps are a variation on this in which a triangular flap is elevated and its sides advanced.

Rotation flaps

Rotation flaps are a type of advancement flap in which the flap is designed as a semicircle. The flap is rotated into a wedge-shaped defect (Figure 25.4). Ideally the circumference of the flap should be at least four times as long as the width of the defect. If the ratio is smaller than this then it may be necessary to form a Burow's triangle to prevent the formation of a 'dog-ear.' Burow's triangles are small triangles of skin which are excised to remove potential 'dog-ears' in the skin. They are also used to equalize the sides of an asymmetrical skin excision.

Rotation flaps should be designed so that their long axis runs along the relaxed skin tension lines. Natural crease lines can be utilized to camouflage the incision line. A large cheek rotation flap can be used in the repair of anteriorly placed cheek defects. These flaps can also often be conveniently used around the nasolabial groove and in the scalp.

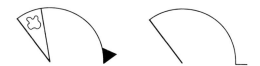

Figure 25.4 Rotation flap. The black shaded area represents a Burow's triangle

Transposition flaps

Transposition flaps are those in which the flap is raised and moved over normal tissue to repair the defect. The flap is usually rotated into the defect. These flaps may be either random or axial. Rhomboid, bilobed and Z-plasty flaps are examples of random flaps, and nasolabial and glabellar flaps are examples of axial transposition flaps.

Rhomboid flaps

The rhomboid flap was described by Limberg in 1966. A rhomboid is a parallelogram with all sides of equal length. In constructing a rhomboid flap, the defect is excised as a rhomboid. A second rhomboid is constructed alongside the first as shown in Figure 25.5.

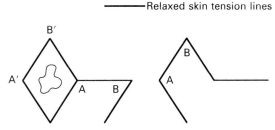

Figure 25.5 The construction of a rhomboid flap. In the diagram on the left the rhomboid flap is constructed around the extended diagonal AB

The second rhomboid is formed around an extended diagonal AB which has the same length as the sides of the first rhomboid. A choice of four flaps exists as can be seen in Figure 25.6.

Bilobed flaps

These were originally described by Esser in 1918, and used as a small flap on the nose. The flap is designed so that the long axis of the larger lobe of the flap is at right angles to the long axis of the defect. The smaller lobe of the flap is designed to be the same length as the first, but half the width. This smaller lobe has its long axis at right angles to that of the larger lobe (Figure 25.7).

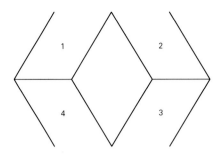

Figure 25.6 The possible flaps which can be constructed around the rhomboid

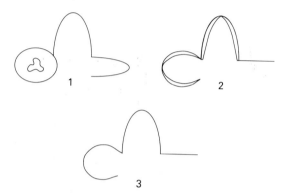

Figure 25.7 The formation of the bilobed flap

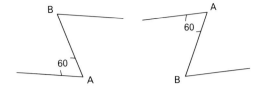

Figure 25.8 'Z'-plasty. The figure on the left shows the flaps before elevation, that on the right after elevation

Bilobed flaps can be used on the nose or as larger flaps on the cheek. They may also be used to good effect for reconstruction of auricular defects as described by Weerda (1983). They are used in situations where there is insufficient soft tissue to close the defect formed by the primary skin flap and where extra tissue is thus needed to close the second defect.

Z-plasty

The Z-plasty has a number of uses in surgery. It consists of a pair of triangular flaps in the form of a 'Z'. The two flaps are interposed. The Z-plasty may simply consist of a pair of flaps or a series of flaps forming a multiple Z-plasty. The flaps are normally designed with angles of 60°. The Z-plasty will rotate the central incision through 90°. It will lengthen the tissues in the direction of the central limb, at the expense of narrowing the tissues on either side of this (Figure 25.8).

The Z-plasty can therefore be used to lengthen an area where there is a shortage of tissue, such as a web across a concavity, e.g. on an inner canthal incision. The procedure may be used to rotate a scar into a more favourable position such as a crease line. It may be utilized to elevate or depress the oral commissure or the outer canthus of the eye.

Axial flaps

Axial flaps are those which have a named vessel or branch of a named vessel running along their length. These flaps can therefore be as long as the supplying vessel. They are local flaps and thus are usually quite a good colour match. They are extremely reliable and rarely fail. Examples of axial flaps used in head and neck surgery are nasolabial flaps, glabellar flaps and forehead flaps.

Nasolabial flap (Figure 25.9)

The nasolabial flap is supplied by branches of the facial artery. The flap may be either superiorly or inferiorly based. It must be designed so that it is entirely superior and lateral to the nasolabial crease. This is so that closure of the donor site does not affect the position of the upper lip. The nasolabial flap may be used for repair of defects on the nose, especially for reconstruction of the alar margins; and for defects of the cheek and upper lip.

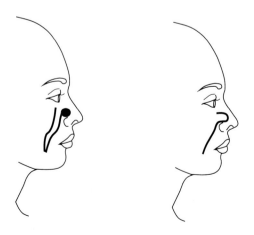

Figure 25.9 Nasolabial flap

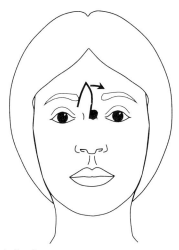 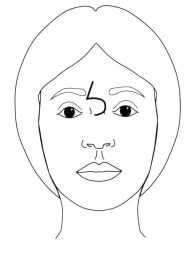

Figure 25.10 Glabellar flap

Glabellar flaps (Figure 25.10)

These are based on the supratrochlear vessels. They are most commonly used to repair defects around the upper part of the nose and inner canthal areas.

Forehead flap

This large flap comprises the whole of the non-hair-bearing skin of the forehead. The flap was most commonly used in the repair of intraoral defects, because it is a lengthy, dependable flap. The main disadvantages are that it needs to be divided when used intraorally, at a second stage, and that it is usually necessary to graft the donor site, with split skin, leaving an ugly scar.

Midline forehead flap

This is a long flap containing the supratrochlear vessels. It is most commonly used for repair of large defects of the nose and is the flap of choice in the reconstruction of the nose.

Myocutaneous flaps

The commonest myocutaneous flap to be used in the neck is the routine skin flap elevated with its layer of platysma. If the skin flaps are elevated without platysma the skin may not be viable.

Other myocutaneous flaps include the pectoralis major (Ariyan, 1979) and trapezius flaps (Demergasso and Piazza, 1979). The pectoralis major flap consists of a pedicle of pectoralis major muscle with its overlying skin from the lower chest wall. Its blood supply is from the pectoral branch of the thoracoacromial artery. The advantages of the myocutaneous flaps, such as the pectoralis major flap, are that they are quite predictable and safe (though not invariably so). They are a one-stage flap, not requiring division at a later procedure. The bulkiness of the flap may be used to advantage in certain circumstances.

These flaps, because they contain skin, subcutaneous tissue and muscle are usually thick, and this may also, in some situations, be a disadvantage. Furthermore, they usually come from distant sites and so skin colour match may not be good.

Complications in facial plastic surgery

Complications occurring in facial plastic surgery are of course the complications of any surgical procedure. These include primary and secondary haemorrhage, infection and scarring. There are some more specific complications however, because of the anatomical area involved. Additional complications during surgery include flap ischaemia from inadvertent damage to the main vessels of the particular flap. Surgical trauma to these vessels may render the flap non-viable and care must be taken to ensure, when dissecting out a skin flap, that its main vessels are not damaged. Haemorrhage and haematoma formation under a flap, especially a random flap, is a cause of ischaemia and subsequent flap loss.

Damage to nerves in the head and neck is common. This may be planned, such as division of the great auricular nerve in the course of a parotidectomy; or it may be unplanned, e.g. damage to the marginal mandibular nerve in surgery around the lower border of the mandible.

Intermediate complications include secondary haemorrhage, and infection and ischaemia of the skin flaps. Ischaemic lesions of flaps and tissue edges may be caused by undue tension from sutures, or by attempts to close defects with inadequate amounts of skin. Undue tissue tension can be avoided by careful planning of flaps, especially with regard to local skin elasticity and extensibility. Some tension may be eased by the use of skin undermining. The skin edges may be undermined for a distance of up to about 1 cm.

Management of lesions in the head and neck

Lesions of the upper, mid- and lower face

Management of lesions in these areas (excluding the nose, eyelids and lip) should be considered along the basic rules that have already been discussed. Excision of tumours must be planned so that the lesion is excised with an adequate margin in all directions and, secondly, the repair of the defect must be planned after consideration of the position, size and dimensions of the defect.

Very small benign lesions such as neurofibromas may simply be removed using a diathermy needle, the diathermized surface of the lesion is then simply scraped gently away with a scalpel blade. Slightly larger lesions of a similar nature may be shaved using a scalpel blade or razor blade. These techniques should be reserved for very small (up to 3 mm) benign lesions. Surgical management of benign lesions greater than this size or of any malignant lesion involves an excisional technique.

Excision of basal cell and squamous cell carcinomas and of malignant melanomas must be performed with an adequate margin of healthy tissue. Traditionally this has been achieved by having a margin of 5 mm or so around the wound edges in a superficial lesion and with an adequate deep margin, usually down to an anatomically defined layer such as a fascial or muscle layer.

In areas of concern, frozen sections should be used. However, the use of Mohs' technique (Mohs, 1941, 1976) has shown that even apparently superficial small basal and squamous cell carcinomas may be surprisingly extensive. Mohs' surgery involves piecemeal excision of tumours using a mapping technique, which allows the surgeon to excise further areas of persistent tumour under frozen section control. This is a very effective technique, albeit extremely time consuming. Having excised the tumour, consideration must then be made for repair of the defect.

Small benign and malignant lesions can be excised using a simple skin ellipse (Figure 25.11). These are

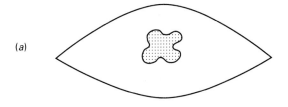

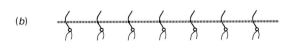

Figure 25.11 Design of a simple skin ellipse

planned so that they are three times as long as they are wide. The ellipse is planned to lie in a skin crease or relaxed skin tension line, for cosmesis. Care must be taken in planning to ensure that tension does not have an unfavourable effect on local structures, e.g. by producing an ectropion from tension around the lower eyelid.

Lesions of the forehead

The relaxed skin tension lines in the forehead run horizontally in the main, but with some running vertically in the glabellar region (see Figure 25.1). The forehead is a large flat area with hair-bearing margins superiorly and inferiorly. Laterally, the temple area is closely situated to the outer canthus of the eye.

The closure of any defect in the forehead region must therefore be planned so that hair-bearing areas are not moved onto the non-hair-bearing areas of the forehead. Similarly the outer canthus of the eye must not be subjected to undue tissue tension which could distort the appearance of the eye. Tissue tension above the eyebrow could elevate one brow compared to the other and provide a cosmetically unacceptable asymmetry. With all these factors in mind, repair of defects on the forehead should, wherever possible, be arranged so that the majority of incisions will lie along the frown lines (within the relaxed skin tension lines). There should be minimal tissue tension in a vertical direction.

Ideally, therefore, the repair of forehead lesions should be performed using skin ellipses for small lesions up to around 1 cm in diameter depending on the age and elasticity of the skin. Larger lesions on the forehead can be closed using an advancement flap, either single or bilateral, where the main incision lines are along the relaxed skin tension lines. However, in most skin flaps there will always be some of the incision lines crossing relaxed skin tension lines.

Lesions of the mid-face

This is essentially the cheek area (excluding the nose). In this part of the face the skin is of medium thickness. The relaxed skin tension lines tend to lie obliquely (see Figure 25.1) and the skin in this area is particularly elastic. Aesthetic and functional problems may arise from tension on the lower eyelid causing an ectropion. Elevation of the oral commissure may also be a complication of inadequate planning.

The temporal branch of the facial nerve is superficially placed over the zygomatic arch and great care must be taken to avoid injury to it in this site.

Any of the various types of skin flaps already described can be used in the cheek and mid-face area. Incisions should lie along the relaxed skin tension lines whenever possible. The cheek is ideally suited for bilobed and rhomboid flap repair. One of the most useful flaps used for large defects in the cheek is the large cheek rotation flap for the repair of anteriorly placed lesions (Figure 25.12). This extensive rotation flap can include most of the cheek and can be rotated to cover anteriorly placed defects of the cheek. It can be designed so that most of the incision lines are in the relaxed skin tension lines.

Lesions of the lower face

This is the area of the face lying below the nasolabial crease. The tissues in this area are quite elastic, although not to the same extent as the cheek, as there is some soft tissue fixation to the underlying mandible in the lower part of this anatomical area. Surgical difficulty may arise because of the proximity of the marginal mandibular division of the facial nerve to the lower border of the mandible. The relaxed skin tension lines in this area run at right angles to the commissure.

Small lesions involving the lip can be excised using a simple wedge excision. Up to 30% of the lip, either upper or lower, may be removed in this fashion.

Larger defects (30–80%) may be repaired using an Abbé-Estlander flap (Estlander, 1848; Abbé, 1898) from the opposite lip (Figure 25.13). An alternative method of repair of these larger defects is to use a rotation flap as described by a number of authors such as Bernard (1853), Gillies and Millard (1957) and Webster (1955).

In defects of the chin itself, use may be made of the curved relaxed skin tension lines around the mental prominence to camouflage elliptical excisions. Lesions around the nasolabial groove are ideally closed using a sliding or island flap (Krupp, Daverio and Brupbacker, 1983) (Figure 25.14) or by the use of a V–Y closure where the limbs of the incision can be disguised around the alar margin and in the nasolabial crease.

Lesions of the nose

Lesions of the nose are perhaps the most difficult of all the facial defects to treat. This is because the nose is such a prominent part of the face, where even small defects or blemishes can be extremely noticeable.

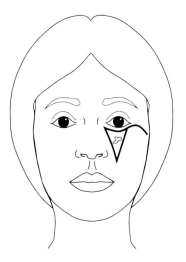 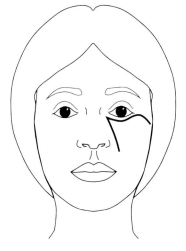

Figure 25.12 Large cheek rotation flap

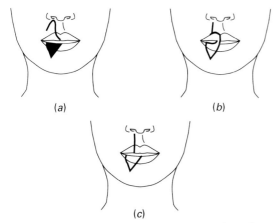

Figure 25.13 Abbé-Estlander flap. (*a*) Excision in lower lip and upper lip flap. (*b*) Rotation of upper flap to lower lip. (*c*) Flap after division after period of delay

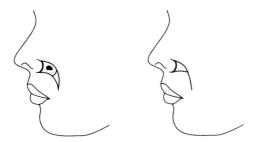

Figure 25.14 Small sliding flap in nasolabial crease

Secondly, repair of defects of the alar margins is one of the most difficult tasks in facial plastic surgery.

Defects of the nose, not including the alar margins, are generally best treated with a local flap. In the upper part of the nose, particularly around the dorsum, glabellar flaps can be extremely useful. In the lateral part of the nose, small rhomboid flaps can be used. Great care must be taken that these do not cross the concavity of the lateral nasal wall as the scar tissue involved in healing will tend to form some degree of webbing. Care must be taken in using transposition flaps that the direction of tension does not produce an ectropion or alter the symmetry of the palpebral fissures. Defects of the lower part of the nose may be managed with the use of nasolabial flaps based as close to the lateral nasal wall as possible. However, lesions involving the alar margin, particularly if fairly small are best dealt with using composite auricular grafts. Care must be used with these grafts to achieve good haemostasis, and also to provide a recipient area with as broad a base as possible to allow early revascularization of the flap.

The midline forehead flap is a safe flap which can be utilized in the reconstruction of the nose. The flap is based on the supratrochlear vessels. It may be as long as the non-hair-bearing area of the forehead, and it can be rotated down as far as the upper lip to reconstruct any part or the whole of the nose. The flap can be folded back on itself to form a double surfaced flap in reconstruction of the nostrils. It is also known as the Indian flap. Amputation of the nose was used in India as a punishment for adultery. The midline forehead flap found popularity among surgeons there in reconstruction of the nose.

Management of skin lesions of the neck

Small lesions of the skin of the neck are by far the easiest to manage in facial plastic surgery. The neck skin is very extensible and the blood supply is excellent. Scars in this area are not quite so prominent as they would be on the face. The range of techniques already described can be used with equal facility in the neck skin.

The ageing face

As skin ages it loses its elasticity, crease lines become more obvious with the passage of time and skin becomes pendulous particularly in dependent areas such as around the chin and in the eyelids. The procedures used in rejuvenation of the ageing face are designed to remove excess skin and by doing so give the impression of tone in the face and neck tissues. They also remove skin creases by stretching the skin. These surgical procedures are only of a temporary nature because clearly the ageing processes in the skin will continue, therefore they should be delayed for as long as possible.

The procedures used include blepharoplasty, to remove excessive skin and herniated fat from the eye lids, rhytidectomy or face lift, and adjunctive procedures such as forehead rhytidectomy or variations on this to elevate the eyebrow and redundant forehead skin.

Blepharoplasty

Indications for this procedure are redundant ptotic skin in either the upper or the lower eyelids. This is often associated with herniation of fat through the orbital septum, particularly in the lower lid area.

Anatomy

The eyelids are formed from skin with an underlying layer of orbicularis muscle. Lying deep to this, in both the upper and lower eyelids, is the tarsal plate. Deep to the orbicularis muscle is the orbital septum. This is a thin fibrous layer in continuity with the periosteum of the orbital rim. Deep to the orbital septum lies the orbital fat. The orbital septum, either with age or as a congenital predisposition may allow herniation of the orbital fat into the eyelid producing a baggy eyelid. Other causes of a bulging eyelid are gravitational folds and orbicularis hypertrophy (Friedman, 1987).

Surgical method

Upper lid blepharoplasty (Figure 25.15)

In this procedure an ellipse of skin and orbicularis muscle is removed. The lower margin of the incision is placed in the upper lid skin crease. This is usually about 10 mm from the lid margin. The upper margin of the ellipse is identified by measuring the amount of redundant skin with the use of forceps such as

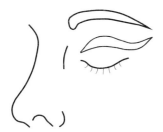

Figure 25.15 Skin/muscle excision in upper lid blepharoplasty

Green's forceps. The skin ellipse is designed so that the lateral part is lateral to the outer canthus and is elevated slightly to prevent inferior rotation of the outer canthus producing 'sad eye'. Any underlying fat, which has herniated through the orbital septum, may be dealt with in a number of ways, including excision, ligation and diathermy. Haemostasis must be meticulously obtained and the wound then closed using fine sutures.

Lower lid blepharoplasty

In this procedure an incision is made just below the lower lid margin and extended out into a crow's foot skin crease. A skin and muscle flap is elevated and herniated fat is dealt with as before. Excess skin is then removed and wound closure obtained. Skin removal must be done judiciously, because, if excess skin is excised, an ectropion may be produced. Skin removal tends to be a narrow margin below the lash line and a small triangle of skin lateral to the outer canthus (Figure 25.16).

Complications of blepharoplasty

The most important and early complications of blepharoplasty include haemorrhage and haematoma within the orbit. This may cause blindness secondary to retinal or optic nerve ischaemia. The cause of this

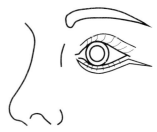

Figure 25.16 Skin/muscle excision in lower lid blepharoplasty

may be related to poor haemostasis, or to vascular ischaemia secondary to the use of adrenalin injections around the eyelids. Permanent late complications include ectropion as a result of excessive skin excision and asymmetry of the palpebral fissure. Temporary complications include dry eye, ecchymosis and lagophthalmos. These usually settle within a short period of time.

Rhytidectomy

This procedure was initially described in 1907 by Miller. The operation is designed to remove excessive and ptotic skin from around the face, and the jowl area of the neck. The operation gives the patient a more youthful appearance by removing the submental 'dewlap', and anterior platysma bands, and by reduction of the majority of crease lines in the face.

Anatomical considerations

The skin of the face in youth remains taut because of inherent skin elasticity, and also because of tone in the subcutaneous musculature – the muscles of facial expression including the platysma.

The superficial muscular aponeurotic system

The superficial muscular aponeurotic system was described by Mitz and Peyronie (1976). This layer divides the subcutaneous fat of the face into a deep and superficial layer. It gives slips to the skin itself. The superficial muscular aponeurotic system forms a fibrous layer from frontalis (posterior part) above to platysma below, in the lower face. Anteriorly, it blends into the investing fascia of the muscles of facial expression. Posteriorly, it attaches to the tragal and mastoid fascia, and to the periosteum of the mandible and the zygomatic arch. The superficial muscular aponeurotic system is most easily identified in the parotid area where it forms a thick fibrous layer. The branches of the facial nerve are deep to the system and in the area of the cheek and zygomatic arch very closely applied. Great care must therefore be taken in dissection in these sites to avoid damage to the underlying nerves. Because the superficial muscular aponeurotic system is applied to the facial muscles it can be used as a tensor of these structures, either in the natural state or in the face-lift operation.

Facial nerve

The facial nerve is particularly vulnerable in rhytidectomy. The nerve is protected by the parotid gland itself. The nerve exits from the gland and it is in these areas where it is most likely to be damaged in flap elevation. The most vulnerable sites are where the frontalis branch crosses the zygomatic arch and where the marginal mandibular branch passes, just deep to platysma, about 1 cm below the lower border of the mandible. The buccal branches may be damaged as they run just deep to the superficial muscular aponeurotic system over the buccal fat pad.

Surgical method

The aim of the surgery is to elevate and reduce sagging cheeks and jowls and thereby produce a more youthful appearance. This is achieved by elevating a skin flap from the temple to the cheek and extending to the neck (Rees, 1980).

Prior to commencing the dissection the operative area is injected with 1/200 000 adrenalin solution. The incision runs in the hairline over the temporalis muscle, it then runs either in the pretragal crease, or just posterior to the tragus, before running around the ear lobe postauricularly to lie horizontally in the occipital, hair-bearing skin (Figure 25.17). The skin flap is then elevated with a thin layer of subdermal fat. Providing one remains superficial to the facial muscles, the facial nerve should be safe, care being taken especially in the danger areas already mentioned. The dissection proceeds as far as the oral commissure and into the neck where the right and left skin flaps may meet.

The dissection of the superficial muscular aponeurotic system is then started. The fascia is divided anterior to the tragus. The superficial muscular aponeurotic system is elevated essentially only over the parotid gland and over temporalis and into the neck. Having elevated the system it is pulled posterosuperiorly to tighten the cheek and neck skin. The superficial muscular aponeurotic system is then shortened and sutured to the tragal perichondrium and mastoid process periosteum.

The skin is similarly elevated. The skin flaps are kept thin with only a thin layer of subdermal fat. The skin flap may be extended as far as the submental region and may be in continuity with the flap on the opposite side. Having elevated the skin flaps the flaps are pulled posterosuperiorly and redundant skin is excised. After trimming the skin flap the skin is closed using skin clips within the hair line, and fine sutures in the more visible areas of the incision.

The face lift procedure does not remove fine lines, particularly around the mouth or the 'crows' feet, wrinkles around the eyelid. It has little effect on the crease lines of the forehead. Its primary function is to tighten skin around the cheeks and neck and will improve the profile of the neck/cheek. The anterior platysma bands may not be dealt with adequately with the face lift procedure and additional surgery to this area such as excision of the bands, suturing of the bands, or a Z-plasty of the anterior platysma bands may be required. This is generally done through a separate submental incision.

Complications of rhytidectomy

The early complications of the face lift procedure include, most importantly, haemorrhage. An extremely large flap will have been elevated, and adequate haemostasis must be secured. Haemorrhage under the flaps may cause at least, unsightly haematoma, and at worst, flap loss to varying degree. A further early complication is damage to the branches of the facial nerve. This may be either temporary or permanent.

Late complications include unfavourable scars and malposition of the incision lines. Of special note in this respect is alteration of the position of the ear lobe in the final suturing.

Brow lift

Segments of the forehead skin may be excised as ellipses in the immediate suprabrow region (direct brow lift) as described by Castanares (1964), or in the midforehead region by Rafaty, Goode and

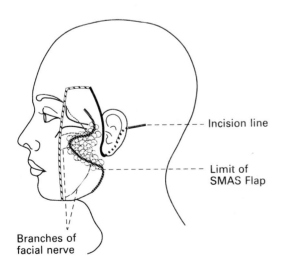

- - - Incision line

- - - Limit of SMAS Flap

Branches of facial nerve

Figure 25.17 Skin incision and superficial muscular aponeurotic system elevated in rhytidectomy

Abrahamson (1978). A more complex procedure, the forehead rhytidectomy (Kaye, 1977) is performed through a scalp incision, just within the hairline. These procedures will elevate the sagging brow, and will reduce frown lines. The direct brow lift is a simple procedure which is particularly useful in the paralysed forehead, to elevate the ptotic brow. The midforehead procedure must only be used in patients with a ptotic brow and frown lines. Otherwise the midforehead scar may remain visible.

Complications of face and brow lifting can be early, intermediate or late. Early complications include ecchymosis, and haematoma formation, as well as neurological trauma to either motor or, more commonly, sensory nerves. Intermediate complications include necrosis of part of the skin flaps; this is most likely to happen around the incision edges. Late complications are hair loss when the flap is too thin or under too much tension; and asymmetry of the face and especially the ear lobes.

Adjunctive procedures in aesthetic plastic surgery

Mentoplasty

Mentoplasty is performed as a simple procedure to augment a weak chin and may be particularly useful in reducing the visual impact of a prominent nose (Millard, 1965; Pitanguy, 1968). Various materials can be used for chin implants, the commonest being Silastic. Other implant materials include hydroxyapatite, Proplast and polyamide mesh.

Chin implants may be inserted either by an external excision in the submental crease or intraorally through the labial mucosa. The former technique is generally preferred because of the decreased likelihood of infection of the implant, but this method is of course associated with a small external scar. Because of the position of the scar it is invisible to the casual observer.

The chin implant is inserted so that the implant lies over the mental prominence. It is convenient usually to keep the implant extraperiosteal, but with the ends of the implant projecting through a slit in the periosteum so that they lie under the periosteum and therefore help retain the implant in a correct position.

Complications of mentoplasty

These include infection and extrusion. It is possible to damage the mental nerve as it exits from the mental foramen. There may be, as a long-term complication, erosion of the bone underlying the implant and associated damage to the dental nerves. Migration of the implant may occur, either superiorly, especially in intraoral implants, or inferiorly in extraoral implants, causing a witch's chin deformity.

Liposuction

This procedure was developed by Kesselring and Meyer (1978), although non-suction methods of lipectomy had been used previously. The method is used to sculpt the underlying tissues by suction of fat deposits thus debulking the area. The subsequent scar tissue causes tightening of the overlying skin, producing a more youthful appearance. The most common procedure in the cervicofacial area is liposuction of the submental fat pad. It is also used to a certain extent in the cheek. Liposuction may be performed under local or general anaesthesia. Great care must be taken to ensure that the liposuction catheter is within the fatty layer of the subcutaneous tissues and does not go deep to platysma, or other muscle layers, for fear of causing damage to the underlying structures. Liposuction is often used as an adjunct to rhytidectomy in the submental area.

The major complication of this procedure is of subcutaneous haematoma formation and skin ecchymosis. If liposuction is performed deep to the muscle layer there is clearly a much greater possibility for damage to the underlying structures.

Chemical peeling

This technique may be used for the treatment of small skin crease lines particularly around the mouth and eyelids, as are often seen in the elderly, and also areas of skin pigmentation. The material normally used is phenol with croton oil and liquid soap in distilled water (Mosienko and Baker, 1978). The basis of the technique is to cause a superficial chemical burn. The healing process subsequently causing rearrangement of the collagen fibres and slight thickening of the skin, thereby obliterating small crease lines.

The complications of the technique may be to cause a deeper chemical burn than planned with a protracted healing period. Scarring is uncommon but may occur particularly in neck skin. Chemical peeling may cause variations in skin pigmentation especially in heavily pigmented skin, and is best reserved for use in fair-skinned individuals.

Dermabrasion

This technique debrides the skin superficially using either small wire brushes or diamond paste burrs (McEvitt, 1950). It is useful for camouflaging small cutaneous scars. Dermabrasion causes partial thickness skin loss which, on healing, obliterates the more obvious underlying scar. This technique may be used for management of acne scars, and as a secondary treatment in scar camouflage after a primary technique such as a W-plasty. It may also be used for the management of rhinophyma in reducing the bulky thickened skin of the nose. It is not generally recommended for the management of fine crease lines where chemical peeling is generally a better technique.

Scar revision and facial plastic surgery

The primary object of scar revision in facial plastic surgery is to disguise a scar or camouflage it so that it is not as visible as previously. Scars may be clearly visible because they are pigmented, because they cross natural skin contour lines or anatomical boundaries, particularly concavities where webbing will tend to occur because they are broad or hypertrophic, or because they cross actual crease lines.

The elements of scar revision are to place the scar, or at least elements of it, within relaxed skin tension lines, and to break up the scar so it is less visible. Generally speaking simple excision of a scar and resuturing without any other technique will not in itself be an effective procedure. It is usually necessary to break up the scar. Two techniques available for this are the W-plasty and the geometric broken-line plasty.

W-plasty

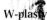

In this procedure the scar is excised as a series of Ws (Figure 25.18). The wound edges are then resutured

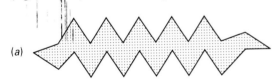

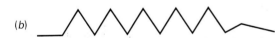

Figure 25.18 'W'-plasty. (*a*) Scar excision. (*b*) Completed suture line

with careful placement of the elements of the W-plasty, so that they form a zig-zag line. Some of the elements of the scar will then lie along relaxed skin tension lines and be less visible than a scar which completely crosses relaxed skin tension lines.

Geometric broken-line plasty

This excises the scar using a series of geometric figures such as half circles, half squares, and triangles (Figure 25.19). This breaks up linear scars and camouflages them.

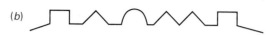

Figure 25.19 Geometric broken-line scar revision. (*a*) Scar excision. (*b*) Completed suture line

Secondary methods of dealing with the scar after scar revision include dermabrasion and chemical peeling which may be highly effective as second stage procedures.

References

ABBÉ, R. (1898) A new plastic operation for the relief of deformity due to double hair lip. *Medical Record*, **53**, 477–488

ARIYAN, S. (1979) The pectoralis major myocutaneous flap. *Plastic and Reconstructive Surgery*, **63**, 73–81

BERNARD, C. (1853) Cancer de la levre inferieure opere par un procede nouveau. *Bulletin Mem Soc Chir (Paris)*, **3**, 357

BORGES, A. F. and ALEXANDER, J. E. (1962) Relaxed skin tension lines. Z-plasties on scars and fusiform excision of lesions. *British Journal of Plastic Surgery*, **15**, 242–254

CASTANARES, S. (1964) Forehead wrinkles, glabellar frown and ptosis of the eyebrows. *Plastic and Reconstructive Surgery*, **34**, 406–413

DEMERGASSO, F. and PIAZZA, M. (1979) Trapezius myocutaneous flap in reconstructive surgery for head and neck cancer. An original technique. *American Journal of Surgery*, **138**, 533–536

ESSER, J. (1918) Gestielte lokale Nasenplastik mit zweizipfligem Lappen, Deckung des sekundaren Defekts vom ersten Zipfel durch den zweiten. *Deutsche Zeitschrift für Chirurgie*, **143**, 385–390

ESTLANDER, J. A. (1848) Methodes d'autoplastic de la joue on d'une ny methode. *Hospitalsmiddelelser (Copenhagen)*, **1**, 212

FRIEDMAN, W. H. (1987) Surgical anatomy of the orbit. *Facial Plastic Surgery*, **4**, 75–81

GILLIES, H. D. and MILLARD, D. R. (1957) *Principles and Art of Plastic Surgery*, vol 1. London: Butterworth and Co. pp. 115–132

KAYE, B. L. (1977) The forehead lift: a useful adjunct to facelift and blepharoplasty. *Plastic and Reconstructive Surgery*, **60**, 161–171

KESSELRING, U. K. and MEYER, R. (1978) Suction curette for removal of excessive local deposits of subcutaneous fat. *Plastic and Reconstructive Surgery*, **62**, 305–306

KRUPP, S., DAVERIO, P. and BRUPBACKER, J. (1983) Island flaps for face and neck repair. *Facial Plastic Surgery*, **1**, 37–50

LANGER, K. (1861) Zur Anatomie und Physiologie der Haur. Uber die Spaltbarkeit der Cutis. *S B Akad. Wiss. Wien*, **44**, 19

LIMBERG, A. A. (1966) Design of local flaps. In: *Modern Trends in Plastic Surgery*, edited by T. Gibson. London: Butterworths. pp. 38–61

MCEVITT, W. G. (1950) Treatment of acne pits by abrasion with sandpaper. *Journal of the American Medical Association*, **142**, 647–648

MILLARD, R. (1965) Adjuncts in augmentation mentoplasty and corrective rhinoplasty. *Plastic and Reconstructive Surgery*, **39**, 48–61

MILLER, C. C. (1907) Subcutaneous section of the facial muscles to eradicate expression lines. *American Journal of Surgery*, **21**, 235–236

MITZ, V. and PEYRONIE, M. (1976) The superficial musculoaponeurotic system (SMAS) in the parotid and cheek area. *Plastic and Reconstructive Surgery*, **58**, 80–88

MOHS, F. E. (1941) Chemosurgery: a microscopically controlled method of cancer excision. *Archives of Surgery*, **42**, 279–295

MOHS, F. E. (1976) Chemosurgery for skin cancer. Fixed tissue and fresh tissue techniques. *Archives of Dermatology*, **112**, 211–215

MOSIENKO, P. and BAKER, T. J. (1978) Chemical peel. *Clinical Plastic Surgery*, **5**, 79–96

PITANGUY, I. (1968) Augmentation mentoplasty. *Plastic and Reconstructive Surgery*, **42**, 460–464

RAFATY, F. M., GOODE, R. L. and ABRAHAMSON, N. R., (1978) The brow lift operation in a man. *Archives of Otolaryngology*, **104**, 69–71

REES, T. D. (1980) *Aesthetic Plastic Surgery*. Philadelphia: W. B. Saunders. pp. 583–683

STUCKER, F. J., BRYARLY, R. C. and SHOCKLEY, N. W. (1986) Reconstructive rhinoplasty. *Otolaryngology – Head and Neck Surgery*, **1**, 799–810

WEBSTER, J. P. (1955) Crescentic peri-alar cheek excision for upper lip advancement with a short history of upper lip repair. *Plastic and Reconstructive Surgery*, **16**, 434–464

WEERDA, H. (1983) Bilobed and trilobed flaps in head and neck defect repair. *Facial Plastic Surgery*, **1**, 51–60

26

Plastic and reconstructive surgery of the head and neck

William R. Panje and Michael R. Morris

'Trivials make perfection but perfection is not trivial.'

Michelangelo

Perhaps the most significant advances in head and neck surgery in the last 20 years have been in the reconstructive field. Advances and discoveries in the uses of regional musculocutaneous and free flaps have revolutionized the surgical management of head and neck defects.

The incision

The cutaneous incision required for many operations is frequently the only significant morbidity for the patient or evidence to others that something has been done. There are three factors under the surgeon's control that affect the acceptability of the final scar: the location, the creation, and the closure of the incision.

Incisions should be placed parallel to the favourable skin tension lines if at all possible. There is an intricate elastic and collagenous fibre network within the skin that creates a very orderly tension force (Figure 26.1). The favourable skin tension lines correspond to the orientation of these tension vectors. By placing the incision along these lines the natural pull of the skin would actually be in direct opposition to the contraction forces of the resultant scar. The net result is a tendency for the scar to contract much less and maintain a more natural appearance.

The face and neck are unique in that there are multiple muscles which insert into the skin. The direction of pull of these muscles happens to be perpendicular to the favourable skin tension lines. This is a fortunate arrangement since the constant contraction and relaxation of the underlying muscles creates sufficient tension vectors as well. When an incision is placed in the direction in which the muscle contracts and relaxes (i.e. perpendicular to the favourable skin tension lines), the force vectors will be constantly changing. This results in unstable healing and a thickening of the ultimate scar. Conversely, the force vectors developed perpendicular to the action of the muscles are relatively static and do not adversely affect the ultimate scar.

Over time skin loses its inherent elasticity and, as the underlying muscles continue to contract, the increasingly lax skin forms wrinkles. Incisions placed parallel to or within a wrinkle will take advantage of the maximum tissue laxity during closure and healing. Incisions running perpendicular to wrinkles will naturally be closed under relatively greater tension which will result in widening of the scar. Once again there is a fortunate situation as the wrinkles of the face and neck correspond closely with the favourable skin tension lines. In other words, an incision placed parallel to or within a wrinkle will take full advantage of the natural pull of the skin, the influence of the underlying muscle action, and the maximum tissue laxity and thus produce the most favourable scar.

A surgeon should also take advantage of the natural camouflage of facial wrinkles and folds, as well as the junctional areas between aesthetic units and the hairline when planning incisions. For more radical head and neck surgical procedures the incisions used must take account of the vascular supply and surface anatomy of the neck. The anterior neck skin has a rich vascular supply with contributions from the facial, the superior thyroid, and the transverse cervical arteries. The posterior triangle neck skin does not have such a robust blood supply and this limits the size of any posteriorly based flaps. Long, superiorly based flaps (apron) are well vascularized but tend to develop venous stagnation and oedema along their

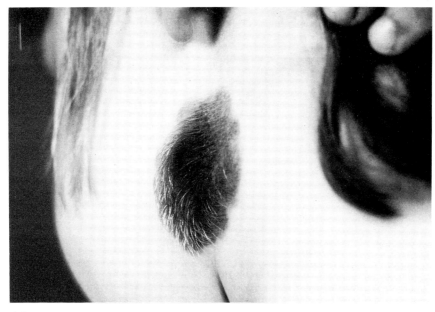

(a)

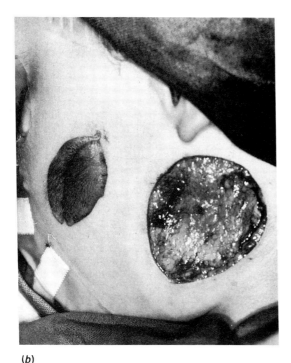

(b)

Figure 26.1 (*a*) Congenital pigmented hairy naevus involving the neck of an 8-year-old girl. (*b*) Appearance of wound following removal of naevus. Note how the wound has become larger because of elastic tissue forces

lower edge. Incisions should not be orientated vertically along the axis of the great vessels and the location of any trifurcations must be carefully thought out. Incisions for less radical neck operations should be placed so that they can be incorporated into a more extensive design if ever needed.

There are three planes to consider in the surface anatomy of the neck: the submental (horizontally orientated), the neck (vertically orientated), and the supraclavicular (horizontally orientated). A good recommendation is to place the incision along a horizontally orientated line running from the mastoid tip and extending between the junction of the submental and neck planes. This will provide about 3–4 cm of cervical skin in the upper flap which is the ideal compromise between adequate length and allowing access to the oral cavity/oropharynx. A second horizontally placed incision along the junction of the neck and supraclavicular planes will allow exposure for neck dissection, while providing the maximum cosmesis for the patient (MacFee, 1960). Any vertically orientated incision in the neck that traverses these planes should be lengthened (i.e. a lazy S pattern) to account for the pull of the platysma and the expected contraction and webbing of the ultimate scar.

After planning and marking out the incision the creation of the wound is the next step. With equal retraction on the opposing skin edges, a scapel blade is used to cut perpendicularly and completely through the skin with a single motion. Bleeding along the wound edges should be minimal and easily controlled with pressure. Persistent, troublesome bleeding can be managed with bipolar cautery. Neck flaps should generally be raised on a subplatysmal plane to reduce the chance of vascular insufficiency at the wound edges.

Prior to closing the wound there must be absolute haemostasis, asepsis, and proper drainage. Closed suction drains are preferred whenever the aerodigestive tract has not been entered. They are brought through the skin away from the incision. The wound edges are minimally debrided if necessary and closure is begun by reapproximating the platysma. Subcutaneous sutures are placed to take all tension off the skin edges. The skin is closed by inserting a sharp, cutting needle through the skin so that it leaves the subcutaneous tissue at a point slightly further from the wound edge than where it entered. After completing a similar bite on the opposite side the suture is loosely tied providing eversion and accurate apposition of the wound edges (Figure 26.2). The surgical trauma will cause a degree of oedema at the wound edges. When suture tension is excessive and does not account for this swelling, strangulation with subsequent necrosis can occur. With regard to the aesthetics of the final scar, the type of suture employed is not nearly as important as the technique employed in closing the wound and the timely removal of the suture material (Table 26.1). Facial skin sutures should be placed every 2–4 mm in most wounds.

Generally, alternate sutures can be removed on day 3 and the remainder on day 5. Neck sutures should be removed on day 7. Skin that has been irradiated takes substantially longer to heal. Generally, the sutures are left in an extra day for every 1000 cGy of radiation received.

Wounds should be reinforced for several days with skin tapes, especially after suture removal. Care and meticulous technique in planning, creating, and closing the incision will generally provide the patient with an acceptable scar.

Scar revision

Patient satisfaction with the aesthetics of a facial or neck scar is quite variable. Some patients are not at all bothered by a poor result, while others demand revision surgery for relatively minor flaws. Patients must have reasonable expectations and a clear understanding of what can be accomplished before proceeding. Photodocumentation is an essential preoperative requirement.

Scar contracture can cause a significant functional handicap. The neck webbing that can occur with vertically orientated scars or inferiorly based musculocutaneous flaps can significantly tether head motion and affect deglutition.

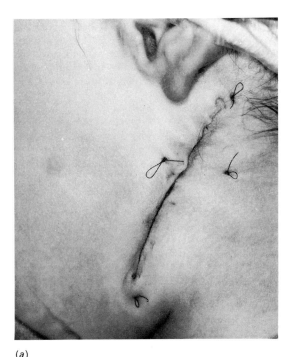

(a)

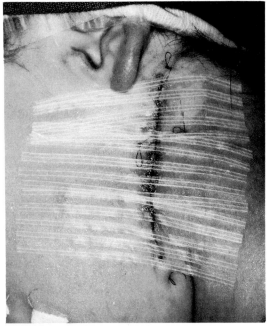

(b)

Figure 26.2 (a) The wound is closed by primary intention. A subcuticular running suture was utilized for the closure. Note the eversion of the skin edges. (b) In order to reduce incision motion and reduce tension small strips of tape are applied perpendicular to the incision

Table 26.1 Absorbable and non-absorbable sutures

Type	Strength (b)	Half-life	Reactivity	Throws required	Comment
Absorbable					
gut	± 3.3	5–20 days	+ + + +	3–4	Low knot security until moist; non-uniform, can fray
collagen	± 3.3	5–20 days	+ + + +	3–4	Low knot security until moist
Dexon	6	10 days	+ +	3–4	Half-life pH dependent
Vicryl	6	10 days	+ +	4–5	Half-life pH dependent
Polydiaxone (PDS)	± 4	4.5 weeks	+	4–5	New, promising monofilament
Non-absorbable					
silk	3	0.5–1 year	+ + +	3–4	Inconsistent strength
cotton	⩽ 3	> 1 year	+ + +	2–3	Drags, cuts tissue
Dacron	4	*	+ + +	2–3	Rough surface causes capillary action
coated Dacron	4	*	+ + +	4–5	Coatings may fragment
nylon monofilament	3.6	0.5–1 year	+	5	Can fracture
nylon braided	4	⩽ 1 year	+ +	3–4	Dead spaces
polypropylene	3.5	*	+	5 +	Can fracture
stainless steel	9.5	*	+	2–3	Poor handling

Scars elsewhere on the body are examined for hypertrophic reaction or keloid formation. Revising scars on these patients may actually worsen the appearance. Time is also an important consideration as most scars settle and improve substantially in appearance after 1 or 2 years. Intervention prior to a prolonged waiting period should only be considered for obviously problematic scars.

The scar is carefully evaluated for why it is considered unsightly (Figure 26.3). This can be related to its overall length, the original amount of tissue loss, the unevenness of the two edges with respect to each other or the surrounding tissues, or the direction the scar takes with respect to the skin tension lines. Longer scars can be subdivided into smaller component parts with the end result of breaking up the eye-catching monotony of the single line and camouflaging the scar. Where contracture has occurred secondary to extensive tissue loss, successful revision will require complete freeing up and mobilization of the scarred area. Adjacent or distant tissue will then have to be used to fill the defect. Unevenness can be easily remedied by dermabrasion or simple excision and proper reapproximation. The relationship of the scar to the tension lines becomes a critical factor in choosing the method of revision.

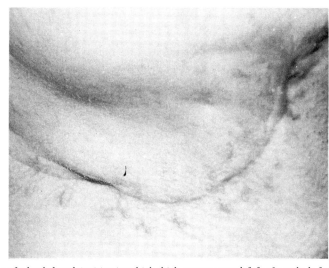

Figure 26.3 Appearance of a healed neck incision in which thick sutures were left for 2 weeks before removal. Note the zipper appearance of the scar

There are three basic revision techniques that must be understood: the fusiform excision, the W-plasty, and the Z-plasty. By applying the principles of these three methods, most facial and neck scars can be altered to provide a more acceptable deformity.

Fusiform excision

By using the techniques previously discussed for making and reapproximating an incision, most unaesthetic linear scars can be improved with simple fusiform excision. This method will not significantly alter the direction of the scar so is best applied to revisions of scars that follow or run very close to (less than 30–35°) the favourable skin tension lines. The ends of the excision should come to a 30° angle or less and it is often not necessary or recommended to remove the scarring below the skin. This will allow for a meticulous closure without tension with only limited undermining.

W-plasty

When the direction of the scar must be reorientated with respect to the tension lines (more than 30–35°), the W-plasty provides the best alternative. This method changes a straight line into an irregular pattern which camouflages the scar. A saw-toothed-shaped complete excision of the width of the scar is the first step. Each of the triangular cuts should be 5–7 mm in length and have an angle of between 55 and 60°. One side of the incision should be the template for the other side. Once the two edges of the excision are mobilized they actually interdigitate with one another to form a broken line closure. The ends of the excision should come to a 30° angle or less to avoid a standing cone. The principles of the W-plasty have been expanded by using a variety of geometrical shapes in addition to the triangle. This allows orientation of many of the lines of the eventual scar with the tension lines and improving the overall aesthetic result.

Z-plasty

The basic Z-plasty consists of two triangular flaps of skin and subcutaneous tissue formed by three connecting incisions of equal length and at a 30–60° angle to one another (McGregor, 1980) (Figure 26.4). Essentially, the two flaps are moved until they have exchanged places which gains length in one direction at the expense of width in the other. Greater elongation is achieved by the use of wider flaps with concomitant larger angles to the vertical axis (Figure 26.5).

The horizontal limbs of the Z-plasty should be along the favourable skin tension lines or a wrinkle line if at all possible. If necessary, the angles formed between the wrinkle line and the triangular flaps may be a good deal less than 60°. Depending on specific conditions, e.g. the skin on one side may be looser and require less elongation, the triangular angles of each flap may be of unequal size (i.e. a 30° and a 60° flap). The 60° Z-plasty is best applied when the direction of the scar is 60° or more away from the lines of tension. When using the Z-plasty to manage scars over 30–35° but less than 60° from the tension lines the surgeon should still cut the horizontal limbs as close to the tension line as possible. When the flaps are transposed the overall effect is to improve the orientation of the scar with the tension lines and produce a more aesthetic scar.

Multiple Z-plasties are useful for improving a variety of deformities. The vertical bowstring scar seen with a pedicled musculocutaneous flap is a good example (Figure 26.6). The central limb of the Z extends for the full length of the contracture. Multiple parallel transverse limbs are placed forming the continuous multiple Z-plasty. The number of transverse limbs depends on the local availability of skin and the dimensional requirements of reorientating the scar. Increasing the number of components reduces the demand on each flap for available laxity. Remember that the gain in scar length comes from mobilizing the tissue and borrowing from the width. The less mobile the surrounding tissue the more Zs required. If the scar traverses all three planes of the neck

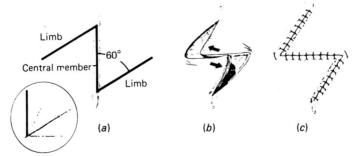

Figure 26.4 Z-plasty: note how the central member of the Z lies along the scar. This area will be elongated by transposing the two triangular flaps

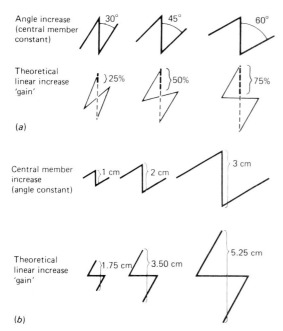

(a)

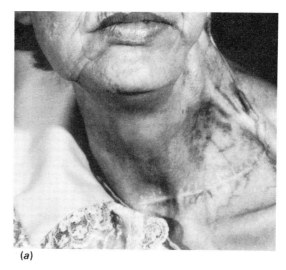

(a)

Figure 26.5 (*a,b*) Increasing the angle between the central member and arms of the Z will result in a theoretical linear increase of the central arm. Similarly keeping the angle constant, but increasing the central member length, will also produce lengthening in the direction of the original central member

(submental, neck, and supraclavicular), it will need a minimum of three components. Each of the planes must be managed independently even though the scar is managed in a continuous fashion. This will allow the resulting scar to lie flat and conform to the dimensions of the neck.

Cutaneous loss

When the extent of the defect means that direct primary closure is impossible, an alternative technique must be used. The surgeon needs to approach these situations logically to provide the patient with the best possible reconstruction. Several factors will need to be considered starting initially with the patient and his general health. A fit 70 year old will no doubt have many more productive years and deserves the best reconstruction possible. Conversely, a 50 year old with significant heart disease has greatly increased perioperative risks so anaesthetic times should be kept to a minimum. Diabetes, peripheral vascular disease, malnutrition, and previous radiation will greatly affect the success rate. A patient with limited mental fortitude may not tolerate the cosmetic deformity of a secondarily healing defect or a skin graft and a flap may prove the best option. On

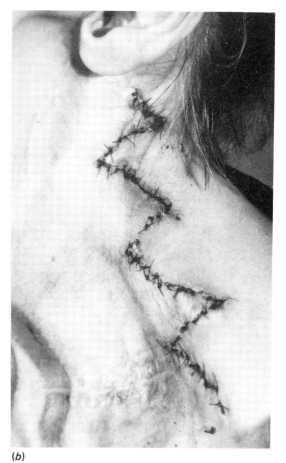

(b)

Figure 26.6 (*a*) Cervical contracture scar following radical neck dissection. (*b*) Contracture released with multiple Z-plasty

the other hand, delaying the reconstruction with some patients can have a beneficial effect on their overall acceptance of the final result. If the reconstruction requires a musculocutaneous or free flap, the surgeon must consider the donor morbidity. Golf, tennis, swimming, etc., all involve different actions of the trunk and shoulder girdle. If a patient has a strong desire to pursue a skill or hobby, every effort should be made to preserve the necessary muscle function. The reason the defect was created can also alter the surgical approach. Fear of tumour recurrence following excision of a cancer would prompt a more conservative management of a defect than if it were the result of trauma.

The size and location of the cutaneous defect also influences the reconstructive requirements. External defects of the ear and nose are usually of cosmetic significance only. So long as the ear and nose can hold spectacles in place, many people will be content with an aesthetically poor reconstruction (Figure 26.7). The eyelids, on the other hand, protect the globe from exposure and help distribute the tear film during blinking. This function must be maintained with the reconstruction or the patient will surely complain (Figure 26.8). The upper eyelid must be thin enough to fold on itself when open where the lower lid must have enough rigidity and support to

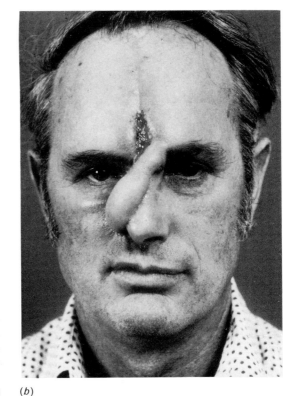
(b)

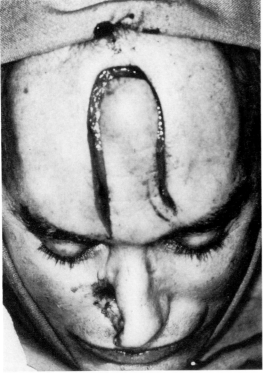
(a)

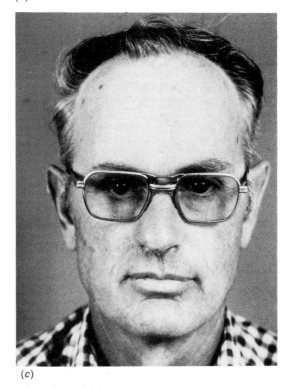
(c)

Figure 26.7 (a,b,c) A midline forehead flap to close a through-and-through nasal defect

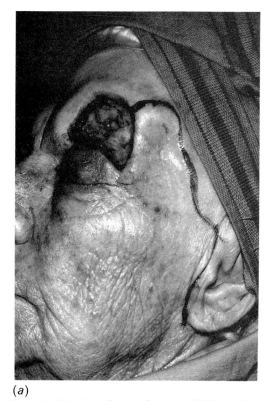
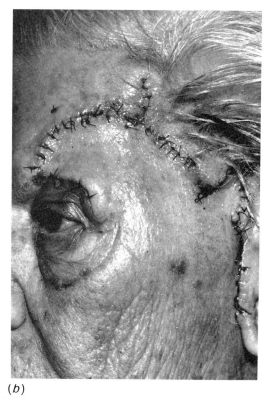

(a)   *(b)*

Figure 26.8 (*a*) Large brow and upper eyelid defect after removal of skin cancer. Proposed rotation advancement temporal cheek flap. (*b*) In order to even the donor flap edge with recipient tissues a wedge of tissue was removed from the recipient circumference as well as a posterior Z-plasty. Note the evenness of closure and lack of tension on the upper eyelid

resist gravity and wound contracture (i.e. ectropion). The lips also have major functional consequences if not appropriately reconstructed. Sphincteric incompetence and/or loss of sensation will result in persistent drooling (Figure 26.9). Primary closure of large defects can cause microstomia and hinder mouth care, intraoral inspection, and the wearing of dentures (Figure 26.10). If the cutaneous loss involves a large portion of an aesthetic facial unit, removing the remaining tissue and reconstructing the entire unit should be considered (Burget and Menick, 1989).

Healing by secondary intention

Healing by secondary intention is an underutilized option in facial reconstruction (Panje, Bumsted and Ceilley, 1980; Zitelli, 1983). Surgeons are often forced to accept delayed healing when dealing with grossly contaminated wounds or following the failure of another method. The advantages of healing by secondary intention include avoiding further surgery, allowing scrutinization of surgical margins, actively involving patients in their own care, and providing

for excellent and predictable cosmetic results (Figure 26.11). Wound contraction begins 4–5 days after injury and will gradually increase over the next few weeks. On or about 24 days after injury there is a marked decrease in wound contraction (Bumsted, Panje and Ceilley, 1983). When a facial cutaneous defect has adjacent tissue that is firmly attached to underlying bone or cartilage the resultant healing will be excellent. This is because there will be minimum contraction of the surrounding skin, allowing granulation tissue to build up, which is then followed by epithelial ingrowth from the edges (James and Newcombe, 1961). The areas where this best applies are the medial canthal region, the temple, the midline forehead, and the nasolabial area. Contraction and scarring are more prominent in areas of loose skin and areas with excessive motion. Since mature scars tend to be hypopigmented and relatively avascular, the best results with healing by secondary intention (as with any other method) are in fair-skinned individuals. Areas of denuded cartilage or bone will not form granulation tissue and must be modified if this technique is employed. Small punches can be taken out of the cartilage to expose

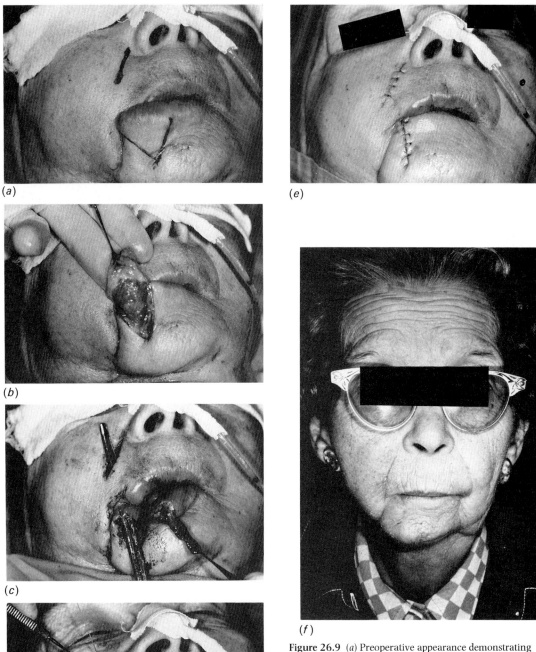

Figure 26.9 (*a*) Preoperative appearance demonstrating labial sphincter incompetence because of oral cancer operation. Patient had poor speech, with drooling and facial disfigurement. Markings indicate planned incisions. (*b*) Orbicularis oris exposed and preserved. Excess labial skin and mucosa were excised. (*c*) A superior labial tunnel was created to allow insertion of the orbicularis muscle remnant. (*d*) Orbicularis muscle was sutured to underlying facial musculature (quadratus labii superioris). (*e*) Immediate postoperative view. (*f*) Appearance 1 year later. Note symmetry and approximation of lips. Oral competency was restored

granulation forming perichondrium from the opposite side. Similarly the outer cortex of bone can be removed to expose the underlying and reparative medullary bone.

The beneficial effects of healing by secondary intention can be used as an adjunct to another reconstructive technique (Goldwyn and Rueckert, 1977). In large midface defects or where surgical margins are not certain, the wound is left to granulate in a semiocclusive environment. After 24 days, maximum contraction will have occurred and the wound bed will have filled in considerably with very vascular tissue. A circumferential strip of granulation tissue and marginal skin are excised to break up the tension forces and the central mass of granulation is debrided to remove any fibrin and crosshatched. A very thick split-thickness or full-thickness skin graft can then be used. If a flap is the more appropriate option, the surgeon will have had ample time for planning. The now contracted wound would not require as large a flap for closure, minimizing the donor defect and the cosmetic results should be much improved.

Skin grafting

A thin split-thickness skin graft will rarely provide the best cosmetic result in reconstructing head and neck defects, however there are some advantages.

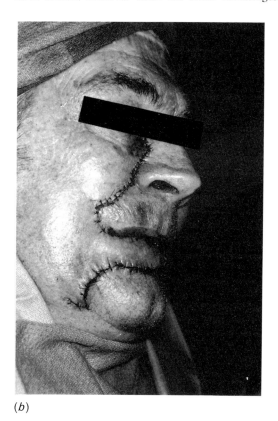

(*b*)

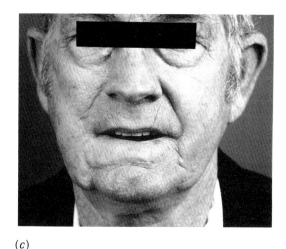

(*a*)   (*c*)

Figure 26.10 (*a*) Appearance following full thickness lip excision. An inferiorly based nasolabial flap has been elevated. (*b*) Following transposition of the nasolabial flap. Note that the medial limb of the flap was extended into the lower lip to provide better approximation of tissues. (*c*) Appearance 2 years following lip reconstruction

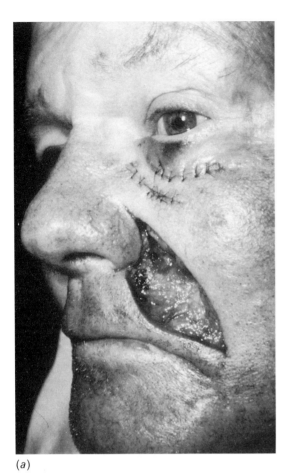

(a)

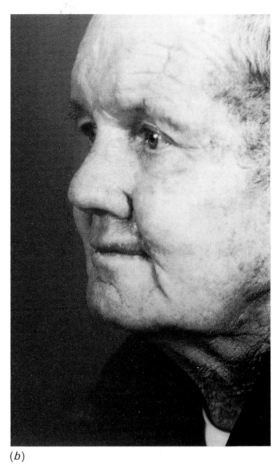

(b)

Figure 26.11 (*a*) Patient following removal of a large skin cancer involving the lip and cheek. (*b*) Four weeks later the wound has completely healed by secondary intention without the use of grafts or flaps

The technique for harvesting and applying grafts is simple and easily learned. The thinner the graft the better the chance of survival during the plasmatic imbibition phase. Because of the abundance of capillaries in the superficial dermis, these thin grafts revascularize rapidly even on relatively poor wound beds. There is generally no hair growth but the thinner grafts tend to contract much more. Split skin grafts will not hide or obscure areas where a cancer recurrence is possible, however, they produce an invariably poor cosmetic result and offer little protection and poor durability. Cosmesis can be substantially improved by using postauricular, neck or supraclavicular skin as the donor tissue and by applying the delayed technique previously described. In darker skinned individuals, hyperpigmentation of split skin grafts can generally be expected. Skin harvested from previous donor areas, if available, does not tend to become hyperpigmented and can be predictably applied to facial defects. Another

alternative is to use a dermal graft. A dermatome is used to cut a thin split skin graft (0.012 in, 0.03 cm), with care to leave the distal end of the graft attached. A new blade is placed on the dermatome and a second graft (0.014–0.016 in, 0.04 cm) is harvested from the exposed area. The split skin graft is then reapplied and fixed to the donor site providing the ideal biological dressing and much less donor morbidity for the patient. The dermal graft will take and survive similarly to a split skin graft and will have less of a tendency to hyperpigmentation (Smiler *et al.*, 1977).

A full-thickness skin graft or a thick split skin graft will not contract as much as a thin split-thickness skin graft and will provide better protection and cushioning to underlying tissues. One alternative for small defects of the nasal tip or lower eyelid is the perichondrial–cutaneous graft (Stucker and Shaw, 1992). Up to 2.5 × 4 cm of tissue can be harvested from each conchal bowl. This composite of full thickness skin, minimal subcutaneous tissue, and perichondrium offers a relatively thick, nicely coloured graft that can be applied just as a full thickness skin graft. The addition of the perichondrial layer allows for rapid revascularization.

The preparation of the recipient bed and the fixation of the graft are crucial to the overall success with any kind of free graft. There must be absolute haemostasis and a relatively level bed so that the chance of a haematoma is very small. The graft is first fixed circumferentially with sutures. Small incisions are made through the graft to allow egress of fluids. Quilting stitches are liberally placed to improve graft contact with the vascular bed, limit graft motion, and reduce the chance of haematoma. The need for a pressure dressing will depend on the size and location of the graft. If used, a bolster of cotton soaked in glycerin is fashioned to conform precisely to the graft site. A layer of bacitracin ointment is applied to the graft first, followed by a strip of non-adherent gauze followed by the bolster. Sutures are placed around the periphery of the graft site (not at the graft–skin junction) and left long to use as ties to secure the bolster. The bolster is kept moist with bacitracin and is removed after 5–7 days.

Flaps

The basic principles of flap dynamics and application apply to all techniques, from the simplest local advancement flap to the most complicated composite free flap transfer. In managing cutaneous loss, flaps offer the advantage of one stage repair with generally excellent colour, bulk and texture. Proper planning can minimize the morbidity caused at the donor area and give the patient the best possible result. An understanding of the vascular anatomy of muscle and skin is essential for a successful flap transfer (Panje, 1984). All skin is supplied by either small perforating branches from named musculocutaneous arteries or by direct (septocutaneous) arteries (Figure 26.12). In humans the vast majority of skin is supplied from musculocutaneous perforators, however, there are several areas where flaps can be designed to take advantage of a major vascular supply. It is the presence of this feeding vessel in the pedicle of the flap that will determine the size or length of transferrable tissue. As Milton clearly stated: 'Flaps made under the same conditions of blood supply survive to the same length, regardless of width. The only effect of decreasing width is to reduce the chance of the pedicle containing a large vessel' (Milton, 1970).

Flaps can be logically split into axial and random patterned (McGregor and Morgan, 1973). Random denotes the vascular supply is dependent solely on the subdermal–dermal plexus, whereas axial means there is an identifiable vessel within the pedicle. The

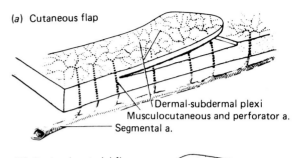

(a) Cutaneous flap

Dermal-subdermal plexi
Musculocutaneous and perforator a.
Segmental a.

(b) Peninsula arterial flap

Dermal-subdermal plexi

Direct cutaneous a. (and vein)

Dermal-subdermal plexi

(c) Island arterial flap
Direct cutaneous a. (and vein)

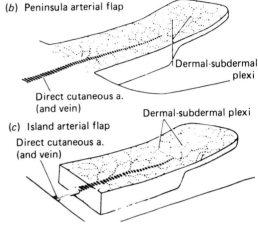

Figure 26.12 Examples of cutaneous and arterial flaps (after Daniel and Williams, 1973)

axial supply can be a large perforating branch from a musculocutaneous artery or from a direct cutaneous artery and there can be both axial and random portions within the same flap. Predicting how much tissue will survive on a certain pedicle design is obviously critical to success. The concept of an angiosome was developed as a way of understanding the macrocirculation of flaps (Taylor and Palmer, 1987). An angiosome represents an anatomical unit with an intrinsic vascular architecture supplied by a major perforator. Adjacent angiosomes are joined by choke areas or transitional zones where the individual vascular supplies merge. Taylor feels that adjacent angiosomes (i.e. one choke zone) can survive on the vascular input of only one perforator, however the perfusion pressure of only one perforator will not reliably supply beyond a second choke zone. Surgeons can use a doppler to map out the major perforators around the defect, design a flap that adheres to the above principle, and expect success.

The skin island on a musculocutaneous flap can be considered axially supplied as long as it overlies the muscle. Once the edge of the muscle is reached, any additional skin is randomly supplied. Predicting how much of this random extension will survive can be quite difficult but will generally be less than 6–7 cm (Haughey and Panje, 1985). Surgical delay can be used with either a random or axially supplied flap to increase the amount of transferable tissue and/or improve the survivability of the flap. Blood flow to a particular area of skin is dynamic and when a flap is lifted a large part of the collateral circulation is suddenly stopped. The vascular supply must re-equilibrate with respect to the input that remains. Delaying implies partially incising and raising a flap then returning it to its original position. The trauma of this initial surgery disrupts many of the sensory nerves and divides portions of the sympathetic innervation. With the loss of sympathetic tone there is a profound vasodilatation, particularly in the arteriovenous shunts. The delayed tissue experiences an increase in vascular volume and flow rates. Most surgeons feel the flap will have an increased tolerance to ischaemia, however, it is the increased nutrient blood flow that gives delayed tissue its ability to survive (Kerrigan and Hjortdal, 1992).

Once a particular flap has been chosen it should be designed so that it will fill the defect precisely. Flaps that are too large will be compressed when inset into the defect. This will have a kinking effect on the subdermal plexus and may increase the haemodynamic microcirculatory resistance leading to skin necrosis (Panje, 1984). There should be virtually no tension on the flap–defect interface. If suture tension is needed to overcome resistance from the vascular base of the flap, then the flap must be repositioned, redesigned, or abandoned in favour of a better alternative. The use of local flaps to close small defects of the face or neck creates a secondary defect that must be closed as well. Being attentive to the lines of maximum tissue extensibility in designing the flap will allow the surgeon to use the laxness of surrounding tissue to his advantage. For example, the surgeon can turn a ragged defect into a parallelogram with 60° and 120° angles (Figure 26.13). If he orientates two of the sides of the defect parallel to the lines of maximum extensibility (i.e. perpendicular to facial wrinkles), the laxness of the surrounding skin will allow the flap to be inset and the donor defect to be closed (Figure 26.14). Absolute haemostasis, adequate drainage and an aseptic technique are always imperative for success.

When a flap looks or becomes ischaemic, the surgeon must be prepared to act. Tolerance to ischaemia varies with the type of tissue involved, with skin being the most resistant (up to 8–10 hours) and intestine being the least (only 2–4 hours) (Panje, 1984). Flap ischaemia generally means a technical problem and obvious factors such as pedicle kinking, constriction, or haematoma must be looked for. The surgeon can look at capillary refilling, flap temperature, turgor, or colour but if it does not bleed when punctured with an 18 gauge needle it is probably not being perfused. Free flaps must be explored at once

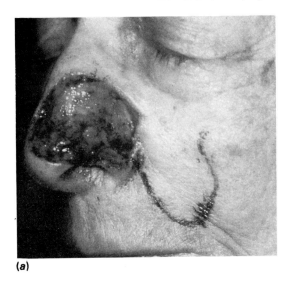

(a)

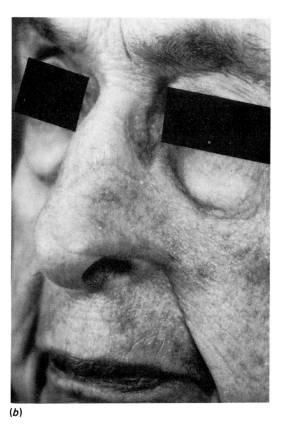

(b)

Figure 26.13 (*a*) A rotation flap is designed so that it takes full advantage of the lines of maximal extensibility to close the donor site. (*b*) Following rotation of flap and healing

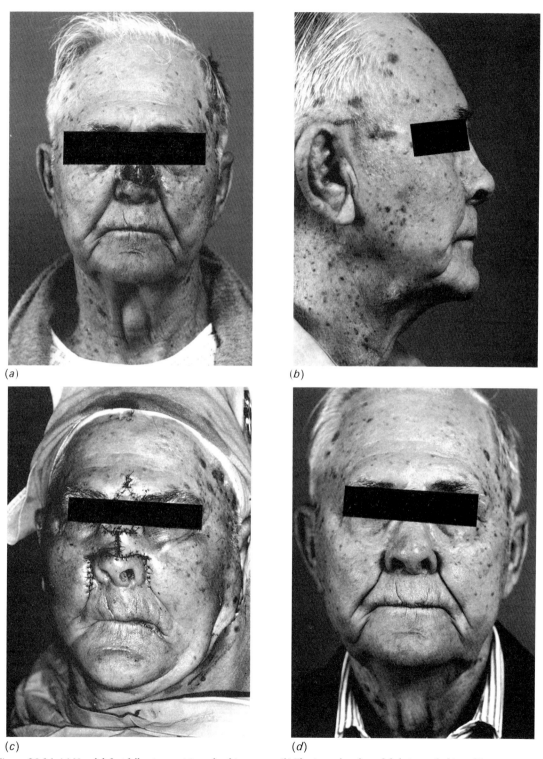

(a)

(b)

(c)

(d)

Figure 26.14 (*a*) Nasal defect following excision of a skin cancer. (*b*) The irregular-shaped defect was fashioned into a rectangular shape and then closed with bilateral nasolabial flaps and a V to Y advancement of nasal glabella skin. (*c*) and (*d*) Appearance 6 months later

as vascular insufficiency means total flap failure. Musculocutaneous and cutaneous flaps can be systematically evaluated. Epidermis is debrided to check for deep dermal bleeding, then dermis and so forth down to the bare muscle if necessary. Debridement stops as soon as viable tissue is encountered. Often, a significant portion of the flap can be salvaged. The vascular pedicle of a flap (including a free flap) should be protected. The position, torsion, and tension of the pedicle should be totally controlled and fixed in the operating room. The surgeon must carefully monitor the transfer of the patient from the operating table to the stretcher, from the stretcher to the bed, and subsequently to the chair to ensure proper head position and support. A beautiful reconstruction in the operating room can easily fail because of overzealous nursing or inattention to detail postoperatively.

Oral cavity and oropharyngeal reconstruction

The surgical defects resulting from the excision of a large oral cavity or oropharyngeal cancer can be physically mutilating and functionally devastating to such actions as eating, breathing, tasting, smelling, hearing and seeing. The reconstructive surgeon is given the task of restoring the functional and aesthetic integrity of the area. With the multitude of techniques currently available, he can choose a refined and individual approach that meets the needs of a particular patient.

Any patient undergoing a large resection of the oral cavity or oropharynx will have some degree of dysphagia and aspiration. Most patients can adapt to losses of up to 50% of any single region without much morbidity but major defects often encompass adjoining regions. The finest reconstruction cannot recreate the complex neuromuscular function necessary for a normal swallow. A systematic analysis of the areas that have been removed or affected by the excision will help the surgeon in managing the expected defect.

Once food is in the mouth it must be transported to the oropharynx. A good lip seal and oral competence are the first considerations. If at all possible, any lip reconstruction should be done with local tissue of the face, maintaining muscular and neural integrity. A sling of facia lata or gortex can be used to suspend an incompetent lower lip. Bolus preparation and transport are a function of the tongue and floor of the mouth. The tongue must be able to contact the hard palate to move food posteriorly. The tongue and the floor of the mouth are reconstructed as separate structures with care to maintain a lingual vestibule, and preserve tongue mobility. Tongue mobility should be a primary goal of any reconstructive technique dealing with this area.

The involuntary aspects of the swallow occur once the food bolus reaches the oropharynx. The hyoid is pulled anteriorly by the submental musculature and the tongue base moves superiorly and posteriorly to contact the posterior pharynx. The larynx follows the pull of the hyoid and tilts up under the tongue base. Tongue bulk is thus an important aim in base of tongue reconstruction and laryngeal suspension from the anterior jaw is a helpful adjunct whenever the submental musculature has been disrupted.

The soft palate will simultaneously elevate to seal off the nasopharynx and prevent nasal reflux. When soft palate competence is lost as a result of surgery, velopharyngeal narrowing via a palatal or pharyngeal flap may be necessary.

The last part of the swallow is cricopharyngeal relaxation. Laryngeal elevation displaces the cricoid anteriorly and superiorly while a pharyngeal reflex relaxes the upper oesophageal sphincter. The cricopharyngeal region thus opens allowing passage of the bolus. The vocal cords have already approximated and the aryepiglottic folds close at the beginning of the oropharyngeal swallow. This contraction pulls the arytenoids up to the base of the epiglottis providing maximum protection of the airway as the bolus passes. This whole action takes place in just over 2 seconds so it is easy to understand how it can become incoordinated (Logemann, 1991). The result is dysphagia, pooling of secretions and aspiration. A cricopharyngeal myotomy is often quite beneficial to patients with an altered swallow.

The success of any reconstruction will be measured primarily by how well the patient ultimately gets on with his day-to-day life. Any surgeon involved with reconstructing these defects must combine his understanding of the expected morbidity with contemporary reconstruction and well-planned rehabilitation. It is not appropriate to undertake these complex operations without the support of a competent radiation therapist, oncologist, dentist, speech pathologist, prosthodontist, nurse and social worker.

Specific guidelines

Reconstruction of the anterior two-thirds of the tongue must aim to maintain the maximum mobility possible. Defects created by a laser can be left to granulate with little worry about slough, infection, pain, or significant scar formation with secondary contracture (Panje, Scher and Karnell, 1989). Wounds produced by the scalpel or diathermy should either be closed primarily or covered with a split skin or dermal graft.

The key to reconstructing through-and-through defects of the oral cavity is to re-establish muscular support for the floor of the mouth and treat the floor of the mouth and tongue as separate structures. When the mandibular arch remains intact all that is required is to replace the missing soft tissue. Primary closure of the mylohyoid is done whenever possible but often a flap will have to be used to replace the defect. Some examples of local flaps are the hyoglossal (Barton and Ucmakli, 1977), platysmal (Coleman, Nahai and Mathes, 1982), and superiorly based sternocleidomastoid flap (Hamaker, 1986), temporoparietal fascia (Panje and Morris, 1991) and nasolabial flap (Mutimer and Poole, 1987). The common thread with these examples is the limited bulk and maximum pliability of the tissue provided. Inferiorly pedicled musculocutaneous flaps, like the pectoralis major, will contract over time as the muscle atrophies. This inferior tethering and pull can adversely affect the mobility of the floor of the mouth and/or tongue and reduce function. Free flaps have been applied with great success to floor of the mouth reconstructions (Panje, 1981). The cutaneous sensation of the radial forearm skin can be re-established by microneural techniques providing a reconstruction with sensation (Urken *et al.*, 1990). This sensory information can be a tremendous help in the oral transport phase of the swallow. Another unique reconstruction is the gastro-omental free flap (Panje, Little and Moran, 1987). This tissue provides the patient with a secreting mucosal surface which can help the dysphagia secondary to radiation xerostomia.

When only one half of the tongue base has been removed and there is good contralateral function, the setback of the anterior tongue into the base defect provides an excellent reconstruction (Panje, 1987). It provides base of tongue bulk and maintains mobility in the anterior tongue. When the function of both hypoglossal nerves is lost along with most of the tongue mass there is a major problem. Any anterior tongue is maintained to provide sensory information important in initiating a swallow. Airway protection becomes the critical determinant on how best to proceed. If a patient is medically unstable, debilitated, handicapped, or alcoholic then a total laryngectomy is in order. This would greatly simplify the overall reconstruction as the surgeon only needs to recreate a funnel. With motivated and healthy patients laryngeal preservation should be a goal of the reconstruction. The reconstructed tongue must then have enough bulk to contact the hard palate. Bone grafts or wire suspension support will provide a scaffolding to help maintain its position. The movements still available to the patient (i.e. cheek retraction, jaw activity) will thus have a stable structure to work against allowing oral transport of the bolus. Laryngeal suspension and cricopharyngeal myotomy are crucial elements of any total tongue reconstruction. A temporary epiglottoplasty (Biller, Lawson and Beck, 1983) or laryngotracheal diversion (Eisele *et al.*, 1989) should also be considered as it will protect the airway while the patient learns to swallow. Again the best success with total or near total tongue reconstruction has come with sensate free flaps such as the radial forearm or the latissimus dorsi.

Mandibular reconstruction

The overall impact that an intact lower jaw has on cosmesis and function means that reconstructive surgeons must be well versed in how to manage mandibular defects. The basic principles of mandibular reconstruction were initially developed for non-vascularized autologous bone grafts. Since these grafts undergo resorption and substitution during healing, strict adherence to an aseptic environment is essential. There must also be rigid fixation so that no movement at the jaw–graft junction occurs. In the past there was an unacceptable degree of osteomyelitis, malunion, and graft failure with primary reconstruction so the prevailing philosophy was to do a secondary reconstruction. Once adequate soft tissue replacement had occurred and there was complete healing, the bone graft could be inserted without exposing it to oral contamination. With the development of modern fixation techniques, vascularized soft tissue flaps, and vascularized bone flaps there has been a great shift to immediate reconstruction of the jaw (Figure 26.15). Since the vascularized bone

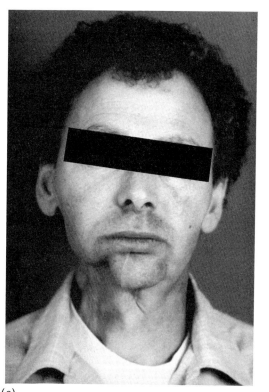

(a)

Figure 26.15 (*a*) Appearance of a patient following composite resection of a floor of the mouth cancer. He had had previous unsuccessful radiation therapy. The midline osteotomy became infected with subsequent osteoradionecrosis.

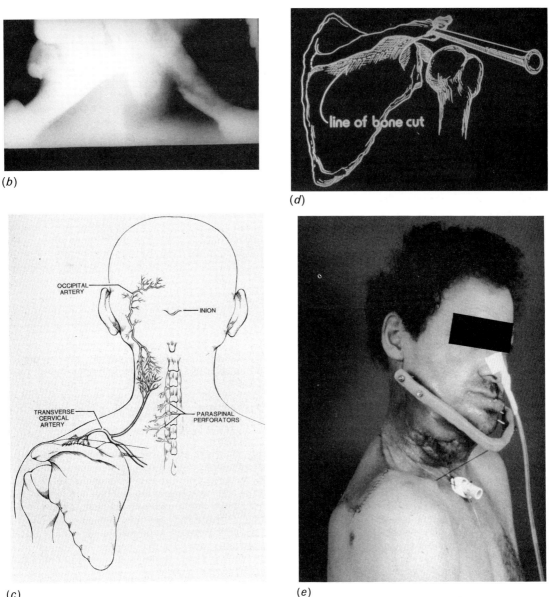

Figure 26.15 (*b*) Radiograph reveals extensive osteoradionecrosis of the jaw and sequestrum. (*c*) Vascular architecture necessary for development of a compound trapezius osteo musculoscapular spine flap based upon the transverse cervical artery. (*d*) Removal of scapular spine. (*e*) Early postoperative appearance – a biphase appliance holds the mandibular fragments in place with scapular spine wired into place.

brings its own blood supply it is much more tolerant of oral contamination and success rates have become acceptable. The surgeon must now decide if reconstructing the jaw is in the best interests of the patient. Several excellent sources of vascularized bone are available to restore the loss of contour and provide a good cosmetic result, however, functional rehabilitation is frequently of greater concern for patients. The added surgical time, risk of failure, and need for multiple operations inherent with any complex recon-

struction must be carefully considered. The reconstruction of mandibular ramus defects common with lateral composite resections may, in fact, be significantly detrimental to postoperative function. The cosmetic defect secondary to these lateral defects can be minimized substantially by providing adequate soft tissue replacement and preventing mandibular drift during healing. This is accomplished by either internal or external fixation for 4–6 weeks and/or isometric exercises.

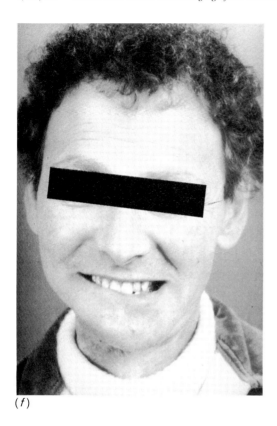

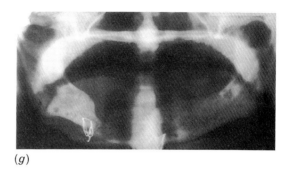

(*g*)

(*f*)

Figure 26.15 (*f*) Appearance 1 year later. Wears dentures with excellent oral rehabilitation. (*g*) Panorex radiograph 1 year later

A composite resection of the anterior floor of the mouth and jaw produces devastating functional and cosmetic morbidity. There are instances when an elaborate reconstruction is not the appropriate option even for these defects. Severely debilitated or elderly patients will not tolerate the extended operating time or degree of postoperative rehabilitation necessary. If tongue function is significantly compromised as well, any hope of oral intake is remote. The lower lip can be suspended from the zygoma to maintain oral competence and the patient is fed with a gastrostomy tube. In most patients, however, these anterior defects need to be reconstructed. It is unreasonable for a single surgeon to manage an extensive resection of an oral cancer and then undertake a complicated reconstruction. The reconstruction with vascularized bone flaps often takes more time and greater attention than the excision. Attempting such an undertaking is certainly unwise and risks serious complications. A team approach is probably the best option with one group of surgeons removing the cancer and another group performing the reconstruction. Another approach would be to delay the reconstruction for a few days during which time the wound is packed. Not only will this provide time for the surgeon and patient to recover from the stress of the first opera-

tion, but will allow the pathologist to study the specimen and confirm adequacy of margins by paraffin sections. The last approach would be to reconstruct the soft tissue defect only and replace the mandibular defect with a metal plate. This plate will stabilize the remaining jaw segments and provide adequate cosmesis for the patient. This is a relatively easier alternative for the surgeon and can be completed in a much shorter operative time (Shockley and Weissler, 1991). A period of surveillance for tumour recurrence can follow after which the defect can be reconstructed with a bone flap or graft. Maximizing success with mandibular metal plating requires some attention to detail. A minimum of three-screw fixation is required on each fragment plated. If possible, plates are always adjusted and set before any bony resection. Titanium or vitallium are preferred because of their excellent tissue compatibility, suitable rigidity, and because they are non-ferromagnetic.

When considering the benefits and drawbacks of the various approaches and techniques for reconstituting a jaw, the surgeon must include the applicability of implants. Osseointegration has greatly enhanced the potential dental rehabilitation for these patients (van Steenbergh *et al.*, 1991). A functioning dental prosthesis is an advantage and by providing one the surgeon can do wonders for the overall self-esteem and well-being of these patients.

Hypopharyngeal and oesophageal reconstruction

The replacement of the pharynx and/or oesophagus can be a very complex undertaking. The circumference and length of the defect is the single most important factor in determining which reconstruction is best suited. As with any situation, a logical approach keeping things simple, will facilitate the success of the operation. Primary closure is the preferred technique for partial pharyngeal defects whenever certain criteria are met. The mucosal edges that will make the anastomosis must be well vascularized. When making the incisions to ablate the tumour, the surgeon should go through the pharyngeal musculature and mucosa cleanly. This will prevent having mucosa with a tenuous blood supply and reduce postoperative infection or fistula. There must be enough mucosa left to provide a minimum of a 34 French conduit. A narrower gullet will have an increased risk of stenosis and cause problems with speech rehabilitation. The mucosal edges are internally everted.

When there is residual mucosa running the full length of a defect but primary closure would create too small a lumen, a split skin or dermal graft can be employed. A salivary bypass stent is inserted to bridge the defect and provide a template for the neopharynx. The graft is sutured to the edges of the mucosa and tented snugly over the stent with the skin/superficial dermal surface facing internally. A well-vascularized flap is placed over the exposed surface of the graft to act as the recipient bed. There are many flaps – levator scapulae (Goodman and Donald, 1990), sternocleidomastoid (Hamaker, 1986), deltopectoral (Chaffoo and Goode, 1988), pectoralis major (Ariyan, 1979), latissimus dorsi (Maves, Panje and Shagets, 1984), trapezius (Panje and Cutting, 1980) – which will provide the adequate vascularized tissue a particular defect might require. An external pressure dressing is kept in place for 5–7 days and the bypass stent removed endoscopically in 6–8 weeks.

When facing a total circumferential defect above the cricopharyngeus, the free jejunal graft gives the best possible reconstruction (McDonough and Gluckman, 1988). It provides a secreting, mucosally-lined tube with peristalsis which comes close to providing an identical tissue replacement. The upper and lower pharyngeal and oesophageal anastomoses will be circumferential so the surgeon must lengthen the scar to help prevent stricture. This can be done by modifying the jejunum to provide an oblique anastomosis. When segments of jejunum longer that 10 cm are

used an end-to-side oesophagojejunal anastomosis is preferred with the end of the flap brought out to the skin as a controlled fistula.

Major pharyngo-oesophageal reconstructions carry a significant morbidity and mortality. Gastric pull-up mortality can be as high as 40%, although most centres report only about a 10% incidence (Harrison, 1986). This high figure is tempered by the fact that a pull-up provides true palliation for a very debilitated group of patients. They are able to swallow effectively and the new gullet is fairly resistant to the ingrowth of recurrent/persistent tumour. Morbidity from an intra-abdominal donor site must be appreciated as well. Peritonitis, intestinal necrosis, diaphragmatic herniation, haemorrhage and anastomotic leaks have all been reported (Harrison, 1986).

References

ARIYAN, S. (1979) The pectoralis major myocutaneous flap. *Plastic and Reconstructive Surgery*, **63**, 73–81

BARTON, R. T. and UCMAKLI, A. (1977) Treatment of squamous cell carcinoma of the floor of mouth. *Surgery, Gynecology and Obstetrics*, **145**, 21–27

BILLER, H. F., LAWSON, W. and BECK, S. (1983) Total glossectomy. A technique of reconstruction eliminating laryngectomy. *Archives of Otolaryngology*, **109**, 69–73

BUMSTED, R. M., PANJE, W. R. and CEILLEY, R. I. (1983) Delayed skin grafting in facial reconstruction. *Archives of Otolaryngology*, **109**, 178–184

BURGET, G. C. and MENICK, F. C. (1989) Nasal support and lining: the marriage of beauty and blood supply. *Plastic and Reconstructive Surgery*, **84**, 189–203

CHAFFOO, R. A. and GOODE, R. L. (1988) Modification of the deltopectoral flap for pharyngoesophageal reconstruction. *Laryngoscope*, **98**, 460–462

COLEMAN, J. J., NAHAL, F. and MATHES, S. J. (1982) Platysmal musculocutaneous flap: clinical and anatomical considerations in head and neck reconstruction. *American Journal of Surgery*, **144**, 477–481

DANIEL, R. K. and WILLIAMS, H. B. (1973) The free transfer of skin flaps by microvascular anastomosis. *Plastic and Reconstructive Surgery*, **52**, 16–31

EISELE, D. W., YARRINGTON, C. T. JR, LINDEMAN, R. C. and LARABEE, W. F. JR (1989) The tracheoesophageal diversion and laryngotracheal separation procedures for treatment of intractable aspiration. *American Journal of Surgery*, **157**, 230–236

GOLDWYN, R. M. and RUECKERT, F. (1977) The value of healing by secondary intention for sizeable defects of the face. *Archives of Surgery*, **112**, 285–292

GOODMAN, A. L. and DONALD, P. J. (1990) Use of the levator scapulae muscle flap in head and neck reconstruction. *Archives of Otolaryngology – Head and Neck Surgery*, **116**, 1440–1444

HAMAKER, R. C. (1986) Oral cavity and oropharyngeal reconstruction. In: *Otolaryngology – Head and Neck Surgery*, edited by C. Cummings, J. H. Frederickson, L. A. Harker, C. J. Krause and D. E. Schuller. St Louis: Mosby Year Book. pp. 1526–1527

HARRISON, D. F. N. (1986) Pharyngolaryngoesophagectomy with pharyngogastric anastomosis for cancer of the hypopharynx. Review of 101 operations. *Head and Neck Surgery*, **8**, 418–428

HAUGHEY, B. H. and PANJE, W. R. (1985) Extension of the musculocutaneous flap by surgical delay. *Archives of Otolaryngology*, **111**, 234–240

JAMES, D. W. and NEWCOMBE, J. F. (1961) Granulation tissue resorption during free and limited contraction of skin wounds. *Journal of Anatomy*, **95**, 247–255

KERRIGAN, C. L. and HJORTDAL, V. E. (1992) Skin flap physiology and pathophysiology. In: *Local Flaps and Free Skin Grafts*, edited by J. Bardach. St Louis: Mosby Year Book. pp. 24–41

LOGEMANN, J. A. (1991) Approaches to management of disordered swallowing. *Clinical Gastroenterology*, **5**, 269–280

MCDONOUGH, J. J. and GLUCKMAN, J. L. (1988) Microvascular reconstruction of the pharyngoesophagus with free jejunal grafts. *Microsurgery*, **9**, 116

MACFEE, W. F. (1960) Transverse incisions for neck dissection. *Annals of Surgery*, **151**, 279–284

MCGREGOR, I. A. (1980) *Fundamental Techniques of Plastic Surgery*. Edinburgh: Churchill Livingstone

MCGREGOR, I. A. and MORGAN, R. G. (1973) Axial and random pattern flaps. *British Journal of Plastic Surgery*, **26**, 202–213

MAVES, M. D., PANJE, W. R. and SHAGETS, F. W. (1984) Extended lastissimus dorsi myocutaneous flap reconstruction of major head and neck defects. *Otolaryngology – Head and Neck Surgery*, **92**, 551–558

MILTON, S. H. (1970) Pedicled skin flaps: the fallacy of the length-width ratio. *British Journal of Surgery*, **51**, 502–508

MUTIMER, K. L. and POOLE, M. D. (1987) A review of nasolabial flaps for intraoral defects. *British Journal of Plastic Surgery*, **40**, 472–477

PANJE, W. R. (1981) Free compound groin flap reconstruction of anterior mandibular defects. *Archives of Otolaryngology*, **107**, 17–22

PANJE, W. R. (1984) Musculocutaneous and free flaps: physiology and practical considerations. *Otolaryngology Clinics of North America*, **17**, 401–412

PANJE, W. R. (1987) Immediate reconstruction of the oral cavity. In: *Comprehensive Management of Head and Neck Tumors*, edited by S. Thawley and W. Panje. London: W. B. Saunders. pp. 563–595

PANJE, W. R. and CUTTING, C. (1980) Trapezius osteomyocutaneous island flap for reconstruction of the anterior floor of mouth and mandible. *Head and Neck*, **3**, 66–71

PANJE, W. R. and MORRIS, M. R. (1991) The temporoparietal fascia flap in head and neck reconstruction. *Ear, Nose and Throat Journal*, **70**, 311–317

PANJE, W. R., BURNSTED, R. M. and CEILLEY, R. I. (1980) Secondary intention healing as an adjunct to the reconstruction of mid-facial defects. *Laryngoscope*, **90**, 1148–1154

PANJE, W. R., LITTLE, A. G. and MORAN, W. J. (1987) Immediated free gastro-omental flap reconstruction of the mouth and throat. *Annals of Otology, Rhinology and Laryngology*, **96**, 15–21

PANJE, W. R., SCHER, N. and KARNELL, M. (1989) Transoral carbon dioxide laser ablation for cancer, tumors and other diseases. *Archives of Otolaryngology – Head and Neck Surgery*, **115**, 681–688

SHOCKLEY, W. W. and WEISSLER, M. C. (1991) Immediate mandibular replacement using reconstruction plates. *Archives of Otolaryngology – Head and Neck Surgery*, **117**, 745–749

SMILER, D., RADACK, K., BILOVSKY, P. and MONTEMARANO, P. (1977) Dermal graft – a versatile technique for oral surgery. *Oral Surgery*, **43**, 342–349

STUCKER, F. J. and SHAW, G. Y. (1992) The perichondrial cutaneous graft. A 12-year clinical experience. *Archives of Otolaryngology – Head and Neck Surgery*, **118**, 287–292

TAYLOR, G. I. and PALMER, J. H. (1987) The vascular territories (angiosomes) of the body: experimental study and clinical applications. *British Journal of Plastic Surgery*, **40**, 113–141

URKEN, M. L., WEINBERG, H., VICKERY, C. and BILLER, H. F. (1990) The neurofasciocutaneous radial forearm flap in head and neck reconstruction: a preliminary report. *Laryngoscope*, **100**, 161–173

VAN STEENBERGH, D., BRANEMARK, P. I., QUIRYNEN, M., DEMARS, G. and NAERT, I. (1991) The rehabilitation of oral defects by osseointegrated implants. *Journal of Clinical Periodontology*, **18**, 488–493

ZITELLI, J. A. (1983) Wound healing by secondary intention. A cosmetic appraisal. *Journal of the American Academy of Dermatology*, **9**, 407–415

27

Terminal care of patients with head and neck cancer

J. R. Hardy

Terminal care in patients with head and neck cancer poses special problems because of the nature of the disease. More than 50% of these patients die from local disease, although the majority will have distant metastases at autopsy (MacDougall, Munro and Wilson, 1993). This chapter discusses the control of pain, the management of oral problems, of nausea and vomiting, wound care and dying in this specific group of patients.

Pain

Pain is the commonest and most feared symptom in patients with advanced malignancy. Pain control in patients with head and neck cancer presents specific problems: the oral route is the preferred route of giving medication to the terminally ill, but is often inappropriate in this group of patients because of difficulty in swallowing secondary to disease or previous treatment. It is therefore necessary to rely on drugs that are either soluble (and therefore more easily swallowed), or those that are able to be delivered by nasogastric or gastrostomy tubes. Alternatively, other routes of drug delivery may be employed, e.g. rectal, sublingual or subcutaneous.

It must be stated that even in this group of patients there is very little indication for giving intramuscular or intravenous drugs to the terminally ill.

World Health Organization (WHO) analgesic ladder

The use of analgesic and adjuvant drugs according to WHO guidelines has been shown to be safe and highly effective for the treatment of pain in head and neck cancer (Grond *et al.*, 1993).

The standard WHO analgesic ladder for the control of cancer pain (WHO, 1986) is shown in Figure 27.1 and is based on oral medications. These guidelines require some modification for head and neck patients as described below, although the basic principles hold: specifically, the regular use of analgesics to maximum dose at each step of the ladder before moving to the next step. It is illogical to try another agent at the same step if the previous agent has failed.

Step 1 – non-opioids

Aspirin and paracetamol are both available as dispersible preparations. Aspirin has more side effects with respect to gastric irritation and therefore should be avoided if possible.

Step 2 – weak opioids

Codeine and dihydrocodeine are weak opioids appropriate for use at step 2 on the analgesic ladder as single agents. Both are available in elixir form.

Many combination analgesics, e.g. co-codamol, co-codaprin and codydramol contain low doses of the opioid component which are subtherapeutic. Combination preparations containing paracetamol 300–500 mg with codeine 30 mg or dextropropoxyphene 32.5 mg are the most frequently employed step 2 analgesics in cancer pain management. Examples are co-proxamol (dextropropoxyphene 32.5 mg, paracetamol 325 mg), or preparations containing paracetamol 500 mg and codeine phosphate 30 mg, e.g. Tylex. Solpadol contains paracetamol 500 mg and codeine phosphate 30 mg and comes in a dispersible preparation.

Aspav comes in a dispersible preparation and contains aspirin 500 mg with mixed opium alkaloids equivalent to papaveretum 10 mg. The papaveretum

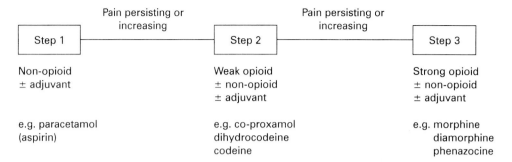

Figure 27.1 Modified WHO-three step analgesic ladder

contains 50% morphine which is the strongest analgesic in the mixture and so there is little advantage over the use of morphine alone, although it can be used as a step 2 analgesic.

Step 3 – strong opioids

Morphine is the WHO strong opioid of choice and comes in several formulations as listed in Table 27.1. The correct dose of morphine is that dose which controls the pain, there being no upper limit. Guidelines for the prescription of morphine are given in Table 27.2. The commonest side effects are nausea, vomiting, drowsiness, constipation and dry mouth. Although side effects tend to resolve after 2–3 days, constipation is an inevitable long-term complication so aperients must always be given in conjunction. Uncommon side effects include confusion, hallucinations, itching and sweating. The respiratory depressant effect of morphine can be used to advantage in patients with advanced malignancy to palliate cough or dyspnoea. This is not usually a problem when using morphine to control pain; pain being a physi-

ological antagonist of the respiratory depressant effects of opioid analgesics (Hanks and Hoskin, 1987).

Care must be taken when titrating morphine in patients with renal impairment. The elimination of one of the active metabolites of morphine (morphine-6-glucuronide) is delayed in this situation such that these patients are likely to require low doses at longer dosage intervals (Portenoy *et al.*, 1991). A few patients (often the elderly) are unable to tolerate morphine. Phenazocine, a strong opioid related to methadone, is the alternative strong opioid of choice in this situation. It is less sedating and has fewer psychotomimetic side effects than morphine and may be given sublingually, although administration by this route is usually avoided because of its bitter taste. One tablet (5 mg) can be considered equivalent to 20–25 mg of morphine. Buprenorphine can also be given sublingually, but has the disadvantage of being a partial-agonist, i.e. has a potential ceiling dose above which increasing the dose will not lead to any further benefit with respect to pain. It also has unpredictable acute side effects in some patients and chronic side effects as with other opioids.

Table 27.1 Morphine formulations commercially available for routine use

1 *Immediate release oral preparations* – duration of action 4 hours	
Morphine sulphate e.g. (Oramorph) oral solution	10 mg/5 ml + taste mask suitable for dose titration
Concentrated oral morphine sulphate solution	100 mg/5 ml (no taste mask)
Morphine sulphate unit dose vials	10 mg/5 ml, 30 mg/5 ml, 100 mg/5 ml
Morphine tablets (Sevredol)	10 mg, 20 mg tablets suitable for those patients intolerant of oral solutions and able to swallow tablets
Morphine suppositories	10, 15, 20, 30, 50, 100 mg
2 *Delayed release oral preparations* – duration of action 12 hours	
Morphine sulphate slow release tablets, e.g. MST, SRM	Available in 5, 10, 30, 60, 100 and 200 mg strength Suitable for patients with good pain control on a stable dose of morphine
Morphine sulphate slow release suspension	Sachet of granules to mix with water
3 *Morphine sulphate injection*	Diamorphine is usually used in preference because of its greater solubility

Table 27.2 Guidelines for the prescription of morphine

1   There is no 'standard dose' of morphine. The dose may range from 5 mg 4-hourly to more than 200 mg 4-hourly (the majority of patients will not need more than 30 mg 4-hourly)

2   Start low and work up using immediate release preparations for dose titration
    A common sequence of dose increments is:
       $10 \rightarrow 15 \rightarrow 20 \rightarrow 30 \rightarrow 40 \rightarrow 60 \rightarrow 80 \rightarrow 100 \rightarrow 120 \rightarrow 150 \rightarrow 200$ mg

3   Prescribe a regular 4-hourly dose

4   Prescribe the same dose for as required (prn) use to be repeated as often as necessary for breakthrough pain

5   A double dose can be prescribed at night to save waking the patient at 03.00 hours (except for doses $\geq$ 300 mg 4-hourly)

6   Review after 24–48 hours and adjust regular dose according to breakthrough requirements

7   Once patients are stable, convert to twice daily slow release morphine preparations

8   Where neither the oral nor rectal route is available, use diamorphine via the subcutaneous route (1/3 oral morphine dose)

9   *Always* prescribe a laxative to be taken concurrently with morphine

10   Prescribe antiemetics on the prn chart

Diamorphine is more soluble than morphine and is therefore the agent of choice when using strong opioids by subcutaneous or intravenous infusion. It should be given at one-third the dose of oral morphine to achieve the same degree of analgesia. The intravenous dose of diamorphine is the same as the subcutaneous dose, but tolerance is thought to develop more rapidly when this route is used. There is never any indication for giving intramuscular opioids.

Co-analgesics

Co-analgesics or adjuvant analgesics often have some primary indication other than pain control but can be used in conjunction with the 'standard' analgesics as listed above for an additive analgesic effect or for special indications.

The non-steroidal anti-inflammatory drugs (NSAIDs) are particularly valuable for the treatment of bone pain or inflammatory lesions. Many of the drugs within this group are available in elixir or suppository form (Table 27.3). Ketoralac and diclofenac can both be given as continuous subcutaneous infusions (Blackwell *et al.*, 1993), but neither is licensed for this indication. Gastrointestinal irritation is the most common side effect and is not avoided by giving the drugs parenterally as this is a systemic effect. There is no evidence that any one agent in this group is any better than the others, but there is considerable variation in individual patient response.

Corticosteroids have both specific indications (e.g. for raised intracranial pressure, cord compression, or the treatment of lymphangitis carcinomatosis) as well as non-specific indications, e.g. mood and appetite stimulation. They can also be very valuable as an adjunct to standard analgesics. Dexamethasone tablets can be crushed and mixed in water and have less mineralocorticosteroid effects than prednisolone and therefore cause less fluid retention. Long-term use results in distressing side effects, however, i.e. proximal weakness, cushinoid habitus and bone demineralization (Twycross, 1992).

Neuropathic pain (that secondary to nerve damage) and nociceptive pain (that caused by ongoing activation of pain receptors) is common in head and neck cancer (Vecht, Hoff and Boer, 1990). Antidepressants, anti-epileptics and some antiarrhythmic agents can all be effective in controlling pain of this type (Dunlop *et al.*, 1988; Glynn, 1989) (Table

Table 27.3 Non-steroidal anti-inflammatory agents (NSAIDs)

	Usual oral dose	*Available in suppository form*	*Elixir or dispersible tablets*
Naproxen	500 mg b.d.	√	√
Diclofenac	50 mg t.d.s.	√	√
Ibuprofen	400 mg t.d.s.	—	√
	–600 mg q.d.s.		
Flurbiprofen	100 mg t.d.s.	√	—
Sulindac	200 mg b.d.	—	—
Indomethacin	50 mg t.d.s.	√	√
Ketoralac	40 mg/day	—	

27.4). The dose required for pain control is usually well below that required for a usual therapeutic effect in their licensed indication and the onset of action is more rapid.

Non-pharmacological analgesia

Palliative chemotherapy or radiotherapy as well as acupuncture, transcutaneous electrical nerve stimulation (TENS), relaxation therapy and massage, can all have a place in the management of pain in some patients. For intractable pain, neurosurgical and anaesthetic techniques, e.g. trigeminal nerve section, high cervical or pontine spinothalamic tractotomy or thalamotomy may be considered (MacDougall, Munro and Wilson, 1993).

Mouth care

Because of the frequency of locally recurrent disease and side effects of treatment, mouth care is of primary importance in patients with head and neck cancer especially when in the terminal phase of illness (Calman and Langdon, 1991). The following are modified from the Royal Marsden Hospital mouth care recommendations.

1 *Routine care/oral hygiene.* Tooth brushing should be encouraged with regular use of a mouth wash, for example chlorhexidine gluconate 0.2%, 5 ml in half a tumbler of water four times a day.
2 *Dry mouth.* This is particularly common in patients who have had radiotherapy. Fluoride appears to stimulate production of saliva in some patients. Fluoride mouth washes and toothpastes are therefore recommended. Many patients find artificial saliva distasteful but may tolerate a lubricant spray. Sucking crushed ice or frozen tonic water can help. Tinned pineapple contains a proteolytic enzyme, ananase, that will stimulate saliva production and also cleanse the mouth.
3 *Coated tongue.* Regular mouth care plus one-quarter of a vitamin C effervescent tablet applied to the tongue four times a day may help.
4 *Fungal infections.* Nystatin suspension 1 ml q.d.s. is a prophylactic dose and 5 ml q.d.s. is required for treatment. Many patients find amphotericin lozenges unpalatable because the tablets are large and sticky. For severe fungal infections fluconazole may be indicated. This can be given intravenously or as an elixir.
5 *Ulcers.* For minor ulcers a choline salicylate dental gel, e.g. Bonjela can give relief. If there is evidence of herpetic infection acyclovir should be prescribed (this is available as a suspension). Sucralfate suspension 5 ml q.d.s. gargled or used as a mouth wash tends to coat ulcers and provides relief in patients with severe ulceration.
6 *Infections.* Anaerobes can often be cultured from infected lesions in the mouth or neck, therefore a suitable penicillin or metronidazole are usually the most appropriate antibiotics.
7 *Halitosis.* The use of a regular mouth wash, for example chlorhexidine mouth wash plus antibiotics (if severe) may help.
8 *Painful mouth.* Adequate systemic analgesia must be given at all times. A paracetamol mouth wash (2 × 500 mg soluble tablets dissolved in water) or aspirin dissolved in lemon mucilage is an appropriate first line medication. For severe local oral pain, for example secondary to extensive painful mucositis, lignocaine 2% gel can be applied. Alternatives include mucaine suspension, lignocaine spray, or sucralfate suspension. In cases such as these intravenous or subcutaneous diamorphine is often required.

Table 27.4 Co-analgesics

			Usual dose	Comments
1	Antidepressants	dothiepin[+] amitriptyline[E]	50–75 mg nocte p.o. 50–150 mg p.o.	Can be useful for control of neuropathic pain at doses well below antidepressant dose
2	Anticonvulsants	carbamazepine[E] sodium valproate[E]	100–200 mg b.d. p.o. 200–800 mg b.d. p.o.	Useful for lancinating and paroxysmal neuropathic pain
3	Antiarrhythmics	flecainide mexiletine	50–200 mg b.d. 150–300 mg t.d.s. o.d.	For neuropathic pain. Use with caution in patients with pre-existing heart disease, rapid onset of action if effective
4	Corticosteroids	dexamethasone[+]	2–8 mg b.d. p.o.	Non-specific plus specific analgesic effect in some patients
5	Benzodiazepines	diazepam[E] lorazepam	2–5 mg b.d.–t.d.s. p.o. 1–2 mg, o.d.–b.d. sublingual, or p.o.	Useful anxiolytic and muscle relaxant effects

[E] Elixir or syrup; [+] tablets that can be crushed or opened; p.o. by mouth

Nausea and vomiting

This is one of the most common symptoms in terminally ill patients and the cause is often multifactorial. Reversible causes, e.g. hypercalcaemia, uraemia, drugs or brain metastases, need to be identified and treated appropriately. In the absence of any obvious cause, any one of the agents listed in Table 27.5 may be appropriate. Drugs from more than one class of antiemetic may be used in combination for nausea and vomiting that is difficult to control.

Metoclopramide, cyclizine and haloperidol can all be given via a subcutaneous infusion. Prochlorperazine is useful in motion or positional sickness. Although the 5HT3 antagonists are very effective for nausea and vomiting induced by chemotherapy or radiotherapy, their use in chronic nausea and vomiting is not established. Methotrimeprazine, a potent antiemetic, is useful in the terminal phase of illness, prior to this its use is limited by a profound sedative effect. Steroids are often the most effective antiemetics and may be the only agents that can give complete control.

Wounds

Appropriate dressings for wounds, e.g. ulcerated tumours or malignant ulcers depend on whether the wound is wet or dry, exudative or malodorous. In the terminal care setting wounds are unlikely to heal so that patient comfort should be the primary aim of any dressing. Each wound requires individual assessment (Table 27.6). The skill of a nurse experienced in this field is often invaluable in finding the dressing best suited to a particular wound. Alginate dressings can help to stop bleeding from fungating wounds especially if the dressing is well moistened prior to a dressing change. Paraffin gauze can be moulded into contours and does not stick to wounds. Itching is often associated with non-broken skin, e.g. superficial nodules. In such cases menthol in aqueous cream has a cooling non-drying effect and can provide relief along with cooled hydrogel sheets. Odorous wounds usually reflect the presence of anaerobic bacteria. Systemic treatment may be indicated but metronidazole gel provides appropriate topical treatment and charcoal dressings can reduce odour. For pain relief during dressing changes, short-acting analgesics, e.g. Entonox gas or dextromoramide tablets may be called for.

The dying patient

The dying patient is often no longer able to take oral medications. Although most medications can usually be phased out at this time it is important to continue analgesics to prevent distress caused by their reduction, especially when the patient has been on opioids. As is discussed above, many analgesics can be given rectally or sublingually, but in this situation, subcutaneous pumps are particularly helpful (Dover, 1987).

Terminal restlessness is distressing to patients and relatives. Midazolam, a water-soluble benzodiazepine is the agent of choice in this situation, although diazepam and chlorpromazine are alternatives. Midazolam can be mixed with diamorphine in a subcutaneous pump and can be titrated until the desired effect is achieved (Bottomley and Hanks, 1990). If nausea and vomiting are significant problems methotrimeprazine is worth considering.

'Death rattles' secondary to retained bronchial secretions are often more distressing to relatives than the patient. These secretions are usually effectively

Table 27.5 Antiemetics

Class		Usual dose	Comments
Gastrokinetics	metoclopramide*E	10–20 mg q.d.s., p.o., i.v. s/c	Avoid in bowel obstruction
	domperidoneE,S	20 mg q.d.s., p.o. or 30–60 mg 4–6 hourly p.r.	
Phenothiazines	chlorpromazineE,S	10–25 mg t.d.s., p.o.	Can cause dry mouth
	prochlorperazineE,S	10 mg t.d.s. p.o., 25 mg t.d.s., p.r.	
	methotrimeprazine*	12.5–25 mg b.d., p.o. 12.5–50 mg 6 hourly s/c	Highly sedative
Butyrophenones	haloperidol*E	1.5–3 mg b.d., p.o. 1.5–4 mg 12 hourly s/c	Sedative, long half-life, can be given once daily
Antihistamines	cyclizine*S	50 mg t.d.s., p.o. 75 mg 12 hourly s/c 100 mg t.d.s., p.r.	Can cause drowsiness and dry mouth
5HT3 antagonists	ondansetron	4–8 mg i.v., p.o., o.d.–b.d.	Effective in chemotherapy and radiotherapy-induced sickness
	granisetron	3 mg i.v. daily	
Corticosteroids	dexamethasone*	2–4 mg t.d.s. p.o., i.v., s/c	

* Can be given subcutaneously (s/c); E elixir or syrup; S suppository available

Table 27.6 Wound management

Type of wound	Appropriate dressing/management
1 Necrotic (with eschar)	Hydrogel, e.g. Intrasite gel (Scherisorb) Enzymes, e.g. Varidase
2 Sloughy	Hydrogel, e.g. Intrasite gel Enzymes, e.g. Varidase Silastic foam + Intrasite gel
3 Infected	Cleaning solutions (sterile sodium chloride) Topical antibiotics (metronidazole gel, silver sulphadiazine) Dressing according to wound type, size, amount of exudate, e.g. alginate products (Sorbsan) Hydrocolloids (Granuflex) Foam dressing (Lyofoam, silastic foam) Hydrogels (Intrasite, Second skin)
4 Granulating and epithelializing	Hydrocolloid sheets or paste or hydrogel sheets for low exudate wounds Alginate ribbon or foam sheets for high exudate wounds

dried with the use of hyoscine hydrobromide 0.4 mg given subcutaneously 4-hourly. In general this should not be given unless the patient is comatose as the drying effect can be distressing.

Massive haemorrhage is not an uncommon terminal event in head and neck patients, e.g. secondary to erosion by tumour into large arteries. If such an event is anticipated it is advisable to have available syringes of midazolam 10 mg and/or diamorphine 10 mg which can be both given subcutaneously or 10 mg of diazepam which could be given rectally. The patient must never be left alone in these circumstances and simple measures such as the use of red towels and a calming presence can help what can be a horrifying situation.

There is considerable controversy with respect to the giving of fluids by intravenous or nasogastric routes to a dying patient (Micetich, Steinecker and Thomasma, 1983; Twycross and Lichter, 1993). Discontinuing these can be distressing to relatives but is often of benefit to the patient, i.e. the resultant dehydration lessens the requirement for suctioning and can reduce pulmonary congestion. The major side effect of dehydration is dry mouth and this can be quite adequately palliated with regular mouth care. To die without lines and tubes allows death with dignity and can break down barriers between patient and family/relatives.

Acknowledgement

The help of J. Mulholland and S. Jones of the Department of Pharmacy, Royal Marsden Hospital is gratefully acknowledged.

References

BLACKWELL, N., BANGHAM, L., HUGHES, M., MELZACK, D. and TROTMAN, I. (1993) Subcutaneous ketorolac – a new development in pain control. *Palliative Medicine*, **7**, 63–65

BOTTOMLEY, D. M. and HANKS, G. W. (1990) Subcutaneous midazolam infusions in palliative care. *Journal of Pain and Symptom Management*, **5**, 259–261

CALMAN, F. and LANGDON, J. (1991) Oral complications of cancer. *British Medical Journal*, **302**, 485–486

DOVER, S. B. (1987) Syringe driver in terminal care. *British Medical Journal*, **294**, 553–555

DUNLOP, R., DAVIES, R. J., HOCKLEY, J. and TURNER, P. (1988) Analgesic effects of oral flecainide. *Lancet*, i, 420

GLYNN, C. (1989) An approach to the management of the patient with deafferation pain. *Palliative Medicine*, **3**, 13–21

GROND, S., ZECH, D., LYNCH, J., DIEFENBACH, C., SCHUG, S. and LEHMANN, K. (1993) Validation of World Health Organisation guidelines for pain relief in head and neck cancer. A prospective study. *Annals of Otology, Rhinology and Laryngology*, **102**, 342–348

HANKS, G. and HOSKIN P. J. (1987) Opioid analgesics in the management of pain in patients with cancer. A review. *Palliative Medicine*, **1**, 1–25

MACDOUGALL, R. H., MUNRO, A. J. and WILSON, J. A. (1993) Palliation in head and neck cancer. In: *Oxford Textbook of Palliative Medicine*, edited by D. Doyle, G. Hanks and N. MacDonald. Oxford: Oxford University Press. pp. 422–433

MICETICH, K. S., STEINECKER, P. H. and THOMASMA, D. C. (1983) Are intravenous fluids morally required for a dying patient? *Archives of Internal Medicine*, **143**, 975–978

PORTENOY, R. K., FOLEY, K. M., STULMAN, J., KHAN, E., ADELHARDT, J. and LAYMAN, M. *et al.* (1991) Plasma morphine and morphine-6-glucuronide during chronic morphine therapy for cancer pain: plasma profiles, steady state concentrations and the consequences of renal failure. *Pain*, **47**, 13–19

TWYCROSS, R. (1992) Corticosteroids in advanced cancer. *British Medical Journal*, **305**, 996–970

TWYCROSS, R. G. and LICHTER, I. (1993) The terminal phase. In: *Oxford Textbook of Palliative Medicine*; edited by D. Doyle, G. W. Hanks and N. MacDonald. Oxford: Oxford University Press, pp. 651–661

VECHT, C. J., HOFF, A. M. and BOER, M. F. (1990) Types and causes of pain in cancer of the head and neck (Abstract). *Pain*, Suppl. 5, 354

WORLD HEALTH ORGANIZATION (1986) *Cancer Pain Relief*. Geneva: WHO

Volume index

Abscesses:
  cervical, 1/11
  mouth, 3/9
  retropharyngeal, 4/5–6, 16/16
  see also Parapharyngeal abscesses;
    Peritonsillar abscesses
Achalasia of the cardia, 2/17
Acquired immune deficiency syndrome
    (AIDS):
  hairy leukoplakia and, 4/14
  neck manifestations, 16/14
  oral manifestations, 3/2
  see also Human immunodeficiency
    virus Actinomycosis, 5/18, 16/14
Adenocarcinoma, 3/16, 23/36
Adenoid cystic carcinoma, 22/5–6,
    23/36
  larynx, 11/37
  salivary glands, 3/16, 21/6–7
  treatment, 3/27
Adenoids, 13/3–4
  radiography, 2/2
Adenolymphoma, 2/18
Adenoma:
  infratemporal fossa, 22/5
  larynx, 11/8
  oxyphil, 20/9
  thyroid gland, 18/17
  see also Pleomorphic adenoma
Adenomatoid odontogenic tumour,
    23/16
Adenovirus, acute tonsillitis and, 4/2
Advancement flaps, 25/4
Aesthesioneuroblastoma, 23/36
Agranulocytosis, 3/2
  pharyngeal symptoms, 4/13
AIDS, *see* Acquired immune deficiency
    syndrome
Air embolism following tracheostomy,
    7/14
Airway obstruction, 7/1–18
  foreign bodies, 1/10

intubation of larynx, 7/1–6
  difficulties, 7/4–5
  indications, 7/2
  positioning of tube, 7/5
  prevention of complications,
    7/5–6
  techniques, 7/2–4
  management options, 7/6–7
  see also Obstructive sleep apnoea;
    Tracheostomy
Alcohol as risk factor, 1/1
  hypopharyngeal cancer, 15/4
  mouth cancer, 3/14
Alkali ingestion, 1/12
Ameloblastic fibro-odontoma, 23/16
Ameloblastic fibrodentinoma, 23/16
Ameloblastic fibroma, 23/15–16
Ameloblastic fibrosarcoma, 23/18
Ameloblastoma, 22/4–5, 23/13–15
  extraosseous, 23/15
  malignant, 23/17
  unicystic, 23/14–15
Amyloidosis, 5/14, 11/4
Anaesthesia, 1/5–6
Analgesics, *see* Terminal care
Aneurysmal bone cyst, 23/12–13
Angina, Ludwig's, 16/17
Angiocentric lymphoma, 23/20–1
Angiofibroma, 12/1–6, 22/4
  behaviour, 12/2–3
  differential diagnosis, 12/4
  investigations, 12/3–4
  pathogenesis, 12/2
  pathology, 12/2
  site of origin, 12/2
  symptoms, 12/3
  treatment, 12/4–6, 22/14–15
    complications of, 12/6
Angiography, 2/21
Angioneurotic oedema, 5/6
Ankyloglossia, 3/2
Antiemetics, 27/5

Aphthous ulceration, 3/5–6
Arytenoid adduction, 9/18–19
Arytenoidectomy, 9/19
Axial flaps, 25/5

Barium swallow, 2/1, 2/14–17, 2/23
Barrett's oesophagus, 24/13–14
Batteries, ingestion of, 1/12, 24/22
Behçet's syndrome, 3/6
Benzocaine, 1/5
Benzodiazepine, 1/5
Besnier–Boeck disease, *see* Sarcoidosis
Bilobed flaps, 25/4–5
Blastomycosis, South American, 5/18
Blepharoplasty, 25/9–10
Bohn's nodule, 23/2–3
Botryoid odontogenic cyst, 23/4
Brain heterotopia, 13/25
Branchial cyst carcinoma, 14/3
Branchial cysts, 16/4–7
  clinical features, 16/6
  embryology, 16/4
  origin, 16/4–5
  pathogenesis, 16/5–6
  terminology, 16/4
  treatment, 16/7
Branchial fistulae, 16/4
  treatment, 16/7
Branchial sinuses, 16/4–7
  clinical features, 16/6
  pathogenesis, 16/5–6
  treatment, 16/7
Branchogenic carcinoma, 16/7
Breathing:
  breath support, 6/3–4
  patterns of, 6/2–3
Bronchial tree, 1/4
  examination of, 1/9
  foreign bodies, 1/10, 1/12–13
Bronchoscopy, 1/3
  complications, 1/10
  laser bronchoscopy, 1/9

Bronchoscopy (*cont.*)
  positioning of patient, 1/5
  rigid, 1/8–9
Brow lift, 25/11–12
Brucellosis, 16/15
Bulimia, parotomegaly and, 19/5
Bullae, 3/6

Calcifying epithelial odontogenic
    tumour, 23/15
Calcifying odontogenic cyst, 23/16–17
Calcitonin, 18/4
Candidiasis, 3/5
  HIV and, 4/14
  laryngeal infection, 5/17
  pharyngeal infection, 4/13
Carcinoma, *see Individual types of
    carcinoma*
Carcinosarcoma, larynx, 11/37
Cardia, achalasia of, 2/17
Carotid body tumours, 16/8, 16/10, 22/7
  treatment, 16/11
Carotid space, 2/11–12
Cat-scratch disease, 16/15
Cavernous lymphangioma, 16/11, 16/12
Cervical spine, endoscopy and, 1/10
Chancre, 3/4, 4/11
Chemical peeling, 25/12
Chemical shift fat suppression, 2/21
Chemodectoma, 22/6–7
Chest pain, 24/3
Chondroma:
  CT scanning, 2/7
  larynx, 11/5–6
Chondrosarcoma, 11/37, 22/8
Chordoma:
  infratemporal fossa, 22/4
  nasopharynx, 13/25
Cigarette smoking, *see* Smoking as risk
    factor
Cineradiography, 2/14–15
Clear cell odontogenic tumour, 23/15
Co-analgesics, 27/3–4
Cocaine, 1/5
Coccidioidomycosis, 5/18
Common cold, 4/8
  laryngitis, 5/1
Communication, non-verbal, 6/1–2
  see also Voice
Composite grafts, 25/3
Computerized tomography, 2/1, 2/5–7,
    2/23
  metastatic neck disease, 17/6
  mouth cancer investigation, 3/17–18
  nodal metastases, 2/13
  oropharynx, 2/20–1
  parapharyngeal region, 2/9–13
  salivary glands, 2/18
Contact granuloma, 5/13–14, 11/3–4
Contact pachydermia, 5/10
Contact ulcers, 5/10, 11/3–4
Cordectomy, 9/19
Corrosives, ingestion of, 1/12
Corticosteroids, 27/3
Coryza, 4/8

Cough, spasmodic, 5/3–4
Coxsackie viruses, 3/3
Craniofacial resections, 23/32–5
Craniopharyngioma, 13/25
Cricoid stenosis, 8/9
Cricopharyngeal myotomy, 10/17–18,
    11/31–2
Cricopharyngeus muscle, 10/2
Cricothyroidotomy, 1/10, 7/7, 7/17–18
  complications, 7/18
  indications, 7/17–18
  techniques, 7/18
Cryotherapy, 3/26
Cystic hygroma, 16/11, 16/12
Cysts, 2/17
  dermoid, 3/8, 16/13
  larynx, 11/1–2
  mouth, 3/8
  nasopharynx, 13/25–6
  salivary gland, 19/11
  tonsils, 4/7
  vocal cords, 6/19
  see also Branchial cysts; Jaws;
    Thyroglossal cysts
Cytomegalovirus, pharyngeal
    infection, 4/10

de Quervain's thyroiditis, 18/13–14
Dental caries, 3/9
Dental plaque, 3/9
Dentigerous cysts, 3/8, 23/5–6
Dermabrasion, 25/12–13
Dermoid cysts, 3/8, 16/13
Dermoids, 13/25
Desmoid tumours, 22/8
Diphtheria, 4/6–7, 9/6–7
  clinical features, 4/6
  diagnosis, 4/6, 9/7
  immunization, 4/6–7
  pathology, 9/6
  prognosis, 9/7
  symptoms, 9/6–7
  treatment, 4/6, 9/7
Diverticula, oesophageal, 10/1, 24/23–4
  see also Pharyngeal diverticula;
    Zenker's diverticulum
Dohlman's operation, 10/13–15
Drug reactions, oral manifestations, 3/2
Dyskeratosis congenita, 3/1
Dysphagia, 24/2–3
  barium swallow demonstration,
    2/14–15
  following tracheostomy, 7/16
  Zenker's diverticulum and,
    10/10–11
Dysphonia:
  habitual, 6/12–13
  hypo- and hyperkinetic forms,
    6/14–15
  spasmodic, 9/11
  see also Voice disorders
Dystonia, laryngeal, 9/11

Earache, following tonsillectomy, 4/22
Electroglottogram, 6/10

Electromyography, 6/10
Endoscopy:
  anaesthesia, 1/5–6
  complications of, 1/9–10, 24/20–1
  flexible, 1/2–4
    sterility, 1/2
  foreign body removal, 1/11–12
  indications, 1/6
  panendoscopy, 1/7
  pharyngoscopy, 1/8
  rigid, 1/4–9
    preparation of patient, 1/4–5
  tumour recording, 1/6
  see also Bronchoscopy;
    Laryngoscopy; Oesophagoscopy
Enteral feeding, 15/13
Epidermoid cyst, 16/13
Epiglottitis, acute, 5/4–5
Epignathus, 13/25
Epstein pearls, 23/10
Epstein–Barr virus:
  acute tonsillitis, 4/2
  infectious mononucleosis, 4/7
  nasopharyngeal carcinoma and,
    13/19–20
Epulis, 3/9–10
Eruption cysts, 3/8, 23/6
Erythema migrans, 3/8
Erythema multiforme, 3/6
Erythroplakia, **mouth cancer and**, 3/15
Eunuchoidism, 6/16–17
Eyelid reconstructive surgery, 26/7–8

Facial plastic surgery, *see* Plastic
    surgery
Fat suppression technique, 2/13
  chemical shift fat suppression, 2/21
Fibroma:
  ameloblastic, 23/15–16
  larynx, 11/7
  nasal, 23/23
  see also Angiofibroma; Neurofibroma
Fish bones, *see* Foreign bodies
Fissural cysts, 23/10–11
Fistulae, 2/17
  branchial, 16/4
    treatment, 16/7
  chylous, 17/11–12
  following tracheostomy, 7/15–16
  salivary gland, 19/11–12
Flap repair:
  oral cavity, 3/24–5
  plastic surgery, 25/3–6, 26/12–15
Fordyces spots, 3/1
Forehead flap, 25/6
Foreign bodies, 1/10–13
  acute foreign body airway
    obstruction, 1/10
  bronchial, 1/10, 1/12–13
  larynx, 1/10, 1/11
  management, 1/11–12
  oesophagus, 1/10–12, 2/15–16,
    24/21–2
  pharynx, 1/11
Fossa of Rosenmüller, 13/1–3

Free flaps, 25/3
Full thickness grafts, 25/2–3
Fusiform excision, 26/5

Ganglioma, 16/8, 22/6
  see also Paraganglioma
Gangrenous stomatitis, 3/4
Gastric transposition, 15/11–12
Gastro-oesophageal reflux, 24/12–16
  Barrett's oesophagus, 24/13–14
  otolaryngological manifestations,
    24/14–16
  pathophysiology, 24/12–13
  symptoms, 24/3
General anaesthesia, 1/5–6
Geographical tongue, 3/8
Gingival cysts, 23/3
  infants, 23/2–3
Gingivitis, 3/9
  acute necrotizing gingivitis, 3/3–4
Glabellar flaps, 25/6
Glandular odontogenic cyst, 23/4–5
Globus pharyngis, 4/10, 9/4–5, 24/25–7
Globus sensation, 24/3, 24/25–7
Glomus tumours:
  carotid space, 2/11–12
  of jugular, 22/7
  of vagus, 16/9, 16/10, 22/7
Glossitis:
  median rhomboid, 3/2
  migratory, 3/8
Glossopharyngeal nerve, 9/1
Glossopharyngeal neuralgia, 9/5–6
Glottic carcinoma, 11/16–19, 11/42
Glottic stenosis, 8/8–9
Glottis, voice generation, 6/4–7
Goitre, 18/7–10
  diffuse non-toxic, 18/7
  diffuse toxic, *see* Grave's disease
  multinodular non-toxic, 18/8–9
  simple, 18/7
  surgery, 18/9–10
  complications of, 18/10
  toxic nodular (Plummer's disease),
    18/12–13
Gonococcal pharyngitis, 4/10
Granular cell myoblastoma, 3/11
Granuloma:
  contact, 5/13–14, 11/3–4
  intubation, 5/13–14, 11/3
  larynx, 11/2–4
  non-healing, 23/18–21
    angiocentric lymphoma, 23/20–1
    Wegener's granulomatosis, 23/19–
      20
Grave's disease, 18/10–12
  pathology, 18/11
  treatment, 18/11–12
    complications of, 18/12
Gumma, 3/4, 4/11

Haemangioma:
  larynx, 11/5
  nasal, 23/23
  oral, 3/10–11

Hairy leukoplakia, AIDS and, 4/14
Hairy tongue, 3/8
Hand, foot and mouth disease, 3/3
  acute pharyngitis and, 4/9
Hashimoto's autoimmune thyroiditis,
  18/13
Head, lymphatic system, 17/2–3
Healing by secondary intention, 26/8–
  10
Heartburn, 24/3
Heimlich manoeuvre, 1/10, 7/6
Hereditary haemorrhagic
  telangiectasia, 3/2
Herpangina, 3/3
  acute pharyngitis and, 4/9
Herpes labialis, 3/3
Herpes simplex, 3/3
  acute pharyngitis, 4/9
Herpes zoster, 3/3
  pharyngeal infection, 4/9, 9/6
Histiocytosis X, 22/8
Histoplasmosis, 3/5
  larynx, 5/18
History, 1/1
HIV, *see* Human immunodeficiency
  virus
Hoarseness:
  following intubation, 7/6
  Zenker's diverticulum and, 10/11
  see also Voice disorders
Hodgkin's disease, 14/5
Hopkins rod, 1/3–4
Human immunodeficiency virus (HIV):
  parotomegaly and, 19/6
  pharyngeal manifestations, 4/14–15
    hairy leukoplakia, 4/14
    lymphoid tissue hyperplasia, 4/15
    neoplasia, 4/15
    opportunistic infections, 4/14–15
Hyperthyroidism, 6/18
Hypopharynx:
  reconstruction, 26/19
  surgical anatomy, 15/1–2
  tumours of, 15/2–15
    benign, 15/2–3, 15/8
    clinical presentation, 15/5
    diagnosis, 15/5–6
    enteral feeding, 15/13
    epidemiology, 15/4–5
    investigation, 15/6
    malignant, 15/3, 15/8
    metastases, 15/3–4
    palliative care, 15/15
    pathology, 15/2–4
    radiotherapy, 15/10, 15/13–14
    rehabilitation, 15/15
    risk factors, 15/4–5
    staging, 15/6–8
    surgery, 15/10–11, 15/14
    surgical reconstruction, 15/11–12
    treatment complications,
      15/13–15
    treatment methods, 15/10–12
    treatment philosophy, 15/8–10
    treatment planning, 15/8

Hypothyroidism, 6/18, 18/3
  following laryngectomy, 11/33

Idiopathic globus, 9/4–5
Incisive canal cyst, 23/9–10
Infantile paralysis, 9/7–9
Infectious mononucleosis, 4/7, 16/15
Influenza, 4/8
  acute tonsillitis, 4/2
Infratemporal fossa:
  anatomy, 22/1–2
  CT scanning, 2/9–11
  tumours of, 22/3–8
    ameloblastomas, 22/4–5
    angiofibroma, 22/4
    chemodectomas, 22/6–7
    chondrosarcomas, 22/8
    chordoma, 22/4
    clinical aspects, 22/8–9
    desmoid tumours, 22/8
    histiocytosis X, 22/8
    lymphoma, 22/8
    meningioma, 22/4, 22/5
    neurogenic tumours, 22/6
    osteoblastomas, 22/8
    parotid gland tumours, 22/5–6
    pleomorphic adenomas, 22/5
    pseudoparotomegaly and, 19/2
    radiology, 22/10–11
    squamous carcinoma, 22/7–8
    tissue diagnosis, 22/11
    treatment, 22/11–19
Intersexuality, voice disorders and, 6/16
Intubation, *see* Airway obstruction
Intubation granuloma, 5/13–14, 11/3
Iridium implants, 3/20
Iron deficiency, and postcricoid
  carcinoma, 15/5

Jaws:
  benign tumours, 23/13–17
    adenomatoid odontogenic tumour,
      23/16
    ameloblastic fibro-odontoma,
      23/16
    ameloblastic fibrodentinoma,
      23/16
    ameloblastic fibroma, 23/15–16
    ameloblastoma, 23/13–15
    calcifying epithelial odontogenic
      tumour, 23/15
    calcifying odontogenic cyst,
      23/16–17
    clear cell odontogenic tumour,
      23/15
    odontoameloblastoma, 23/16
    squamous odontogenic tumour,
      23/15
  cysts of, 23/1–2
    aneurysmal bone cyst, 23/12–13
    botryoid odontogenic cyst, 23/4
    classification, 23/1
    dentigerous cyst, 3/8, 23/5–6
    eruption cyst, 3/8, 23/6
    fissural cyst, 23/10–11

Jaws *(cont.)*
  gingival cyst, **23**/2–3
  glandular odontogenic cyst,
    23/4–5
  lateral periodontal cyst, **23**/3–4
  midpalatal cysts of infants, **23**/10
  naevoid basal cell syndrome,
    23/7–9
  nasolabial cyst, **23**/10
  nasopalatine cyst, **3**/8, **23**/9–10
  odontogenic keratocyst, **23**/6–7
  radicular inflammatory cyst, **23**/11
  solitary bone cyst, **23**/11–12
  malignant tumours, **23**/17–18
    ameloblastic fibrosarcoma, **23**/18
    ameloblastoma, **23**/17
    odontogenic cysts, malignant
      change, **23**/18
    primary intraosseous carcinoma,
      23/18
  surgical treatment of tumours,
    23/28–36
Jugular foramen lesions, **9**/2–3
Jugular glomus tumours, **22**/7

Kaposi's sarcoma, **4**/15
Keratosis, **5**/10
  grading, **5**/11–12
  larynx, **11**/14
Kiel classification, **14**/5
Killian's dehiscence, **10**/2, **10**/8

Language, use of voice, **6**/2
Laryngeal dystonia, **9**/11
Laryngeal mask, **1**/6, **7**/4
Laryngeal nerves, **9**/1–2
  palsies, **9**/12–15
    aetiology, **9**/13
    bilateral abductor paralysis, **9**/14–15
    bilateral adductor paralysis, **9**/15
    investigations, **9**/13–14
    Semon's law, **9**/12
    superior laryngeal nerve, **9**/12
    symptoms, **9**/13
    treatment, **9**/14–15
    unilateral abductor paralysis, **9**/14,
      9/19
    unilateral adductor paralysis, **9**/14
    Wagner and Grossman theory, **9**/12–
      13
Laryngeal spasm, **1**/9
Laryngectomy, **11**/26–37, **11**/38–41
  emergency, **11**/26
  partial:
    lateral, **11**/28–30
    supraglottic, **11**/30–1
    subtotal, **11**/32
    total, **11**/32–7
      complications, **11**/33–5
      disabilities, **11**/36–7
      voice rehabilitation, **6**/21–4,
        11/35–6
Laryngitis:
  acute, **5**/1–5
    aetiology, **5**/1

diagnosis, **5**/1–2
pathology, **5**/1
symptoms, **5**/1
treatment, **5**/2
acute epiglottitis, **5**/4–5
acute laryngotracheobronchitis,
  5/2–3
atrophic, **5**/13
chronic, **5**/8–13
  aetiology, **5**/8–9
  clinical features, **5**/9–10
  grading system, **5**/11–12
  histology, **5**/10–12
  malignant transformation, **5**/12
  treatment, **5**/12
hyperplastic, **6**/15
membranous, **5**/4
reflux and, **24**/15–16
subglottic, **5**/3–4
Laryngocoele, **16**/17–18
  clinical features, **16**/17–18
  pathology, **16**/17
  radiography, **2**/2
  tomography, **2**/3
  treatment, **16**/18
Laryngopathia gravidarum, **6**/18
Laryngoscopy:
  direct, **1**/7, **11**/13
  indirect, **1**/2, **11**/13
  microlaryngoscopy, **1**/7–8
  nasolaryngoscopy, **1**/2–3
Laryngospasm, following endoscopy,
  1/9
Laryngotracheobronchitis, acute,
  5/2–3
Larynx:
  actinomycosis, **5**/18
  adenoid cystic carcinoma, **11**/37
  adenoma, **11**/8
  amyloidosis, **5**/14, **11**/4
  artificial, **6**/24
  barium swallow, **2**/14–15
  cancer of, **11**/9–43
    aetiology, **11**/12
    biopsy, **11**/14
    chemotherapy, **11**/24
    classification, **11**/11, **11**/14–15,
      11/42
    diagnosis, **11**/12–14
    examination, **11**/12–14
    incidence, **11**/10
    keratosis, **11**/14
    metastases, **11**/13
    palliation, **11**/22–4
    pathology, **11**/14–16
    presentation, **11**/10–11
    radiology, **11**/13
    radiotherapy, **11**/24–5, **11**/37–38–
      41
    spread of, **11**/16–22
    staging, **11**/11–12, **11**/42–3
    surgery, **11**/23–4, **11**/25–37, **11**/38–
      41
    symptoms, **11**/12
    treatment, **11**/22–41

see also Laryngectomy
candidiasis, **5**/17
carcinosarcoma, **11**/37
chondroma, **11**/5–6
chondrosarcoma, **11**/37
coccidioidomycosis, **5**/18
congenital abnormalities, **6**/18
contact ulcers, **5**/10, **11**/3–4
CT scanning, **2**/5–7, **2**/23
cysts, **11**/1–2
examination of, **1**/1–8, **11**/13
  flexible endoscopy, **1**/2–3
  Hopkins rod, **1**/3–4
  photography, **1**/4
  stroboscopy, **1**/4
fibroma, **11**/7
foreign bodies, **1**/10, **1**/11
fractures of, **2**/6
granular cell tumours, **11**/7
granulomas, **11**/2–4
  contact granuloma, **5**/13–14,
    11/3–4
haemangioma, **11**/5
histoplasmosis, **5**/18
injection techniques, **9**/16–18
  collagen, **9**/17–18
  steroids, **9**/18
  teflon, **9**/16–17
intubation, *see* Airway obstruction
leiomyoma, **11**/6–7
leprosy, **5**/17
lipoma, **11**/7
lymphatic drainage, **17**/3
magnetic resonance, **2**/7–9
melanoma, **11**/37
mycotic infections, **5**/17–18
myogenic tumours, **11**/6–7
neurogenic tumours, **11**/8
neurological lesions, **9**/11–15
  aetiology, **9**/2–3
  anatomy, **9**/1–2
non-Hodgkin's lymphoma, **11**/37
oedema, **5**/5–6
  angioneurotic oedema, **5**/6
  Reinke's oedema, **5**/5–6
papillomatosis, **6**/19
paracoccidioidomycosis, **5**/18
paraganglioma, **11**/8–9
paralysis of, **9**/11
parasitic infections, **5**/18
perichondritis, **5**/6–7
phonosurgery, **6**/20–1, **9**/15–19
polyps, **6**/14–15
radiography, **2**/2–3
relapsing polychondritis, **5**/7–8
retention cysts, **11**/1–2
rhabdomyoma, **11**/7
sarcoidosis, **5**/15
scleroma, **5**/16–17
spastic, **9**/11
squamous cysts, **11**/1–2
stenosis, **8**/6–10
  assessment, **8**/7–8
  cricoid, **8**/9
  epidemiology, **8**/6

glottic, 8/8–9
pathological considerations, 8/6–7
prognosis, 8/10
supraglottic, 8/8
tracheal, 8/9–10
treatment, 8/7, 8/8–10
suspension of, 6/5
syphilis, 5/16
tomography, 2/3–5
trauma, 6/19–20, 8/1–6
    assessment, 8/4–5
    biomechanics, 8/1–3
    epidemiology, 8/1
    high velocity blunt injuries, 8/6
    low velocity blunt injuries, 8/6
    pathological consequences, 8/3
    penetrating injuries, 8/5–6
    treatment, 8/3–4, 8/5–6
tuberculosis, 5/14–15
vascular neoplasms, 11/4–5
ventricular cysts, 11/2
verrucous carcinoma, 11/16, 11/37
Laser bronchoscopy, 1/9
Laser surgery:
    mouth cancer, 3/26
    tonsillectomy, 4/20
Lateral periodontal cyst, 23/3–4
Lateral pharyngeal space, see
    Parapharyngeal space
Leiomyoma, laryngeal, 11/6–7
Leprosy:
    larynx, 5/17
    pharynx, 4/12–13
Leukemia:
    oral manifestations, 3/2
    pharyngeal symptoms, 4/13
Leukoplakia, 3/7, 5/10
    candidal, 3/5
    hairy, AIDS and, 4/14
    mouth cancer and, 3/15
Lichen planus, 3/7
    mouth cancer and, 3/15
Lignocaine, 1/5–6
Lingual thyroid, 3/2
Lingual tonsillitis, 4/6
Lip split, 3/22–3
Lipoma:
    computerized tomography, 2/7
    larynx, 11/7
Liposuction, 25/12
Lips:
    cancer of, 3/27–8
        metastases, 3/27–8
        staging, 3/28
        treatment, 3/28
    protection during endoscopy, 1/5
    reconstructive surgery, 26/8
Local anaesthesia, 1/5
Ludwig's angina, 16/17
Lugol's solution, 1/3
Lupus vulgaris, 4/12
Lymph nodes:
    head and neck, 17/2–3
        deep system, 17/3
        superficial system, 17/3

see also Metastases; Metastatic neck
    disease
Lymphangioma, 3/11, 16/11–13
    clinical features, 16/12
    embryology, 16/11
    pathology, 16/11–12
    terminology, 16/11
    treatment, 16/12–13
Lymphoepithelioma, 14/4
Lymphoid tissue hyperplasia, HIV and,
    4/15
Lymphoma, 14/5
    aetiology, 14/5
    angiocentric, 23/20–1
    classification, 14/5, 14/6
    histology, 14/7
    HIV and, 4/15
    infratemporal fossa, 22/8
    nasopharynx, 13/24
    non-Hodgkin's, 11/37
        treatment, 14/17–18
    parapharyngeal space, 22/8
    salivary glands, 21/8–9
    site incidence, 14/7
    staging, 14/8
    thyroid gland, 18/17
    treatment, 14/7–8

Macroglossia, 3/2
Magnetic resonance, 2/1–2, 2/7–9, 2/23
    fast gradient echo techniques, 2/20
    larynx, 2/7–9
    mouth cancer investigation, 3/18
    nodal metastases, 2/13, 17/6
    oropharynx, 2/20–1
    parapharyngeal region, 2/11–12,
        2/22
    salivary glands, 2/18–19
Mandible:
    tumours of, 3/13
        ameloblastoma, 22/4–5
        management, 3/23
        pseudoparotomegaly and, 19/2
        reconstruction, 3/25–6, 26/16–19
Masseter hypertrophy, 19/1–2
Mastoiditis, pseudoparotomegaly and,
    19/2
Maxillectomy, 23/28, 23/29–32
    completion of resection, 23/29–31
    osteotomies, 23/29
    rehabilitation, 23/31
    soft tissue approach, 23/29
Medialization laryngoplasty, 9/18
Median rhomboid glossitis, 3/2
Melanoma:
    larynx, 11/37
    nasal, 23/35–6
    oral cavity, 3/16
        treatment, 3/27
Membranous laryngitis, 5/4
Meningioma, 22/4, 22/5
Mentoplasty, 25/12
Metastases:
    hypopharyngeal tumours, 15/3–4
        pyriform fossa tumours, 15/9

laryngeal carcinoma, 11/13, 11/20
lip cancer, 3/27–8
mouth cancer, 3/18–19
nodal, imaging, 2/13
oropharynx, 14/2–3, 14/13–14
pharyngeal space, 22/8
pyriform fossae, 15/9
Metastatic neck disease:
    bilateral, 17/14
    lymph node assessment, 17/5–7
        clinical examination, 17/5–6
        computerized tomography, 17/6
        fine needle aspiration cytology,
            17/6–7
        fixation, 17/14
        history, 17/5
        imaging, 2/13
        magnetic resonance imaging, 17/6
        radioisotopes, 17/6
        ultrasound, 17/6
    management, 3/21
    patterns of cancer spread, 17/3–5
        histological differentiation, 17/4
        host factors, 17/4–5
        primary tumour site, 17/4
        primary tumour size, 17/4
    prognosis, 17/14
    prophylactic treatment, 3/22
    pyriform fossa tumours and, 15/9
    radiotherapy, 17/7–8
    staging, 17/5
    surgery, 17/8–9
    TNM classification, 17/5
    treatment, 17/7
    unknown primary tumour, 17/14–15
    see also Metastases; Neck
Microlaryngoscopy, 1/7–8
Midfacial degloving, 23/29, 23/32
Midline forehead flap, 25/6
Migratory glossitis, 3/8
Minitracheostomy, 7/17
Mirror examination, 1/2
Moniliasis, see Candidiasis
Morphine, 27/2–3
Motor neuron disease, 9/10
Mouth:
    anatomy, 3/1, 3/12–13
    benign tumours, 3/10–11
        granular cell myoblastoma, 3/11
        haemangioma, 3/10–11
        neurogenic tumours, 3/11
        papilloma, 3/10
        pleomorphic adenoma, 3/10
    cancer of, see Mouth
    cancer care in terminally ill patients,
        27/4
    congenital conditions, 3/1–2
    cysts, 3/8
    examination of, 1/2
    imaging, 2/20–1
    infective conditions, 3/3–5
        bacteria, 3/3–5
        fungi, 3/5
        viruses, 3/3
    inflammatory swellings, 3/8–10

Mouth (*cont.*)
  epulis, 3/9–10
  lymphatic drainage, 3/13, 17/3
  pigmentation, 3/3
  reconstruction, 26/15–16
  stomatitis, 3/2
  systemic disease manifestations,
    3/2–3
  ulceration, 3/2, 3/5–8
    aphthous, 3/5–6
    Behçet's syndrome, 3/6
    benign mucous membrane
      pemphigoid, 3/6
    erythema multiforme, 3/6
    leukoplakia, 3/7
    lichen planus, 3/7
    necrotizing sialometaplasia, 3/6–7
    pemphigus vulgaris, 3/6
    traumatic, 3/5
    xerostomia, 3/11
  Sjögren's syndrome, 3/11
  see also Lips; Mandible; Salivary
    glands; Tongue
Mouth cancer, 3/12–27
  aetiology, 3/14–15
  applied anatomy, 3/12–13
  clinical features, 3/16–18
  diagnosis, 3/16–18
    examination, 3/17
    radiology, 3/17–18
  epidemiology, 3/14
  metastases, 3/18–19
  pathology, 3/15–16
    melanoma, 3/16
    spindle cell carcinoma, 3/16
    squamous cell carcinoma, 3/15
    verrucous carcinoma, 3/15–16
  sites of, 3/17
  staging, 3/18
  treatment of, 3/19–27
    early lesions, 3/20
    later stages, 3/21–2
    mandible management, 3/23,
      3/25–6
    melanoma, 3/27
    radiotherapy, 3/20–1, 3/26
    reconstruction, 3/23–5
    sarcoma, 3/27
    surgery, 3/20, 3/22–3
Mucoepidermoid carcinoma, 3/16
Mucosal haemorrhage following
  endoscopy, 1/9
Myasthenia gravis, 9/9–10
Myocutaneous flaps, 25/6
Myotomy, cricopharyngeal, 10/17–18,
  11/31–2

Naevoid basal cell syndrome, 23/7–9
Nasal tumours, 23/21–8
  fibroma, 23/23
  haemangioma, 23/23
  malignant tumours, 23/23–8
    aetiology, 23/24
    classification, 23/25
    investigation, 23/25

melanoma, 23/35–6
  pathology, 23/24
  presentation, 23/24–5
  treatment, 23/25–8
  nasal cavity, 23/36
  neurofibroma, 23/23
  osteoma, 23/23
  papilloma, 23/21–3
Nasendoscopy, 1/2–3
Nasoalveolar cyst, 23/10
Nasolabial cyst, 23/10
Nasolabial flap, 25/5
Nasolaryngoscopy, 1/2–3
Nasopalatine cysts, 3/8, 23/9–10
Nasopharynx:
  cancer of, 13/4–13
    chemotherapy, 13/16
    clinical presentations, 13/10–13
    environmental factors, 13/7–9
    epidemiology, 13/4–7
    histopathology, 13/9
    immunogenetics, 13/22–4
    immunology, 13/19–22
    natural history, 13/9–10
    paediatric, 13/26
    radiotherapy, 13/15–16
    stage-classification, 13/14–15,
      13/26–8
    surgical treatment, 13/16–19
  cysts, 13/25–6
  examination of, 13/13–14
  radiography, 2/2–3
  surgical anatomy, 13/1–4
    epithelial lining, 13/3
    lymphatic drainage, 13/3, 17/3
    lymphoid tissue, 13/3–4
    pharyngeal bursa, 13/4
    pharyngeal hypophysis, 13/4
  tumours of, 13/4–6
    basal encephalocoeles, 13/25
    chordoma, 13/25
    craniopharyngioma, 13/25
    malignant lymphoma, 13/24
    paediatric, 13/24–5
    plasmacytoma, 13/24
    teratoid, 13/25
  see also Angiofibroma
Neck:
  actinomycosis, 16/14–15
  AIDS manifestations, 16/14
  anatomy, 17/1–3
    divisions of, 17/1–2
    fascia, 17/2
    lymphatic system, 17/2–3
  benign diseases of, 16/1–18
    branchial fistulae, 16/4–7
    branchial sinuses, 16/4–7
    branchogenic carcinoma, 16/7
    thyroglossal carcinoma, 16/4
    see also Branchial cysts;
      Thyroglossal cysts
  brucellosis, 16/15
  cat-scratch disease, 16/15
  dissection:
    complications, 17/10–12

conservational, 17/12–13
    elective, 17/13
    history, 17/7
    non-malignant conditions, 17/15
    non-squamous malignancy, 17/15
    operative procedure, 17/9–10
    second radical neck dissection,
      17/14
  examination of, 1/2, 11/13
  infectious mononucleosis, 16/15
  lymphangiomas, *see* Lymphangioma
  metastases, *see* Metastatic neck
    disease
  neck space infections, 16/15–17
    Ludwig's angina, 16/17
    parapharyngeal abscess, 16/16–17
    retropharyngeal abscess, 16/16
  neurogenous tumours, 16/8–11
    clinical features, 16/9–10
    pathogenesis, 16/9
    terminology, 16/8–9
    treatment, 16/10–11
  plastic surgery, *see* Plastic surgery
  sarcoidosis, 16/14
  toxoplasmosis, 16/14
  tuberculosis, 16/13–14
Neck disease, *see* Metastatic neck
    disease
Necrotizing sialometaplasia, 3/6–7
Neoglottis, 11/36
Neuralgia, glossopharyngeal, 9/5–6
Neuroblastoma, olfactory, 23/36
Neurofibroma, 16/8, 22/6
  nasal, 23/23
Neurogenic tumours:
  infratemporal fossa, 22/6
  larynx, 11/8
  mouth, 3/11
  neck, 16/8–11
  parapharyngeal space, 22/6
Neuroma:
  carotid space, 2/11–12
  postoperative, 16/8, 16/10
Nodal metastases, *see* Metastases
Non-Hodgkin's lymphoma, 11/37
  treatment, 14/17–18
Non-steroidal anti-inflammatory drugs,
  27/3
Nose, non-healing granulomas, 23/18–
  21
  see also Nasal tumours

Obesity, parotid gland and, 19/5
Obstructive sleep apnoea, 4/15–17
  clinical features, 4/16
  treatment, 4/16–17
Odontoameloblastoma, 23/16
Odontogenic keratocyst, 23/6–7
Oesophageal voice, 6/21–3, 11/36
Oesophagitis, 1/3
Oesophagogastroduodenoscopy, 1/3
Oesophagoscopy, 1/8
  positioning of patient, 1/4–5
Oesophagus:
  barium swallow, 2/15–17

cancer of, 24/16–20
  demography, 24/16
  diagnosis, 24/17–18
  palliative treatment, 24/19–20
  pathology, 24/17
  predisposing factors, 24/16–17
  radical treatment, 24/18–19
  staging, 24/18
diseases of:
  clinical features, 24/2–3
  investigations, 24/3–9
diverticula, 10/1, 24/23–4
foreign bodies, 1/10–12, 2/15–16, 24/21–2
globus pharyngis, 24/25–7
motility disorders, 24/9–12
  lower oesophageal sphincter, 24/11–12
  oesophageal body, 24/10–11
  upper oesophageal sphincter, 24/9–10
physiology:
  lower sphincter barrier function, 24/2
  motility, 24/1–2
  upper sphincter function, 24/1
reconstruction, 26/19
traumatic lesions, 24/20–3
  chemical injury, 24/22–3
  perforation during endoscopy, 1/9, 24/20–1
  rupture, 24/20
tumours, 24/23
webs, 24/24–5
see also Gastro-oesophageal reflux

Olfactory neuroblastoma, 23/36
Oncocytoma, 20/9
Operating microscope, 1/7–8
Opioids, 27/1–3
Oral cavity, *see* Mouth
Oropharynx, 14/1–2
  divisions of, 14/1–2
  imaging, 2/20–1
  lymphatic drainage, 17/3
  lymphoepithelioma, 14/4
  lymphoma, *see* Lymphoma
  reconstruction, 26/15–16
  salivary gland tumours, 14/5–7
    treatment, 14/18
  squamous cell carcinoma, 14/2–4
    aetiology, 14/4
    chemotherapy, 14/16
    classification, 14/4
    cryosurgery, 14/17
    incidence, 14/2
    laser therapy, 14/17
    metastases, 14/2–3, 14/13–14
    nodal classification, 14/4
    radiotherapy, 14/11–12, 14/14
    reconstruction following surgery, 14/14–16
    surgery, 14/12–14
    treatment, 14/10–17
  tumours of, 14/1–2

clinical examination, 14/8–9
epithelial tumours, 14/2–4
investigations, 14/9–10
pathology, 14/2
symptoms, 14/8
Osler–Weber–Rendu disease, 3/2
Ossification, 2/3
Osteoblastoma, 22/8
Osteoma, 23/23
Oswald–Unton tube, 1/6
Oxyphil adenoma, 20/9

Pachydermia, 5/10
Pain relief, *see* Terminal care
Palatal fenestration, 23/32
Palate:
  myoclonus, 9/10
  paralysis of, 9/3–4
    diphtheria and, 9/6–7
    management, 9/10
Palliative care:
  hypopharyngeal tumours, 15/15
  laryngeal cancer, 11/22–4
  oesophageal cancer, 24/19–20
  tracheostomy, 11/23
Panendoscopy, 1/7
Papilloma, 3/10
  HIV and, 4/15
  nasal, 23/21–3
Papillomatosis, laryngeal, 6/19
Paracoccidioidomycosis, 5/18
Paraganglioma, 16/8–9
  larynx, 11/8–9
Parapharyngeal abscesses, 4/4–5, 16/16–17
  clinical features, 4/5
  complications, 4/5
  treatment, 4/5
Parapharyngeal region, soft tissue imaging, 2/9–13
Parapharyngeal space:
  anatomy, 16/16, 22/2–3
  CT scanning, 2/11
  tumours of, 22/3–8
    ameloblastomas, 22/4–5
    chemodectomas, 22/6–7
    clinical aspects, 22/9–10
    investigation, 2/12–13
    lymphoma, 22/8
    meningioma, 22/4, 22/5
    metastatic carcinoma, 22/8
    neurogenic tumours, 22/6
    pleomorphic adenomas, 22/5
    pseudoparotomegaly and, 19/2
    radiology, 22/10–11
    squamous carcinoma, 22/7–8
    tissue diagnosis, 22/11
    treatment, 22/11–19
Paraspinal space, 2/12
Parathyroid glands, 18/3–4
  insufficiency following thyroidectomy, 11/33
Parotid gland:
  imaging, 2/18–20
  intraparotid lesions, 19/3

malignant tumours, 22/5–6
  treatment, 22/12–14
obesity and, 19/5
origin of parapharyngeal masses, 2/11
pleomorphic adenoma, 2/19–20, 22/5
  carcinoma in, 21/8
  treatment, 22/11–12
radiotherapy and, 19/6
surgical anatomy, 20/2–5
see also Salivary gland tumours; Salivary glands
Parotidectomy, 20/12–15, 21/11–12
  complications, 20/17
  partial, 20/12–13
Parotitis, 19/3–5
  clinical features, 19/4
  conservative treatment, 19/4–5
  fine needle aspiration biopsy, 19/4
  investigations, 19/4
  pathogenesis, 19/3–4
  radiology, 19/4
  surgical treatment, 19/5
Parotomegaly:
  drug–induced, 19/5–6
  HIV infection and, 19/6
  metabolic, 19/5
  see also Pseudoparotomegaly
Pemphigoid, oral, 3/6
Pemphigus vulgaris, 3/6
Perichondritis, laryngeal, 5/6–7
Periodontal disease, 3/9
Peritonsillar abscesses (quinsy), 4/3–4
  bacteriology, 4/3
  clinical features, 4/3–4
  complications, 4/4
  differential diagnosis, 4/4
  indications for tonsillectomy, 4/17
  treatment, 4/4
Pharyngeal bursa, 13/4
Pharyngeal diverticula, 10/1–19
  classification, 10/2, 10/3
  lateral pouches, 10/2–5
    acquired, 10/3–5
    congenital, 10/3
    pharyngocoeles, 10/4–5
  posterior pouches, 10/5–6
    acquired, 10/6
    congenital, 10/5
  see also Zenker's diverticulum
Pharyngeal hypophysis, 13/4
Pharyngitis:
  acute, 4/1, 4/8–10
    gonococcal, 4/10
  chronic infections, 4/10–13
    candidiasis, 4/13
    leprosy, 4/12–13
    non-specific, 4/10–11
    scleroma, 4/13
    syphilis, 4/11–12
    toxoplasmosis, 4/12
    tuberculosis, 4/12
  viral, 4/8–9
    cytomegalovirus, 4/10

Pharyngitis (*cont.*)
　　hand, foot and mouth disease, 4/9
　　herpangina, 4/9
　　herpes simplex, 4/9
　　herpes zoster, 4/9, 9/6
Pharyngocoeles, 10/4–5
Pharyngoscopy, 1/8
Pharynx:
　　acute anterior poliomyelitis, 9/7–9
　　anatomy, 10/1–2
　　barium swallow, 2/14–15
　　blood diseases and, 4/13–14
　　　　acute leukaemia, 4/13
　　　　agranulocytosis, 4/13
　　　　Vincent's angina, 4/14
　　diphtheria, *see* Diphtheria
　　diverticula, *see* Pharyngeal
　　　　diverticula; Zenker's diverticulum
　　divisions of, 14/1
　　embryology, 10/1–2
　　examination of, 1/1–2, 1/8
　　foreign bodies, 1/11
　　globus pharyngeus, 9/4–5
　　glossopharyngeal neuralgia, 9/5–6
　　HIV infection and, 4/14–15
　　　　hairy leukoplakia, 4/14
　　　　lymphoid tissue hyperplasia, 4/15
　　　　neoplasia, 4/15
　　　　opportunistic infections, 4/14–15
　　lymphatic drainage, 17/3
　　motor neuron disease, 9/10
　　myasthenia gravis, 9/9–10
　　neurological affections:
　　　　aetiology, 9/2–3
　　　　anatomy, 9/1–2
　　palatal myoclonus, 9/10
　　paralysis of, 9/3–4
　　　　management, 9/10
　　posterior wall, 15/2
　　　　tumours, 15/9
　　pouches, *see* Pharyngeal diverticula;
　　　　Zenker's diverticulum
　　rabies, 9/9
　　radiography, 2/2–3
　　stenosis, 4/14
　　see also Hypopharynx; Nasopharynx;
　　　　Oropharynx
Phonetogram, 6/9
Phonosurgery, 1/8, 6/20–1, 9/15–19
　　arytenoid adduction, 9/18–19
　　arytenoidectomy, 9/19
　　cordectomy, 9/19
　　laryngeal injection techniques, 9/16–
　　　　18
　　　　collagen, 9/17–18
　　　　steroids, 9/18
　　　　Teflon, 9/16–17
　　medialization laryngoplasty, 9/18
　　reinnervation procedures, 9/19
Photography, 1/4
Plasmacytoma, 13/24
　　CT scanning, 2/7
Plastic surgery, 25/1–13, 26/1–19
　　aesthetic procedures, 25/12–13
　　　　chemical peeling, 25/12

　　　　dermabrasion, 25/12–13
　　　　liposuction, 25/12
　　　　mentoplasty, 25/12
　　ageing face rejuvenation, 25/9–13
　　　　blepharoplasty, 25/9–10
　　　　brow lift, 25/11–12
　　　　rhytidectomy, 25/10–11
　　complications, 25/6–7
　　cutaneous loss, 26/6–15
　　healing by secondary intention,
　　　　26/8–10
　　incision, 26/1–3
　　lesion management, 25/7–9
　　　　forehead, 25/7–8
　　　　lower face, 25/8
　　　　mid-face, 25/8
　　　　neck, 25/9
　　　　nose, 25/8–9
　　scar revision, 25/13, 26/3–6
　　　　fusiform excision, 26/5
　　　　W-plasty, 26/5
　　　　Z-plasty, 26/5–6
　　skin replacement, 25/2–6
　　　　grafts, 25/2–3, 26/10–12
　　　　skin flaps, 25/3–6, 26/12–15
　　suturing, 25/2, 26/3, 26/4
　　tissue handling, 25/2
　　wound closure, 26/3
Pleomorphic adenoma, 2/19–20,
　　20/7–9
　　carcinoma in, 21/8
　　mouth, 3/10
　　parapharyngeal space, 22/5
　　recurrent, 20/15–16
　　removal from hard palate, 20/16–17
　　treatment, 22/11–12, 22/17–18
Plummer's disease, 18/12–13
Pneumomediastinum, following
　　tracheostomy, 7/14–15
Pneumothorax:
　　as complication of neck dissection,
　　　　17/12
　　following tracheostomy, 7/14–15
Poliomyelitis, 9/7–9
Polychondritis, relapsing, 5/7–8
Polyps:
　　hairy, 13/25
　　laryngeal, 6/14–15
Postcricoid area, 15/2
　　tumours of, 15/4
　　treatment, 15/9
Posterior fossa lesions, 9/2–3
Primary herpetic gingivostomatitis, 3/3
Primary intraosseous carcinoma,
　　23/18
Primordial cyst, 23/6–7
Progressive bulbar palsy, 9/10
Pseudocroup, 5/3–4
Pseudoparotomegaly, 19/1–3
　　ageing, 19/2
　　dental causes, 19/2
　　hypertrophy of the masseter, 19/1–2
　　infratemporal fossa tumours, 19/2
　　intraparotid lesions, 19/3
　　mandibular tumours, 19/2

　　mastoiditis, 19/2
　　parapharyngeal space tumours, 19/2
　　see also Parotomegaly
Pterygomaxillary fissure, 2/10, 22/2
Pterygopalatine fossa, 2/9–11
Pull-through procedure, 3/22
Pyriform fossae, 15/1–2
　　barium swallow, 2/14
　　CT scanning, 2/6
　　tumours of, 15/3
　　　　metastases, 15/9
　　　　treatment, 15/8–9

Quinke's disease, 4/10
Quinsy, *see* Peritonsillar abscesses

Rabies, 9/9
Radicular inflammatory cysts, 23/11
Radiography, 2/2–3
Random flaps, 25/3
Ranula, 3/8
Reconstructive surgery, *see* Plastic
　　surgery
Regurgitation, Zenker's diverticulum
　　and, 10/11
Reinke's oedema, 5/5–6
Relapsing polychondritis, 5/7–8
Relaxed skin tension lines, 25/1
Retention cysts, 3/8
　　larynx, 11/1–2
Retrograde intubation, 7/4, 7/7
Retropharyngeal abscess, 4/5–6, 16/16
Retropharyngeal space, 16/16
Rhabdomyoma, laryngeal, 11/7
Rhinoscleroma, *see* Scleroma
Rhinotomy, 23/28–9, 23/31–2, 23/33
Rhomboid flaps, 25/4
Rhytidectomy, 25/10–11
Rotation flaps, 25/4

Salivary gland tumours, 3/16, 14/5–7,
　　21/1–13
　　aetiology, 20/6
　　benign lymphoepithelial lesion, 20/9
　　biopsy, 21/11
　　carcinomas, 21/4–8
　　　　acinic cell carcinoma, 21/5–6
　　　　adenocarcinoma, 3/16, 21/7
　　　　adenoid cystic carcinoma, 3/16,
　　　　　　21/6–7
　　　　in pleomorphic adenoma, 21/8
　　　　mucoepidermoid carcinoma, 3/16,
　　　　　　21/4–5
　　chemotherapy, 21/12
　　classification, 21/1, 21/2, 21/9
　　distribution, 21/1–3, 21/4
　　epidemiology, 21/3, 21/4
　　examination, 20/10–11
　　historical perspective, 20/1–2
　　incidence, 20/6
　　investigations, 20/12
　　lymphatic malformations, 20/7
　　lymphomas, 21/8–9
　　management, 3/26–7, 14/18,
　　　　21/9–12

oxyphil adenoma, **20**/9
pleomorphic adenoma, **2**/19–20,
　　3/10, **20**/7–9, **22**/5
　　carcinoma in, **21**/8
　　predisposing factors, **21**/3–4
　　prognosis, **21**/13
　　radiology, **21**/10–11
　　radiotherapy, **21**/12
　　surgical pathology, **20**/6–7
　　surgical treatment, **20**/12–15, **21**/11–
　　　12
　　complications, **20**/17–18
　　symptoms, **20**/10
　　vascular malformations, **20**/7
　　Warthin's tumour, **20**/9
Salivary glands:
　　cysts, **19**/11
　　fistulae, **19**/11–12
　　imaging, **2**/18–20
　　sialectasis, **19**/6–9
　　　clinical features, **19**/6–7
　　　investigations, **19**/7–8
　　　pathogenesis, **19**/6
　　　treatment, **19**/8–9
　　structure, **21**/1
　　see also Parotid gland; Salivary gland
　　　tumours; Sjögren's syndrome;
　　　Sublingual gland; Submandibular
　　　gland
Sarcoidosis:
　　laryngeal, **5**/15
　　neck manifestation, **16**/14
Sarcoma:
　　Kaposi's, **4**/15
　　oral cavity, treatment of, **3**/27
Sarcomatoid carcinoma, **3**/16
Scar revision in facial plastic surgery,
　　25/13, **26**/3–6
　　fusiform excision, **26**/5
　　W-plasty, **26**/5
　　Z-plasty, **26**/5–6
Scarlet fever, **4**/2
Schirmer's test, **19**/10
Schwannoma, **3**/11, **16**/8, **22**/6
Scleroma:
　　larynx, **5**/16–17
　　pharynx, **4**/13
Semon's law, **9**/12
Sexual orientation, voice
　　　characteristics and, **6**/17
Sialectasis, *see* Salivary glands
Sialo-odontogenic cyst, **23**/4–5
Sialography, **2**/18
Sialometaplasia, necrotizing, **3**/6–7
Sinography, **2**/17
Sinuses, **2**/17
　　non-healing granulomas,
　　　23/18–21
　　thyroglossal, **16**/1
　　　treatment, **16**/4
　　tumour classification, **23**/27
　　see also Branchial sinuses
Sjögren's syndrome, **3**/11, **19**/9–11
　　clinical features, **19**/9–10
　　epidemiology, **19**/9

investigations, **19**/10–11
natural history, **19**/11
treatment, **19**/11
Skin flaps in plastic surgery, **25**/3–6,
　　26/12–15
Skin grafts, **25**/2–3, **26**/10–12
　　split skin grafts, **3**/23
Smoking as risk factor, **1**/1
　　hypopharyngeal cancer, **15**/4
　　mouth cancer, **3**/14
　　nasopharyngeal cancer, **13**/8
Snoring, **4**/16
Solitary bone cyst, **23**/11–12
South American blastomycosis, **5**/18
Spasmodic cough, **5**/3–4
Spasmodic dysphonia, **9**/11
Spastic larynx, **9**/11
Speech, **1**/2
　　oesophageal, **6**/21–3, **11**/36
　　see also Voice
Spindle cell carcinoma, **3**/16
Split skin grafts, **25**/2
Squamous cell carcinoma:
　　CT scanning, **2**/7
　　HIV and, **4**/15
　　oral cavity, **3**/15–16
　　　grading, **3**/15
　　　verrucous carcinoma, **3**/15–16
Squamous cell hyperplasia, **5**/10
　　grading, **5**/11–12
Squamous odontogenic tumour,
　　23/15
Stevens–Johnson syndrome, **3**/6
Stomatitis, **3**/2
　　gangrenous, **3**/4
　　primary herpetic gingivostomatitis,
　　　3/3
Streptococci, acute tonsillitis and, **4**/2
Stroboscopy, **1**/4, **6**/9–10
Subglottic carcinoma, **11**/19, **11**/42
Subglottic laryngitis, **5**/3–4
Subglottic stenosis, **8**/9–10
　　cricoid, **8**/9
　　tracheal, **8**/9–10
Sublingual gland, **20**/5
　　surgical removal, **20**/16
Submandibular gland, **20**/5
　　surgical removal, **20**/16
　　complications, **20**/17–18
Submandibular space, **16**/16
Subtraction technique, **2**/8
Supraglottic carcinoma, **11**/19, **11**/42
Supraglottic stenosis, **8**/8
Surgical emphysema, **2**/2
　　following tracheostomy, **7**/14
Suturing, **25**/2, **26**/3, **26**/4
Swallowing, **1**/2, **26**/14
　　endoscopy, **1**/2
　　following laryngectomy, **11**/34–5
　　mechanism, **10**/7–8
　　see also Dysphagia
Syphilis:
　　laryngeal, **5**/16
　　mouth cancer and, **3**/14
　　oral manifestations, **3**/4–5

pharyngeal, **4**/11–12
　　primary, **3**/4, **4**/11
　　secondary, **3**/4, **4**/11
　　tertiary, **3**/4–5, **4**/11
　　tests for, **3**/4

Teeth:
　　damage during endoscopy, **1**/9–10
　　dental caries, **3**/9
　　dental plaque, **3**/9
　　protection during endoscopy, **1**/5
　　see also Jaws
Teratoid cyst, **16**/13
Teratomas, **13**/25
Terminal care, **27**/1–6
　　mouth care, **27**/4
　　nausea and vomiting, **27**/5
　　pain management, **27**/1–4
　　　co-analgesics, **27**/3–4
　　　non-opioids, **27**/1
　　　non-pharmacological analgesia,
　　　　27/4
　　　strong opioids, **27**/2–3
　　　weak opioids, **27**/1–2
　　　WHO analgesic ladder, **27**/1, **27**/2
　　the dying patient, **27**/5–6
　　wound management, **27**/5, **27**/6
Thornwaldt's cyst, **13**/4
Throat, functions of, **1**/1
Thyroglobulin, **18**/4
Thyroglossal carcinoma, **16**/4
Thyroglossal cysts, **16**/1–4
　　clinical features, **16**/2–3
　　embryology, **16**/1
　　pathogenesis, **16**/1–2
　　terminology, **16**/1
　　treatment, **16**/3–4
Thyroglossal sinuses, **16**/1
　　treatment, **16**/4
Thyroid crisis, **18**/12
Thyroid gland, **18**/1–22
　　anaplastic carcinoma, **18**/17
　　　treatment, **18**/21
　　anatomy, **18**/1–3
　　　lymphatics, **18**/2
　　　nerves, **18**/2–3
　　　vascular supply, **18**/1–2
　　　veins, **18**/2
　　cancer of, **18**/14–22
　　　aetiology, **18**/14
　　　classification, **18**/15
　　　complications of treatment, **18**/22
　　　diagnosis, **18**/18–19
　　　incidence, **18**/14
　　　postoperative management, **18**/22
　　　prognostic factors, **18**/17
　　　symptoms, **18**/17–18
　　　treatment, **18**/19–22
　　enlargement, **18**/7–10
　　　diffuse non-toxic goitre, **18**/7
　　　multinodular non-toxic goitre,
　　　　18/8–9
　　　simple goitre, **18**/7
　　　surgery, **18**/9–10
　　fine needle aspiration biopsy, **18**/7

Thyroid gland (*cont.*)
  follicular adenoma, 18/17
  follicular carcinoma, 18/15–16
    treatment, 18/20–1
  function tests, 18/5–6
  Grave's disease, 18/10–12
    pathology, 18/11
    treatment, 18/11–12
  hyperthyroidism, 6/18
  hypothyroidism, 6/18, 18/3
  imaging, 18/6–7
  lingual, 3/2
  lymphoma, 18/17
    treatment, 18/21
  medullary carcinoma, 18/16
    treatment, 18/21
  papillary carcinoma, 18/15
    treatment, 18/20
  physiology, 18/4–5
    calcitonin, 18/4
    thyroid antibodies, 18/4–5
  Plummer's disease, 18/12–13
  solitary hot nodules, 18/13
Thyroid hormones, 18/4
Thyroiditis:
  acute, 18/13
  de Quervain's, 18/13–14
  Hashimoto's autoimmune, 18/13
Thyropharyngeus muscle, 10/2
Tinnitus, nasopharyngeal carcinoma
    and, 13/12
Tomography, 2/3–5
  see also Computerized tomography
Tongue:
  cancer of, 3/13, 3/17
  congenital lesions, 3/2
  examination of, 1/2
  geographical tongue, 3/8
  hairy tongue, 3/8
  imaging, 2/20–1
  lymphatic drainage, 17/3
  reconstruction, 26/15–16
  squamous cell carcinoma, 14/3
Tongue tie, 3/2
Tonsillectomy, 4/17–23
  complications, 4/20–3
    haemorrhage, 4/20, 4/21
    infection, 4/22
    malignancy, 4/22–3
    oedema of the uvula, 4/21–2
    pain, 4/22
  contraindications, 4/18
  for biopsy, 4/17–18
  indications, 4/17–18
  postoperative care, 4/20
  preoperative considerations, 4/18
  surgical procedure, 4/18–20
    laser tonsillectomy, 4/20
Tonsillitis:
  acute, 4/1–3
    causative organisms, 4/2
    clinical features, 4/2
    complications, 4/3
    differential diagnosis, 4/2
    lingual, 4/6

    treatment, 4/2–3
    recurrent, 4/17
Tonsils:
  cysts, 4/7
  lymphatic drainage, 17/3
  squamous cell carcinoma, 14/3
  tonsillar debris, 4/7
  ulceration, 4/7–8
  unilateral enlargement, 4/7
Toxoplasmosis:
  neck manifestations, 16/14
  pharyngeal infection, 4/12
Trachea:
  fistulae, following tracheostomy,
    7/15–16
  necrosis, following tracheostomy,
    7/15
  radiography, 2/2–3
  stenosis, 8/9–10
    following intubation, 7/5
    following tracheostomy, 7/16
Tracheostomy, 7/7–18
  complications, 7/13–16
  emergency, 7/9–10
  history of, 7/7–8
  indications for, 7/8
  long-term, 7/16–17
  minitracheostomy, 7/17
  palliative, 11/23
  percutaneous, 7/17
  postoperative management,
    7/11–12
    accidental decannulation, 7/12
    haemorrhage, 7/12
    obstruction, 7/11–12
    self-care, 7/12–13
  surgical technique, 7/8–9
  tubes, 7/10–11
Transposition flaps, 25/4
Transtracheal ventilation, 7/4, 7/7
Trench mouth, *see* Vincent's angina
Tuberculosis, 1/3
  laryngeal, 5/14–15
  neck, 16/13–14
  oral infection, 3/5
  pharyngeal infection, 4/12
Tuberculous otitis media, 4/12

Ulcers:
  contact ulcers, 5/10, 11/3–4
  larynx, 11/3–4
  tonsils, 4/7–8
  see also Mouth
Ultrasound:
  metastatic neck disease, 17/6
  thyroid gland imaging, 18/6, 18/19
Uvula:
  oedema of, 4/10
  as complication of tonsillectomy,
    4/21–2

Vagus nerve, 9/1–2
  glomus tumours, 16/9, 16/10
Venturi jet system, 1/6
Verrucous carcinoma, 3/15–16

    larynx, 11/16, 11/37
Videography, 1/4
Vincent's angina, 3/3–4
  pharyngeal symptoms, 4/14
Vitamin deficiency, oral manifestations,
    3/2
Vocal cords, 11/11
  cancer of, 6/20
  cysts, 6/19
  fixation, 11/18
  glottic carcinoma, 11/16–19
  oedema, 6/14–15
  paralysis, 6/15–16
    treatment, 6/15–16
    with hypopharyngeal tumours,
      15/3
  see also Phonosurgery
  tomography, 2/3
Vocal nodules, 6/14
Voice:
  activating air-stream, 6/2–4
  control, 6/2, 6/7
  generator, 6/4–7
  non-language use, 6/1–2
  rehabilitation following
    laryngectomy, 6/21–4, 11/35–6
    artificial larynx, 6/24
    neoglottis, 11/36
    oesophageal voice, 6/21–3, 11/36
    surgical methods, 6/24
    valves, 11/36
  resonator, 6/6–7
  use in language, 6/2
Voice disorders:
  adolescence and, 6/13
  diagnosis, 6/10–11
  endocrine causes, 6/16–18
    eunuchoidism, 6/16–17
    hyperthyroidism, 6/18
    hypothyroidism, 6/18
    intersexuality, 6/16
    laryngopathia gravidarum, 6/18
    sexual orientation and, 6/17
    virilization in women, 6/17–18
  examination of, 6/7–10
    airflow recording during
      phonation, 6/10
    electroglottogram, 6/10
    electromyography, 6/10
    functional assessment, 6/8
    history, 6/7–8
    indirect laryngoscopy, 6/8–9
    magnetic tape recording, 6/9
    phonetogram, 6/9
    stroboscopy, 6/9–10
    wave motion pattern, 6/10
  laryngeal papillomatosis, 6/19
  laryngeal trauma, 6/19–20
  psychogenic, 6/11–13
  senile atrophy, 6/18–19
  vocal cord cancer, 6/20
  vocal cord cysts, 6/19
  vocal cord paralysis, 6/15–16
  see also Dysphonia
von Recklinghausen's disease, 3/11

W-plasty, **26**/5
Wagner and Grossman theory, **9**/12–13
Warthin's tumour, **2**/18, **20**/9
Weber–Fergusson approach, **23**/29
Webs, oesophageal, **24**/24–5
Wegener's granulomatosis, **23**/19–20
    autoantibody estimation, **23**/20
    clinical features, **23**/19–20
    laryngeal manifestations, **5**/17
    treatment, **23**/20
White sponge naevus, **3**/1–2
WHO analgesic ladder, **27**/1, **27**/2
Wolfe grafts, **25**/2–3

Xeroradiography, **2**/1, **2**/2
Xerostomia, **3**/11

Z-plasty, **25**/5, **26**/5–6
Zenker's diverticulum, **5**/10–19
    aetiology, **10**/8–10
        anatomical, **10**/8–9
        electromyography, **10**/10
        manometry, **10**/9–10
        radiological, **10**/9
    carcinoma of, **10**/19
    history of, **10**/7
    incidence, **10**/10

    investigations, **10**/11–12
    pathogenesis, **10**/12–13
    signs, **10**/11
    symptoms, **10**/10–11
    treatment, **10**/13–18
        complications of, **10**/18–19
        cricopharyngeal myotomy,
            10/17–18
        endoscopy, **10**/13–15
        inversion, **10**/16
        one-stage diverticulectomy,
            10/15–16